Emergency Vascular and Endovascular Surgical Practice

Emergency Vascular and Endovascular Surgical Practice

Second Edition

Edited by

Aires A B Barros D'Sa OBE MD FRCS FRSCEd

Honorary Professor of Vascular Surgery, The Queen's University of Belfast

Consultant Vascular Surgeon, Regional Vascular Surgery Unit

Royal Victoria Hospital, Belfast, UK

and

Anthony D B Chant BA BSC MS FRCS

Medical Director, British Vascular Foundation

London, UK

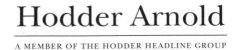

Hodder Arnold

A MEMBER OF THE HODDER HEADLINE GROUP

First published in Great Britain in 2005 by
Hodder Education, a member of the Hodder Headline Group,
338 Euston Road, London NW1 3BH

http://www.hoddereducation.com

Distributed in the United States of America by
Oxford University Press Inc.,
198 Madison Avenue, New York, NY10016
Oxford is a registered trademark of Oxford University Press

Whilst the advice and information in this book are believed to be true and
accurate at the date of going to press, neither the author[s] nor the publisher
can accept any legal responsibility or liability for any errors or omissions
that may be made. In particular, (but without limiting the generality of the
preceding disclaimer) every effort has been made to check drug dosages;
however it is still possible that errors have been missed. Furthermore,
dosage schedules are constantly being revised and new side effects
recognised. For these reasons the reader is strongly urged to consult the
drug companies' printed instructions before administering any of the drugs
recommended in this book.

British Library Cataloguing in Publication Data
A catalogue record for this book is available from the British Library

Library of Congress Cataloging-in-Publication Data
A catalog record for this book is available from the Library of Congress

ISBN-10: 0 340 81012 2
ISBN-13: 978 0 340 81012 5

1 2 3 4 5 6 7 8 9 10

Commissioning Editor: Sarah Burrows
Project Editor: Naomi Wilkinson
Production Controller: Joanna Walker
Cover Design: Sarah Rees
Indexer: Indexing Specialists (UK) Ltd.
                           Website: www.indexing.co.uk

Typeset in 10/12 Minion by Charon Tec Pvt. Ltd, Chennai, India
www.charontec.com
Printed and bound in the UK by CPI Bath

What do you think about this book? Or any other Hodder Arnold
title? Please visit our website at www.hoddereducation.com

To
Elizabeth, Vivienne, Lisa, Miranda and Angelina Barros D'Sa
and
Ann, Ben, Harvey and Thomas Chant

Contents

Contributors

Cameron M Akbari MD MBA FACS
Senior Vascular Surgeon
Director Vascular Diagnostic Laboratory
Washington Hospital Center
Washington, DC
USA

Sebastián F Ameriso MD
Professor of Neurology
Austral University School of Medicine
Chief, Vascular Neurology Division
Fundación para la Lucha contra las Enfermedades Neurológicas de la Infancia (FLENI)
Buenos Aires
Argentina

Juan A Asensio MD FACS FCCM
Professor and Chief
Division of Clinical Research in Trauma Surgery
Trauma Surgery and Surgical Critical Care
University of Medicine and Dentistry of New Jersey
The University Hospital
New Jersey
USA

A Aulich MD
Institute of Diagnostic Radiology
Heinrich Heine University
Duesseldorf
Germany

Daryll M Baker FRCS
Department of Vascular Surgery
Royal Free and St Mary's Hospital
London
UK

Aires AB Barros D'Sa OBE MD FRCS FRCSEd
Honorary Professor of Vascular Surgery
The Queen's University of Belfast, and
Consultant Vascular Surgeon
Regional Vascular Surgery Unit
Royal Victoria Hospital
Belfast
UK

Iris Baumgartner MD
Professor, Division of Angiology
Department of Internal Medicine
University of Berne
Berne
Switzerland

David K Beattie FRCS
Consultant Surgeon
Department of Surgery
Charing Cross Hospital
London
UK

Peter RF Bell KBE MD FRCS
Professor of Surgery
Department of Surgery
University of Leicester
Leicester Royal Infirmary
Leicester
UK

David Bergqvist MD PhD FRCS
Professor of Vascular Surgery
Department of Surgery
University Hospital
Uppsala
Sweden

Ramon Berguer MD PhD
Chief, Division of Vascular Surgery
Harper University Hospital
Detroit Medical Center and Wayne State University
Detroit, MI
USA

Martin Björck MD PhD
Associate Professor
Consultant Vascular Surgeon
Department of Surgery
University Hospital
Uppsala
Sweden

Paul HB Blair MD FRCS
Consultant Vascular Surgeon and Director of Trauma
Vascular Surgery Unit
Royal Victoria Hospital
Belfast
UK

Amman Bolia MBChB FRCR
Consultant Vascular Radiologist
Department of Vascular Radiology
Leicester Royal Infirmary
Leicester
UK

Charles W Bouch MD
Vascular Surgery Fellow
Division of Vascular Surgery
University of Florida College of Medicine
Gainesville, FL
USA

Michael D Brennen FRCS
Consultant Plastic Surgeon
Department of Plastic Surgery
Ulster Hospital
Belfast
UK

Kevin G Burnand ChM FRCS
Professor of Vascular Surgery
Department of Surgery
St Thomas's Hospital
London
UK

Bruce Campbell MS FRCP FRCS
Professor and Consultant Surgeon
Royal Devon and Exeter Hospital
Exeter
UK

Sandra C Carr MD
Assistant Professor
Division of Vascular Surgery
University of Wisonsin Clinical Sciences
Madison, WI
USA

Brian Chambers
Associate Director and Head of Ultrasound Research
National Stroke Research Institute
Austin Hospital
Heidelberg, Victoria
Australia

Anthony DB Chant BA BSc MS FRCS
Medical Director, British Vascular Foundation
London
UK

Harvey J Chant BSc MD FRCS
Consultant Vascular Surgeon
Peninsular Medical School
Royal Cornwall Hospital
Truro
UK

Michael D Dake MD
Associate Professor of Radiology and Medicine
Chief, Division of Interventional Radiology
Stanford University School of Medicine
Stanford, CA
USA

Simon G Darke MS FRCS
Consultant Vascular Surgeon
Royal Bournemouth Hospital
Bournemouth
UK

Alun H Davies MA DM FRCS
Reader and Consultant Surgeon
Department of Surgery
Charing Cross Hospital
London
UK

Thomas Diamond BSc MD FRCS
Consultant Surgeon and Honorary Senior Lecturer
Mater Hospital
Belfast
UK

Do Dai Do MD
Professor, Division of Angiology
Department of Internal Medicine
University of Berne
Berne
Switzerland

Geoffrey A Donnan MD FRACP
Director, National Stroke Research Institute
Professor of Neurology, University of Melbourne
Director of Neurosciences, Austin and Repatriation Medical Centre
Heidelberg, Victoria
Australia

Alasdair Dow FRCA
Consultant Anaesthetist
Royal Devon and Exeter Hospital
Exeter
UK

Jonothan J Earnshaw DM FRCS
Consultant Surgeon
Gloucestershire Royal Hospital
Gloucester
UK

Bo GH Eklof MD PhD
Clinical Professor
John A Burns School of Medicine
University of Hawaii
Chief, Vascular Center
Straub Clinic and Hospital
Honolulu, HI
USA

Peter K Ellis FRCR
Consultant Radiologist
Department of Radiology
Royal Victoria Hospital
Belfast
UK

Luis M Ferreira MD
Staff, Vascular Surgery Department
Fundación para la Lucha contra las Enfermedades Neurológicas de la Infancia (FLENI)
Buenos Aires
Argentina

Roy M Fujitani MD FACS
Associate Professor of Surgery
Chief, Division of Vascular Surgery
UCI Medical Center
Orange, CA
USA

David J Gerrard FRCS
Specialist Registrar
Department of Surgery
Guy's & St Thomas' Hospital Trust
London
UK

Alastair Graham MD FRCS
Consultant Cardiothoracic Surgeon
Department of Thoracic Surgery
Royal Victoria Hospital
Belfast
UK

Per-Ola Granberg MD PhD
Emeritus Professor of Endocrine Surgery
Karolinska Hospital
Stockholm
Sweden

George Hamilton MD FRCS
Professor of Vascular Surgery
University Department of Surgery
Royal Free Hospital
London
UK

Denis W Harkin MD FRCS
Consultant Vascular Surgeon
Regional Vascular Surgery Unit
Royal Victoria Hospital
Belfast
UK

Peter L Harris MD FRCS
Director and Consultant Vascular Surgeon
Regional Vascular Unit
Royal Liverpool University Hospital
Liverpool
UK

Peter K Henke MD
Associate Professor of Surgery
University of Michigan Medical Center
Ann Arbor, MI
USA

Robert J Hinchliffe MB FRCS
Department of Vascular and Endovascular Surgery
University Hospital
Nottingham
UK

John M Hood MPhil FRCS
Consultant Vascular Surgeon
Regional Vascular Surgery Unit
Royal Victoria Hospital
Belfast
UK

Brian R Hopkinson MB ChM FRCS
Emeritus Professor of Vascular Surgery
Department of Surgery
University Hospital
Nottingham
UK

R Huber MD
Department of Vascular Surgery and Kidney Transplantation
Heinrich Heine University
Duesseldorf
Germany

Elaine Imoto MD
Department of Chest Diseases
Straub Clinic and Hospital
Honolulu, HI
USA

Krassi Ivancev MD PhD
Professor and Chief, Endovascular Centre
Department of Radiology
Malmö University Hospital
Malmö
Sweden

Michael P Jenkins BSc MS FRCS
Consultant Vascular Surgeon
Regional Vascular Unit
St Mary's and Chelsea & Westminster Hospitals
London
UK

Dhanesh Kamerkar MB MS(Surgery)
Consultant Vascular Surgeon
Ruby Hall Clinic, and
Associate Honorary Vascular Surgeon
Department of Surgery
KEM Hospital
Pune
India

Curtis B Kamida MD
Clinical Assistant Professor
John A Burns School of Medicine
University of Hawaii
Department of Radiology
Straub Clinic and Hospital
Honolulu, HI
USA

Barry Kelly FRCR
Consultant Radiologist
Department of Radiology
Royal Victoria Hospital
Belfast
UK

Peter Kennedy FRCR
Consultant Radiologist
Department of Radiology
Royal Victoria Hospital
Belfast
UK

Ronald A Kline MD FACS FAHA
Arizona Endovascular Center
Medical Director, St Joseph Wound Care Center
Tucson, AZ
USA

S Ram Kumar MD
Resident, Division of Vascular Surgery
Kech School of Medicine
University of Southern California
Los Angeles, CA
USA

Mauri Lepäntalo MD PhD
Professor of Vascular Surgery, Helsinki University
Chief, Department of Vascular Surgery
Helsinki University Central Hospital
Helsinki
Finland

Bengt LT Lindblad MD PhD
Associate Professor
Department of Vascular Diseases
University Hospital Malmö
Malmö
Sweden

Christer Ljungman MD PhD
Assistant Professor of Vascular Surgery
Department of Surgery
University Hospital
Uppsala
Sweden

Frank W LoGerfo MD FACS
Professor and Chief, Division of Vascular Surgery
Beth Israel Deaconess Medical Center
Harvard Medical School
Boston, MA
USA

Felix Mahler
Professor and Chief, Division of Angiology
Department of Internal Medicine
University of Berne
Berne
Switzerland

Averil O Mansfield CBE ChM FRCS
Former Professor of Surgery
Imperial College of Science, Technology and Medicine
St Mary's Hospital
London
UK

James A McGuigan FRCS
Consultant Thoracic Surgeon
Department of Thoracic Surgery
Royal Victoria Hospital
Belfast
UK

Kieran G McManus BMedSc FRCS
Consultant Thoracic Surgeon
Department of Thoracic Surgery
Royal Victoria Hospital
Belfast
UK

Colin M Morrison FRCS
Department of Plastic Surgery
Ulster Hospital
Belfast
UK

Kenneth A Myers MS FRACS FACS
Consultant Surgeon
Monash Medical Centre and Epworth Hospital
Melbourne, Victoria
Australia

Bernard H Nachbur MD FMH
Emeritus Professor of Surgery
University of Berne
Berne
Switzerland

Sekar Natarajan MB MS MCh(Vascular) FICS
Professor and Senior Vascular Surgeon
Department of Vascular Surgery
Madras Medical College and Research Centre
Chennai
India

Anh Nguyen MD
Surgical Resident, John A Burns School of Medicine
University of Hawaii
Straub Clinic and Hospital
Honolulu, HI
USA

Thang D Nguyen MD
Department of General Surgery
University of California, Irvine
Irvine, CA
USA

Lars Norgren MD FRCS
Professor of Surgery
Chairman, Department of Surgery
Örebro University Hospital
Örebro
Sweden

William Paaske MD DrMedSci FRCS FRCSEd FACS
Professor of Vascular Surgery, Chief Vascular Surgeon
Department of Cardiothoracic and Vascular Surgery T
Skejby Hospital
Aarhus University Hospital, Skejby Sygehus
Aarhus
Denmark

Rowan W Parks MD FRCSI FRCSEd
Senior Lecturer in Surgery and Honorary Consultant Surgeon
Department of Clinical & Surgical Sciences
University of Edinburgh
Royal Infirmary
Edinburgh
UK

Juan C Parodi MD
Chief of the Department of Angiology and Vascular Surgery
Fundación para la Lucha contra las Enfermedades
Neurológicas de la Infancia (FLENI)
Buenos Aires
Argentina; and
Professor of Surgery and Radiology
Washington University School of Medicine
Saint Louis, MO
USA

Jonathon Refson MS FRCS
Consultant Surgeon
Princess Alexandra Hospital
Harlow
UK

Linda M Reilly MD
Professor, Department of Surgery
University of California San Francisco
San Francisco, CA
USA

Hans–Beat Ris MD PhD
Professor and Director
Department of Thoracic Surgery
University of Lausanne
Lausanne
Switzerland

John V Robbs ChM(CT) FRCS(Ed) FRCPS(Glas) FCS(SA)
Professor and Head, Division of Surgery
Head, Metropolitan Vascular Services and
School of Clinical Sciences
Nelson R Mandela School of Medicine
Durban
South Africa

David Rosenthal MD
Professor of Surgery, Medical College Georgia
Chief of Vascular Surgery, Atlanta Medical Center
Atlanta, GA
USA

Vincent L Rowe MD
Division of Vascular Surgery
Department of Surgery
Keck School of Medicine
University of Southern California
Los Angeles, CA
USA

John P Royle FRACS FRCSEd
Former Director, Vascular Surgery Unit
Austin & Repatriation Medical Center
Heidelberg, Victoria
Australia

Wilhelm Sandmann MD
Professor and Chief
Department of Vascular Surgery and Kidney Transplantation
University of Duesseldorf
Duesseldorf
Germany

James M Seeger MD
Vascular Surgeon
Professor and Chief, Division of Vascular Surgery
University of Florida College of Medicine
Gainsville, FL
USA

RJ Seitz MD
Department of Neurology
Heinrich Heine University
Duesseldorf
Germany

Gregory W Self MB FRACS
Consultant Vascular Surgeon
Monash Medical Centre and Epworth Hospital
Melbourne, Victoria
Australia

Clifford P Shearman MS FRCS
Professor of Vascular Surgery
University of Southampton
Southampton General Hospital
Southampton
UK

M Siebler
Department of Neurology
Heinrich Heine University
Duesseldorf
Germany

Henrik Sillesen MD DMSc
Chairman, Department of Vascular Surgery
Gentofte University Hospital
Hellerup
Denmark

Malcolm H Simms MB FRCS
Consultant Vascular Surgeon
Department of Vascular Surgery
University Hospital
Birmingham
UK

James C Stanley MD
Professor of Surgery
University of Michigan Medical Center
Ann Arbor, MI
USA

Peter R Taylor MA MChir FRCS
Consultant Vascular Surgeon
London Bridge Hospital
London
UK

John F Thompson MS FRCSEd FRCS
Consultant Surgeon
Royal Devon & Exeter Hospital
Exeter
UK

Thomas J Troëng MD PhD
Associate Professor
Department of Surgery
Blekinge Hospital
Karlskrona
Sweden

J Tsui MA MRCS
Vascular Research Fellow
Royal Free Hospital
London

Lynne Tudhope MBChB Mmed
Consultant Vascular Surgeon
Unit for Peripheral Vascular Surgery
Pretoria Academic Hospital
University of Pretoria
South Africa

William D Turnipseed MD
Division of Vascular Surgery
University of Wisconsin Clinical Sciences
Madison, WI
USA

S Rao Vallabhaneni FRCS
Endovascular Research Fellow
Regional Vascular Unit
The Royal Liverpool University Hospital
Liverpool
UK

Jacobus van Marle MBChB Mmed FCS(SA)
Consultant Vascular Surgeon
Unit for Peripheral Vascular Surgery
Pretoria Academic Hospital
University of Pretoria
South Africa

Matthew Waltham MA FRCS
Surgical Lecturer
Guy's, King's and St Thomas' School of Medicine
London
UK

Fred A Weaver MD
Professor of Surgery
Division of Vascular Surgery
Department of Surgery
Keck School of Medicine
University of Southern California
Los Angeles, CA
USA

Eric D Wellons MD
Department of Vascular Surgery
Atlanta Medical Centre
Atlanta, GA
USA

Samuel E Wilson MD
Division of Vascular Surgery
UCI Medical Center
Orange, CA
USA

John HN Wolfe FRCS
Consultant Vascular Surgeon
Regional Vascular Unit
St Mary's Hospital
London
UK

Foreword

War and strife have long since set the scene for advances in the urgent care of the wounded. Galen, when serving as surgeon to the school of gladiators at Pergamon, near Troy, cured a traumatic brachial aneurysm by the simple expedient of prompt and securely maintained local compression. Ambroise Paré and Baron Larrey both recognised the opportunity of the 'golden hour' after injury. Writing from the battle zone, Norman Rich documented the memorable achievements of the mobile forward vascular teams in Vietnam, their bounty being that for hundreds of young men the otherwise certain prospect of limb loss was avoided.

The emergence of terrorism and violence in Northern Ireland provided new opportunities for acute, definitive repair of life-threatening vascular wounds. The challenges faced were quickly appreciated at the Royal Victoria Hospital, Belfast, where Aires Barros D'Sa, heading the next generation of modern vascular surgeons, applied novel and effective strategies, particularly in the testing scenario of complex limb vascular injuries. In one of the first dedicated

regional vascular surgical centres established in the British Isles, his use of early perfusion operative techniques enabled more accurate and reliable vascular repairs, and better end results have been the dividend. The second edition of this book sets new standards for our specialty.

Endovascular surgery is here to stay, though, predictably, along with its own problems. The potential indications and techniques for such intervention seem to proliferate. This new edition gives authoritative help with these. Today's professional emphasis on risk assessment, the mandatory measurement of treatment outcomes and the growing awareness of medico-legal consequences and their avoidance are given consideration. New material on stroke makes a welcome appearance, as does a rearranged section on the acutely swollen limb. The greatly expanded authorship, with increased international input, adds further merit to this distinguished book.

H H G Eastcott

Foreword to the 1st edition

Medical and surgical emergencies involving the vascular system continue to challenge clinicians and vascular surgeons worldwide. Life as well as limb can be threatened by a wide variety of diseases or injuries of arteries and veins. Emerging new technologies have been associated with both diagnostic and therapeutic complications.

The editors, also contributors to the volume, are leading vascular surgeons with an international reputation in current vascular surgical practice and research. In this book they have mobilized the aggregated experience of other distinguished contributors from Europe, Australia and the United States. They have addressed numerous emergency clinical situations which require a mandated emergency response by those with an interest in and an expertise for managing vascular disease and injury.

The emergency vascular services and the general support required in treating the patient are identified. Disease processes associated with a threat to life ranging from a ruptured aneurysm to a cardiovascular accident are included. Space is given over to post-surgical complications, including infected grafts and the appropriate emergency vascular response. A combination of medical as well as surgical therapy is incorporated within the armamentarium of response to various vascular emergencies. Challenging clinical emergencies involving the venous system, ranging from thrombosis and pulmonary embolism to portal hypertension with variceal bleeding have a place in this book. In tackling vascular injuries, a regional focus is conveniently provided. Iatrogenic vascular injuries as well as limb replantation which fall within the realm of emergency vascular practice all receive coverage.

Some of the subject matter contained in this most welcome book may be found scattered piecemeal in large volumes on vascular surgery or may be omitted altogether. During this century there have been few efforts to provide within one volume the comprehensive range of acute vascular material which has been collected here. The book contains a unique and valued reference for doctors of all disciplines engaged in the management of vascular emergencies. The contributions of internationally renowned and experienced physicians and surgeons will ensure its survival as a unique resource. It is a book which will not be relegated to gather dust on the bookshelf, rather it will be a manual for frequent perusal by those engaged in emergency vascular practice.

Norman M Rich MD FACS
Professor and Chairman,
Department of Surgery,
Uniformed Services
University of the Health Sciences,
Bethesda, Maryland, USA

Preface

Patients presenting with emergency vascular problems, often during antisocial hours, form a substantial percentage of the caseload of a vascular surgeon. Ruptured aortic aneurysms, acute limb ischaemia and stroke represent the core of that emergency practice but the spectrum varies from one country to another. In some populations, as has been true of Northern Ireland for at least a quarter of a century of terrorist violence, vascular surgeons have also had to deal with life-threatening penetrating injuries. In other societies they have had to cope with grave vascular emergencies generated by substance abuse, HIV/AIDS or cold injury.

Between the covers of this book is to be found a comprehensive range of vascular emergencies affecting the entire body, if one excludes those of intracranial and cardiac origin. Full consideration is given to current practice, evidence-based or otherwise, as well as to anticipated developments particularly in the field of minimally invasive intervention. Endovascular interventions for some emergency vascular conditions seem to offer, long-term trial results pending, speedy resolution, shortened hospital stay and rapid return to an active life. In most centres in the UK a collaborative team approach, with vascular surgeons and radiologists sharing specialist skills, has proved effective and has largely averted the turf wars with cardiologists and neurologists reputedly plaguing those across the Atlantic.

Each chapter begins by defining the nature and extent of 'the problem' when confronted with a particular emergency, emphasising clinical presentation and prudence in resorting to time-consuming investigations. In terms of treatment, 'hands-on' practical advice is imparted based on fundamental principles, identifying pitfalls, offering guidelines and giving helpful tips assisted by algorithms on available management strategies. The reader will find 'boxed' key points within the text where appropriate, and from the extensive bibliography of all chapters, selected references are recommended for further reading.

The text is divided conveniently into nine broad sections, the first on 'General Considerations' leading off with introductory chapters outlining the provision of vascular services in different countries. Focused chapters on the pathophysiology of acute limb ischaemia and colonic ischaemia, and the systemic sequelae to these insults, precede others on critical care, risk assessment and current imaging techniques in refining diagnosis. Indicators of 'best practice' being absolutely central to modern management of vascular emergencies, this section ends with chapters on outcomes of treatment gleaned from the three prestigious Scandinavian registries and a more recent UK database, followed by an important review of relevant medico-legal considerations.

Three further clinical sections follow under the headings of acute cerebrovascular syndromes, the acutely swollen limb and acute lower limb ischaemic states, the latter including a superb chapter on the diabetic foot from a well recognised centre. The sheer wealth of topics within the section on thoracoabdominal catastrophes is exemplified by an authoritative contribution on stenting in acute aortic dissection, a modality of treatment positioned to virtually displace both the relatively ineffectual conservative medical approach as well as the more perilous surgical option. Further important sections cover acute complications of endovascular aortic repair (EVAR), regional vascular trauma and iatrogenic injuries, the last section including first rate chapters on catheterisation and peripheral endovascular injuries. Fresh chapters by recognised world experts on substance abuse, HIV/AIDS and cold injury give added weight to the concluding section on special acute vascular challenges.

With a book such as this devoted solely to the management of vascular emergencies, the vascular specialist looking for information is spared the laborious exercise of delving through burgeoning tomes on vascular surgery in general. For the vascular trainee this book represents essential reading; for the established vascular surgeon, radiologist and angiologist it is a source to be consulted profitably from time to time; for general surgeons, traumatologists, emergency physicians and other specialists it contains pertinent chapters of interest.

Distinguished vascular surgeons, radiologists and other specialists around the world have enriched this book with their personal expertise and enthusiasm tempered by sound evidence and mature reflection. I am grateful to them for generously taking time in the course of their busy professional lives to contribute invaluably to this book. I must thank Tony Chant, co-editor to the first edition, for staying on board and for his assistance with the preliminary editing of a few chapters. I would like to register my appreciation to the publishers for encouraging a second edition, in particular Jo Koster, Director of Health Sciences Subdivision of Hodder Arnold, for moving the project forward. I am indebted most of all to Sarah Burrows, Senior Development Editor and latterly Commissioning Editor, for her unfailing kindness, diligent support and professional expertise during every phase of preparation of the book. I also thank Naomi Wilkinson, current Project Editor, for ensuring that the production of this book is of the highest quality. To that end the superb artwork by Simon Lindo, Oxford Designers and Illustrators, and the meticulous scrutiny by Lotika Singha, copy editor, and Andy Anderson, proofreader, are acknowledged.

Aires A B Barros D'Sa

Preface to the 1st edition

Arteries and veins disrupt or occlude, and if they do so suddenly an emergency situation arises. Rapid deterioration will threaten the viability of a limb or organ, and indeed the survival of the patient. These emergency vascular situations call for an attitude of urgency, fine judgement and decisiveness if optimal results are to be achieved.

Vascular surgical techniques directed at minimizing the effects of these acute events have been available since the early 1960s, and many of the treatment options have changed little during that time. Even relatively new concepts such as thrombolysis have been documented since the late 1960s. What has changed, however, is the manner in which these techniques have been employed: whereas general surgeons previously applied them in a relatively *ad hoc* manner with occasional spectacular successes, it is now increasingly common for a patient who suffers a vascular catastrophe to come under the care of a vascular team.

Our objectives in editing this book were to collect all the important vascular emergencies within one volume, the chapters of which represent a pooling of intercontinental expertise in each of the topics. The very nature of the subject means that the authors recruited are very busy clinicians with a special personal experience of the problems they discuss. We are extremely grateful to them, and to Arnold for their help in co-ordinating such an ambitious venture. Following the three general introductory chapters, the emergency vascular problems covered in subsequent chapters are subdivided into three further sections, namely arteries, veins and trauma. These contributions come from prominent centres responsible for significant advances in their respective areas.

The authors were especially encouraged to approach their topics by first outlining the problem confronting the clinician, and then by examining the pathophysiological sequelae of a particular vascular emergency. Having established this starting point, each contributor then outlined the various strategies employed in the practical management of the condition. Many of these vascular emergencies involve other medical specialties and therefore require a multidisciplinary approach. It is hoped that access to the broad range of specialties fused within the volume will be of value not only to vascular, general and trauma surgeons, but also to radiologists, angiologists, physicians and emergency personnel.

Anthony D B Chant
Aires A B Barros D'Sa

General Considerations

Emergency Vascular Services in the UK

ANTHONY DB CHANT

THE PROBLEM

A patient suffering a vascular emergency is best served when under the care of a vascular team working in an appropriately equipped hospital. The reality, however, is often very different. The reasons for this are partly due to demographic and socioeconomic conditions but also partly the medical culture of the country in question (see Chapters 1B and 1C). Perhaps equally important has been our difficulty, as vascular physicians, surgeons and scientists, in establishing vascular surgery as specialty in its own right and in providing hard evidence with which to convince our administrations and the myriad healthcare managers that such specialisation is necessary. So-called 'level 1' proof, the kind that is sometimes obtained from the meta-analysis of prospective trials is, in the vast majority of vascular emergencies, unlikely to be obtained. There have been and will be opportunities for this approach, particularly in adjuvant or supporting therapies. On the whole, however, information has been achieved in a different way. Retrospective and prospective audits have all played an important role in furthering our knowledge, and reflection on the dramatic improvements achieved even over the last 20 years bears witness to their value.[1] Neither should we be apologetic about the lack of trials. As any aeronautical scientist will tell you, there is no requirement necessary to run a controlled trial in order to produce a new aeroplane. A priori thinking, computer modelling, animal experiments together with excellence in the area of audit, both individual and in combination with other groups, should give us the evidence we need in order to argue the case for resources necessary to maintain high standards.[2]

EVOLUTION OF EMERGENCY VASCULAR SERVICES

Vascular surgery as a specialty in its own right started to emerge in 1966 when the Vascular Society of Great Britain and Ireland was founded. Gradually, over a period of some 40 years this specialty has almost detached itself from general surgery. The peculiarity of the economics of the British National Health Service (NHS), however, has encouraged generalism rather than specialisation and this, in turn, slowed down the development of the specialty. This was true with the exception of cities such as Glasgow, Edinburgh and Belfast where, during the early 1980s, individual surgeons forged ahead independently to establish dedicated regional vascular units – the one in Belfast being located at the main teaching hospital in which also resides a level IA trauma centre, with the advantage that patients sustaining vascular injuries also received optimal vascular care. Nevertheless, in the overall environment, surgeons trained in vascular surgery found themselves on general surgical emergency intake rotas. Conversely, patients with ruptured aneurysms were operated on by, for example gastroenterologists or even urologists.

In an effort to paper over this ridiculous divide, serious papers have been published attempting to justify this solution. Indeed, as recently as July 2000, in the *Annals of the Royal College of Surgeons of England*, there were no less than three papers discussing this very topic. The first by Cook *et al.*,[3] argued that 'patient outcome alone does not justify the centralisation of vascular services'. The second, by Sutton *et al.*,[4] describes the evolution of vascular surgery at a district hospital and asks 'is specialisation inevitable?'.

This particular paper is interesting because it demonstrates quite clearly the inevitable rise of the specialty: in 1984 the total number of vascular cases comprised only 3.4 per cent of all operations on this particular unit and rose to 33.4 per cent by 1998, leading to the firmly stated conclusion that 'with such a rapidly growing arterial caseload, specialisation to vascular surgery is inevitable'. The third paper in this particular volume of the journal[5] discusses regional variations in varicose vein operations across England. A similar disparity was revealed in the provision of carotid endarterectomy in Wessex.[6] The results again confirm the inconsistency between subregions in the numbers of operations done. In other words, despite the relatively uniform prevalence of vascular disease across the UK, the actual number of patients treated depends very much on local circumstances.

The kind of arguments that have been previously advanced by those wishing to retain the status quo and remain generalists as well as doing 'a bit of vascular surgery' go as follows. First, that all but a few pregangrenous legs can be treated with analgesics and rehydration overnight and that angiograms ought to be done only in daylight hours. A further simplistic but plausible argument has also been forwarded regarding abdominal aortic aneurysms: as 50 per cent of these patients die before entering hospital, and as an expert vascular surgeon can salvage only 60 per cent of the remaining 50 per cent, namely 30 patients, not much is to be gained by having an expert vascular surgeon; further, because an experienced general surgeon might salvage 40 per cent of the remaining 50 per cent, in other words, 20 patients, the extra spending on the retention of specialist vascular surgeons and resources results in a net gain of only 10 lives; the money, therefore, could be better spent in managing other illnesses.

RECOMMENDATIONS FROM THE SPECIALTY

In October 1998 the Vascular Surgical Society published the first recommendation in respect of the provision of vascular surgery services.[1] This very comprehensive document details the problems faced by the British NHS at that time in terms of providing emergency vascular services and goes on to suggest the following solutions.

Major vascular units

Wherever possible, vascular services should be provided on a single site. The recommendation was that four or more consultant surgeons should staff these centres, a number allowing for a workable on-call rota. These consultants, in turn, should be supported by interventional radiologists and vascular anaesthetists and by facilities such as an intensive therapy unit, a high-dependency unit and a vascular laboratory. The workload figures at that time suggested

that such a unit could care for a population of at least 500 000. The benefits, of course, would be the concentration of clinical experience and the provision of excellent supervision for training.

Intermediate vascular units

These units would service populations of between 300 000 and 400 000, but in truth, were they to run efficiently, would still require four consultant surgeons plus support staff. It was thought, perhaps, that this was not an economically viable arrangement.

Remote vascular units

This description was applied to geographically isolated hospitals serving small populations of between 100 000 and 250 000. At this point the concept of 'hub and spoke' was discussed. The problems associated with this approach have been discussed elsewhere.[7] The main criticism of this concept is that those specialists at the end of the 'spoke', although on appointment well trained in modern vascular surgical techniques, in time, and because of the lack of elective operating, inevitably would become less efficient and less tuned in to best practice. Moreover, it is hard to justify, economically, the duplication of support services in these peripheral units, when for much of the time the 'plant' would remain unused.

These initial fairly simple recommendations were further complicated by the fact that the Royal College of Surgeons changed their Fellowship requirements so that even quite senior trainees required supervision at all times. The European Working Time Directive 'Department of Health, Hours of Work for Doctors in Training'[8] was then published, this 'New Deal' limited the hours that doctors, both senior and junior, could either work or remain on-call. Trainee vascular surgeons will now receive even less exposure to vascular emergencies. It was considered wrong, for example for a surgeon to be on a more than one in five emergency rota. Given the complexity of the government rules and their economic consequences for individual hospitals, it is perhaps not surprising that in a few areas in the UK general surgeons still have to look after vascular patients. That said, things have improved markedly and there is now much closer liaison between both specialist interventional radiology[9] and anaesthetic services. The repeated emphasis over the years by the National Confidential Enquiry into Postoperative Deaths (NCEPOD) of the need for vascular emergencies to be treated by a specialist vascular team[10] is probably being achieved but probably more so as a product of other influences. That objective, undoubtedly, will be accelerated by the absolutely unanimous desire of the members of the Vascular Surgical Society, expressed in November 2003, to seek independent specialty status outside general surgery.

The most recent recommendations from the Vascular Surgical Society, the *Provision of Emergency Vascular Services*, were published in November 2001[11] and, realising that the scene was constantly shifting, it was agreed that the document should be reviewed in 2004. Much of the rationale for the management of vascular emergencies by vascular surgeons is described above, but two significant new items have been added. First, it notes the introduction of so-called 'clinical governance' and goes on to state 'general surgeons who are not vascular specialists undertake no active emergency arterial surgery, and it is difficult for them to justify treating vascular emergencies under the scrutiny of clinical governance'. In other words, if a general surgeon in the UK now performed an operation for a vascular emergency, and were that patient to die or perhaps lose a leg unnecessarily, then that surgeon may well be open to litigation. It cannot be emphasised enough just how important a shift of opinion this is in service terms. The second important change is that there is at last an admission that 'there is an accumulation of evidence that outcomes are better when vascular patients are treated by vascular specialists'.[12,13] Moreover the document[11] goes on to state quite dogmatically that 'the modern generation of newly appointed consultant general surgeons is insufficiently trained and experienced to manage complex emergencies outside their own specialist field'.

While this was all accepted in theory, political negotiations aimed at actually amalgamating units have proved extremely difficult, because, quite certainly, some of the smaller hospitals would lose their vascular services completely. Important situations such as 'in-house emergencies' might be difficult to deal with. Does one, for example, transfer a diabetic patient who requires a simple ray amputation of a toe, 30 or 40 miles (48 or 64 km) to a major unit? And how does one deal with the dilemma of a patient, who, in the process of undergoing a general or other non-vascular surgical operation, sustains an iatrogenic vascular injury (see Chapter 40). These and other questions demand sensible, workable and current solutions. Therefore, after a two-year period of consultation with the membership, the Vascular Surgical Society, in liaison with, and the approval of, the departments of health of the four regions of the UK, published *Provision of Vascular Services 2004* in November 2003.[14] This document supports local collaborative strategies which achieve a preferred minimum emergency on-call rota of one in six, which goes a long way to providing that 24-hour cover necessary in dealing with the kind of situations illustrated above in this paragraph. Emergency work is onerous and time consuming and these facts deserve recognition by a government now committed to the strategies laid down in this document and by hospitals negotiating new contracts with consultant vascular surgeons. In due course, with increasing participation in the National Vascular Database[2] by the membership of the Vascular Society, solid data should emerge which will assist in refining existing arrangements for the management of vascular emergencies in the UK.

Conclusion

The, perhaps slightly optimistic, conclusion to the management of emergencies is that the gradual evolution of comprehensive vascular services in the UK may be in the process of being accomplished now that the government has given its tacit approval and accepted a measure of co-responsibility in the most recent provisions.[14] Arriving at this juncture has been a painful process in many respects but, to an extent, it illustrates the complexity of having to please everyone. Advancement of the specialty in the UK has been hampered, partly by the remoteness of some parts of these islands, but mainly by under resourcing of the NHS and the encouragement, until very recently, of generalism rather than specialisation. If you choose to live or work in a remote area, then it is unlikely that you will get the very best of medical treatment. That is a reality of life.

Key references

Department of Health. *New Deal Doctor Training the European Working Hour Directive*. London: DHSS, 2002.

Earnshaw JJ, Ridler BMF (eds). *National Vascular Database Report 2000*. London: The Vascular Society of Great Britain and Ireland.

The Royal College of Radiologists and the Vascular Society of Great Britain and Ireland. *Provision of Vascular Radiological Services. Combined Recommendations*. London: VSS, April 2003.

The Provision of Emergency Vascular Services. A document prepared for the Vascular Society of Great Britain and Ireland. London: VSS, November 2001.

The Provision of Vascular Services. A document prepared for the Vascular Society of Great Britain and Ireland by the Surgical Advisory Committee. London: VSS, October 1998.

REFERENCES

1   *The provision of vascular services*. A document prepared for the Vascular Society of Great Britain and Ireland by the Surgical Advisory Committee. London: VSS, October 1998.

2   Earnshaw JJ, Ridler BMF (eds). *National vascular database report 2000*. London: The Vascular Society of Great Britain and Ireland.

3   Cook SJ, Rocker MD, Jarvis MR, Whitely MD. Patient outcome alone does not justify the centralisation of vascular services. *Ann R Coll Surg Engl* 2000; **82**: 268–71.

4   Sutton CD, Gilmour JP, Berry DP, Lewis MH. The evolution of a vascular surgeon in a district general hospital. *Ann R Coll Surg Engl* 2000; **82**: 272–4.

5   Galland RB, Whatling PJ, Crook TJ, Magee TR. Regional variation in varicose veins operations in England 1989–1996. *Ann R Coll Surg Engl* 2000; **82**: 275–9.

6   Ferris G, Roderick P, Smithies A, *et al*. An epidemiological needs assessment of carotid endarterectomy in an English health region. *BMJ* 1998; **317**: 447–51.

7   Chant A. Emergency vascular services. In: Chant A, Barros D'Sa AAB. (eds). *Emergency Vascular Practice*. London: Arnold,1997.

8   Department of Health. *New deal doctor training the European Working Hour Directive*. London: DHSS, 2002.

9   The Royal College of Radiologists and the Vascular Society of Great Britain and Ireland. *Provision of vascular radiological services. Combined recommendations*. London: VSS, April 2003.

10 Gallimore SC, Hoile RW, Ingram GS, Sherry KM. *The Report of the National Confidential Enquiry into Perioperative Deaths, 1994/95*. London: Royal College of Surgeons of England, 1997.

11 *The Provision of Emergency Vascular Services*. A document prepared for the Vascular Society of Great Britain and Ireland. London: VSS, November 2001.

12 Michaels J, Brazier J, Palfreys, *et al*. Cost and outcome implications of the organisation of vascular services. *Health Technol Assess* 2000; **4**.

13 Wolfe J. The delivery of vascular services in the United Kingdom. *Cardiovasc Surg* 1999; **7**: 692–3.

14 *The provision of vascular services 2004*. Document prepared by the Working Group of the Vascular Surgical Society of Great Britain and Ireland. London: VSS, November 2003.

Emergency Vascular Services in Denmark

HENRIK SILLESEN

THE PROBLEM AND THE NEED FOR EMERGENCY VASCULAR SERVICES

Vascular surgery is a field of expertise demanding some degree of specialisation and therefore in many countries it is recognised as a monospecialty. In most of these countries, specialisation within vascular surgery requires a number of years training within vascular surgery following two to three years in general surgical training. It should follow, therefore, that, in general, results are superior in larger hospitals with access to vascular surgery rather than in smaller hospitals.[1,2] The results of emergency vascular surgery should also be better if conducted by specialists. This difference may be more difficult to observe because of a number of factors, including that of smaller numbers and the difficulty in comparing cases. In Denmark, however, where all vascular surgery is performed within only 10 units staffed solely by specialists in vascular surgery, the results of surgical treatment of ruptured abdominal aortic aneurysms (RAAAs) speak for themselves: the mortality in treating more than 1400 cases of RAAA was 42 per cent (Table 1B.1).

STAFFING AND STRUCTURING OF THE UNIT AND HOSPITAL REQUIREMENTS

In order to provide expert emergency vascular service 24 hours a day, 365 days a year, the specialist unit needs to be staffed accordingly. Taking all duties into account, in addition to vacation and holidays, continuing medical education, scientific meetings and so forth, a minimum of three, and preferably four to five vascular surgical specialists are needed in each unit. Looking at the organisation in Denmark, a total of only 10 vascular surgical units/departments serves the population of 5.5 million. All elective as well as emergency cases are treated in these 10 units, staffed, in total, by approximately 45 consultants.

Depending on whether the hospital is a university or a regional hospital, the departments may have their own junior staff or share them with a general surgical unit. In most university hospitals the vascular surgical unit will have its own staff on call represented by an intern/resident in-house and a fellow/consultant on call, the latter available within 30 minutes. When the vascular fellow is on call a consultant is also similarly committed. Thus, when dealing with an RAAA, an operating team of two to three

Table 1B.1 *Thirty-day mortality following emergency operation for ruptured abdominal aortic aneurysm (RAAA) in Denmark (www.karbase.dk). With a population of 5.5 million the average number of RAAAs is 4.3 per 100 000 per year*

	1997	1998	1999	2000	2001	Total
No. of cases	259	264	230	205	232	1190
Mortality (n)	93	120	105	92	102	512
Mortality (per cent)	36	46	46	45	44	42

surgeons is available, including a vascular surgical consultant and fellow. Having staff on call leads to long working hours and the need for compensatory absence. In Denmark the official working week is 37 hours, and even though some time on call may be compensated financially, a senior fellow/consultant will be on compensatory leave, often for 1 week out of a 4- to 6-week period. With a shortage of consultants in almost all specialties in Denmark this poses a problem, especially for staffing the more 'remotely' located units. Consequently, a new kind of intercounty collaboration is being developed where a university/large regional hospital may cover the neighbouring counties for emergency/ acute cases after 4 pm. Vascular surgical activity being fairly limited beyond daylight hours, more effective use is made of a consultant's skills, but the potential catchment population covered may well be a million or more inhabitants.

Naturally, access to an operation room (OR) is mandatory and a large theatre is preferable. As in many cases there is no time for preoperative radiological investigation, the surgeon has to resort to intraoperative angiography in treating lower limb emergencies. Physical space for mobile or permanently installed X-ray equipment is necessary, along with staff capable of using it at any hour of day or night. The nurses and staff in the OR assisting the vascular surgeon should have a thorough knowledge of the instruments and the common vascular reconstructive procedures. Obviously, the provision of a complete vascular surgical team of assistants, available 24 hours a day, would be the ideal situation but this is probably only achievable in very few units. Having a core of nurses mainly in support of the vascular surgeons, makes it possible for at least one of them to be on call most of the time. With a surgical volume of a minimum of 400–600 vascular cases per year, vascular surgical operations are performed daily, providing sufficient numbers for training OR staff.

This caseload also allows anaesthesia personnel to gain the necessary experience in dealing with patients with both central and peripheral arterial disease (PAD). Patients with PAD generally suffer from other diseases such as concomitant coronary heart disease and chronic obstructive lung disease. These risk factors in turn account for a high perioperative morbidity and mortality even in elective lower limb surgery. The Danish National Register of Vascular Surgery (www.karbase.dk)[3] recorded a 30-day mortality of approximately 4 per cent in 5012 peripheral bypass operations performed during 1996–99. Of course, these patients did not die directly from the operation as from the consequences of other competing circulatory or respiratory diseases. In general, first it should be assumed that any patient with PAD also suffers from coronary heart disease even though there are no cardiac symptoms. Second, managing the major haemodynamic changes during aortic surgery following cross-clamping of the aorta requires skill and experience. Furthermore, the great volume losses during RAAA surgery create demanding situations. Vascular

surgery is ideally performed in hospitals where other major operations on patients with significant competing diseases are undertaken, and therefore, where all the personnel working in the vicinity of the vascular surgeon are cognisant of the common challenges.

A well-equipped intensive case unit (ICU) is mandatory when performing vascular surgery. Both in elective as well as emergency vascular cases, major complications result in failure of almost any organ, most notably the lung, kidney and heart. Similarly, for the staff of the ICU, regular contacts, preferably daily or at least weekly, with vascular surgical patients is mandatory. Access to dialysis is also important as renal failure is a common complication in major vascular surgical emergency cases, in particular ruptured aneurysms. Transfer of vascular surgical patients to other hospitals for dialysis, where vascular surgeons are not in attendance, may result in less intensive surveillance of coexisting vascular surgical problems. In general, the need for dialysis may be a significant prognostic factor for a vascular patient and, although difficult to document, it is the experience of the author that moving a vascular surgical patient to another hospital for dialysis is a strong predictor of death. This, of course, is reflected in the high mortality of patients with renal failure following major vascular surgery. Having the patient in another hospital where there is no vascular surgical expertise, however, may result in decisions being made which might not be the best for the patient.

A ward caring only for vascular surgical patients is of course the ideal solution. In a number of Danish hospitals this is the case. These are relatively small units of 14–20 beds staffed with personnel taking care of only vascular surgical patients. This allows for special training of the nursing staff, in turn improving the quality of surveillance and care of vascular surgical patients. These skills include experience with ischaemic and venous ulcers, supervision of newly operated patients, ability to measure ankle pressures, evaluate whether or not a bypass graft is patent and functioning well, experience with the continuous infusion of thrombolytic agents and management of patients with high comorbidities. If a unit solely dedicated to vascular surgery is not attainable, a section within a surgical ward can be a good start. For nursing staff dedicated to vascular patients, however, it is vitally necessary in order to maintain continued and optimal surveillance and care.

The radiological department should have a dedicated angio-suite and one or preferably two vascular radiologists whose duties are mainly vascular. Whether or not access to an expert radiological vascular service is necessary at all times is debatable, however, day-to-day contact is. On the other hand, a round-the-clock facility for computed tomography (CT) is mandatory. It is also advantageous to have ultrasound expertise available if the vascular surgeon cannot perform this examination on his or her own.

Finally, having a vascular laboratory, ideally located within the vascular surgical unit is of great value. Although, many emergency vascular cases may utilise the skills of the radiological department, some of the complications can be investigated in the vascular laboratory. The advantages of a vascular laboratory are discussed further below.

WHAT CAN AN EXPERT UNIT DO?

In addition to treating emergency vascular cases, vascular surgical staff at an expert unit can also provide elective services to a region. Units covering an area with 400 000–500 000 inhabitants, staffed by three or four consultants, should generally have an activity level of around 400–600 arterial cases, 75 per cent being open surgical cases and 25–35 per cent percutaneous transluminal angioplasties, although the proportion of the latter may be higher in some countries. Added to the 'real' arterial cases is an average of 0.2–0.3 additional, usually secondary operations per arterial reconstruction, mainly minor amputations, wound revisions and so on, thereby increasing the operative caseload by 20–30 per cent.

Vascular surgical activity includes the entire spectrum of preoperative work-up, diagnostic studies, the operation itself, the care provided during hospitalisation and finally, but very importantly, postoperative monitoring and indeed follow-up. In Denmark, most departments/units offer 30-day and one-year follow-up for all patients. In addition, patients undergoing bypass surgery are often also seen at intervals between the standard re-visits, usually at 6–12-week intervals during the first year. Venous disease, especially the more complex cases of redo varicose vein surgery, secondary varicose veins and chronic venous obstruction can also be treated by vascular surgeons. Although not within the scope of this chapter, we find it increasingly important that vascular surgeons ensure patients are treated adequately with respect to secondary prevention.[4] A special outpatient clinic dedicated to the organisation of risk factor reduction by means of lifestyle changes and medication allows well-trained and supervised vascular nurses to take the responsibility of improving the total care of the vascular patient.

The volume of emergency work is of a reasonable size with an average of 20–25 RAAAs, within a range of 10–35 cases treated per unit depending on the size of the catchment area.

With a staff of at least three or four consultant vascular surgeons per unit, continuing education of staff is possible in the knowledge that vascular surgical expertise is always available during meetings and courses. Given that all vascular surgical operations in Denmark are performed in the aforementioned 10 vascular surgical units/departments, it follows that no Danes are treated by anyone other than full-time vascular surgical consultants. An organisation in which all vascular activity is concentrated within a few centres ensures that vascular surgeons are solely responsible. It may be argued that vascular surgeons should keep their general surgical skills up to date at all times, but as all vascular surgical units/departments in Denmark are either in university hospitals or regional hospitals, where general surgical staff are also to be found, a gastroenterological or urological consultant surgeon, for example, can be called upon if necessary. An indepth devotion to the specialty, concentrating on vascular cases only, sharpens a consultant's expertise and certainly makes for better outcomes.

The surgical throughput in the vascular surgical units described is sufficient to offer a broad range of experience in keeping the skills of the consultants and associated staff up to date. Depending on the size of the unit/department, it also allows for one or more resident/fellow appointments. In Denmark, a 'small' unit with three or four consultants provides one of the three years of training required by a fellow for specialisation in vascular surgery. The larger units, wherein all kinds of vascular surgical treatments are undertaken, provide the remaining two years of training. The larger units also offer resident positions for 6 months which are very important in the recruitment of future vascular surgeons.

A consultant is always on call in support of a vascular fellow and to whom the trainee has access for advice and supervision in the management of emergency cases. During daylight hours, one vascular trainee working under three or four consultants will generally receive very good supervision in the management of elective cases.

Large units facilitate the establishment of a vascular laboratory located within a vascular surgical unit or outpatient clinic which not only means that patients do not have to attend another clinic but also increases use of expensive equipment. For instance, a duplex scan is more frequently performed if it can be done immediately and without the time-consuming administrative measures in having it performed elsewhere, or even worse, on another day. A vascular laboratory immediately available within a unit also offers important educational as well as research opportunities for the vascular surgical trainee.

A senior vascular surgical trainee represents the availability of vascular expertise not only for 'in-house' emergencies but also for those in another hospital within the unit's intake area. Injured patients brought into the emergency room may turn out to have vascular problems or, occasionally, an iatrogenic vascular injury may complicate a non-vascular surgical procedure. If a vascular surgeon is not available to deal with such cases, the outcome may be less than favourable.

On approximately 10 occasions annually, vascular surgeons at Gentofte University Hospital perform emergency operations at one of the other three hospitals within Copenhagen County, which has a population of 630 000 inhabitants. For example, the time taken for a vascular surgeon to travel to a patient with a ruptured aneurysm in circulatory shock is much less than that needed to stabilise the patient for transportation and effect the actual transfer of the patient to Gentofte. Using this strategy, the results of emergency RAAA operations performed in other hospitals on 19 patients from 1996 to 1999 by Gentofte staff show a 30-day survival of 47 per cent.[5] When compared with the results in-house at Gentofte or with those of the whole country, these results are almost as good, despite the fact that in these particular cases the worst possible outcome might otherwise have been expected. This raises the question as to what is most important when treating a ruptured aneurysm: is time or the organisation of the vascular surgical unit the key issue? It is well recognised that the patient with an RAAA represents a challenge for anaesthetists and it has also been argued that, unless both they and the ICU staff are experienced, results may suffer. In Copenhagen County, the patients operated outside Gentofte Vascular Surgical Department are almost always transferred to Gentofte Hospital as soon as possible, that is, immediately after surgery or the day after. Similarly, for trauma cases dealt within Copenhagen County, the availability of a 'travelling' expert is important especially as these other hospitals are all university hospitals with large teaching anaesthesia departments and well-equipped ICUs.

It is of course debatable as to whether a 'travelling service' will produce good results in all cases. For example, when operating on hypotensive patients with RAAAs in remote small hospitals inexperienced in major surgical work the outcome is usually poor. A recent Danish study from a less densely populated area presented the results of emergency RAAA surgery undertaken in remote hospitals by a 'travelling vascular surgeon': the 30-day mortality in this small series was 70 per cent, and although the authors concluded that such operations were worthwhile, it could be argued that the results contradicted this view and that patients should be transferred to the expert unit under all circumstances.[6] The experience from southern Sweden shows that the on-table mortality from RAAA is similar whether patients are operated in a university hospital (12 per cent) or a county hospital (15 per cent), nevertheless, there was a difference in the 30-day mortality, being 26 and 41 per cent, respectively.[2]

The organisation of vascular services in Denmark, in general, has encouraged good results in treating emergencies, if the 30-day survival of operations for ruptured aneurysms is taken as an indicator. Looking at the results of all cases treated over 5 years (1997–2001), a 30-day mortality rate is 42 per cent in 1190 cases treated (see Table 1B.1), with only minor variations from one year to another.[3]

Comparison between departments is difficult on an annual basis due to the numbers being treated. Over six years, however, experience reveals quite similar results in the 10 Danish centres. The difference between the department with the best results and that with the highest mortality is 14 per cent (39–53), but using 95 per cent confidence intervals this difference is not statistical significant. Even if it were, the differences in mortality might simply reflect differences in the performance of the attending

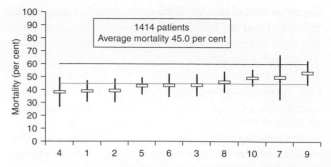

Figure 1B.1 *Thirty-day mortality in 10 Danish vascular surgical departments over a 6-year period (1996–2001); 95 per cent confidence intervals are shown. The numbers below the figure indicate department number and these are kept confidential; each centre knows its result and what number they are on this figure; however, they are unaware of other departments' numbers (source: www.karbase.dk[3])*

surgeons, case selection and not necessarily the capabilities of an individual department or hospital (Fig. 1B.1).

The five-year mortality rate of 42 per cent, derived from all RAAA surgery undertaken in Denmark, compares well with similar analyses from other countries. Of the 10 Danish hospitals performing vascular surgery, only five are university based and the other five are regional hospitals. In the USA an analysis of 13 887 cases from 20 per cent of a random sample of all hospital activity during 1996–97 showed an overall RAAA mortality of 47 per cent. A meta-analysis of all English literature quoting RAAA mortality during 1995–98 revealed an overall operative mortality of 48 per cent.[7]

POLITICAL ISSUES

An understanding of the Danish organisation of emergency services is based on the recognition of the following issues. Almost all healthcare is socialised and paid for by public services. The country is divided into 19 counties, each responsible for its own organisation and the economics of healthcare within it. A central administrative authority is answerable to a political county council elected by the inhabitants of that county every four years. Virtually all vascular surgery is performed within public hospitals. The cost of healthcare in Copenhagen County is paid for by its inhabitants. In total, Denmark has 19 counties, 10 of which decided to have their own vascular surgical service.

The decision to establish a specialised unit or not is a local decision for a particular county. If it chooses not to have its own specialist unit, it has to transfer vascular surgical patients to a hospital in another county and pay for their treatment. Given the system of reimbursement between counties implemented by the year 2000, and using diagnosis related groups (DRGs), the price for treating the individual case is a little higher than the 'cost' price, which makes it fairly attractive to hospitals receiving patients from another county.

The service a county wishes to provide has a political dimension. Some counties, despite being relatively small, may have a political majority favouring the provision of all medical speciality services and, consequently, in some small specialties the cost per case may be very high. In other counties a more pragmatic attitude may be evident where economical considerations rule decision making.

National health authorities define a disease requiring specialist attention by, for example, stating that aortic abdominal aneurysms need vascular surgical attention. Within vascular surgery itself, certain procedures are considered so rare that they ought to be concentrated in a few tertiary units. These cases would include mesenteric and renal artery obstruction, infected abdominal vascular prosthesis and certain supra-aortic emergencies.

LOCATION OF AND DISTANCE BETWEEN VASCULAR SURGICAL SERVICES

Ideally, in the majority of cases, the time needed to transport a patient from home, or from another hospital lacking a specialist vascular service, should not exceed 1–2 hours. In Denmark, this is the case almost anywhere in the country, with the exception of people living on small remote islands. Even then the possibility of providing transport by helicopter exists. In these cases, however, it is often a matter of transporting a patient to the right hospital rather than just the nearest one. This, of course, is dependent on someone making the correct diagnosis which may not happen until the patient is actually in a hospital which has a vascular surgical service.

Conclusion

Vascular surgery is a specialty which benefits from centralisation, partly with respect to quality of treatment, but also with regard to cost. This is especially important with regard to patients presenting as emergency cases in the care of whom the availability of an experienced vascular surgeon is crucial; equally so is the hospital's ability and experience in dealing with emergency vascular surgical cases.

Key references

Brown MJ, Sutton AJ, Bell PR, Sayers RD. A meta-analysis of 50 years of ruptured aortic aneurysm repair. *Br J Surg* 2002; **89**: 714–30.

Dimick JB, Stanley AC, Axelrod DA, *et al.* Variation in death rate after abdominal aortic aneurysmectomy in the United States: impact of hospital volume, gender and age. *Ann Surg* 2002; **235**: 579–85.

Karbase Landsregister. Website of The Danish Vascular Registry, www.karbase.dk (accessed 11 December 2004).

Sillesen H. Who should treat patients with peripheral atherosclerosis – the vascular specialist [editorial]. *Eur J Vasc Endovasc Surg* 2002; **24**: 1–3.

Zdanowski Z, Danielsson G, Jonung T, *et al.* Outcome of treatment of ruptured abdominal aortic aneurisms depending on the type of hospital. *Eur J Surg* 2002; **168**: 96–100.

REFERENCES

1   Dimick JB, Stanley AC, Axelrod DA, *et al.* Variation in death rate after abdominal aortic aneurysmectomy in the United States: impact of hospital volume, gender and age. *Ann Surg* 2002; **235**: 579–85.

2   Zdanowski Z, Danielsson G, Jonung T, *et al.* Outcome of treatment of ruptured abdominal aortic aneurisms depending on the type of hospital. *Eur J Surg* 2002; **168**: 96–100.

3   Karbase Landsregister. Website of The Danish Vascular Registry, www.karbase.dk (accessed 11 December 2004).

4   Sillesen H. Who should treat patients with peripheral atherosclerosis – the vascular specialist [editorial]. *Eur J Vasc Endovasc Surg* 2002; **24**: 1–3.

5   Vammen S, Fasting H, Henneberg EW, Lindholdt JS. Karkirurgisk assisterede operationer for rumperet abdominalt aortaaneurisme udført på primært modtagende sygehus. *Ugeskrift for Læger* 1999; **161**: 4868–70.

6   Jensen LP, Bækgaard N, Sillesen H. Ruptured aneurysms can be treated by assisted surgery in local hospitals if the condition does not allow transportation. *Ugeskrift for Læger* 2000; **162**: 198–9.

7   Brown MJ, Sutton AJ, Bell PR, Sayers RD. A meta-analysis of 50 years of ruptured aortic aneurysm repair. *Br J Surg* 2002; **89**: 714–30.

Emergency Vascular Services in the USA

VINCENT L ROWE, JUAN A ASENSIO, FRED A WEAVER

THE PROBLEM

Emergency vascular surgery services encompass a wide variety of disorders, including aortic aneurysm disease, acute lower limb ischaemia, symptomatic carotid occlusive disease and vascular trauma, to name but a few. The variety of disorders encountered in the emergency rooms of hospitals in the USA necessitates familiarity with evaluation and management of vascular disorders in order that the patient can be cared for expeditiously.

Delivery of emergency vascular services requires a diverse group of healthcare professionals including vascular and trauma surgeons, emergency room (ER) physicians, nursing personnel, emergency medical technicians, radiological and operating room personnel. Organising services into a co-ordinated functioning unit requires co-operation between surgery, radiology and emergency medicine personnel.

This chapter reviews the manner in which vascular services are facilitated and organised in the USA using one large public hospital as an example. The most common emergency vascular problems are ruptured abdominal aortic aneurysms (RAAAs), vascular trauma, acute limb ischaemia and stroke.

EPIDEMIOLOGY

The overall incidence of acute vascular surgical emergencies in the USA is difficult to quantify. Owing to the catastrophic consequences of delay in correct diagnosis and treatment of such acute circulatory problems, numerous patients will succumb to vascular emergencies outside hospital and remain unaccounted for by our current methods of medical record keeping. An estimate of activity at our medical centre may provide some insight in this matter.

The vascular surgery service at Los Angeles County and University of Southern California (LAC + USC) Medical Centre annually admits over 250 patients and provides consultations on over 300 inpatients. Approximately 25 per cent of these admissions are of an emergency nature and come through the ER or clinic. Over the past three years, our vascular service has performed an average of 355 operations, 21 per cent of these cases being emergencies. Interestingly, the same distribution applies to the average number of surgical hours spent on vascular elective and emergency operations.

The most common vascular emergency at our institution is that of acute upper and lower extremity ischaemia, constituting almost 20 per cent of all emergency vascular operations undertaken. While the aetiology of ischaemia in the upper extremity is most frequently due to an embolic source, acute ischaemia of the lower extremity encompasses embolic as well as thrombotic complications in atherosclerotic patients. Given the lower rate of limb salvage in the latter group of patients, the number of amputations performed for ischaemic disease may provide a rough estimate of this problem throughout the USA.[1–3]

Despite improvement in care and technological advancements, the incidence of RAAAs continues to be a persistent and common problem.[4,5] The relative incidence of ruptured to elective aortic aneurysm repairs for a particular medical centre is difficult to quantify given that multiple variables are involved. Referral patterns from primary care practitioners, technological advancements and indeed the reputation of surgical staff, all have an impact on the incidence of elective aneurysms treated at a particular institution. Similarly, the urgency of the patient's condition and the proximity of the nearest medical facility have an effect on the incidence of RAAAs seen at each medical centre. At the majority of large urban hospitals, a ratio of elective to ruptured aortic aneurysm repairs is approximately 4:1. Here at LAC + USC Medical Centre, however, the distribution of major vascular procedures is heavily weighted towards reconstructions for aortic occlusive disease. As such, our centre manages an even mix of ruptured and elective abdominal aortic aneurysm repairs, essentially unchanged over the past five years.

The management of patients sustaining vascular injuries caused by firearms and motor vehicle accidents continues to pose a significant challenge to our institution. Over the past 10 years, the LAC + USC Trauma Centre has admitted 967 patients with 1399 vessels injured, a mean revised trauma score (RTS) of 5.44 and a mean injury severity scores (ISS) of 23. Most of these patients were admitted in haemorrhagic shock with a mean systolic blood pressure of 92. The majority of them underwent operative treatment of their vascular injuries sustaining a mean estimated blood loss of 3862 mL of blood. Clearly the special resources at our level I trauma centre contributed to the excellence in the provision of care for both critically injured trauma patients as well as for patients presenting with vascular emergencies.

Cerebrovascular accidents are the third leading cause of death in the USA. At our medical centre, approximately 750 patients with newly diagnosed strokes are managed annually. Of these patients, the aetiology of the stroke is ischaemia in over 60 per cent of cases. This is not to mention the additional number of unaccounted patients experiencing transient cerebral ischaemia who are treated and then discharged from the emergency room. To improve the timely treatment of this devastating entity, integration of emergency room personnel, radiology staff, specialty neurologists and vascular surgeons to form a dedicated acute stroke team is currently in action at our medical centre.

REQUIREMENTS

The American College of Surgeons (ACS) founded in 1913, along with its oldest standing committee, the ACS Committee on Trauma (ACS-COT) established in 1922, have been the leaders in the provision and standardisation of care for injured patients. Amongst some of the most important steps taken by the ACS-COT was the creation of a document entitled *Optimal Hospital Resources for Care of the Injured Patient*, which, over the years, has evolved with the contributions of many trauma surgeons into the monograph *Resources for Optimal Care of the Injured Patient*, first published in 1990 and revised in 1993 and 1999.[6,7] This publication is periodically updated by the members of the ACS-COT and strives to set guidelines for the verification of trauma centres. Simultaneously, the designation of trauma centres by 'levels' has evolved into the development of a comprehensive trauma care system, which, in geographical terms, provides care for injured patients throughout the USA.

The LAC + USC Trauma Centre is a level I trauma centre and considered a regional resource facility caring for the citizens of Los Angeles County, the most populous county in the USA. It is one of the largest trauma centres in the USA admitting on a yearly basis between 7500 and 8200 injured patients. Being of level I status, in-house trauma surgery specialists are available 24 hours a day, along with 24-hour availability of operating rooms, surgical intensive care units and a full complement of other surgical and non-surgical specialists needed for optimal provision of trauma care.

The special expertise and resources available to maintain a verified level I trauma centre are both easily applicable and transportable to the management of vascular emergencies. Both injured patients and those admitted with vascular emergencies may arrive at the ER in profound shock and severe physiological compromise, requiring a rapid mobilisation of all resources. This includes resuscitation, immediate transport to a surgical suite for definitive lifesaving interventions and immediate availability of large quantities of blood. Immediately postoperatively, individuals trained in surgical critical care continue the process of resuscitation and administer advanced technological support to patients decompensating into single and/or multiple system organ failure.

Trauma patients and those with vascular emergencies also may have need for multiple staged procedures which require 'bail out/damage control'. Consequently, the presence of a well established ACS verified level I trauma centre with its multidisciplinary approach to the management of complex injuries can also serve a dual purpose in the provision of excellent care to patients presenting with vascular emergencies.

Physicians in most emergency rooms make an initial assessment of a vascular emergency. They provide the initiative in pursuing an aggressive approach involving appropriate specialists and the vascular surgeon in particular. Familiarity with common vascular emergencies and the ability to perform a thorough vascular examination is therefore critical to an emergency physician's expertise in providing an initial assessment and diagnosis on these patients.

Emergency physicians are very dependent on emergency services and emergency medical technicians. In the USA, these individuals are trained to stabilise and move the patient rapidly from the scene of a non-traumatic problem to the hospital where treatment can be provided with the highest degree of sophistication and equipment.

The diagnostic approach to extremity trauma has changed dramatically over the past few decades. Initially, the influences from combat experience led to the aggressive approach of mandatory exploration for all penetrating trauma to an extremity.[8,9] The application of this policy to civilian injuries, however, resulted in negative exploration rates as high as 84 per cent in cases of penetrating trauma. After intense evaluation at our institution, we currently recommend angiography only in patients with signs of vascular injury such as a pulse deficit, bruit or an ankle:brachial index of less than 1.00.[8-10]

Colour-flow duplex (CFD) is gaining widespread acceptance as an initial tool in the diagnostic work-up of vascular trauma. Being non-invasive and lacking side effects makes it an extremely attractive tool in evaluating patients with potential vascular injuries. With improvements in resolution as well as in operator skills, many authors have proposed CFD as a replacement or supplement to angiography. Reported sensitivities and specificities have ranged from 50 to 100 per cent and 99 to 100 per cent, respectively, when compared with angiography.[11-13] We are currently evaluating the role of CFD in the management of patients with extremity trauma at our institution, accepting that angiography still remains the gold standard.

In those instances where an RAAA is being considered, an expedient history and physical examination are necessary. Currently emergency room physicians and trauma surgeons have the capability of performing fast and rapid real time ultrasound assessments of the abdominal aorta in those patients in whom the suspicion of rupture is low but nevertheless has to be excluded. By the same token ultrasound assessment can also provide rapid confirmation of aneurysm rupture as the patient moves to the operating room (OR).

Immediate and 24-hour availability of computed tomographic (CT) scanning and angiography are essential components in the management of vascular emergencies. Technological advances with helical CT scanning configurations have shortened scanning times while providing enhanced resolution and reconstruction capabilities. At the LAC + USC Medical Centre, 24-hour availability of these services provides prompt scanning and feedback on the presence or absence of many vascular disorders.

The need for a second surgeon to assist the vascular surgeon during a complex vascular reconstruction cannot be underestimated. In those instances where the surgeon is working within a university construct with resident training, which may be in general surgery or a combination of general surgery and vascular surgery, valuable surgical assistance should readily be available 24 hours a day. For those surgeons in a community setting, however, the need for assistance in the operating room is critical when faced with an entity such as an RAAA. Support from a surgical partner, trained physician's assistant, or a certified nurse first assistant is invaluable. A call schedule ensuring the availability of such personnel within the community for support is essential.

OPERATING ROOM

The availability of OR personnel familiar with emergency vascular procedures, particularly RAAAs, is crucial. Familiarity with the fundamentals of graft types and vascular instrumentation is necessary for an expeditious operation. With level 1 trauma designation, anaesthesiologists and OR staff are present in the hospital 24 hours a day. Operating room staff not only include OR nurses and technicians but also perfusionists in cases where significant haemorrhage is anticipated. Similarly, an OR, with staff competent in most areas of management of surgical emergencies, should be accessible 24 hours a day. During the procedure, care should be taken to ensure maintenance of core body temperature by warming the OR and by using warm fluid intravenously or intracorporeally. The anaesthesia service should also be well versed in the care of the critically ill patient, able to intubate patients with full stomachs safely and, in hypotensive patients, provide rapid vascular access using large bore central venous lines and arterial lines (see Chapter 7B). In the OR such staffing and policies expedite surgical treatment of vascular emergencies.

Conclusions

What has been presented above is the ideal set up for emergency vascular services. In our own institution, 'level 1' trauma centre designation has made such provisions possible. Our medical centre is a very large busy public facility with the experience of a huge number of ER admissions and emergency vascular procedures. Even in a city as populous as Los Angeles, however, our type of facility is the exception and not the norm. Hospitals which are smaller and without trauma centre designation have difficulty providing and executing care for the critically ill vascular patient. In these instances, local community hospitals may attempt to transfer critical vascular patients from their ER to a hospital facility with 24-hour availability of the type of resources cited above. Transfers of this nature do occur but only sporadically due to a variety of factors, the most important of which is the absence of a recognised system facilitating transfer. This trauma centre, overseen by the ACS, is a successful example of such a system. Expansion of this concept to include vascular surgical emergencies as well as other acute life-threatening conditions would substantially improve outcomes.

Key references

Committee on Trauma. *Resources for the optimal care of the injured patient: 1999*. Chicago, IL: American College of Surgeons 1999; 23–26.

Committee on Trauma. *Resources for the optimal care of the injured patient: 1999*. Chicago, IL: American College of Surgeons 1999; 43–46.

Graves EJ. Detailed Diagnosis and Procedures, National Hospital Discharge Survey: National Center for Health Statistics. *Vital Health Stat* 1989; **100**: 72.

Schwartz MR, Weaver FA, Yellin, *et al*. Refining the indications for arteriography in penetrating extremity trauma: a prospective analysis. *J Vasc Surg* 1993; **17**: 166.

Weaver FA, Papanicolaou G, Yellin AE. Difficult peripheral vascular injuries. *Surg Clin North Am* 1996; **76**: 843–59.

REFERENCES

1 Malone JM, Moore WS, Goldstone J, Malone SJ. Therapeutic and economic impact of a modern amputation program. *Ann Surg* 1979; **189**: 798–802.

2 Krupski WC, Skinner HB, Effeney DJ. Amputation. In: Way LW (ed). *Current Surgical Diagnosis and Treatment*. San Mateo, CA: Appleton and Lange, 1988; 704–14.

3 Bunt TJ, Malone JM. Revascularization or amputation in the over 70 year old. *Am Surg* 1994; **60**: 349–52.

4 Graves EJ. Detailed Diagnosis and Procedures, National Hospital Discharge Survey: National Center for Health Statistics. *Vital Health Stat* 1989; **100**: 72.

5 Department of Health and Human Services, Office of Health Research, Statistics and Technology. *Detailed Diagnosis and Surgical Procedures for Patients Discharged from Short Stay Hospitals*. Hyattsville, MD: National Center for Health Statistics, 1982; **30**.

6 Committee on Trauma. *Resources for Optimal Care of the Injured Patient: 1999*. Chicago, IL: American College of Surgeons 1999; 23–26.

7 Committee on Trauma. *Resources for Optimal Care of the Injured Patient: 1999*. Chicago, IL: American College of Surgeons 1999; 43–46.

8 Schwartz MR, Weaver FA, Yellin, *et al*. Refining the indications for arteriography in penetrating extremity trauma: a prospective analysis. *J Vasc Surg* 1993; **17**: 166.

9 Weaver FA, Yellin AE, Bauer M, *et al*. Is arterial proximity a valid indication for arteriography in penetrating extremity trauma? A prospective analysis. *Arch Surg* 1990; **125**: 1256.

10 Weaver FA, Papanicolaou G, Yellin AE. Difficult peripheral vascular injuries. *Surg Clin North Am* 1996; **76**: 843–59.

11 Bynoe RP, Miles WS, Bell RM, *et al*. Noninvasive diagnosis of vascular trauma by duplex ultrasonography. *J Vasc Surg* 1991; **14**: 346.

12 Fry WR, Smith RS, Sayes DV, *et al*. The success of duplex ultrasonographic scanning in diagnosis of extremity vascular proximity trauma. *Arch Surg* 1993; **128**:1368.

13 Meissner M, Paun M, Johansen K. Duplex scanning for arterial trauma. *Am J Surg* 1991; **161**: 552.

2

Pathophysiology of Acute Vascular Insufficiency

AIRES AB BARROS D'SA, DENIS W HARKIN

THE PROBLEM

Acute vascular insufficiency of the limb is a commonly encountered surgical emergency. Presenting typically in elderly patients with widespread atherosclerotic disease, it threatens not only the viability of the limb but also the life of the patient if treatment is delayed or unsuccessful. The incidence of acute limb ischaemia (ALI) has been estimated to be approximately 14 episodes per 100 000 population and represents 10–16 per cent of the total vascular workload.[1] In most instances the lower limb is affected, either *de novo* or against a background of chronic arterial disease, and therefore failed treatment with subsequent amputation carries substantial social and economic costs for the individual and society at large. Despite modern advances in investigation and treatment, patients presenting with ALI have a particularly severe short term outlook in terms of limb loss, with 30-day amputation rates of 10–30 per cent and mortality rates of around 15 per cent.[1] This high mortality reflects the degree of comorbidities and associated increased risks from coronary and cerebrovascular events in these patients.[2,3] Therefore, when managing acute vascular insufficiency of the limb, overzealous attempts at revascularisation in the elderly or infirm must be tempered by the knowledge that they may precipitate systemic deterioration and fatality (see Chapters 9A and 9B).

AETIOLOGY

Acute vascular insufficiency of the limb is most commonly caused by thrombosis or embolic occlusion. However, an extensive range of aetiologies may be involved, especially

Table 2.1 *Potential causes of acute vascular insufficiency*

Embolism	Cardiac diseases
	Extracardiac arterial diseases
Intrinsic arterial diseases	Occlusive atherosclerosis
	Atherosclerotic aneurysms
	Arteritis and autoimmune diseases
	Fibromuscular dysplasia
Haematological disorders	Clotting factor deficiencies
	Antiphospholipid antibodies
	Red cell, white cell and globulin disorders
	Malignant diseases
	Heparin induced thrombosis syndrome
	Oral contraceptive
Repetitive external trauma	Thoracic outlet syndrome
	Athletic injuries
	Axillary crutch injury
	Trauma to the hands and fingers
Iatrogenic injury	Arterial catherisation
	Anaesthetic arm blocks
	Intra-arterial injections
	Thrombosed axillofemoral bypass
	Irradiation arteritis
	Ergotism
	Radial artery fistula steal
Self-inflicted injury	Intra-arterial narcotic injection
	Deliberate self-harm
Acute external trauma	Blunt injuries
	Penetrating injuries

when the presentation is atypical or in a young adult, as listed in Table 2.1. In this section the important features of the commonest aetiologies pertaining to acute vascular insufficiency of the limb are discussed.

Acute thrombosis

A variety of pathological processes may lead to thrombosis in the intact vascular system representing the final common pathway to vessel occlusion (see Chapters 15, 16 and 20). Normal vascular homoeostasis requires integrity of the vessel wall, a balance between procoagulant and anticoagulant factors in the blood and adequate blood flow. These factors, individually, may each induce thrombosis, but more often they act in combination, and for the purpose of clarity they are discussed separately as those affecting the wall, the blood and miscellaneous extrinsic factors.

VESSEL WALL FACTORS PREDISPOSING TO THROMBOSIS

Intrinsic arterial disease, most importantly atherosclerosis, is by far the commonest predisposing factor in acute vascular insufficiency and may have a long progressive subclinical phase prior to acute presentation. Also discussed here are the much less common cystic medial necrosis and inflammatory arteritis.

Atherosclerosis and atherothrombosis

Atherosclerosis, previously thought to be the preserve of old age, is now recognised in increasingly younger individuals, indeed autopsy studies have demonstrated that some degree of lower limb atherosclerosis is present in most of the adult population.[4] By late middle age, almost 8 per cent of males demonstrate significant disease on non-invasive testing and 5 per cent experience symptoms related to lower limb arterial insufficiency in the form of intermittent claudication.[5] More seriously, studies of hospital patients with claudication suggest that 25 per cent ultimately require bypass surgery or amputation.[6,7] In the upper limb a similar pattern exists,[8] although symptoms requiring surgery are less frequent.

The central pathology in the development of atherosclerosis, namely, the accumulation of plasma lipoproteins, particularly low density lipoproteins (LDLs) in the arterial wall, brings about gradual narrowing of the vessel lumen producing vascular insufficiency. These LDLs undergo oxidation (oxLDLs) and are believed to generate and release products chemotactic to circulating monocytes and smooth muscle cells (SMCs) in the vessel wall. Monocytes attracted to the vessel wall then migrate across the endothelium and differentiate to macrophages in the tissues, phagocytose the oxLDLs and become lipid laden foam cells as depicted in Fig. 2.1. Multiple growth factors, cytokines and other substances produced by endothelial cells, SMCs, macrophages and T lymphocytes encourage cellular accumulation, proliferation and inflammatory injury.[9] The accumulating atherosclerotic plaque, which is covered by a fibrous cap of connective tissue (type I and III collagen, elastin and proteoglycans) synthesised by the SMCs, may then extrude into the vessel lumen compromising cross-sectional diameter and blood flow. Subsequent alterations in blood flow,

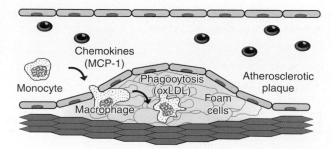

Figure 2.1 *The pathological development of an atherosclerotic plaque. MCP-1, monocyte chemoattractant protein-1*

and consequently vessel wall shear stress, also influence the occurrence and progression of these atherosclerotic plaques.[10]

Acute ischaemic events appear to be related to plaque rupture rather than progressive plaque enlargement and stenosis.[11] The vulnerability of a plaque is dependent on a variety of factors including the size of the lipid pool, the thickness of fibrous cap, the content and metabolic activity of lipids[12] and finally the activity of macrophages and matrix metalloproteinases.[13] Disruption of advanced plaques with exposure of the highly thrombotic lipid core, combined with high intraluminal levels of tissue factor and platelet derived vasoconstrictors, combine to trigger intravascular thrombosis.[14]

Cystic medial necrosis

This relatively rare pathological process primarily affects the aorta and is characterised by myxoid accumulations in the aortic media, accompanied by fragmentation of the elastica, the significance being that cystic medial necrosis can predispose to intimal tears and so precipitate aortic dissection. This outcome is thought to represent the endpoint of a variety of injuries but, in particular, is associated with severe or prolonged hypertension. Interestingly, it is also observed in **Marfan's disease** and may be seen to represent a connective tissue disorder.

Arteritis, autoimmune and associated disorders

Arteritis includes a range of inflammatory processes, which affect the arterial system and lead to acute limb ischaemia (see Chapter 43). These conditions, listed in Table 2.2, are often broadly subdivided on the basis of the vessel size they affect, although significant overlap exists. As systemic inflammatory disorders they commonly present as a non-specific 'rheumatic-like' illness with features such as fever, weight loss, malaise, anaemia, arthralgia, myalgia and arthritis.[15] **Temporal (giant cell) arteritis**, is the commonest of the arterititides and is characterised by focal granulomatous inflammation of medium and small arteries, chiefly the cranial vessels. It most commonly presents clinically in the temporal arteries of older white women.[16] Headache and ocular symptoms predominate and may be accompanied by fever, myalgia, and arthralgia, a syndrome known as

Table 2.2 *Some causes of acute vascular insufficiency associated with arteritis or autoimmune diseases*

Disease	Vessels involved	Distribution
Takayasu's disease	Aorta, arteries	Extremities, head and neck, viscera
Buerger's disease	Arteries, veins, nerves	Extremities
Giant cell arteritis	Muscular arteries	Cranial arteries
Polyarteritis nodosa	Muscular arteries	Any extra-pulmonary site, viscera
Hypersensitivity angiitis	Small venules, capillaries, arterioles	All organs and tissues
Kawasaki's disease	Arteries	Coronary arteries

polymyalgia rheumatica. **Takayasu's disease** is an idiopathic systemic inflammatory disease typically involving large arteries such as the aorta and its main branches, and sometimes the coronary and pulmonary arteries. Typically it affects children and young adults, with a marked female preponderance and geographically more commonly seen in the Far East.[17] Granulomatous vasculitis progresses to medial fibrosis with resultant stenosis or occlusion. The prognosis is poor, with severe hypertension, retinopathy, aortic regurgitation and aneurysm formation being the four main complications.[18] **Kawasaki's disease (mucocutaneous lymph node syndrome)** is a disease which is endemic in Japan, but occurs much less commonly in Europe. Typically it affects infants and children and presents with fever, lymphadenopathy, skin rash, oral and conjunctival erythema and, in 20 per cent of cases, it leads to coronary arteritis. Morbidity and even mortality is associated with coronary arteritis, which can lead to aneurysm formation, thrombosis and acute myocardial injury.

Buerger's disease or **thromboangiitis obliterans** is an inflammatory occlusive disease of the medium- and small-sized arteries of the extremity presenting with segmental thrombotic occlusions of multiple distal arteries.[19] Its prevalence is high in Japan, Israel, and other Asiatic countries and most commonly affects young males who are smokers. Angiography reveals the pathognomonic features of tapering of vessels, abrupt occlusions and classically the corkscrew configuration of collaterals. The prognosis for the limbs is generally poor but their chance of survival is improved in those who stop smoking (see Chapter 42).

Polyarteritis nodosa is a systemic disease characterised by necrotising inflammation of the medium- and small-sized arteries throughout the body, sparing the pulmonary circulation. The lesions are usually sharply demarcated and often induce thrombosis, causing distal ischaemia. Typically affecting young adults, especially men, the condition is accompanied by fever, malaise and weight loss but when the renal vessels are involved morbidity is severe.

Aneurysmal disease and acute arterial dissection

Acute vascular insufficiency of the limb may result from dilating and dissecting arterial diatheses. Aneurysms, the vast majority of which are **atherosclerotic** in nature, but occasionally may be mycotic, post-traumatic or congenital, cause acute vascular insufficiency due to thrombosis, embolism and rupture. Aneurysms must be considered a potential source of acute or chronic embolism compromising the distal circulation, especially if a cardiac source is not identified. Moreover, acute intra-abdominal catastrophes such as ruptured abdominal aortic aneurysm and the resultant low flow state may be confused with primary acute limb ischaemia, therefore systemic assessment of the patient is essential in all cases. The commonest peripheral aneurysm, that of the popliteal artery, constitutes a limb-threatening lesion in that it can be the site of acute thrombo-embolism or the source of chronic low grade embolism which progressively occludes the distal arterial network.[20]

Acute aortic dissections often cause life-threatening ischaemia of peripheral arterial territories and the vital end organs they supply. Stanford type B dissections, which commence beyond the left subclavian artery origin and extend distally, affect the iliac vessels either directly by occlusion of their true lumen or indirectly when a dissecting flap closes off the origin of the artery. Compromise of the true aortic lumen by an expanding high pressure false lumen may lead to the phenomenon of **pseudocoarctation** resulting in a resultant low flow state in the distal organs and limbs. Much more rarely, primary dissections of the iliofemoral segment may cause acute vascular insufficiency of the limb, and are usually associated with underlying pathology such as **fibromuscular dysplasia**.

BLOOD FACTORS PREDISPOSING TO THROMBOSIS

Hypercoagulability or **thrombophilia** represents a state of increased risk of developing arterial or venous thrombosis.[21] Normally a delicate balance between the natural pro-coagulant and anticoagulant pathways prevents unwanted clot formation but a variety of defects, either inherited or acquired, may disturb that equilibrium and cause acute thrombosis. Although most available evidence of thrombogenesis pertains to the venous system, the same underlying defects are thought to be responsible for thrombosis of the native artery or a bypass graft.

Inherited thrombophilia

Inherited defects, either in the procoagulant, anticoagulant or fibrinolytic pathways, as shown in Table 2.3, combined with exposure to common risk factors represent a potentially increased risk for thrombosis. For instance, although the risk of venous thromboembolism below 40 years of age is less than 0.5 per cent in the general population, in certain families, that risk in the same age group rises to 5 per cent.[22] One large study of patients with *idiopathic* venous thrombosis found that 18 per cent of affected individuals were

Table 2.3 *The known inherited thrombophilias arising from defects in the procoagulant, anticoagulant or fibrinolytic pathways*

Type	Specific defect
Deficiencies	Antithrombin
	Protein C
	Protein S
	Plasminogen
	Heparin cofactor II
Defects	Antithrombin
	Protein C
	Protein S
	Factor V Leiden (activated protein C resistance)
	Dysfibrinogenaemias
	Prothrombin mutation 20210
	Thrombomodulin
Elevated procoagulants	Prothrombin
	Hyperhomocysteinaemia
	Plasminogen inhibitor activator type 1
	Histidine-rich glycoprotein

heterozygous for factor V Leiden gene point mutation (activated protein C resistance) and 1.5 per cent of them were homozygous.[23] Much interest has also focused on the presence of prothrombin mutation 20210, which has been reported to be present in up to 18 per cent of patients with thrombosis.[24] Once initiated, coagulation must be controlled by the fibrinolytic system if widespread intravascular thrombosis is to be avoided. Defects in precursor proteins involved in the generation of plasmin, and indeed deficiencies in plasminogen and plasmin action, have been identified. Metabolic defects, such as hyperhomocysteinaemia, are known to be associated with an increased incidence of arterial disease[25] and recently have also been found to be associated with both arterial and venous thromboembolism.[26]

Acquired thrombophilia

Several systemic factors, as shown below, are associated with increased thrombogenicity of the blood, and these include changes in hormonal metabolism, smoking, hyperlipidaemia, hyperglycaemia, disseminated cancer, nephrotic syndrome, trauma, oral contraceptives, pregnancy and the postpartum state.[27] Increased plasma fibrinogen, in particular, is an independent risk factor for thrombotic complications in patients with atherosclerotic disease[28] and trauma.[29] Diabetic patients may have a range of defects which increase blood thrombogenicity, due in part to glycosylation of collagen and proteins, increased levels of plasma fibrinogen and plasminogen activator inhibitor-1[30] and platelet hyperaggregability.[31] Recently increased levels of circulating tissue factor antigen have been observed in patients with cardiovascular disease[32] and consumptive coagulation disorders.[33] Thrombosis is also more common

in a variety of hyperviscosity syndromes such as **polycythaemia**, **macroglobulinaemia**, **cryoglobulinaemia** and **sickle cell anaemia**.

Acquired thrombophilia

- Lupus anticoagulant
- Antiphospholipid antibody
- Myeloproliferative disorders
- Malignancy
- Prolonged immobilisation
- Postoperative states
- Nephrotic syndrome
- Birth control pills
- The known acquired thrombophilias arising from excessive loss or underproduction of anticoagulant or fibrinolytic factors or secretion of procoagulant factors

---

Phlegmasia caerulea dolens

In certain instances venous thrombosis may directly induce acute vascular insufficiency. Phlegmasia caerulea dolens, due to massive iliofemoral deep venous thrombosis, may present with a suddenly painful swollen leg (see Chapter 20). Arterial inflow may be so acutely compromised, due to the venous outflow obstruction, that it threatens the vascular integrity of the limb as is the case with **phlegmasia alba dolens**.

MISCELLANEOUS EXTRINSIC FACTORS PREDISPOSING TO THROMBOSIS

A variety of extrinsic factors which cause acute or chronic vessel injury and luminal compromise may induce arterial thrombosis and lead to acute vascular insufficiency. Acute arterial trauma, perhaps the most dramatic extrinsic injury caused by either blunt or penetrating injury, is discussed in detail elsewhere (see Chapter 33). A range of less dramatic but just as significant chronic injuries, however, may culminate in acute vascular insufficiency and are discussed here briefly.

Repetitive external trauma

Repetitive vessel injury in a few specific syndromes may result in acute vascular insufficiency, often against a background of chronic symptoms.

Thoracic outlet syndrome describes a variable group of symptoms arising from neurovascular compression from either bone or soft tissue structures in the root of the neck, resulting in a clinical picture of chronic pain, neurological disturbance and, more rarely, vascular symptoms[34] (see Chapter 41). Furthermore, the accompanying post-stenotic dilation may progress to an aneurysm and either by embolism or acute thrombosis[35] present clinically as acute arm ischaemia. Thoracic outlet syndrome may have acute vascular manifestations due to scalene muscle trauma in association with hyperextension arm injuries. Furthermore, repeated external trauma to the axillary artery from a shoulder crutch, although rare nowadays, may present as acute thrombosis or secondary thrombosis complicating aneurysmal change.[36] **Popliteal artery entrapment syndrome** describes a developmental defect in which the popliteal artery, and occasionally the popliteal vein, is compressed either beneath the medial head of the gastrocnemius muscle, a slip of that muscle or more rarely the popliteus muscle. The most widely accepted classification recognises five types of popliteal entrapment.[37] It may be responsible for up to 40 per cent of cases in those patients aged less than 30 years presenting with lower limb claudication.[38]

Traumatic vessel injury

Major trauma resulting in acute vascular insufficiency may be blunt or penetrating and the vessel injury can range from subclinical intimal injury to complete vessel disruption. Compounding factors often include associated multisystem injury, haemorrhage, exposure and delayed presentation.[39] Although acute traumatic vessel injury is dealt with in subsequent chapters, a few specific situations require further mention here.

The incidence of **iatrogenic injury** has matched the increasing use of invasive monitoring and endovascular therapy. Catheterisation of a peripheral artery in the critically ill is standard practice[40] and responsible for acute vascular insufficiency in up to 4 per cent of cases,[41] while bleeding and pseudoaneurysm formation may occur, especially if coagulopathy coexists. The increasing use of larger diameter catheters and devices such as intra-aortic balloon pumps has inevitably heralded a mounting frequency of iatrogenic problems in the femoral area (see Chapters 38 and 39).

Endovascular therapy such as angioplasty may produce large areas of intimal–medial dehiscence, commonly at the site of junction between plaque and disease-free wall.[42] However, only rarely do these dissections result in acute vessel closure, and if identified early can be remedied by additional angioplasty or stent placement (see Chapter 39). Angioplasty also significantly stimulates the production of hydroperoxy acids, which are known to mediate vessel spasm and inflammation, in turn leading to arterial thrombosis.[43]

Osseofascial compartment hypertension (compartment syndrome) describes a self-propagating cycle, which occurs within the confines of the osseofascial compartments of the extremities (see Chapter 33). This syndrome may complicate limb trauma, with or without arterial injury, as well as after reconstructive arterial surgery for severe or prolonged ischaemia.[44] Following a period of ischaemia, reperfusion causes capillary endothelial injury which leads to interstitial oedema and an increase in compartment pressure, further compounding tissue hypoxia. Untreated it may lead to permanent neurovascular damage, myoglobinuria, renal failure, sepsis and death.[45] Patients with peripheral vascular disease are much more susceptible to injury from compartment syndrome as their lower resting

Table 2.4 *Aetiology of acute arterial embolic occlusion*

Source	Aetiology
Cardiac	Atrial fibrillation
	Myocardial infarction (mural thrombus)
	Infective endocarditis (mycotic vegetations)
	Prosthetic valve (thrombus)
	Atrial myxoma
	Paradoxical embolus (septal defect)
Major vessels	Atherosclerotic plaque
	Proximal aneurysm
	Mycotic aneurysm
Iatrogenic	Arterial catheterisation
	Postangioplasty/stenting
	Intra-arterial injection

arterial pressure cannot withstand even small increases in compartment pressure.

Finally, **exertional compartment syndromes** may arise due to severe or unaccustomed exercise, most commonly involving the lower extremity and, in particular, the anterior compartment of the lower leg. Rarely, an exertional compartment syndrome may present as an emergency.

Embolic disease

Embolic disease is the second commonest cause of acute vascular insufficiency of the limb. An embolus is a blood clot or other foreign body which is formed in or gains access to the vascular system in one location and is carried by the flow of blood to another site where it produces vascular obstruction (see Chapters 15, 16 and 21). The lower extremity vessels are involved approximately five times as frequently as the upper extremities.[46] The commonest lower limb target site is the common femoral bifurcation, which is also the commonest overall site accounting for 35–50 per cent of instances, whereas the commonest upper limb site is the brachial artery.[47] The majority of emboli originate in the heart, either in patients with atrial fibrillation or in those with mural thrombosis complicating recent myocardial infarction. Less common predisposing cardiac causes are rheumatic heart disease, aortic valve prosthesis, mycotic emboli from subacute bacterial endocarditis and, rarely, atrial myxoma (Table 2.4). A significant proportion of arterial emboli originate from primary arterial diseases proximal to their site of impaction,[47] and they include **atherosclerosis**, **aortitis** and **aneurysmal disease**.

Once present, the clinical outcome of any embolic event depends primarily upon the territory of the vessel involved, the completeness of obstruction and the collateral circulation available. Skeletal muscle is relatively resistant to ischaemic injury but periods beyond 6 hours will usually result in progressive permanent injury. The combination of a paralysed and insensate limb and the onset of ischaemic neuropathy are ominous signs and demand immediate revascularisation if the limb is to be salvaged. The early use of therapeutic anticoagulation with heparin helps prevent secondary clotting or clot propagation, a phenomenon which causes significant deterioration in untreated embolic occlusions. Furthermore, the clinician must be alert to the fact that embolic events are often multiple and may involve several arterial territories. Occult compromise of the splanchnic circulation must be suspected early in a patient who deteriorates systemically if an adverse outcome is to be avoided. A combination of age, high myocardial risk and late presentation contribute to high rates of amputation and mortality.[46,48]

Graft failure

Failure of an existing arterial bypass graft is a common cause of acute vascular insufficiency. Most patients with graft occlusion present with a recurrence of previous symptoms and a smaller number are identified by routine graft surveillance;[49] unfortunately, a significant proportion go on to develop critical ischaemia. Factors within the wall, in the blood and extrinsic factors may all contribute to graft failure. Graft failure can be broadly categorised as immediate (within 30 days), intermediate (between 1 and 18 months), and late (after 18 months). Graft failures in the immediate phase account for 5–20 per cent of cases, and most failures can be attributed to imperfections in surgical technique and in patient selection. Occasionally, in low-flow states, in situ thrombosis reflects the thrombogenicity of the graft. Intermediate phase graft failures, accounting for 5–10 per cent of cases, are largely caused by neointimal hyperplasia. Late failures account for the remaining cases and are usually the result of progression of atherosclerotic disease of inflow and outflow vessels (see Chapter 17).

PATHOPHYSIOLOGY OF ACUTE LIMB ISCHAEMIA

Skeletal muscle ischaemia followed by reperfusion produces several functional and morphological changes including impaired ability to develop tension, mitochondrial swelling, disruption of sarcomere organisation, leakage of cytosolic enzymes into the circulation, endothelial cell swelling and denudation, and the development of the 'no-reflow' phenomenon. In sublethal skeletal muscle ischaemia-reperfusion (I/R) injury most of the tissue abnormalities occur not during ischaemia but on reperfusion.[50] Fortunately, skeletal muscle is relatively resistant to ischaemic injury for a time but when it exceeds 2–7 hours,[51] the opportunity for salvage diminishes. Chronically ischaemic limbs with peripheral vascular disease will tolerate substantially longer periods of ischaemia, in part due to collateralisation but also due to the poorly understood phenomenon of ischaemic tolerance, a sustained ischaemic preconditioning effect, which, of course, when induced acutely, can be shown to prevent reperfusion injury and its systemic effects.[52]

Ischaemic injury

Adenosine triphosphate (ATP), essential in nearly all body processes requiring the output of energy, is depleted during the period of ischaemia,[53] and persistently low tissue levels of ATP can lead directly to cellular death.[54] During the ischaemic period depletion of ATP is associated with the conversion of xanthine dehydrogenase to xanthine oxidase, provoking elevations in purine metabolites, hypoxanthine and xanthine, an environment richly conducive to the production of reactive oxygen species.[55,56] With more prolonged periods of ischaemia severe fibre damage consisting of myofibrillar derangement, loss of organisation of myofilaments or frank myonecrosis ensues.[57]

Oxidative injury

Reperfusion of ischaemic muscle tissue initiates a complex sequence of events which includes the generation of reactive oxygen metabolites, liberation of proinflammatory mediators and granulocyte adherence, infiltration and activation, which result in microvascular and parenchymal cell injury.[58] The influx of a large amount of molecular oxygen at reperfusion generates the production of oxygen-derived free radicals (OFR) which play an important role in inducing postischaemic tissue injury. Oxygen free radicals, including superoxide anions (O_2^-), hydrogen peroxide and hydroxyl radicals (OH^-), arise as byproducts of the enzyme xanthine-xanthine oxidase system, the mitochondrial electron transport system, and the nicotinamide adenosine dinucleotide phosphate (reduced form) (NADPH) oxidase system of neutrophils. These oxygen-free radicals have a direct lytic effect on cellular membranes through lipid peroxidation. Endothelial cell membrane injury is associated with increased microvascular permeability,[59] indeed leg oedema is a common complication after reconstructive vascular surgery.[60] Evidence from animal experiments shows that skeletal muscle injury following ischaemia is attenuated by hypoxic reperfusion rather than by oxygenated blood,[61] or by the use of free radical scavengers.[62]

ANTIOXIDANT DEFENCE AND OXIDATIVE STRESS

Skeletal muscle has several endogenous defences against oxidative injury caused by reactive oxygen metabolites, including, but not limited to the intracellular enzymes superoxide dismutase (SOD), catalase (CAT) and glutathione peroxidase. Superoxide dismutase catalyses the dismutation of superoxide and hydrogen peroxide to water and molecular oxygen, while glutathione peroxidase can also reduce hydrogen peroxide by catalysing its reaction with reduced glutathione (GSH) to form oxidised glutathione disulphide and water. The protective effect of exogenous SOD and catalase in attenuating ischaemia-reperfusion induced skeletal muscle injury has been demonstrated.[63,64] Unfortunately, to be clinically effective they must be given prior to the ischaemic period, which limits their clinical

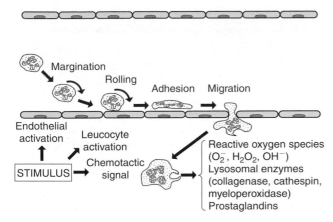

Figure 2.2 *The interaction between circulating neutrophils and the endothelial walls leads to transendothelial migration and inflammatory tissue injury*

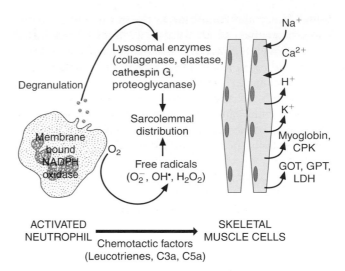

Figure 2.3 *The process of oxidative cellular injury by an activated neutrophil chemoattracted to an ischaemia-reperfusion injured monocyte. CPK, creatine phosphate kinase; GOT, glutamic oxaloacetic transferase; GPT, glutamic pyruvic transferase; LDH, lactose dehydrogenase; NADPH, nicotinamide adenosine dinucleotide phosphate (reduced form)*

usefulness.[65] Antioxidant vitamins, such as C and E, may also act as free radical scavengers, and have been shown to prevent experimental ischaemia-reperfusion injury when given prior to the ischaemic injury.[66]

POLYMORPHONUCLEAR LEUCOCYTE–ENDOTHELIAL INTERACTION

The influx of activated polymorphonuclear leucocytes (PMNs) into postischaemic tissues is one of the hallmarks of ischaemia-reperfusion injury. Polymorphonuclear leucocyte adherence to the endothelium is a requirement for these cells to alter the endothelial barrier and so to allow PMN transmigration to the site of injury. The process of cell adherence, cell activation and cell migration involves an interplay between the expression of adhesion molecules by the endothelial cell, leucocyte activation and local cytokine activity[67,68] as illustrated in Fig. 2.2.

Sequestration of circulating neutrophils in the microvessels of skeletal muscle begins with constitutively expressed neutrophil L-selectin receptors binding to the postcapillary venule endothelial P-selectin and E-selectin receptors. This is the first phase of neutrophil adhesion, and is manifested by 'neutrophil rolling' along the venular luminal surface. The second phase of neutrophil adhesion occurs after activation or 'upregulation' of the CD11/CD18 integrins and shedding of L-selectin from the neutrophil surface, caused by release of proinflammatory cytokines, platelet activating factor (PAF) and eicosanoids from the damaged endothelial cell. This halts neutrophil rolling by providing strong neutrophil–endothelial cell adhesion through the interaction of the CD11b/CD18 integrin with the endothelial receptor, intercellular adhesion molecule-1 (ICAM-1). Finally transmigration occurs, which involves both chemotactic stimuli, such as interleukin-8, and binding to the platelet–endothelial cell adhesion molecule-1 (PECAM-1).[69] Attenuation of neutrophil accumulation in postischaemic tissues using antibodies directed against the neutrophil surface adherence complex in skeletal muscle[70] has been successfully demonstrated. After reperfusion of postischaemic tissue the accumulation of PMN is associated with severe morphological injuries manifested as large and numerous intramitochondrial dense bodies, mitochondrial swelling and intermyofibillar oedema.[71] While adhering to the endothelium, neutrophils damage endothelial cells and the basement membrane by releasing superoxide anions via the NADPH oxidase system, secreting myeloperoxidase which catalyses the production of hypochlorus acid (HOCL), and releasing granular enzymes including elastase, collagenase and cathepsin G,[72] as shown in Fig. 2.3. Enhanced neutrophil adhesion to endothelium is seen in postcapillary venules during ischaemia with a more pronounced response following reperfusion.[73]

'NO-REFLOW' PHENOMENON

After an extended period of ischaemia in skeletal muscle, some capillaries fail to perfuse on reinstitution of blood flow.[74,75] This 'no-reflow' phenomenon results in incomplete and maldistributed perfusion and contributes to injury by prolonging hypoxia and exposure of the tissues to toxic metabolites.[76]

Maldistribution of blood flow due to the failure of local vascular autoregulation is understood to be the cause of the 'no-reflow' phenomenon noted after ischaemic injury and tends to compound ischaemic damage in underperfused areas. This maldistribution of flow is not simply based on vasoconstriction but represents a failure of vascular smooth muscle responsiveness to the usual vasoactive mediators such as PO_2, PCO_2, pH, lactate, potassium, adenine nucleotides, bradykinin, prostaglandins, nitric oxide and changes in osmolality.[77]

Mechanical obstruction of small vessels due to entrapment of enlarged adherent leucocytes 'plugging' the capillary lumen[74] may also contribute to the 'no-reflow' phenomenon. Oxidative endothelial damage leads to endothelial cell swelling which reduces the diameter of the vascular lumen adding to vascular resistance[70] and capillary neutrophil plugging.[78] The adhesion of neutrophils to the venular endothelial cells in turn increases capillary pressure and fluid filtration, through an already damaged endothelial barrier, compounding interstitial oedema and compression of the microcirculatory system.[58]

UPREGULATION OF GENE EXPRESSION

As our understanding of the intracellular events during ischaemia-reperfusion injury improves with advances in molecular biology, we shall soon understand why different tissues have such disparate tolerances to ischaemic injury. Early work has confirm enhanced gene expression or 'upregulation' during ischaemia and perhaps more importantly in early reperfusion.[79] Experimental work is already in progress exploring the benefits of new genetic therapies in skeletal muscle ischaemia-reperfusion injury.[80] Improved understanding of the role of these genes and their sequence of upregulation may well open a new arena for therapeutic intervention.

Systemic response to reperfusion

Reperfusion of the acutely ischaemic limb not only causes local effects but, with revascularization, also carries a variety of proinflammatory stimuli into the systemic circulation. Products of oxidative injury, namely, reactive oxygen species, arachidonic acid metabolites and hydroperoxides, interact with activated endothelial cells and leucocytes in an environment rich in proinflammatory cytokines. These proinflammatory mediators and activated leucocytes initiate an intravascular cascade of pro- and anti-inflammatory responses resulting in remote vital organ injury.[81] This systemic inflammatory response syndrome (SIRS), which may lead to multiple organ dysfunction syndrome (MODS), is dealt with in Chapter 4.

CLINICAL ASSESSMENT OF ACUTE VASCULAR INSUFFICIENCY

The clinician must interpret the patient's history and clinical signs to determine the extent and duration of the underlying injury, the feasibility of revascularisation and the wisdom of doing so in a particular setting. A variety of clinical grading systems aid the clinician in the decision making process, perhaps the most widely accepted being that adopted by the Society for Vascular Surgery and the International Society of Cardiovascular Surgery (SVS/ISCVS) and given in Table 2.5. These systems, at best, only provide

Table 2.5 *The Society for Vascular Surgery/International Society of Cardiovascular Surgery (SVS/ISCVS) grading system for limb ischaemia*

Grade	Description	Treatment
Class I	Viable leg, without impairment of sensory or motor function and audible Doppler signals	Heparin is given and elective treatment, either conservative or interventional, is arranged
Class IIa	Marginally threatened with symptoms limited to a mild sensory loss (usually in the toes)	A delay of 9 hours is acceptable to attempt treatment by lysis
Class IIb	Immediately at risk with pronounced sensory loss, mild to moderate motor loss but audible Doppler signals	Delay is unacceptable and urgent clot extraction by aspiration or embolectomy is required Accelerated thrombolysis may be used
Class III	Absent Doppler flow, paralysis, total sensory loss and irreversible tissue damage	Attempts to restore blood flow would lead to hyperkalaemia and myoglobinuria, so delayed amputation should be performed after resuscitation

guidance because the treatment for each patient has to be individualised by an experienced vascular surgical team.

Conclusions

It is clear that acute vascular insufficiency is a common surgical emergency in a high risk patient population inherently predisposed to cardiovascular and cerebrovascular risk. Despite advances in management it is a condition which continues to be associated with high amputation and mortality rates. Diagnosis and treatment require a multidisciplinary approach involving interventional radiologists, haematologists, immunologists, clinical biochemists and vascular technicians under the supervision of an experienced vascular surgeon. When revascularisation is indicated the extent and duration of ischaemia time is the major determinant of outcome. The clinician must also recognise the settings in which revascularisation is detrimental to the patient and in these instances it may be wiser to adopt a suitably palliative approach. The rapid advances in endovascular therapies and our increasing understanding of genetic and environmental factors predisposing to acute vascular insufficiency will combine to ensure that this remains an interesting and evolving clinical field.

Key references

Campbell WB, Ridler BM, Szymanska TH. Current management of acute leg ischaemia: results of an audit by the Vascular Surgical Society of Great Britain and Ireland. *Br J Surg* 1998; **85**: 1498–503.

Carden DL, Smith JK, Korthuis RJ. Neutrophil-mediated microvascular dysfunction in postischemic canine skeletal muscle. Role of granulocyte adherence. *Circ Res* 1990; **66**: 1436–44.

Dormandy J, Heeck L, Vig S. The natural history of claudication: risk to life and limb. *Semin Vasc Surg* 1999; **12**: 123–37.

Smith JK, Carden DL, Korthuis RJ. Role of xanthine oxidase in postischemic microvascular injury in skeletal muscle. *Am J Physiol* 1989; **257**: H1782–H1789.

Smith JK, Grisham MB, Granger DN, Korthuis RJ. Free radical defense mechanisms and neutrophil infiltration in postischemic skeletal muscle. *Am J Physiol* 1989; **256**: H789–H793.

REFERENCES

1 Dormandy J, Heeck L, Vig S. Acute limb ischemia. *Semin Vasc Surg* 1999; **12**: 148–53.

2 Dormandy J, Heeck L, Vig S. The natural history of claudication: risk to life and limb. *Semin Vasc Surg* 1999; **12**: 123–37.

3 Leng GC, Fowkes FG, Lee AJ, *et al.* Use of ankle brachial pressure index to predict cardiovascular events and death: a cohort study. *BMJ* 1996; **313**: 1440–4.

4 Sternby NH. Atherosclerosis in a defined population. An autopsy survey in Malmo, Sweden. *Acta Pathol Microbiol Scand* 1968; Suppl.

5 Fowkes FG, Housley E, Cawood EH, *et al.* Edinburgh Artery Study: prevalence of asymptomatic and symptomatic peripheral arterial disease in the general population. *Int J Epidemiol* 1991; **20**: 384–92.

6 Fowkes FG. The measurement of atherosclerotic peripheral arterial disease in epidemiological surveys. *Int J Epidemiol* 1988; **17**: 248–54.

7 Fowkes FG. Epidemiology of atherosclerotic arterial disease in the lower limbs. *Eur J Vasc Surg* 1988; **2**: 283–91.

8 Bergqvist D, Ericsson BF, Konrad P, Bergentz SE. Arterial surgery of the upper extremity. *World J Surg* 1983; **7**: 786–91.

9 Varela O, Martinez-Gonzalez J, Badimon L. The response of smooth muscle cells to alpha-thrombin depends on its arterial origin: comparison among different species. *Eur J Clin Invest* 1998; **28**: 313–23.

10 Turitzto VT, Hall CL. Mechanical factors affecting hemostasis and thrombosis. Thromb Res 1998; 92: S25–S31.

11 Badimon L, Meyer BJ, Badimon JJ. Thrombin in arterial thrombosis. *Haemostasis* 1994; **24**: 69–80.

12 Felton CV, Crook D, Davies MJ, Oliver MF. Relation of plaque lipid composition and morphology to the stability of human aortic plaques. *Arterioscler Thromb Vasc Biol* 1997; **17**: 1337–45.

13 Libby P. Molecular bases of the acute coronary syndromes. *Circulation* 1995; **91**: 2844–50.

14 Fernandez-Ortiz A, Badimon JJ, Falk E, *et al.* Characterization of the relative thrombogenicity of atherosclerotic plaque components: implications for consequences of plaque rupture. *J Am Coll Cardiol* 1994; **23**: 1562–9.

15 Hoffman GS. Takayasu arteritis: lessons from the American National Institutes of Health experience. *Int J Cardiol* 1996; **54**(suppl): S99–S102.

16 Paice EW. Giant cell arteritis: difficult decisions in diagnosis, investigation and treatment. *Postgrad Med J* 1989; **65**: 743–7.

17 Rizzi R, Bruno S, Stellacci C, Dammacco R. Takayasu's arteritis: a cell-mediated large-vessel vasculitis. *Int J Clin Lab Res* 1999; **29**: 8–13.

18 Morales E, Pineda C, Martinez-Lavin M. Takayasu's arteritis in children. *J Rheumatol* 1991; **18**: 1081–4.

19 Shionoya S. Buerger's disease: diagnosis and management. *Cardiovasc Surg* 1993; **1**: 207–14.

20 Dawson I, Sie RB, van Bockel JH. Atherosclerotic popliteal aneurysm. *Br J Surg* 1997; **84**: 293–9.

21 Miletich JP. Thrombophilia as a multigenic disorder. *Semin Thromb Hemost* 1998; **24**(suppl 1): 13–20.

22 Koster T, Rosendaal FR, Briet E, *et al.* Protein C deficiency in a controlled series of unselected outpatients: an infrequent but clear risk factor for venous thrombosis (Leiden Thrombophilia Study). *Blood* 1995; **85**: 2756–61.

23 FR, Koster T, Vandenbroucke JP, Reitsma PH. High risk of thrombosis in patients homozygous for factor V Leiden (activated protein C resistance). *Blood* 1995; **85**: 1504–8.

24 Poort SR, Rosendaal FR, Reitsma PH, Bertina RM. A common genetic variation in the 3′-untranslated region of the prothrombin gene is associated with elevated plasma prothrombin levels and an increase in venous thrombosis. *Blood* 1996; **88**: 3698–703.

25 De S, V, Finazzi G, Mannucci PM. Inherited thrombophilia: pathogenesis, clinical syndromes, and management. *Blood* 1996; **87**: 3531–44.

26 den Heijer M, Koster T, Blom HJ, *et al.* Hyperhomocysteinemia as a risk factor for deep-vein thrombosis. *N Engl J Med* 1996; **334**: 759–62.

27 Fowkes FG, Housley E, Riemersma RA, *et al.* Smoking, lipids, glucose intolerance, and blood pressure as risk factors for peripheral atherosclerosis compared with ischemic heart disease in the Edinburgh Artery Study. *Am J Epidemiol* 1992; **135**: 331–40.

28 Yarnell JW, Baker IA, Sweetnam PM, *et al.* Fibrinogen, viscosity, and white blood cell count are major risk factors for ischemic heart disease. The Caerphilly and Speedwell collaborative heart disease studies. *Circulation* 1991; **83**: 836–44.

29 Dalmon J, Laurent M, Courtois G. The human beta fibrinogen promoter contains a hepatocyte nuclear factor 1-dependent interleukin-6-responsive element. *Mol Cell Biol* 1993; **13**: 1183–93.

30 Meigs JB, Mittleman MA, Nathan DM, *et al.* Hyperinsulinemia, hyperglycemia, and impaired hemostasis: the Framingham Offspring Study. *JAMA* 2000; **283**: 221–8.

31 Rauch U, Crandall J, Osende JI, *et al.* Increased thrombus formation relates to ambient blood glucose and leukocyte count in diabetes mellitus type 2. *Am J Cardiol* 2000; **86**: 246–9.

32 Soejima H, Ogawa H, Yasue H, *et al.* Heightened tissue factor associated with tissue factor pathway inhibitor and prognosis in patients with unstable angina. *Circulation* 1999; **99**: 2908–13.

33 Gando S, Nanzaki S, Sasaki S, Kemmotsu O. Significant correlations between tissue factor and thrombin markers in trauma and septic patients with disseminated intravascular coagulation. *Thromb Haemost* 1998; **79**: 1111–15.

34 Roos DB. The thoracic outlet syndrome is underrated. *Arch Neurol* 1990; **47**: 327–8.

35 Scher LA, Veith FJ, Samson RH, *et al.* Vascular complications of thoracic outlet syndrome. *J Vasc Surg* 1986; **3**: 565–8.

36 Lee AW, Hopkins SF, Griffen WO Jr. Axillary artery aneurysm as an occult source of emboli to the upper extremity. *Am Surg* 1987; **53**: 485–6.

37 Rich NM, Collins GJ Jr, McDonald PT, *et al.* Popliteal vascular entrapment. Its increasing interest. *Arch Surg* 1979; **114**: 1377–84.

38 Hamming JJ, Vink M. Obstruction of the popliteal artery at an early age. *J Cardiovasc Surg (Torino)* 1965; **6**: 516–24.

39 Barros D'Sa AAB. Twenty five years of vascular trauma in Northern Ireland. *BMJ* 1995; **310**: 1–2.

40 Clark VL, Kruse JA. Arterial catheterization. *Crit Care Clin* 1992; **8**: 687–97.

41 Frezza EE, Mezghebe H. Indications and complications of arterial catheter use in surgical or medical intensive care units: analysis of 4932 patients. *Am Surg* 1998; **64**: 127–31.

42 Uchida Y, Hasegawa K, Kawamura K, Shibuya I. Angioscopic observation of the coronary luminal changes induced by percutaneous transluminal coronary angioplasty. *Am Heart J* 1989; **117**: 769–76.

43 Cragg A, Einzig S, Castaneda-Zuniga W, *et al.* Vessel wall arachidonate metabolism after angioplasty: possible mediators of postangioplasty vasospasm. *Am J Cardiol* 1983; **51**: 1441–5.

44 Barros D'Sa AAB. Complex vascular and orthopaedic limb injuries. *J Bone Joint Surg Br* 1992; **74**: 176–8.

45 Matsen FA, III, Winquist RA, Krugmire RB Jr. Diagnosis and management of compartmental syndromes. *J Bone Joint Surg Am* 1980; **62**: 286–91.

46 Panetta T, Thompson JE, Talkington CM, *et al.* Arterial embolectomy: a 34-year experience with 400 cases. *Surg Clin North Am* 1986; **66**: 339–53.

47 Davies MG, O'Malley K, Feeley M, *et al.* Upper limb embolus: a timely diagnosis. *Ann Vasc Surg* 1991; **5**: 85–7.

48 Campbell WB, Ridler BM, Szymanska TH. Current management of acute leg ischaemia: results of an audit by the Vascular Surgical Society of Great Britain and Ireland. *Br J Surg* 1998; **85**: 1498–503.

49 Moody P, de Cossart LM, Douglas HM, Harris PL. Asymptomatic strictures in femoro-popliteal vein grafts. *Eur J Vasc Surg* 1989; **3**: 389–92.

50 Sjostrom M, Neglen P, Friden J, Eklof B. Human skeletal muscle metabolism and morphology after temporary incomplete ischaemia. *Eur J Clin Invest* 1982; **12**: 69–79.

51 Karpati G, Carpenter S, Melmed C, Eisen AA. Experimental ischemic myopathy. *J Neurol Sci* 1974; **23**: 129–61.

52 Harkin DW, Barros D'Sa AAB, McCallion K, *et al.* Ischemic preconditioning before lower limb ischemia–reperfusion protects against acute lung injury. *J Vasc Surg* 2002; **35**: 1264–73.

53 Hinshaw DB, Armstrong BC, Beals TF, Hyslop PA. A cellular model of endothelial cell ischemia. *J Surg Res* 1988; **44**: 527–37.

54 Lindsay TF, Liauw S, Romaschin AD, Walker PM. The effect of ischemia/reperfusion on adenine nucleotide metabolism and xanthine oxidase production in skeletal muscle. *J Vasc Surg* 1990; **12**: 8–15.

55 Grisham MB, Hernandez LA, Granger DN. Xanthine oxidase and neutrophil infiltration in intestinal ischemia. *Am J Physiol* 1986; **251**: G567–G574.

56 Smith JK, Carden DL, Korthuis RJ. Role of xanthine oxidase in postischemic microvascular injury in skeletal muscle. *Am J Physiol* 1989; 257: H1782–9.

57 Kuzon WM Jr, Walker PM, Mickle DA, *et al.* An isolated skeletal muscle model suitable for acute ischemia studies. *J Surg Res* 1986; **41**: 24–32.

58 Korthuis RJ, Granger DN, Townsley MI, Taylor AE. The role of oxygen-derived free radicals in ischemia-induced increases in canine skeletal muscle vascular permeability. *Circ Res* 1985; **57**: 599–609.

59 Kupinski AM, Shah DM, Bell DR. Permeability changes following ischemia-reperfusion injury in the rabbit hindlimb. *J Cardiovasc Surg (Torino)* 1992; **33**: 690–4.

60 Persson NH, Takolander R, Bergqvist D. Lower limb oedema after arterial reconstructive surgery. Influence of preoperative ischaemia, type of reconstruction and postoperative outcome. *Acta Chir Scand* 1989; **155**: 259–66.

61 Korthuis RJ, Smith JK, Carden DL. Hypoxic reperfusion attenuates postischemic microvascular injury. *Am J Physiol* 1989; **256**: H315–19.

62 Smith JK, Grisham MB, Granger DN, Korthuis RJ. Free radical defense mechanisms and neutrophil infiltration in postischemic skeletal muscle. *Am J Physiol* 1989; **256**: H789–93.

63 Reikeras O, Ytrehus K. Oxygen radicals and scavenger enzymes in ischaemia-reperfusion injury of skeletal muscle. *Scand J Clin Lab Invest* 1992; **52**: 113–18.

64 Ytrehus K, Semb AG, Myhre ES. Ibuprofen abolishes the increase in leucocyte chemiluminescence observed during ischemic myocardial failure, but fails to improve hemodynamic function. *Basic Res Cardiol* 1992; **87**: 385–92.

65 Faust KB, Chiantella V, Vinten-Johansen J, Meredith JH. Oxygen-derived free radical scavengers and skeletal muscle ischemic/reperfusion injury. *Am Surg* 1988; **54**: 709–19.

66 Harkin DW, Barros D'Sa AAB, Yassin MMI, *et al.* Reperfusion injury is greater with delayed restoration of venous outflow in concurrent arterial and venous limb injury. *Br J Surg* 2000; **87**: 734–41.

67 Adams DH, Shaw S. Leucocyte-endothelial interactions and regulation of leucocyte migration. *Lancet* 1994; **343**: 831–6.

68 Davies MG, Hagen PO. The vascular endothelium. A new horizon. *Ann Surg* 1993; **218**: 593–609.

69 Smith CW, Marlin SD, Rothlein R, *et al.* Cooperative interactions of LFA-1 and Mac-1 with intercellular adhesion molecule-1 in facilitating adherence and transendothelial migration of human neutrophils *in vitro. J Clin Invest* 1989; **83**: 2008–17.

70 Carden DL, Smith JK, Korthuis RJ. Neutrophil-mediated microvascular dysfunction in postischemic canine skeletal muscle. Role of granulocyte adherence. *Circ Res* 1990; 66: 1436–44.

71 Formigli L, Lombardo LD, Adembri C, *et al.* Neutrophils as mediators of human skeletal muscle ischemia-reperfusion syndrome. *Hum Pathol* 1992; **23**: 627–34.

72 Weiss SJ. Tissue destruction by neutrophils. *N Engl J Med* 1989; **320**: 365–76.

73 Granger DN, Kvietys PR, Perry MA. Leukocyte-endothelial cell adhesion induced by ischemia and reperfusion. *Can J Physiol Pharmacol* 1993; **71**: 67–75.

74 Bagge U, Amundson B, Lauritzen C. White blood cell deformability and plugging of skeletal muscle capillaries in hemorrhagic shock. *Acta Physiol Scand* 1980; **108**: 159–63.

75 Strock PE, Majno G. Microvascular changes in acutely ischemic rat muscle. *Surg Gynecol Obstet* 1969; **129**: 1213–24.

76 Allen DM, Chen LE, Seaber AV, Urbaniak JR. Pathophysiology and related studies of the no reflow phenomenon in skeletal muscle. *Clin Orthop* 1995; **314**: 122–33.

77 Forrest I, Lindsay T, Romaschin A, Walker P. The rate and distribution of muscle blood flow after prolonged ischemia. *J Vasc Surg* 1989; **10**: 83–8.

78 Walden DL, McCutchan HJ, Enquist EG, *et al.* Neutrophils accumulate and contribute to skeletal muscle dysfunction after ischemia-reperfusion. *Am J Physiol* 1990; **259**: H1809–12.

79 Paoni NF, Peale F, Wang F, *et al.* Time course of skeletal muscle repair and gene expression following acute hind limb ischemia in mice. *Physiol Genomics* 2002; **11**: 263–72.

80 Brevetti LS, Sarkar R, Chang DS, *et al.* Administration of adenoviral vectors induces gangrene in acutely ischemic rat hindlimbs: role of capsid protein-induced inflammation. *J Vasc Surg* 2001; **34**: 489–96.

81 Harkin DW, Barros D'Sa AAB, McCallion K, *et al.* Circulating neutrophil priming and systemic inflammation in limb ischaemia-reperfusion injury. *Int Angiol* 2001; **20**: 78–89.

3

Intestinal Ischaemia in Aortic Surgery

MARTIN G BJÖRCK

THE PROBLEM

Intestinal ischaemia in the postoperative period after aortoiliac surgery represents a major challenge to the vascular surgeon. This complication constitutes a lethal threat to the patient and occurs so frequently that the ability to manage it will affect the overall outcome.

The cardinal symptoms, namely, early bloody diarrhoea and peritonitis, are more often absent than present. If the complication is diagnosed merely on the basis of these clinical symptoms and signs over half of these patients would suffer an unnecessary and potentially lethal delay in treatment. On the other hand, benign mucosal ischaemic lesions are common, especially after emergency surgery, and an unnecessary re-laparotomy in such cases would represent a threat to the patient. Timely recognition and proper grading of the ischaemic lesion, therefore, are essential ingredients for a favourable outcome.

Understanding the pathophysiology of this condition is helpful if it is to be prevented. The correlation between intestinal ischaemia, ischaemia-reperfusion injury (IRI) (detailed in Chapter 2), systemic inflammatory response syndrome (SIRS) and multiple organ dysfunction syndrome (MODS) (see Chapter 4) and intra-abdominal hypertension poses a number of questions regarding the general treatment of patients after major abdominal surgery or trauma.

INCIDENCE AND GRADING OF THE ISCHAEMIC LESION

Although colonic ischaemia was reported just a year after the very first successful repair of an abdominal aortic aneurysm (AAA),[1] its true incidence has long remained unclear. Differences in case-mix may explain why, during the very same year of 1960, one group[2] reported an incidence of 10 per cent (12 of 120) while another[3] of 0.2 per cent (2 of 931); the latter report from Houston of operations on a highly selected group of patients has never been reproduced over the decades right up to the introduction of endovascular repair (EVAR) and illustrates the continued failure to recognise the existence of colonic ischaemia. The largest retrospective study from a single centre[4] reported an incidence of 1.1 per cent among 2137 patients, only 147 (6.8 per cent) of whom required surgery for rupture. The frequency of emergency operations performed and postmortem examinations undertaken, the latter being included in only three publications,[5–7] has a profound impact on the reported incidence of the complication.

Colonic ischaemia accounts for approximately 95 per cent of cases of intestinal ischaemia complicating aortoiliac surgery.[6,8] The resulting ischaemic lesions can be divided into three grades, namely, mucosal ischaemia, mucosal plus muscular ischaemia and transmural gangrene (Fig. 3.1).[9]

> **Grades of ischaemia**
>
> - Grade I – mucosal ischaemia
> - Grade II – mucosal plus muscular ischaemia
> - Grade III – transmural gangrene

Prospective studies, in which all patients were examined postoperatively by sigmoidoscopy[10–12] or by pH$_i$-guided sigmoidoscopy,[5,13] reported incidences of colon ischaemia of 5–11 per cent after elective AAA surgery and 15–60 per cent after operation for rupture. Most of these patients, however, had superficial mucosal lesions the clinical relevance of which is a matter of controversy.

The definition of normal or of pathological appearances at sigmoidoscopy varies. If the findings of diffuse hyperaemia, submucosal haemorrhagic spots and solitary erosions are to be defined as pathological, then no patient undergoing aortic surgery should be regarded as having normal colonic mucosa.[14] When colonoscopy was combined with biopsy 1 week after elective aortic surgery (28 for AAA and 28 for occlusive disease) histological signs of colonic ischaemia were observed in 30 per cent of patients.[15]

The introduction of vascular registries has permitted analyses of the incidence of colonic ischaemia in large non-selected patient populations, undergoing surgery for both elective and ruptured AAA (Table 3.1). In these reports only those patients with clinically relevant ischaemia were included, and most of them (80 per cent) had bowel gangrene. Patients with grade II lesions often develop ischaemic strictures and diarrhoea whereas patients with grade III lesions may advance to the clinically problematic manifestation of bloody stools.

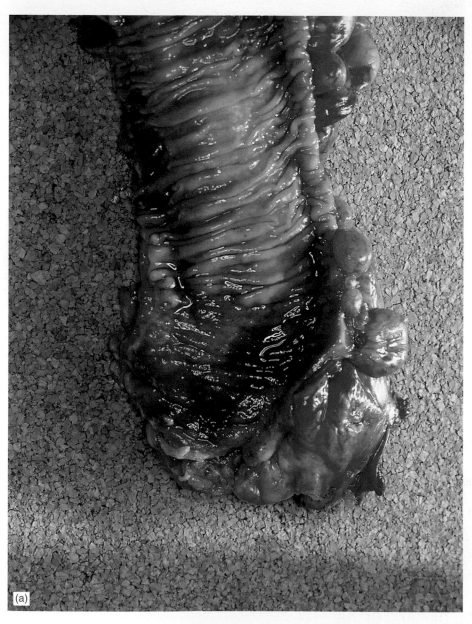

Figure 3.1   *(a) Specimen of resected sigmoid colon showing a grade II lesion with distinct differences between normal and ischaemic mucosa. After a combined operation for abdominal aortic aneurysm (AAA) and renal artery stenosis the patient developed colonic ischaemia and mucosal gangrene was confirmed on colonoscopy postoperatively. When anuria developed on the fifth day, the patient's sigmoid colon was resected. (b) Postmortem specimen of the left colon revealing a grade III lesion with distinct differences between normal and ischaemic colon at the left flexure. The 80-year-old patient arrived in shock due to a ruptured AAA and 4 hours after the operation developed bloody diarrhoea; colonic ischaemia was confirmed at sigmoidoscopy and 2 days later the patient died in multiple organ failure*

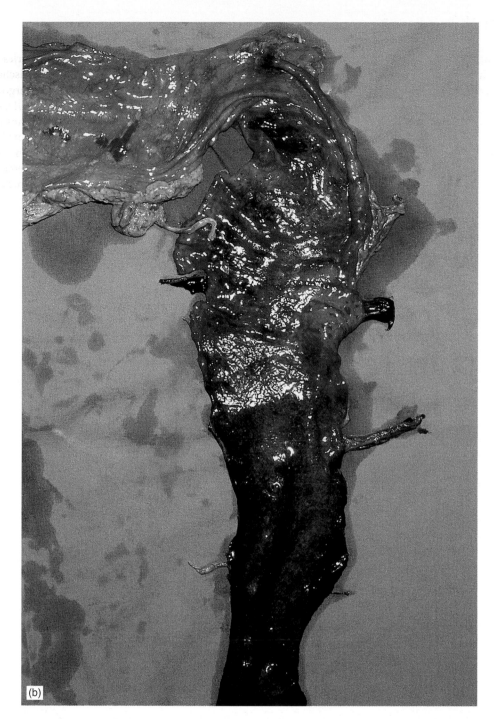

Figure 3.1 *(Cont'd)*

Table 3.1 *Incidence of intestinal ischaemia after aortic surgery in vascular registries*

Source	Registry	Time period	Number of patients	Incidence (per cent)		
				Overall	Elective operation	Rupt. AAA
Amundsen *et al.*[16]	All of Norway	1981–1983	444	3.4	2	10
Longo *et al.*[17]	VA Registry, USA	1987–1991	4957	1.2	?	?
Björck *et al.*[6]	Swedvasc, Sweden	1987–1993	2930	2.8	1.1	5.9
Järvinen *et al.*[18]	Finnvasc, Finland	1991–1993	1752	1.2	0.8	3.1
Norgren*	Eurostar	1994–2001	3558	0.2	0.2	–

*L Norgren, personal communication. Data from the Eurostar Registry, August 2001.

Incidence after endovascular repair

Most reports of series of endovascular stent graft repair (EVAR) refer to elective rather than ruptured AAA. The incidence of bowel ischaemia following open surgery is approximately 1 per cent and more than 5000 patients would have to undergo EVAR in order to demonstrate a fall in the complication rate to 0.5 per cent.

By August 2001, nine of 3658 patients in the Eurostar Registry developed colonic ischaemia, an incidence of 0.2 per cent (L. Norgren, personal communication; data from the Eurostar Registry, August 2001), which, within 95 per cent confidence limits, is lower than the 0.9 per cent (11 cases of 1160 open elective AAA operations) observed in the Swedvasc Registry.[6] Nevertheless, it is important to point out that the Swedvasc data were extensively validated and that the autopsy rate was 66 per cent; in contrast, such valuable and pertinent information does not exist in the Eurostar Registry.

Importance

The clinical importance of colonic ischaemia in AAA surgery is evident from an analysis of data available in the Swedvasc Registry. We found that 9 per cent of the patients who died after an elective operation and 23 per cent of those who died after operation of a ruptured AAA suffered this complication.[19]

AETIOLOGY AND PATHOPHYSIOLOGY

The aetiology of intestinal ischaemia is complex with confounding factors. For instance, operations for ruptured AAA are associated with prolonged cross-clamping and substantial bleeding. We studied 62 patients who suffered the complication in a case–control study nested in a cohort of 2824 patients.[20] For the first time it was possible to study the risk factors using multivariate analysis. The **independent risk factors** identified are shown in Table 3.2.

Risk factors, such as preoperative shock or renal insufficiency are not easily controlled, while others depend on surgical decision making. Intestinal ischaemia following surgery was more prevalent in regional than in district hospitals and is probably attributable to the sustained treatment provided in the former resulting in better survival at 30 days. However, no difference in survival was noted between the two groups after 1 year. It appears that in district hospitals staff are more inclined to withdraw treatment when patients deteriorate in the early postoperative period.

Patients with an occluded **inferior mesenteric artery** (IMA) had an elevated, though insignificant, risk of developing bowel ischaemia, relative risk (RR) = 1.64 (0.62–4.31), compared with those whose IMA was ligated at surgery. In 1978 Ernst *et al.* published a report[21] on 52 patients undergoing elective AAA surgery, 13 of whom had an occluded IMA and 39 in whom pre- and post-reconstruction

Table 3.2 *Independent risk factors for intestinal ischaemia, identified by multivariate analysis in a cohort of 2824 patients*[20]

Risk factor	Relative risk/odds ratio
Blood loss >10 L	6.3
Patient in shock due to a ruptured AAA	3.2
Ligation of one or both internal iliac arteries	2.6
Emergency surgery	2.4
Aorto-bifemoral graft	2.4
Renal insufficiency (creatine >150 μmol/L)	2.3
Operation at a regional hospital	1.9
	Hazard rate
Age	3.5% per year
Aortic cross-clamp time	1.2% per minute
Operating time	0.9% per minute

IMA stump pressures were measured. One patient suffered mild, subclinical, ischaemic colitis diagnosed on routine sigmoidoscopy which resolved completely by the eighth day. This patient had the lowest post-reconstruction stump pressure of 33 mmHg, and in nine patients pressures of between 40 and 50 mmHg were recorded. From this single observation far-reaching conclusions were made: it was claimed that if the IMA had thrombosed or if IMA stump pressure exceeded 40 mmHg, ischaemic colitis would not occur and therefore ligation of the IMA could be safely carried out.

Two other case–control studies[13,22] evaluated ligation of a patent IMA as a risk factor for intestinal ischaemia and both concluded that it was not a significant factor. In a prospective study using sigmoid colon pH_i measurements, patients with an occluded IMA prior to surgery had lower pH_i values than those with a patent IMA at all stages, and the difference became significant on the third postoperative day.[5] Occlusion of the IMA was associated with increasing age, larger aneurysms, longer operations and greater volumes of blood loss. In conclusion, occlusion of the IMA prior to surgery is a marker for advanced arterial disease and there are no data to support reimplantation of a patent IMA in an attempt to prevent colonic ischaemia.

The fact that the left colon is the segment most liable to be affected when bowel ischaemia follows aortoiliac surgery is explained by the **watershed phenomenon**. The combination of aortic cross-clamping, low cardiac output, the low priority given to the colon in terms of critical oxygen delivery and the loss of important collateral pathways due to atherosclerosis or surgical ligation results in the left colon becoming the segment of that organ most vulnerable to ischaemia. This mechanism is supported by the actual findings of preoperative shock in ruptured AAA and the ligation of internal iliac arteries is strongly associated with the complication.

Oxygen delivery to the intestine may become critical as a consequence of two different **primary events**. The collateral circulation may well be adequate initially, but oxygen delivery may become deficient as a result of central events such as postoperative myocardial infarction. Alternatively, even though the patient may be haemodynamically stable, the collateral circulation may be compromised by the degree of atherosclerosis and/or the level of surgical intervention. Ischaemic bowel injury is the primary event, and organ impairment may develop as a result of bacterial translocation and endotoxin migration through the injured intestinal wall, but in the clinical situation it is difficult to establish which mechanism precedes the other.

In this context the effects of different **vasoactive drugs** should be evaluated. Patients are subjected to polypharmacy after aortoiliac surgery, especially after operation for ruptured AAA. In a randomised trial,[23] patients treated with low dose dopamine had significantly lower sigmoid colon pHi values than controls.

In the knowledge that ischaemic intestine is vulnerable to undue pressure, **trauma** from retractors, especially of the self-retaining variety, should be avoided.

Although first described by paediatric surgeons in the 1940s[24] the importance of **intra-abdominal hypertension** and of the abdominal compartment syndrome (see Chapters 4 and 6) has received little recognition until recently.[25–27] We monitored intra-abdominal pressure in all patients operated on for aortoiliac disease since 1998 and there are indications of a correlation between intra-abdominal hypertension and colonic ischaemia.

Aetiology of bowel ischaemia after endovascular repair

The pathophysiological mechanism of colonic ischaemia in the first reported case history after the advent of EVAR[28] was attributed to multiple embolism to the foot and via the internal iliac artery, sometimes designated 'trash colon'. The latter is a rare cause of bowel ischaemia having been identified as a possible cause in only one of 63 cases of embolism following aortoiliac surgery.[6] Although embolism may be more common after EVAR than after open repair it does not seem to raise the overall incidence of intestinal ischaemia (L. Norgren, personal communication; data from the Eurostar Registry, August 2001). Sigmoid colon pH$_i$ fell less after EVAR than after open repair in one prospective study,[29] probably because haemodynamic impairment using the endovascular technique is less of a problem. As EVAR becomes increasingly used in the treatment of patients with ruptured AAA, in whom the retroperitoneal haematoma remains unevacuated, it would be wise to monitor the intra-abdominal pressure. Whether the incidence of colonic ischaemia rises or falls as EVAR continues to be applied to patients with ruptured AAA remains an open question.

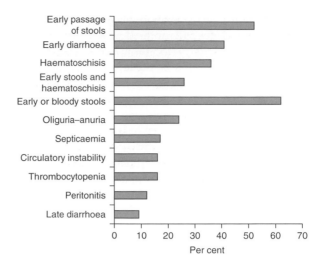

Figure 3.2 *Frequency of presenting symptoms of intestinal ischaemia (Swedvasc)[6]*

DIAGNOSIS

Clinical

The classic clinical triad of intestinal ischaemia is early bloody diarrhoea and signs of peritonitis. Very few publications report on sufficient numbers of patients to permit meaningful discussion on the prevalence of presenting symptoms and signs. Longo *et al.*,[17] reporting to the national Veterans Administration (VA) Registry on the outcome in 4957 patients, identified 49 with bowel ischaemia. The predominant symptom was postoperative hypotension (<90 mmHg) in 15 patients, diarrhoea in 14, bloody stools in 11, fever in eight and abdominal pain in one. Thus, in 23 patients (47 per cent), none of the three classic symptoms was a predominant feature.

In a report from Swedvasc[6] the picture was similar (Fig. 3.2). A third of the patients lacked all three classic symptoms and signs. In a five-year prospective study we identified six patients with bowel ischaemia and in two of them the clinical triad was absent altogether.[7] Signs of peritonitis develop late, at which point the patients may be beyond salvage. It is also difficult to evaluate the abdomen in the postoperative period, especially if epidural anaesthesia has been used. Therefore, if one relies on clinical symptoms and signs alone, many patients will be lost.

Investigations

Many different investigations have been recommended in the detection of colonic ischaemia during the primary surgical intervention. The problem, however, is that colonic ischaemia usually manifests itself in the postoperative period and is a product of the depth and duration of the ischaemic insult. Of the 63 patients identified in the Swedvasc study[6] only five (8 per cent) of the cases of ischaemic bowel were evident at the primary operation, all these patients having been in deep shock due to a ruptured AAA. In a study involving pH measurements of the distal colon in 34 patients undergoing aortoiliac surgery[5] the lowest pH_i values, representing the most severe degree ischaemia, were observed, not during the operation, but 4–24 hours postoperatively.

An elevated concentration of plasma **lactate** (>2.5 mmol/L) has been shown to be a sensitive indicator of bowel gangrene,[30] but the specificity was very low. In one study D-lactate was more specific than L-lactate.[31] It has been hypothesised, though never been tested in this specific context, that sustained high lactate levels, sometimes referred to as lact-time, might be a better pointer to bowel gangrene. An elevated **D-dimer** was found to have a good sensitivity and specificity in a preliminary study on patients suspected of having acute thromboembolic occlusion of the superior mesenteric artery,[32] but it has not been investigated in patients operated on for aortoiliac disease. **Leucocytosis** is prevalent early in the development of bowel gangrene and is followed by leucocytopenia, but these are non-specific indicators. That coagulopathy in general, and **thrombocytopenia** in particular, are more common among patients with this complication,[33] is probably a result of confounding risk factors such as major bleeding and pre-operative shock. When taken as a whole the above estimations can be of some value in the sense that a patient with normal lactate, D-dimer and white cell count is unlikely to have developed bowel gangrene.

Perioperative intestinal mucosal blood flow has been measured using a laser Doppler probe[34] and theoretically, if the probe is left inside the colon with its light beam in close contact with the mucosa, it can be monitored postoperatively, but bowel movement and faecal content represent major practical problems.

Colonoscopy is eminently repeatable and the findings have been extensively reported[14] but caution is required to avoid perforation and abdominal hypertension due to excessive gas insufflation. Faecal contents constitute a practical problem, especially after emergency operations. The flushing of large amounts of saline may be necessary to visualise the mucosa. The investigation should be performed by an experienced endoscopist, but it is important that the vascular surgeon is present in order to evaluate the findings. The distribution of lesions on endoscopy among the 63 patients studied[6] is illustrated in Fig. 3.3; an isolated small bowel ischaemic lesion was present in only one case but the left colon and/or rectum were affected in 95 per cent of cases. Colonoscopy up to the left flexure would have been diagnostic in most cases. It must be acknowledged, however, that although colonoscopy will pick up ischaemic lesions, it cannot differentiate transmural from mucosal ischaemia.[35]

Sigmoid colon pH_i monitoring, developed by Fiddian Green *et al.* (see Schiedler *et al.*,[13]) relies on the use of a gas-permeable balloon placed in contact with the mucosa of the sigmoid colon where it detects increased carbon dioxide production caused by ischaemia. The original method of

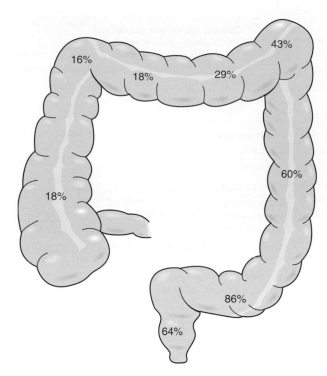

Figure 3.3 *Distribution of ischaemic lesions in the colon and rectum in 63 patients studied.[6] As more than one segment of the colon can be affected in the same patient the sum exceeds 100 per cent. In 95 per cent of patients some part of the left colon and/or rectum was affected*

saline-filled balloons has been displaced by continuous air tonometry (Tonocap; Datex-Ohmeda, Helsinki, Finland) offering practical online measurements.[36,37] Several investigators have studied this diagnostic method in elective aortoiliac surgery, a situation in which bowel ischaemia occurs in only 1 per cent of cases and, not surprisingly, no conclusion on its validity been made. On the other hand, three studies of patients operated for ruptured AAA,[5,7,13] did include patients who developed the complication.

It is hardly justifiable to monitor sigmoid colon pH_i after routine elective surgery. Since 1992 we have used pH_i monitors on all patients operated for ruptured AAA, occlusive or aneurysmal disease of the internal iliac arteries or in those carrying potentially high risk factors for colonic ischaemia.[7] In addition to monitoring perfusion of this very vulnerable organ, pH_i monitoring can be used to prevent further ischaemic injury and when it occurs to recognise it in time and properly grade it so as to avoid unnecessary re-laparotomies.

MANAGEMENT

Management options in the prevention of bowel ischaemia are summarised below and the sequence of actions to be taken when ischaemia is suspected is illustrated in Fig. 3.4.

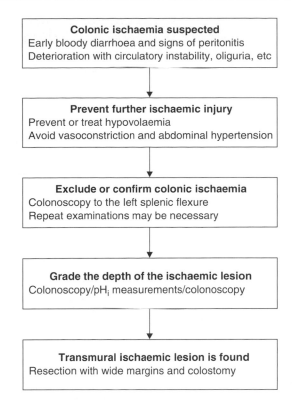

Colonic ischaemia suspected
Early bloody diarrhoea and signs of peritonitis
Deterioration with circulatory instability, oliguria, etc

↓

Prevent further ischaemic injury
Prevent or treat hypovolaemia
Avoid vasoconstriction and abdominal hypertension

↓

Exclude or confirm colonic ischaemia
Colonoscopy to the left splenic flexure
Repeat examinations may be necessary

↓

Grade the depth of the ischaemic lesion
Colonoscopy/pH$_i$ measurements/colonoscopy

↓

Transmural ischaemic lesion is found
Resection with wide margins and colostomy

Figure 3.4 *Algorithm for management of suspected colonic ischaemia after aorto-iliac surgery*

Of course, when this complication has occurred, timely confirmation and grading of the lesion are prerequisites to a successful outcome. Effective collaboration with anaesthetists and the staff in the intensive care unit is important. Excessive fluid administration will lead to prolonged mechanical ventilation and increased abdominal pressure, effects which are as dangerous to a vulnerable colonic circulation as are hypovolaemia and the indiscriminate use of inotropic drugs. Once the complication has manifested itself as transmural gangrene of the colon, the choice is clear, namely, immediate bowel resection with wide margins and colostomy.

Measures to prevent colonic ischaemia in aortoiliac surgery

- Intraoperative measures
  - Avoid excessive blood loss, prolonged cross-clamping and operating time
  - Avoid aortobifemoral reconstruction
  - Preserve blood flow to the internal iliac arteries
  - Avoid embolisation to the internal iliac arteries
  - Avoid pressure on the colon from retractors
- Postoperative measures
  - Prevent hypovolaemia and hypotension
  - Avoid unnecessary vasoactive drugs
  - Prevent or treat intra-abdominal hypertension

RESULTS

In retrospective reviews from single centres the mortality among those who develop bowel ischaemia has varied between 50 and 100 per cent. When reviewing this complication within the Swedvasc Registry we found that among those who suffered the complication in a mixed group of patients who underwent emergency or elective aortoiliac surgery, the overall 30-day mortality had risen from 12 to 41 per cent, and the one-year rate from 18 to 59 per cent.[6] In this group of patients institutional mortality or one-year mortality are far more valid measures of outcome than classic surgical mortality. Among patients with transmural colonic gangrene following surgery for ruptured AAA, the one-year mortality had reached 90 per cent. Results from a prospective study with pH$_i$ monitoring suggest that mortality can be reduced by timely recognition and treatment.[7]

Conclusions

Colonic ischaemia is a major complication of open repair of a ruptured AAA. A reduction in its incidence will improve the overall survival in this group of patients. After elective open repair the frequency is approximately 1 per cent, but 9 per cent of the patients who die after elective surgery will have suffered the complication. The incidence may be lower after elective endovascular repair. Shock, major blood loss and the sacrifice of blood flow to the internal iliac arteries are the most important risk factors. Investigations performed during the operation offer no solution because 90 per cent of patients develop colonic ischaemia in the postoperative period. The classic clinical triad of early bloody diarrhoea and signs of peritonitis cannot be relied upon, all these three cardinal features being absent in a third of patients. Colonoscopy up to the left flexure will identify colonic ischaemia in 95 per cent of patients affected, and therefore it is an investigation which should be carried out liberally. Sigmoid colon pH monitoring offers the advantages of possible prevention, timely recognition and proper grading of the ischaemic lesions. Treatment of transmural gangrene is immediate resection with wide margins and colostomy.

Key references

Björck M, Broman G, Lindberg F, Bergqvist D. pH$_i$-monitoring of the sigmoid colon after aortoiliac surgery. A five-year prospective study. *Eur J Vasc Endovasc Surg* 2000; **20**: 273–80. This study shows that pH$_i$-monitoring can detect the complication early and grade the ischaemic lesion properly. Despite that six patients suffered colonic ischaemia, no mortality was associated with the complication.

Björck M, Troëng T, Bergqvist D. Risk factors for intestinal ischaemia after aortoiliac surgery. A combined cohort and case-control study of 2824 operations. *Eur J Vasc Endovasc Surg* 1997; **13**: 531–9. In this combined cohort and case-control study independent risk-factors are identified by multivariate analysis.

Björck M, Bergqvist D, Troëng T. Incidence and clinical presentation of bowel ischaemia after aortoiliac surgery – 2930 operations from a population-based registry in Sweden. *Eur J Vasc Endovasc Surg* 1996; **12**: 139–49. This study analyses the incidence and clinical presentation in a non-selected population.

Moore SW. Resection of the abdominal aorta with defect replaced by homologous graft. *Surg Gyn Obst* 1954; **99**: 745–55. In this first intelligent case report, the basis of scientific medicine, the clinical picture is described and many of the risk factors are identified.

Soong CV, Halliday MI, Barros D'Sa AAB, *et al.* Effect of low-dose dopamine on sigmoid colonic intramucosal pH in patients undergoing elective abdominal aortic aneurysm repair. *Br J Surg* 1995; **82**: 912–15. This well performed, randomised, controlled trial shows that routine administration of dopamine results in sigmoid colon ischaemia.

REFERENCES

1 Moore SW. Resection of the abdominal aorta with defect replaced by homologous graft. *Surg Gyn Obst* 1954; **99**: 745–55.

2 Smith RH, Szilagyi DE. Ischemia of the colon as a complication in the surgery of the abdominal aorta. *Arch Surg* 1960; **80**: 806–21.

3 Ochsner JL, Cooley DA, DeBakey ME. Associated intra-abdominal lesions encountered during resection of aortic aneurysms. *Dis Colon Rectum* 1960; **3**: 485–90.

4 Brewster DC, Franklin DP, Cambria RP, *et al.* Intestinal ischemia complicating abdominal aortic surgery. *Surgery* 1991; **109**: 447–54.

5 Björck M, Hedberg B. Early detection of major complications after abdominal aortic surgery: predictive value of sigmoid colon and gastric intramucosal pH monitoring. *Br J Surg* 1994; **81**: 25–30.

6 Björck M, Bergqvist D, Troëng T. Incidence and clinical presentation of bowel ischaemia after aortoiliac surgery – 2930 operations from a population-based registry in Sweden. *Eur J Vasc Endovasc Surg* 1996; **12**: 139–49.

7 Björck M, Broman G, Lindberg F, Bergqvist D. pHi-monitoring of the sigmoid colon after aortoiliac surgery. A five-year prospective study. *Eur J Vasc Endovasc Surg* 2000; **20**: 273–80.

8 Johnson WC, Nabseth DC. Visceral infarction following aortic surgery. *Ann Surg* 1974; **180**: 312–18.

9 Tollefson DJF, Ernst CB. Colon ischemia following aortic reconstruction. *Ann Vasc Surg* 1991; **5**: 485–9.

10 Hagihara PF, Ernst CB, Griffen WO. Incidence of ischemic colitis following abdominal aortic reconstruction. *Surg Gyn Obst* 1979; **149**: 571–3.

11 Bast TJ, van der Biezen JJ, Scherpenisse J, Eikelboom BC. Ischaemic disease of the colon and rectum after surgery for abdominal aortic aneurysm: a prospective study of the incidence and risk factors. *Eur J Vasc Surg* 1990; **4**: 253–7.

12 Meissner MH, Johansen KH. Colon infarction after ruptured abdominal aortic aneurysm. *Arch Surg* 1992; **127**: 979–85.

13 Schiedler MG, Cutler BS, Fiddian-Green RG. Sigmoid intramural pH for prediction of ischemic colitis during aortic surgery. *Arch Surg* 1987; **122**: 881–6.

14 Scherpenisse J, van Hees PAM. The endoscopic spectrum of colonic mucosal injury following aortic aneurysm resection. *Endoscopy* 1989; **21**: 174–6.

15 Welch M, Baguneid MS, McMahon RF, *et al.* Histological study of colonic ischaemia after aortic surgery. *Br J Surg* 1998; **85**: 1095–8.

16 Amundsen S, Trippestad A, Viste A, Søreide O. Abdominal aortic aneurysms – a national multicentre study. *Eur J Vasc Surg* 1988; **2**: 239–43.

17 Longo WE, Lee TC, Barnett MG, *et al.* Ischemic colitis complicating abdominal aortic aneurysm surgery in the US Veteran. *J Surg Res* 1996; **60**: 351–4.

18 Järvinen O, Laurikka J, Salenius JP, Lepentalo M. Mesenteric infarction after aortoiliac surgery on the basis of 1752 operations from the National Vascular Registry. *World J Surg* 243–7.

19 Björck M. On intestinal ischaemia after aortoiliac surgery. Epidemiological, clinical and experimental studies. Comprehensive summaries of Uppsala dissertations from the faculty of medicine 740. Uppsala: Acta Universitatis Upsaliensis,1998.

20 Björck M, Troëng T, Bergqvist D. Risk factors for intestinal ischaemia after aortoiliac surgery. A combined cohort and case-control study of 2824 operations. *Eur J Vasc Endovasc Surg* 1997; **13**: 531–9.

21 Ernst CB, Hagihara PF, Daugherty ME, Griffen WO. Inferior mesenteric artery stump pressure: a reliable index for safe IMA ligation during abdominal aortic aneurysmectomy. *Ann Surg* 1978; **187**: 641–6.

22 Piotrowski JJ, Ripepi AJ, Yuhas JP, *et al.* Colonic ischemia: the Achilles heel of ruptured aortic aneurysm repair. *Am Surg* 1996; **62**: 557–61.

23 Soong CV, Halliday MI, Barros D'Sa AAB, *et al.* Effect of low-dose dopamine on sigmoid colonic intramucosal pH in patients undergoing elective abdominal aortic aneurysm repair. *Br J Surg* 1995; **82**: 912–15.

24 Gross R. A new method for surgical treatment of large omphaloceles. *Surgery* 1948; **24**: 277–92.

25 Schein M, Ivatury R. Intra-abdominal hypertension and the abdominal compartment syndrome. *Br J Surg* 1998; **85**: 1027–8.

26 Loftus IM, Thompson MM. The abdominal compartment syndrome following aortic surgery [review]. *Eur J Vasc Endovasc Surg* 2003; **25**: 97–109.

27 Rasmussen TE, Hallet JW, Noel AA, *et al.* Early abdominal closure with mesh reduces multiple organ failure after ruptured abdominal aortic aneurysm repair: guidelines from a 10-year case-control study. *J Vasc Surg* 2002; **35**: 246–53.

28 Sandison AJP, Edmondson RA, Panayitopoulos YP, *et al.* Fatal colonic ischaemia after stent graft for aortic aneurysm. *Eur J Vasc Endovasc Surg* 1997; **13**: 219–20.

29 Syk I, Brunkwall J, Ivancev K, *et al.* Postoperative fever, bowel ischaemia, and cytokine response to abdominal aortic aneurysm repair – a comparison between endovascular and open surgery. *Eur J Vasc Endovasc Surg* 1998; **15**: 398–405.

30 Lange H, Jäckel R. Usefulness of plasma lactate concentration in the diagnosis of acute abdominal disease. *Eur J Surg* 1994; **160**: 381–4.

31 Poeze M, Froom AH, Greve JW, Ramsay G. D-lactate as an early marker of intestinal ischaemia after ruptured abdominal aortic aneurysm repair. *Br J Surg* 1998; **85**: 1221–4.

32 Acosta S, Nilsson IK, Björck M. Elevated D-dimer level could be a useful early marker for acute bowel ischaemia. A preliminary study. *Br J Surg* 2001; **88**: 385–8.

33 Lannerstad O, Bergentz SE, Bergqvist D, Takolander R. Ischemic intestinal complications after aortic reconstructive surgery. *Acta Chir Scand* 1985; **151**: 599–602.

34 Krohg-Sørensen K, Line PD, Haaland T, *et al.* Intraoperative prediction of ischaemic injury of the bowel: a comparison of laser Doppler flowmetry and tissue oximetry to histological analysis. *Eur J Vasc Surg* 1992; **6**: 518–24.

35 Houe T, Thorböll JE, Sigild U, *et al.* Can colonoscopy diagnose transmural ischaemic colitis after abdominal aortic surgery? An evidence-based approach. *J Vasc Endovasc Surg* 2000; **19**: 304–7.

36 Heinonen PO, Jousela IT, Blomqvist KA. Validation of air tonometric measurement of gastric regional concentrations of CO_2 in critically ill septic patients. *Intensive Care Med* 1997; **23**: 524–9.

37 Lebuffe G, Decoene C, Raingeval X, *et al.* Pilot study with air-automated sigmoid capnometry in abdominal aortic aneurysm surgery. *Eur J Anaesth* 2001; **18**: 585–92.

4

Ischaemia-Reperfusion Injury, SIRS and MODS

DENIS W HARKIN, AIRES AB BARROS D'SA

INTRODUCTION

The humoral and cell-mediated immune responses to tissue injury represent the first stages of repair, but if it is excessive local tissue injury may extend to a potentially lethal systemic inflammatory response syndrome (SIRS). In certain individuals a heterogeneous variety of insults, including trauma, haemorrhage, major surgery and ischaemia-reperfusion injury (IRI), may provoke an overwhelming inflammatory response ultimately leading to multiple organ dysfunction syndrome (MODS), organ failure and, ultimately, death. While the inflammatory response to tissue injury bears many similarities to the sepsis syndrome, a septic focus is not a prerequisite to SIRS. Paradoxically, when systemic inflammation becomes established, the essentially sterile IRI often exhibits a septic component which plays a crucial role in the propagation rather than the resolution of inflammation. In this chapter the pathophysiological processes involved in the evolution of SIRS and MODS in vascular patients are discussed.

THE PROBLEM

Despite modern advances in perioperative care, emergency vascular surgery continues to exact a severe toll on this patient population in terms of morbidity and mortality. In its most florid presentation, surgery for a ruptured abdominal aortic aneurysm (AAA), despite initial success, continues to register in-hospital mortality rates of 50–75 per cent in specialist units.[1–3] Of greater concern, however, is the fact that emergency limb salvage procedures in patients presenting with acute vascular insufficiency of the limb also inflict a substantial mortality of 10–20 per cent.[4] Although the majority of early deaths in these patients is due to cardiovascular disease, which reflects the systemic nature of atherosclerosis, late deaths are mostly due to MODS, which remains the leading cause of death in surgical intensive care units[5] (see Chapters 9A and 9B).

Clinical implications of premorbid risk factors

Perhaps the most important factor influencing outcome in emergency cases is the recognition that vascular surgical procedures typically involve the elderly patient in whom either occult disease or overt signs of pre-existing organ dysfunction raise the likelihood of perioperative morbidity and mortality. It is now recognised that peripheral vascular disease is a strong pointer to systemic atherosclerosis and therefore coronary and cerebrovascular events occur much more frequently in vascular patients.[6,7] Renovascular disease, associated with diabetes, hypertension or atherosclerotic renal artery stenosis, is relatively more likely to precipitate postoperative renal dysfunction in vascular patients, and once established it substantially heightens the risk of mortality, especially after AAA repair.[8] Although, advanced chronological age is predictive of high mortality in some patients,[9] good results can be achieved even in octogenarians if they are otherwise physiologically healthy.[8] Local ischaemic injury to the limb can, under certain circumstances, evolve into SIRS potentially leading to MODS and death.

ISCHAEMIA-REPERFUSION INJURY

Lower limb IRI is a common clinical sequela of thromboembolism, trauma, bypass surgery and low-flow states, classically observed in ruptured AAAs. A vascular emergency becomes life threatening if accompanied by physiologically stressful situations: haemorrhage in association with a ruptured AAA, multisystem injuries in cases of vascular trauma, pre-existing vital organ dysfunction especially in the elderly arteriopath. Deoxygenation (ischaemia) and

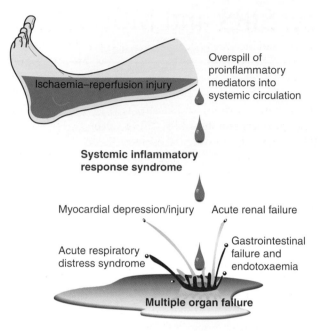

Figure 4.1 *Pictorial representation of the evolution of systemic inflammation and multiple organ dysfunction after limb ischaemia-reperfusion injury*

reoxygenation (reperfusion) of the tissues is characterised by local endothelial activation, membrane lipid peroxidation, cellular oedema, capillary leak and leucocyte recruitment, activation and tissue infiltration. This local tissue injury develops into a systemic phenomenon as metabolic byproducts, oxygen reactive species, arachidonic acid derivatives, cytokines, mediators and activated leucocytes are flushed into the systemic circulation where they can be harmful to vital organ systems, as depicted in Fig. 4.1. The pathophysiology of acute limb vascular insufficiency, and IRI which accompanies it, is covered elsewhere (see Chapter 2), and therefore the discussion here is focused on systemic inflammation and organ dysfunction which evolve in this setting.

SYSTEMIC INFLAMMATORY RESPONSE SYNDROME

As proinflammatory mediators overcome native anti-inflammatory pathways a SIRS ensues. Products of oxidative injury, namely, reactive oxygen species, arachidonic acid metabolites and hydroperoxides, interact with activated endothelial cells and leucocytes in an environment rich in proinflammatory cytokines causing vital organ injury. In response to IRI the complex cascade of proinflammatory

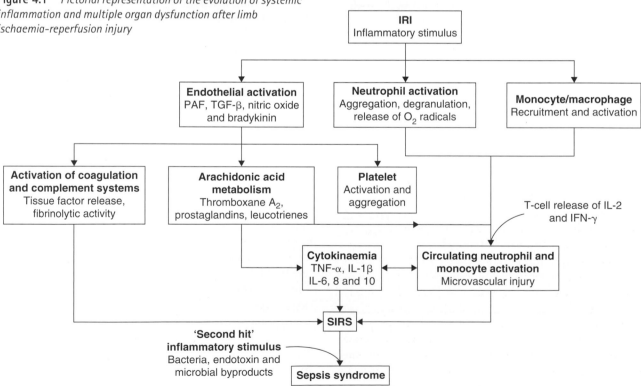

Figure 4.2 *The development of the systemic inflammatory response syndrome (SIRS) after the inflammatory stimulus of ischaemia-reperfusion injury (IRI) represents a complex cascade of proinflammatory mediator and immune cell interactions, which may be further complicated by the development of a sepsis syndrome. IL, interleukin; IFN, interferon; PAF; platelet activating factor; TGF, transforming growth factor; TNF, tumour necrosis factor*

mediator and immune cell interactions leads to the development of SIRS, and not infrequently it is complicated by the sepsis syndrome, as illustrated in Fig. 4.2.

Intravascular response to reperfusion

At its most severe the intravascular response to limb IRI involves the establishment of cytokine and immune cell interactions propagating an inflammatory cascade which causes generalised capillary dysfunction and ultimately leads to organ failure. Major vascular surgery has been shown to initiate a systemic inflammatory response characterised by increased plasma levels of proinflammatory cytokines[10] and circulating polymorphonuclear (PMN) leucocyte, or neutrophil, activation.[11] Experimental studies have shown that activated neutrophils accumulate within remote organs in proportion to the severity of tissue injury[12,13] caused by an acute microvascular insult.[14–17] Plasma factors augment neutrophil and endothelial cell activation after revascularisation of ischaemic tissue by the activation, or 'upregulation', of neutrophil surface adhesion receptor integrins (CD11b/CD18) and endothelial cell adhesion molecules (ICAM-1),[18] in turn leading to degranulation and tissue injury.[12]

Antioxidant defence mechanisms, normally protecting tissues against harmful oxygen reactive species created as byproducts of metabolism, respiration or immune mediated microbial killing are overwhelmed by uncontrolled oxidant production. Consumptive systemic depletion of antioxidants has been demonstrated both during ischaemia and after reperfusion in AAA repair.[19] The resultant oxidative cell membrane injury leads to the creation of **eicosanoids** such as prostaglandins, thromboxanes and leucotrienes, which are oxygenated products of 20-carbon fatty acids such as arachidonic acid. Agonist–receptor mediated activation of membrane phospholipase A_2 leads to specific release of arachidonic acid, the substrate for cyclooxygenase or lipoxygenase enzymes. **Thromboxane (TX) A_2**, a potent vasoconstrictor and platelet aggregator, is a product of the cyclo-oxygenase initiated pathway and is produced rapidly following aortic clamp release at which point it is related, temporally, to the onset of pulmonary hypertension.[20] **Leucotriene (LT) B_4**, a product of the lipoxygenase initiated pathway is derived from neutrophils, mast cells, macrophages and endothelial cells. Both these eicosanoids have been shown to be highly chemotactic for neutrophils contributing to their endothelial adherence and transmigration.[21] **Nitric oxide**, normally produced in basal amounts by the vascular endothelium is critical to normal vascular homoeostasis,[21,22] by mediating vascular smooth muscle relaxation and inhibiting platelet aggregation and neutrophil adherence.[23] Endothelial cell production of nitric oxide is decreased during reperfusion,[24] and that is compounded by superoxide anion induced inactivation of nitric oxide.[25] This intravascular proinflammatory milieu

then converts the local inflammatory injury into a systemic inflammatory response.

Definition of systemic inflammatory response syndrome

Despite the varied initiating stimuli, SIRS, once established, follows a common, if often chaotic, pathway leading to widespread increased microvascular permeability and organ injury. The systemic inflammatory response to injury essentially represents a spectrum of responses which can be mild and self-limiting or severe, leading rapidly to multiple organ failure (MOF) and death. This is reflected in the descriptive criteria shown in Table 4.1 proposed by Baue.[26] It is recognised, however, that the more innocuous first insult is often aggravated by another in the form of sepsis eventually ushering in MOF and death.[27]

SIRS: the propagation or resolution of inflammation

A complex cascade of events depicted in Fig. 4.3 leads from the initial inflammatory stimulus to MOF, which is lethal. Bone[28] classifies SIRS further into the compensatory anti-inflammatory response syndrome (CARS) and the mixed antagonistic response syndrome (MARS), which suggests that weighting the process in one direction or the other decides the outcome. As Baue[26] points out, however, that despite the desire to represent inflammation as an orderly response, it is in fact neither organised and sequential, nor coordinated but a rather chaotic process. While the early rise in circulating cytokine concentrations could be beneficial to the host by initiating the acute phase response, their uncontrolled production undoubtedly contributes to the development of MODS.[29] Paradoxically, depression of the cytokine response does not improve outcome; indeed, it is associated with increased mortality.[30] Systemic inflammatory response syndrome, once established, is propagated by

Table 4.1 *Criteria for the determination of the systemic inflammatory response syndrome (SIRS)* *

Condition[†]	Criterion
Temperature	A temperature lower than 36 °C or higher than 38 °C
Cardiac	A heart rate more than 90 beats per minute
Pulmonary	A respiratory rate more than 20 breaths per minute or a $PaCO_2$ less than 32 mmHg, *which usually means hypoxic hyperventilation*
Haematological	A white blood cell count more than 12.0×10^9/L or less than 4.0×10^9/L or the presence of greater than 10 per cent immature or band forms

*Data from Baue.[26]
[†]SIRS requires two or more of the conditions be met.

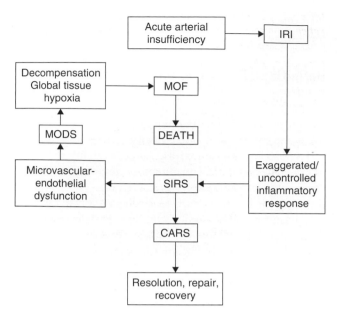

Figure 4.3 *A schematic representation of the progressive spiral from a severe inflammatory stimulus to lethal multiple organ failure. CARS, compensatory anti-inflammatory response syndrome; MODS, multiple organ dysfunction syndrome; MOF, multiple organ failure; IRI, ischaemia-reperfusion injury; SIRS, systemic inflammatory response syndrome*

a variety of mediators, perhaps most importantly by the balance between pro- and anti-inflammatory cytokines. Similarly, the development of a secondary septic injury or sepsis syndrome, from either exogenous or endogenous bacterial pathogens, is often a grave indicator of relentless progression to organ failure and death.

CYTOKINES

Cytokines, originating from monocytes, neutrophils, mast cells, lymphocytes, tissue macrophages and vascular endothelial cells[31] have myriad pro- and anti-inflammatory properties and play a key a role in an evolving SIRS. Postischaemic extremities have been shown to exhibit the immediate release of tumour necrosis factor alpha (TNF-α).[32] In animal studies TNF elicits many key features of SIRS including fever, proteolysis, shock and organ dysfunction.[33] This is in part due to its role in upregulating neutrophil surface adhesion receptors (integrin CD11b/CD18).[34]

The interleukin (IL) family of cytokines has a variety of pro- and anti-inflammatory effects. Interleukin-1β is an early proinflammatory cytokine, often synergistically potentiating TNF-α effects, and is produced by macrophages, monocytes and vascular endothelium.[35] Interleukin-6 is a pleiotropic cytokine, produced by a wide variety of immune reactive cell types[36] and found in high concentrations in association with morbidity after AAA repair;[37] post-traumatic elevated IL-6 levels also correlate closely with injury severity scores (ISS) and mortality.[38] In an experimental

model of lower limb IRI we have shown that high plasma levels of IL-6 are associated with MOF and high mortality.[39] *In vitro* studies have shown that IL-6 delays PMN apoptosis, which may explain why PMNs may exhibit increased functional longevity and a potential for oxidative tissue injury.[36] However, IL-6 also has an important immunomodulatory role – by directly inhibiting expression of proinflammatory TNF-α and IL-1β[40] and stimulating macrophage expression of IL-1β receptor antagonist and soluble TNF-α receptor. Interleukin-8, produced by a variety of cell types, is a potent leucocyte chemoattractant and activator[41] and highest levels of this interleukin have been recorded in patients who developed MOF after trauma.[42] In addition IL-8 has been demonstrated in the bronchoalveolar lavage fluid of patients with acute respiratory distress syndrome (ARDS).[43] Interleukin-10 is produced by immunoregulatory cells[44] and has the potential to inhibit the production of various cytokines, including TNF-α and IL-6.[45] Despite this an increase in plasma IL-10 levels has been associated with septicaemia.[46]

GASTROINTESTINAL BARRIER DYSFUNCTION

The concept of gut origin sepsis, in which dysfunction of the intestinal barrier results in the passage of bacteria and their toxins from the lumen to normally sterile extraintestinal sites, is attributable to Fine.[47] Intestinal barrier failure has been implicated in the pathogenesis of complications following thermal injury,[48] trauma[49] and major vascular surgery.[30]

Bacterial translocation

The gastrointestinal tract is normally inhabited by a large collection of microbial species most notably Gram-negative bacteria.[50] Corson *et al.*[51] showed a link between limb IRI, remote gut injury and increased systemic endotoxin concentrations. Increased intestinal permeability was demonstrated after major vascular surgery.[30] Subsequently, at our centre, lower limb IRI was confirmed to be associated with remote gut mucosal injury and increased permeability.[52] Indeed, research has shown that bacterial translocation can be provoked by a variety of injurious stimuli including burns,[53] endotoxaemia[54] and haemorrhage.[55] Predisposing factors include bacterial overgrowth,[54] gut mucosal barrier disruption[56] and abnormal host defences.[57]

Endotoxaemia

Abdominal aortic aneurysm repair is associated with portal and systemic endotoxaemia.[58,59] Endotoxin, a lipopolysaccharide (LPS) component of the cell wall of Gram-negative bacteria, is a potent stimulus to cytokine generation, coagulation and complement activation[60] as well as leucocyte activation.[61] In humans endotoxin has been implicated in the pathogenesis of SIRS and the development of acute lung injury[61,62] but its precise role after vascular surgery remains controversial.[63] In experimental studies at our centre it has been demonstrated that lower limb IRI is associated with endotoxaemia[64] and that the resulting SIRS is associated with a rise in mortality.[65]

Colonic ischaemia

Colonic ischaemia is a feared complication of aortic surgery, with an incidence ranging from 7 per cent after repair of a ruptured AAA to 0.6 per cent after bypass for aortoiliac occlusive disease.[66] The inferior mesenteric artery, the main blood supply to the left colon, is often sacrificed at AAA repair and important collateral channels from the hypogastric vessels may be lost if internal iliac arteries are excluded during the implantation of a bifurcated aortic graft. The combination of vascular interruption, hypotension and prolonged aortic clamp time magnify the risk to the colon.[67] The damage may range from mild self-limiting mucosal ischaemia to frank ischaemic infarction, perforation and sepsis.

HEPATIC RETICULOENDOTHELIAL DYSFUNCTION

The vast hepatic sinusoidal network is lined with fixed tissue macrophages, or Kupffer cells, which are strategically located to interact with gut derived endotoxin. In addition to clearing bloodborne endotoxin (LPS)[68] the Kupffer cells are a rich source of inflammatory mediators such as TNF, interleukins, platelet activating factor (PAF), and arachidonic acid metabolites. Accordingly, the intestinal–hepatic axis may be crucial in the development of systemic inflammation in patients undergoing major vascular surgery. In the critically ill, impairment of Kupffer cell function is associated with overwhelming sepsis and poor prognosis.

Sepsis syndrome

The sepsis syndrome, defined in Table 4.2, results from activation of the host's defence mechanisms in response to invading microorganisms and their products, including endotoxin.[69] The development of sepsis syndrome is a grave prognostic indicator, regardless of the origin of the bacterial pathogen, whether from an endogenous source such as the intestine or exogenous foci such as ventilatory acquired pneumonia or intravascular catheter sepsis. Severe sepsis is a major cause of death in patients admitted to the intensive care unit (ICU) and continues to be responsible for the high mortality of 25–58 per cent.[70]

MULTIPLE ORGAN DYSFUNCTION SYNDROME

Classical definitions of MOF as an 'all-or-nothing' phenomenon,[71] have been displaced by the consensus view that MOF, the criteria for which are shown in Table 4.3, is more accurately portrayed as an extension of MODS.[73] It remains the leading cause of death in the surgical ICU,

Table 4.2 *Criteria for determination of sepsis syndrome.** * Patients clinically suspected to be septic fulfilled the following criteria for sepsis syndrome*

System	Criteria[+]
Temperature	Hyperthermia ($>38\,°C$)
	Hypothermia ($<35.5\,°C$)
	A proved site of infection
Heart rate	Tachycardia (>90 beats per minute in the absence of β-blockade)
Respiratory rate	Tachypnoea (>20 breaths per minute)
	A requirement for mechanical ventilation
Organ function	Evidence of dysfunction of one or more end organs, defined as follows:
	(a) Plasma lactate greater than 1.2 mmol/L, base deficit greater than 5 mmol/L, or systemic vascular resistance less than 800 dyne.s.cm^{-5};
	(b) PaO$_2$/fraction inspired oxygen less than 30 kPa or PaO$_2$ less than 9.3 kPa;
	(c) Less than 120 mL urine output during 4 hours; or
	(d) Glasgow Coma Scale score less than 15 in the absence of a neurological lesion.

* Data from Bone.[28]
+ Each category requires one or more criteria.

with overall mortality rates exceeding 70 per cent,[74] the rate rising with the number of organs failing.[71] Clinical studies have shown that *all* patients undergoing aortic reconstruction suffer transient organ dysfunction affecting the lung, gut and kidney.[75] Mortality rates of 5 per cent after elective, and 50 per cent after ruptured AAA repair, are still common[76] and at least 20 per cent of these deaths are attributable to MODS.[77] In the past MODS was assumed to be a complication of uncontrolled infection or a manifestation of an occult septic focus, but it is now clear that it can develop in the absence of an identifiable focus of infection.[78] This supports the hypothesis that bacteria or endotoxin from the gut lumen may translocate into the circulation at times of systemic stress and drive the inflammatory response.[79] As described, an uncontrolled SIRS is implicated in the aetiology of MODS.[80] The common cellular abnormality in all these organs is increased microvascular permeability with sequestration of activated inflammatory cells in the microvessels of systemic organs.

Immune system

Deficiencies of the immune system after surgery, burns and trauma are well documented and may occur in a variety of ways. Adverse postinjury events include:

- inhibition of the phagocytic cellular response[81]
- decreased lymphokine (particularly IL-2) generation[35]
- increased complement activation[82]

Table 4.3 *Criteria for the determination of multiple organ failure* *

Organ system	Criteria [†]
Cardiac	Heart rate <54 beats/min
	Mean arterial blood pressure <49 mmHg
	Ventricular tachycardia or fibrillation
	Serum pH <7.24 with $PaCO_2$ <49 mmHg
Haematological	White blood cells <1.0×10^9/L
	Platelets <20.0×10^9/L
	Haematocrit <0.20
Hepatic	Prothrombin time >4 seconds over control (in the absence of anticoagulation)
	Bilirubin >103 μmol/L (>6 mg/dL)
Central nervous system	Glasgow Coma Scale <6 (in the absence of sedation)
Renal	Urine output <479 mL/24 hours (<159 mL/8 hours)
	Urea nitrogen >35.7 mmol/L (>100 mg/dL)
	Creatinine >309 μmol/L (3.5 mg/dL) (excluding long term dialysis)
Pulmonary	Respiratory rate <5 or >49/min
	$PaCO_2$ >50 mmHg
	Alveolar–arterial oxygen difference >350 mmHg
	Ventilator dependence >3 d with another organ failed

* Data from Knaus *et al*.[72]
[†] Each category requires one or more criteria.

- raised prostaglandin production (PGE_2)[83]
- appearance of immunosuppressive serum factors[84]
- alterations in T cell functions including decreased proliferation[57]
- relative increase in suppressor cells[85]
- alterations in B cell functions such as decreased immunoglobulin production.[86]

These effects, in combination, render the patient more susceptible to sepsis and associated complications which contribute to the general proinflammatory milieu.

Haematological system

Critical illness is associated with various haematological abnormalities, a mild anaemia being common along with abnormalities in red cell deformability,[87] a high or inappropriately low leucocyte count and in some cases even an absolute lymphopenia. Reductions in platelet count are common in patients undergoing elective repair of an AAA[88] and perhaps more dramatically that of a ruptured AAA.[89] Later, patients develop hyperfibrinogenaemia and thrombocytosis, which may persist for several weeks.[88] Activation of the fibrinolytic system, haemorrhage, hepatic dysfunction and massive blood transfusion contribute to the risk of

coagulopathy.[89] Another important haematological pathway activated after major vascular surgery is that of the complement system, the creation of small antigen–antibody complexes in the circulation and the appearance of altered cell surface epitopes which activate the classic and alternative complement pathways, respectively. Activated products of the complement pathway are potent inflammatory mediators with myriad effects that include alteration of blood vessel permeability and tone, leucocyte chemotaxis and the activation of multiple inflammatory cell types.

Cardiovascular system

Depressed cardiac function is common in the critically ill and contributes to global hypoperfusion. Supraventricular arrhythmia and impaired myocardial contractility are the most readily evident alterations in cardiac function in the critically ill. Right ventricular function is particularly affected as a consequence of increased pulmonary vascular resistance[90] and an interplay of multiple depressive influences, including catecholamine excess, hypoxia, acidosis[91] and myocardial depressant factors.[92,93] A dilated peripheral vascular bed coupled with widespread capillary leakage aggravates cardiac workload and may ultimately leads to myocardial ischaemia. This added cardiovascular strain may be critical in those with pre-existing coronary artery disease.

Respiratory system

Acute non-cardiac pulmonary oedema after major vascular surgery, in particular aneurysm repair, is well recognised. Experimental lower torso ischaemia-reperfusion induces acute pulmonary injury which is characterised by increased microvascular permeability and neutrophil infiltration,[94] a phenomenon which can be effectively prevented experimentally by neutrophil depletion.[95] Damage to the capillary endothelium resulting in leakage of fluid and protein is produced by an interaction of inflammatory cells and mediators including leucocytes, cytokines, oxygen radicals, complement and arachidonate metabolites. The picture is clinically inseparable from ARDS, which can be of varying intensity as shown in Table 4.4, and is characterised by diffuse pulmonary capillary leak, a common complication in the critically ill. The lungs become stiff and less compliant, lung volumes are reduced and as a consequence of alveolar atelectasis an extreme level of intrapulmonary shunting occurs with characteristic bilateral pulmonary interstitial infiltrates on chest X-ray. Pulmonary hypertension is associated with ARDS[96] and may be improved, in part, by locally delivered vasodilators such as nitric oxide. Septic patients are at greater risk of developing ARDS,[97] indeed experimental infusion of LPS elicits a syndrome of acute lung injury which closely resembles ARDS.[98] Abdominal distension contributes to the loss of pulmonary compliance,

Table 4.4 *Postinjury acute respiratory distress syndrome socre (ARDS)*

	Variables	Grade 1	Grade 2	Grade 3	Grade 4
A	Pulmonary/radiographic	Diffuse, mild interstitial markings/opacities	Diffuse, marked interstitial/ mild air space opacities	Diffuse, moderate air space consolidation	Diffuse, severe air space consolidation
B	PaO$_2$/FiO$_2$ (mmHg)	175–250	125–174	80–124	<80
C	Minute ventilation (L/min)	11–13	14–16	17–20	>20
D	PEEP (cmH$_2$O)	6–9	10–13	14–17	>17
E	Static compliance	40–50	30–39	17–20	<20

ARDS SCORE = A + B + C + D + E when PCWP ≤18 mmHg or when there is no clinical reason to suspect hydrostatic pulmonary oedema.
PEEP, peak end expiratory pressure; PCWP, Pulmonary capillary wedge pressure.

compounding respiratory failure in those who have sustained acute intra-abdominal catastrophes.[99]

Renal system

Acute renal failure (ARF) complicates both emergency and elective aortic aneurysm surgery.[100] Renal parenchymal ischaemic injury is a common sequela of suprarenal aortic clamping and is exacerbated in some by atheroembolism.[101] Postoperatively, renal hypoperfusion brought about by preferential shunting and falling central arterial blood pressure compounds the effects of renal ischaemia. Furthermore, the release of oxygen free radicals, systemic vasoconstrictors, toxic metabolites, myoglobin and activation of neutrophils as a consequence of limb reperfusion, act in concert to produce acute tubular dysfunction.[102] Common radiological contrast agents also induce renal dysfunction in all too many vascular patients. Despite advances in providing support for the critically ill patient the development of ARF remains quite common and carries a grave prognosis with a mortality of around 45 per cent, and in those with sepsis it may be as high as 75 per cent.[103]

Hepatic system

The liver may sustain direct ischaemic injury during supracoeliac aortic clamping and also indirectly in association with perioperative hypotension. Hepatocellular injury impairs the liver's ability to manufacture clotting factors necessary to satisfy the demands of a hypercoagulopathy, to produce albumin sufficient to maintain intravascular volume in the presence of capillary leak and finally to metabolise mediators and metabolic byproducts in the presence of ongoing inflammation. Although transient moderate rises in hepatocellular enzymes are common after major aortic surgery, a large or sustained rise must be regarded as a grave sign.

Gastrointestinal tract

A variety of factors contribute to gut injury including direct ischaemia by supracoeliac aortic clamping and remote injury mediated by inflammatory mediators, activated leucocytes and hypoperfusion.[80] The crucial role of gut ischaemia in the pathogenesis of MODS is indicated by the improved survival of shocked patients in whom gut ischaemia, as determined by gastric tonometry, can be reversed.[104] Naturally, the gut has been described as the 'motor' driving the systemic inflammatory response.[27] Sustained acidosis of the gastric and sigmoid mucosa has been shown to be a highly sensitive predictive indicator of mortality and morbidity in elective and emergency AAA surgery patients.[105] For this reason the clinician must remain vigilant to the possible development of non-occlusive mesenteric ischaemia (see Chapters 3 and 29). Furthermore, gut mucosal atrophy during critical illness damages its absorptive ability, though that can be prevented, in part, by early enteral feeding.

Neuroendocrine system

Plasma catecholamine concentrations increase during conventional surgery,[106] and during open AAA repair are associated with cardiovascular instability.[107] The acute phase response to injury brings with it a catecholamine surge as the body tries to maintain its essential functions. Glucocorticoids initially provide a welcome anti-inflammatory response, inhibiting the production of cytokines TNF-α[108] and IL-6,[109] but their influence, if prolonged, becomes deleterious. Failure to satisfy the sustained hypermetabolic demands of critical illness is associated with a poor outcome.[110]

General metabolism

The systemic inflammatory response brings with it a hypercatabolic state and as the immune system and major organs attempt to cope with that increased demand the body switches from aerobic to anaerobic respiration on a massive scale. If tissue hypoxia persists, markers of intermediary metabolism, such as ketone body ratio, point to a process of decompensation heralding MOF and mortality in the critically ill.[111] Postoperative hypermetabolism, as estimated by an increase in baseline oxygen consumption, is manifested experimentally by higher circulating levels of endotoxin, TNF and IL-6.[112] Paradoxically, cytokines such as IL-6 also have a role in depressing cellular metabolic activity and that will induce cachexia.[113]

MONITORING OF ORGAN DYSFUNCTION IN SIRS

Although mortality rates from MODS remain high, historical comparisons of critically ill surgical patients suggest the incidence of ARF, ARDS, gastrointestinal stress haemorrhage and abdominal abscess formation have decreased. The key reason for organ dysfunction in the critically ill is global tissue hypoxia. Central shunting attempts to maintain vital organ perfusion, often at the cost of sacrificing splanchnic and peripheral circulation. Historically, clinicians have directed their treatment so as to avert oxygen debt by optimising systemic haemodynamics and tissue oxygenation. Shoemaker et al.[114] have gone further and proposed targeted therapy to achieve 'supranormal' oxygen delivery in critically ill patients to improve survival.

Monitoring of global haemodynamics

The pulmonary artery catheter, introduced by Swan et al.,[115] remains the clinical standard for monitoring macrohaemodynamic variables such as cardiac output, pulmonary artery occlusion pressure, mixed venous oxygen saturation and derived variables of oxygen delivery. However, concerns have been raised since Connors et al.[116] showed a rise in mortality, prolonged stay in intensive care and increased treatment costs for those being monitored invasively. Non-invasive methods for assessing cardiac output remain largely experimental and include transthoracic and transoesophageal bioimpedance monitoring, carbon dioxide and soluble gases rebreathing methods and Doppler echocardiography.

Monitoring of tissue oxygenation

Falls in either cardiac output or arterial oxygen content lead to an imbalance whereby oxygen consumption exceeds oxygen delivery. This tissue hypoxia in the critically ill patient is compounded by a heightened catabolic state and anaerobic metabolism ensues. Therefore careful assessment of the quality of tissue oxygenation in these patients is essential. Global tissue oxygenation is often assessed indirectly by measuring plasma lactate levels which rise in response to excessive anaerobic metabolism. Elevated lactate levels, however, may reflect either impaired elimination, due to hepatic failure and renal failure, or increased production,

as observed in a variety of conditions such as sepsis, myeloproliferative disease, pancreatitis, short bowel syndrome or induced by drugs such as catecholamines, biguanides, methanol, ethanol and ethylene glycol. In the critically ill, high lactate levels have been shown to be predictive of morbidity and mortality.[117]

INDICATORS OF REGIONAL TISSUE OXYGENATION

Hollow viscus tonometry is increasingly used to monitor the adequacy of splanchnic tissue perfusion either via the gastric or the sigmoid route.[118] Sustained acidosis of intestinal mucosa has been shown to be highly sensitive in predicting mortality and morbidity in elective and emergency aortic aneurysm surgery.[105]

MONITORING PULMONARY GAS EXCHANGE

Arterial blood gas samples with a known fraction of inspired oxygen remains the clinical standard for monitoring pulmonary gas exchange. Pulse oximetry is useful but does not detect impaired tissue oxygenation attributable to a leftward shift of the oxygen–haemoglobin dissociation curve. The continued development of fibreoptic blood gas and pH sensors, at present still experimental, may further refine continuous monitoring of high risk patients.

Monitoring of renal function

Diuresis and creatinine clearance currently represent the clinically most important variables in monitoring global renal function. The goal must be to detect and correct renal hypoperfusion before the development of overt signs of renal failure such as anuria, hyperkalaemia, acidaemia and azotaemia. In general, renal blood flow is hard to predict using simple systemic haemodynamic variables because of complex renal-based blood pressure maintaining compensatory mechanisms, namely, sympathetic activity and the renin–angiotensin–aldosterone system. Unfortunately, newer imaging techniques such as greyscale and duplex ultrasonography and magnetic resonance imaging provide little assistance in predicting ARF in the critically ill patient.[119]

Predictive scores in critically ill vascular patients

Vascular surgery patients with marked atherosclerotic disease and underlying comorbidities represent a high risk group when compared with most other patients undergoing surgery. In many reports over half of those patients undergoing elective AAA repair suffer one or more atherosclerosis related complications.[120] Multiorgan failure is the most important cause of late death,[121,122] the mortality rising with increasing number of failing organ systems.[72] Postoperative complications have been attributed to preoperative risk factors such as advancing age, poor ventricular function, ischaemic heart disease, chronic pulmonary disease, renal failure and diabetes mellitus.[76,123] Therefore, extensive efforts are being made, using scoring systems, to predict the risk of morbidity and mortality in patients prior to commitment to a surgical procedure.

THE APACHE SCORE

Acute Physiology And Chronic Health Evaluation (APACHE) II score[72] is perhaps the most widely accepted predictive score used to assess the severity of critical illness in ICUs. It is based on 12 physiological and laboratory based factors (temperature, mean arterial pressure, heart rate, respiratory rate, PO_2, arterial pH, serum sodium, serum potassium, serum creatinine, haematocrit, white cell count and Glasgow Coma Score), as well as on age and previous health status. In general, APACHE II is a good predictor of outcome in ruptured AAA repair but its power to predict outcome in any individual patient is limited.[124]

THE POSSUM SCORE

Physiological and Operative Severity Score for the enUmeration of Mortality (POSSUM) was designed specifically for patients undergoing surgical intervention. It is based on 12 readily available physiological and laboratory variables (age, cardiac signs, respiratory history, systolic blood pressure, pulse rate, Glasgow Coma Score, haemoglobin, white cell count, urea, serum sodium, serum potassium electrocardiogram) as well as on six operative severity parameters. The original POSSUM[125] failed to predict outcome sufficiently reliably after ruptured AAAs,[124] but the modified Portsmouth POSSUM or P-POSSUM[126] would appear to have greater relevance to vascular patients.

Therapeutic strategies in MODS

The management of the critically ill patient with SIRS, sepsis and evolving MODS is complex and best undertaken in the ICU. The aim of initial resuscitation and supportive therapies is to achieve and maintain adequate tissue oxygenation. Hypoxaemia should be managed by increased inspired oxygen, where appropriate, to assist non-compliant and failing lungs by means of mechanical ventilation and regular monitoring by blood gas analysis. Cardiovascular support using a combination of intravenous fluid, inotropes and vasoconstrictors may require invasive haemodynamic monitoring. Antibiotic therapy should be instituted early where signs of sepsis exist, initially with broad spectrum antibiotics, and then in a more focused manner depending on microbiological results. Renal support can be achieved by optimising renal perfusion, and where this fails, by means of haemodialysis. Nutrition should be maintained

during this intensely catabolic process, and ideally via the enteral route. Recent advances in molecular biology have enhanced our understanding of the various actions and interactions which represent the systemic inflammatory response to tissue injury. Beyond standard support of the critically ill patient, attention has focused on the use of either natural or synthetic therapeutic agents aimed at promoting or inhibiting various components of the inflammatory response. These are outlined in Table 4.5 and are discussed briefly below.

Anticytokine therapies

The balance between pro- and anti-inflammatory cytokines is crucial to the promotion or resolution of inflammation. Therapeutic interventions have ranged from purified concentrates of natural endogenous antibodies and stimulated donor hyperimmune globulins to monoclonal antibodies directed against specific cytokines. In both animal experiments and human trials attention has focused on modulation of the potent proinflammatory cytokine TNF-α. Its normal biological activity is usually counterbalanced by

Table 4.5   *Novel potential therapeutic targets for the modulation of systemic inflammatory response syndrome (SIRS) and prevention of multiple organ dysfunction syndrome (MODS)*

Therapies	Target	Potential mode of action
Cytokine	TNF-α and receptor	Anti-inflammatory
	IL-1β, 6, 8, and 10 and receptors	Anti-inflammatory
Antiendotoxin	Gut decontamination	Reduced septic challenge
	LPS binding protein (LBP)	Improved endotoxin clearance
	LPS	Direct inhibition endotoxin
	BPI, recombinant BPI	Reduced inflammatory response to endotoxin
Immune cell	Leucocyte integrins	Inhibits leucocyte adhesion
	Endothelial ICAM-1	Inhibits leucocyte adhesion
	Steroids	Anti-inflammatory
Complement	C1, sCR1	Inhibits classical pathway
	C3	Inhibits alternative pathway
	C5, C5a, C5aR	Inhibits leucocyte activation
	C5b-9 (MAC)	Inhibits cytolysis

TNF, tumour necrosis factor; IL, interleukin; LPS, lipopolysaccharide; BPI, bactericidal permeability increasing protein; ICAM, intercellular adhesion molecule.

natural inhibitors known as TNF-α binding proteins and identified as soluble forms of extracellular fragments of the TNF-α receptors.[127] In high risk patients early postoperative rises in plasma levels of soluble TNF-α receptors, a hallmark of excessive TNF-α production, are associated with a high complication rate and a poor prognosis.[128] Despite encouraging animal studies showing a lowering of mortality from sepsis,[129] in one phase II trial a dose dependent increase in mortality was reported using the potent antagonist soluble TNF p75 receptor.[130] Another proinflammatory cytokine and potential target is IL-1β, but animal experiments here are also inconclusive with antibodies directed against its receptor: in small doses protecting those animals from *Klebsiella pneumoniae* but in larger doses increasing the lethal power of those organisms.[131] The pleiotropic cytokine IL-6 has also been investigated, and the monoclonal antibodies directed against both IL-6 and its receptor having been shown to protect against lethal injury from TNF-α, LPS and sepsis.[132,133] Interestingly, plasma levels of an anti-inflammatory cytokine IL-10 also rise in patients with septic shock[134] and are correlated with an adverse outcome.[135] Currently, IL-10 inhibition therapy is being explored in a phase I study in patients undergoing thoracoabdominal aneurysm repair,[136] the results of which are awaited.

Antiendotoxin therapy

The sepsis syndrome, secondary to bacteraemia or endotoxaemia, remains a leading cause of morbidity and mortality, despite antibiotics and intensive care support. **Gut decontamination** has been shown to cause a dramatic reduction in colonisation and effectively prevents bacterial translocation from the gut, but it does not significantly reduce the mortality rate or hospital stay in critically ill patients.[137]

Lipopolysaccharide binding protein (LBP) is an essential factor in the immune system responsible for meeting bacterial or septic challenges. Initial optimism based on the finding that mice, injected with high concentrations of LBP, could survive an otherwise lethal septic challenge[138] was tempered by studies in LBP-knockout mice which showed that they fare no worse than their wild-type littermates in response to septic challenge.[139] **Antiendotoxin immunoglobulins** have also been explored in several studies which demonstrated that normal pooled γ-globulin or immunoglobulins can improve outcome in sepsis related conditions.[140] The *Escherichia coli* J5-immune plasma and γ-globulin study[141] revealed some benefit using immune plasma but it was minimal when immune γ-globulin was used.[142] There was more convincing evidence of protection from exogenous γ-globulins in a clinical study using 'natural' antiendotoxin antibodies.[143] **Endotoxin neutralising protein** antilipopolysaccharide factor isolated from the amoebocytes of horseshoe crabs, *Limulus polyphemus* and *Limulus tachypleus*, is known to bind various endotoxins,[144] and is protective in animal models of meningococcal sepsis[145] and *E. coli* sepsis.[146] **Bactericidal/permeability-increasing protein** (BPI) prevents LPS induced PMN activation, TNF-α production and, in addition to its ability to neutralise LPS, BPI has been shown to alter bacterial membrane permeability and kill Gram-negative organisms.[147,148] Recently, recombinant BPI has been shown to attenuate systemic inflammation and acute lung injury after experimental lower limb IRI.[149–151]

Modulation of immune cell function

As the key effectors of tissue injury, and the source of many of the proinflammatory mediators present in SIRS, immune cells or leucocytes represent an obvious therapeutic target. **Polymorphonuclear leucocyte depletion** has been shown in animal studies to reduce reperfusion injury effectively.[94,95,152] In humans, however, global inhibition of leucocyte function is not a viable clinical option so that attempts to reduce their endothelial interaction and transmigration seem a more realistic goal than limiting tissue injury. **Inhibition of PMN leucocyte adherence and migration**, using monoclonal antibodies directed against the β-chain of the CD11/CD18 glycoprotein adherence complex, decreases PMN adherence to the endothelium and attenuates the microvascular dysfunction associated with reperfusion of skeletal muscle.[153] More recently anti-CD18 monoclonal antibodies have been used to reduce multiple organ injury in an animal model of ruptured AAA.[154]

Complement inhibition

The complement system is activated in a range of inflammatory states and has various potentially deleterious vasoactive and inflammatory effects. However, it also has many beneficial effects, especially in the ability of the host to resist septic challenge, and therefore, in order to be effective, inhibition must be targeted. Encouraging results have been obtained using anti-C5 antibody, and C5a receptor (C5aR) antagonist, and the results of ongoing human trials are awaited.

Genetic therapies

Quite recently it has become apparent that genetic polymorphisms to many of the previously described cytokines and inflammatory mediators do exist. Some of these polymorphisms are functional in that it is possible to demonstrate differing cytokine responses to a standard stimulus. This would suggest the possibility of genetic predisposition to increased mortality from sepsis or SIRS in some individuals. The first such polymorphism to be described in this field was in relation to TNF, but they have also been noted in regard to IL-1β, IL-1 receptor antagonist and IL-10.[155]

Conclusions

The lack of improvement in mortality rates in those vascular patients who develop MODS probably reflects an increase in the number and complexity of vascular interventions in an increasingly elderly and unfit patient population rather than a failure of modern intensive care support. It is expected that a more enlightened understanding of the mechanisms involved in the development of IRI and its progression via SIRS to MODS will contribute to improve outcomes. Finally, it cannot be sufficiently emphasised that prevention of MOF by optimising tissue oxygen delivery at all stages is crucial to achieving better results. Careful assessment of a patient's general medical condition and risk factors allows suitable patient selection and preventive treatment strategies to be put in place.

Key references

Baigrie RJ, Lamont PM, Whiting S, Morris PJ. Portal endotoxin and cytokine responses during abdominal aortic surgery. *Am J Surg* 1993; **166**: 248–51.

Baue AE. Multiple organ failure, multiple organ dysfunction syndrome, and systemic inflammatory response syndrome. Why no magic bullets? *Arch Surg* 1997; **132**: 703–7.

Groeneveld AB, Raijmakers PG, Rauwerda JA, Hack CE. The inflammatory response to vascular surgery-associated ischaemia and reperfusion in man: effect on postoperative pulmonary function. *Eur J Vasc Endovasc Surg* 1997; **14**: 351–9.

Halpern VJ, Kline RG, D'Angelo AJ, Cohen JR. Factors that affect the survival rate of patients with ruptured abdominal aortic aneurysms. *J Vasc Surg* 1997; **26**: 939–45.

Marshall JC, Christou NV, Meakins JL. The gastrointestinal tract. The 'undrained abscess' of multiple organ failure. *Ann Surg* 1993; **218**: 111–19.

REFERENCES

1 Adam DJ, Mohan IV, Stuart WP, et al. Community and hospital outcome from ruptured abdominal aortic aneurysm within the catchment area of a regional vascular surgical service. *J Vasc Surg* 1999; **30**: 922–8.

2 Campbell WB, Ridler BM, Szymanska TH. Current management of acute leg ischaemia: results of an audit by the Vascular Surgical Society of Great Britain and Ireland. *Br J Surg* 1998; **85**: 1498–503.

3 Henderson A, Effeney D. Morbidity and mortality after abdominal aortic surgery in a population of patients with high cardiovascular risk. *Aust N Z J Surg* 1995; **65**: 417–20.

4 Go LL, Healey PJ, Watkins SC, et al. The effect of endotoxin on intestinal mucosal permeability to bacteria *in vitro*. *Arch Surg* 1995; **130**: 53–8.

5 Campbell WB, Collin J, Morris PJ. The mortality of abdominal aortic aneurysm. *Ann R Coll Surg Engl* 1998; **68**: 275–8.

6 Dormandy J, Heeck L, Vig S. The natural history of claudication: risk to life and limb. *Semin Vasc Surg* 1999; **12**: 123–37.

7 Leng GC, Lee AJ, Fowkes FG, et al. Incidence, natural history and cardiovascular events in symptomatic and asymptomatic peripheral arterial disease in the general population. *Int J Epidemiol* 1996; **25**: 1172–81.

8 Halpern VJ, Kline RG, D'Angelo AJ, Cohen JR. Factors that affect the survival rate of patients with ruptured abdominal aortic aneurysms. *J Vasc Surg* 1997; **26**: 939–45.

9 Hardman DT, Fisher CM, Patel MI, et al. Ruptured abdominal aortic aneurysms: who should be offered surgery? *J Vasc Surg* 1996; **23**: 123–9.

10 Groeneveld AB, Raijmakers PG, Rauwerda JA, Hack CE. The inflammatory response to vascular surgery-associated ischaemia and reperfusion in man: effect on postoperative pulmonary function. *Eur J Vasc Endovasc Surg* 1997; **14**: 351–9.

11 Barry MC, Kelly C, Burke P, et al. Immunological and physiological responses to aortic surgery: effect of reperfusion on neutrophil and monocyte activation and pulmonary function. *Br J Surg* 1997; **84**: 513–19.

12 Welbourn CR, Goldman G, Paterson IS, et al. Pathophysiology of ischaemia reperfusion injury: central role of the neutrophil. *Br J Surg* 1991; **78**: 651–5.

13 Salzman AL, Wang H, Wollert PS, et al. Endotoxin-induced ileal mucosal hyperpermeability in pigs: role of tissue acidosis. *Am J Physiol* 1994; **266**: G633–46.

14 Anner H, Kaufman RP Jr, Valeri CR, et al. Reperfusion of ischemic lower limbs increases pulmonary microvascular permeability. *J Trauma* 1988; **28**: 607–10.

15 Welbourn R, Goldman G, Kobzik L, et al. Role of neutrophil adherence receptors (CD 18) in lung permeability following lower torso ischemia. *Circ Res* 1992; **71**: 82–6.

16 Gadaleta D, Fantini GA, Silane MF, Davis JM. Neutrophil leukotriene generation and pulmonary dysfunction after abdominal aortic aneurysm repair. *Surgery* 1994; **116**: 847–52.

17 Klausner JM, Anner H, Paterson IS, et al. Lower torso ischemia-induced lung injury is leukocyte dependent. *Ann Surg* 1988; **208**: 761–7.

18 Barry MC, Wang JH, Kelly CJ, et al. Plasma factors augment neutrophil and endothelial cell activation during aortic surgery. *Eur J Vasc Endovasc Surg* 1997; **13**: 381–7.

19 Murphy ME, Kolvenbach R, Aleksis M, et al. Antioxidant depletion in aortic crossclamping ischemia: increase of the plasma alpha-tocopheryl quinone/alpha-tocopherol ratio. *Free Radic Biol Med* 1992; **13**: 95–100.

20 Paterson IS, Klausner JM, Goldman G, et al. Thromboxane mediates the ischemia-induced neutrophil oxidative burst. *Surgery* 1989; **106**: 224–9.

21 Doukas J, Hechtman HB, Shepro D. Endothelial-secreted arachidonic acid metabolites modulate polymorphonuclear leukocyte chemotaxis and diapedesis *in vitro*. *Blood* 1988; **71**: 771–9.

22 Kuo PC, Schroeder RA. The emerging multifaceted roles of nitric oxide. *Ann Surg* 1995; **221**: 220–35.

23 McMillen MA, Huribal M, Sumpio B. Common pathway of endothelial-leukocyte interaction in shock, ischemia, and reperfusion. *Am J Surg* 1993; **166**: 557–62.

24   Summers RW, Hayek B. Changes in colonic motility following abdominal irradiation in dogs. *Am J Physiol* 1993; **264**: G1024–G1030.

25   McCall TB, Boughton-Smith NK, Palmer RM, *et al.* Synthesis of nitric oxide from L-arginine by neutrophils. Release and interaction with superoxide anion. *Biochem J* 1989; **261**: 293–6.

26   Baue AE. Multiple organ failure, multiple organ dysfunction syndrome, and systemic inflammatory response syndrome. Why no magic bullets? *Arch Surg* 1997; **132**: 703–7.

27   Moore FA, Moore EE. Evolving concepts in the pathogenesis of postinjury multiple organ failure. *Surg Clin North Am* 1995; **75**: 257–77.

28   Bone RC. Immunologic dissonance: a continuing evolution in our understanding of the systemic inflammatory response syndrome (SIRS) and the multiple organ dysfunction syndrome (MODS) [see comments]. *Ann Intern Med* 1996; **125**: 680–7.

29   Froon AH, Greve JW, Van der Linden CJ, Buurman WA. Increased concentrations of cytokines and adhesion molecules in patients after repair of abdominal aortic aneurysm. *Eur J Surg* 1996; **162**: 287–96.

30   Roumen RM, Hendriks T, van der Ven-Jongekrijg J, *et al.* Cytokine patterns in patients after major vascular surgery, hemorrhagic shock, and severe blunt trauma. Relation with subsequent adult respiratory distress syndrome and multiple organ failure. *Ann Surg* 1993; **218**: 769–76.

31   May LT, Santhanam U, Tatter SB, *et al.* Phosphorylation of secreted forms of human beta 2-interferon/hepatocyte stimulating factor/interleukin-6. *Biochem Biophys Res Commun* 1988; **152**: 1144–50.

32   Sternbergh WC 3rd, Tuttle TM, Makhoul RG, *et al.* Postischemic extremities exhibit immediate release of tumor necrosis factor. *J Vasc Surg* 1994; **20**: 474–81.

33   Tracey KJ, Lowry SF, Fahey TJ 3rd, *et al.* Cachectin/tumor necrosis factor induces lethal shock and stress hormone responses in the dog. *Surg Gynecol Obstet* 1987; **164**: 415–22.

34   Witthaut R, Farhood A, Smith CW, Jaeschke H. Complement and tumor necrosis factor-alpha contribute to Mac-1 (CD11b/CD18) up-regulation and systemic neutrophil activation during endotoxemia *in vivo*. *J Leukoc Biol* 1994; **55**: 105–11.

35   Abraham E. Effects of stress on cytokine production. *Methods Achiev Exp Pathol* 1991; **14**: 45–62.

36   Biffl WL, Moore EE, Moore FA, Peterson VM. Interleukin-6 in the injured patient. Marker of injury or mediator of inflammation? *Ann Surg* 1996; **224**: 647–64.

37   Baigrie RJ, Lamont PM, Whiting S, Morris PJ. Portal endotoxin and cytokine responses during abdominal aortic surgery. *Am J Surg* 1993; 166: 248–51.

38   Svoboda P, Kantorova I, Ochmann J. Dynamics of interleukin 1, 2, and 6 and tumor necrosis factor alpha in multiple trauma patients. *J Trauma* 1994; **36**: 336–40.

39   Yassin MM, Harkin DW, Barros D'Sa AAB, *et al.* Lower limb ischaemia-reperfusion injury triggers a systemic inflammatory response and multiple organ dysfunction. *World J Surg* 2002; **26**: 115–21.

40   Ulich TR, del Castillo J, Yin SM, Egrie JC. The erythropoietic effects of interleukin 6 and erythropoietin *in vivo*. *Exp Hematol* 1991; **19**: 29–34.

41   Shalaby MR, Halgunset J, Haugen OA, *et al.* Cytokine-associated tissue injury and lethality in mice: a comparative study. *Clin Immunol Immunopathol* 1991; **61**: 69–82.

42   Botha AJ, Moore FA, Moore EE, *et al.* Early neutrophil sequestration after injury: a pathogenic mechanism for multiple organ failure. *J Trauma* 1995; **39**: 411–17.

43   Cohen AB, MacArthur C, Idell S, *et al.* A peptide from alveolar macrophages that releases neutrophil enzymes into the lungs in patients with the adult respiratory distress syndrome. *Am Rev Respir Dis* 1988; **137**: 1151–8.

44   Nickoloff BJ, Fivenson DP, Kunkel SL, *et al.* Keratinocyte interleukin-10 expression is upregulated in tape-stripped skin, poison ivy dermatitis, and Sezary syndrome, but not in psoriatic plaques. *Clin Immunol Immunopathol* 1994; **73**: 63–8.

45   Bogdan C, Vodovotz Y, Nathan C. Macrophage deactivation by interleukin 10. *J Exp Med* 1991; **174**: 1549–55.

46   Marchant A, Bruyns C, Vandenabeele P, *et al.* Interleukin-10 controls interferon-gamma and tumor necrosis factor production during experimental endotoxemia. *Eur J Immunol* 1994; **24**: 1167–71.

47   Fine J. Endotoxaemia in man. *Lancet* 1972; **ii**: 181.

48   LeVoyer T, Cioffi WG Jr, Pratt L, *et al.* Alterations in intestinal permeability after thermal injury. *Arch Surg* 1992; **127**: 26–9.

49   Pape HC, Dwenger A, Regel G, *et al.* Increased gut permeability after multiple trauma. *Br J Surg* 1994; **81**: 850–2.

50   van Deventer SJ, ten Cate JW, Tytgat GN. Intestinal endotoxemia. Clinical significance. *Gastroenterology* 1988; **94**: 825–31.

51   Corson RJ, Paterson IS, O'Dwyer ST, *et al.* Lower limb ischaemia and reperfusion alters gut permeability. *Eur J Vasc Surg* 1992; **6**: 158–63.

52   Yassin MMI, Barros D'Sa AAB, Parks TG, *et al.* Lower limb ischaemia-reperfusion injury alters gastrointestinal structure and function. *Br J Surg* 1997; **84**: 1425–9.

53   Deitch EA, Maejima K, Berg R. Effect of oral antibiotics and bacterial overgrowth on the translocation of the GI tract microflora in burned rats. *J Trauma* 1985; **25**: 385–92.

54   Deitch EA, Ma L, Ma WJ, *et al.* Inhibition of endotoxin-induced bacterial translocation in mice. *J Clin Invest* 1989; **84**: 36–42.

55   Deitch EA, Bridges W, Baker J, *et al.* Hemorrhagic shock-induced bacterial translocation is reduced by xanthine oxidase inhibition or inactivation. *Surgery* 1988; **104**: 191–8.

56   Ambrose NS, Johnson M, Burdon DW, Keighley MR. Incidence of pathogenic bacteria from mesenteric lymph nodes and ileal serosa during Crohn's disease surgery. *Br J Surg* 1984; **71**: 623–5.

57   O'Gorman RB, Feliciano DV, Matthews KS, *et al.* Correlation of immunologic and nutritional status with infectious complications after major abdominal trauma. *Surgery* 1986; **99**: 549–56.

58   Soong CV, Blair PH, Halliday MI, *et al.* Endotoxaemia, the generation of the cytokines and their relationship to intramucosal acidosis of the sigmoid colon in elective abdominal aortic aneurysm repair. *Eur J Vasc Surg* 1993; **7**: 534–9.

59   Woodcock NP, Sudheer V, el Barghouti N, *et al.* Bacterial translocation in patients undergoing abdominal aortic aneurysm repair. *Br J Surg* 2000; **87**: 439–42.

60   van Deventer SJ, Buller HR, ten Cate JW, *et al.* Experimental endotoxemia in humans: analysis of cytokine release and coagulation, fibrinolytic, and complement pathways. *Blood* 1990; **76**: 2520–6.

61   Foulds S, Cheshire NJ, Schachter M, *et al.* Endotoxin related early neutrophil activation is associated with outcome after thoracoabdominal aortic aneurysm repair. *Br J Surg* 1997; **84**: 172–7.

62   Roumen RM, Frieling JT, van Tits HW, *et al.* Endotoxemia after major vascular operations. *J Vasc Surg* 1993; **18**: 853–7.

63   Roumen RM, Hendriks T, Wevers RA, Goris JA. Intestinal permeability after severe trauma and hemorrhagic shock is increased without relation to septic complications. *Arch Surg* 1993; **128**: 453–7.

64   Yassin MMI, Barros D'Sa AAB, Parks TG, *et al.* Lower limb ischaemia-reperfusion injury causes endotoxaemia and endogenous antiendotoxin antibody consumption but not bacterial translocation. *Br J Surg* 1998; **85**: 785–9.

65   Yassin MM, Barros D'Sa AAB, Parks TG, *et al.* Mortality following lower limb ischemia-reperfusion: a systemic inflammatory response? *World J Surg* 1996; **20**: 961–7.

66   Van Damme H, Creemers E, Limet R. Ischaemic colitis following aortoiliac surgery. *Acta Chir Belg* 2000; **100**: 21–7.

67   Welch M, Baguneid MS, McMahon RF, *et al.* Histological study of colonic ischaemia after aortic surgery. *Br J Surg* 1998; **85**: 1095–8.

68   Dobbins WO, III. Gut immunophysiology: a gastroenterologist's view with emphasis on pathophysiology. *Am J Physiol* 1982; **242**: G1–8.

69   Glauser MP, Zanetti G, Baumgartner JD, Cohen J. Septic shock: pathogenesis. *Lancet* 1991; **338**: 732–6.

70   Bone RC. Why sepsis trials fail. *JAMA* 1996; **276**: 565–6.

71   Fry DE, Pearlstein L, Fulton RL, Polk HC, Jr. Multiple system organ failure. The role of uncontrolled infection. *Arch Surg* 1980; **115**: 136–40.

72   Knaus WA, Draper EA, Wagner DP, Zimmerman JE. APACHE II: a severity of disease classification system. *Crit Care Med* 1985; **13**: 818–29.

73   Bone RC. The sepsis syndrome. Definition and general approach to management. *Clin Chest Med* 1996; **17**: 175–81.

74   Carrico CJ, Meakins JL, Marshall JC, *et al.* Multiple-organ-failure syndrome. *Arch Surg* 1986; **121**: 196–208.

75   Paterson IS, Klausner JM, Pugatch R, *et al.* Noncardiogenic pulmonary edema after abdominal aortic aneurysm surgery. *Ann Surg* 1989; **209**: 231–6.

76   Huber TS, Harward TR, Flynn TC, *et al.* Operative mortality rates after elective infrarenal aortic reconstructions. *J Vasc Surg* 1995; **22**: 287–93.

77   Harris LM, Faggioli GL, Fiedler R, *et al.* Ruptured abdominal aortic aneurysms: factors affecting mortality rates. *J Vasc Surg* 1991; **14**: 812–18.

78   Goris RJ, te Boekhorst TP, Nuytinck JK, Gimbrere JS. Multiple-organ failure. Generalized autodestructive inflammation? *Arch Surg* 1985; **120**: 1109–15.

79   Marshall JC, Christou NV, Meakins JL. The gastrointestinal tract. The 'undrained abscess' of multiple organ failure. *Ann Surg* 1993; **218**: 111–19.

80   Deitch EA. Multiple organ failure. Pathophysiology and potential future therapy. *Ann Surg* 1992; **216**: 117–34.

81   Bjornson AB, Bjornson HS, Altemeier WA. Serum-mediated inhibition of polymorphonuclear leukocyte function following burn injury. *Ann Surg* 1981; **194**: 568–75.

82   Rubin BB, Smith A, Liauw S, *et al.* Complement activation and white cell sequestration in postischemic skeletal muscle. *Am J Physiol* 1990; **259**: H525–H531.

83   Wood JJ, Grbic JT, Rodrick ML, *et al.* Suppression of interleukin 2 production in an animal model of thermal injury is related to prostaglandin synthesis. *Arch Surg* 1987; **122**: 179–84.

84   Hakim AA. An immunosuppressive factor from serum of thermally traumatized patients. *J Trauma* 1977; **17**: 908–19.

85   Munster AM. Post-traumatic immunosuppression is due to activation of suppressor T cells. *Lancet* 1976; **1**: 1329–30.

86   Munster AM, Hoagland HC, Pruitt BA Jr. The effect of thermal injury on serum immunoglobulins. *Ann Surg* 1970; **172**: 965–9.

87   Hurd TC, Dasmahapatra KS, Rush BF Jr, Machiedo GW. Red blood cell deformability in human and experimental sepsis. *Arch Surg* 1988; **123**: 217–20.

88   Bradbury A, Adam D, Garrioch M, *et al.* Changes in platelet count, coagulation and fibrinogen associated with elective repair of asymptomatic abdominal aortic aneurysm and aortic reconstruction for occlusive disease. *Eur J Vasc Endovasc Surg* 1997; **13**: 375–80.

89   Davies MJ, Murphy WG, Murie JA, *et al.* Preoperative coagulopathy in ruptured abdominal aortic aneurysm predicts poor outcome. *Br J Surg* 1993; **80**: 974–6.

90   Hoffman MJ, Greenfield LJ, Sugerman HJ, Tatum JL. Unsuspected right ventricular dysfunction in shock and sepsis. *Ann Surg* 1983; **198**: 307–19.

91   Levison M. Myocardial failure. *Surg Clin North Am* 1982; **62**: 149–56.

92   Lefer AM. Role of a myocardial depressant factor in the pathogenesis of circulatory shock. *Fed Proc* 1970; **29**: 1836–47.

93   Haglund U. Systemic mediators released from the gut in critical illness. *Crit Care Med* 1993; **21**: S15–S18.

94   Klausner JM, Anner H, Paterson IS, *et al.* Lower torso ischemia-induced lung injury is leukocyte dependent. *Ann Surg* 1988; **208**: 761–7.

95   Korthuis RJ, Grisham MB, Granger DN. Leukocyte depletion attenuates vascular injury in postischemic skeletal muscle. *Am J Physiol* 1988; **254**: H823–H827.

96   Leeman M. Pulmonary hypertension in acute respiratory distress syndrome. *Monaldi Arch Chest Dis* 1999; **54**: 146–9.

97   Parsons PE, Worthen GS, Moore EE, *et al.* The association of circulating endotoxin with the development of the adult respiratory distress syndrome. *Am Rev Respir Dis* 1989; **140**: 294–301.

98   Wollert PS, Menconi MJ, O'Sullivan BP, *et al.* LY255283, a novel leukotriene B4 receptor antagonist, limits activation of neutrophils and prevents acute lung injury induced by endotoxin in pigs. *Surgery* 1993; **114**: 191–8.

99   Gilroy RJ Jr, Lavietes MH, Loring SH, *et al.* Respiratory mechanical effects of abdominal distension. *J Appl Physiol* 1985; **58**: 1997–2003.

100   Barratt J, Parajasingam R, Sayers RD, Feehally J. Outcome of Acute Renal Failure Following Surgical Repair of Ruptured Abdominal Aortic Aneurysms. *Eur J Vasc Endovasc Surg* 2000; **20**: 163–8.

101   Gelman S. The pathophysiology of aortic cross-clamping and unclamping. *Anesthesiology* 1995; **82**: 1026–60.

102   Grace PA. Ischaemia-reperfusion injury. *Br J Surg* 1994; **81**: 637–47.

103   Neveu H, Kleinknecht D, Brivet F, *et al.* Prognostic factors in acute renal failure due to sepsis. Results of a prospective multicentre study. The French Study Group on Acute Renal Failure. *Nephrol Dial Transplant* 1996; **11**: 293–9.

104   Gutierrez G, Palizas F, Doglio G, *et al.* Gastric intramucosal pH as a therapeutic index of tissue oxygenation in critically ill patients. *Lancet* 1992; **339**: 195–9.

105 Bjorck M, Hedberg B. Early detection of major complications after abdominal aortic surgery: predictive value of sigmoid colon and gastric intramucosal pH monitoring. *Br J Surg* 1994; **81**: 25–30.

106 Derbyshire DR, Smith G. Sympathoadrenal responses to anaesthesia and surgery. *Br J Anaesth* 1984; **56**: 725–39.

107 Thompson JP, Boyle JR, Thompson MM, *et al.* Cardiovascular and catecholamine responses during endovascular and conventional abdominal aortic aneurysm repair. *Eur J Vasc Endovasc Surg* 1999; **17**: 326–33.

108 Zuckerman SH, Bendele AM. Regulation of serum tumor necrosis factor in glucocorticoid-sensitive and -resistant rodent endotoxin shock models. *Infect Immun* 1989; **57**: 3009–13.

109 Ray A, LaForge KS, Sehgal PB. On the mechanism for efficient repression of the interleukin-6 promoter by glucocorticoids: enhancer, TATA box, and RNA start site (Inr motif) occlusion. *Mol Cell Biol* 1990; **10**: 5736–46.

110 Slag MF, Morley JE, Elson MK, *et al.* Free thyroxine levels in critically ill patients. A comparison of currently available assays. *JAMA* 1981; **246**: 2702–6.

111 Ozawa K. [Clinical and biological significance of arterial blood ketone body ratio in hepatic surgery] (Article in Japanese). *Nippon Geka Gakkai Zasshi* 1983; **84**: 753–7.

112 Oudemans-van Straaten HM, Scheffer GJ, *et al.* Oxygen consumption after cardiopulmonary bypass – implications of different measuring methods. *Intensive Care Med* 1993; **19**: 105–10.

113 Oldenburg HS, Rogy MA, Lazarus DD, *et al.* Cachexia and the acute-phase protein response in inflammation are regulated by interleukin-6. *Eur J Immunol* 1993; **23**: 1889–94.

114 Shoemaker WC, Appel PL, Kram HB. Tissue oxygen debt as a determinant of lethal and nonlethal postoperative organ failure. *Crit Care Med* 1988; **16**: 1117–20.

115 Swan HJ, Ganz W, Forrester J, *et al.* Catheterization of the heart in man with use of a flow-directed balloon-tipped catheter. *N Engl J Med* 1970; **283**: 447–51.

116 Connors AF Jr, Speroff T, Dawson NV, *et al.* The effectiveness of right heart catheterization in the initial care of critically ill patients. SUPPORT Investigators. *JAMA* 1996; **276**: 889–97.

117 Shoemaker WC, Appel PL, Kram HB. Tissue oxygen debt as a determinant of lethal and nonlethal postoperative organ failure. *Crit Care Med* 1988; **16**: 1117–20.

118 Fiddian-Green RG, Amelin PM, Herrmann JB, *et al.* Prediction of the development of sigmoid ischemia on the day of aortic operations. Indirect measurements of intramural pH in the colon. *Arch Surg* 1986; **121**: 654–60.

119 Mucelli RP, Bertolotto M. Imaging techniques in acute renal failure. *Kidney Int Suppl* 1998; **66**: S102–S105.

120 Crawford ES, Saleh SA, Babb JW 3rd, *et al.* Infrarenal abdominal aortic aneurysm: factors influencing survival after operation performed over a 25-year period. *Ann Surg* 1981; **193**: 699–709.

121 Gloviczki P, Pairolero PC, Mucha P Jr, *et al.* Ruptured abdominal aortic aneurysms: repair should not be denied. *J Vasc Surg* 1992; **15**: 851–7.

122 Harris KA, Ameli FM, Lally M, *et al.* Abdominal aortic aneurysm resection in patients more than 80 years old. *Surg Gynecol Obstet* 1986; **162**: 536–8.

123 Bjerkelund CE, Smith-Erichsen N, Solheim K. Abdominal aortic reconstruction. Prognostic importance of coexistent diseases. *Acta Chir Scand* 1986; **152**: 111–15.

124 Lazarides MK, Arvanitis DP, Drista H, *et al.* POSSUM and APACHE II scores do not predict the outcome of ruptured infrarenal aortic aneurysms. *Ann Vasc Surg* 1997; **11**: 155–8.

125 Copeland GP, Jones D, Walters M. POSSUM: a scoring system for surgical audit. *Br J Surg* 1991; **78**: 355–60.

126 Prytherch DR, Whiteley MS, Higgins B, *et al.* POSSUM and Portsmouth POSSUM for predicting mortality. Physiological and Operative Severity Score for the enUmeration of Mortality and morbidity. *Br J Surg* 1998; **85**: 1217–20.

127 Seckinger P, Isaaz S, Dayer JM. A human inhibitor of tumor necrosis factor alpha. *J Exp Med* 1988; **167**: 1511–16.

128 Pilz G, Kaab S, Kreuzer E, Werdan K. Evaluation of definitions and parameters for sepsis assessment in patients after cardiac surgery. *Infection* 1994; **22**: 8–17.

129 Tracey KJ, Fong Y, Hesse DG, *et al.* Anti-cachectin/TNF monoclonal antibodies prevent septic shock during lethal bacteraemia. *Nature* 1987; **330**: 662–4.

130 Fisher CJ Jr, Agosti JM, Opal SM, *et al.* Treatment of septic shock with the tumor necrosis factor receptor:Fc fusion protein. The Soluble TNF Receptor Sepsis Study Group. *N Engl J Med* 1996; **334**: 1697–702.

131 Mancilla J, Garcia P, Dinarello CA. The interleukin-1 receptor antagonist can either reduce or enhance the lethality of *Klebsiella pneumoniae* sepsis in newborn rats. *Infect Immun* 1993; **61**: 926–32.

132 Libert C, Vink A, Coulie P, *et al.* Limited involvement of interleukin-6 in the pathogenesis of lethal septic shock as revealed by the effect of monoclonal antibodies against interleukin-6 or its receptor in various murine models. *Eur J Immunol* 1992; **22**: 2625–30.

133 Gennari R, Alexander JW. Anti-interleukin-6 antibody treatment improves survival during gut-derived sepsis in a time-dependent manner by enhancing host defense. *Crit Care Med* 1995; **23**: 1945–53.

134 Derkx B, Marchant A, Goldman M, *et al.* High levels of interleukin-10 during the initial phase of fulminant meningococcal septic shock. *J Infect Dis* 1995; **171**: 229–32.

135 Neidhardt R, Keel M, Steckholzer U, *et al.* Relationship of interleukin-10 plasma levels to severity of injury and clinical outcome in injured patients. *J Trauma* 1997; **42**: 863–70.

136 Huber TS, Gaines GC, Welborn MB 3rd, *et al.* Anticytokine therapies for acute inflammation and the systemic inflammatory response syndrome: IL-10 and ischemia/reperfusion injury as a new paradigm. *Shock* 2000; **13**: 425–34.

137 Blair P, Rowlands BJ, Lowry K, *et al.* Selective decontamination of the digestive tract: a stratified, randomized, prospective study in a mixed intensive care unit. *Surgery* 1991; **110**: 303–9.

138 Lamping N, Dettmer R, Schroder NW, *et al.* LPS-binding protein protects mice from septic shock caused by LPS or Gram-negative bacteria. *J Clin Invest* 1998; **101**: 2065–71.

139 Jack RS, Fan X, Bernheiden M, *et al.* Lipopolysaccharide-binding protein is required to combat a murine Gram-negative bacterial infection. *Nature* 1997; **389**: 742–5.

140 Pilz G, Appel R, Kreuzer E, Werdan K. Comparison of early IgM-enriched immunoglobulin vs polyvalent IgG administration in score-identified postcardiac surgical patients at high risk for sepsis. *Chest* 1997; **111**: 419–26.

141 Ziegler EJ, Fisher CJ Jr, Sprung CL, *et al.* Treatment of Gram-negative bacteremia and septic shock with HA-1A human

monoclonal antibody against endotoxin. A randomized, double-blind, placebo-controlled trial. The HA-1A Sepsis Study Group. *N Engl J Med* 1991; **324**: 429–36.

142 Cometta A, Baumgartner JD, Lew D, *et al.* Prospective randomized comparison of imipenem monotherapy with imipenem plus netilmicin for treatment of severe infections in nonneutropenic patients. *Antimicrob Agents Chemother* 1994; **38**: 1309–13.

143 Fomsgaard A, Baek L, Fomsgaard JS, Engquist A. Preliminary study on treatment of septic shock patients with antilipopolysaccharide IgG from blood donors. *Scand J Infect Dis* 1989; **21**: 697–708.

144 Muta T, Miyata T, Tokunaga F, *et al.* Primary structure of anti-lipopolysaccharide factor from American horseshoe crab, *Limulus polyphemus* [published erratum appears in *J Biochem (Tokyo)* 1987; **102**:443]. *J Biochem (Tokyo)* 1987; **101**: 1321–30.

145 Alpert G, Baldwin G, Thompson C, *et al. Limulus* antilipopolysaccharide factor protects rabbits from meningococcal endotoxin shock. *J Infect Dis* 1992; **165**: 494–500.

146 Saladino RA, Stack AM, Thompson C, *et al.* High-dose recombinant endotoxin neutralizing protein improves survival in rabbits, with *Escherichia coli* sepsis. *Crit Care Med* 1996; **24**: 1203–7.

147 Marra MN, Wilde CG, Griffith JE, *et al.* Bactericidal/permeability-increasing protein has endotoxin-neutralizing activity. *J Immunol* 1990; **144**: 662–6.

148 Weiss J, Elsbach P, Shu C, *et al.* Human bactericidal/permeability-increasing protein and a recombinant NH_2-terminal fragment cause killing of serum-resistant gram-negative bacteria in whole blood and inhibit tumor necrosis factor release induced by the bacteria. *J Clin Invest* 1992; **90**: 1122–30.

149 Harkin DW, Barros D'Sa AAB, Yassin MM, *et al.* Recombinant bactericidal/permeability-increasing protein attenuates the systemic inflammatory response syndrome in lower limb ischaemia-reperfusion injury. *J Vasc Surg* 2001; **33**: 840–6.

150 Harkin DW, Barros D'Sa AAB, McCallion K, *et al.* Bactericidal/permeability-increasing protein attenuates systemic inflammation and acute lung injury in porcine lower limb ischaemia-reperfusion injury. *Ann Surg* 2001; **234**: 233–44.

151 Harkin DW, Barros D'Sa AAB, Yassin MM, *et al.* Gut mucosal injury is attenuated by recombinant bactericidal/permeability-increasing protein in hind limb ischaemia-reperfusion injury. *Ann Vasc Surg* 2001; **15**: 326–31.

152 Belkin M, LaMorte WL, Wright JG, Hobson RW. The role of leukocytes in the pathophysiology of skeletal muscle ischemic injury. *J Vasc Surg* 1989; **10**: 14–18.

153 Carden DL, Smith JK, Korthuis RJ. Neutrophil-mediated microvascular dysfunction in postischemic canine skeletal muscle. Role of granulocyte adherence. *Circ Res* 1990; **66**: 1436–44.

154 Boyd AJ, Rubin BB, Walker PM, *et al.* A CD18 monoclonal antibody reduces multiple organ injury in a model of ruptured abdominal aortic aneurysm. *Am J Physiol* 1999; **277**: H172–82.

155 Vincent JL. Microvascular endothelial dysfunction: a renewed appreciation of sepsis pathophysiology. *Crit Care* 2001; **5**(suppl 2): S1–5.

5

Pathophysiology of Stroke

HARVEY J CHANT

THE PROBLEM

Stroke can be defined as a rapid onset neurological deficit of presumed vascular origin lasting for more than 24 hours and which may result in death.[1] Each year in the UK, over 100 000 people are affected by this disease[2] and on a worldwide scale, it is estimated that there are 4.5 million deaths from stroke per year.[3] Furthermore, with the increasing size of the elderly population anticipated over the next few years, this number is likely to rise.[3,4] The prevalence of stroke is dependent upon case fatality and incidence. In the USA, stroke affects 550 000 people per year; of these 150 000 die, approximately 350 000 are disabled and there are an estimated 3 million survivors from stroke.[5] A study of the pathophysiology of stroke suggests that it is likely that both the survival and the quality of life of stroke survivors might be improved by early reperfusion of the area of brain immediately adjacent to the core of cerebral infarction.

The aetiology of stroke depends on the age of the patient so that although stroke in the young is rare, and stroke caused by atherosclerosis is exceedingly rare. However, with increasing age, it becomes the predominant cause and because of the greater number of strokes occurring in the elderly, atherosclerosis overtakes all other causes of stroke.[6] It can be difficult to establish the cause of cerebral infarction and in up to 40 per cent of cases a cause is never identified. Furthermore, the relative contribution of each risk factor is difficult to ascertain, for example ischaemic heart disease and atrial fibrillation often coexist making the diagnosis unclear.[6] Cerebral infarction accounts for approximately 85 per cent of strokes and the mechanism of infarction is small and large vessel atherosclerosis (45 per cent), cardiogenic embolism (20 per cent), and cryptogenic and unusual causes (35 per cent).[7]

The Oxfordshire Community Stroke Project (OCSP) investigated incidence and cause of first-time strokes and transient ischaemic attacks (TIAs) in the community.[2] Using clinical assessment this project classified ischaemic stroke into four groups: total anterior circulation infarction (TACI), partial anterior circulation infarction (PACI), lacunar infarction and posterior cerebral infarction. This classification system is a valuable tool for the studies of stroke subtype and incidence. In a large epidemiological survey based in Manchester, UK, Mead et al.[8] investigated the prevalence of carotid atherosclerosis in the four OCSP stroke categories. Of 305 patients with cerebral infarction, 201 (66 per cent) were classified as either PACI or TACI. Furthermore, in the TACI group (100 patients) four patients had ipsilateral severe (70–99 per cent) internal carotid artery (ICA) stenosis and 25 had ipsilateral ICA occlusion. In the PACI group, 16 had ipsilateral severe ICA stenosis and 11 had ICA occlusion.[8] ICA atherosclerosis is a well recognised cause of stroke.[9] Mead's study quantifies the contribution of severe ICA stenosis and ICA occlusion to the epidemiology of stroke and confirms ICA disease as a major target for stroke prevention and treatment (Fig. 5.1).

In patients surviving stroke, the personal cost is often considerable. In the OCSP, 92 of 543 patients with cerebral infarction were classified as TACIs. Of this subgroup only 4 per cent of patients were independent and 56 per cent were still dependent at 30 days following stroke.[10] The number of patients remaining independent was unchanged at one year. Although stroke is primarily a disease of the elderly, a significant proportion of cases occur in patients under retirement age. For example in an American study the annual incident rate for first ever or recurrent stroke in men between the ages of 55 and 64 years was 458 per

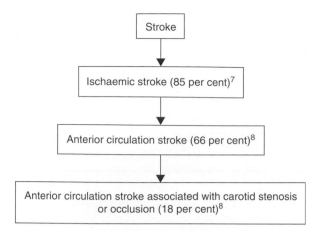

Figure 5.1 *Relative proportions of patients presenting with ischaemic stroke associated with carotid disease*

100 000.[11] This puts great strain on patients and relatives, with loss of earnings, possible change in lifestyle and dependency on others. In 1988, Isard and Forbes estimated that the cost to the health service in Scotland for one stroke was £6000 but they only considered the cost to the hospital and local doctors.[12] This is similar to a more recent European study finding the total cost per patient treated in London of approximately £5000.[13] However, when other associated factors are included, such as community care and loss of productivity, the cost, in the USA, is estimated to be the equivalent of £70 000 at 1990 prices.[14] The difficulties in assessing the cost of stroke to the community are perhaps a reflection of the protean manifestations of this disease, and that patients often present with other pathologies that may compound the problems of stroke.[15] Overall, it is estimated that 4 per cent of UK National Health Service resources are consumed in treating and managing stroke each year.[4,16] The NHS budget for 2002–2003 was in excess of £60 billion and therefore the total expenditure on stroke can be estimated to total some £2.4 billion.

RATIONALE FOR ACUTE TREATMENT OF ISCHAEMIC STROKE

Until recently stroke was considered the least treatable of all neurological conditions, however, it has become increasingly recognised that in certain circumstances, appropriate therapy instituted promptly will reduce the overall impact of stroke. There are three mechanisms by which this may occur:

Measures to reduce the impact of acute stroke

- by preventing further strokes
- by salvaging ischaemic but not infarcted brain
- by limiting the damage caused by stroke.

It is well recognised that carotid stenosis predisposes to recurrent stroke[9,17] and there are series that suggest patients with severe carotid stenosis may be at a particularly high risk of early stroke recurrence.[18–20] The potential benefit of early carotid surgery in preventing acute stroke has now been demonstrated in a trial of 25 patients with PACI and carotid stenosis (70–99 per cent) randomised to surgery either within 1 week of stroke or at 2 months. The reinfarction rate was significantly lower in the group undergoing urgent surgery.[21] (See Chapters 12 and 13.)

In carotid artery occlusion the situation is less clear. It has previously been assumed that once an ICA has occluded it will be unlikely to cause further embolisation. It is clear, however, that such patients do have an increased risk of subsequent stroke either from extension of the original thrombus/embolus or by 'watershed infarction'. Studies of the natural history of ICA occlusion are complicated by the fact that it may present as a unilateral or bilateral phenomenon. Furthermore, there is a variable contribution to cerebral blood flow arriving via the vertebral arteries and other collaterals.[22,23] There is evidence to suggest that embolism occurs distal to an occluded segment of the ICA[24] but it is not easy to determine whether the emboli originate from the thrombus or arrive via the collateral circulation. In the Joint Study of Extracranial Arterial Occlusion, of 368 patients identified as having unilateral ICA occlusion and having survived the initial stroke, new strokes occurred in at least 25 per cent within the ensuing 44 months.[25] Several other studies confirm these findings and not surprisingly the outlook for bilateral ICA occlusion is worse.[26] However, all of these studies are subject to selection bias towards poor collateral circulation as many patients with good collateral circulation may not present to clinicians in the event of ICA occlusion.

In the remainder of this chapter, the pathophysiology of cerebral reperfusion will be described in relation to the problems faced by clinicians attempting to provide a cerebral reperfusion service (see Chapters 12 and 13).

THE PATHOGENESIS OF CEREBRAL INFARCTION: CELL DEATH AND APOPTOSIS

'Ischaemia' implies complete cessation of blood flow, but in stroke, blood flow is rarely completely absent. The infarction occurs in a nebulous area which ranges between hypoxia and total ischaemia. In the following discussion the term ischaemia will be used to denote a reduction in the supply of oxygen and nutrients of sufficient severity and duration to cause cerebral infarction. Furthermore, cerebral infarction involves pan-necrosis where all the elements of neural tissue, glial and endothelial cells as well as neurones, are involved. Complicating the issue of cerebral infarction is the fact that the extent of injury is dependent on both the degree and the duration of hypoxia. In the following sections the mechanisms of cell death will be briefly described followed by a discussion of the effects of depth and duration of ischaemia. This sets the scene for the introduction of the concept of the **ischaemic penumbra**.

The brain is extremely sensitive to reductions in oxygen delivery as it depends almost entirely on oxidative phosphorylation for energy production. An impairment in the supply of oxygen (and other nutrients, especially glucose) leads to a failure in maintenance of ionic homoeostasis. This is followed by cellular depolarisation and the release of excitatory amino acid transmitters from presynaptic terminals. This damage in turn leads to an increase in cytosolic sodium and chloride producing intracellular oedema followed by brain swelling and further reductions in cerebral perfusion. In addition, a rise in intracellular calcium concentration causes the activation of proteolytic enzymes and the generation of free radical species by cyclooxygenase and phospholipase A_2. Further structural cellular damage follows and eventually cell death ensues.[27] The above events describe the process of cell necrosis, however, some cells are killed by a different mechanism termed **apoptosis**. This is an active process of cell death characterised by the maintenance of cell membrane and mitochondrial integrity. The cells reduce in volume and become susceptible to phagocytosis. This occurs prior to membrane rupture and prevents the content of the cell from being discharged into the surrounding milieu.[28] Both apoptosis and necrosis occur in the brain: it appears that necrosis occurs with catastrophic reductions in blood flow, but at times of more controlled flow reduction, or 'relative ischaemia', apoptosis occurs as a method of 'damage limitation'.

Brief periods of cerebral ischaemia lasting a few minutes cause little or no evidence of histological damage. Ischaemia lasting more than 5 minutes but less than 1 hour results in the progressive death of selectively vulnerable neurones. Certain groups of neurones are more sensitive than others; hippocampal CA1 neurones and cerebellar Purkinje fibres are more vulnerable to ischaemia compared with other cells, as demonstrated by their susceptibility to even brief periods of cardiac arrest.[29] The process whereby some brain tissue dies before other areas has been called 'selective neuronal necrosis'. However, after 1 hour, depending upon the species, infarction ensues within the zone of lowest blood flow progressively enlarging to a maximum volume over 3–4 hours in rodents,[30] and 6–8 hours in non-human primates.[31] Until recently it has been hard to define this critical time interval in humans. Observations of anaesthetised patients undergoing carotid surgery and neurosurgery can be misleading as general anaesthetic reduces cerebral metabolic activity. This has the potential of increasing neuronal survival times. Moreover, with the advent of trials of thrombolysis it seems clear that in certain circumstances normal brain function and morphology can be restored up to and possibly beyond a 3-hour time window.[32]

As well as the duration of ischaemia, several studies have demonstrated thresholds of cerebral blood flow upon which neuronal function and survival are critically dependent. These are referred to as the **threshold of electrical failure** and the **threshold of membrane failure**, respectively. The former refers to the rate of blood flow at which neuronal function ceases and the latter to the point at which neuronal death ensues.

The threshold of electrical failure

In primates, normal cerebral blood flow is in the range of 50–60 mL per 100 g of brain per minute.[33] As flow is gradually reduced, the threshold of electrical failure is approached and physiological function is impaired. In a cat model of reversible middle carotid artery (MCA) occlusion, Heiss *et al.* simultaneously recorded single (neuronal) cell activity and local blood flow and were able to demonstrate that spontaneous electrical activity ceased at flow levels of about 18 mL per 100 g per minute and that normal function returned after restoration of flow.[34,35] In the baboon, Branston *et al.* demonstrated that evoked cortical responses disappeared at similar flow thresholds and reappeared on reperfusion.[36,37] These findings were subsequently corroborated by the results of clinical studies on patients undergoing carotid surgery.[38,39] Because electroencephalographic activity in the patients undergoing carotid endarterectomy returned to precross-clamp levels following restoration of blood flow, it was assumed that the neurones were not irreversibly damaged. Clearly, however, these results need to be interpreted in the light of the fact that anaesthetic agents reduce cerebral metabolic requirements.

The threshold for membrane failure

The lower limit for cell survival, the threshold for membrane failure, was initially estimated by recording the extracellular potassium concentration at varying flow rates.[40,41] Elevation of extracellular potassium, indicative of the collapse of transmembrane potentials, pointed to membrane failure at flow rates below 10–12 mL/100 g per minute. The demonstration that hypoxic cell death involved the coupled uptake of calcium and efflux of potassium at similar low flow rates was taken as further evidence indicative of membrane failure.[42] These thresholds are slightly higher in rats and gerbils perhaps correlating with the higher cerebral metabolic rate of these animals.[43]

THE CONCEPT OF THE ISCHAEMIC PENUMBRA

From the preceding discussion it is clear that focal cerebral infarction is highly dependent upon both the duration and severity of ischaemia. The studies of ischaemic thresholds

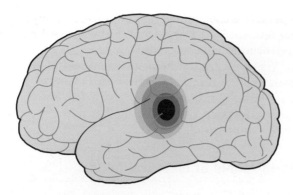

Figure 5.2 *Schematic representation of the ischaemic penumbra – a central core of cerebral infarction surrounded by an area of hypoperfused but viable brain*

discussed above have important implications in the development of cerebral infarction in humans. In 1981, Astrup suggested that the ischaemic core of focal infarction is surrounded by a rim of tissue with reduced blood supply, sufficient to maintain transmembrane potentials but insufficient to maintain electrical activity.[44] It was suggested that the cells in the central core of an infarct were dead but were surrounded by a zone of cells in a twilight zone between electrical failure and membrane failure. The term 'ischaemic penumbra' was based on the Greek word for partial shadow (Fig. 5.2).[44]

Since this initial description, the ischaemic penumbra has become the focus of intense research efforts, both in establishing its existence and in verifying it as a target for therapeutic intervention in stroke. Evidence for the existence of the penumbra came originally from animal studies and later from human studies.

Animal studies

Several animal studies have shown that the tissue surrounding a core of infarction is biochemically distinct from both the normal brain and the infarct. In a rat model of focal reversible ischaemia, Kristian *et al.* demonstrated that calcium homoeostasis is abolished soon after the insult at the core of the infarction but takes up to 6 hours to disappear at the periphery.[45] Positron emission tomography (PET) is a useful tool in the study of brain pathology as it enables direct measurement of cerebral blood flow and metabolic parameters such as cerebral glucose, oxygen consumption and cerebral oxygen extraction. In a nonreversible feline model of MCA occlusion, Heiss *et al.* performed serial PET scans up to 24 hours following occlusion.[46] At the onset of infarction the oxygen extraction was greatest at the centre of the focus of ischaemia but as the central cells gradually died, oxygen extraction fell at the centre and then increased towards the periphery of the lesion. This process took up to 24 hours suggesting that in

this model the cells in the penumbral region took up to 24 hours to die.[46] In a shorter term experiment using permanent ischaemia in rats, Kohno *et al.* compared reductions in blood flow, measured by diffusion-weighted magnetic resonance imaging (DWI), with areas of biochemical abnormality, manifested by acidosis and adenosine triphosphate (ATP) depletion: after 30 minutes of ischaemia the area of acidosis and low perfusion was larger than the area of ATP depletion.[47] Over the following two hours, however, ATP depletion progressed towards the periphery of the lesion. The authors interpreted this finding as a gradual depletion of energy in the zone surrounding a central infarction core of established infarction.

Patient studies

Computed tomography (CT) is commonly used in the clinical investigation of stroke and is able to demonstrate haemorrhage, oedema and parenchymal necrosis. Unfortunately, it lacks sensitivity for the structural changes in the acute stage of stroke. For this reason, and unless haemorrhage has to be excluded, CT scanning is usually delayed for 24 hours or more to ensure a hypodense, i.e. visible, infarct is identified if present. Olsen *et al.* performed CT and xenon clearance studies on patients with acute stroke, demonstrating that blood flow abnormalities make up a significantly larger area than that measured by CT.[48] They interpreted this finding as evidence that the tissue surrounding an infarct, i.e. the penumbra, may not take on the CT appearances of infarction but is physiologically abnormal and, importantly, a potential therapeutic target.

Using single photon emission computed tomography (SPECT) Wise *et al.* studied the metabolic changes occurring in the tissue surrounding an infarct and found that there was evidence of continuing neuronal death up to 1 week following infarction.[49] More comprehensive PET studies, using a shorter time interval, have subsequently confirmed these findings demonstrating metabolically active tissue at 17 hours following infarction. In the absence of treatment, this tissue subsequently became metabolically inert.[50] In a more comprehensive study, Baron described three patterns of blood flow in untreated stroke patients in whom an ischaemic penumbra was present.[51] Firstly, some patients develop early extensive cortical damage, indicated by a rapid decline in the cerebral metabolic rate of oxygen, and have no evidence of recovery. A second group showed evidence of hyperperfusion, with preserved cerebral metabolic rate of oxygen, indicating complete or almost complete recovery. In the third pattern, patients develop severe cortical ischaemia with a relatively well preserved cerebral metabolic rate of oxygen, consistent with the two threshold flow rates already discussed. These patients have a very variable outcome consistent with the presence of hypoperfused but viable tissue.[51]

Conventional magnetic resonance imaging (MRI) measures alterations in tissue water content. This makes the technique of limited value in the early investigation of stroke as urgent treatments should aim to prevent damage which results in fluid shifts. However, there are several modifications of the technique that have provided a valuable insight into the existence of the ischaemic penumbra. Diffusion-weighted magnetic resonance imaging measures the diffusion of water in 'regions of interest' and in areas of cerebral ischaemia there is a detectable reduction in the rate of diffusion of water molecules. In patients with stroke of less than 2 hours duration, well circumscribed lesions relating to the decrease in molecular water diffusion have been demonstrated.[52] Contrast studies also appear useful. Perfusion-weighted scanning obtains images (PWI) by measuring the rate of appearance of contrast in a volume of brain tissue. Because the rate of appearance of contrast is dependent on blood flow, this technique accurately measures blood flow at the capillary level. By combining PWI and DWI it is possible to measure the volume of the initial infarction (using DWI), the volume of hypoperfused brain (PWI) and the final infarction volume (using conventional MRI). Fisher and Garcia used this technique to show that the volume of hypoperfused brain is larger than the volume of infarcted brain, as would be expected with an infarct surrounded by penumbra, and that the eventual infarction volume corresponds to the volume of hypoperfused brain, as would be expected if the penumbra slowly died to become complete infarction.[53]

Finally, magnetic resonance spectroscopy studies complement all of the above studies: with this technique serial measurements of various key metabolites can be taken throughout the time course of stroke. Lactate (a marker of anaerobic metabolism), N-acetylaspartate (a neuronal marker) and creatinine/phosphocreatinine ratio (present in both glia and neurones) can be measured spectroscopically. Abnormal or ischaemic regions can be compared with contralateral healthy brain, and it can be demonstrated that neurones die faster than glia. Furthermore, this technique provides evidence of neuronal death occurring up to 10 days following the initial insult,[54] in agreement with the earlier findings of Wise et al. in 1983.[49]

It is clear from the above studies that there is strong evidence for the existence of an ischaemic penumbra. It appears to be a dynamic process which, with time, eventually disappears and is replaced by infarction. Although many of these studies have indicated that the penumbra may last for up to several days, it would appear, intuitively, that prompt treatment would salvage more brain.

However, in order to accept the premise that the presence of the penumbra justifies attempts at cerebral reperfusion, we require proof that reperfusion alters the nature of the penumbra; in other words, that restoration of blood flow converts inactive neurones at risk of death back to electronically functional tissue. There is, in fact, a wealth of evidence to indicate that early reperfusion reduces the eventual infarction volume, however there are comparatively few data confirming the restoration of normal homoeostasis in tissue which was previously 'penumbral'.

The quiescent cells within the penumbra are precariously balanced and in the absence of reperfusion the cells eventually die. An increase in local blood flow or perfusion pressure may be sufficient to restore function but an increase in adjacent energy demand or an increase in intracranial pressure may reduce the supply of oxygen and glucose to a level below that required to maintain transmembrane potentials.[55]

Clearly the reperfusion of the brain must be set against the disadvantage of delayed reperfusion causing 'reperfusion injury'. This phenomenon is well described in the peripheral vascular system (see Chapter 4) and is now known to be highly relevant in the brain.[56]

When brain becomes ischaemic, there is an initial elevation in intracellular calcium, activating proteases and phospholipases which in turn lead to the breakdown of membrane lipids and the production of damaging reactive oxygen species. In the absence of reperfusion, much of the initial damage occurs in this fashion. However, following reperfusion and the restoration of oxygen supply the production of free radicals is greatly increased. This allows the production of further free radicals by a process of amplification from several intracerebral sources: the sudden upsurge in mitochondrial activity following restoration of blood flow brings about the production of arachidonic acid released by the phospholipases activated during ischaemia. This fatty acid is converted by cyclo-oxygenase generating free reactive oxygen species. These molecules cause lipid peroxidation, leading to neuronal, glial and endothelial membrane dysfunction. The blood–brain barrier becomes more permeable and results in the development of 'vasogenic' oedema (see Chapter 13). The neurones, glia and endothelial cells develop 'cellular' oedema as a result of cell wall dysfunction. Furthermore, the breakdown of the blood–brain barrier allows the migration of macrophages into the cerebral extravascular space and this induces a further cascade of neurotoxic events.[27] The understanding of these events at cellular level is helpful in the interpretation of findings from clinical studies of cerebral reperfusion.

CLINICAL CONSEQUENCES OF REPERFUSING ISCHAEMIC BRAIN

There are several features of cerebral physiology and anatomy which make the reperfusion of the brain a complex process. These factors include the blood–brain barrier, the collateral blood supply, the ventriculo-cisternal system containing cerebrospinal fluid, the skull and dura forming a rigid external boundary, the high metabolic rate of brain tissue and its almost total dependence upon aerobic metabolism. Each factor has a crucial impact on the specific problems associated with cerebral reperfusion.

Complications of reperfusing ischaemic brain

- Haemorrhagic stroke
- Ischaemic stroke
- Cerebral oedema

In broad terms however, there are two pathological processes that can complicate the reperfusion of ischaemic brain: oedema and haemorrhage. Both have been demonstrated to contribute to the mortality and morbidity of stroke in the presence of physiological (i.e. spontaneous) and therapeutic reperfusion.

Cerebral oedema

Cerebral metabolic disturbances caused by ischaemia and subsequent reperfusion can lead to the development of both cellular and vasogenic oedema.

Cellular oedema is similar to that seen in other organs. Maintenance of the normal cell volume is an energy dependent mechanism based on the 'pump–leak' model.[57] Both neurones and glia control their volume by the active extrusion of sodium ions against a concentration gradient favouring inward flux of sodium. Failure of the energy supply results in a net increase in intracellular sodium followed by osmotically obliged water, leading to an increase in volume. The increase in volume may be clinically unnoticed (compensated for by a reduction in extracellular fluid volume) but is physiologically desirable (i.e. glial swelling in compensation for increased local neuronal activity), or it may be manifested as a mass effect.

Vasogenic oedema occurs when the integrity of the blood–brain barrier is interrupted; the flux of water from the plasma into the cerebral extracellular fluid results in tissue oedema and consequent brain swelling. The causes of blood–brain barrier disruption are not clear: at the cellular level free radicals, bradykinin and histamine have been implicated, as have infection, cranial trauma and stroke.[58] In practice, vasogenic and cellular cerebral oedema often coexist and in the context of stroke, this is usually the case. Vasogenic oedema necessarily involves an increase in flow of plasma from the blood. This contains many substances toxic to the brain, such as glutamate and potassium, and that in turn leads to further cerebral damage. As damage continues to progress, the microcirculation is disrupted, the tissue swells further to the point at which intracranial pressure rises and cerebral perfusion is compromised. As the mass expands, the cerebrospinal fluid (CSF) and venous volume decrease and healthy parts of brain become compressed to accommodate the expanding oedematous mass. Once these compensatory mechanisms fail, the contents of the cranial vault become non-compliant and intracranial pressure increases. Eventually, cerebral tissue is forced through the openings of the skull and, in the absence of treatment, the brainstem is forced through the foramen magnum, so called 'coning', and death rapidly ensues.

Haemorrhagic transformation of ischaemic infarction

Between 10 and 20 per cent of strokes are primarily due to subarachnoid or intraparenchymal haemorrhage. However, some ischaemic strokes may undergo **haemorrhagic transformation**.[59] This phenomenon ranges from a few petechial haemorrhages across the surface of the brain to extensive intracranial haematoma formation.[60] Postmortem studies give high rates of haemorrhagic transformation, presumably because they are biased towards more severe strokes. However, prospective radiological studies of patients presenting with stroke tend to underestimate the incidence of such transformation because, at the time when the research was carried out, many scanners did not have the resolution to identify the smaller bleeds.[60] Furthermore, to investigate the possibility that haemorrhagic transformation may be underdiagnosed, and hence primary haemorrhage overdiagnosed, Bogousslavsky et al. describe a series of 15 patients with an admission CT demonstrating no cerebral haemorrhage; subsequent clinical deterioration and CT scanning within 18 hours revealed the appearances of intracranial haemorrhage arising as haemorrhagic transformation.[61] Although they did not state the size of the population from which the sample was taken, the work suggests that studies of the aetiology of haemorrhagic stroke may overestimate the incidence of primary haemorrhage as the cause.

Clearly, the timing of the CT scan is important, and the use of serial CT scanning has now enabled researchers to establish the rate of haemorrhagic transformation over time after onset of stroke. Okada et al. found that of 160 patients with well documented cerebral embolism, 65 (41 per cent) underwent haemorrhagic transformation within one month of the ictus.[62] In a series of 65 patients Hornig et al. reached similar conclusions; 28 patients (43 per cent) developed haemorrhagic transformation within four weeks of stroke with a peak incidence during the second week.[63] Although there are no reports of studies in this area it seems possible that late *spontaneous* reperfusion may result in an increased risk of haemorrhagic transformation.

The aetiology of haemorrhagic transformation is not well understood but the theory proposed by Fisher and Adams in the 1950s is generally accepted: an embolus lodges in a vessel causing downstream infarction. Subsequently, the embolus autolyses, fragments and, with the force of the blood behind it, is driven downstream exposing the ischaemic vessels to blood flow at high pressure which ruptures the vessel and causes bleeding.[64] This hypothesis appears applicable to haemorrhagic transformation, both spontaneous and that complicating stroke therapies.

In favour of this theory is the fact that cardioembolism increases the rate of haemorrhagic transformation.[65] This suggests that emboli from the heart are able to undergo lysis and migrate distally as opposed to thromboembolic causes of occlusion.

Two studies have found that haemorrhagic transformation is significantly more frequent in large areas of infarction and in patients with severe neurological deficits.[62,63] Furthermore, Okada *et al.* found that elderly patients (over 70 years) were especially at risk.[62] Interestingly, in both of the above studies hypertension *was not* related to the risk of haemorrhage whereas the two available animal studies, designed to assess the role of hypertension in haemorrhagic transformation, both found that increased blood pressure *was* related to an increase in cerebral haemorrhage.[66,67] Unfortunately, the species differences between cats, rabbits and humans make direct comparison of these results impossible. Bowes *et al.* used a rabbit model of stroke and simply controlled the hypertension caused by induction of stroke[66] whereas Saku *et al.* induced hypertension by aortic occlusion.[67]

Iatrogenic haemorrhage

The risk of drug induced haemorrhagic transformation is relevant to potential new therapies because until the advent of thrombolysis for stroke, haemorrhagic transformation held little significance. Now, however, it is seen as a major risk factor for thrombolysis and consequently a great deal of research effort has been channelled into to the cause of haemorrhagic transformation following deliberate cerebral reperfusion.

In a baboon model of reperfusion, del Zoppo *et al.* found that there was no difference in the incidence of haemorrhage and volume of infarction and that none of the three doses of recombinant tissue plasminogen activator (rtPA) given in the study had any increased tendency to haemorrhage when given at three hours.[68] In a Cochrane review of randomised controlled, mainly intravenous, trials of thrombolysis for stroke, death and dependency are reduced at the expense of an increased risk of intracerebral haemorrhage.[69] However, the important principle from the thrombolysis experience seems to be that the risk of bleeding increases with the time delay to reperfusion, again supporting the rationale of early reperfusion, by whatever means (see Chapters 12 and 13).

Cerebral haemorrhage is a feared complication of carotid reconstruction for stroke and many studies of emergency carotid surgery for stroke include carotid endarterectomy and thromboendarterectomy. The conclusions of early studies lean towards avoiding surgery in patients with extensive neurological deficits, and it was inferred that the mechanism for haemorrhagic transformation in these patients is similar to that proposed by Fisher and Adams.[64] However, most of these studies were from the pre-CT era

where patients underwent reperfusion regardless of the possibility that they had presented with a cerebral haemorrhage. Most of the later studies of emergency carotid surgery for stroke use CT in the selection criteria to exclude haemorrhage and find surgery advantageous.[70]

Future directions in cerebral reperfusion

- Strategies to reduce the time delay between stroke and treatment
- Strategies to avoid the complications of reperfusion

The extent of injury following cerebral reperfusion clearly relates to the duration and severity of the initial ischaemic insult, such that the sooner reperfusion is established the less severe the injury. The twofold rationale for early reperfusion of brain following stroke is therefore clear: first, blood flow must be promptly restored in order to salvage viable penumbral brain tissue, and second, the extent of reperfusion injury avoided or reduced.

LOGISTICAL PROBLEMS

All of the above evidence suggests that the traditional, dogmatic stance against the treatment of acute stroke is no longer tenable. There is a wealth of evidence both from animal and human studies to indicate that timely reperfusion of the brain is possible and may bring reductions in morbidity and mortality from this disease. However, cerebral reperfusion carries significant risks and approaches to reperfusion have been hampered by difficulties in delivering the care, the complications of which can be catastrophic. From the onset of stroke, cerebral tissue is dying and as time progresses the risks associated with reperfusion appear to increase. Safe and effective cerebral reperfusion requires detailed consideration of the following important stages: recognition of the stroke by the patient, rapid transfer to hospital, investigation and treatment.

Many studies have investigated the pre-hospital delay of patients presenting with stroke. Clearly, patients living alone and unable to make contact to seek help are in a grim position. Suffering a stroke in the presence of people with a knowledge of stroke decreases the time delay from stroke to hospital[71,72] whereas the involvement of primary care has been associated with increased delays in arrival at hospital.[73–75] Education appears to be the key issue here and efforts to increase stroke awareness have reduced stroke-to-hospital times in some American centres.[74]

The mode of transport to hospital is important. In the UK, unpublished audits from Bristol and Manchester showed that the transport used by stroke patients attending hospital ranged from emergency ambulance transfer to the local bus service! Emergency ambulance 'blue light' transfer in the UK takes less than 8 minutes in 75 per cent of patients. If all patients attended via such a service the delay may be minimised but there are other potential 'spin-offs'. A recent study has demonstrated that ambulance paramedics have a high diagnostic accuracy for strokes.[75] Paramedics are in an ideal position to forewarn hospital staff of the imminent arrival of patients who may benefit from early stroke treatment.

A major delay in the management of stroke patients is in the availability of appropriate investigations. Over the last 20 years CT scanning has become commonplace in the management of stroke. However, outside the setting of clinical trials in which strict protocols are observed, there is great variability of access to scanning for stroke patients. This is, in part, due to the differences in opinion about the usefulness the timing of the scans. An early CT scan, i.e. within 24 hours, is of value in excluding haemorrhagic stroke, but it can also identify thrombus in the middle cerebral artery. The extent of infarction, however, is not clear at this stage and later scans are required to define the boundaries of infarction, seen as hypodense areas on CT. Other reasons for delay in CT scanning are a simple lack of resources and, importantly, a pessimistic attitude as to the value of the investigation.

More sophisticated scanning modalities such as MRI and PET are more sensitive in detecting early ischaemic changes but are even less available than CT scanning. Assuming that patients have reached hospital rapidly and have been imaged immediately, they then require access to treatment. Again, outside the context of major trials this is a problem: emergency carotid endarterectomy or thrombo-endarterectomy is possible, as is thrombolysis, but both involve the use of intensive care or high dependency facilities which, in many countries, are scarce. Furthermore, the entire population of the UK is not currently served by vascular specialists willing to undertake such complex cases. These problems should be set against the broader picture of stroke care: an increase in stroke-free or independent stroke survivors has clear long term benefits for both society and the individual.

Conclusions

Acute ischaemic stroke is common and has wide ranging implications for the individual and society. The benefit of early treatment of selected patients by intravenous thrombolysis has been established and, contrary to the nihilistic surgical attitude in most quarters, surgery may also have a role to play. This is a developing area and technical advances will need to be paralleled by improvements in the treatment of stroke patients at all levels from primary to tertiary care.

Key references

Bamford J, Sandercock P, Dennis M, *et al.* A prospective study of acute cerebrovascular disease in the community: Oxfordshire Community Stroke Project 1981–86. 1. Methodology, demography and incident cases of first-ever stroke. *J Neurol Neurosurg Psychiatry* 1988; **51**: 1373–80.

Bamford J, Sandercock P, Dennis M, *et al.* Classification and natural history of clinically identifiable subtypes of cerebral infarction. *Lancet* 1991; **337**: 1521–6.

Dirnagl U, Iadecola C, Moskowitz M. Pathobiology of ischaemic stroke: an integrated view. *Trends Neurosci* 1999; **22**: 391–7.

Okada Y, Yamaguchi T, Minematsu K, *et al.* Haemorrhagic transformation in cerebral embolism. *Stroke* 1989; **20**: 598–603.

Wise R, Bernadi S, Frackowiak R, *et al.* Serial observations on the pathophysiology of acute stroke. The transition form ischaemia to infarction as reflected in regional oxygen extraction. *Brain* 1983; **106**: 197–222.

REFERENCES

1   Warlow C, Dennis M, van Gijn J, *et al. Stroke: A Practical Guide to Management.* Oxford: Blackwell Scientific, 1996.

2   Bamford J, Sandercock P, Dennis M, *et al.* A prospective study of acute cerebrovascular disease in the community: Oxfordshire Community Stroke Project 1981–86. 1. Methodology, demography and incident cases of first-ever stroke. *J Neurol Neurosurg Psychiatry* 1988; **51**: 1373–80.

3   Wolfe C. The impact of stroke. *Br Med Bull* 2000; **56**: 275–86.

4   Bergman L, van der Meulin J, Limburg M, Halbema T. Cost of medical care after first ever stroke in the Netherlands. *Stroke* 1995; **26**: 1830–6.

5   Becker R. Incidence of stroke may be on the rise. *Stroke* 1997; **28**: 1657–9.

6   Chant H, McCollum C. Stroke in young adults: The role of paradoxical embolism. *Thromb Haemost* 2001; **85**: 23–9.

7   Sherman D, Lalonde D. Anticoagulants in stroke treatment. In: Welch KMA, Kaplan LR, Reis DJ, *et al.* (eds) *Primer on Cerebrovascular Diseases.* London: Academic Press,1997.

8   Mead G, Shingler H, Farrell A, *et al.* Carotid disease in acute stroke. *Age Ageing* 1998; **27**: 677–82.

9   European Carotid Surgery Trialists' Collaborative Group. Randomised trial of endarterectomy for recently symptomatic carotid stenosis: final results of the MRC European Carotid Surgery Trial (ECST). *Lancet* 1991; **351**: 1379–87.

10 Bamford J, Sandercock P, Dennis M, *et al.* Classification and natural history of clinically identifiable subtypes of cerebral infarction. *Lancet* 1991; **337**: 1521–6.

11 Williams G, Jiang J, Matchar D, Samsa G. Incidence and recurrence of total (first-ever and recurrent) stroke. *Stroke* 1999; **30**: 2523–8.

12 Isard P, Forbes J. The cost of stroke to the National Health Service in Scotland. *Cerebrovasc Dis* 1992; **2**: 47–50.

13 Grieve R, Hutton J, Bhalla A, *et al.* on behalf of the Biomed II European study of stroke care. A comparison of the costs and survival of hospital-admitted stroke patients across Europe. *Stroke* 2001; **32**: 1684–91.

14 Taylor T, Davis P, Torner J, *et al.* Lifetime cost of stroke in the United States. *Stroke* 1996; **27**: 1459–66.

15 Warlow C. Epidemiology of stroke. *Lancet* 1998; **352** (suppl III): 1–4.

16 Wade DT. Stroke (acute cerebrovascular disease). In: Stevens A, Raftery J. (eds) *Health Care Needs Assessment Vol 1.* Oxford: Radcliffe Medical Press, 1994.

17 Burn J, Dennis M, Bamford J, *et al.* Long term risk of recurrent stroke. The Oxfordshire community stroke project. *Stroke* 1994; **25**: 333–7.

18 Dosick S, Whalen R, Gale S, Brown O. Carotid endarterectomy in the stroke patient. Computerised axial tomography to determine timing. *J Vasc Surg* 1985; **2**: 214–19.

19 Piotrowski J, Bernhard V, Rubin J, *et al.* The timing of carotid endarterectomy after stroke. *J Vasc Surg* 1990; **11**: 45–52.

20 Blaser T, Hofmann K, Buerger T, *et al.* Risk of stroke, transient ischaemic attack, and vessel occlusion before carotid endarterectomy in patients with symptomatic severe carotid stenosis. *Stroke* 2002; **33**: 1057–62.

21 Welsh S, Mead G, Chant H, *et al.* Early carotid surgery in acute stroke: a multicentre randomised pilot study. *Cerebrovasc Dis* 2004; **18**: 200–5.

22 Margolis M, Newton T. Collateral pathways between the cavernous portion of the internal carotid artery and external carotid arteries. *Radiology* 1969; **93**: 834–6.

23 Norris J, Krajewski A, Bornstein N. The clinical role of the cerebral collateral circulation in carotid occlusion. *J Vasc Surg* 1990; **12**: 113–18.

24 Castaigne P, Lhermitte F, Gautier J-C, *et al.* Internal carotid artery occlusion. A study of 61 instances in 50 patients with post mortem data. *Brain* 1970; **93**: 231–58.

25 Blaisdell F, Hall A, Thomas A. Surgical treatment of chronic internal carotid artery occlusion by saline endarterectomy. *Ann Surg* 1966; **163**: 103–11.

26 Freidman S. Current management of the patient with internal carotid artery occlusion. *Eur J Vasc Surg* 1989; **3**: 97–101.

27 Dirnagl U, Iadecola C, Moskowitz M. Pathobiology of ischaemic stroke: an integrated view. *Trends Neurosci* 1999; **22**: 391–7.

28 Leist M, Nictera P. Cell death: Apoptosis versus necrosis. In: Welch K, Kaplan L, Reis D, *et al.* (eds) *Primer on Cerebrovascular Diseases.* London: Academic Press, 1997: 101–4.

29 Graham D. Hypoxia and vascular disorders. In: Adams J, Duchen L (eds) *Greenfield's Neuropathology.* Oxford: Oxford University Press, 1992.

30 Kaplan B, Brint S, Tanabe J, *et al.* Temporal thresholds for neocortical infarction in rats subjected to reversible focal cerebral ischaemia. *Stroke* 1991; **22**: 1032–9.

31 Jones T, Morawetz R, Crowell R, *et al.* Thresholds of focal cerebral ischaemia in awake monkeys. *J Neurosurg* 1981; **54**: 773–82.

32 Hill M, Hachinski V. Stroke treatment. Time is brain. *Lancet* 1998; **352**(suppl III): 10–14.

33 Pulsinelli W. Pathophysiology of acute ischaemic stroke. *Lancet* 1992; **339**: 533–6.

34 Heiss W, Hayakawa T, Waltz A. Cortical neuronal function during ischaemia. Effects of occlusion of one middle cerebral artery on single unit activity in cats. *Arch Neurol* 1976; **33**: 813–20.

35 Heiss W, Rosner G. Functional recovery of cortical neurones as related to the degree and duration of ischaemia. *Ann Neurol* 1983; **14**: 294–301.

36 Branston N, Symon L, Crockard H, Pasztor E. Relationship between the cortical evoked potential and local cortical blood flow following acute middle cerebral artery occlusion in the baboon. *Exp Neurol* 1974; **45**: 195–208.

37 Symon L, Branston N, Strong A, Hope T. The concepts of thresholds of ischaemia in relation to brain structure and function. *J Clin Pathol* 1977; (suppl: Roy Coll Pathol)**11**: 149–54.

38 Sharbrough F, Messick J Jr, Sundt T Jr. Correlation of continuous electroencephalograms with cerebral blood flow measurements during carotid endarterectomy. *Stroke* 1973; **4**: 674–83.

39 Sundt T Jr, Sharbrough P, Anderson R, Michenfelder J. Cerebral blood flow measurements and electroencephalograms during carotid endarterectomy. *J Neurosurg* 1974; **41**: 310–20.

40 Astrup J, Symon L, Branston N, Lassen N. Cortical evoked potentials and extracellular K^+ and H^+ at critical levels of brain ischaemia. *Stroke* 1977; **8**: 51–7.

41 Branston N, Strong A, Symon L. Extracellular potassium activity evoked potential and tissue blood flow: relationship during progressive ischaemia in baboon cerebral cortex. *J Neurol Sci* 1977; **32**: 305–21.

42 Harris R, Symon L, Branston N, Bayhan M. Changes in extracellular calcium activity in cerebral ischaemia. *J Cereb Blood Flow Metab* 1981; **1**: 203–9.

43 Siesjo B. Pathophysiology and treatment of focal cerebral ischaemia. Part 1. Pathophysiology. *J Neurosurg* 1992; **77**: 169–84.

44 Astrup J. Thresholds in cerebral ischaemia – the ischaemic penumbra. *Stroke* 1981; **12**: 723–5.

45 Kristian T, Gido G, Kuroda S, *et al.* Calcium metabolism of focal and penumbral tissues in rats subjected to transient middle cerebral artery occlusion. *Exp Brain Res* 1998; **120**: 503–9.

46 Heiss W, Graf R, Weinhard K, *et al.* Dynamic penumbra demonstrated by sequential multitracer pet after middle cerebral artery occlusion in cats. *J Cereb Blood Flow Metab* 1994; **14**: 892–902.

47 Kohno K, Hoehn-Berlage M, Mies G, *et al.* Relationship between diffusion-weighted MR images, cerebral blood flow, and energy state in experimental brain infarction. *Mag Res Imag* 1995; **13**: 73–80.

48 Olsen T, Larsen B, Herning M, *et al.* Blood flow and vascular reactivity in collaterally perfused brain tissue: evidence of an ischaemic penumbra in patients with acute stroke. *Stroke* 1983; **14**: 332–41.

49 Wise R, Bernadi S, Frackowiak R, *et al.* Serial observations on the pathophysiology of acute stroke. The transition form ischaemia to infarction as reflected in regional oxygen extraction. *Brain* 1983; **106**: 197–222.

50 Marchal G, Beaudouin V, Rioux P, *et al.* Prolonged persistence of substantial volumes of potentially viable brain tissue after stroke. *Stroke* 1996; **27**: 599–606.

51 Baron J. Pathophysiology of acute cerebral ischemia: PET studies in humans. *Cerebrovasc Dis* 1991; **1**(suppl 1): 22–31.

52 Warach S, Chien D, Li W, *et al.* Fast magnetic resonance diffusion-weighted imaging of acute human stroke. *Neurology* 1992; **42**: 171–3.

53 Fisher M, Garcia J. Evolving stroke and the ischaemic penumbra. *Neurology* 1996; **47**: 884–8.

54 Saunders D, Howe F, van den Boogaart A, *et al.* Continuing ischaemic damage after acute middle cerebral artery infarction in humans demonstrated by short-echo proton spectroscopy. *Stroke* 1995; **26**: 1007–13.

55   Obrenovitch T, Urenjak J, Richards D, *et al.* Extracellular neuroactive amino acids in the rat brain striatum during moderate and severe transient ischaemia. *J Neurochem* 1993; **61**: 178–86.

56   Hallenbeck J, Dutka A. Background review and current concepts of reperfusion injury. *Arch Neurol* 1990; **47**: 1245–54.

57   Baethmann A, Staub F. Cellular oedema. In: Welch K, Kaplan L, Reis D, *et al.* (eds) *Primer on Cerebrovascular Diseases.* London: Academic Press, 1997: 153–6.

58   Betz L. Vasogenic oedema. In: Welch K, Kaplan L, Reis D, *et al.* (eds) *Primer on Cerebrovascular Diseases.* London: Academic Press, 1997: 156–9.

59   Lyden P, Zivin J. Hemorrhagic transformation after cerebral ischemia: Mechanisms and incidence. *Cerebrovasc Brain Metab Rev* 1993; **5**: 1–16.

60   Teal P, Pessin M. Haemorrhagic transformation. The spectrum of ischaemia-related brain haemorrhage. *Neurosurg Clin North Am* 1992; **3**: 601–10.

61   Bogousslavsky J, Regli F, Uske A, Maeder P. Early spontaneous haematoma in cerebral infarct: is primary cerebral haemorrhage overdiagnosed? *Neurology* 1991; **41**: 837–40.

62   Okada Y, Yamaguchi T, Minematsu K, *et al.* Haemorrhagic transformation in cerebral embolism. *Stroke* 1989; **20**: 598–603.

63   Hornig C, Dorndorf W, Agnoli A. Haemorrhagic cerebral infarction – a prospective study. *Stroke* 1986; **17**: 179–85.

64   Fisher C, Adams R. Observations on brain embolism with special reference to the mechanism of haemorrhagic infarction. *J Neuropathol Exp Neurol* 1951; **10**: 92–4.

65   Lodder J, Krijne-Kubat B, Broekman J. Cerebral haemorrhagic infarction at autopsy: cardiac embolic cause and the relationship to the cause of death. *Stroke* 1986; **17**: 626–9.

66   Bowes M, Zivin J, Thomas G, *et al.* Acute hypertension, but not thrombolysis, increases the incidence and severity of hemorrhagic transformation following experimental stroke in rabbits. *Exp Neurol* 1996; **141**: 40–6.

67   Saku Y, Choki J, Waki R, *et al.* Hemorrhagic infarct induced by arterial hypertension in cat brain following middle cerebral artery occlusion. *Stroke* 1989; **21**: 589–95.

68   del Zoppo G, Copeland B, Anderchek K, *et al.* Hemorrhagic transformation following tissue plasminogen activator in experimental cerebral infarction. *Stroke* 1990; **21**: 596–601.

69   Wardlaw J, del Zoppo G, Yamaguchi T. Thrombolysis for acute ischaemic stroke. In: *Cochrane Library*, Issue 1, 2002.

70   Mead G, O'Neill P, McCollum C. Is there a role for carotid surgery in acute stroke? *Eur J Vasc Endovasc Surg* 1997; **13**: 112–21.

71   Feldmann E, Gordon N, Brooks J, *et al.* Factors associated with early presentation of acute stroke. *Stroke* 1993; **24**: 1805–10.

72   Rosamond W, Gorton R, Hinn A, *et al.* Rapid response to stroke symptoms: the delay in accessing stroke healthcare (DASH) study. *Acad Emerg Med* 1998; **5**: 45–51.

73   Ferro J, Melo T, Oliveira V, *et al.* An analysis of the admission delay of acute strokes. *Cerebrovasc Dis* 1994; **4**: 72–5.

74   Barsan W, Brott T, Broderick J, *et al.* Urgent therapy for acute stroke. Effects of a stroke trial on untreated patients. *Stroke* 1994; **25**: 2132–7.

75   Harbison J, Massey A, Barnett L, *et al.* Rapid ambulance protocol for acute stroke. *Lancet* 1999; **353**: 1935.

6

Assessing the Risk in Vascular Emergencies

PETER R TAYLOR, DAVID J GERRARD

THE PROBLEM

Successful surgical intervention depends on striking a balance between the potential benefit from the procedure and the possibility of harm. The majority of elective vascular operations are performed to prevent possible adverse events from lesions which may be asymptomatic or may have only caused transient symptoms. Elective abdominal aortic aneurysm surgery is performed to prevent rupture, and the majority of patients will have no symptoms related to their aneurysm. Similarly, internal carotid artery stenoses may have caused amaurosis fugax or transient ischaemic attacks (TIAs) which have no lasting effect on the patient, but may well be the portent of a major stroke. The operations of abdominal aortic aneurysm repair and carotid endarterectomy are both associated with life-threatening complications such as death and stroke, and therefore some assessment has to be undertaken to identify the risk:benefit ratio. Unfortunately, there is a scarcity of good quality publications on this very important subject. The majority of papers which can be used for such an analysis come from randomised clinical trials which almost always involve elective operations. Very few vascular and endovascular non-elective procedures are performed on the basis of level 1 evidence, indeed, such trials may be unethical.

THE CONCEPT OF RISK:BENEFIT RATIO

Randomised clinical trials have a great advantage in that the risk involved in one treatment can be compared with another, or indeed with the natural history of the disease under investigation. Vascular surgery usually lends itself well to clinical trials because of the clearly defined nature of the clinical endpoints such as death, stroke or limb loss. Comparison of the outcome following the experimental event rate and the control event rate allows the absolute risk reduction rate to be calculated. The number of patients 'needed to treat' is defined as the number of patients who would have to be treated over a specific period of time to prevent one bad outcome and this is the inverse of the absolute risk reduction.[1]

The concept has been well demonstrated in the case of surgery for symptomatic carotid stenoses with regard to any disabling stroke, fatal stroke or death from any cause following surgery. The impact of surgery on outcome has been shown by both the European Carotid Surgery Trial (ECST) and the North American Symptomatic Carotid Endarterectomy Trial (NASCET).[2,3] The results have recently been combined in a meta-analysis which showed that for internal carotid artery stenoses causing a diameter reduction of between 70 and 99 per cent there is an absolute risk reduction of 6.7 per cent with a 95 per cent confidence limit of 3.2 to 10 per cent when surgery is compared with best medical therapy.[4] The number needed to treat is therefore 15, with confidence limits between 10 and 31. The concept is easy to understand: 15 patients have to undergo carotid endarterectomy in order to prevent one from having a stroke. The converse is therefore obvious: 14 patients will have no benefit from the procedure. The paper also showed that patients with 50–69 per cent diameter reduction had an absolute risk reduction of 4.7 per cent (confidence limits 0.8 to 8.7) with the number needed to treat being 21 (confidence limits 11 to 125). Finally, those with a stenosis of less than 49 per cent had an absolute risk increase of 2.2 per cent (confidence limits 0 to 4.4) and the number needed to harm was 45 (confidence limits 22 to infinity). This last category showed that surgery was harmful in this group of patients, and gives an example of an intervention which is associated with a worse outcome than those patients treated medically. Such an increase is termed the absolute risk increase, and the number needed to harm is the number of patients, who if they had surgery, would lead to one additional patient being harmed (i.e. the inverse of the absolute risk increase).

There were other factors which were found to be important in assessing the risk:benefit ratio of surgery. In the NASCET study group of patients with 70–99 per cent stenoses, those who were male had an increased benefit as did those over 70 years of age. Other groups who derived more benefit from surgery were those with hemispheric symptoms compared with those who had retinal events, and those with angiographic evidence of plaque ulceration. The ECST data showed that patients with lacunar infarcts, which may not be due to embolism from the internal carotid artery plaque, had a relative risk increase from surgery of 22 per cent (confidence limits 51 to 200 per cent).

This chapter will concentrate on the evidence for assessing risk in the three index operations for arterial surgery: carotid endarterectomy, abdominal aortic aneurysm repair and lower limb arterial reconstruction. In the absence of good evidence an attempt will be made in each case to extrapolate valid conclusions from the elective to the emergency situation.

Index operations

- Carotid endarterectomy
- Abdominal aortic aneurysm repair
- Lower limb arterial reconstruction

CAROTID ENDARTERECTOMY

There are many other factors which influence the reported outcome following carotid endarterectomy[5] and these are elaborated elsewhere (see Chapters 12–14). The following summary gives an indication of the difficulties encountered in an emergency situation. These include the number and specialty of the surgeons, the type of hospital in which the operation takes place and the number of operations performed by both the hospital and the surgeon each year. However, the presenting symptoms and the findings on preoperative computed tomography (CT) scans have also been found to be predictive of outcome.[6]

There is some evidence on the factors involved in poor outcome after carotid endarterectomy undertaken for urgent indications (see Chapter 13). One paper has shown that urgent surgery for crescendo transient ischaemic attacks (TIAs) has a worse outcome compared with elective operation.[7] The comparison of the final outcome, however, can be difficult, as the comparator may be a patient who is not neurologically normal. Operations undertaken for acute strokes have this difficulty. Should the final outcome be the status of the patient before the stroke occurred or that immediately before surgery? As some recovery after stroke is not unusual, should the comparison be made between two groups of patients with stroke, one of which had undergone carotid surgery and the other not? This question clearly muddies the waters in that clearly defined endpoints are not being used.

There is some evidence on the minimum number of operations which should be undertaken either by a hospital or by an individual surgeon each year in order to achieve low morbidity and mortality from carotid endarterectomy. A retrospective study of 9918 carotid operations undertaken in Maryland, USA, over 6 years was reported by Perler et al.[8] In this series hospitals which performed more than 10 but fewer than 50 operations per year had a mortality of 1.1 per cent and a neurological event rate of 1.3 per cent per year. This compared favourably with hospitals performing 50–100 procedures per year with a death rate of 0.8 per cent but a slightly higher neurological event rate of 1.8 per cent. Those hospitals performing fewer than 10 carotid endarterectomies per year had a mortality of 1.9 per cent but a neurological event rate of 6.1 per cent. Another review of 1280 carotid endarterectomies performed by eight hospitals in Toronto looked at the number of cases performed per surgeon each year.[9] If more than 12 operations were performed the death rate was 1.2 per cent, the stroke rate 4.2 per cent and the stroke and death rate 5.4 per cent. The equivalent figures for those surgeons performing between six and 12 operations per year were 4.2 per cent, 3.8 per cent and 8 per cent, respectively. Those surgeons doing fewer than six cases per year had no deaths but a high stroke rate of 18.4 per cent. Figures of 10–50 carotid endarterectomies per year and the individual vascular surgeon responsible for over 12 of these are probably better than most vascular surgeons would have predicted. One further piece of evidence suggests that operations performed by board certified surgeons carry a 15 per cent lower risk of death or complications compared with those undertaken by uncertified surgeons.[10] A review of 45 744 carotid endarterectomies in Florida, USA, also suggests that a doubling of the operative workload reduced the adverse event outcome by 4 per cent.

The technique of carotid endarterectomy is probably important in reducing complications. Most of the data come from elective operations, as there is so little evidence from non-elective procedures. In a large meta-analysis patching was found to be important in reducing ipsilateral stroke, perioperative carotid thrombosis, and ipsilateral stroke and death during follow-up.[11] The evidence for shunting was less strong.[12] The importance of avoiding carotid occlusion is well known to surgeons performing the operation as was shown by Radak et al.[13] reporting a series of 2250 operations: 41 patients had an intraoperative stroke with a mortality of

49 per cent whereas 18 had a postoperative stroke and a mortality of 22 per cent.

Why not, therefore, patch all patients undergoing carotid endarterectomy? First, vein patches can rupture; second, synthetic patches can become infected; third, the operation takes longer; and finally patching may not abolish technical error. Up to 12 per cent of patched vessels have major problems, detectable by duplex scanning, which require revision.[14] The carotid arteries of women seem to be more likely to restenose following primary closure, and therefore may benefit more from patch angioplasty.[15] Duplex has the advantage of revealing both anatomical and functional lesions which may require revision,[16] and is very useful as a teaching tool in making instant feedback available to junior staff.[17] Some authorities rely on other forms of completion imaging such as arteriography or inspection by angioscopy.[18]

The replacement of routine preoperative angiography by duplex scan, the abandonment of the routine preoperative CT brain scan and the use of high dependency nursing rather than intensive care postoperatively and early discharge, within 24 hours, even after general anaesthesia, can all be achieved without compromising patient safety.[19] These then are the complicated issues relating to risk–benefit analysis in the elective situation. Generalisations about these issues in the emergency situation, therefore, are even more difficult. Any understanding of the subject will largely depend on carefully documented series from busy units such as the Cleveland Clinic in which a series of 314 patients had undergone non-elective carotid endarterectomy.[20] Unfortunately the definition of 'non-elective' was wide and included asymptomatic patients (9 per cent). Only 14 per cent had completed strokes and a further 2 per cent developed unstable strokes. The median interval between presentation and surgery was 2 days with 48 per cent of operations being performed within 24 hours. The best results were in the asymptomatic group with a combined stroke and mortality rate of 3.4 per cent; the worst results of 14 per cent were found, predictably, in those patients with unstable strokes. Women were more likely to have ipsilateral strokes in the follow-up period (risk ratio 2.38, 95 per cent confidence limits 1.02 to 5.56). Unfortunately, this study typifies the poor quality of papers on vascular emergencies and the inclusion of asymptomatic patients within a non-elective group is difficult to comprehend.

ABDOMINAL AORTIC ANEURYSM REPAIR

The Small Aneurysm Study performed in the UK, showed that there was no benefit from early surgery for infrarenal abdominal aortic aneurysms (AAAs) measuring between 4 cm and 5.5 cm on ultrasound.[21] This study was conducted on elective patients, and one of the criteria used to remove patients from the surveillance arm was the development of symptoms such as tenderness over the aneurysm and the development of back pain. Unfortunately, there is no good randomised trial of treatment for symptomatic aneurysms and the natural history of such aneurysms is unknown. Traditional teaching suggests that infrarenal AAAs associated with pain should be operated on within 24 hours. Experienced vascular surgeons know that many patients who have tender aneurysms have a contained retroperitoneal haematoma. Others may have oedema present in the surrounding tissues and some turn out to be inflammatory in nature. Current smoking and poor lung function were associated with an increased risk of rupture and a higher mortality following surgery in the Small Aneurysm Study.[21]

The Vascular Surgical Society of Great Britain and Ireland produced a national outcome audit report which attempted to predict outcome based upon the patient's risk factors, the degree of urgency and the vascular procedure.[22] The most important factor in determining outcome was the degree of urgency of the admission, with emergency operations carrying the most risk. The patient's physiology seemed to be of more importance than the factors encountered at surgery. The ability to compare vascular units and individual vascular surgeons is likely to be based upon such analyses. The Portsmouth group devised P-POSSUM (Portsmouth predictor modification of the Physiological and Operative Severity Score for the enUmeration of Mortality and morbidity) for determining outcome following arterial surgery.[23] When this methodology was developed further (V-POSSUM) and applied to the Vascular Surgical Society database it accurately predicted both mortality and morbidity.[24] Further analysis, however, suggests that different models should be used to predict outcome following elective and ruptured AAAs,[25] as there was a failure of prediction of outcome in ruptured AAAs using both the P-POSSUM and the V-POSSUM models.

Other studies have looked at specific aspects of the emergency situation. For example, a prospective study of AAA repair found a high incidence of multiple sequential organ failure and colonic ischaemia in non-elective operations[26] (also see Chapters 3 and 4). A randomised study on the effect of dopexamine on colonic mucosal ischaemia after elective aortic surgery suggests that it may provide significant histological protection to the colonic mucosa.[27] Further studies are required to see if this drug can improve the mortality in non-elective AAA surgery. There is some evidence that the placement of pulmonary artery catheters and the use of goal directed therapy may adversely influence the outcome after non-elective AAA surgery.[28] In another report a consecutive series of patients was admitted to two different hospitals under the care of a single vascular surgeon: one unit used pulmonary artery catheters in 96 per cent of patients and large volumes of fluid to achieve specified targets. The other used catheters in only 18 per cent of cases and achieved a significantly lower mortality and a lower incidence of acute renal failure. There has been, therefore, a move away from goal directed therapy in many intensive care units. A randomised study showed that the use of pulmonary artery catheters with optimisation of the patient's haemodynamic status provided no benefit in terms of outcome in patients undergoing elective vascular surgery.[29]

Various other factors may be important in predicting outcome following ruptured AAA surgery and these include the avoidance of raised intra-abdominal pressure. This increased pressure is associated with oedema of the bowel, retroperitoneum and the abdominal wall and is recognised as the abdominal compartment syndrome[30] (see Chapters 3, 4 and 23). Closing the abdominal wound with a mesh and delayed primary closure of the wound has been found to be associated with a better outcome. The incidence of multiple sequential organ failure is lower, but the definitive trial has not yet been performed. A recent non-randomised study has confirmed that patients who had a mesh-based early abdominal closure had a better outcome than those requiring a second operation for abdominal compartment syndrome following primary closure.[31] This is an important aspect of management which deserves consideration in Chapter 23.

Factors which have been associated with a poor outcome after ruptured AAA repair include soluble tumour necrosis factor (TNF) receptors,[32] a low platelet count at the end of the operation[33] and low endothelin-1 levels[34] (see Chapters 3 and 4). A study of coagulation and fibrinolysis factors showed that rupture is associated with an inhibition of systemic fibrinolysis and the generation of thrombin.[35] This procoagulant state has been postulated to be the cause of myocardial infarction, multiple organ failure and thromboembolism following surgery.

Age has been postulated to be a factor in poor outcome after a ruptured AAA but there is some evidence that good results can be obtained if biological rather than chronological age is used to determine fitness for surgery.[36] The distance travelled by patients remains a controversial subject. Patients surviving the journey to the regional centre performing the surgery are likely to survive the operation, while those who are at higher risk select themselves out by dying *en route*, as was clearly shown in a Northern Ireland series.[37] Distance, therefore probably does not make a huge difference to the outcome.[38]

The role of endovascular repair for elective infrarenal AAA is currently under investigation in the EndoVascular Aneurysm Repair (EVAR) trials being performed in the UK. The use of an aorto-uni-iliac device has been shown to reduce the mortality of rupture significantly, although this view is based on small numbers.[39] Control can be achieved by the use of aortic occlusion balloons or by the deployment of the proximal stent into the neck of the aneurysm. Revascularisation of the contralateral limb is carried out by a femoro-femoral crossover bypass graft. The problems with this technique include the availability and durability of stent grafts and the logistical difficulties of mobilising both radiological and surgical staff.

LOWER LIMB ARTERIAL RECONSTRUCTION

A number of risk factors need to be considered in patients presenting with acute lower limb ischaemia who require urgent reconstruction. The viability of a limb must be established before any attempt is made to revascularise it. The absence of capillary return or the presence of fixed staining of the tissues are features indicative of irreversible ischaemia. Severe neurological damage sustained in an accident also causing ischaemia may be a relative contraindication to vascular surgery. The duration of ischaemia and ischaemia-reperfusion injury (IRI) is crucial to outcome (see Chapter 2). The tolerance of different tissues to ischaemia also determines outcome, for instance, peripheral nerves and muscle have less resistance than skin to ischaemia. Muscle which has been completely ischaemic for 4–6 hours is probably damaged irreparably. The presence of a collateral circulation, however, may help in extending the period of ischaemia.

Local changes may impair restoration of normal flow after the circulation has been restored. This has been called the 'impaired reflow' or 'no-reflow' phenomenon (see Chapter 2). Swollen cells occluding the lumen, capillary spasm and the trapping of red and white cells all contribute to occlusion of the microcirculation. Restoration of the circulation following acute ischaemia leads to the formation of free radicals and other metabolites which then pass into the systemic circulation where they can damage normal tissues by the activation of neutrophils.[40] These neutrophils interact with the endothelium and cause damage to distant organs, such as the lungs and kidneys through the release of free radicals and proteases. Cytokines, including TNF and interleukins (ILs) such as IL-1, IL-6 and IL-8, are thought to be implicated in the development of multiple organ failure in vascular patients (see Chapter 4). Therapeutic measures to counteract these changes include the administration of free radical scavengers such as mannitol and allopurinol[41,42] (see Chapters 2, 4 and 33).

Unfortunately, many compounds effective either in theory or in the experimental situation do not translate into the clinical scenario. Monoclonal antibodies against IL-1 were shown to be ineffective in a randomised controlled trial despite initial enthusiasm.[43] Experimental studies which may help in managing the clinical situation in future include the use of technetium-99m-glucarate to identify muscle damage,[44] prostaglandins and iloprost to enhance muscle blood flow,[45] and the technique of thermal preconditioning does seem encouraging.[46] There is some human evidence supporting the use of ischaemic preconditioning in the prevention of IRI.[47] There is currently much interest in the use of recombinant human activated protein C for severe sepsis.[48] In a randomised, double blind, placebo controlled multicentre trial, patients with systemic inflammation and organ failure secondary to sepsis had a significantly lower mortality when treated with drotrecogin alfa (activated) (activated protein C) with an absolute risk reduction of 6.1 per cent.

The use of thrombolysis is contraindicated in the patient with multiple injuries, but may be useful in the acutely ischaemic limb, especially if it is secondary to graft thrombosis, but the risk:benefit equation must take into account the serious complications associated with thrombolysis. These include a 3–5 per cent risk of death, a 2 per cent risk of stroke and an incidence ranging from 5 to 12.5 per cent of major haemorrhage.[49–52] The use of thrombolysis for claudication is contraindicated because of an adverse risk:benefit ratio. The incidence of major amputation of 7 per cent, deaths 14 per cent and major haemorrhage 5 per cent in a reported series is much worse than the natural history of claudication.[53] Age is also associated with a poor outcome for patients with acute limb ischaemia treated with thrombolysis.[54]

There is evidence that techniques which re-establish blood flow to ischaemic tissues are beneficial and this is clearly important in acute limb ischaemia caused by trauma. Plastic shunts placed in both arteries and veins in order to arrest tissue hypoxia have been shown to be effective in the Northern Ireland experience[55] (see Chapter 33). Experimental studies at that centre have confirmed the importance of restoring venous outflow when both artery and vein are damaged.[56]

Acute limb ischaemia occurring in a young patient without an obvious cause should arouse concern. Hypercoaguable states may well be responsible, and any attempt at reconstruction may result in amputation. Deficiencies of protein C, protein S, activated protein C or antithrombin III are all responsible for the hypercoaguable state.[57] The presence of antiphospholipid antibodies and the prothrombin gene variant (20210 G to A) are also causes of arterial thrombosis. Hyperhomocysteinaemia has also been associated with poor outcome in arterial reconstruction.[58–60] The risk:benefit ratio can be altered in favour of a successful outcome if conditions such as these are diagnosed and treated before arterial intervention is undertaken.

Conclusions

All interventions carry a risk, particularly those involving the arterial circulation in the emergency setting. Surgeons must be aware of the risk:benefit ratio involved in treating patients with vascular emergencies. The clinical picture is often complex and the outcome is dependent upon many factors, some of which may be within the control of the surgeon. Inevitably, others will have been established well before the surgeon is involved, and will remain outside the therapeutic sphere. Surgeons who deal with such emergencies need to be up to date with the latest literature to optimise patient care. The evidence for the efficacy of various interventions is slowly being accrued but there is much scope for further trials to produce convincing evidence in the treatment of vascular emergencies.

Key references

Bernard GR, Vincent JL, Laterre PF, et al. Efficacy and safety of recombinant human activated protein C for severe sepsis. N Engl J Med 2001; **3444**: 699–709.

Counsell C, Salinas R, Warlow C, Naylor R. Patch angioplasty versus primary closure for carotid endarterectomy. Cochrane Database Syst Rev 2000; **2**: CD000160.

European Carotid Surgery Trialists' Collaborative Group. MRC European Carotid Surgery Trial: interim results for symptomatic patients with severe (70–99%) or with mild (0–29%) carotid stenosis. Lancet 1991; **337**: 1235–43.

North American Symptomatic Carotid Endarterectomy Trial Collaborators. Beneficial effect of carotid endarterectomy in symptomatic patients with high-grade carotid stenosis. N Engl J Med 1991; **325**: 445–53.

The UK Small Aneurysm Participants. Mortality results for randomised controlled trial of elective surgery or ultrasonographic surveillance for small abdominal aortic aneurysms. Lancet 1998; **352**: 1649–55.

REFERENCES

1 Legemate DA, Tijssen JG. Definitions and analysis of complications in relation to the benefits of treatment. In: Branchereau A, Jacobs M (eds). Complications in Vascular and Endovascular Surgery, Part 1. New York: Futura Publishing Company, 2001: 1–5.

2 European Carotid Surgery Trialists' Collaborative Group. MRC European Carotid Surgery Trial: interim results for symptomatic patients with severe (70–99%) or with mild (0–29%) carotid stenosis. Lancet 1991; **337**: 1235–43.

3 North American Symptomatic Carotid Endarterectomy Trial Collaborators. Beneficial effect of carotid endarterectomy in symptomatic patients with high-grade carotid stenosis. N Engl J Med 1991; **325**: 445–53.

4 Cina CS, Clase CM, Haynes BR. Refining the indications for carotid endarterectomy in patients with symptomatic carotid artery stenosis: a systematic review. J Vasc Surg 1999; **30**: 606–17.

5 McGuinness CL, Taylor PR. Difficulties interpreting the reported results of carotid endarterectomy: the importance of prospective independent audit. Int J Clin Pract 2000; **54**: 484–485.

6 Blohme L, Sandstrom V, Hellstrom G, et al. Complications in carotid endarterectomy are predicted by qualifying symptoms and preoperative CT findings. Eur J Vasc Endovasc Surg 1999; **17**: 213–18.

7 Gollege J, Cuming R, Beattie DK, et al. Influence of patient variables on the outcome of carotid endarterectomy. J Vasc Surg 1996; **24**: 120–6.

8 Perler BA, Dardik A, Burleyson GP, et al. Influence of age and hospital volume on the results of carotid endarterectomy: a statewide analysis of 9918 cases. J Vasc Surg 1998; **27**: 25–31.

9 Kucey DS, Bowyer B, Iron K, et al. Determinants of outcome after carotid endarterectomy. J Vasc Surg 1998; **28**: 1051–8.

10 Pearce WH, Parker MA, Feinglass J, et al. The importance of surgeon volume and training in outcomes for vascular surgical procedures. J Vasc Surg 1999; **29**: 768–76.

11 Counsell C, Salinas R, Warlow C, Naylor R. Patch angioplasty versus primary closure for carotid endarterectomy. *Cochrane Database Syst Rev* 2000; **2**: CD000160.

12 Counsell C, Warlow C, Naylor R. Patches of different types for carotid patch angioplasty. *Cochrane Database Syst Rev* 2000; **2**: CD000071.

13 Radak D, Popovic AD, Radicevic S, *et al.* Immediate reoperation for perioperative stroke after 2250 carotid endarterectomies: differences between intraoperative and early postoperative stroke. *J Vasc Surg* 1999; **30**: 245–51.

14 Seelig MH, Oldenburg WA, Chowla A, Atkinson EJ. Use of intraoperative duplex ultrasonography and routing patch angioplasty in patients undergoing carotid endarterectomy. *Mayo Clinic Proc* 1999; **74**: 870–6.

15 Anderson A, Padayachee TS, Sandison AJP, *et al.* The results of routine primary closure in carotid endarterectomy. *Cardiovasc Surg* 1999; **7**: 50–5.

16 Padayachee TS, Brooks MD, Modaresi KB, *et al.* Intraoperative high resolution duplex imaging during carotid endarterectomy: which abnormalities require surgical correction? *Eur J Vasc Surg Endovasc Surg* 1998; **15**: 387–93.

17 Padayachee TS, Brooks MD, McGuinness CL, *et al.* Value of intraoperative duplex imaging during supervised carotid endarterectomy. *Br J Surg* 2001; **88**: 389–92.

18 Naylor AR, Hayes PD, Allroggen H, *et al.* Reducing the risk of carotid surgery: a 7-year audit of the role of monitoring and quality control assessment. *J Vasc Surg* 2000; **32**: 750–9.

19 Sandison AJP, Wood CH, Padayachee TS, *et al.* Cost effective carotid endarterectomy. *Br J Surg* 2000; **87**: 323–7.

20 Tretter JF, Hertzer NR, Mascha EJ, *et al.* Perioperative risk and late outcome of nonelective carotid endarterectomy. *J Vasc Surg* 1999; **30**: 618–31.

21 The UK Small Aneurysm Participants. Mortality results for randomised controlled trial of elective surgery or ultrasonographic surveillance for small abdominal aortic aneurysms. *Lancet* 1998; **352**: 1649–55.

22 Earnshaw JJ, Ridler BMF, Kinsman R on behalf of the Audit Committee of the Vascular Surgical Society of Great Britain and Ireland. *National Outcome Audit Report.* London: Vascular Surgical Society of Great Britain and Ireland, May 2000.

23 Prytherch DR, Whiteley MS, Higgins B, *et al.* POSSUM and Portsmouth POSSUM for predicting mortality. *Br J Surg* 1998; **85**: 1217–20.

24 Prytherch DR, Beard JD, Ridler BF, Earnshaw JJ. Vascular Surgical Society operative outcome study: preoperative physiology predicts outcome. *Br J Surg* 2000; **87**: 507–8.

25 Prytherch DR, Sutton GL, Boyle JR. Portsmouth POSSUM models for abdominal aortic aneurysm surgery. *Br J Surg* 2001; **88**: 958–63.

26 Sandison AJP, Panayiotopoulos YP, Edmondson RC, *et al.* A four year prospective audit of the cause of death after infrarenal aortic aneurysm surgery. *Br J Surg* 1996; **83**: 1386–9.

27 Baguneid MS, Welch M, Bukhari M, *et al.* A randomized study to evaluate the effect of a perioperative infusion of dopexamine on colonic mucosal ischemia after aortic surgery. *J Vasc Surg* 2001; **33**: 758–63.

28 Sandison AJP, Wyncoll DLA, Edmondson RC, *et al.* ICU protocol may affect the outcome of non-elective abdominal aortic aneurysm repair. *Eur J Vasc Surg Endovasc Surg* 1998; **16**: 356–61.

29 Bender JS, Smith-Meek MA, Jones CE. Routine pulmonary artery catheterization does not reduce morbidity and mortality after elective vascular surgery: results of a prospective randomised trial. *Ann Surg* 1997; **226**: 229–36.

30 Oelschlager BK, Boyle EM Jr, Johansen K, Meissner MH. Delayed abdominal closure in the management of ruptured abdominal aortic aneurysms. *Am J Surg* 1997; **173**: 411–15.

31 Rasmussen TE, Hallett JW, Noel AA, *et al.* Early abdominal closure with mesh reduces multiple organ failure after ruptured abdominal aortic aneurysm repair: guidelines from a 10-year case-controlled study. Society for Vascular Surgery Abstract Booklet 2001: 86.

32 Adam DJ, Lee AJ, Ruckley CV, *et al.* Elevated levels of soluble tumor necrosis factor receptors are associated with increased mortality rates in patients who undergo operation for ruptured abdominal aortic aneurysm. *J Vasc Surg* 2000; **31**: 514–19.

33 Bradbury AW, Bachoo P, Milne AA, Duncan JL. Platelet count and the outcome of operation for ruptured abdominal aortic aneurysm. *J Vasc Surg* 1995; **21**: 484–91.

34 Adam DJ, Evans SM, Webb DJ, Bradbury AW. Plasma endothelin levels and outcome in patients undergoing repair of ruptured infrarenal abdominal aortic aneurysm. *J Vasc Surg* 2001; **33**: 1242–6.

35 Adam DJ, Ludlam CA, Ruckley CV, Bradbury AW. Coagulation and fibrinolysis in patients undergoing operation for ruptured and nonruptured infrarenal abdominal aortic aneurysms. *J Vasc Surg* 1999; **30**: 641–50.

36 Robson AK, Currie IC, Poskitt KR, *et al.* Abdominal aortic aneurysm repair in the over eighties. *Br J Surg* 1989; **76**: 1018–20.

37 Barros D'Sa AAB. Optimal travel distance before ruptured aortic aneurysm repair. In: Greenhalgh RM, Mannick JA (eds). *The Cause and Management of Aneurysms.* London: WB Saunders 1990; 409–31.

38 Adam DJ, Mohan IV, Stuart WP, *et al.* Community and hospital outcome from ruptured abdominal aortic aneurysm within the catchment area of a regional vascular service. *J Vasc Surg* 1999; **30**: 922–8.

39 Ohki T, Veith FJ. Endovascular grafts and other image-guided catheter-based adjuncts to improve the treatment of ruptured aortoiliac aneurysms. *Ann Surg* 2000; **232**: 466–79.

40 Pararajasingam R, Nicholson ML, Bell PRF, Sayers RD. Non-cardiogenic pulmonary oedema in vascular surgery. *Eur J Vasc Endovasc Surg* 1999; **17**: 93–105.

41 Nicholson ML, Baker DM, Hopkinson BR, Wenham PW. Randomised controlled trial of the effects of mannitol on renal reperfusion injury during aortic aneurysm surgery. *Br J Surg* 1996; **83**: 1230–3.

42 Soong CV, Young IS, Lightbody JH, *et al.* Reduction of free radical generation minimises lower limb swelling following femoropopliteal bypass surgery. *Eur J Vasc Surg* 1994; **8**: 435–40.

43 Opal SM, Fisher CJ Jr, Dhainaut JF, *et al.* Confirmatory interleukin-1 receptor antagonist trial in severe sepsis: a phase III, randomised, double-blind, placebo-controlled, multicenter trial. The Interleukin-1 Receptor Antagonist Sepsis Investigator Group. *Crit Care Med* 1997; **25**: 1115–24.

44 Wiersema AM, Oyen WJG, Verhofstad AAJ, *et al.* Early assessment of skeletal muscle damage after ischaemia-reperfusion using Tc-99m-glucarate. *Cardiovasc Surg* 2000; **8**: 186–91.

45 Rowlands TE, Gough MJ, Homer-Vanniasinkam S. Do prostaglandins have a salutary role in skeletal muscle ischaemia-reperfusion injury? *Eur J Vasc Endovasc Surg* 1999; **18**: 439–44.

46 McLaughlin R, Kelly CJ, Kay E, Bouchier-Hayes D. Diaphragmatic dysfunction secondary to experimental lower torso ischaemia-reperfusion injury is attenuated by thermal preconditioning. *Br J Surg* 2000; **87**: 201–5.

47 Kharbanda RK, Peters M, Walton B, Kattenhorn M, *et al.* Ischemic preconditioning prevents endothelial injury and systemic activation during ischemia-reperfusion in humans *in vivo*. *Circulation* 2001; **103**: 1624–30.

48 Bernard GR, Vincent JL, Laterre PF, *et al.* Efficacy and safety of recombinant human activated protein C for severe sepsis. *N Engl J Med* 2001; **3444**: 699–709.

49 Ouriel K, Veith FJ, Sasahara AA for the Thrombolysis or Peripheral Arterial Surgery (TOPAS) Investigators. A comparison of recombinant urokinase with vascular surgery as initial treatment for acute arterial occlusion of the legs. *N Engl J Med* 1998; **338**: 1105–11.

50 Weaver FA, Comerota AJ, Youngblood M, *et al.* and the STILE Investigators. Surgical revascularization versus thrombolysis for nonembolic lower extremity native artery occlusions: results of a prospective randomized trial. *J Vasc Surg* 1996: **24**: 513–23.

51 Berridge DC, Makin GS, Hopkinson BR. Local low dose intra-arterial thrombolytic therapy: the risk of stroke or major haemorrhage. *Br J Surg* 1989; **76**: 1230–3.

52 Comerota AJ, Weaver FA, Hosking JD *et al.* Results of a prospective, randomised trial of surgery versus thrombolysis for occluded lower extremity bypass grafts. *Am J Surg* 1996; **172**: 105–12.

53 Braithwaite BD, Tomlinson MA, Walker SR, *et al.* Peripheral thrombolysis for acute-onset claudication. Thombolysis Study Group. *Br J Surg* 1999; **86**: 800–4.

54 Braithwaite BD, Davies B, Birch PA, *et al.* Management of acute leg ischaemia in the elderly. *Br J Surg* 1998; **85**: 217–20.

55 Barros D'Sa AAB. Shunting in complex lower limb vascular trauma. In: Greenhalgh RM, Hollier LH (eds). *Emergency Vascular Surgery.* London: WB Saunders, 1992; 331–44.

56 Harkin DW, Barros D'Sa AAB, Yassin MMI, *et al.* Reperfusion injury is greater with delayed restoration of venous outflow in concurrent arterial and venous limb injury. *Br J Surg* 2000; **87**: 734–41.

57 Bontempo FA, Kibbe MR, Makaroun MS. Hypercoaguable states and unexplained vascular thrombosis. In: Branchereau A, Jacobs M (eds). *Complications in Vascular Surgery and Endovascular Surgery, Part I.* New York: Futura Publishing Company, 2001; 13–22.

58 Neilsen TG, Nordestgaard BG, von Jessen F, *et al.* Antibodies to cardiolipin may increase the risk of failure of peripheral vein bypasses. *Eur J Vasc Endovasc Surg* 1997; **14**: 177–84.

59 Doggen CJ, Cats VM, Bertina RM, Rosendaal FR. Interaction of coagulation defects and cardiovascular risk factors: increased risk of myocardial infarction associated with factor V Leiden or prothrombin 20210 A. *Circulation* 1998; **97**: 1037–41.

60 Taylor LM Jr, Moneta GL, Sexton GJ, *et al.* Prospective blinded study of the relationship between plasma homocysteine and progression of symptomatic peripheral arterial disease. *J Vasc Surg* 1999; **29**: 8–19.

Perioperative Care in Emergency Vascular Practice

ALASDAIR DOW, JOHN F THOMPSON

THE PROBLEM

Vascular teams are frequently confronted by patients who are rapidly losing blood or have already lost it. Ruptured aortic aneurysms or trauma involving major vessels are obvious examples but the bleeding may be iatrogenic, for example, vascular injury during interventional radiological procedures. This chapter concerns immediate resuscitation of the shocked patient, blood transfusion and component therapy, intraoperative autotransfusion and blood management in the perioperative period.

Intensive care units (ICUs) and high dependency units (HDUs) may improve outcomes for patients with a wide variety of surgical conditions. Recent data suggest that high risk surgical patients who receive such care *prior* to surgery may have reduced mortality rates and a shorter hospital stay.

A number of current topics, including the choice of fluids, timing of surgery, estimation of cardiac output and β-blockade are relevant and important. The postoperative care of patients after emergency vascular surgery will also be considered in this chapter. These problems represent the most vexing issues for the surgical team and suggestions for dealing with them will be discussed.

INITIAL MANAGEMENT

Attention to the airway, breathing and circulation must be emphasised. The shocked patient has undergone profound peripheral vasoconstriction and venous access may be difficult to obtain. The best way to be certain is to *anticipate* and to insert wide bore cannulae before initiating procedures which may be associated with unexpected blood loss such as thrombolysis.

During the management of major trauma lines should *not* be inserted in the lower half of the body. There are good reasons for this, such as occult venous injury in the pelvis or the need to use lower limb veins for bypass grafting. Most texts recommend the use of arm veins for emergency venous access, but modern catheter systems allow central venous lines to be inserted with speed and reliability (see Chapter 7B). Cannulation of the internal jugular vein with the patient in a head-down tilt avoids the risk of pneumothorax and is the best approach in patients who are already profoundly hypovolaemic. A large introducer sheath may then be used for volume resuscitation or a central venous or pulmonary artery catheter may be inserted. Once intravenous access is established a urinary catheter should be inserted.

'PREOPTIMISATION' OF EMERGENCY VASCULAR PATIENTS

High dependency units and ICUs provide a level of treatment not available on the majority of general wards, so-called 'augmented care', requiring a number of resources. Improved staffing, often a 1:1 staff to patient ratio is crucially important. Invasive monitoring, such as measurement of left atrial filling pressure and cardiac output, is also essential. More recently, mixed venous oxygen saturation (SvO_2) monitoring has been used as an early detector of changes in cardiac output and haemoglobin concentration following aortic surgery.[1] This technique is also useful in critically ill patients following cardiac surgery.[2] The use of complex ventilatory strategies, including invasive and non-invasive ventilation, makes a significant difference to the quality of care afforded to these patients. Inevitably, the development of these modern units will prove to be of great benefit.

Features of 'augmented care'

- 1:1 staff: patient ratio
- Invasive monitoring
- Advanced ventilatory strategies

There has been considerable debate as to the cost-effectiveness of such units, but augmented care may improve outcome and shorten hospital stay.[3] The problem is to select those who will benefit and whether time is available to do that. The ruptured aneurysm is usually too urgent a condition to allow anything other than transfer to theatre, even though patients with leaking/expanding aortic aneurysms could be considered good candidates. Compared with general surgical emergencies, these patients have a higher incidence of cardiovascular disease, spend a prolonged time in theatre and are at risk of renal and cardiac complications.

There is no agreement on the best method of selecting patients who might benefit from 'preoptimisation'. Echocardiography, either resting or during induced stress, has the advantage that it is quicker and less invasive than thallium perfusion scans and is effective in detecting wall motion defects in patients with vascular disease.[4] Dobutamine echocardiography is a good predictor of cardiac risk.[5,6] An alternative is the use of a scoring system such as POSSUM (Physiological and Operative Severity Score for the enUmeration of Mortality and Morbidity).[7] In London, 101 preoperative general/vascular surgical patients were studied. They were ill enough to warrant admission to ICU, but resources did not permit it. The outcome was predicted by POSSUM, and the actual outcomes in those admitted to ICU preoperatively were compared with those admitted postoperatively: mortality was reduced in patients admitted preoperatively.[8]

Which therapies are beneficial in the HDU/ICU? Most studies are difficult to interpret; and even in emergency vascular surgery mortality is low, so that the study size needs to be large. However, a theme emerges. Measurement of right or left heart filling and improvement in oxygen tissue delivery may confer benefit. Berlauk et al. showed that preoperative improvement of haemodynamic variables reduced cardiac morbidity and graft thrombosis in peripheral vascular surgery.[9] Others, however, were unable to support this finding.[10] Ziegler et al. studied 72 patients undergoing aortic or limb salvage surgery.[11] All were admitted to ICU preoperatively and randomised to treatment or control. The 32 patients in the treatment group had their physiological variables adjusted to improve their SvO_2 to above 65 per cent after pulmonary artery catheter insertion. The control group had a similar catheter inserted, but no attempt was made to adjust their SvO_2. Mortality was 9 per cent in the treatment group and 5 per cent in the control group, there being no significant difference. It is difficult to draw conclusions from this small series and there is a pressing need for a large well-powered study to guide the use of such expensive preoperative care.

PERIOPERATIVE CARDIAC PROTECTION

Vascular surgery involves changes in systemic vascular resistance (SVR), resulting in alteration in cardiac output. A rise in SVR increases afterload against which the left ventricle has to contract may induce left ventricular failure. Conversely, a reduction in SVR may lead to diastolic hypotension, precipitating myocardial ischaemia in patients with narrowed coronary arteries. Thus, the manipulation of SVR and cardiac output may be beneficial for emergency vascular surgery patients, particularly those with low intravascular volume.

The gold standard over the past two decades for the estimation of cardiac output has been the Swan–Ganz pulmonary artery catheter which uses thermodilution to estimate cardiac output and software to calculate SVR and other variables. Recent work, however, indicates that the pulmonary artery catheter may not improve outcome and may actually contribute to morbidity.[12,13]

There has been recent interest in non-invasive measurement of cardiac output. Doppler ultrasound probes do not require central venous cannulation, but their accuracy may be more operator dependent. Nevertheless, there is good correlation between values obtained from a pulmonary artery catheter and those calculated by Doppler.[14] The probe is passed into the oesophagus until a mark on the sheath reaches the teeth. The sheath is then adjusted until the 'best' signal of descending thoracic aortic velocity is obtained. To reduce operator error some machines will assist in indicating when that has occurred.

Transoesophageal Doppler measures stroke volume, cardiac output and systolic flow time corrected for heart rate (FTc), which is an indication of contractility. The majority of studies have looked at the improvement in FTc using fluids and/or inotropes. In patients undergoing elective cardiac surgery, Mythen and Webb aimed to show that fluid optimisation would be better using Doppler, as demonstrated by better gut perfusion.[15] Patients were randomised to a control group receiving standard fluid therapy or to the protocol group in which therapy was based on Doppler derived variables. The protocol group had a shorter ICU and hospital stay with no serious complications, though six in that group did suffer some complications. Gan et al. studied 100 patients predicted to have a blood loss of greater than 500 mL.[16] All underwent Doppler probe insertion and were then randomised to standard or therapy groups. The standard group received fluid boluses according to deviations from baseline variables not measured by the Doppler. The therapy group received fluid based on their stroke volume and FTc. The therapy group had a shorter stay, earlier time to diet and less nausea and vomiting. Although this work has not been repeated in vascular surgery specifically, the lower complication rate associated with Doppler makes it an attractive option in high risk cases.

There is great interest in the use of β-adrenergic blockade to reduce the risk of perioperative myocardial infarction in vascular surgery. Following several positive observational studies, Poldermans reported a randomised trial in 112 patients undergoing aortic reconstruction, who had a positive dobutamine stress test and were not already taking a β-blocker. Fifty-nine were randomly assigned to treatment with bisoprolol and 53 to standard care. The combined cardiac death/non-fatal myocardial infarction rate was 3.4 per cent with bisoprolol compared to 34 per cent with standard care ($P = 0.001$).[17] A prospective trial is underway, but many surgeons are already convinced.

INITIAL RESUSCITATION

The precise fluid used for resuscitation is relatively unimportant. Colloidal solutions, which are starch or gelatin derivatives, are relatively expensive and contain potential allergens. Hydroxyethyl starch has an average molecular weight of 450 000 and a half-life of 26 hours. Polygelines have a molecular weight of 35 000 and a half life of 2.5 hours. Hetastarch is the most effective when packed cells are transfused in view of its longer half-life. Albumin is no longer regarded as a suitable plasma expander in view of cost and the danger of transmissible disease. With regard to clear fluids, normal saline contains an excess of chloride, so that there is a theoretical risk of hyperchloraemia; also Ringer's solution contains lactate which may worsen acidosis.

The 'crystalloid versus colloid' argument is based on highly controlled experiments where subjects, usually dogs or pigs, were venesected to induce hypotension and then resuscitated. It has now become clear that shock increases microvascular permeability allowing large molecules to cross into the interstitial space. During recovery they may be difficult to remove and may exert an osmotic effect which draws fluid from the intravascular compartment.

The fashion then swung to high volume crystalloid resuscitation. Experimental studies involving a more 'realistic'

bleed caused by an aortic tear,[18] however, demonstrated the detrimental postoperative effects of high volumes of saline.

The redistribution of crystalloids through the extravascular compartment means that they are usually required in volumes five times that of colloid. This ratio increases further in situations of trauma including ruptured aneurysms.[19] This redistribution, or 'third spacing', is more common after crystalloid rather than colloid use and can lead to pulmonary oedema.[20] Hydrostatic pressure is more important than colloid osmotic pressure in the movement of water across the pulmonary capillary membrane.

There is little evidence to indicate that colloids reduce mortality or morbidity, despite their theoretical advantages. Indeed, doubts were expressed that the use of albumin solutions in critically ill patients might be associated with a *higher* mortality. A meta-analysis, however, showed that albumin was not associated with alteration in survival.[21] The studies included in the analysis were not all surgical, but a more complex meta-analysis from the Australian Cochrane Centre looked at colloid solutions in patients with trauma, burns or after surgery.[22] The authors concluded that there was no benefit attributable to any of the colloids over crystalloids and it was suggested that their extra cost could not be justified.

A recent Australian study adds further uncertainty as to the choice of fluid type. The Saline versus Albumin Fluid Evaluation (SAFE) study used a multicentre prospective randomised trial method to allocate patients to receive either 4 per cent albumin or saline for fluid resuscitation.[23] The chosen fluid was employed exclusively during the 28-day study period for intravascular resuscitation of 6997 patients recruited, of whom 3497 received albumin. The results showed that there were 726 deaths in the albumin group as against 729 in the saline group (risk ratio 0.99; 95 per cent confidence interval 0.91 to 1.09; $P = 0.87$). Further, there was no significant difference between the number of days spent in the ICU ($P = 0.44$), days in hospital ($P = 0.30$) or days of renal replacement therapy ($P = 0.41$). The power of this study is sufficiently great to justify the conclusion that in a broad cross-section of ICU patients there is a similar outcome following the use of either 4 per cent albumin or saline as a resuscitation fluid.

The vascular team is faced with a wealth of data that does not support one fluid type over the other. Until a large-scale trial favours one type of fluid, it is likely that personal or institutional preference will predominate.

RESUSCITATION FLUIDS: HOW MUCH IS ENOUGH?

The Advanced Trauma Life Support (ATLS) scheme and the American College of Surgeons Committee on Trauma emphasise the importance of aggressive volume resuscitation in hypotensive patients, and this has been amplified by recent reports in patients with ruptured abdominal aortic aneurysms.[24] Nevertheless, as long ago as 1928, Canon et al.[25] concluded, 'Haemorrhage in the case of shock may not have occurred to a marked degree because blood pressure has been too low and flow too scant to overcome the obstacle offered by a clot. If the pressure is raised before the surgeon is ready to check any bleeding that may take place, blood that is sorely needed may be lost'.

The 'leaky bucket' syndrome, where injudicious resuscitation leads to further bleeding by disrupting haemostatic clots within constricted vessels has been demonstrated by Blair et al. who showed an increased rate of re-bleeding after upper gastrointestinal haemorrhage in transfused patients.[26] Aggressive resuscitation was questioned by Kaweski et al.[27] who studied 6855 trauma patients and found no correlation between survival and preoperative fluid resuscitation in patients with similar probabilities of survival as assessed by TRISS criteria, TRISS being a trauma scoring method based on a combination of the Revised Trauma Score (RTS) and the Injury Severity Score (ISS). Although hypotension was an overall predictor of poor outcome, the administration of fluids had no influence on it. Further evidence that intravenous fluids may not be beneficial, but could be harmful, was provided by Bickell et al.[28] A total of 300 consecutive patients with gunshot or stab wounds with a systolic blood pressure of 90 mmHg or less were randomised to either immediate intravenous resuscitation by a paramedic team ($n = 96$) or delayed resuscitation ($n = 81$). The latter received no intravenous fluid until 'knife to skin'. There were no differences in the rate of postoperative complications, but if the data are analysed to only include strict protocol adherents, i.e. absolutely *no* fluid resuscitation, there was a survival advantage.

In conclusion, there is convincing evidence against the use of routine blood pressure elevation by the aggressive administration of intravenous fluids before surgical haemostasis in patients with trauma.[29]

INTRAOPERATIVE VOLUME REPLACEMENT

Loss of 20 per cent of the blood volume can generally be replaced with clear fluids (Table 7A.1), but in the emergency situation it may be impossible to estimate blood loss on clothing or drapes and since rapid haemorrhage involves simultaneous loss of red cells and plasma, the peripheral venous haemoglobin concentration or haematocrit do not fall immediately.

Pulse, blood pressure and urine output reflect the high pressure side of the circulation, which contains only a fraction of the blood volume and is maintained by well-known neurohormonal reflexes. The greatest part of the intravascular volume resides in the venous capacitance vessels of the splanchnic circulation. Adrenergic venoconstriction leads to contraction of this compliant reservoir to maintain right atrial filling pressure. Thus, central venous pressure may not reflect the state of the blood volume. In the ventilated patient, even pulmonary artery wedge pressure may be difficult to determine if positive end expiratory pressure is used and may not reflect left ventricular filling pressure.[30] In shocked patients the vascular space is contracted and is not re-expanded even by large quantities of clear fluid and blood. This was demonstrated well by Simmons et al.[31] in 29 combat victims, ^{51}Cr-labelled autologous red cells were used to estimate red cell mass and plasma volume was measured using ^{125}I-labelled albumin. [125]I albumin leaves the circulation in shocked patients and therefore blood volumes were overestimated. Despite this, 13 of the 29 patients had significantly reduced red cell volume after they had been 'adequately' resuscitated by conventional criteria; reductions in the red cell volume did not correlate well with haemodynamic measurements in shocked patients.

In practice, clinical judgement, in other words 'educated guesswork', and a combination of 'hard' measurements must be used to gauge the volume required to be transfused. A good technique is to assess the effect of a fluid challenge by rapidly infusing boluses of 200 mL and monitoring the effect on various parameters.

Table 7A.1 *Pathophysiological features of hypovolaemia*

	Class I	Class II	Class III	Class IV
Per cent loss	<15	15–30	30–40	>40
Volume (mL)	750	750–1500	1500–2000	>2000
Systolic	Unchanged	Normal	Reduced	Low
Pulse (beats per minute)	<100	>100	>120	>140
Diastolic	Unchanged	Raised	Reduced	Very low
Capillary fill	Normal	Slow	Slow	Undetectable
Respiratory rate (per minute)	14–20	20–30	30–40	>40
Urine output (mL)	>30	20–30	30–40	>40
Mental	Apprehensive	Anxious	Confused	Lethargic

Red cell transfusion   77

RED CELL TRANSFUSION

Red cell transfusion restores oxygen carrying capacity to maintain tissue oxygen delivery. Red cells should not be used for volume expansion and indeed the adage that blood loss must be replaced with whole blood is simplistic and dangerous.

As with all other aspects of trauma management, communication is vital. The haematology technician on call must be notified of the arrival of the patient and given an estimate of blood which will be required and of the time scale involved. He or she will usually be involved with other patients and must plan their laboratory work accordingly. Adequate samples should include 5 mL of blood in EDTA for full blood count and preferably two 10 mL plain glass tubes for crossmatch. If there is any doubt regarding pre-existing coagulopathy, a 5 mL citrate sample should be sent. Coagulopathy is a poor prognostic indicator in patients with ruptured abdominal aortic aneurysm[32] and this probably applies to other cases of vascular trauma. Results of coagulation tests may guide early and appropriate component therapy.

Accurate labelling is vital, especially in the emergency situation. The name, date of birth and hospital number should be checked with wrist band identification whenever possible, as clerical error is still the leading cause of fatal transfusion reactions. It is helpful if previous potentially sensitising episodes such as blood transfusion and pregnancy are mentioned on the request form.

Blood volume replacement

- Clear fluid infusion – crystalloids versus colloids? How much?
- Whole blood transfusion – type specific/O Rhesus negative (Rh−ve) in an emergency
- Red cell transfusion – packed cells
- Component therapy – platelets/fresh frozen plasma/cryoprecipitate
- Autologous blood transfusion

It is well known that group O Rh−ve blood is the universal donor but there is a reluctance to use it[33] despite prospective studies demonstrating its effectiveness.[34] As anti A, B or AB antibodies are present in plasma, packed cells are safer than whole blood.

In a rapidly bleeding patient, the transfusion of uncrossmatched blood is not nearly as important as the speed of the transfusion. The compatibility of uncrossmatched randomly selected blood is 64 per cent. If blood is ABO compatible, this rises to 99.4 per cent, only autologous red cells being 100 per cent compatible. Thus, type specific blood is

very safe in an emergency. O Rh−ve blood is not always available and it is permissible to give male patients O Rh+ve blood and accept the risk of seroconversion. If female Rh−ve patients are given Rh+ve blood they can be given anti-D serum if they plan to have children in the future. The principal reason for avoiding universal group O transfusion in trauma is that group O blood is often in short supply. There is often a surplus of group A blood; group AB patients can be transfused with group A or B blood, especially if this is in the form of packed cells.

Crossmatching detects reactions between an antibody present in the recipient's blood and rare antigens present on donor cells. It takes 15–20 minutes to crossmatch blood using modern techniques and it is almost always possible to wait before transfusion. Testing of the donor serum against the patient's red cells is no longer necessary, especially if plasma-reduced blood is transfused.

Red cell concentrates are now cleared of most of their leucocyte content by a process of sedimentation and may be further leucodepleted by filtration. This is to reduce the possibility of transmitting leucocyte-associated viruses such as cytomegalovirus, other DNA herpes viruses and the human T cell group. At the time of writing it is known that prion protein has been demonstrated on lymphocytes, monocytes and platelets and so there is a theoretical risk of transmission of variant Creutzfeldt–Jakob disease by blood transfusion. The message for surgical practice is that blood transfusion is life saving but should be carefully monitored to avoid undue exposure to infective risk.

Blood should be infused through sterile giving sets containing a standard 170 μm filter. The set is calibrated so that there are 20 drops of blood to 1 mL. Further filtration of blood is unnecessary. In trauma, rapid transfusion is probably more important than the benefits of filtration.

Intraoperative transfusion

The decision to transfuse blood must be taken with regard to the overall clinical picture, especially the presence of coexisting cardiac and respiratory disease, and whether bleeding is continuing. The *optimum* haemoglobin level for tissue oxygen delivery is 10 g/dL because blood viscosity falls with the haematocrit and intracapillary red cell flow increases.

Portable devices such as the Stat-Crit (Unipath Ltd, Bedford, UK) or Haemocue (Angelholm, Sweden) enable repeatable, rapid haematocrits or haemoglobin concentrations to be determined in theatre to guide blood transfusion (Fig. 7A.1). The accepted teaching that a single unit transfusion is anathema has been challenged by the use of this equipment. Repeated estimations enable the response to a single unit transfusion to be measured; if the agreed trigger is exceeded, transfusion is stopped.

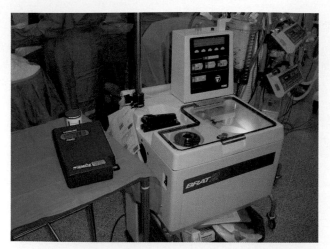

Figure 7A.1 *Haemocue device (Angelholm, Sweden) for in-theatre haemoglobin estimations can be used to direct blood transfusions. Seen here next to the Cobe BRAT II cell salvage equipment (Cobe Cardiovascular, Arvada, CO, USA) during aneurysm repair*

Postoperative transfusion

Two important factors lead to an artificially low haemoglobin level after operation. 'Preloading' the circulation with clear fluid dilutes the red cells and epidural anaesthesia leads to sympathetic blockade in the lower half of the body. Subsequent vasodilation increases intravascular volume, which is filled by fluid shift from the interstitial space and by exogenous fluid transfusion. In the postoperative period this excess intravascular fluid is excreted and redistributed, resulting in a rise in the haemoglobin concentration of 1.5–2.0 g/dL.

In trauma the true preoperative haemoglobin concentration is unknown and the red cell mass can only be estimated from body mass. In the clinical situation hypovolaemic anaemia can be identified by assessing the response to red cell transfusion. Hypovolaemic patients accommodate both resuscitation fluids and red cells so that the proportion of red cells, that is the haematocrit, and the concentration of haemoglobin do not change significantly. If blood volume is normal, transfused blood raises the red cell mass and the plasma volume. Redistribution and subsequent diuresis of the 'excess' plasma raises both the haematocrit and haemoglobin concentrations. Laboratory determination of these parameters may be inaccurate if performed too soon after transfusion, i.e. before redistribution has taken place.

Guidelines for red cell transfusion are available on several websites such as http://transfusionguidelines.org.uk and all follow the general recommendations given in the box below.

Guidelines for red cell transfusion

- No transfusion if haemoglobin >10 g/dL
- Transfuse if haemoglobin <7 g/dL
- Haemoglobin 8–10 g/dL is safe if euvolaemic, even with cardiopulmonary disease
- Transfuse symptomatic anaemic patients

Chronic anaemia is well tolerated when there are no other complicating factors. Patients with renal failure frequently have haematocrits between 20 and 30 per cent and patients with hookworm infestations have survived haematocrits below 10 per cent. Czer and Shoemaker investigated perioperative mortality based on pretransfusion haematocrit: at a haematocrit of less than 21 per cent, 68 per cent of a group of 94 critically postoperative patients died; at a haematocrit of between 27 and 33 per cent, 87 per cent survived, and yet at a haematocrit of greater than 33 per cent only 50 per cent survived.[35] In a case–control study of 125 Jehovah's Witnesses, operative mortality was inversely related to preoperative haemoglobin level.[36] Mortality was 7.1 per cent for patients with haemoglobin levels above 10 g/dL but rose sharply to 61.5 per cent for those with levels below 6 g/dL. Mortality was also, not surprisingly, related to perioperative blood loss. In this study no patient with a haemoglobin above 8 g/dL and an operative blood loss below 500 mL died.

At haematocrit levels greater than 25 per cent the heart rate is normal. Stroke volume and therefore cardiac output increase as long as normovolaemia is maintained. Coronary blood flow increases due to coronary vasodilatation and increased blood fluidity. Direct electrode studies have shown that the tissue oxygen concentration of the gut, kidney, muscle, brain and heart remains normal at haematocrits greater than 20 per cent. Both in animals and patients wound healing is not impaired by haematocrits of 15–20 per cent provided that blood volume is normal and tissue perfusion is kept at near normal levels.[37] In practice this means that it is probably safe to err on the side of undertransfusion and to use repeated haematocrit estimations to guide careful replacement of operative blood loss.

This strategy of conservative postoperative transfusion, studied by Hebert *et al.*[38] showed that both a survival advantage as well as a lower complication rate could be anticipated in ICU patients.

PROBLEMS ASSOCIATED WITH MASSIVE TRANSFUSION

There are serious problems associated with high volume blood transfusion (also see Chapter 4). Incompatibility and volume overload have been discussed. Hypothermia is common if blood is used straight from the refrigerator. Countercurrent heat exchangers such as the Level 1 device (Level 1, Inc., Rockland MA, USA) enable fluid to be infused rapidly at near normal temperature.

A unit of blood contains 67.5 mL of citrate but only 35 mL is required to chelate calcium to prevent coagulation. Thus, in cases of rapid transfusion, free citrate may be present and may cause myocardial irritability and even ventricular fibrillation in hypothermic patients. Calcium gluconate is used if transfusion is very rapid.

As greater volumes of bank blood are transfused, mixed venous oxygen tension falls as a consequence of the increased

Table 7A.2 *Blood components for the bleeding patient; indications and doses. Remember to warm the patient and transfuse fluids*

Blood component	Indication	Dose
Platelets	Platelet count $<50 \times 10^9$ and bleeding Count $<100 \times 10^9$ and serious bleeding	250×10^9 (adult)
Fresh frozen plasma	>1.0 blood volumes transfused INR >1.5 *and* continued bleeding	four packs for average adult (15 mL/kg)
Cryoprecipitate	Only if fibrinogen <1.0 g/L Use fresh frozen plasma first	10 units initially

INR, international normalised ratio.

oxygen affinity of bank blood. This is manifest as a decrease in the *in vivo* P_{50}. Although animal experiments have always shown that this does not affect myocardial performance, Weisel *et al.* demonstrated that arteriopaths are unable to increase cardiac index due to their impaired heart muscle function. The mechanism may involve decreased inorganic phosphate or decreased ionised calcium associated with blood transfusion.[39]

Coagulopathy following massive transfusion generally occurs after more than 15 units have been given. Miller *et al.* studied the effect on battle casualties in Vietnam and observed only one episode of clinical bleeding before 20 units were given.[40] All of their patients developed coagulopathy after 30 units. The mechanism was multifactorial and bleeding was corrected by fresh blood and platelets but *not* fresh frozen plasma.

Following massive transfusion some patients develop coagulopathy whereas others do not. The volume of blood transfused does not always correlate with the extent of the coagulopathy but it does correlate very well with the duration and depth of the shock period.[41] It is the disease, namely, hypoperfusion, and not the treatment, i.e. transfusion, that causes coagulopathy. Even after an exchange transfusion, clotting factor levels remain at 30 per cent of their original value and several studies emphasise the relative unimportance of fresh frozen plasma transfusion.[42]

Septicaemia remains one of the greatest challenges in the postoperative patient. Patients who have undergone emergency vascular surgery are at particular risk, because of associated gut ischaemia and also because of acute lung injury/adult respiratory distress syndrome complicating massive transfusion. The recognition that some patients with septic shock may have low levels of protein C resulted in the introduction of recombinant human activated protein C, drotrecogin alpha. This recent advance in biotechnology has provided some impressive results in the reduction of mortality from septic shock, and it is gaining rapid acceptance in ICU practice.

One of the most recent evaluations, under the acronym ENHANCE US (Extended evaluation of recombinant human activated protein C United States Trial), compared the effect on mortality of activated protein C with that in previous studies.[43] The study was a prospective single arm multicentre trial in the USA and Puerto Rico, and looked at the 28-day all-cause mortality in patients receiving activated protein C. The study recruited 273 patients and showed that the 28-day mortality was 26.4 per cent. This was 6 per cent lower than the mortality of the placebo group in the Protein C Worldwide Evaluation in Severe Sepsis (PROWESS) and Secretory Phospholipase A2 Inhibitor (sPLA2I) trials, two trials studying similar groups of patients who had been randomised to activated protein C or placebo. Further, the PROWESS trial had a treatment group mortality of 24.4 per cent, similar to the figure for the ENHANCE study. The ENHANCE trial serves to confirm previous data and suggests that activated protein C is a beneficial therapy in patients with septic shock. The major side effect with reference to vascular patients is that of excessive bleeding, and the current advice is that activated protein C should not be given until 12 hours following surgery. Further, if unexpected surgery is required during treatment, the infusion should be stopped, and recommenced 12 hours after return from the operating theatre.

COMPONENT THERAPY

The separation of blood into its components of red cells, plasma and platelets has enabled clinicians to undertake specific therapy aimed at the treatment of deficiencies of any one of these factors. The indications are summarised in Table 7A.2.

Platelet concentrates are either prepared from whole blood, with a volume of 50–70 mL and platelet count of $0.5–1.1 \times 10^{11}$/L, or by using a continuous flow cell separator which yields a volume of 20–500 mL and a platelet content of $2.6–3.0 \times 10^{11}$/L. Indications for platelet transfusion in surgical patients are either dilutional thrombocytopenia or acquired platelet dysfunction. Dilutional thrombocytopenia secondary to massive transfusion should be treated with platelet transfusions only if the platelet count is less than about 50×10^9/L in association with active oozing from capillaries. Platelet function is highly dependent on temperature and it may be necessary to warm the patient to achieve adequate haemostasis.

Ideally, ABO and Rh specific platelet concentrates should be transfused but in an emergency incompatible platelets may be given for the reasons discussed above in relation to red cell transfusion. Giving group O platelet concentrates to group A or B subjects may result in an acute haemolytic reaction and rhesus sensitisation is possible via red cells present in platelet concentrate.

During cardiopulmonary bypass and high volume salvage autotransfusion, platelet function is depressed due to platelet activation in the extracorporeal circuit. Platelet transfusion may be necessary in these situations.

There are very few indications for fresh frozen plasma transfusion. In the surgical patient it is useful for emergency reversal of oral anticoagulants. There is no evidence to support the routine use of fresh frozen plasma in severe liver disease, disseminated intravascular coagulation (DIC) and notably massive transfusion. There is no justification for the use of plasma as a volume expander as colloids are more effective, cheaper and much safer. When transfusion exceeds 1–1.5 blood volumes *and there is clinical non-surgical bleeding*, plasma may be required.

The haemostatic system is extraordinarily resilient to loss of clotting factors during haemorrhage. Counts *et al.* studied 27 massively transfused patients prospectively during resuscitation, using modified whole blood which had the platelets and cryoprecipitate removed.[44] Despite high volume haemorrhage and transfusion, it was unusual for measured coagulation factors to decrease to dangerous levels. Non-surgical bleeding was found to be due to thrombocytopenia and also DIC. There was no justification for the routine administration of supplemental plasma in this and other studies.

AUTOLOGOUS BLOOD TRANSFUSION

The perceived dangers of third party blood transfusion and the cost of screening donor blood have rekindled interest in blood conservation. Autologous blood can be pre-deposited, withdrawn using isovolaemic haemodilution in the anaesthetic room, salvaged during surgery with immediate reinfusion or collected from wound drains. The last two techniques are relevant to trauma surgery.

Blood which collects in serosal cavities such as the chest or peritoneum is exposed to tissue plasminogen activator, undergoes clotting and then lysis. Reinfusion of chest drainage in trauma patients with haemothoraces was first reported in 1917.[45] This technique is still useful if chest drains are inserted while in the field. The blood can be reinfused during transfer to the trauma centre.

Postoperatively, blood which has been collected from wound drains may be reinfused without processing. Despite theoretical worries about the consequence of infusing activated clotting and other factors, there have been no reports of adverse consequences using this method. The Solcotrans orthopaedic system (CR Bard, NJ, USA) uses a moderate vacuum to drain blood and is useful following arthroplasty. Various devices such as the Sorensen system can be used to collect chest drain or mediastinal drainage blood for reinfusion. The utility of these devices depends on the rate of bleeding and the haematocrit of the salvaged blood. If blood loss is rapid it has no time to be lysed and therefore clots. If blood loss is very slow the transfusate is mainly tissue fluid with a low red cell content.

During the Vietnam war, Klebanoff and Watkins developed a roller pump technique to reinfuse blood aspirated from the surgical field.[46] Unfortunately, reports of air embolism led to its withdrawal from the market. The Cell Saver was a descendent of centrifugal blood separators used to produce γ-globulin and albumin from whole blood for the treatment of burns. Originally the process was discontinuous but the invention of a rotary seal by Latham in 1947 enabled continuous flow separation to be used. The operating principle of the Cell Saver (Haemonetics UK Ltd, Leeds, UK) is now well known: a centrifuge is used to separate the red cells while anticoagulant and plasma are eluted. The technique is particularly useful in trauma (Fig. 7A.2a) because the patient does not have to be heparinised. Modern equipment can be set up in minutes and the equipment does not require a specialised perfusionist (Fig. 7A.2b).

There are few studies reporting the use of cell centrifuge devices in trauma. Goulet *et al.* reported a 42 per cent reduction in homologous blood requirement for revision hip arthroplasty and found that autotransfused patients who had sustained spinal trauma required 33 per cent less blood than historical controls.[47] Cell salvage devices are very useful in ruptured aortic aneurysm surgery, but, having said that, small contained retroperitoneal ruptures may result in a hypercoagulable state. Platelets and clotting factors have not been consumed to a great degree and the patient has activated platelets and elevated factor VIII as a result of the stress. This may make salvage impossible as the machinery fills with clot. If, on the other hand, there has been a large bleed and platelet and clotting factors have been consumed the patient becomes auto-anticoagulated and salvage is particularly useful.

A further area of concern is the use of cell washing in a contaminated field. Although the process does not eliminate bacterial contamination, reinfusion of contaminated blood has been reported without significant complications.[48] In trauma surgery intraoperative autotransfusion combined with broad spectrum antibiotic cover can be life saving if no other source of blood is available. The only absolute contraindication to cell saving is faecal contamination because of the danger of physical blockage of the filters. There is no evidence that the use of intraoperative autotransfusion devices leads to acquired bleeding tendencies either due to thrombocytopenia or disseminated intravascular coagulopathy.[49]

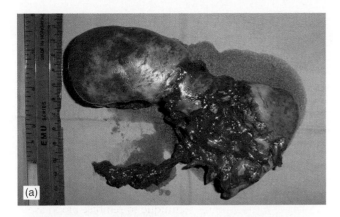

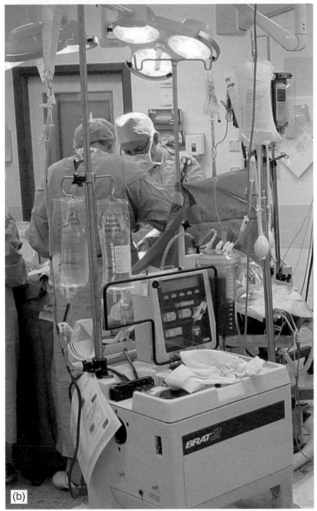

Figure 7A.2 *Life-saving cell salvage devices can be life saving in vascular emergencies (a) A motor cyclist in a road accident presented with a right kidney avulsed at the renal artery and vein and tearing the vena cava. (b) Six litres of blood were recycled during surgery and he made a good recovery*

PHARMACOLOGICAL AGENTS

There are no clear data to support the use of pharmacological agents in the reduction of traumatic blood loss. However,

there has been a surge of interest in the serine protease inhibitor, aprotinin (Trasylol, Baylor, UK). Although aprotinin reduces blood loss following cardiopulmonary bypass, a double blind placebo-controlled study showed it to be ineffective during elective aortic surgery.[50] A similar trial in ruptured aortic aneurysm patients failed to show benefit[51] and it is likely that aprotinin is only of benefit in hyperfibrinolytic states. Recombinant factor VII is at present undergoing randomised clinical trials and although there are a few anecdotal case reports from enthusiasts there is no convincing evidence to support this very expensive drug.

REGIONAL BLOCK OR NOT FOR VASCULAR EMERGENCIES

The role of regional blocks in elective vascular surgery is either as an adjunct to general anaesthesia or as the sole method of anaesthesia for limb surgery or carotid endarterectomy. Regional techniques are just as applicable to emergency as well as elective situations, provided that time and normal coagulation variables permit. Two questions have to be considered in the application of regional anaesthesia:

- Is there a benefit of regional block in addition to general anaesthesia?
- How does abnormal coagulation influence the timing of such blocks?

Yeager *et al.* studied 53 high risk patients undergoing elective vascular surgery: they were randomised to receive either general anaesthesia + epidural ($n = 28$) or general anaesthesia + postoperative intravenous opiates ($n = 25$).[52] Patients were matched for surgical risk and there were no other major differences between the groups. The epidural group had a lower incidence of postoperative complications, cardiac failure, major infectious complications and lower hospital costs; all differences were significant at $P < 0.05$. Subsequent studies have confirmed improved cardiovascular and pulmonary function in patients receiving epidural analgesia following vascular surgery but have not shown an improvement in morbidity. This may be because of an inadequate number of small studies, which prevented closer interpretation by meta-analysis.[53] However, a large-scale trial currently in progress is addressing the question of cardiac morbidity and mortality with epidural analgesia.

There are other benefits of epidural anaesthesia, either as a sole technique or combined with general anaesthesia. A meta-analysis showed that patients undergoing surgery for hip fracture had a lower incidence of venous thromboembolism under regional block, than with general anaesthesia alone.[54] However, this benefit did not extend to reduced mortality. In lower limb revascularisation procedures, there is a reduction in early graft thrombosis in patients receiving epidural analgesia.[55,56]

Abdominal procedures are complicated by deterioration in pulmonary function in the postoperative period. Epidural analgesia reduces this problem and improves oxygenation.[57] A large meta-analysis of randomised controlled trials found that an opioid/local anaesthetic mixture via a thoracic epidural decreased atelectasis, pulmonary infection and hypoxaemia when compared with systemic opioids.

The dilemma with the emergency vascular patient is no longer whether an epidural be performed, but when. In ruptured aortic aneurysms, those patients who are unstable and require volume expansion should have their epidural insertion delayed until after surgery has been completed. All others should have a brief explanation about the benefits and disadvantages of epidural analgesia, and if agreed, an epidural catheter should be placed before surgery.

The issue with those who have not had an epidural catheter placed before surgery relates mostly to placement and coagulopathy. This is particularly relevant in emergency vascular patients, who may have received large volumes of fluids and heparin intraoperatively. No large-scale trial has considered this issue and it is unlikely that such a trial would be feasible because of the low incidence of the most feared complication, namely, epidural haematoma. An audit of 912 vascular patients with an indwelling epidural catheter, and who received full anticoagulation peroperatively, found no occurrence of symptomatic epidural haematomas.[58] The main criticisms of this study, apart from the design and small sample size, are that the catheter was already sited and also that asymptomatic haematomas were not excluded. A second study in patients who had received low molecular weight heparin thromboprophylaxis prior to spinal or epidural analgesia found no cases of epidural haematoma,[59] and concluded that the practice was safe.

In emergency practice the patient will usually require an epidural *after* surgery. The evidence suggests that this is still likely to be very safe, but platelet function and coagulation studies should be normalised before the introduction of such a block. This may delay extubation after surgery, but it is justified by the benefits of epidural analgesia.

Conclusions

Recent studies have provided new evidence that closely monitored limited early resuscitation, early surgical control of bleeding and careful use of blood transfusion can improve the outlook in patients with massive bleeding. Preoptimising patients, if time allows, and the use of HDU/ICU is essential. Epidural anaesthesia and techniques for avoiding postoperative coagulopathy, especially warming, and the use of autologous blood, are further refinements which should be part of routine emergency surgical practice.

Key references

Christopherson R, Beattie C, Frank SM, *et al*. Peri-operative morbidity in patients randomised to epidural or general anaesthesia for lower limb vascular surgery. *Anaesthesiology* 1993; **79**: 422–34.

Finfer S, Bellomo R, Boyce N *et al*. A comparison of albumin and saline for fluid resuscitation in the intensive care unit. *N Engl J Med* 2004; **350**: 2294–6.

Gan TJ, Soppitt A, Maroof M, *et al*. Goal-directed intraoperative fluid administration reduces length of hospital stay after major surgery. *Anesthesiology* 2002; **97**: 820–6.

Ranaboldo CJ, Thompson JF, Davies JN, Shutt A, *et al*. Aprotinin in elective aortic reconstruction: a double blind randomised control trial. *Br J Surg* 1997; **84**: 1110–13.

Treasure T, Bennett D. Reducing the risk of major elective surgery. *BMJ* 1999; **318**: 1087–8.

REFERENCES

1 Pestana D, Garcia de Lorenzo A, Madero R. Relationship between mixed venous saturation and cardiac index, haemoglobin and oxygen consumption in aortic surgery. *Rev Esp Anesthesiol Reanim* 1998; **45**: 136–40.

2 Vedrinne C, Bastien O, De Varax R, *et al*. Predictive factors for usefulness of fibreoptic pulmonary artery catheter for continuous oxygen saturation in mixed venous blood monitoring in cardiac surgery. *Anaesth Analg* 1997; **85**: 2–10.

3 Treasure T, Bennett D. Reducing the risk of major elective surgery. *BMJ* 1999; **318**: 1087–8.

4 Henein MY, Anagnostopoulos C, Das SK, *et al*. Left ventricular long axis disturbances as predictors for thallium perfusion defects in patients with known peripheral vascular disease. *Heart* 1988; **79**: 295–300.

5 Shafritz R, Ciocca RG, Gosin JS, *et al*. The utility of dobutamine echocardiography in preoperative evaluation for elective aortic surgery. *Am J Surg* 1997; **174**: 121–5.

6 Ryckwaert F, Leclerq F, Colson P. Dobutamine echocardiography for the pre-operative evaluation of patients for surgery of the abdominal aorta. *Ann Fr Anaesth Reanim* 1998; **17**: 13–18.

7 Copeland GP, Jones D, Walters M. POSSUM. A scoring system for surgical audit. *Br J Surg* 1991; **78**: 355–60.

8 Curran JE, Grounds RM. Ward versus intensive care management of high-risk surgical patients. *Br J Surg* 1998; **85**: 956–61.

9 Berlauk JF, Abrams JH, Gilmour IJ, *et al*. Preoperative optimisation of cardiovascular haemodynamics in improves outcome in peripheral vascular surgery. *Ann Surg* 1991; **214**: 289–97.

10 Bender JS, Smith-Meek MA, Jones CE. Routine pulmonary artery catheterisation does not reduce morbidity and mortality of elective vascular surgery: results of a prospective randomised trial. *Ann Surg* 1997; **226**: 229–36.

11 Ziegler DW, Wright JG, Choban PS, Flancbaum L. A prospective randomised trial of preoperative optimisation of cardiac function in patients undergoing elective peripheral vascular surgery. *Surgery* 1997; **122**: 584–92.

12 Dalen JE, Bone RC. Is it time to pull the pulmonary artery catheter? [editorial] *JAMA* 1996; **276**: 916–18.

13 Robin ED. Death by pulmonary artery flow-directed catheter. Time for a moratorium? *Chest* 1987; **92**: 727–31.

14 DiCorte CJ, Latham P, Greilich P. Pulmonary artery catheter vs. esophageal Doppler monitor: measurement of cardiac output and left ventricular filling during cardiac surgery [abstract]. *Anaesth Analg* 1999; **88**: SCA37.

15 Mythen MG, Webb AR. Peri-operative plasma volume expansion reduces the incidence of gut mucosal hypoperfusion during cardiac surgery. *Arch Surg* 1995; **130**: 423–9.

16 Gan TJ, Soppitt A, Maroof M, *et al*. Goal-directed intraoperative fluid administration reduces length of hospital stay after major surgery. *Anesthesiology* 2002; **97**: 820–6.

17 Poldermans D for the Dutch Echocardiographic Cardiac Risk Evaluation Applying Stress Echocardiography Study Group. The effect of bisoprolol on perioperative mortality and myocardial infarction in high risk patients undergoing vascular surgery. *N Engl J Med* 1999; **341**: 1789–94.

18 Bickel WH, Bruttig SP, Millnamov GA, *et al*. The detrimental affects of intravenous crystalloid after aortotomy in swine. *Surgery* 1991; **110**: 529–36.

19 Bock JC, Barker BC, Clinton AG, *et al*. Post-traumatic changes in, and effect of colloid oncotic pressure on the distribution of body water. *Ann Surg* 1989; **210**: 395–405.

20 Astiz ME, Galera-Santiago A, Rackow EC. Intravascular volume and fluid therapy for severe sepsis. *New Horizons* 1993; **1**: 127–36.

21 Wilkes MM, Navickis RJ. Patient survival after human albumin administration. A meta-analysis of randomised, controlled trials. *Ann Intern Med* 2001; **135**: 205–8.

22 Alderson P, Schierhout G, Roberts I, Bunn F. Colloids versus crystalloids for fluid resuscitation in critically patients. *Cochrane Database Syst Rev* 2000; **2**.

23 Finfer S, Bellomo R, Boyce N *et al*. A comparison of albumin and saline for fluid resuscitation in the intensive care unit. *N Engl J Med* 2004; **350**: 2294–6.

24 Johansen K, Kohler TR, Nicholls SC, *et al*. Ruptured abdominal aortic aneurysm: the Harborview experience. *J Vasc Surg* 1991; **13**: 245–7.

25 Cannon WB, Fraser J, Kelwell EM. The preventative treatment of wound shock. *JAMA* 1928; **70**: 618–21.

26 Blair SD, Janverin SB, McCollum CN, Greenhalgh RM. Effects of early blood transfusion on gastrointestinal haemorrhage. *Br J Surg* 1986; **73**: 783–5.

27 Kaweski SM, Sise MJ, Virgilio RW. The effect of pre hospital fluids on survival in trauma patients. *J Trauma* 1990; **30**: 1215–19.

28 Bickell WH, Shafton GW, Mattox KL. Intravenous fluid administration and uncontrolled haemorrhage. *J Trauma* 1989; **29**: 409.

29 Assalia A, Schein M. Resuscitation for haemorrhagic shock. *Br J Surg* 1993; **80**: 213.

30 Shippey CR, Appel PL, Shumaker WC. Reliability of clinical monitoring to assess blood volume in critically ill patients. *Crit Care Med* 1984; **12**: 107–12.

31 Simmons RL, Heisterkamp CA, Mosely RV, Doty DB. Post resuscitative blood volumes in combat casualties. *Surg Gynecol Obstet* 1969; **128**: 1193–201.

32 Davies MJ, Murphy WG, Murie JA, *et al*. Pre-operative coagulopathy in ruptured abdominal aortic aneurysm predicts poor outcome. *Br J Surg* 1993; **80**: 974–6.

33 Barnes A. Transfusion of universal donor and uncrossmatched blood. *Bibl Haematol* 1980; **46**: 132–42.

34 Schwab CW, Shayne JP, Turner J. Immediate trauma resuscitation with type O uncrossmatched blood: a two year prospective experience. *J Trauma* 1986; **26**: 897–902.

35 Czer SC, Shumaker WC. Optimal haematocrit value in critically ill post-operative patients. *Surg Gynecol Obstet* 1978; **147**: 363–8.

36 Carson JL, Poses RM, Spence RK, Bonavita G. Severity of anaemia and operative mortality and morbidity. *Lancet* 1988; **i**: 727–9.

37 Hunt TK, Rabkin J, Von Smitten K. Effects of oedema and anaemia on wound healing and infection. *Curr Stud Haematol Blood Transf* 1986; **53**: 101–11.

38 Hebert PC, Wells G, Blajchman MA, *et al*. A multicenter, randomized, controlled clinical trial of transfusion requirements in critical care. Transfusion Requirements in Critical Care Investigators, Canadian Critical Care Trials Group. *N Engl J Med* 1999; **340**: 409–17.

39 Weisel RD, Dennis RC, Manny J, *et al*. Adverse effects of transfusion therapy during abdominal aortic aneurysetomy. *Surgery* 1978; **83**: 682–90.

40 Miller RD, Robins TO, Tong MJ, Barton SL. Coagulation defects associated with massive blood transfusion. *Ann Surg* 1971; **174**: 781–94.

41 Harke H, Rahman S. Haemostatic disorders in massive transfusion. *Bibl Haematol* 1980; **46**: 179–88.

42 Collins JA. Recent developments in the area of massive transfusion. *World J Surg* 1987; **11**: 75–81.

43 Bernard GR, Margolis BD, Shanies HM, *et al*. Extended evaluation of recombinant human activated protein C United States Trial (ENHANCE US): a single-arm, phase 3B, multicenter study of drotrecogin alfa (activated) in severe sepsis. *Chest* 2004; **125**: 2206–16.

44 Counts RB, Haeisch C, Simon TL, *et al*. Haemostasis in massively transfused trauma patients. *Ann Surg* 1979; **190**: 91.

45 Elmendorf A. Uber wieder infusion nach punktion eines frischen hamathorax. *Munch Med Wochenschr* 1917; **64**: 36–7.

46 Klebanoff G, Watkins D. A disposable auto-transfusion unit. *Ann J Surg* 1968; **116**: 475–6.

47 Goulet JA, Bray TJ, Timoman LA, *et al*. Intraoperative auto-transfusion in orthopaedic patients. *J Bone Joint Surg* 1989; **71a**: 3–7.

48 Timberlake GA, McSwain NE. Auto-transfusion of blood contaminated by enteric contents: a potentially life saving measure in the massively haemorrhaging trauma patient. *J Trauma* 1988; **28**: 855–7.

49 Thompson JF. Intra-operative auto-transfusion. *Curr Pract Surg* 1993; **5**: 137–41.

50 Ranaboldo CJ, Thompson JF, Davies JN, Shutt A, *et al*. Aprotinin in elective aortic reconstruction: a double blind randomised control trial. *Br J Surg* 1997; **84**: 1110–13.

51 Robinson J, Nawaz S, Beard J. Randomised multi centre double blind placebo controlled trial of the use of aprotinin in ruptured abdominal aortic aneurysm. *Br J Surg* 2000; **87**: 754–7.

52 Yeager MP, Glass DD, Neff RK, Brinck-Johnson T. Epidural anaesthesia and analgesia in high-risk surgical patients. *Anaesthesiology* 1987; **66**: 729–36.

53 Buggy DJ, Smith G. Epidural anaesthesia and analgesia: better outcome after major surgery? *BMJ* 1999; **319**: 530–1.

54 Sorenson RM, Pace NL. Anaesthetic techniques during surgical repair of femoral neck fractures. A meta-analysis. *Anaesthesiology* 1992; **77**: 1095–104.

55 Tuman KJ, McCarthy RJ, March RJ, *et al.* Effects of epidural anaesthesia and analgesia on coagulation and outcome after major vascular surgery. *Anaesth Analg* 1991; **73**: 696–704.

56 Christopherson R, Beattie C, Frank SM, *et al.* Peri-operative morbidity in patients randomised to epidural or general anaesthesia for lower limb vascular surgery. *Anaesthesiology* 1993; **79**: 422–34.

57 Dahl JB, Rosenberg J, Hansen B, *et al.* Differential analgesic effects of low-dose epidural morphine and morphine-bupivacaine at rest and during mobilization after major abdominal surgery. *Anaesth Analg* 1992; **74**: 362–5.

58 Baron HC, LaRaja RD, Rossi G, Atkinson D. Continuous epidural anaesthesia in the heparinized vascular surgical patient: a retrospective review of 912 patients. *J Vasc Surg* 1987; **6**: 144–6.

59 Bergqvist D, Lindblad B, Matzsch T. Low molecular weight heparin for thromboprophylaxis and epidural/spinal anaesthesia – is there a risk? *Acta Anaesthesiol Scand* 1992; **36**: 605–9.

7B

Emergency Vascular Access

THANG D NGUYEN, ROY M FUJITANI, SAMUEL E WILSON

THE PROBLEM

Intravenous (IV) catheters have become essential tools in the management of hospital patients. Over the years, developments in catheters and insertion techniques have allowed reliable and rapid access to the central venous system. Techniques have become simplified to the point that bedside insertions are now commonplace. Indications for central line access have evolved to encompass parental nutrition, administration of irritating or caustic solutions, haemodynamic monitoring and temporary haemodialysis. The ability to attain rapid central access without the need for operating suites makes these types of access useful tools during medical and surgical emergencies. In spite of the simplified techniques and the high frequency with which we use them, complications ranging from minor to fatal can occur.[1–9] Respect for central access and understanding its limitations remain essential when seeking central access.

The subject of emergency vascular access encompasses a wide array of clinical settings. During a critical injury where the priority of IV access ranks second only to securing airway, two large-bore peripheral IVs are often sufficient. In the setting of a hypotensive patient in vascular collapse peripheral IVs can be challenging. These patients require two large calibre central catheters, one on either side of the diaphragm to facilitate resuscitation. Similarly, patients who require rapid fluid resuscitation may require multilumen central catheters to accommodate multiple IV medications. In these circumstances the central venous catheter may be inserted in any available site. Haemodialysis patients, on the other hand, require additional considerations. When these patients present for emergency access, strategic planning is

required to preserve potential access sites. A poorly planned 'quick fix' in these patients can ruin an entire limb for future dialysis.

In this chapter we will discuss the vascular access options available during emergencies. Selected procedures, particularly central line placements along with the insertion techniques and the management of their complications will be discussed. Emergency vascular access for the purpose of haemodialysis requires specific evaluation and this subject deserves special consideration.

THE HAEMODIALYSIS PATIENT

Chronic renal insufficiency: patients anticipating haemodialysis

The chronic renal failure patient who anticipates haemodialysis is usually referred by nephrologists and is frequently encountered in outpatient settings. These patients are medically stable and do not commonly require immediate access. They will, however, require a permanent arteriovenous (AV) fistula. The preferred site is the non-dominant distal upper extremity, typically the radial artery to the nearest suitable vein. Whenever possible, an autologous fistula of the Brescia–Cimino type is preferred over the synthetic polytetrafluoroethylene (PTFE) graft because of its superior primary patency and lower revision rate[10] (see Chapter 41). Since native vein shunts typically require a 2–4-week maturation period, autologous fistulae frequently require the simultaneous placement of an indwelling haemodialysis catheter in the contralateral internal jugular vein. This allows the patient to undergo haemodialysis while the fistula matures. The catheter can be removed after the functional status of the Cimino fistula is established. In the event that the native vein fistula is not possible due to a small calibre or tortuous radial vein, a PTFE straight graft from the radial artery to the antecubital vein should be considered. Given that PTFE grafts do not customarily require a maturation period, the simultaneous placement of a temporary catheter is not necessary.

Acute renal failure and the thrombosed arteriovenous graft

End stage renal patients require lifelong haemodialysis. Unfortunately, AV grafts do not last a lifetime. There are a number of modalities available to address failed AV grafts, but none can be considered superior. Interventional radiology offers a variety of percutaneous techniques which achieve satisfactory thrombolysis and thrombectomy under fluoroscopic guidance. In appropriate circumstances, interventional radiologists can perform percutaneous transluminal (balloon) angioplasty of compromised outflow or inflow vessels. Several series report promising results which rival surgical outcome.[11,12] Secondary patency rates, however, remain similar. For many patients with acutely thrombosed AV grafts, this modality offers a minimally invasive alternative to surgical revisions. Grafts with multiple revisions or extensive intimal hyperplasia require surgical intervention.

When these patients present for surgical repair it is important to determine the relative urgency of the matter. In the presence of fluid overload, uraemic encephalopathy or hyperkalaemia, the need for AV access should be considered as an emergency. The proper evaluation of patients in this condition mandates a thorough history and physical examination. Important historical elements include a history of previous central catheter placements, hypercoagulable states, immune compromise conditions and the date of the last dialysis. A thrombosed graft identified 1 day after effective dialysis would not require emergency repair whereas one identified 3 days later may do so. Physical examination must include the patient's vital signs, weight, mental status and neurological status. If a new graft involving the radial artery is contemplated, an evaluation of the ipsilateral ulnar artery supply is warranted. A weak or absent ulnar artery can be demonstrated by Allen's test (see Chapter 41). A graft involving the radial artery in the presence of a weak or absent ulnar pulse may result in a steal phenomenon causing ischaemia in the ipsilateral hand. Fever and leucocytosis are signs of infection precluding the placement of a PTFE graft. A thrombosed AV graft site should be examined for evidence of infection necessitating graft removal. The ipsilateral extremity should be examined for evidence of venous hypertension, the presence of which warrants a duplex ultrasound of the axillary–subclavian venous system

to evaluate outflow obstruction. In the presence of proximal stenosis a distal AV graft will be at risk for early failure. Some vascular surgeons advocate a duplex ultrasound study whenever an AV graft in the distal extremity thromboses.

Pertinent laboratory studies include a basic metabolic panel and a complete blood count. Marked elevation in blood urea nitrogen can result in uraemic encephalopathy as well as platelet dysfunction. The latter may be an important consideration when contemplating surgery or temporary catheter placement. Marked fluid overload or severe hyperkalaemia requires emergency haemodialysis. This may be necessary prior to the availability of a functional graft. In these circumstances, the placement of a temporary haemodialysis catheter is appropriate. The site for permanent access should be assessed prior to percutaneous cannulation. When using the internal jugular vein for temporary access, the catheter should be inserted contralateral to the site of the planned permanent access.[13]

In general, acute vascular access can be accommodated in one of two ways: a double lumen central venous catheter and a bridge graft AV shunt. Whereas the former is appropriate for haemodialysis commencing immediately, the latter can be available for dialysis commencing within 24 hours. If dialysis is deemed an emergency, and will be needed for two or more weeks, a soft tunnelled silastic catheter with a Dacron cuff should be used. A soft catheter carries a lower incidence of vein stenosis and the Dacron cuff decreases the likelihood of line sepsis by serving as a barrier against bacterial migration. Whereas bridge graft AV shunts must be placed in the operating room (OR), the percutaneous and tunnelled catheters can be inserted in the OR or in the interventional radiology suite. Only the percutaneous catheter can be inserted at the bedside.

INDICATIONS FOR HAEMODIALYSIS

With the exception of complete renal failure, no two patients have the same degree of renal insufficiency. Furthermore, the susceptibility to renal failure complications varies from patient to patient. One factor which can be fatal in all renal failure patients, however, is hyperkalaemia. The elderly patient with pre-existing heart disease may be more susceptible to cardiac arrhythmias from hyperkalaemia than one without a cardiac history. Additionally, a patient with chronic renal failure may tolerate a higher degree of hyperkalaemia than one in acute renal failure (ARF). Consequently, there is no consensus on the laboratory values which ought to trigger emergency haemodialysis. Most physicians will agree that symptomatic uraemia or abnormal potassium levels along with electrocardiographic (ECG) changes warrant urgent dialysis. Frequently, medical management of hyperkalaemia must be initiated while awaiting haemodialysis. This is particularly important in the hyperkalaemic patient with metabolic acidosis. This combination is potentially fatal and necessitates immediate intervention.

When failing kidneys lose the ability to excrete bodily acids, blood pH must be maintained by other compensatory means. One mechanism involves the uptake of excess extracellular hydrogen in exchange for intracellular potassium; the result is homoeostatic pH at the expense of worsening hyperkalaemia. This can be further exacerbated in an

Table 7B.1 *Electrocardiographic (ECG) changes in hyperkalaemia*

ECG changes	Potassium levels
T waves tenting	5.7–6.9 mEq/L
P wave amplitude decreases, widen PR interval	7.0–8.3 mEq/L
P wave flat	8.4–8.9 mEq/L
QRS widening	9.0–11 mEq/L
Ventricular fibrillation	>12 mEq/L

Table 7B.2 *Signs and symptoms of uraemia*

Signs	Symptoms
Pericardial friction rub	Nausea/vomiting
Refractory pulmonary oedema	Anorexia
Metabolic acidosis	Fatigue
Foot/wrist drop	Diminished sensorium
Asterixis	

Table 7B.3 *Indications for haemodialysis*

Relative indications	Absolute indications
Blood urea nitrogen >100 mg/dL	Volume overload
Total parental nutrition or blood transfusions in acute renal failure	Hyperkalaemia
Uraemic coagulopathy	Metabolic acidosis
Drug intoxication	Uraemia

intubated patient who cannot compensate for metabolic acidosis by respiratory efforts. The threshold for arrhythmia arising from hyperkalaemia depends on the patient and can occur abruptly without uraemic symptoms. Thus, dialysis access in these patients may be more urgent than symptoms would suggest. The priority of management in these patients must be directed toward protecting the heart. An ECG must be obtained to evaluate hyperkalaemia induced changes. Table 7B.1 lists the ECG signs of hyperkalaemia. Calcium infusion must be administered to stabilise the myocardium. Serum potassium can be reduced by the following manoeuvres: intravenous administration of glucose and insulin, intravenous bicarbonate and enteral Kayexalate. The use of loop diuretics, such as furosemide, can often be effective, but may not be useful in the setting of renal failure. These therapeutic options are initiated in addition to establishing vascular access in preparation for haemodialysis.

Table 7B.2 lists signs and symptoms of uraemia. Table 7B.3 lists absolute and relative indications for haemodialysis. In general, chronic dialysis therapy is indicated when glomerular filtration rate falls below 10 mL/min. More acute indications include fluid overload, congestive heart failure, hyperkalaemia, metabolic acidosis, hypertension uncontrolled by conservative measures and uraemia induced conditions such as encephalopathy, neuropathy, pericarditis and bleeding diathesis. Occasionally a fluid-restricted anuric patient requires blood transfusions or parenteral feeds. Haemodialysis may be the only means of removing excess fluids in these patients. Patients with ARF who may not require haemodialysis are those developing ARF from reversible conditions. Such conditions include dehydration, urinary tract infection, urinary obstruction, hypercatabolic states, hypercalcaemia and low cardiac output states. The decision to initiate haemodialysis therapy requires an evaluation of the patient's clinical condition as well as of serum potassium levels. The urgency with which dialysis is required will determine whether temporary or permanent access is more appropriate.

Types of catheter

Table 7B.4 lists the various types of central venous catheter and their sizes. There are a multitudes of catheters available and not all are appropriate for haemodialysis.

Table 7B.4 *Types of catheters*

Type	Indications	Insertion site	Size
Cordis, triple lumen	Acute blood loss, dehydration	Femoral, internal jugular, subclavian	9 Fr cordis/7 Fr triple lumen
HD Catheter	Haemodialysis	Femoral	12–13 Fr/16–19 cm
HD Catheter	Haemodialysis	Internal jugular vein	12–13 Fr/13–16 cm
HD Catheter	Plasmaphoresis	Femoral	12–13 Fr/16–19 cm

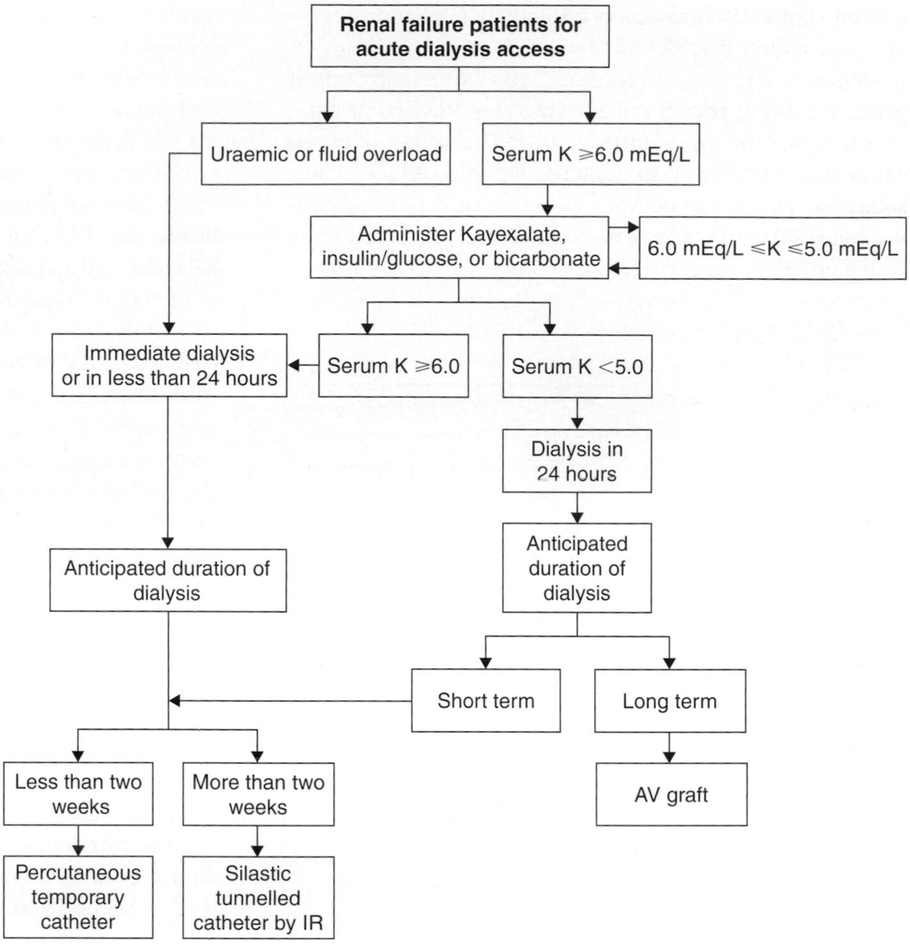

Figure 7B.1 *Algorithm for acute vascular access for haemodialysis. Temporary catheters are appropriate for haemodialysis commencing immediately. A bridge graft arteriovenous (AV) shunt should be placed if dialysis commences in 24 hours. If the immediate need for haemodialysis is anticipated to exceed two weeks, a soft tunnelled silastic catheter with a Dacron cuff should be used. In asymptomatic patients, serum potassium (K) levels of 6 mEq/L or greater requires immediate medical intervention in the form of Kayexalate, insulin/glucose infusion or bicarbonate. Potassium levels between 5 and 6 mEq/L may be treated medically. More than one dose may be necessary. Refractive hyperkalaemia (≥6 mEq/L) necessitates immediate dialysis. IR, interventional radiography*

When contemplating a temporary catheter for haemodialysis, both diameter and length must be considered. The unit known as French (Fr) describes the catheter diameter, and three Fr units are equivalent to 1 mm. The length of central venous catheters is measured in centimetres. Catheters specifically designed for haemodialysis are typically 12 or 13 Fr (4 mm). Whereas the femoral vein can accommodate a long catheter, the internal jugular catheter length is limited by the position of the heart. In the femoral vein a 16–19 cm catheter is required whereas in the internal jugular vein a 13–16 cm catheter would be appropriate for most patients. On an upright chest X-ray the internal jugular catheter tip situated at the junction of the superior vena cava (SVC) and the right atrium would be considered ideal.

Figure 7B.1 provides an algorithm for acute vascular access for haemodialysis.

ACUTE ACCESS

At the bedside, central access is attained percutaneously. This method relies on anatomical landmarks to identify suitable veins. Occasionally, anatomical variation or pre-existing thrombosis makes the 'blind' insertion of central catheters exceedingly difficult and even dangerous. In recent years, portable real time ultrasound has made the identification of suitable targets easier and increased the rate of successful cannulation. Not surprisingly, central line placement under ultrasound guidance is associated with fewer complications.[14–19] When central access is contemplated for patients with previous multiple central lines, real time ultrasound is recommended.

SELDINGER TECHNIQUE

In principle, the Seldinger technique provides a reliable method for locating and percutaneously cannulating a vessel. This method makes use of a soft guidewire threaded through an 18 gauge needle placed in a vein. The wire then serves as a guide over which a softer catheter can be inserted. As with any procedure, proper preparation helps to minimise complications. The site of insertion must be prepped widely with povidone iodine. The patient as well as the surrounding work area is draped with sterile towels. The physician is capped, masked, gowned and gloved in a sterile fashion. All components of the catheter must be confined to a sterile field and readily accessible.

The skin and subcutaneous tissue at the insertion site are anaesthetised with 3–5 mL of 1 per cent lidocaine (Xylocaine) using a 25 gauge needle. A thin walled 18 gauge needle is introduced into the vein guided by landmarks and/or real time ultrasound. The needle enters at a 45 degree angle with the skin, aspirating as the needle advances. The return of dark non-pulsatile blood indicates venepuncture. The syringe is then removed with the needle still in place. The hub of the needle should be covered at this point to avoid introducing air into the vascular system. A sterile guidewire is passed into the vein through this needle which is then removed over the wire. A number 11 scalpel blade extends the insertion site by 2–3 mm at the skin. A dilator is passed over the wire through the cutaneous tissue into the vein and subsequently removed. A catheter is then placed over the wire into the vein. The wire is withdrawn with the catheter still in place. The functions of all ports are evaluated by withdrawing blood from each of them, followed by a sterile heparinised saline flush. The catheter is ultimately sutured in place and dressed in sterile fashion.

FEMORAL VEIN

The femoral vein lies medial to the usually palpable femoral artery located in the femoral triangle (Fig. 7B.2). The insertion site is approximately 1 cm medial to the femoral artery and 3–4 cm below the inguinal ligament. The patient is positioned supine with the lower extremity slightly externally rotated. The Seldinger technique is then used to complete the insertion. Resistance at the femoral site suggests either that the wire has failed to enter the vein or that the patient is not supine. In the former case, the wire must be withdrawn and the femoral vein is sought again with a needle and syringe, whereas in the latter the patient is repositioned lying supine but avoiding flexion at the hip so that the wire does not have difficulty negotiating a bend. Ascites can sometimes cause resistance at the femoral site. In no circumstances should the wire be forced. An alternative site should be considered if resistance persists despite the above manoeuvres.

Advantages of the femoral site

The femoral veins are relatively far from the heart and lungs. This makes the femoral site ideal when a central line is required during cardiopulmonary resuscitation (CPR). From a technical viewpoint, the femoral vein is easily accessible and its landmarks are readily apparent. Alternative sites such as the internal jugular or subclavian vein increases the risk of pulmonary injury. Thus, patients with poor ventilation, pulmonary oedema or congestive heart failure may be better served with femoral line access.[1,2] The femoral catheter does not require a postprocedural X-ray to verify position. A successfully placed femoral line is therefore immediately functional and extremely useful during emergencies.

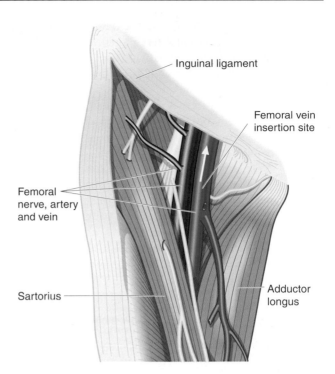

Figure 7B.2 *The femoral triangle is defined by the inguinal ligament superiorly, the sartorius muscle laterally and the adductor longus medially. The femoral nerve, artery and vein course through this triangle. The femoral vein lies medial to the artery. The palpable artery in this triangle helps to identify the vein. The arrow indicates site of catheter insertion*

Disadvantages of the femoral line

The femoral site is in close proximity to the rectum and genitalia. Bacteria migration facilitated by bodily fluids from this region increases the likelihood of line infections. In non-emergency settings, femoral access may interfere with mobility and is itself thrombogenic. Nonetheless, femoral lines are used in ambulatory dialysis settings and have been reported safe and effective for as long as 14 days.[14] In the setting of trauma where hip fracture is a possibility the femoral site may not be the best choice. Local oedema and tenderness interfere with proper positioning and exposure. If the line is placed for the purpose of haemodialysis, the femoral site is not always practical. The sitting position produces a bend in the femoral catheter thereby reducing flow during dialysis. The patient is thus required to remain supine for the duration of the haemodialysis session lasting 2–4 hours. Furthermore, the femoral IV can be particularly cumbersome in the OR because anesthesiologists, positioned at the head of bed, may find it difficult to gain access to the catheter.

Complications associated with femoral access

While the placing of femoral lines is technically simple, and provides a rapid means of establishing vascular access, it is not without complications. Femoral **pseudoaneurysms** can result from attempted femoral vein catheterisation and is attributed to inadvertent artery puncture, the risk being higher in the anticoagulated patient (see Chapter 38). The patient commonly presents with local pain with an associated palpable mass at the site of puncture. Auscultation over the mass may reveal a bruit. Ultrasound shows extravasated blood contained within the surrounding tissues. Direct pressure usually results in total resolution but can be painful and may take up to 37 minutes to resolve.[20,21] In a small percentage of cases, compression therapy fails, requiring ultrasound guided thrombin injection. Obliteration of these false aneurysms with thrombin injections is reportedly immediate and pain free. Failure of thrombin therapy may be related to the size of the pseudoaneurysm. The principal concern is the rupture of the pseudoaneurysm resulting in uncontained blood loss.[13] Surgical repair may be necessary.

Another femoral catheter complication is the formation of an **AV fistula** (see Chapter 38). Diversion of blood from artery to vein has the potential of causing ipsilateral venous hypertension, distal arterial insufficiency and high output heart failure.[13] A possible mechanism involves inadvertent arterial puncture during attempts at central access. The subsequent venepuncture on the ipsilateral side sets up an AV communication. Duplex ultrasound is often diagnostic but an angiogram may be warranted in the presence of arterial insufficiency and inconclusive ultrasound. Large symptomatic fistulae usually require surgical repair.

Another reported complication of the femoral catheter is the **entanglement of the guidewire** with an existing inferior vena cava (IVC) filter[22] (see Chapter 20). Careful attention to the history helps avoid this particular complication. Guidewire entanglement with an IVC filter has also been reported during catheter placement in the right internal jugular vein[6] and subclavian vein.[22–26] The interventional radiologist can, under fluoroscopic guidance, facilitate removal of the wire. In the presence of an IVC filter, it is probably best to perform central access under fluoroscopic guidance.

Potential complications at sites used in venous access

- Femoral
  - Pseudoaneurysm
  - AV fistula
  - Guidewire entanglement in IVC filter
- Internal jugular
  - Pneumothorax
  - Arrhythmias
  - Thrombosis
  - Guidewire migration
- Subclavian
  - Stenosis
  - Venous hypertension and thrombosis

THE INTERNAL JUGULAR VEIN

Catheterising the internal jugular vein is also achieved by the Seldinger technique. When possible, the patient should be adequately sedated, and placed under external cardiac monitoring. The patient is place in a 15–20 degree Trendelenburg position with the head turned away from the insertion side. A towel roll placed horizontally behind the shoulders extends the neck and accentuates landmarks. The internal jugular can be accessed either by a middle or posterior approach[2] (Figs 7B.3 and 7B.4). The safest method to locate the IJ vein is by way of a 25 gauge seeker needle. Once found, an 18 gauge needle can be introduced into the vein following a course parallel to that of the seeker needle.

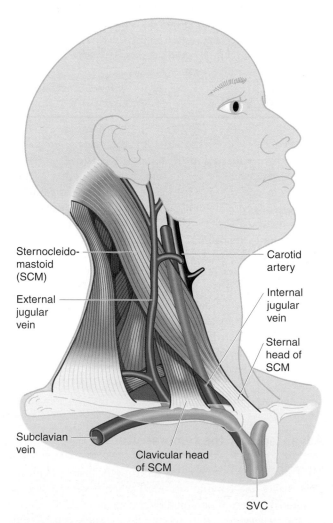

Figure 7B.3 *Muscles and vasculature of the neck. The vessel coloured red represents the carotid artery whereas those coloured blue represent the internal jugular vein, the subclavian vein and the superior vena cava (SVC). The clavicular and sternal heads of the sternocleidomastoid (SCM) join superior to the clavicle and serve as a landmark in locating the internal jugular vein. The clavicle and suprasternal notch are landmarks for the subclavian approach*

The middle approach

The internal jugular lies deep to the sternocleidomastoid (SCM), approximately 1 cm posterolateral to the palpable internal carotid artery, coursing most superficially between the clavicular and sternal heads of the SCM[2] (see Figs 7B.3 and 7B.4). The middle approach cannulates the internal jugular at this site. With one finger on the carotid pulse and a 25 gauge needle attached to a 5 ml syringe in the opposite hand, the internal jugular vein is sought by penetrating the skin lateral to the pulse in the direction of the ipsilateral nipple, aspirating as the needle advances. If redirection is required, the needle should be withdrawn and reinserted in a more lateral direction. Once found, the

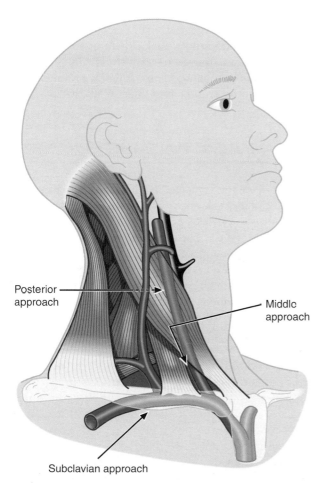

Posterior approach

Middle approach

Subclavian approach

Figure 7B.4   *Central line insertion sites at the neck. The arrows indicate sites of insertion. Two widely used sites for the internal jugular vein are illustrated, namely, the middle and the posterior approach. The middle approach uses the most superficial segment of the internal jugular vein, which lies at the junction of the two heads of the sternocleidomastoid (SCM). The posterior method approaches the internal jugular from behind the lateral edge of the SCM just superior to its junction with the external jugular vein. Whereas risks of arterial puncture are higher from the posterior approach, the middle approach is associated with a higher incidence of pneumothorax. Also illustrated is the subclavian site. The risk of pneumothorax is greatest with this approach*

syringe is removed with the needle remaining in place. An 18 gauge thin wall needle then follows a parallel course entering the skin at a 30–45 degree angle. When dark non-pulsatile blood returns, the Seldinger technique is used to complete catheter insertion.

The posterior approach

The posterior approach enters the internal jugular from the posterior edge of the SCM superior to the point where it meets the external jugular vein. A seeker needle is directed deep to the SCM and towards the suprasternal notch. Once located, an introducer needle follows the course of the seeker needle in parallel fashion. The internal jugular vein can then be cannulated as described by the Seldinger technique.

An upright chest X-ray is essential to verify catheter tip position and to rule out pulmonary injury. The preferred tip position is in the SVC approximately 1–2 cm above the SVC–atrium junction. Most catheters have depth markers that help guide proper placement. In a 70 kg patient, the catheter should be inserted to the 17 cm mark from the left internal jugular vein. When cannulating the right internal jugular vein, the catheter should be inserted to the 14 cm mark. Soft catheters can be placed as far as the right atrium. Stiff catheters such as those used for temporary haemodialysis will irritate the myocardium causing arrhythmia.[1]

Advantages of the internal jugular catheter

In the vast majority of cases the internal jugular site is readily accessible. The landmarks are readily apparent, and the carotid artery can be easily compressed should it be nicked during the search for the vein. Central catheters in this position are well tolerated. Mobility of the neck is minimally affected, and the patient may walk without affecting the function or position of the catheter. Being relatively remote from the rectum and genitalia keeping this site clean is less problematic than it is for femoral catheters, thus allowing the line to be kept in place for a relatively longer period of time. The right internal jugular leads directly to the SVC without much curvature so that a rigid catheter can be placed easily without provoking the stenosing effect associated with subclavian central lines.[1–3,13,27,28]

Disadvantages of internal jugular catheters

Insertion of a large bore needle into the anterior triangle of the neck in search of a carotid sheath structure carries inherent risks. Local injuries ranging from haematomas, infections and nerve injuries to ipsilateral lung collapse are all documented complications. In addition, there are a variety of conditions that can make the internal jugular vein virtually inaccessible. In the trauma setting, a hard cervical collar often precludes the placement of a central line at this site. In an obese patient with a short neck the anatomical landmarks may be distorted making identification of the internal jugular vein difficult. A patient in pulmonary oedema or congestive heart failure would not tolerate the Trendelenburg position required for the cannulation of vessels in the neck. Cardiopulmonary resuscitation in progress, particularly chest compressions, makes it virtually impossible to place a line in the internal jugular vein. Compared with other central sites, the internal jugular carries the highest rate of anatomical variability resulting in difficult venous access. In a patient without previous central lines, anatomical variability can be as high as 5 per cent.[1] In a patient who has not previously had a central line inserted thrombosis or variability ranges from 16 to 27 per cent.[1,8,9,14,15,17] Whereas real time ultrasound can guide the operator toward a suitable vein in 41 per cent of these cases, in the remaining cases the veins were found to be either too small for cannulation, thrombosed or nonexistent.[9] When confronted with a difficult access it is important to keep in mind the fact that the risk of pneumothorax increases with the number of attempts. An ultrasound guided technique may therefore be helpful.

Complications of internal jugular catheters

The lung apex is in the direct path of the introducer needle as it penetrates the internal jugular from either side and therefore **pneumothorax** represents an inherent risk of internal jugular vein catheterisation. The rate of this complication in association with internal jugular insertions is within the range of 0 to 1.8 per cent,[1] occurring much more frequently with the **middle approach**.[2] Pneumothorax may be recognised during the procedure by the aspiration of air, respiratory distress and decreased ipsilateral breath sounds. Contralateral tracheal shift and hypotension are signs of a tension pneumothorax requiring immediate decompression. An upright chest X-ray confirms the diagnosis, and in most patients, particularly those on positive pressure ventilation, air has to be evacuated via thoracostomy tubes.

The risk of pneumothorax can be minimised by attention to a few technical considerations. First, the introducer needle should enter the skin at a 30–45 degree angle to the neck, particularly when using the middle approach. A lower angle places the needle in the direct path of the lung apex. Second, the incidence of pneumothorax rises with the number of attempts. Given the high anatomical variability and abnormality in patients, repeated blind attempts are never recommended. Real time sonographic guidance can be a useful adjunct when landmarks fail.

Cardiac problems are not infrequently encountered during attempts at central access on patients in the intensive care unit. Continuous cardiac monitoring reveals premature ventricular contractions which occasionally lead to ventricular tachycardia. The cause is often myocardial irritation caused by the guidewire. When this occurs, the wire is partially withdrawn until the arrhythmia subsides. Sometimes, infusion of 1 mg/kg of injectable lidocaine is necessary to abort this arrhythmia. Consequently, some institutions advocate continuous cardiac monitoring during all internal jugular and subclavian central access procedures.

Central vein **thrombosis** and thrombosis within the atrium have been described in association with central venous catheters.[1] Although not often symptomatic, central vein thrombosis presents with swelling of the ipsilateral extremity with associated pain and tenderness. Ultrasound venography is diagnostic and the treatment is catheter removal and anticoagulation. A thrombus in the right atrium is rare but life threatening. Removal of the catheter under real time sonography with lytic therapy may be necessary to avoid large scale pulmonary embolism.[1]

A less frequent but real complication of the internal jugular line is **losing control of the wire** and allowing it to be dislodged entirely into the vascular system.[29] Retrieval requires the help of interventional radiology using real time ultrasound guidance. Migration of the 'out of control' wire into the heart can result in fatal arrhythmias. The inability to remove the inciting factor quickly in this situation is potentially life threatening. The solution is prevention and therefore the wire must be kept under control at all times.

SUBCLAVIAN LINE PLACEMENT

The union of the cephalic and axillary veins marks the beginning of the sublcavian vein. It enters the thorax, coursing deep to the clavicle and superficial to the anterolateral aspect of the first rib. The subclavian artery lies deep to the vein. The anterior scalene muscle separates the two vessels, and the lung apex lies medial and posterior to the subclavian vein. Landmarks for subclavian vein access include the *clavicle, acromioclavicular joint* and *suprasternal notch*[2] (see Figs 7B.3 and 7B.4).

The patient is placed in a 20–30 degree Trendelenburg position with the head turned away from the side of insertion. A towel roll is placed vertically between the scapulae to accentuate landmarks. The insertion site is widely prepped with antiseptic solution and the surrounding work area is draped in a sterile fashion. As with any central access procedure, the physician is capped, gowned and gloved in sterile fashion.

The **insertion site** is 1–2 cm below the inferior margin of the clavicle at the junction of its distal and medial thirds. The skin, subcutaneous tissue and the clavicular periosteum are anaesthetised with 1 per cent lidocaine using a 25 gauge needle. With the index finger on the sternal notch and the thumb on the clavicle, an 18 gauge introducer needle enters the anaesthetised skin with the bevel cephalad, aiming at the sternal notch and intentionally hitting the clavicle. When the clavicle is encountered, march down the clavicle until the needle is flush with the inferior surface of the clavicle. The needle is advanced slowly with the needle 'hugging' the inferior margin of the clavicle and aspirating simultaneously. When dark non-pulsatile blood returns, the needle is rotated 180 degrees so that the needle bevel now faces caudal to facilitate guidewire insertion. The Seldinger method is used to complete the cannulation.

Advantages of subclavian catheters

Although potentially dangerous and clearly requiring skill, many physicians favour the subclavian site because it offers constant anatomy. The clavicle serves as a landmark regularly directing the physician to the subclavian vein. This landmark is usually palpable even in obese patients, regardless of the length of the neck. In the trauma setting where cervical collars preclude internal jugular placement, subclavian catheterisation remains a viable option. Once in place, the catheter can be secured below the clavicle, hidden away from visible areas. The mobility of the patient is entirely unaffected, and this site can be kept clean with relative ease.

Disadvantages of subclavian catheters

Along with the many advantages of subclavian catheters, there are definite pitfalls. Like internal jugular lines, subclavian catheters are difficult if not impossible to place during chest compressions. Like the internal jugular site, subclavian line placements are most successful when patient is in the Trendelenburg position. Patients unable to tolerate the flat or head-down position may not be suitable candidates for subclavian central lines. Also as with internal jugular catheterisation, pneumothorax is an associated risk. The risk of pneumothorax is higher during subclavian line placement (2–5 per cent)[2] compared with that that of internal jugular catheterisation. In addition, the clavicle is an effective rigid barrier over the subclavian vessels making direct compression impossible should the subclavian artery be punctured inadvertently.

Complications of subclavian catheters

Subclavian and internal jugular access procedures share many common complications but those unique to the subclavian catheter deserve separate discussion. Subclavian haemodialysis catheters are associated with subclavian vein **stenosis** ranging from 42 to 50 per cent.[1,2,30] Significantly, the same type of catheter in the internal jugular site is associated with a markedly reduced internal jugular stenosis rate (0 to 10 per cent),[1,22,31] thought to be attributable to stresses exerted by the rigid haemodialysis catheter on the subclavian vein as it negotiates the brachiocephalic trunk. The point of insertion becomes a focal point of stress aggravated by transmitted irritation from the beating heart[13] and endothelial irritation eventually developing into a stenotic lesion. The relatively direct path from the right internal jugular vein to the SVC requires no bend in the catheter. The result is that less stenosis is observed with haemodialysis catheters at the internal jugular vein.[1]

This is particularly important to the chronic renal dialysis patient whose continued dialysis depends on availability of vascular access. Stenosis at this central site can compromise outflow from the ipsilateral arm. Consequently, AV shunts distal to the lesion ultimately fail secondary to **venous hypertension**. This observation led to a strategic approach in the management of dialysis patients who require temporary catheters. Clearly, the first choice for a temporary catheter site should be the right internal jugular vein. Equally clear is the site of last resort, namely, the subclavian vein. Choices falling in between are the left internal jugular and the femoral site. Whereas the left internal jugular has a tortuous path to the SVC, the femoral veins are associated with higher risks of line infection.

Conclusions

The need for emergency vascular access is encountered in a wide array of clinical settings. In recent years, temporary venous catheters have become indispensable tools within hospital. The ease of insertion has made these devices useful during resuscitation efforts in cases of trauma, dehydration, haemorrhage and 'code blue' situations. For patients requiring emergency haemodialysis, these catheters have become life-saving temporising measures.

In spite of the many short term advantages, immediate and life-threatening complications such as haemopneumothorax, haemorrhage, infection, arterial laceration, as well as the long term consequences of thrombosis and stenosis are associated with temporary catheters. These complications can occur even in the hands of experienced physicians. Respect for the potential complications and an understanding of the physician's own limits are essential when seeking central access.

Key references

Agee R, Kim, Balk AR. Central venous catheterization in the critically ill patient. *Crit Care Clin* 1992; **8**: 677–86.

Bambauer R, Inniger R, Pirrung KJ, *et al.* Complications and side effects associated with large-bore catheters in the subclavian and internal jugular veins. *Artificial Organs* 1993; **18**: 318–21.

Cameron LJ. *Current Surgical Therapy*, 6th edn. Vascular Access, 833–7.

McIntyre AS, Levison RA, Wood S, *et al.* Duplex Doppler ultrasound identifies veins suitable for insertion of central feeding catheters. *J Parenter Enteral Nutr* 1992; **16**: 264–7.

Schwab S, Beathard G. The hemodialysis catheter conundrum: hate living with them, but can't live without them. *Kidney Int* 1999; **53**: 1–17.

REFERENCES

1 Schwab S, Beathard G. The hemodialysis catheter conundrum: hate living with them, but can't live without them. *Kidney Int* 1999; **53**: 1–17.

2 Agee R, Kim, Balk AR. Central venous catheterization in the critically ill patient. *Crit Care Clin* 1992; **8**: 677–86.

3   Bambauer R, Inniger R, Pirrung KJ, *et al*. Complications and side effects associated with large-bore catheters in the subclavian and internal jugular veins. *Artificial Organs* 1993; **18**: 318–21.

4   Barrera R, Mina B, Huang Y, Groeger JS. Acute complications of central line placement in profoundly thrombocytopenic cancer patients. *Cancer* 1996; **78**: 2025–30.

5   De Moor B, Vanholder R, Ringoir S. Subclavian vein hemodialysis catheters: advantages and disadvantages. *Artificial Organs* 1993; **18**: 293–7.

6   Duong MH, Jensen WA, Kirsch CM, *et al*. An unusual complication during central catheter placement. *J Clin Anesth* 2001; **13**: 131–2.

7   Wood KE, Reedy JS, Pozniak MA, Coursin DB. Phlegmasia cerulea dolens with compartment syndrome: a complication of femoral vein catheterization. *Crit Care Med* 2000; **28**: 1626–30.

8   Farrell K, Walshe J, Gellens M, Martin KJ. Complications associated with insertion of jugular venous catheters for hemodialysis: the value of postprocedural radiograph. *Am J Kidney Dis* 1997; **30**: 690–2.

9   Denys BG, Uretsky BF. Anatomical variations of internal jugular vein location: Impact on central venous access. *Crit Care Med* 1991; **19**: 1516–19.

10 Gibson KD, Gillen DL, Kohler TR, *et al*. Vascular access survival and incidence of revisions: A comparison of prosthetic grafts, simple autogenous fistulas, and venous transposition fistulas from the United States Renal Data System Dialysis Morbidity and Mortality Study. *J Vasc Surg* 2001; **34**: 694–700.

11 Schwartz CI, McBrayer CV, Sloan JH, *et al*. Thrombosed dialysis graphs: comparison of treatment with transluminal angioplasty and surgical revision. *Radiology* 1995; **194**: 337–41.

12 Beathard GA. Thrombolysis versus surgery for the treatment of thrombosed dialysis access grafts. *J Am Soc Nephrol* 1995; **6**: 1619–24.

13 Cameron LJ. *Current Surgical Therapy*, 6th edn. Vascular Access, 833–7.

14 McIntyre AS, Levison RA, Wood S, *et al*. Duplex Doppler ultrasound identifies veins suitable for insertion of central feeding catheters. *J Parenter Enteral Nutr* 1992; **16**: 264–7.

15 Funaki B, Zaleski GX, Leef JA, *et al*. Radiologic placement of tunneled hemodialysis catheters in occluded neck, chest, or small thyrocervical collateral veins in central venous occlusion. *Ann Emerg Med* 1999; **34**: 711–14.

16 Sadler DJ, Gordon AC, Klassen J, *et al*. Image-guided central venous catheters for apheresis. *Bone Marrow Transplant* 1999; **23**: 179–82.

17 Hatfield A., Bodenham A. Portable ultrasound for difficult central venous access. *Br J Anaesth* 1999; **83**: 964.

18 Farrell J, Gellens M. Ultrasound guided cannulation versus the landmark-guided technique for acute haemodialysis access. *Nephrol Dial Transplant* 1997; **12**: 1234–7.

19 Kwon TH, Kim YL, Cho DK. Ultrasound guided cannulation of the femoral vein for acute haemodialysis access. *Nephrol Dial Transplant* 1997; **12**: 1009–12.

20 Taylor BS, Rhee RY, Muluk S, *et al*. Thrombin injection versus compression of femoral artery pseudoaneurysms. *J Vasc Surg* 1999; **30**: 1052–9.

21 Eisenberg L, Paulson EK, Kliewer MA, *et al*. Sonographically guided compression repair of pseudoaneurysms: further experience from a single institution. *AJR Am J Roentgenol* 2000; **174**: 1788–9.

22 Loesberg A, Taylor FC, Awh MH. Dislodgment of inferior vena caval filters during 'blind' insertion of central venous catheters. *AJR Am J Roentgenol* 1993; **161**: 637–8.

23 Granke K, Abraham FM, McDowell DE. Vena cava filter disruption and central migration due to accidental guide-wire manipulation: a case report. *Ann Vasc Surg* 1996; **10**: 49–53.

24 Marelich GP, Tharratt RS. Greenfield inferior vena cava filter dislodged during central venous catheter placement. *Chest* 1994; **106**: 957–9.

25 Ellis PK, Deutsch LS, Kidney DD. Interventional radiological retrieval of a guide-wire entrapped in a greenfield filter – treatment of an avoidable complication of central venous access procedure. *Clin Radiol* 2000; **55**: 238–9.

26 Uppot RN, Garcia M, Gheyi V, *et al*. Entanglement of guide wires by vena cava filters during central venous catheter insertion: report of three cases and a review of the literature. *Del Med J* 2000; **72**: 69–73.

27 Wendt RJ. Cannulation of the right internal jugular vein is preferable to that of the left internal jugular vein. *JAMA* 1986; **255**: 1140.

28 Rello J, Campistol JM, Almirall J, Revert LI. Vascular access for haemodialysis. *Lancet* 1989; **i**: 379.

29 Akazawa S, Nakaigawa Y, Hotta K, *et al*. Unrecognized migration of an entire guide-wire on insertion of a central venous catheter into the cardiovascular system. *Anesthesiology* 1996; **84**: 241–2.

30 Beenen L, van Leusen R, Deenik B, Bosch FH. The Incidence of subclavian vein stenosis using silicone catheters for hemodialysis. *Artificial Organs* 1993; **18**: 289–92.

31 Schillinger F, Schilleinger D, Montagnag R, Milcent T. Post catheterization vein stenosis in haemodialysis: comparative angiographic study of 50 subclavian and 50 internal jugular accesses. *Nephrol Dial Transplant* 1991; **6**: 722–4.

Imaging for Vascular Emergencies

PETER K ELLIS, BARRY KELLY, PETER KENNEDY, PAUL HB BLAIR

INTRODUCTION

Vascular imaging techniques have improved significantly in the past decade and a wide range of invasive and non-invasive modalities are now available to the clinician. It should be remembered that when dealing with vascular emergencies, time is of critical importance in preventing life-threatening haemorrhage and restoring vascular continuity and tissue perfusion. Although there has been an overall reduction in the time required to obtain high quality images, significant delays during investigations still occur which may have a disastrous consequence for the patient. Liberal use of radiological investigations is never a substitute for good clinical acumen. A careful history and detailed examination should facilitate selection of the appropriate imaging technique.

In certain situations, unstable patients in the accident and emergency department benefit from direct transfer to the operating room for life- or limb-saving surgery. Recent developments in endovascular surgery have improved the quality and range of imaging techniques available in the operating room for such patients.

Alternatively, following diagnostic imaging, some patients may benefit from radiological intervention such as vessel embolisation or stent placement. In this situation it is important that patients are monitored appropriately in the imaging suite while retaining easy access for possible anaesthetic and surgical intervention. A patient presenting with a vascular emergency is best served by the early involvement of both a senior vascular surgeon and radiologist. In addition to established skills in performing complex interventional procedures an experienced radiologist can often detect subtle signs from initial plain films or non-invasive tests. Similarly, during an evolving vascular emergency, the presence of an experienced vascular surgeon will help in establishing priorities, particularly if an imaging procedure has to be abandoned and the patient taken to the operating theatre expeditiously.

As a result of recent endovascular developments, some centres have excellent imaging facilities in the operating theatre. This can reduce delays and facilitate endovascular intervention.

It is important that a good working relationship is maintained between vascular surgeons and radiologists and that multidisciplinary guidelines based on local resources and clinical expertise are agreed and implemented in the management of vascular emergencies.

This chapter provides a broad overview of the range of imaging techniques available in managing vascular emergencies. The advantages and disadvantages of imaging techniques in specific anatomical areas are discussed. Individual authors outline their preferred imaging techniques in managing specific vascular emergencies in the relevant chapters of this volume.

VASCULAR IMAGING TECHNIQUES

Digital subtraction angiography

The modern angiographic suite is equipped with a large diameter image intensifier which offers excellent real time fluoroscopic image quality with a minimised radiation dose. Many strategies are employed to keep the radiation dose to the operator to a minimum such as pulsed fluoroscopy, last image hold, undertable lead curtains and ceiling hung lead glass which can be positioned optimally for each acquisition. The suite will often provide an operating theatre environment with at least 20 air exchanges per hour, quality floor and wall coverings and a minimum of horizontal surfaces. Image acquisition can be achieved at high frame rates, typically up to 12 frames per second with a 1024 matrix. Postprocessing tools such as automatic pixel shift, rewindow and remask will often enable diagnostic images to be retrieved from series acquisition even following significant patient movement. An example of a peripheral leg run-off study is shown in Fig. 8.1a.

Duplex ultrasound

Duplex ultrasonography is the combination of grey scale ultrasound imaging with Doppler sonography allowing an evaluation of vessel morphology and blood flow characteristics. The technique is particularly useful in the diagnosis of carotid artery disease and deep vein thrombosis (DVT). The modality is somewhat operator dependent, however,

and some detailed vascular studies can be time consuming, thus limiting its role in emergency situations. Its advantages include the lack of ionising radiation, the relatively low cost of equipment and its mobility. The recent development of small portable scanners is likely to increase the role of emergency duplex sonography.

Computed tomography

Computed tomography (CT) is widely available and in the context of vascular imaging is relatively easy to carry out and to interpret. Imaging is performed in the arterial phase following intravenous injection of contrast (approximately 20–50 seconds). Multiplanar reconstruction and various display techniques such as surface shaded display and maximum intensity projection provide different formats with which to view the acquired data. Computed tomography

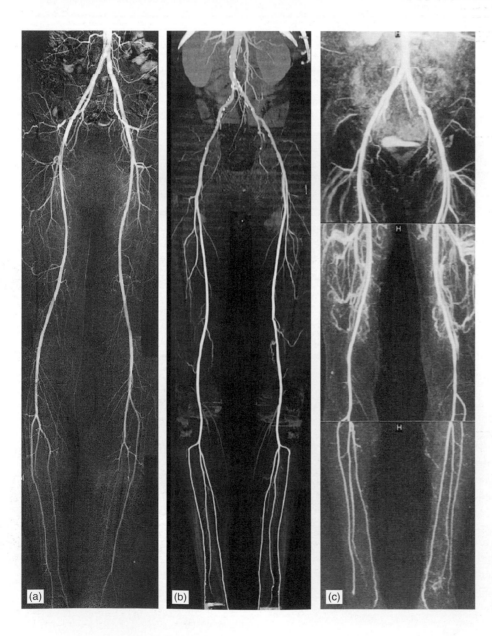

Figure 8.1 *Normal lower limb angiogram: (a) digital subtraction angiogram, (b) computed tomography angiogram and (c) magnetic resonance angiogram*

provides superb contrast resolution and visualisation of adjacent non-vascular structures thus giving a multisystem evaluation from one acquisition and is particularly useful in the evaluation of a trauma patient. The development of multislice technology has further expanded the indications for CT angiography (CTA) as accurate images of run-off vessels (Fig. 8.1b) are now also available with the advantages of reduced examination time, reduced contrast load and increased contrast and spatial resolution.[1] There is a radiation dose penalty but advances in detector technology have minimised this disadvantage. The occasional drawbacks are the requirement for long and cumbersome post-processing and the presence of calcified plaques which further complicate the evaluation.[2]

Magnetic resonance angiography

Magnetic resonance imaging (MRI) has some drawbacks in the acute setting: emergency access is limited in many institutions due to a large scheduled workload; it may be difficult to determine the presence of any contraindications to imaging for each patient; transfer of the intubated patient into the magnetic field requires MRI compatible anaesthetic equipment.[3] Intravenous injection of gadolinium-based contrast reduces the T1 value of blood so that short TR (time of repetition) imaging results in high signal from the blood, providing excellent contrast resolution.[4] Most sequences used are three-dimensional gradient recalled echo techniques with heavy T1 weighting. Low TR values ensure suppression of background structures, while high intra-arterial concentration of contrast material ensures good vessel-to-background contrast.[5] Short imaging sequences obtained during a single breath-hold minimise respiratory artefact. The use of contrast to directly image the blood avoids the limitations encountered when the imaging signal is derived from blood flow, such as long imaging times, in-plane saturation effects and loss of signal at sites of stenosis due to turbulent flow.[6] This last limitation often results in an overestimation of the degree of vessel stenosis, although the presence of occlusion is detected very accurately by both methods. When higher doses of gadolinium are used results can match those of intra-arterial digital subtraction angiography (DSA), even for the clinically important stenoses of 70–99 per cent.[7]

Additional techniques are being developed constantly to improve image quality. Several authors have reported the value of image subtraction, comparable to DSA, in which an image is obtained immediately before administration of gadolinium and used as a mask image to subtract from that obtained after gadolinium is injected (Fig. 8.1c). Thus background tissues, in particular fat, are removed and as a result the quality of the image is improved.[8] Magnetic resonance angiography (MRA) has replaced invasive preoperative imaging in many centres, and it has been used as the imaging modality for planning endovascular interventions.[9]

IMAGING IN SPECIFIC VASCULAR TERRITORIES

Head and neck

The gold standard technique for imaging the carotid and vertebral arteries is selective angiography. The most important complication of cerebral angiography is stroke occurring as a result of emboli dislodged from atherosclerotic plaques or the accidental injection of thrombus or air. The incidence of permanent cerebral ischaemic episodes is approximately 0.5 per cent.[10] Other complications include vessel dissection and puncture site haematoma.

Duplex ultrasonography of the extracranial carotid arteries provides exquisite images of the carotid bifurcation but falls short in the evaluation of high internal carotid artery lesions and in characterising very high grade stenoses. Recent advances in MRA have resulted in high quality, high resolution, non-invasive imaging which is likely to replace catheter directed angiography.

Imaging of thoracic vessels

The thoracic aorta can be studied using a catheter passed to the level of the ascending aorta. Several images per second should be obtained using a number of radiographic projections, in particular the steep right posterior oblique which unfolds the aortic arch and the great vessels best (Fig. 8.2). Complications (1–3 per cent) are rare and are most

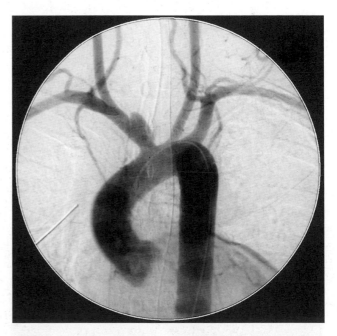

Figure 8.2 *Flush arch angiogram in right posterior oblique projection demonstrating the aortic arch and origins of great vessels in a patient with blunt chest trauma. There is a pseudoaneurysm indicating injury of the proximal innominate artery*

commonly seen at the puncture site. Others include arterial dissection, embolisation resulting in cerebral ischaemia and major artery thrombosis. In general terms, inexperience on the part of the operator and prolonged procedure times compound the risk of complications.

Transoesophageal echocardiography (TOE) in the management of the critically injured patient is of value in detecting possible injury to the thoracic aorta and in excluding the presence of blood in the pericardial sac. This is a particularly useful investigation in unstable patients in the operating room or intensive care unit who cannot be transported to the radiology suite.

Spiral CT images, derived during the pulmonary arterial phase in a single breath-hold following the administration of intravenous contrast, have been shown to be useful in the diagnosis of pulmonary embolism.[11] The options for reconstruction and display, and the more rapid imaging afforded by multislice scanning, will no doubt increase the utility of this modality in coming years. Magnetic resonance imaging can also be used to visualise the pulmonary arteries, (Fig. 8.3) and, in addition, MR velocity mapping can confirm reverse diastolic flow in patients with pulmonary hypertension.

Pulmonary angiography today is a safe and simple procedure and is still considered the gold standard for imaging these vessels. Access is usually obtained via a femoral vein although the jugular or brachial routes are alternatives. Complications are rare and usually involve cardiac arrhythmias while the catheter is within the heart. Acute cor pulmonale may occur in patients with pulmonary

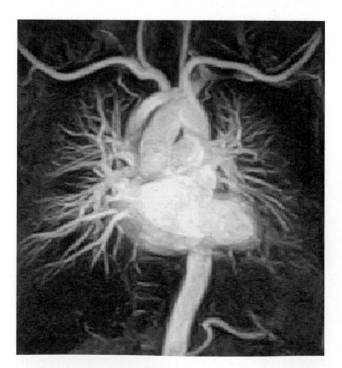

Figure 8.3 *Three-dimensional gadolinium-enhanced magnetic resonance angiogram of the chest demonstrating pulmonary and systemic vessels (courtesy of Siemens Medical Imaging)*

hypertension but the overall mortality from this complication is around 0.3 per cent.

Abdominal aorta

Where possible angiography of the aorta is performed via a transfemoral approach, although in the situation of aortic stenosis or occlusion a 4 Fr catheter placed via the brachial or axillary artery is effective. In current practice direct translumbar aortography is very rarely performed.

Volumetric CT scanning is the most commonly used technique in the evaluation of aortic aneurysms as it provides accurate information concerning the size of the aneurysm and in cases of rupture by demonstrating with high sensitivity the presence of retroperitoneal haemorrhage. The use of multiplanar reconstruction allows accurate measurement of aneurysm dimensions essential in planning for aortic stent grafting.

In the assessment of aortic aneurysms MR imaging can provide excellent depiction without the requirement for iodinated contrast, again multiplanar reformatting is possible providing advantages similar to those with CT scanning. Ultrasound is useful particularly in screening for aortic aneurysms; its sensitivity in the detection of retroperitoneal haemorrhage, however, is significantly less than that of CT scanning. The use of Doppler ultrasound, particularly when combined with ultrasound contrast agents, has been shown to be extremely sensitive in the detection of endoleaks post-aortic stent grafting.[12]

Renal arteries

The renal arteries can be assessed angiographically by the placement of a flush catheter within the aorta just above their origins. More than one view is normally obtained as renal arteries have a variable site of origin from the aortic wall. Carbon dioxide is a useful adjunct to the procedure in a setting in which the patient has renal impairment and where radiographic contrast is relatively contraindicated.

Contrast-enhanced MRA now offers an alternative. Early sequences using time-of-flight (TOF) methods or phased-contrast techniques were unfortunately limited by poor spatial resolution and in-plane flow saturation. Three-dimensional acquisitions using gadolinium enhancement with a single breath-hold overcome these problems and allow satisfactory imaging in most instances (Fig. 8.4). Sensitivities of 95–100 per cent have been regularly reported.[13]

Visceral aortic branches

Angiography is still the gold standard for assessment of the coeliac axis and mesenteric arteries. Vessel origins are best displayed using a lateral or lateral oblique projection of a flush aortogram. Selective injections can be undertaken, particularly when looking for distal pathology such as acute bleeding (Fig. 8.5). A variety of precurved catheters are available for this purpose and the optimal choice will depend on the configuration of a vessel. Very distal positions within the mesenteric or coeliac territories can be achieved using coaxial catheters where, for example, a 3 Fr catheter is passed through the lumen of the 4 or 5 Fr catheter placed in the origin of the vessel. This technique is particularly useful where acute distal bleeding points are identified in various settings: trauma, acute gastrointestinal haemorrhage and wherever embolisation is contemplated.

Doppler ultrasound can be used to assess the volume of flow in the superior mesenteric artery by measuring the luminal area and the mean velocity of flow. In general, the waveform in this vessel demonstrates high impedance flow with reversal of flow in diastole. Doppler ultrasound is particularly useful in the assessment of the portal vein, angiographic definition of which is generally achieved indirectly. It is also useful in the assessment of hepatic arterial flow volumes and in liver transplantation where stenosis of the hepatic arterial anastomosis can lead to loss of the graft.

Computed tomography arteriography is also useful and the various methods of image reconstruction described above can be used to demonstrate very adequately the proximal branches of the superior mesenteric artery and coeliac axis. Distal active bleeding points can also be detected as a blush of contrast extravasation. Mesenteric occlusive disease can also be assessed using MR angiography. A single breath-hold, three-dimensional gradient echo sequence using intravenous gadolinium can be used to avoid the artefacts produced using older techniques. In addition, real time imaging of up to 20 images per second can be achieved.[14] Quantification of blood flow is also achievable using several MR techniques.

Pelvic imaging

Haemorrhage is a common complication of pelvic trauma. Computed tomography can very adequately delineate pelvic haematoma and with dynamic scanning extravasation of contrast will point to an arterial bleeding source. Frequently CT fails to show the exact source of bleeding but that objective is best achieved using arteriography. Flush angiography from a site just above the aortic bifurcation will frequently demonstrate an actively bleeding source in the pelvic vessels (Fig. 8.6). Should that fail, selective

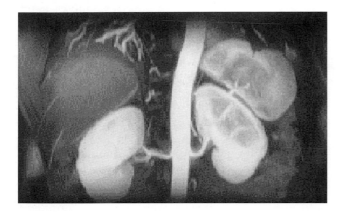

Figure 8.4 *Three-dimensional gadolinium-enhanced magnetic resonance angiogram of renal arteries (courtesy of Siemens Medical Imaging)*

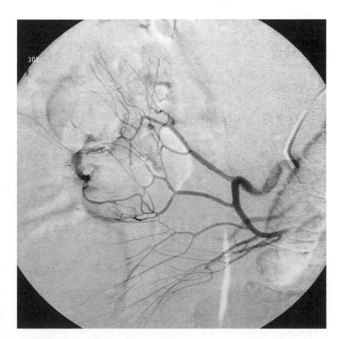

Figure 8.5 *Selective arteriogram of distal jejunal arcade in a patient with acute gastrointestinal haemorrhage. Note active extravasation from a jejunal bleeding point*

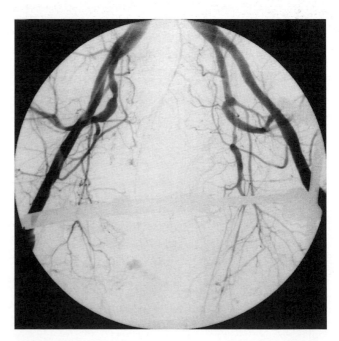

Figure 8.6 *Flush arteriogram in a patient with multiple pelvic fractures. Note extravasation from an actively bleeding right obturator artery*

injection, particularly of both internal iliac arteries, will be helpful using a variety of precurved catheters. This should allow identification of bleeding sites and subsequently haemorrhage control by transcatheter embolisation using a variety of embolic materials.[15]

The decision to attempt pelvic embolisation can be extremely difficult and requires an informed discussion between the clinicians involved. It is important to exclude other sources of abdominal haemorrhage and to achieve some form of pelvic bony stability before embarking on attempts at embolisation.

Lower limb vessels

The imaging gold standard for the assessment of lower limb arteries is probably angiography (Fig. 8.7). A non-invasive method of assessment is duplex ultrasonography. This technique is time consuming and requires considerable experience, but it has a sensitivity and specificity exceeding 90 per cent in the detection of arterial lesions.[16]

A wide variety of MR angiographic pulse sequences can be used to demonstrate adequate blood flow. Two-dimensional time-of-flight imaging (with saturation banding) can be employed to detect flow in a single direction but it normally takes a relatively long time and currently gadolinium-enhanced three-dimensional angiography is preferred in many centres. The latter technique, however, demands the exact timing of contrast enhancement and a moving table is also necessary. Magnetic resonance angiography may well replace catheter directed angiography but to do that it must

provide equivalent, if not superior, diagnostic information. Studies have shown comparable, or in some cases, slightly better visualisation of distal vessel patency using MR angiography.[17]

Upper extremity

Angiographic studies of the upper extremity are normally performed via a transfemoral approach. Injection in the aortic arch is necessary for the evaluation of the origins of the subclavian arteries. In order to visualise the more distal vasculature, selective catheterisation of the artery and its branches can be carried out. Direct catheterisation is associated with a higher complication rate.

The distal vasculature of the upper extremity, superficially located as it is, is eminently suited to Doppler ultrasound examination. The peripheral arteries of the arm show the same triphasic pattern as the lower extremity arteries. Magnetic resonance angiography using various techniques can provide excellent images of the upper extremity, including detailed angiography of the hand and wrist. In addition, in the diagnosis of thoracic outlet syndrome, MRI offers the capability of providing angiographic imaging as well as useful anatomical detail of cervical ribs or bands and the associated deviation or distortion of the brachial plexus and subclavian artery.

VENOUS IMAGING

Lower limb deep venous thrombosis

The two commonly used imaging methods for identifying lower limb DVT are ascending venography and ultrasound.

Ascending venography

Ascending venography is a method of delineating the venous anatomy of a territory by opacifying the vessels with iodinated contrast, typically a low osmolar water-soluble contrast agent. After placing a tourniquet around the ankle, a vein on the dorsum of the foot is cannulated with a 21 gauge needle and a further tourniquet is placed above the level of the knee. The function of both tourniquets is to divert venous return from the superficial veins into the deep veins so as to opacify them with contrast.

The patient is placed on a tilting fluoroscopic table and 50 mL of contrast is injected. Fluoroscopic imaging of the leg is performed from the level of the ankle joint, through the knee, thigh and then the pelvis. The progress of the contrast is screened and 'spot-films' are taken; in normal circumstances the veins opacify uniformly. When veins are

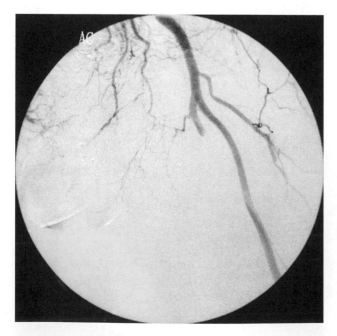

Figure 8.7 *Arteriogram of the left femoral arteries. Note abrupt 'cut-off' of the profunda femoris artery due to transection by a bullet*

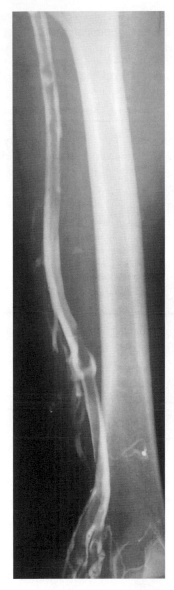

Figure 8.8 *Leg venogram: thrombus within the femoral vein*

thrombosed a small track of contrast is seen at the margins of the vessel while the central thrombosed section of the vessel remains unopacified, an appearance which is termed 'tramlining' (Fig. 8.8).

As a rule the imaging proceeds cranially to the level of the iliac vein and the lower part of the inferior vena cava. Streaming of contrast at the level of the iliac vein can reduce resolution and therefore a key observation in the diagnosis of iliac thrombosis is the demonstration of an extensive collateral network from the affected side across to the contralateral normal side as small venous channels enlarge to permit venous drainage.

Contrast ascending venography is still recognised as the gold standard for obtaining images of lower limb DVT but it requires patient exposure to ionising radiation in addition to intravenous injection of iodinated contrast. Consequently,

ultrasound is now routinely used as the primary imaging method for suspected DVT.

Ultrasound venography

Ultrasound imaging utilises the production of high frequency sound waves, typically of megahertz frequency, to identify tissue planes spatially within the body. Ultrasound is particularly effective in the evaluation of non-osseous, non-gaseous soft tissues and also fluid-filled structures. These attributes render it particularly effective in the evaluation of venous anatomy. A piezoelectric crystal is used to generate the sound waves and the image generated can be displayed on a television monitor, providing a two-dimensional view of the veins: this is known as real time or B-mode sonography. Not only can the physical dimensions of veins be estimated but, using the principle of Doppler ultrasound, information on the presence, speed, and direction of blood flow can also be derived.

The Doppler principle utilises red blood cells as reflectors of pulses of sound waves emitted and received by the ultrasound probe. The blood's speed and direction can be encoded as either a spectral trace or a colour image. In the latter case the colour denotes the direction of blood flow away from or towards the probe and the hue and brightness correspond to the speed of the flow. Absence of colour-coded flow or persistent underfilling of a venous segment with isoechoic or echogenic thrombus is clear evidence of thrombus.[18]

The combination of the real time image and spectral trace or colour map represents duplex ultrasound and all three appearing on the same image is known as triplex ultrasound.

Ultrasound imaging in deep venous thrombosis

Essentially, two components are incorporated in the ultrasound evaluation of the lower limb with DVT. The first of these is venous compression, and the second, a series of adjunctive manoeuvres to provide supplementary information based on the phasic flow of blood in the veins.

VEIN COMPRESSIBILITY

When the soft tissues overlying normal healthy veins are compressed with an ultrasound probe, their thin walls are brought together obliterating the vein lumen completely. The walls of an artery, however, being more muscular, cannot be easily compressed, which is a useful differentiating feature.

In the presence of thrombosis the vein lumen will not compress fully (Fig. 8.9), and this failure is an important finding. Although established thrombus is echogenic and easily visualised, a recent thrombus may be sonolucent, i.e. black, and, on real time ultrasound examination, may be indistinguishable from normal sonolucent blood within a vein. The normal vein is, of course, easily compressible.

Imaging begins at the level of the groin. Three vessels, the long saphenous vein, common femoral vein and common femoral artery are identified as three black overlapping circles (Fig. 8.10). This makes a convenient reference point. The two veins should compress freely but the artery will not.[19] Transverse compression is therefore applied from the level of the groin to the knee at 1 cm intervals. Cranial to the level of the knee joint, the femoral vessels enter the adductor canal and move posteriorly. Direct compression in this area can be problematic. It may be necessary to turn the patient into the decubitus or erect

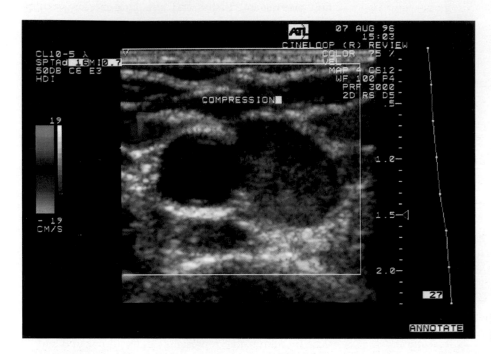

Figure 8.9 *Transverse ultrasound of groin: deep venous thrombosis*

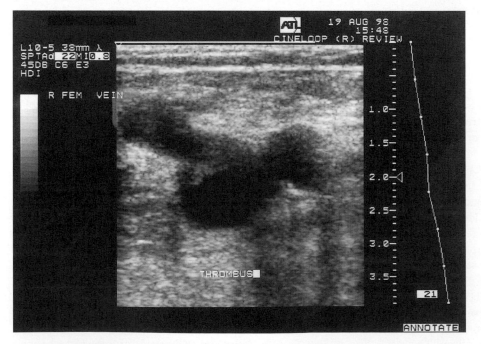

Figure 8.10 *Transverse ultrasound image of groin: normal vascular structures*

position to evaluate the venous segments in the adductor canal and indeed the popliteal fossa.

The sensitivity for diagnosing venous thrombus from the popliteal venous level upwards is of the order of 98 per cent.[20] Studies have demonstrated that the sensitivity falls below popliteal level and therefore calf veins are not often formally evaluated with ultrasound. Currently there is significant inter-physician variability on the treatment algorithm for infrapopliteal DVT and, in addition, because of the lack of ionising radiation, it is perfectly feasible to perform serial ultrasound examinations of the lower limb to exclude the possibility of thrombus propagation extending from the calf into the popliteal veins.[21]

SUPPLEMENTARY ULTRASOUND TECHNIQUES

Unlike the pulsatile arterial system, flow within the venous system is phasic, i.e. flow which varies with the phases of respiration. This phasic flow can be observed by imaging a venous segment and using Doppler ultrasound to identify either colour or spectral frequency changes as the patient breathes normally.

Clearly, if cessation of normal phasic activity can be demonstrated, for example, by asking the patient to breath-hold, this will demonstrate that there is no obstruction to normal venous return between the area being evaluated, e.g. the groin, and the right side of the heart. It is therefore possible to indirectly ascertain whether or not there is occlusion of the inferior vena cava and iliac veins. In addition, if the patient actively increases intra-abdominal pressure, e.g. with a Valsalva manoeuvre, further proof is provided that there is no venous obstruction or thrombosis proximally.

When the deep veins are imaged between the femoral and popliteal levels and the calf is squeezed distally by the sonologist, blood is propelled forward in a cephalad direction. This sudden relatively high velocity venous blood is detectable again either by using colour flow or spectral Doppler. Confirming a normal calf squeeze response indicates that there is a patent venous system distal to the point of the ultrasound probe. The inclusion of the calf squeeze and Valsalva manoeuvres allows the complete evaluation of the venous system from the level of the calf veins to the inferior vena cava.

Venous thrombosis in the upper limbs

ISOLATED ARM VEIN THROMBOSIS

Once again the same imaging methods are used. With contrast venography, a tourniquet is placed at the level of the elbow to occlude the superficial cephalic vein and allow the contrast to be directed preferentially through the deeper upper limb veins. With Doppler sonography, compressibility,

augmented by demonstration of phasic flow, will exclude significant thrombus.

CENTRAL AND CAVAL THROMBUS

In a significant number of cases thrombosis of the superior vena cava and brachiocephalic veins is associated with sinister underlying pathology. Lymphadenopathy and neoplasia, particularly bronchogenic carcinoma and lymphoma should be excluded. Formal evaluation of the frontal chest radiograph is essential to ensure that the mediastinal contours are normal.

When the superior vena cava and the brachiocephalic veins are being evaluated, ultrasound has only a very limited role. The imaging method of choice is contrast venography. To opacify the brachiocephalic veins and the superior vena cava, synchronous injections of contrast are performed by simultaneously injecting 50 mL of water-soluble contrast medium through 21 gauge needles positioned at the level of the elbow. Fluoroscopic evaluation of the veins is then performed and spot images taken.

Cross-sectional imaging in central venous thrombosis

COMPUTED TOMOGRAPHY

Computed tomography is very accurate at identifying mediastinal masses which are causing compression or effacement of the superior vena cava. Low attenuation within the SVC, however, can result from the mixing of contrast enhanced blood draining from the arm which has been cannulated, and unopacified blood from the contralateral limb. This artefact can be mistaken in normal individuals for thrombus. The presence of delayed or collateral venous filling provides further evidence of central thrombus. Computed tomography also has the added advantage in that if an associated underlying malignancy is present, it can be accurately staged simultaneously.[22]

Helical and multidetector CT angiography enable volumetric acquisition of data in a single breath-hold and this reduces motion artefact and respiratory misregistration, improving accuracy of detection of venous thrombosis.[23]

MAGNETIC RESONANCE ANGIOGRAPHY

Magnetic resonance angiography has an increasing role in the first line investigation of vascular pathology – MR has the advantages of multiplanar imaging and does not use ionising radiation. Like CT, MRA can also delineate the underlying aetiological process.

Magnetic resonance venography may also permit the assessment of vascular flow patterns and thereby determine the evolution of thromboembolic events.[24]

Conclusions

Imaging of vascular disease continues to evolve. Increasingly non-invasive alternatives to percutaneous angiographic and venographic techniques such as duplex ultrasound, CT and MRI are used in the management of vascular emergencies and are gaining acceptance in most vascular centres. It is likely that these imaging modalities will eventually replace invasive diagnostic imaging, the latter being largely reserved for therapeutic intervention. The principles, advantages and drawbacks of these techniques when applied to specific anatomical areas have to be considered. In addition, the field of vascular radiology is evolving and now exercises a rapidly expanding therapeutic role. Continued innovation can only be of benefit to patients and those involved in the treatment of vascular diseases.

Key references

Baum RA, Rutter CM, Sunshine JH, et al. Multicenter trial to evaluate magnetic resonance angiography of the lower extremity. JAMA 1995; 174: 875–80.

Baxter GM. The role of ultrasound in deep venous thrombosis. Clin Radiol 1997; 52: 1–3.

Miller N, Satin R, Tousignant L, Sheiner NM. A prospective study comparing duplex scan and venography for the diagnosis of lower-extremity deep venous thrombosis. Cardiovasc Surg 1996; 4: 505–8.

Prokop M. Multislice CT angiography. Eur J Radiol 2000; 36: 86–96.

Remy-Jardin M, Remy J, Wattine L, et al. Central pulmonary thromboembolism: diagnosis with spiral volumetric CT with single breathhold technique – comparison with pulmonary angiography. Radiology 1992; 185: 381–7.

REFERENCES

1　Rubin GD, Shiau MC, Leung AN, et al. Aorta and iliac arteries: single versus multiple detector-row helical CT angiography. Radiology 2000; 215: 670–6.

2　Prokop M. Multislice CT angiography. Eur J Radiol 2000; 36: 86–96.

3　Chaljub G, Kramer LA, Johnston RF, et al. Projectile cylinder accidents resulting from the presence of ferromagnetic nitrous oxide or oxygen tanks in the MR suite. AJR Am J Roentgenol 2001; 177: 27–30.

4　Prince MR. Contrast-enhanced MR angiography: theory and optimization. Magn Reson Imaging Clin N Am 1998; 6: 257–67.

5　Ho KY, Leiner T, de Haan MW, van Engelshoven JM. Peripheral MR angiography. Eur Radiol 1999; 9: 1765–74.

6　Mitsuzaki K, Yamashita Y, Sakaguchi T, et al. Abdomen, pelvis and extremities: diagnostic contrast-enhanced turbo MR angiography compared with conventional angiography – initial experience. Radiology 2000; 216: 909–15.

7　Loewe C, Schoder M, Rand T, et al. Peripheral vascular occlusive disease: evaluation with contrast-enhanced moving-bed MR angiography versus digital subtraction angiography in 106 patients. Am J Roentgenol 2002; 179: 1013–21.

8　Ho KYJAM, Haan MW de, Kessels AGH, et al. Peripheral vascular tree stenoses: detection with subtracted and nonsubtracted MR angiography. Radiology 1998; 206: 673–81.

9　Mistretta CA. Relative characteristics of MR angiography and competing vascular imaging modalities. J Magn Reson Imag 1993; 3: 685–98.

10　Willinsky RA, Taylor SM, terBrugge BAK, et al. Neurologic complications of cerebral angiography: prospective analysis of 2899 procedures and review of the literature. Radiology 2003; 227: 522–8.

11　Remy-Jardin M, Remy J, Wattine L, et al. Central pulmonary thromboembolism: diagnosis with spiral volumetric CT with single breathhold technique – comparison with pulmonary angiography. Radiology 1992; 185: 381–7.

12　McWilliams RG, Martin J, White D, et al. Use of contrast-enhanced ultrasound in follow up after endovascular aortic aneurysm repair. J Vasc Interv Radiol 1999; 10: 1107–14.

13　Bakker J, Beek FJ, Beutler JJ, et al. Renal artery stenosis and accessory renal arteries: accuracy of detection and visualisation with gadolinium enhanced breath-hold MR angiography. Radiology 1998; 207: 497–504.

14　Kerr AB, Pauly JM, Hu BS, et al. Real-time interactive MRI on a conventional scanner. Magn Reson Med 1997; 38: 355–67.

15　Ayella RJ, DuPriest RW Jr, Khanega SC, et al. Transcatheter embolisation of autologous clot in the management of bleeding associated with fractures of the pelvis. Surg Gynecol Obstet 1978; 147: 849.

16　Cossman DV, Ellison JE, Wagner JH, et al. Comparison of contrast arteriography to arterial mapping with colour-flow duplex imaging in the lower extremities. J Vasc Surg 1989; 10: 522–9.

17　Baum RA, Rutter CM, Sunshine JH, et al. Multicenter trial to evaluate magnetic resonance angiography of the lower extremity. JAMA 1995; 174: 875–80.

18　Baxter GM. The role of ultrasound in deep venous thrombosis. Clin Radiol 1997; 52: 1–3.

19　Kelly BE, McArdle CS. Imaging the Acutely Ill Patient: A Clinician's Guide. London: WB Saunders, 2001; 112–15.

20　Miller N, Satin R, Tousignant L, Sheiner NM. A prospective study comparing duplex scan and venography for the diagnosis of lower-extremity deep venous thrombosis. Cardiovasc Surg 1996; 4: 505–8.

21　Baud JM, Stephas L, Ribadeau-Dumas C, et al. Short and medium term duplex sonography follow up of deep venous thrombosis of the lower limbs. J Clin Ultrasound 1998; 26: 7–13.

22　Webb WR, Brant WE, Helms CA. Fundamentals of Body CT, 2nd edn. Philadelphia: WB Saunders, 1998: 35–7.

23　Bradbury MS, Kavanagh PV, Bechtold RE, et al. Mesenteric venous thrombosis: diagnosis and non-invasive imaging. Radiographics 2002; 22: 527–41.

24　Butty S, Hagspiel KD, Leung DA, et al. Body MR venography. Radiol Clin North Am 2002; 40: 899–919.

Outcomes of Emergency Vascular Procedures.
A View from the British Isles

JONOTHAN J EARNSHAW

INTRODUCTION

The results of elective arterial procedures are well documented, but that is not the case in emergency vascular surgery. Yet, out-of-hours operating constitutes a large proportion of the workload of a vascular surgeon, in contrast to the other specialties grouped under 'general surgery'. Reports are sparse because the data are harder to collect. It is generally believed that the outcome from emergency arterial surgery is worse than for elective operation which might explain the natural reluctance to detail those results. Much of the emergency surgery in the UK and Ireland used to be performed by trainees, though this is changing as a result of recent training reforms.

Arterial surgery falls into three broad categories: carotid disease, which is seldom performed urgently, aortic aneurysms, where up to 50 per cent of the workload of an individual unit may include urgent or ruptured aneurysms, and the management of leg ischaemia, the traumatic causes of which will not be discussed here. The management of acute leg ischaemia represents one of the most difficult challenges for a vascular surgeon. Management decisions are complex and treatment selection can significantly affect outcome, which is often poor, with high amputation and mortality rates. Although a large proportion of vascular operations are performed out of hours, it is often possible to avoid doing so under emergency conditions. Only true ruptured aortic aneurysms and acute total leg ischaemia demand immediate intervention; other conditions may permit a period of observation and semi-elective surgery. Although this sounds attractive and suggests that a vascular

surgeon may plan to deal with urgent operations in daylight hours, the fact is that they often have to be squeezed into a schedule that is already busy. In many hospitals where the vascular services are under pressure, it could be argued that emergency patients receive less than ideal care.

In the UK, arrangements for the care of vascular patients remain varied. Increasingly vascular surgeons are gathering into major units where 24-hour cover is offered with on-call specialist staff. This has only been possible in large conurbations with populations of over 600 000, where four or five surgeons can manage an on-call rota. Other models, including cross-cover between adjacent units, have enabled an increasing number of vascular on-call rotas.[1] This does mean that a patient with a vascular emergency may need to travel some distance for specialist treatment. For most vascular patients, the delay is immaterial; indeed several studies have suggested that even for those with a ruptured aortic aneurysm, there is no correlation between distance travelled to hospital and outcome.[2] Many surgeons believe that this is a process of natural selection, because only those likely to survive the operation survive the journey.

There is some evidence that the outcome of vascular surgery is better when carried out by a specialist, particularly for acute leg ischemia, the results of which improved with the establishment of a regional vascular unit.[3] In the UK, there remain a number of units with insufficient surgeons to man an on-call vascular rota. Although most elective arterial operations in the UK are performed by trained vascular surgeons, the arrangements for emergency cover are variable. In some hospitals, dedicated vascular surgeons provide *ad hoc* cover, but in others, general surgeons provide emergency care. As might be expected this can exaggerate the variation in the outcome from emergency vascular surgery, though this may not simply be the result of surgical skill. In a study from Wales, the outcome of patients with a ruptured aneurysm was similar if they had surgery by a general or a vascular surgeon, but general surgeons were more likely to turn a patient down for operation.[4]

RESULTS OF EMERGENCY ARTERIAL SURGERY IN THE BRITISH ISLES

Most publications on outcome derive from the practices of enthusiasts or major centres. In general, only good results are reported and that imparts a degree of bias to the true outcome for any disease or treatment. Outcomes derived from prospectively collected data, preferably from several sources in a multicentre trial, or results from randomised trials are more likely to be nearer the truth. Some Scandinavian countries have large incident databases from which both process and outcome data can be obtained (Swedvasc and Finnvasc). In the UK, a few multicentre studies have been carried out. The Audit and Research Committee of the Vascular Society of Great Britain and Ireland (VSGBI) has conducted prospective and retrospective audits on some of the principal vascular operations.

Carotid surgery

Most carotid surgery is done electively. In the audit performed by the VSSGBI, there were no emergency procedures.[5] Urgent carotid endarterectomy for recent stroke became unpopular in the 1970s following the publication of dismal results.[6] This may be explained by the fact that a proportion of the operations were done on patients with cerebral hemorrhage rather than embolic disease. Recently, it has been argued that a more selective approach using computed tomography to identify appropriate patients with a thromboembolic stroke means that more patients could be offered urgent surgery. In a pilot trial, however, few suitable patients were identified (16 from 593 reviewed), although surgical results were reasonable.[7] Perhaps the most frequent indication for emergency intervention is when a patient develops a stroke after carotid endarterectomy (see Chapter 14). Most surgeons reoperate for an early carotid occlusion as it is felt intuitively that this should improve outcome. There is little evidence, even in recent studies, that this is the case.[8]

Aortic surgery

Although ruptured aortic aneurysm is the most frequent reason for an emergency vascular operation, it is very difficult to define a clear outcome for this condition. One reason is that most patients never actually reach hospital, and once there, a significant number are rejected as unfit. It is estimated that only 15 per cent of patients with a ruptured abdominal aortic aneurysm (AAA) survive. Surgeons may have less influence over the outcome of the condition than they think. It is often difficult to obtain complete data on patients with a ruptured AAA. Those who die in the accident and emergency department or in the preoperative bay usually end up with scanty hospital records and the data somehow never seem to reach a surgical database.

Classification difficulties can also confuse the issue. A shocked patient with a ruptured aneurysm is a clear clinical entity, however, some patients with a contained rupture may remain well for hours or even days. Some patients present with a tender aneurysm and have an urgent operative repair. It is clear that there is a spectrum of outcomes for these different situations. Surgeons may influence the results they report by choosing which groups to include.[9] For example, the best results for aortic surgery are obtained by including only patients who have an elective admission and operation. Results for emergency AAA repair can be improved by counting all those who have an out-of-hours operation, including patients with a tender non-ruptured aneurysm.

There are few good reports of outcome from ruptured AAA. Meta-analysis of all English language publications suggested that the average mortality rate was 48 per cent and that the results have improved slowly over the last 50 years.[10] In the UK, the VSGBI pilot national database included 276 patients who had AAA surgery, but only 43 who had emergency surgery. The mortality rate was 23 per cent for urgent AAA repair and 51 per cent for rupture.[11] In Wales a prospective audit of operations performed by both general and vascular surgeons revealed a survival rate of only 36 per cent.[4] The results for the two groups were similar, though vascular surgeons operated on 82/92 (89 per cent) of patients admitted under their care with a 39 per cent survival rate, compared with general surgeons who operated on 51/141 (36 per cent) patients with a 31 per cent survival rate.[4] Longitudinal data from large vascular units such as the one in Edinburgh have shown little change in survival over the last 20 years.[12] Mortality rates after ruptured AAA actually rose in the second decade from 35 to 40 per cent.

Operative outcome can be improved by case selection. The more unfit patients are refused surgery, the better will be the results of an individual surgeon. Surgeons have agonised about the indications for repair of a ruptured AAA in an unfit patient. Hardman et al. described a number of criteria that can help make this difficult decision.[13] There is also the possibility that the Physiological and Operative Severity Score for the enUmeration of Mortality and morbidity (POSSUM) physiology scoring could give a preoperative prediction of outcome.[14] The Portsmouth POSSUM model was developed from 213 emergency aneurysm repairs, with a mortality rate of 40 per cent.[15]

As the published results have barely changed in a generation, it may be time to think of alternative means of reducing the community mortality of aneurysm disease. One way would be to commence a screening programme to detect AAAs while asymptomatic and to perform elective repair before rupture occurs.[16] An alternative might be to consider endovascular repair for ruptured AAAs. Small series reports of this treatment exist,[17] but regular interventions would require an investment in infrastructure and a change in culture. On the other hand, that might be the only way of bringing about a significant improvement in outcome for ruptured AAAs.

Acute leg ischaemia

A prospective audit of acute leg ischaemia in Gloucestershire suggested that a county with a population of half a million would treat approximately 75 patients a year.[18] The overall 30-day outcome was limb salvage 67 per cent, amputation 7 per cent and deaths 26 per cent. A number of patients were not suitable for intervention and when they were excluded, the results for patients treated actively were limb salvage 78 per cent, amputation 6 per cent and deaths 16 per cent.[18]

The VSGBI also completed a prospective audit on acute ischaemia: 539 episodes were reported in 474 patients.[19] At 30 days 70 per cent of legs were definitely viable, 16 per cent had been amputated and the overall mortality was 22 per cent, these results confirming the high risk attached to the treatment of acute leg ischaemia.[19] A subsequent paper demonstrated the poor intermediate term outcome for this condition, a further 35 per cent of initial survivors having died within 2 years.[20] Recurrent leg ischaemia and subsequent amputation risk appeared to be reduced by warfarin anticoagulation. The study also highlighted the variety of different methods of treatment available. This difficult condition requires decisions to be taken at senior level, such as making the choice between surgery or thrombolytic therapy. An easy embolectomy can be done by an experienced trainee, but when the operation is not proceeding well a consultant's experience is needed, particularly if a full range of vascular procedures may have to be considered. Thrombolytic therapy is a high risk option and demands the active involvement of trained radiology staff (see Chapters 8, 16 and 39).

The Thrombolysis Study Group has collected data on intra-arterial thrombolysis over the past decade.[21] Over 1000 episodes of lysis have been evaluated. The initial outcome after intra-arterial lysis was a complete lysis rate of 41 per cent, a partial lysis rate of 28 per cent, and a failed lysis, or lysis but no run-off, rate of 29 per cent. At 30 days the outcome was amputation-free survival in 75.2 per cent, major limb amputation 12.5 per cent and deaths 12.4 per cent. Although most of this work has been observational, the Group is now in a position to try to define the patients most likely to benefit from thrombolytic therapy. Factors affecting amputation-free survival included the severity of leg ischaemia and the type of vessel occluded, namely native artery (72 per cent) or graft (78 per cent). The main anxiety in thrombolysis is the risk of stroke which occurred in 2.4 per cent of patients on the database although only half of these were haemorrhagic, and many occurred several days after initiating thrombolysis.

TOWARDS A NATIONAL VASCULAR DATABASE IN THE UK AND IRELAND

With the exception of Northern Ireland, which has had a vascular database (Northern Ireland Vascular Registry or NIVASC) for the last seven years, surgeons in the rest of the UK have looked enviously at the well ordered national databases of Scandinavian countries. There remains a problem of scale, however, in that expectations of collecting routine data from over 400 individual consultant members of the VSGBI would require resources beyond any current medical organisation. Existing databases, however, have really only collected data on process and mortality, and surgeons in tertiary referral centres or deprived inner city areas may feel disadvantaged if their clinical performance were to be judged solely on the basis of crude mortality rates. In fact such assessments might influence the surgeon offering surgical treatment to a patient. A surgeon worrying about personal results may be reluctant to operate on a high risk patient. Finally, there is the problem of verification. Most registries rely on the honesty of their participants. A follow-up of patients who had surgery but were not included in the database, whether accidentally or deliberately, revealed that these are a very high risk group.[22]

The VSGBI has adopted the attitude that any national database should take account of the case-mix of patients. For the past few years there has been an investigation into various scoring systems that could be used to incorporate an allowance for case-mix into a comparison of outcomes among individual surgeons. UK vascular surgeons have performed two large trials collecting POSSUM data items on their patients. POSSUM scoring involves 12 preoperative physiological data items and eight operative items. It has been shown that both POSSUM and Bayes analytical techniques used on this dataset can predict outcome. The first VSGBI study involved nearly 1500 patients from 121 surgeons in 93 hospitals.[23] They collected data on consecutive arterial procedures over a two-month interval in 1998. The statisticians introduced a new POSSUM regression equation, known as V-POSSUM, which predicted outcome across the range of arterial procedures and hospitals. Indeed it was possible to do so based on the preoperative physiology scores alone, meaning that in future, a preoperative outcome prediction might be possible for an individual patient.[23]

Table 9A.1   *Results of POSSUM analysis on abdominal aortic aneurysms (AAA) from the Vascular Surgical Society of Great Britain and Ireland (VSGBI) Pilot National Vascular Database 2001*

Per cent range predicted risk	Mean per cent predicted risk	No.	Predicted	Reported	χ^2
(a) All abdominal aortic aneurysms*					
Mortality: V–POSSUM physiology and operative scores					
>0 to ≤ 7	3.84	352	14	19	2.33
>7 to ≤ 15	10.61	204	22	31	4.52
>15 to ≤ 30	20.91	118	25	31	2.05
>30 to ≤100	48.47	99	48	35	6.82
>0 to ≤100	13.95	773	108	116	15.72
$\chi^2 = 15.720$	P(4 df) = 0.00		Evidence of lack of fit		
Mortality: V–POSSUM physiology only scores					
>0 to ≤7	3.89	446	17	48	56.42
>7 to ≤15	9.91	196	19	31	7.67
>15 to ≤30	20.54	85	17	16	0.15
>30 to ≤100	43.15	46	20	21	0.12
>0 to ≤100	9.58	773	74	116	64.36
$\chi^2 = 64.360$	P(4 df) = 0.00		Evidence of lack of fit		
(b) Ruptured abdominal aortic aneurysms†					
Mortality: physiology data only					
>0 to ≤30	22.61	30	7	11	3.39
>30 to ≤40	35.01	34	12	16	2.17
>40 to ≤50	45.04	23	10	11	0.07
>50 to ≤100	64.93	35	23	19	1.74
>0 to ≤100	42.44	122	52	57	7.37
$\chi^2 = 7.369$	P(4 df) = 0.12		No evidence of lack of fit		
Mortality: physiology data only					
>0 to ≤30	24.20	24	6	10	3.99
>30 to ≤40	34.22	31	11	11	0.02
>40 to ≤50	44.54	24	11	13	0.90
>50 to ≤100	64.33	43	28	23	2.20
>0 to ≤100	44.89	122	55	57	7.12
$\chi^2 = 7.117$	P(4 df) = 0.13		No evidence of lack of fit		

*Using the V–POSSUM score, statistical analysis shows 'lack of fit', i.e. the method does not predict outcome accurately.
†Analysed using Portsmouth ruptured AAA equation (Portsmouth data excluded from VSGBI data). There is no 'lack of fit', i.e. the method predicts outcome accurately.
POSSUM, physiological and Operative Severity Score for the EnUmeration of Mortality and Morbidity.

These results were translated into a second phase. It was decided to refine the data collection to include just three index vascular procedures – carotid endarterectomy, aortic aneurysm repair (divided into ruptured and non-ruptured) and infrainguinal bypass. Participating vascular surgeons were asked to include all patients having these procedures under their care. A decision was made to collect data only electronically using the POSSUM dataset. Although electronic data collection has limited the number of surgeons able to participate thus far, a package of supporting devices including an Access database, Excel spreadsheet and bespoke data collection software has been made available to encourage them. The most recent work involved over 12 000 procedures collected from 149 VSGBI

surgeons.[24] The analysis has shown that it is possible to predict outcomes for individual surgeons performing quite small numbers of index procedures; data from the 1999 registry indicate that the average VSGBI member performs 71 index procedures per annum (18 carotid endarterectomies, 25 aneurysms (9 ruptured, 16 non-ruptured) and 28 infrainguinal bypass procedures). The best models for predicted versus expected outcome were gained by using procedure specific databases and formulae. For example, formal POSSUM analysis worked best for ruptured aneurysms using a specific POSSUM regression equation developed in Portsmouth[15] (Table 9A.1). Mortality for the 122 ruptured aneurysms in this latest series was 47 per cent. It was also possible to produce comparative data for all

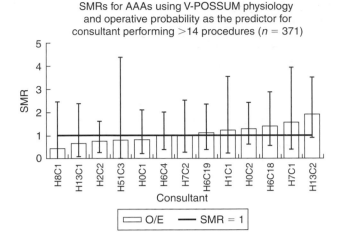

Figure 9A.1 *Data from the Pilot National Vascular Database of the Vascular Society of Great Britain and Ireland (2001). Standardised mortality ratios (SMRs) for individual consultant vascular surgeons who have entered at least 14 procedures onto the Database. Includes both ruptured and non-ruptured aneurysms. If the vertical error bars include the SMR of one, the individual surgeon's results are not significantly better or worse than the whole group. AAA, abdominal aortic aneurysm*

aneurysms, both ruptured and non-ruptured, using Bayes analysis of the same dataset. Cardiac surgeons in the UK currently publish an annual report including outcomes after cardiac surgery,[25] and this could soon also be done by vascular surgeons (Fig. 9A.1).

Conclusions

Results of emergency vascular procedures are worse than for elective operations. It might be anticipated that this is where the skill of a vascular surgeon could make a real difference. However, these are often sick patients, nearing the end of life and decisions as to whether to intervene or not are complex. More data are required so that patients and their surgeons can make informed choices about management.

A good surgeon guide has already been published in a UK national newspaper using nationally available statistics. Cardiac units were ranked by outcome. Indeed, it has also been possible to do this analysis for aortic surgery.[26] Unless surgeons are closely involved in data collection and analysis, comparison among surgeons and units will be done using crude mortality rates based on unreliable hospital information systems. In the UK, surgeons can now submit their data for central comparison against their peers and expect to receive a formal acknowledgement from their Vascular Society.

The system should prove invaluable for surgeons who wish to pass this information on to their patients. It is suspected that the results of some procedures are worse

than those commonly quoted in the scientific literature. These figures are often used to justify surgical procedures. Accurate data about the general risks of surgery can help place the value of a procedure to society. Accurate data about the specific risks of surgery to an individual are crucial to obtaining informed consent from a patient.

Key references

Bown MJ, Sutton AJ, Micholson ML, *et al.* A meta-analysis of 50 years of ruptured abdominal aortic aneurysm repair. *Br J Surg* 2002; **89**: 714–30.

Neary WD, Crow P, Foy C, *et al.* Comparison of POSSUM scoring and the Hardman Index in selection of patients for repair of ruptured abdominal aortic aneurysm. *Br J Surg* 2003; **90**: 421–5.

Elfstrom J, Stubberod A, Troeng T. Patients not included in medical audit have a worse outcome than those included. *Int J Qual Health Care* 1996; **8**: 153–7.

Prytherch DR, Ridler BMF, Beard JD, Earnshaw JJ on behalf of the Audit and Research Committee of the Vascular Surgical Society of Great Britain and Ireland. A model for national outcome audit in vascular surgery. *Eur J Vasc Endovasc Surg* 2001; **21**: 477–83.

The Vascular Society of Great Britain and Ireland. *Fourth National Vascular Database Report 2004.* Oxford: Dendrite Clinical Systems, 2005.

REFERENCES

1 Baird RN, Baker AR, Hine C, *et al.* Interhospital provision of emergency vascular services for a large population: early outcomes and clinical results. *Br J Surg* 2001; **88**: A620–1.

2 Cassar K, Godden DJ, Duncan JL. Community mortality after ruptured abdominal aortic aneurysm is unrelated to the distance from the surgical centre. *Br J Surg* 2001; **88**: 1341–3.

3 Clason AE, Stonebridge PA, Duncan AJ, *et al.* Acute ischaemia of the lower limb: the effect of centralizing vascular surgical services on morbidity and mortality. *Br J Surg* 1989; **76**: 592–3.

4 Basnyat PS, Biffin AHB, Moseley LG, *et al.* Mortality from ruptured abdominal aortic aneurysm in Wales. *Br J Surg* 1999; **86**: 765–70.

5 McCollum PT, da Silva A, Ridler BD, de Cossart L. Carotid endarterectomy in the UK and Ireland: audit of 30 day outcome. The Audit Committee for the Vascular Surgical Society. *Eur J Vasc Endovasc Surg* 1977; **14**: 386–91.

6 Wylie EJ, Hein MF, Adams JE. Intracranial haemorrhage following surgical revascularization for treatment of acute strokes. *J Neurosurg* 1964; **21**: 212–15.

7 Mead GE, Murray H, Farrell A, *et al.* Pilot study of carotid endarterectomy for acute stroke. *Br J Surg* 1997; **84**: 990–2.

8 Stewart AHR, Cole SAE, Smith FCT, *et al.* Re-operation for neurological complications following carotid endarterectomy. *Br J Surg* 2003; **90**: 832–7.

9 Campbell WB. Mortality statistics for elective aortic aneurysms. *Eur J Vasc Surg* 1991; **5**: 111–13.

10 Bown MJ, Sutton AJ, Micholson ML, *et al*. A meta-analysis of 50 years of ruptured abdominal aortic aneurysm repair. *Br J Surg* 2002; **89**: 714–30.

11 The Vascular Surgical Society of Great Britain and Ireland. *National Outcome Audit Report 1999*. Oxford: Dendrite Clinical Systems, 1999.

12 Bradbury AW, Adam DJ, Makhdoomi KR, *et al*. A 21-year experience of abdominal aortic aneurysm operations in Edinburgh. *Br J Surg* 1998; **85**: 645–7.

13 Hardman DT, Fisher CM, Patel MI, *et al*. Ruptured abdominal aortic aneurysms: who should be offered surgery? *J Vasc Surg* 1996; **23**: 123–9.

14 Neary WD, Crow P, Foy C, *et al*. Comparison of POSSUM scoring and the Hardman Index in selection of patients for repair of ruptured abdominal aortic aneurysm. *Br J Surg* 2003; **90**: 421–5.

15 Prytherch DR, Sutton GL, Boyle JR. Portsmouth POSSUM models for abdominal aortic aneurysm surgery. *Br J Surg* 2001; **88**: 958–63.

16 Beard JD. Screening for abdominal aortic aneurysm. *Br J Surg* 2003; **90**: 515–16.

17 Hinchcliffe RJ, Braithwaite BD, Hopkinson BR. The endovascular management of ruptured aortic aneurysm. *Eur J Vasc Endovasc Surg* 2003; **25**: 191–201.

18 Davies B, Braithwaite BD, Birch PA, *et al*. Acute leg ischaemia in Gloucestershire. *Br J Surg* 1997; **84**: 504–8.

19 Campbell WB, Ridler BMF, Szymanska TH on behalf of the Audit Committee of the Vascular Surgical Society of Great Britain and Ireland. Current management of acute leg ischaemia: results of an audit by the Vascular Surgical Society of Great Britain and Ireland. *Br J Surg* 1998; **85**: 1498–503.

20 Campbell WB, Ridler BM, Szymanska T on behalf of the Audit Committee of the Vascular Surgical Society of Great Britain and Ireland. Two year follow-up after acute thromboembolic limb ischaemia: the importance of anticoagulation. *Eur J Vasc Endovasc Surg* 2000; **19**: 169–73.

21 Earnshaw JJ, Whitman B, Foy C on behalf of the Thrombolysis Study Group. National Audit of Thrombolysis for Acute Leg Ischaemia database: final clinical analysis. *Br J Surg* 2003; **90**: A504.

22 Elfstrom J, Stubberod A, Troeng T. Patients not included in medical audit have a worse outcome than those included. *Int J Qual Health Care* 1996; **8**: 153–7.

23 Prytherch DR, Ridler BMF, Beard JD, Earnshaw JJ on behalf of the Audit and Research Committee of the Vascular Surgical Society of Great Britain and Ireland. A model for national outcome audit in vascular surgery. *Eur J Vasc Endovasc Surg* 2001; **21**: 477–83.

24 The Vascular Society of Great Britain and Ireland. *Fourth National Vascular Database Report 2004*. Oxford: Dendrite Clinical Systems, 2005.

25 The Society of Cardiothoracic Surgeons of Great Britain and Ireland. *National Adult Cardiac Surgical Database Report 2000–2001*. Oxford: Dendrite Clinical Systems, 2001.

26 Rigby KA, Palfreyman S, Michaels JA. Performance indicators from routine hospital data: death following aortic surgery as a potential measure of quality of care. *Br J Surg* 2001; **88**: 964–8.

Outcomes of Emergency Vascular Procedures in Scandinavia

WILLIAM P PAASKE, MAURI LEPÄNTALO, THOMAS TROËNG

INTRODUCTION: VASCULAR SURGERY AND VASCULAR REGISTRIES IN SCANDINAVIA

Norway, Finland and Sweden are countries characterised by widely varying regional population densities, which has implications for the organisation of vascular surgical services. That is less true of Denmark where the population is more evenly distributed. Another Scandinavian feature is the ageing population: in Denmark on New Year's Day 2001, 1.06 million (19.8 per cent) were over 60 years of age with a projected increase of 18.5 per cent to 1.25 million by 2010. The corresponding figures for those over 65 years of age in Finland are 0.77 rising to 0.90 million by 2010 and 1.35 million by 2030. Table 9B.1 presents selected data on demographics and organisation of vascular registries.

Table 9B.1 *Vascular surgery in Denmark, Finland and Sweden*

	Denmark	Finland	Sweden
Population (million)	5.35	5.19	8.9
Vascular centres	11	23	50
Vascular surgeons*	41	42	130
Registrars	12	12	NA
Monospecialty	1983	1999	–
Registry initiated	1990	1989	1985
Registry covering the whole country	1996	1991–1995	1994

*In Finland mostly thoracic and vascular surgeons; in Sweden general surgeons with a vascular profile; in Denmark all are specialists in vascular surgery.
NA, data not available.

Denmark

WORKFORCE

Vascular surgery was recognised as a monospecialty in 1983. Currently, serving in the 11 services of vascular surgery, are 41 specialists in vascular surgery employed as consultants supported by four staff specialists and 12 senior registrars or vascular fellows (see Chapter 1B).

VASCULAR REGISTRY

The Danish Vascular Registry (Karbase) has been operational since 1990. Complete national data are available from 1996 onwards: in 1996, 5798 procedures were carried out of which 4129 (71.2 per cent) were primary operations and 484 (8.3 per cent) reoperations. The corresponding figures for 2000 were: 6508 procedures, 4106 (63.1 per cent) primary and 545 (8.3 per cent) reoperations, which translates into a frequency of 77 primary procedures in a population of 100 000 ($77/10^5$).

Arterial reconstructions are not performed outside vascular surgical departments and in 2000 were responsible for 891 venous procedures. During that year one department with a single surgeon performed 49 procedures while other institutions, staffed with three to five consultants, had an arterial and endovascular surgery volume ranging from 303 to 998. Also during 2000, Karbase registered 1107 percutaneous transluminal angioplasties (PTAs) and 192 arterial thrombolysis treatments. The number of index procedures in 1999 as defined by the European Board of Vascular Surgery[1] has been published,[2] the contributors being those with established registries, namely the

Scandinavian countries, Northern Ireland, Slovakia, New Zealand and single regions in Spain and Russia.

Finland

WORKFORCE

Finland has 21 central hospital regions served by five university and 16 central hospitals. Within central hospital regions there are a number of district hospitals but their role as active vascular units is diminishing; currently, 23 hospitals provide an arterial surgery service.

In conjunction with harmonising Finnish specialist training within the European Union, the previously allied specialty of thoracic and vascular surgery was divided into independent specialties, namely, vascular surgery and cardiothoracic surgery. The vascular workload is borne by 36 thoracic and vascular surgeons, 29 of them with a strong vascular profile, six formally trained vascular surgeons, three staff specialists and 12 vascular surgical trainees. In smaller centres most of these surgeons also perform lung surgery while others also practice general surgery. At the end of year 2003 there were six formally trained vascular surgeons and 12 vascular surgical trainees. The anticipated population growth by 2010 will demand an estimated increase in the number of vascular surgeons to 60 and an expansion of resources required for the diagnosis and treatment of venous disease.

VASCULAR REGISTRY

The Finnvasc registry commenced in 1989 and a pilot scheme progressing to systematic data collection was initiated in 1991. All hospitals with a vascular surgical service participated fully in this exercise up to 1995, but thereafter their involvement fluctuated between 68 and 81 per cent. The diminution in interest is attributable to the extra workload for which there was no remuneration, no support from health authorities and data collection and reporting were delayed. Most significantly, the very strict interpretation of the new personal registry law at the beginning of 2000 paralysed this important activity. At present, registration practices are being reviewed with the aim of establishing computerised real time recording and reporting systems, at least at local level.

In comparing Finnvasc registry figures with those from hospital records the mean percentage of missing vascular procedures in the former was 19 per cent.[3] Similarly, a comparison of data from Statistics Finland, the national statistical bureau, and the Finnvasc registry showed that 18 per cent of patients operated for ruptured abdominal aortic aneurysm (RAAA) and subsequently died were missing from the Finnvasc registry.[4]

The vascular units were staffed with between one and eight consultants with an annual arterial and endovascular throughput ranging from 12 to 1755. According to the 1999 data from registries and other sources 11 835 operations were performed for peripheral vessels, both arteries and veins, and 4846 day-case procedures for simple venous problems. As for endovascular activity, 4160 procedures were recorded in 2000, 292 of these being thrombolysis treatments.

Sweden

WORKFORCE

Vascular surgery used to be performed in 92 units, but the number of vascular centres has fallen to 50. Sweden has nine university hospitals and four of these have separate departments of vascular surgery or combined cardiovascular departments. The 22 county hospitals all have vascular surgical units. There is also vascular activity in some 15 of the smaller district hospitals. Vascular surgery is not a specialty in its own right in Sweden as it is in Denmark and Finland; it remains the responsibility of 130 general surgeons with a vascular profile of whom around 30 are accredited as vascular surgeons by the Swedish Society for Vascular Surgery.

VASCULAR REGISTRY

Sweden has pioneered the development of vascular registries in Scandinavia. Inspired by American experiences during the 1970s the planning for a regional vascular registry began in southern Sweden in late 1985.[5]

The aims of the registry were to monitor practice, changes and outcomes of vascular surgery undertaken in the routine care of a population, to safeguard a high level of data quality, to establish a basis and a starting point for scientific studies, and to develop techniques for quality development. An additional aim was to compare the results of emerging vascular units in county hospitals with those of established centres at university level.

After a year of preparation, including a month of pilot testing, the Vascular Registry in Southern Sweden (VRISS) started regular activities in January 1987 in the South Health Care Region of Sweden and some neighbouring areas. The initial 17 participating centres, including two university, six county and nine district hospitals, covered a population of 1.9 million.

Over the years increasing numbers of surgeons found it useful to participate but by 1990, when half the country's surgeons had joined in, the registry was renamed the Swedish Vascular Registry (Swedvasc). From early 1994 surgeons at all 50 hospitals performing peripheral vascular surgery were members of the registry, covering practically the whole Swedish population of 8.8 million and included the 10 university/regional centres and the 25 county hospitals in the country. Around 130 surgeons take part regularly in this completely volunteered, professional and non-authoritarian exercise. The day to day work of the registry is led by a steering committee representing both academic and community hospitals. Each year more than 9000 procedures are registered and, to date, close to 100 000 cases have been registered.

EMERGENCY ANEURYSM SURGERY

Denmark

During the 5-year period 1996–2000, a total of 1242 patients were admitted to Danish specialist departments with RAAA and underwent surgery. This corresponds to an operation frequency of 4.9 per 10^5 inhabitants of all ages per year. The male:female ratio was 7:4 (1094 men, 88.1 per cent; 148 women, 11.9 per cent) and the median age was 72 years (range 29–91). Although a total of 1276 patients were recorded with this diagnosis, most centres had excluded patients who had not been operated. Not all patients with RAAA were admitted to hospitals with vascular surgical departments, especially those in whom the diagnosis was unclear, and there were cases where, in consultation with a vascular surgeon, the emergency procedure was deemed unreasonable or hopeless.

The circumstances associated with the admission of a RAAA do not permit detailed preoperative questioning of risk factors, comorbidities and social circumstances, and in around a quarter or more of all admissions this information is not available. Given that limitation the data elicited were as follows: cerebrovascular history 29.6 per cent, hypertension 52.3 per cent, cardiac problems 51.3 per cent, pulmonary complaints 41.5 per cent, smoking 9.3 per cent, retired, old age pensioners or on sick leave 66.0 per cent, previous vascular surgery 8.9 per cent, previous amputation 1.1 per cent.

Statistics on the operation itself were as follows: a midline laparotomy was used in 91.4 per cent, duration of procedure was 164 minutes (maximum 480 minutes), blood loss 4.6 L (maximum 42 L), hospital stay 10.3 days (range 0–119). In terms of outcome these were the figures: total hospital mortality 55 per cent, 30-day operative mortality 43 per cent (Table 9B.2). The causes of death were judged to be: cardiac 15.3 per cent, cerebrovascular 0.5 per cent, renal 1.1 per cent, haemorrhage 8.6 per cent, multiorgan failure 10.5 per cent, bowel ischaemia 1.2 per cent, other 1.8 per cent, unknown 15.7 per cent.

The complications directly related to the operation were: amputations 1 per cent, wound infection 6.2 per cent (deep 1.8 per cent), bleeding necessitating a further procedure 7.5 per cent, wound dehiscence 3.3 per cent, intestinal obstruction 1.1 per cent, bowel ischaemia requiring surgery 5.7 per cent, surgery for peripheral embolisation 2.3 per cent. In all, 23.2 per cent of patients had a complication demanding operative treatment. General complications observed were: cardiac (myocardial infarction, pump failure, arrhythmia)

Table 9B.2 *Emergency aneurysm surgery in Scandinavian vascular registry data*

	Denmark	Finland	Sweden
Data from years	1996–2000	1991–1997	1996–2001
Number of patients	1242	1152	1905
Mortality (per cent)			
Symptomatic but not ruptured	NA	11.6	7.6
RAAA/stable	NA	24.8	22.0
RAAA/shock	NA	59.8	45.7
30-day mortality	43	46	38
Total hospital mortality	55*	68*	NA

*Includes 2.5 per cent of non-operated patients from Denmark and 30 per cent non-operated patients from Finland.
NA, data not available; RAAA, ruptured abdominal aortic aneurysm.

14 per cent, pneumonia or atelectasis 12.5 per cent, assisted ventilation for more than 2 days 9.9 per cent, double or higher rises in creatinine 9.5 per cent, dialysis required 8.0 per cent and intensive care unit stay of more than 3 days 11.1 per cent. A 're-do' or additional surgical procedure or arterial reconstruction was necessary in 17.7 per cent. Half of the patients were discharged to their own homes and the other half to another institution.

Finland

In Finland, the reporting format allowed differentiation between three categories of emergency AAAs: emergency, stable with rupture and unstable or in shock with rupture. In the seven years from 1991 to 1997, the 30-day mortality rates were as follows: 474 symptomatic cases without confirmation of rupture, 55 deaths (11.6 per cent); 270 with stable rupture, 67 deaths (24.8 per cent); 418 patients with shock due to rupture, 250 deaths (59.8 per cent) (see Table 9B.2). The exact frequency of the various conditions expressed in per cent per population unit per year, however, is difficult to estimate for this 7-year period due to decreasing and varying reporting activity from 1996 and 1997. Based on the 1995 figures, which cover the entire country, the frequency of procedures per 10^5 inhabitants per year for the three presentations was 1.6 symptomatic non-ruptured, 0.9 ruptured and stable, and 1.2 ruptured and shock, or $3.7/10^5$ in all.

A detailed analysis of mortality in RAAA for the years 1991–94 was undertaken as a cross-sectional study based on Finnvasc and the national cause of death registry.[4] A total of 610 emergency repairs for RAAA were identified in Finnvasc corresponding to 2.9 procedures per 10^5 inhabitants per year (2.9/10^5 per year). Of these, 454 operations were for rupture (2.2/10^5 per year) and 156 for emergency cases without rupture (0.8/10^5 per year). In addition, it was possible to identify 293 operations for rupture in an additional 18 of the 23 hospitals performing operations for rupture. The true frequency of surgery for rupture was found to be around 3.6–$3.8/10^5$ per year, accounting for 75 per cent of the activity in Denmark. A projected increase of at least 50 per cent in RAAA interventions can be expected in Finland during the next two decades.[6]

The 30-day postoperative mortality as registered in Finnvasc was 46 per cent after surgery for rupture and 13.5 per cent for acute non-ruptured cases. Based on national statistics, the mortality was 54 per cent. Total hospital mortality including all patients brought alive to the emergency unit was 68 per cent. The total number of deaths from rupture based on national statistical information was 1004, and as 245 had survived rupture, the overall survival frequency was 19.6 per cent. The death rate of rupture was $4.9/10^5$ per year. If the $1.2/10^5$ per year patients surviving from Finnvasc are added, the total incidence of RAAA comes to $6.1/10^5$ per year. It is noteworthy that there was no correlation between hospital volume and operative mortality in rupture repair, but there was an inverse association between hospital volume and total hospital rupture mortality. The operative activity of RAAA ranged from 37 to 88 per cent among Finnish centres.[4]

The quality of life (QoL) after survival following repair of a RAAA has been an issue. A recent study by Korhonen et al.[7] showed that survivors after repair of RAAA had almost the same QoL as the norms of an age and sex adjusted general population. This further justifies an aggressive operative policy in RAAA. The Glasgow Aneurysm Score, as a potential predictor of the immediate outcome after surgery for RAAA, could only provide information which is supplementary to clinical decision making.[8]

Sweden

The total number recorded in Swedvasc increased rapidly during 1987–93, but during 1994–98 that figure stayed at a fairly constant level with the 1999 data. It is noteworthy that since Swedvasc began, emergency procedures, as a proportion of all operations for AAAs, have, with some regional variations, remained unchanged at around 40 per cent. Interestingly, postoperative mortality has not improved significantly since 1994 when all centres had become participants of Swedvasc (Fig. 9B.1).

The clinical features and outcomes of emergency surgery for AAAs registered during 1996–2001 are presented in detail in Tables 9B.2–9B.6. For two decades AAAs in Sweden treated by surgery have been classified according to Eriksson.[9] Elective procedures can be done for asymptomatic or for symptomatic aneurysms. Emergency procedures are done for non-ruptured, ruptured without shock, or rupture including shock. These five groups differ considerably in terms of postoperative 30-day mortality.

The 30-day mortality for non-ruptured cases was 8.7 per cent and it rose with the degree of complexity of the graft implanted: aortic tube graft 6.3 per cent, aortoiliac

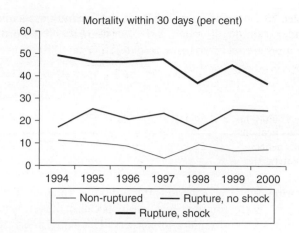

Figure 9B.1 *Mortality within 30 days in emergency abdominal aortic surgery in Sweden*

Table 9B.3 *Characteristics of patients operated for aortic aneurysms as emergency procedures in Sweden. Except for age all data are percentages*

	Emergency not ruptured	RAAA stable	shock	
Males	78.1	84	85.6	$P = 0.002$
Median age, years				
Males	72	73	74	NS
Females	76	77	77	NS
Cerebrovascular disease	15.3	11.6	13.6	NS
Diabetes	6.4	6.4	5.8	NS
Cardiac disease	51.4	45.4	44.8	NS
Hypertension	46.1	51.7	38.9	001
Hyperlipidaemia	6.1	4.6	4.3	NS
Pulmonary disease	16.0	19.9	13.1	$P = 0.003$
Renal disease	9.7	10.6	11.4	NS
Previous vascular surgery	16.3	11.2	9.7	$P = 0.002$
Recorded smoker	31.0	34.9	25.0	$P < 0.001$

NS, not significant. RAAA, ruptured abdominal aortic aneurysm;

graft 12.5 per cent, aortobifemoral graft 20 per cent; for rupture without shock it was 20 per cent and for the three types of graft 19.1, 11.5 and 45.5 per cent, respectively; for rupture with shock it was 40.1 per cent and the breakdown was 37.6, 34.9 and 54.2 per cent, respectively. It is obvious that the clinical presentation has an important bearing on the outcome and this dimension of case-mix ought to be included in comparisons between centres.

Patient characteristics differ little among these groups but in the more urgent cases such data are often missing; interestingly, women seem to arrive in time for surgery before AAA rupture more frequently than do men.

Table 9B.4 *Complications after emergency aneurysm surgery in Sweden as related to the severity of the preoperative state (per cent)*

	Emergency not ruptured	RAAA		
		stable	shock	
Any surgical complications	15.8	24.3	32.4	$P < 0.0001$
Any general complication	25.4	41.5	70.4	$P < 0.001$
Any non-vascular reoperation	5.9	9.3	14.3	$P < 0.001$

RAAA, ruptured abdominal aortic aneurysm.

Table 9B.5 *Complications after emergency surgery in Sweden*

Complications	Per cent
Most common surgical complications	
Haemorrhage/haematoma	9.0
Intestinal ischaemia	3.2
Occlusion/thrombosis	2.5
Superficial infection	2.2
Wound rupture	1.7
Deep/graft infection	1.2
Distal embolisation	0.9
Most common general complications	
ICU >5 days	14.3
Cardiac	12.7
Multiorgan	11.13
Pulmonary	10.8
Renal	8.8
Cerebrovascular	2.2
Sepsis	1.9
Most common non-vascular reoperations	
Intestinal resection	3.2
Laparotomy	3.1
Fasciotomy	2.8
Amputation (above knee)	0.9
Amputation (below knee)	0.2

ICU, intensive care unit.

Complications are common after emergency AAA surgery (Tables 9B.4 and 9B.5), and are clearly associated with the severity of presentation (Table 9B.4). A targeted analysis of 1999 data disclosed 336 patients who had open repairs, of whom 182 presented with shock, 85 without shock and 69 without rupture. The total 30-day mortality was 28.6 per cent and the corresponding subgroup mortality rates were: non-rupture 8.7 per cent, rupture without shock 20 per cent, and rupture with shock 40.1 per cent.

Table 9B.6 *The age distribution of 30-day mortality expressed in per cent in Sweden, 1999*

Age (years)	No rupture	RAAA	
		stable	shock
50–59		33.3	10.0
60–69	10.5	20.8	20.0
70–79	5.0	15.0	46.2
80–89	33.3	27.8	55.0

RAAA, ruptured abdominal aortic aneurysm.

These outcomes were further affected by age (Table 9B.6). The results are better than those in other Scandinavian reports, but the total hospital mortality is not available.

SURGERY FOR ACUTE ISCHAEMIA

Denmark

The database structure allows identification of patients who were admitted to the specialist departments and underwent surgery for acute ischaemia. During the 5-year period 1996–2000, 2808 patients were admitted 3438 times for various procedures (Table 9B.7). The male:female ratio was 0.98 (male 1390 (49.5 per cent):female 1418 (50.5 per cent)) with a median age of 70 years (2–100) and an incidence of $11.0/10^5$ per year.

In contrast to patients with RAAA, information on risk factors and social history for acute ischaemia was elicited in over 95 per cent of cases: diabetes 15.4 per cent, cerebrovascular disease 17 per cent, hypertension 33.2 per cent, cardiac disease 47.2 per cent, pulmonary disease 25.1 per cent, previous vascular surgical procedures in 42.5 per cent, previous amputation 3.7 per cent, smoking 77.6 per cent, retired or old age pensioners 73.6 per cent. The median delay from admission to procedure was 1.2 days (0–76) and median length of hospital stay was 7.1 days (0–101).

The most frequent procedure was embolectomy/thrombectomy in 47.2 per cent of cases: 14.8 per cent in previously implanted grafts and 85.2 per cent in native arteries. The 30-day occlusion frequency was 14.8 per cent in grafts and 10.6 per cent in native arteries. Amputation was necessary in 5.9 per cent of those with occluded grafts and 3.8 per cent of those with blocked native arteries. The other outcomes of graft thrombectomy were: wound problems 11.3 per cent, wound infection 3.5 per cent, vascular surgical complications 2.3 per cent, general complications 8.6 per cent; 30-day mortality was 5.5 per cent. Similarly, outcomes of operations on native arteries were: wound problems 4.1 per cent, wound infection 0.9 per cent, vascular surgical complications 2.3 per cent, general complications 10.1 per cent; 30-day mortality was 16.6 per cent.

Table 9B.7   *Characteristics of patients treated for acute limb ischaemia in Denmark and Sweden. The Danish data are from 2808 patients treated during 1996–2000 and underwent 3438 procedures. The Swedish data are from 7496 primary lower limb procedures carried out during 1987–2000. All data are percentages except for age*

Number of procedures/ 100 000 per year	Denmark 11.0	Sweden 7.8 Embolism	Thrombosis	Comparison between Swedish E *v* T data
Males	49.5	43.1	55.7	P < 0.0001
Median age	70 years	80 years	75 years	P < 0.0001
Cerebrovascular disease	17	26.4	17.7	P < 0.0001
Diabetes	15.4	16.6	19.5	P = 0.002
Cardiac disease	47.2	76.6	55.9	P < 0.0001
Hypertension	33.2	35.0	37.8	P – 0.014
Hyperlipidaemia	–	3.0	4.5	P < 0.0001
Pulmonary disease	25.1	10.3	11.2	NS
Renal disease	–	5.7	7.1	P = 0.013
Previous vascular surgery	42.5	14.8	39.6	P < 0.0001
Previous amputation	3.7	–	–	
Recorded smoker	77.6	15.1	34.7	P < 0.0001

NS, not significant.

Arterial thrombolysis was the second most common procedure accounting for 488 treatments (13.4 per cent) with the following outcomes: 30-day occlusion 13.1 per cent, amputations 11.3 per cent, wound complications 6.8 per cent, wound infection 0.4 per cent, vascular surgical complications requiring surgery 3.5 per cent, general complications 8.4 per cent; 30-day mortality was 4.9 per cent. Percutaneous transluminal angioplasty was the primary procedure in 4.8 per cent carrying a 30-day occlusion rate of 14.9 per cent, an amputation rate of 10.3 per cent and a 30-day mortality of 4.6 per cent.

Finland

A total of 2108 surgical revascularisations were performed for acute ischaemia in Finland during 1991–97 with a mean annual throughput of 387 cases with complete data ($7.6/10^5$ per year). These cases represented 9.8 per cent of the total vascular surgical workload. At the same time only 363 endovascular procedures, mainly thrombolysis, were performed which represent 3.2 per cent of the endovascular workload. The use of thrombolysis, however, has increased threefold during the last five years. Operations most often missing from the Finnvasc database were emergencies and endovascular procedures;[3] detailed analysis of Finnish data on acute ischaemia would therefore be misleading.

Sweden

Patients treated for acute ischaemia of the leg constitute a heterogeneous group. Most patients treated for acute arterial occlusion are old and often have other complicating diseases. The traditional distinction between embolic and thrombotic occlusion has been questioned but the clinical classification used by surgeons seems to define disparate populations with differences between countries.

The frequency of occurrence of risk factors in patients defined as having had an embolus on the one hand and thrombosis on the other differs significantly in several aspects (see Table 9B.7).

The classic treatment for acute ischaemia is an emergency thromboembolectomy. Around 20 per cent of arterial occlusions occur in the upper extremity, and a small proportion involve the visceral arteries; in both instances surgical embolectomy still appears to be the first option. The choice of procedure in the lower extremity, however, has changed considerably during the past decade with endovascular techniques, notably thrombolysis, being chosen increasingly (Fig. 9B.2). During the five years 1996–2000, 28 per cent of the procedures used were endovascular with a significant difference between indications for treatment: embolism 16.9 per cent, thrombosis 34.7 per cent. It also appears as if different therapeutic techniques were chosen for different patient groups (Table 9B.8). According to an analysis using logistic regression of risk factor differences, the endovascular technique was preferred in younger patients with a lower prevalence of cerebrovascular disease. In patients with thrombosis the picture is more complex in that individual risk factors have distinct influences, for example, age was less important while a history of previous vascular surgery was of greater significance.

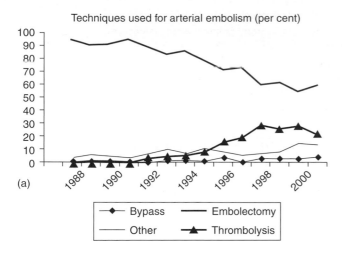

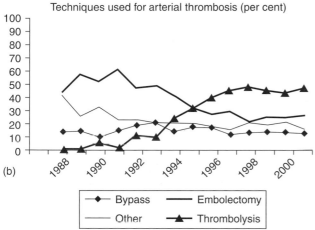

Figure 9B.2 *Proportions (per cent) of different therapies for (a) arterial embolism and (b) arterial thrombosis in Sweden*

Not surprisingly, outcome in the short term is also different between the two groups (Table 9B.9). The 30-day outcome was better (P < 0.001) after endovascular intervention in managing embolism and thrombosis. Most impressive, however, is the difference in mortality: in both groups the risk is at least halved when the endovascular technique is used. Whether this is a true difference in outcome, or simply due to differences in patient selection or degrees of operative trauma, remains to be studied. In those patients for whom thrombolysis is considered possible or suitable, the outcome is certainly not worse than that after open surgery.

VASCULAR TRAUMA

The incidence and spectrum of vascular trauma has changed in Scandinavia during the past 10 years. The rising rate of iatrogenic vascular injuries is directly related to the mounting number of interventional vascular procedures, and, to a lesser degree, of laparoscopic techniques. The majority of blunt injuries are caused by traffic accidents. In penetrating trauma the most common wounding agents are knives and shards of glass, gunshot wounds being rare in Scandinavia, whereas in Finland at least, most patients when injured are under the influence of alcohol.[10]

A striking feature in Scandinavian practice is that most surgeons on call handling emergency vascular trauma have little or no experience in vascular surgery. This is true of all hospitals with the exception of those in Swedish and Finnish university hospitals and larger vascular centres.

Table 9B.8 *Univariate comparison of risk factors among patients presenting with acute ischaemia and treated by different techniques in Sweden*

	Embolism			Thrombosis		
	Endo	Open	Difference	Endo	Open	Difference
Number	428	2108		1114	1861	
Males	49.1	39.5		51.1	53.9	
Median age, years	78	81		75	74	
Cerebrovascular disease	19.2	26.8	0.001	15.5	18.9	0.02
Diabetes	16.4	14.9	NS	20.8	17.3	0.018
Cardiac disease	76.2	77.7	NS	54.3	56.0	NS
Hypertension	42.5	37.4	0.048	41.0	34.8	NS
Hyperlipidaemia	5.1	3.6	NS	7.1	5.0	0.018
Pulmonary disease	9.1	10.6	NS	10.0	13.6	0.004
Renal disease	6.5	6.0	NS	4.8	8.2	0.0001
Previous vascular surgery	19.6	23.2	NS	39.4	57.3	0.0001
Recorded smoker	18.5	13.5	0.007	33.6	32.6	NS

Endo, endovascular; NS, not significant; open, open surgery.

Table 9B.9   *30-day outcome in patients presenting with acute ischaemia in Sweden (per cent)*

| | Embolism | | Thrombosis | |
	Open surgery	Endovascular	Open surgery	Endovascular
Alive, improved	65.5	77.1	54.7	69.2
Alive, unchanged	16.9	13.8	20.4	17.6
Alive, amputated	4.2	2.3	10.5	6.6
Dead	13.4	6.8	14.4	6.6
Number	2108	428	1863	1114

Table 9B.10   *Mechanisms of vascular injuries in Finland and Sweden*

| Country | Years | No. of patients | Trauma mechanism (per cent) | | |
			Penetrating	Blunt	Iatrogenic
Finland	1991–1999	503	39	19	42
Sweden	1987–2000	1000	31	23	46

Denmark

Arterial trauma is rare and during the five-year period 1996–2000, 140 patients (male 100 (71.4 per cent), female 40 (28.6 per cent), median age 35 years (3–90)), 57.3 per cent actively employed, underwent 146 treatment procedures, and taking all ages together represented an incidence of only $0.5/10^5$ per year; the median hospital stay was 3.6 days and 89.5 per cent survived.

Finland and Sweden

The accuracy of emergency case data in the Finnish and Swedish vascular registries is limited by underreporting,[3] a fact especially true of vascular injuries which are not always treated by vascular surgeons. Based on Finnvasc covering the years 1991–99, the annual incidence of vascular injuries was $1.3/10^5$ per year (range 0.9–2.0). During the past 30 years the total incidence in Sweden had increased from 1.1 to $2.26/10^5$ per year, mainly due to the rise in iatrogenic vascular injuries.[11]

In many European countries iatrogenic injuries, as a proportion of vascular trauma, exceeds 40 per cent.[12] In Sweden, the increase in iatrogenic vascular trauma seems to be associated with the introduction of PTA.[13] No iatrogenic injuries were reported in Helsinki in 1985, that being the preangioplasty era,[10] but 10 years later the incidence was 42 per cent.[12] The incidence of iatrogenic vascular injuries in gynaecological interventions was found to be $0.76/10^4$ per year for laparotomies and $0.93/10^4$ per year for laparoscopies, together responsible for 3 per cent of all vascular injuries in Sweden during the reported period.[14]

The incidence of penetrating trauma exceeds blunt injuries in both Finland (39 *v* 19 per cent) and Sweden

(31 *v* 23 per cent) (Table 9B.10). In Scandinavia, aortic and inferior vena cava injuries are caused by stabbing rather than by gunshot wounds, in Finland three times more commonly.[15,16]

The anatomical location of vascular injuries in Finland and Sweden was similar (Table 9B.11). The relative distribution of injuries of vessel injuries was: lower and upper extremity arteries 45 per cent and 33 per cent, respectively; great thoracic vessels 4 per cent; abdominal vessels including the iliac arteries 10 per cent; cervical vessels 3 per cent; veins of the limbs and neck 7 per cent.

The five most common vascular repairs according to Finnvasc (n = 597) were suture repair or ligation 41 per cent, interposition graft 21 per cent, end-to-end anastomosis 10 per cent, thromboembolectomy 6 per cent, patch repair 4 per cent. The corresponding figures for Swedvasc (n = 999) were 32, 33, 9, 6 and 8 per cent, respectively. The mortality rates for Swedvasc (n = 931) were: penetrating trauma 1.7 per cent, blunt 1.4 per cent, iatrogenic injuries 4.5 per cent. The overall mortality in Finnvasc (n = 503) was 2.8 per cent.

In Finland the majority of patients with vascular injuries are managed by vascular surgeons in university and central hospital emergency departments, by general surgeons in smaller hospitals and by cardiothoracic or vascular surgeons in larger hospitals. In Finland the historic association of orthopaedics and traumatology might have hampered the recognition of vascular injuries and caused delay in treatment. A new training programme initiated at the University of Helsinki Medical School is aimed at producing general surgeons capable of managing traumatic and other surgical emergencies of soft tissues. The trend in Sweden, applying the generally accepted Advanced Trauma Life Support (ATLS) concept, is to centralise management of major trauma in county or university hospitals, a principle also valid for endovascular procedures. Only university

Table 9B.11 *Anatomic location of civilian vascular injuries in Finland and Sweden. Data are number (per cent)*

	Finland (n = 510)	Sweden (n = 998)	Total (n = 1508)
Carotid artery	17 (3)	29 (3)	46 (3)
Vertebral artery	–	2 (0.2)	2 (0.1)
Axillary artery	23 (5)	39 (4)	62 (4)
Brachial artery	53 (10)	138 (14)	191 (13)
Radial or ulnar artery	65 (13)	107 (11)	172 (11)
Thoracic great vessel	17 (3)	37 (4)	54 (4)
Abdominal great vessel	13 (3)	29 (3)	42 (3)
Iliac artery	33 (6)	83 (8)	116 (7)
Femoral artery	159 (31)	304 (30)	463 (31)
Popliteal artery	32 (7)	84 (8)	116 (8)
Crural artery	56 (11)	41 (4)	97 (6)
Venous injuries	42 (8)	90 (9)	132 (9)
Miscellaneous	–	15 (2)	15 (1)

hospitals have specialised vascular surgeons on call, but by voluntary agreements, surgeons who have vascular experience can be summoned to the emergency departments of county hospitals when vascular trauma is encountered.

In recent years vascular trauma, in some instances, has been the subject of malpractice claims. Most of these cases have concerned vascular occlusion or disruption associated with orthopaedic or endovascular interventions, the injury having been either overlooked or a diagnosis delayed.

Conclusions

Scandinavian vascular registries depend on information voluntarily submitted and managed by committees under national vascular societies. Contributing vascular surgeons are, in principle, civil servants employed by hospital authorities, and although the legal position of ownership of and access to the database has to be clarified, it remains open to scrutiny by national data inspectorates. Although national reporting formats differ, data conforming to index procedures, as defined by the European Board of Vascular Surgery (Eurovasc),[1] can be extracted. The new collaborative working group, Vascunet, representing established registries in Europe,[2] should contribute to a convergence of structures and formats as essential requirements for scientifically valid comparative studies.

Data collection on risk factors in RAAA are prone to be erroneous and incomplete but that on operative procedures and outcome are much more reliable. The true efficacy of surgery in these cases cannot be assessed if data on the fate of patients not reaching the operating theatre are omitted from the registries. Overall case fatality, that is including all patients with RAAA, was 80 per cent in Finland,[4] 67 per cent in Viborg County, Denmark, and 88 per cent in Sweden.[17] Total hospital mortality, which includes patients entering the emergency room alive, is an objective indicator of the ability of any given hospital to handle RAAA. Finland's high volume centres with an active repair policy had better results than did smaller units. Similarly, the Danish experience[18] of improved results with RAAAs reflects the establishment of vascular centres, centralised emergency vascular services and standard criteria for RAAA repair. The potential of mass AAA screening in improving overall mortality is dominating the literature.

Endovascular techniques have improved outcome and lowered short term mortality in comparison with open surgery in acute ischaemic states. Whether this is the effect of patient selection or of thrombolysis, with or without PTA, remains to be seen. In differentiating between embolic and thrombotic aetiology Swedvasc data may be overdiagnosing embolism; this is not attempted in Karbase. From a clinical point of view, acute ischaemia should be assumed to be thrombotic unless proved otherwise, and that stance is reflected in the increased use of thrombolysis.

Almost half of the vascular injuries in Scandinavia are iatrogenic, affecting older patients with complex coexisting diseases, and carry a higher mortality (4–5 per cent) than injuries from other causes (1–2 per cent). It underlines the need for better teamworking between vascular surgeons and interventional radiologists.

ACKNOWLEDGEMENTS

We are grateful to the following: from Denmark, Leif Panduro Jensen and Jesper Laustsen, Karbase; from Finland, Juha-Pekka Salenius and Maarit Heikkinen, Finnvasc, and Ari Leppäniemi, Helsinki University Central Hospital for trauma expertise, Anita Mäkelä for secretarial assistance; from Sweden, David Bergqvist, Martin Björck, Claes Forssell, Johan Elfström, Tommy Skau, Lars Norgren, K-G Ljungström.

Key references

Bengtsson H, Bergqvist D. Ruptured abdominal aortic aneurysm: a population-based study. *J Vasc Surg* 1993; **18**: 74–80.

Kantonen E, Lepäntalo M, Brommels M, Luther M, Salenius J-P, Ylönen K and the Finnvasc Study Group. Mortality in ruptured abdominal aortic aneurysms. *Eur J Vasc Endovasc Surg* 1999; **17**: 208–212.

Kantonen I, Lepäntalo M, Salenius JP, Forström E, Hakkarainen T, *et al.* Auditing a nationwide vascular registry – the 4-year Finnvasc experience. *Eur J Vasc Endovasc Surg* 1997; **14**: 468–74.

Paaske WP. Eurovasc Report 1999: Vascular and endovascular surgical activity in Denmark, Finland, Galicia Region Spain, New Zealand, Northern Ireland, Slovakia, St Petersburg Region Russia, and Sweden. *Eur J Vasc Endovasc Surg* 2001; **22**: 282.

Swedvasc. Auditing Surgical outcome. Ten years with The Swedish Vascular Registry-Swedvasc. *Eur J Surg* 1998; **164**(suppl 581): 1–48.

REFERENCES

1 Paaske WP. Index operations for procedural activity in vascular surgery. In: Bastounis EA. (ed.) *Proceedings of the 13th Congress of the European Chapter of the International Union of Angiology.* Milan: Monduzzi 1999; 241–4.

2 Paaske WP. Eurovasc Report 1999: Vascular and endovascular surgical activity in Denmark, Finland, Galicia Region Spain, New Zealand, Northern Ireland, Slovakia, St Petersburg Region Russia, and Sweden. *Eur J Vasc Endovasc Surg* 2001; **22**: 282.

3 Kantonen I, Lepäntalo M, Salenius JP, *et al.* Auditing a nationwide vascular registry – the 4-year Finnvasc experience. *Eur J Vasc Endovasc Surg* 1997; **14**: 468–74.

4 Kantonen E, Lepäntalo M, Brommels M, *et al.* and the Finnvasc Study Group. Mortality in ruptured abdominal aortic aneurysms. *Eur J Vasc Endovasc Surg* 1999; **17**: 208–12.

5 Swedvasc. Auditing surgical outcome. Ten years with The Swedish Vascular Registry – Swedvasc. *Eur J Surg* 1998; **164**(suppl 581): 1–48.

6 Heikkinen M, Salenius JP, Auvinen O. Ruptured abdominal aortic aneurysm in a well defined geographical area. *J Vasc Surg* 2002: **36**: 191–296.

7 Korhonen SJ, Kantonen I, Pettilä V, *et al.* Long-term survival and health-related quality of life of patients with ruptured abdominal aortic aneurysm. *Eur J Vasc Endovasc Surg* 2003; **25**: 350–3.

8 Korhonen SJ, Ylonen K, Biancari F, *et al.* Finnvasc Study Group. Glasgow Aneurysm Score as a predictor of immediate outcome after surgery for ruptured abdominal aortic aneurysm. *Br J Surg* 2004; **91**: 1449–52.

9 Eriksson I, Hallén A, Simonsson N, Aberg T. Surgical classification of abdominal aortic aneurysms. *Acta Chir Scand* 1979; **145**: 455–8.

10 Lepäntalo M, Tukiainen E, Böstman O, *et al.* Peripheral vascular injuries in Helsinki 1985. *Finn J Orthop Traumatol* 1987; **10**: 38–9.

11 Bergqvist D, Helfer M, Jensen N, Tägil M. Trends in civilian vascular trauma during 30 years. *Acta Chir Scand* 1987; **153**: 417–22.

12 Fingerhut A, Leppäniemi AK, Androulakis GA, *et al.* The European experience with vascular injuries. *Surg Clin North Am* 2002; **82**: 175–88.

13 Bergqvist D, Jonsson K, Weibull H. An analysis of complications to percutaneous transluminal angioplasty (PTA) of extremity and renal arteries. *Acta Radiol* 1987; **28**: 3–12.

14 Bergqvist D, Bergqvist A. Vascular injuries during gynecologic surgery. *Acta Obstetr Gynecol Scand* 1987; **66**: 19–23.

15 Jousi M, Leppäniemi A. Management and outcome of traumatic aortic injuries. *Ann Chir Gynaecol* 2000; **89**: 89–92.

16 Leppäniemi AK, Savolainen HO, Salo JA. Traumatic inferior vena caval injuries. *Scand J Thorac Cardiovasc Surg* 1994; **28**: 103–8.

17 Bengtsson H, Bergqvist D. Ruptured abdominal aortic aneurysm: a population-based study. *J Vasc Surg* 1993; **18**: 74–80.

18 Lindholt JS, Henneberg EW, Fasting H. Decreased mortality of abdominal aortic aneurysms in a peripheral county. *Eur J Vasc Endovasc Surg* 1995; **10**: 466–9.

10

Medico-Legal Aspects of Emergency Vascular Care in the UK

BRUCE CAMPBELL

INTRODUCTION

There has been a burgeoning of medico-legal activity in the UK[1] and Europe in recent years, which has followed, but by no means caught up with, a similar trend in the USA. This has affected vascular surgery rather less than many other disciplines such as obstetrics, and these differences are reflected in professional insurance premiums. The area of vascular work most often associated with medico-legal problems is the treatment of varicose veins,[2,3] but such cases are invariably elective, rather than emergencies, and have often been dealt with by surgeons who are not vascular specialists.[4]

Arterial surgery is associated with substantial numbers of adverse events, and these often follow emergency or urgent presentations. In the USA, the Harvard Medical Practice Study,[5] involving 30 121 hospital records, found a higher proportion of adverse events in vascular surgery, largely arterial, than any other specialty (16 per cent), although a smaller percentage of these were judged to be due to negligence than in other specialties (18 per cent). A study of 15 000 hospital admissions in Utah and Colorado,[6] documented aortic aneurysm repair and lower limb bypass grafting as the two operations with the highest adverse event rates of all, 19 per cent and 14 per cent, respectively, with 8 per cent and 11 per cent of these adverse events judged as preventable. In Australia, the Quality in Australian Healthcare Study[7] on 14 000 admissions claimed that 49 per cent of the adverse events observed in vascular surgical practice were potentially preventable. Despite the variation in these figures, there is a clear message that many clinical problems after arterial operations may be preventable.

With regard to the incidence of medico-legal claims, collated figures from the National Health Service Litigation Authority (which has indemnified Health Service hospitals in England and Wales since 1995) and from the Medical Defence Union (MDU) (reflecting private practice in the UK from 1990 to 1999) include 36 claims against surgeons for failure to diagnose or treat ischaemia, and 45 for complications of aortic surgery.[4] The MDU database for general practice for the same period contained 299 claims, all related either to alleged mismanagement of limb ischaemia (n = 197) or diagnosis and treatment of aneurysms (n = 102).

In elective arterial practice there is usually ample opportunity for assessment, counselling and record keeping, which are particularly important in guarding against subsequent complaints or litigation.[8] Emergency vascular practice poses a greater chance of medico-legal problems: decisions often need to be made quickly and without all the information clinicians would like; there may be little opportunity for counselling and the immediate writing of good notes; and the potential for loss of life or limb is high. In addition, these patients frequently present to doctors who are not vascular specialists, and the diagnosis may be missed or delayed, with serious consequences for the patient and difficulties for the receiving vascular consultant.

This chapter presents a number of aspects of emergency vascular practice which may be associated with complaints or litigation, and proposes suggestions about how to avoid being sued. It certainly does not provide all the answers, but hopefully offers food for thought.

THE BASIS OF MEDICO-LEGAL ACTIONS

It is important, briefly, to rehearse the law of negligence, which governs medico-legal action against doctors in the UK. There are three fundamental principles:

1 To establish that the doctor had a duty of care to the patient: as a rule this poses no problems, although it may do so in the setting of emergency vascular practice.
2 To show that the doctor has breached that duty of care to the patient: therefore he has been negligent (**liability**).
3 To prove that the doctor's actions, or omissions, have caused damage to the patient (**causation**).

A longstanding and important precedent exists from the case of Bolam (Bolam *v* Friern Hospital Management Committee 1957), namely, 'a doctor is not guilty of negligence if he acted in accordance with the practice accepted as proper by a responsible body of medical men skilled in that particular art', but the professional opinion called to support him must be capable of 'withstanding logical analysis' (from Bolitho *v* City and Hackney Health Authority 1997). Judgments about what was, or was not, likely to have happened are based on the **balance of probabilities** (greater or lesser than 50 per cent probability) and not on the principle of 'beyond reasonable doubt' used in criminal cases. Increasingly in medico-legal judgments, the concept is being used of what a 'reasonable man' would have done rather than simply considering the views of medical specialists.

It is important to remember that only a small proportion of complaints against doctors develop into medico-legal claims: proceedings are issued in only a few of these cases, and fewer still go to court. However, the stress and emotional impact of medical errors[9] and medico-legal threats can be oppressive for those involved, and the time involved in dealing with the issues may be considerable.

MISSED OR DELAYED DIAGNOSIS

This is a major cause of medico-legal activity. The doctors held responsible for missing emergency vascular conditions are most often not vascular surgeons, but vascular surgeons may then find themselves presented with difficult late presentations and may also become targets for the general dissatisfaction about the management of the patient. Certain conditions have special potential for delayed or missed diagnosis.

Spontaneous acute ischaemia due to embolism or thrombosis may be confused with other causes of limb pain, for example sciatica, or may simply not be noticed in uncommunicative or bedridden patients who are in hospital wards or nursing homes. Traumatic arterial damage may escape detection in a setting of multiple trauma or after injuries which are not typically associated with vascular involvement. The swelling and generalised pallor often associated with trauma can make assessment difficult, and a high index of suspicion is the key to diagnosis. Late complications such as false aneurysms can also result in accusations of negligence. Failing to recognise compartment syndromes associated with acute trauma and/or acute ischaemia is a matter of particular concern for vascular surgeons.

The diagnosis of leaking abdominal aneurysm is not infrequently delayed or missed by doctors both in primary care and in hospital. Leaking aneurysms are well known to present with atypical features, being easily confused with other conditions causing abdominal pain such as ureteric colic or diverticular disease, with acute back problems or with conditions causing hypotension such as myocardial infarction. Aortoenteric fistula is another condition which may be rapidly fatal but which is sometimes not recognised: even when suspected in a patient with an aortic graft the diagnosis may be difficult to prove.

If there is concern about the possibility of any of these conditions, but the diagnosis is not clear, then good record keeping is fundamental from the risk management point of view. Written notes that a particular diagnosis was considered, the reasons for uncertainty and the steps taken to investigate, are a powerful defence if that diagnosis was later found to have been 'missed'. It is equally important not to accuse or condemn other doctors in writing after a referral has been made with a delayed diagnosis: the full circumstances may not be known to the receiving specialist, and written accusations of negligence can be the cause of serious and needless problems.

WHO SHOULD BE RESPONSIBLE FOR EMERGENCY VASCULAR PROBLEMS?

This question has assumed importance with the increasing specialisation in general surgery. The days have long gone when acute ischaemia was dealt with by any general surgeon and associated trainees,[10] and decreasing numbers of non-vascular consultants feel competent to operate on leaking aortic aneurysms. In addition, there is a rising public expectation fuelled by the press that all treatment will be delivered by 'specialists'. When all does not go well with emergency vascular cases, 'generalists' may become increasingly vulnerable to medico-legal criticism. The underlying problem, particularly apparent in the healthcare system of the UK, is one of insufficient vascular specialists in many hospitals, especially those outside large urban areas. The history and reasons for this are complex, but the result is that many hospitals do not have a formal emergency vascular surgical, or vascular radiology rota, and as a consequence general surgeons with little or no regular experience of elective vascular work may have to take on emergency cases.

Where formal vascular rotas do not exist, there may be a special medico-legal threat for vascular surgeons, who frequently make themselves available as much as they are able for emergencies.[11] If they are contacted by telephone and are unable or unwilling to attend because they are not formally 'on call', what would be their liability if the outcome is unfavourable for a patient who is dealt with by generalist colleagues or trainees, or who is transferred to another hospital? What is their clinical responsibility and duty of care if they are not contractually on call? Offering advice over the telephone is usually taken to imply clinical responsibility, at least to some degree. This is a difficult area but one which surgeons and managers need to consider. Each hospital should have clear understandings about which consultant is in charge of the patient's care at any given time: admitting general surgeons should not assume that their vascular colleagues have taken over care of an emergency admission until this has been explicitly agreed. This is also important medico-legally with regard to the question of who supervises trainees dealing with the patient, particularly when the duty trainees are not part of the vascular team, currently a common situation.

Another potentially difficult medico-legal issue relates to transfer of patients, which may be required if there is no vascular specialist available in a hospital, or if adequate facilities are not available, for example, no intensive care bed for a leaking aneurysm. Might there be a medico-legal challenge if the treatment of such a patient is delayed, and they die or lose a limb as a result? It is a legal principle that hospitals should not offer services which they cannot provide to a good standard, and this could be taken to imply that it is better to transfer an emergency vascular patient, rather than to treat them in a substandard way. The principles of transfer should be the subject of agreement by health authorities and hospital trusts, following discussion from a 'public health' perspective.

DECISIONS ABOUT WITHHOLDING TREATMENT

Decisions about withholding active treatment are required quite often in emergency vascular practice, for example, in patients with leaking aortic aneurysms[12] or unsalvageable acute limb ischaemia,[13] who are very elderly, who have serious, and often multiple, comorbidities and poor quality of life. This is an area of potential medico-legal concern, although, in response to a questionnaire in 1998,[12] only 22 per cent of vascular surgeons in the UK and Ireland stated that medico-legal concerns ever influenced their decisions about not operating on patients with leaking aortic aneurysms. Quite a different response would probably have been received from surgeons in the USA, where there are generally higher expectations from both patients and relatives for heroic treatment of the very elderly with little chance of survival.

When deciding on palliative care rather than surgical intervention, it is vital that all staff caring for the patient are in tune with the decision, and that they are invited to voice any concern or disagreement. Not only is this part of teamwork and common sense, but it also guards against any disaffected member of the care team later claiming to have been an unwilling party to a wrong or negligent decision. The patient's family must be counselled sensitively, and must concur with the decision, but not be made to feel responsible for it: it is they who might later take legal action if the situation was not dealt with well. Whenever practical, patients themselves should be involved in the decision. These discussions should always involve a senior member of the vascular surgical team.[13]

A particular problem in emergency situations is that little may be known about the patient's pre-existing medical condition, and relatives may not be immediately to hand; patients with leaking aortic aneurysms who have housebound spouses with disabilities are a case in point. When a decision about palliative care is particularly difficult it may be an advantage to involve a senior anaesthetist, both to give an opinion and to record their opinion in the notes; this can be especially helpful when relatives press for active treatment in a patient whose anaesthetic risks are excessive.

With sensitive explanation and counselling, as well as good written records, thoughtful decisions to withhold active surgical treatment will hopefully remain an area which seldom gives rise to medico-legal action, but the potential for problems needs to be kept clearly in mind.

INFORMED CONSENT

Treatment of vascular emergencies is fraught with potential complications, but the urgency of the situation and the condition of many patients can make thorough counselling about risks both impractical and unkind. For example, the collapsed patient with a ruptured aortic aneurysm is in no state to receive any amount of information, except the message that he needs major emergency surgery for a leaking artery. The patient's condition may be so grave that signing of a consent form is not a sensible expectation, but this should never deter surgeons from doing what they believe to be in the patient's best interests as this is their duty from both an ethical and a legal point of view.

When the situation permits more explicit informed consent, then there is a medico-legal expectation that patients should be told about relevant risks, both very serious problems which occur occasionally, and lesser problems which occur more frequently.[14–18] Just how fully the frightened elderly patient should be confronted with any risks beyond the threat to an acutely ischaemic limb is a matter of individual judgement. Whatever they, and their close relatives and especially carers, are told, it is important that the conversation is documented and this is dealt with further below. While it is very helpful, and I believe essential, to have a good standard information booklet about each common operation in the elective setting, this is more difficult for emergency procedures. However, when there is the opportunity to give the patient a booklet, for example about 'thrombolysis' or 'bypass grafts to the limb', then this should certainly be done.

Occasionally patients may say that they do not want to be informed in detail about proposed procedures or risks. That is their right, but if they are not informed because of this kind of request then this should be recorded clearly. It should always be the presumption that every patient wants to be well informed.

THE TEAM APPROACH AND GUIDELINES

Although the vascular surgeon bears ultimate responsibility for the vascular surgical patient, other specialists and disciplines are also important, not only for their contributions to management of the patient, but also in the risk management process and avoidance of litigation. This is particularly true of vascular radiologists who play the leading role in thrombolysis for acute ischaemia, and there needs to be very clear communication between them and their surgical colleagues about the decision for thrombolysis, who counsels and consents the patient, and their specific responsibilities while lysis is in progress. There is a potential for serious medico-legal consequences if a patient has a stroke during thrombolysis without a record of explicit informed consent, or if they develop bleeding which is not dealt with appropriately because of poorly defined responsibilities.

Thrombolysis is a particular area of emergency vascular practice in which written guidelines are very valuable, particularly for trainees and nursing staff, and they should describe the action to be taken if problems occur. Many doctors worry about the medico-legal disadvantages of guidelines,[19] but thrombolysis is a good example of a treatment for which their advantages far outweigh any possible disadvantage. It is relatively complex treatment which involves several disciplines, with which trainees and less experienced nurses may not be very familiar, and which requires efficient monitoring with a clear understanding of what to do if things go wrong. It may be helpful to use published consensus documents[20] when constructing guidelines, but for practical purposes they must reflect local circumstances and preferences.

OMISSION OF PROPHYLAXIS IN THE EMERGENCY SETTING

It is easy for important prophylactic measures to be forgotten in the turmoil of emergency treatment. Prophylactic antibiotics are especially important when grafting ruptured aortic aneurysms: there can be no defence if they are not given at the time of aortic grafting and the graft becomes infected. The need is especially great in the context of aseptic precautions which may be less rigorous than usual, as is sometimes the case when dealing with collapsed patients, and extra doses of antibiotics are wise at the end of the operation when there has been massive blood loss.

Failure to provide prophylaxis against venous thromboembolism has become a regular cause of medico-legal action. In the treatment of acute ischaemia there may also be a need to consider special measures to prevent further arterial thromboembolism, using anticoagulants or dextran 40. Tetanus prophylaxis should not be forgotten in cases of trauma.

WRITTEN RECORDS AND NOTES

The importance of good records cannot be overemphasised in any discussion about medico-legal matters.[3,8,18,21] When dealing with vascular emergencies, for example, ruptured aneurysms, pressure of time often makes writing of thorough preoperative notes impossible. Written notes may be confined to bare working details when time is pressing, but after an emergency operation there is no excuse for the absence of an adequate record of everything that happened. I always dictate an operation note, which is then typed, and this is a good opportunity to describe the initial presentation, the discussions and the reasons for decisions. The typed note is also a useful place to record personal thoughts about the case, prognosis and plans, together with what has been said to the patient's relatives about the likely outcome. The details are not only helpful to those subsequently involved in the patient's care, but they are also invaluable if there is any subsequent complaint or medico-legal claim.

It is vital for doctors to understand that the records they write or dictate provide the *only* evidence of what was thought, said and done. A patient or relatives may make assertions later which are completely untrue, but if no record exists to contradict them then it is difficult to refute their claims. It is worth remembering the cynical point of view: 'If you didn't write it down, it didn't happen'. It is tediously basic, but absolutely mandatory from the medico-legal standpoint, that each page of the clinical record has the patient's name and reference number on it, that each entry is properly dated including the year and not just the month, and that entries, especially for emergency and urgent records, have a time, the 24-hour clock being best.

INCIDENT REPORTING

All hospitals should now have systems in place for immediate reporting of any incidents which might result in complaint or medico-legal proceedings.[18,21,22] If clinicians do this conscientiously, then problems may be averted or minimised. Incident reporting is a huge subject in its own right but all doctors need to know about their local incident reporting systems and how to use them.

CLINICAL AUDIT

There are two particular medico-legal implications of clinical audit. First, it is probably advantageous to be able to report that any case with an adverse outcome was discussed at a peer group audit meeting. Second, audit of individual results may help to support a surgeon's reputation and credibility in a particular area of work. The National Vascular Database being developed by the Vascular Society of Great Britain and Ireland may well come to represent an important tool by which vascular specialists can confirm that their results conform to national norms.[23] Contributing data about procedures to national and international registries, for example aortic stent grafts used to treat leaking aneurysms, is a hallmark of good practice and may help support a clinician, particularly in the context of relatively new procedures.

The extent to which the results of past performance should be required or offered in medico-legal proceedings is a matter for debate. Clinical governance now demands that such records be made, and it seems inevitable that lawyers will increasingly ask for the figures. Demonstration of regular, careful audit, with appropriate changes in practice is likely to contribute to the defence to a surgeon accused of negligence, particularly if the results are good. By the same token surgeons are understandably worried that audit might also be used against them. Their results might be compared unfavourably with published series, which often describe much better outcomes than the norm.[16] In addition, audit data might be used to criticise them for doing a specific procedure infrequently: for example a surgeon who had had poor outcomes from just two or three cases of vascular trauma might find this fact used against them despite good reasons for these results, and a good track record of elective arterial reconstructions. Although regular audit and involvement in national registries certainly are important, these considerations may discourage recourse to audit figures as a routine in medico-legal proceedings.

Clinicians involved in research on procedures for emergency vascular conditions should take particular care in advising patients and their relatives, in record keeping, and in all aspects of research governance. Medico-legal action resulting from an 'experimental' procedure requires particularly robust defence.

Conclusion

Emergency vascular work poses many possibilities for medico-legal challenge. However, the surgeon who makes thoughtful decisions, who communicates them sympathetically to patients and their relatives, and who keeps thorough records stands a good chance of avoiding both complaints and successful claims.

Key references

Campbell B, Callum K, Peacock N. *Operating Within the Law.* Kemberton: tfm publishing, 2001.

Campbell B, France F, Goodwin H, on behalf of the Research and Audit Committee of the Vascular Surgical Society of Great Britain and Ireland. An analysis of medico-legal claims in vascular surgery for the National Health Service and private sector in the United Kingdom. *Ann R Coll Surg Engl* 2002; **84**: 181–4.

Fenn P, Diacon S, Gray A, *et al.* Current cost of medical negligence in NHS hospitals: analysis of claims database. *BMJ* 2000; **320**: 1567–71.

NHS Executive. *Risk Management in the NHS.* London: Department of Health, 1994.

Seeking Patients' Consent: The Ethical Considerations. London: General Medical Council, 1998.

REFERENCES

1 Fenn P, Diacon S, Gray A, *et al.* Current cost of medical negligence in NHS hospitals: analysis of claims database. *BMJ* 2000; **320**: 1567–71.

2 Giordano JM. Malpractice and the vascular surgeon. *J Vasc Surg* 1993; **18**: 901–4.

3 Goodwin H. Litigation and surgical practice in the UK. *Br J Surg* 2000; **87**: 977–9.

4 Campbell B, France F, Goodwin H, on behalf of the Research and Audit Committee of the Vascular Surgical Society of Great Britain and Ireland. An analysis of medico-legal claims in vascular surgery for the National Health Service and private sector in the United Kingdom. *Ann R Coll Surg Engl* 2002; **84**: 181–4.

5 Brennan TA, Leape LL, Laird NM, *et al.* Incidence of adverse events and negligence in hospitalized patients. *N Engl J Med* 1991; **324**: 370–6.

6 Gawande AA, Thomas EJ, Zinner MJ, Brennan TA. The incidence and nature of surgical adverse events in Colorado and Utah in 1992. *Surgery* 1999; **126**: 66–75.

7 Wilson RM, Runciman WB, Gibberd RW, *et al.* The Quality in Australian Health Care Study. *Med J Aust* 1995; **163**: 458–71.

8 Baird RN. The vascular patient as litigant. *Ann R Coll Surg Engl* 1996; **78**: 278–82.

9 Wu AW. Medical error: the second victim. *BMJ* 2000; **320**: 276–7.

10 Nachbur B. Treatment of acute ischaemia: every general surgeon's business? *Eur J Vasc Surg* 1988; **2**: 281–2.

11 Campbell WB, Ridler BMF, Thompson JF. Providing an acute vascular service: two years experience in a district general hospital. *Ann R Coll Surg Engl* 1996; **78**: 185–9.

12 Hewin DF, Campbell WB. Ruptured aortic aneurysm: the decision not to operate. *Ann R Coll Surg Engl* 1998; **80**: 221–5.

13 Campbell WB, Verfaillie P, Ridler BMF, Thompson JF. Non-operative treatment of advanced limb ischaemia: the decision for palliative care. *Eur J Vasc Endovasc Surg* 2000; **19**: 246–9.

14 Marshall JE, Baker PN. Informed consent – legal and ethical issues. Health Care Risk Report 1999: 12–14.

15 Gladstone J, Campbell B. A model for auditing informed consent. *J Clin Effectiveness* 2000; **1**: 247–50.

16 *Seeking patients' consent: the ethical considerations*. London: General Medical Council, 1998.

17 *Reference guide to consent for examination or treatment.* London: Department of Health, 2001.

18 Campbell B, Callum K, Peacock N. *Operating Within the Law.* Kemberton: tfm publishing, 2001.

19 Hurwitz B. Legal and political considerations of clinical practice guidelines. *BMJ* 1999; **318**: 661–4.

20 Working Party on Thrombolysis in the Management of Limb Ischemia. Thrombolysis in the management of lower limb peripheral arterial occlusion – a consensus document. *Am J Cardiol* 1998; **81**: 207–18.

21 NHS Executive. *Risk Management in the NHS.* London: Department of Health, 1994.

22 Roberts G. Untoward incident reporting: quality improvement and control. *Clin Risk* 1995; **1**: 168–70.

23 Campbell B, Earnshaw J. Getting governance to work in surgery. *Ann R Coll Surg Engl* 2001; **83**(suppl): 56–7.

Acute Cerebrovascular Syndromes

11

The Developing Stroke

SEBASTIÁN F AMERISO

THE PROBLEM

Stroke is defined as the acute onset of a focal neurological deficit caused by alterations in blood circulation in the vascular territory of the central nervous system. Cerebral ischaemia can also affect the brain diffusely during prolonged systemic hypotension thereby causing extensive infarcts.

Stroke is the third leading cause of death in North America and the most common cause of prolonged disability in the industrialised world.[1] The absolute number of stroke patients is likely to increase in ageing populations. Until recently, the management of acute cerebral infarction was restricted to supportive measures and control of risk factors in secondary stroke prevention. Acute ischaemic stroke is now viewed as a medical emergency with a narrow therapeutic window clinically comparable to acute myocardial infarction.[2] In the vast majority of patients neuronal damage occurs within a few hours of the initial event and the term 'brain attack' emphasises the need for rapid diagnosis and treatment.

The purpose of this chapter is to discuss the diagnosis and management of acute ischaemic stroke, beginning in an emergency room setting. The supportive and ancillary treatment measures will be underlined and the strategies aimed at reperfusing and protecting the brain while limiting the area of infarction discussed. Special attention will also be given to the prevention of common iatrogenic complications of these patients.

AETIOLOGY/PATHOPHYSIOLOGY

Classification

There are two types of stroke: ischaemic and haemorrhagic. Ischaemic strokes or cerebral infarcts account for approximately 85 per cent of all strokes.[3,4]

Stroke classification

- Ischaemic strokes
  - Large artery atherosclerosis
  - Cardioembolism
  - Small vessel occlusion
  - Other aetiologies (some unknown)
- Haemorrhagic strokes
  - Intraparenchymal haemorrhages: hypertensive; amyloid angiopathy; other causes, such as tumours, blood dyscrasias, etc.
  - Subarachnoid haemorrhage: aneurysmal; traumatic; other causes
  - Rupture of arteriovenous malformations

Athero-thromboembolic or large vessel strokes originate in atheromatous lesions localised within the large cerebral vessels, both extracranial and intracranial. Typically infarcts are large cortical and subcortical lesions in the territory of one of the major cerebral vessels. Cardioembolic strokes occur in conditions such as atrial fibrillation, myocardial infarction, congestive failure, valve disease, congenital malformations and aortic arch plaque.[5,6] The role of mitral valve prolapse and patent foramen ovale in embolism remains controversial. Lacunar or small vessel strokes are small subcortical infarcts caused by occlusion of small, deeper placed vessels affected by the pathological process of lipohyalinosis. Other aetiologies are vasculitis, procoagulant conditions, drug use and venous occlusion.[7] Haemorrhagic strokes comprise approximately 15 per cent of acute cerebrovascular events, including intracerebral haemorrhage and rupture of aneurysms and arteriovenous malformations.

Strokes can also be classified according to the temporal evolution of symptoms. Transient ischaemic attacks (TIAs) are focal neurological deficits with complete resolution within 24 hours. In most cases TIAs last less than a minute or two and certainly well below 1 hour. A reversible ischaemic neurological deficit (RIND) or minor stroke is an event lasting more than 24 hours with complete or near complete resolution within 3–7 days. Infarcts with transient neurological symptoms (ITNS) cannot be distinguished clinically from TIAs, but computed tomography (CT) or magnetic resonance imaging (MRI) will demonstrate a recent ischaemic lesion in the affected territory. Strokes in evolution are neurological events that progress after onset. The deterioration usually occurs during the initial hours of the episode and is caused, at least in part, by progression of the underlying thrombotic process. Completed strokes are permanent neurological deficits without major changes occurring after the initial assessment.

Temporal evolution of acute ischaemic cerebrovascular events

- Transient ischaemic attacks
- Reversible ischaemic neurological deficit or minor stroke
- Infarcts with transient neurological symptoms
- Stroke in evolution
- Completed stroke

Stroke risk factors

Similar to patients with coronary disease, stroke patients usually have conditions that predispose them to the occurrence of strokes.[8] These stroke risk factors can be modifiable or non-modifiable.

Stroke risk factors

- Non-modifiable risk factors
  - Advanced age
  - Male sex
  - Genetic factors
- Modifiable risk factors
  - Hypertension
  - Smoking
  - Diabetes mellitus
  - Dyslipidaemia
  - Cardiac disease
  - History of stroke/TIA
  - Other factors: haemorrheological factors (i.e. elevated haematocrit and fibrinogen), procoagulant conditions, hyperhomocysteinaemia, genetic factors, recent infection/inflammation

---

Pathophysiology

The basic mechanisms of cerebral ischaemia are: (i) *in situ* thrombosis resulting in narrowing of the vessel lumen and reduction in flow or (ii) fragmentation and dislodgement of a clot in the heart or in an artery with subsequent embolisation to a cerebral vessel. When blood flow to an area of the brain is reduced to a critical level through either one of these mechanisms the result is infarction[9] (see Chapter 5).

ISCHAEMIC PENUMBRA

Experimental and clinical evidence have demonstrated the existence of an area surrounding the infarcted tissue in which blood flow is maintained by collateral circulation at a level below 50 per cent of normal. This viable area, known as the ischaemic penumbra, remains in danger of sustaining progressive damage and necrosis.[10] The fact that irreversible damage can occur within a short period of time provides the rationale for early treatment of stroke either by prompt reperfusion or by administering agents which protect the brain from further damage, in other words pharmacological neuroprotection. The time between the initial insult and the completion of neuronal death in the penumbra represents the therapeutic window of opportunity for treatment of ischaemic stroke.[11] The duration of this time window is probably no longer than 3–6 hours and the response to different therapeutic modalities may vary from patient to patient.

CEREBROVASCULAR AUTOREGULATION

This is a normal physiological mechanism which allows for constant maintenance of cerebral blood flow (CBF) through a wide range of perfusion pressures.[12] The normal range of mean arterial pressure (MAP) regulation is 60–130 mmHg and when it goes outside that range autoregulation is lost and cerebral blood flow follows changes in MAP. Chronic hypertension is associated with displacement of the autoregulatory curve to the right. Cerebrovascular autoregulation is defective immediately after a stroke and the ischaemic brain tissue is entirely dependent on available collateral surrounding flow.

Cerebral autoregulation normally maintains CBF at a constant level across a wide range of mean perfusion pressures (mean arterial pressure 60–150 mmHg). Autoregulation is impaired following stroke, and ischaemic brain tissue becomes passively dependent on surrounding collateral blood supply.[12] Rapid reduction of blood pressure to normotensive levels may compromise collateral supply and precipitate acute neurological deterioration.[13]

CLINICAL ASPECTS/DIAGNOSIS

Acute ischaemic stroke is a medical emergency. Early evaluation of patients allows the proper planning of management strategies. Patients with new onset focal neurological deficit, either transient or established, should be admitted to institutions with the resources capable of managing acute cerebrovascular events. That would include the rapid availability of neurologists, vascular surgeons, neurosurgeons, internists and radiologists, backed up by appropriate diagnostic devices available on a 24-hour basis.

Elements raising suspicion of stroke
• Focal neurological deficit reaching maximal severity within minutes to hours • Subject older than 55 years • Presence of vascular risk factors

Patients should be evaluated immediately upon arrival. A detailed medical history will often require help from relatives or other witnesses, particularly if there are signs of language disturbance or a diminished level of awareness. Those with severe deficits or other serious medical conditions should be admitted to an intensive care unit. It is important to determine promptly the need for orotracheal intubation. Careful and frequent evaluation of clinical and neurological status is of value in prevention, diagnosis and treatment of complications.

Special attention should be given to ascertaining the timing and characteristics of symptoms at onset, past neurological status, medication and history of important stroke risk factors such as hypertension, diabetes, smoking, heart disease, previous stroke or TIAs, drug abuse and family history. A complete physical examination is necessary keeping in mind cardiac arrhythmias and murmurs, carotid bruits and evidence of pulmonary aspiration. Neurological examination will determine the characteristics of the deficit and the localisation of the lesion. The affected vascular territory can usually be established based on the spectrum of symptoms and signs.

After a brief but thorough initial physical and neurological examination a non-contrast brain CT should be obtained. This study is often normal during the first

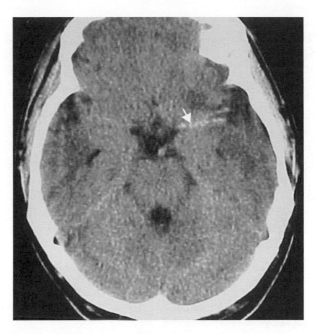

Figure 11.1 *Non-contrast brain computed tomography in a patient with acute onset of right hemiparesis and aphasia. Note hyperdense middle cerebral artery signal suggesting acute occlusion in the vessel (arrow)*

24 hours after an ischaemic stroke but permits the diagnosis of haemorrhagic stroke and other conditions sometimes misdiagnosed as ischaemic strokes.[14] The use of fibrinolytic drugs in the first few hours of stroke and their potential for severe haemorrhagic complications has stimulated the identification of early changes on CT which suggest the presence of infarcted tissue (see box and Fig. 11.1).

Early CT changes in acute ischaemic stroke
• Hyperdense middle cerebral artery signal • Acute hypodensity • Mass effect • Loss of grey/white matter interface • Loss of sulci • Obscured basal ganglia • Loss of insular ribbon

In recent years, MRI using the diffusion/perfusion technique (DWI/PWI) has helped in the early identification of ischaemic changes and, in cases with DWI/PWI mismatch, the delineation of an area of penumbra which will recover if reperfusion can be initiated promptly[15] (Fig. 11.2).

Basic laboratory studies, namely, blood count, coagulation assays, electrolytes, glucose, renal, and liver function tests, electrocardiogram and chest X-ray should be undertaken on admission.

After initial evaluation a strategy of management should be established, with diagnostic evaluation focused on

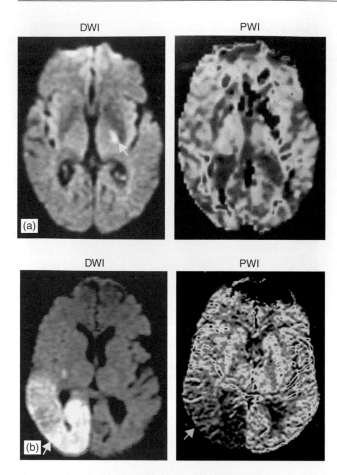

Figure 11.2 *Brain magnetic resonance imaging with diffusion/perfusion weighted (DWI/PWI) technique. (a) DWI/PWI mismatch. Perfusion defect (light blue arrow) is larger than the diffusion defect (yellow arrow). (b) Perfusion and diffusion defects are similar suggesting absence of a penumbra area*

assessing the aetiology of the event and locating disease in large or small vessels, identifying cardioembolic sources, prothrombotic states and other conditions. This process will refine acute management and facilitate planning the most appropriate strategy for secondary prevention. Vascular ultrasound and magnetic resonance angiography have proved useful in the detection of severe stenosis and occlusion in the carotid artery. Cerebral angiography is performed transarterially when intra-arterial thrombolysis is planned or when the information to be obtained is likely to influence therapeutic decisions. The possibility of a cardiac embolic source is excluded by detailed cardiological examination, chest X-ray and electrocardiogram (ECG) and if still suspected by transthoracic and/or trans-oesophageal echocardiography, 24-hour Holter-ECG, myocardial perfusion studies and coronary angiography. Transoesophageal echocardiography allows the determination of size and motility of cardiac chambers, presence of intracavitary thrombi (a negative study does not rule out their existence), valvular disease and atheromatous disease of the aortic arch. Prothrombotic disorders associated with

stroke include antiphospholipid antibodies, elevated fibrinogen, erythrocytosis, hyperhomocysteinaemia, activated protein C resistance and, less frequently, protein C and S congenital deficiencies and antithrombin III deficiency. Cerebrospinal fluid examination is presently reserved for cases of dubious aetiology, especially in young subjects and when there is suspicion of some infectious or inflammatory brain process.

Approximately one-third of patients with ischaemic stroke deteriorate after the initial event: during the first 24 hours (or later in posterior circulation strokes) it represents a progression of the thrombotic process, in other words, stroke in evolution.[16] Cerebral oedema usually accounts for the deterioration occurring between the second and fifth day, especially when patients have sustained large infarcts.

Neurological deterioration can also be related to a haemorrhagic transformation of the infarct, a particular danger in patients treated with fibrinolytic or anticoagulant drugs, but it may follow fresh episodes of embolism in patients with embolic sources, or medical complications such as infection, metabolic disturbance and haemodynamic failure.

GENERAL MANAGEMENT

The principles of emergency management of stroke, i.e. control of potential life-threatening complications and specific treatment of the vascular event,[17] are summarised in the algorithm given in Fig. 11.3.

Bed rest

Bed rest is recommended for the first 48 hours, especially for those with orthostatic hypotension, commonly observed among diabetics, elderly patients and those receiving antihypertensive medication. Neurological deterioration may result from premature mobilisation of patients with orthostatic hypotension and impaired cerebral autoregulation.

Airway and breathing

Ensure airway patency, particularly in patients with decreased alertness. Hypoxia may alter neurological status and contribute to the neurological deficit but supplemental oxygen is not needed routinely. Pulse oximetry will identify the patient with obstructive breathing patterns or desaturation during sleep.[18] Hypercapnia can also be detrimental because it raises intracranial pressure.

Circulation

The management of hypertension following acute ischaemic stroke remains a somewhat controversial issue.[19] Over two-thirds of patients with acute stroke have elevated initial

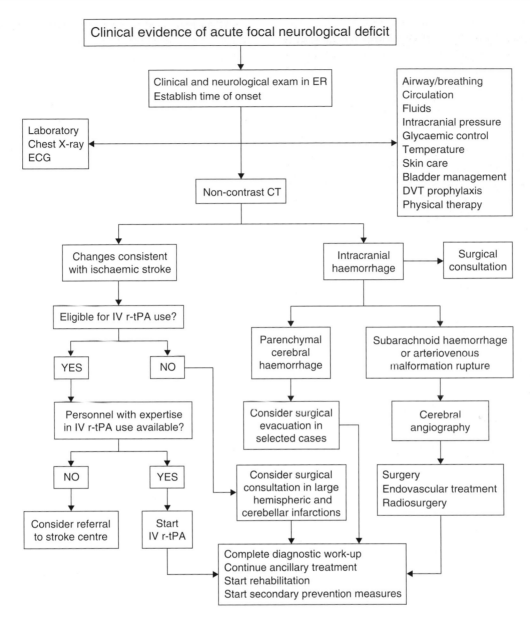

Figure 11.3   *Algorithm of the principles of emergency management of stroke. CT, computed tomography; DVT, deep vein thrombosis; ECG, electrocardiogram; ER, emergency room; IV, intravenous; r-tPA, recombinant tissue plasminogen activator*

blood pressures (>170/100 mmHg), yet there is no clear relation between hypertension and neurological worsening or outcome.[20] Blood pressures tend to normalise spontaneously following stroke, with decreases of about 20 mmHg systolic and 10 mmHg diastolic during hospitalisation.[20] The rate of decline is most rapid during the initial four days and greatest in subjects with higher initial values. Moderate hypertension followed by normalisation is thus expected following ischaemic stroke; moderate hypertension may even be beneficial early on, as has been demonstrated in some animal models.[21]

Certain individuals are particularly susceptible to the dangers of rapid blood pressure reduction, including those with prior chronic hypertension or high grade arterial stenosis and of course the elderly.[22,23] Chronic hypertension is common in stroke patients and may be associated with an upward shift of the lower autoregulatory limit for CBF, say a mean of 85–150 mmHg; thus even modest blood pressure reductions may compromise collateral supply to dependent regions of the brain.[24]

Knowledge of stroke pathophysiology and the benign course of post-stroke hypertension support the axiom that hypertension should be left untreated early on, unless it is dangerously elevated or sustained[25] (Fig. 11.1). Strokes in the setting of aortic dissection, symptomatic congestive heart failure, acute myocardial infarction or other hypertensive organ failure represent exceptions which require more rapid management.

Treatment of hypertension, a cornerstone of secondary stroke prevention, should therefore be initiated cautiously maintaining vigilance for orthostatic side effects. While a graduated reduction of blood pressure is of greater importance than the antihypertensive medication selected, we generally avoid nifedipine, diuretics and clonidine which cause rapid and sharp falls in blood pressure, volume contraction, lowered CBF and changes in mental status.[26] Labetalol, a combined αβ-adrenergic blocker, has proved to be safe and effective in accelerated hypertension when administered orally or intravenously to patients as long as they do not have asthma, chronic obstructive pulmonary disease, bradycardia, heart block or failure.[27]

Hypotension may occur in patients with severe coexistent heart disease marked by arrhythmias, heart failure or acute myocardial infarction, or if they are dehydrated or septic. Cerebral blood flow may be impaired in this situation and urgent correction is advised.

Fluids

An intravenous line is required for management of fluids and electrolytes and for drug administration. We recommend normal saline infusion for most patients, the total fluid intake not exceeding 2500 mL/day for the first four days; fluid restriction minimises the development of brain oedema in those with suspected or proved large infarcts.

Approximately 15 per cent of patients develop hyponatraemia with or without dehydration. Sodium correction must be timely and executed with caution if central nervous system lesions, for example central pontine myelinolysis, are to be avoided. Hypernatraemia is less common but it too must also be corrected cautiously to avoid cerebral oedema.

Raised intracranial pressure

Oedema is caused by intracellular retention of fluid in the ischaemic area and reaches its peak 48–72 hours after the stroke.[28] In patients with large hemispheric and cerebellar infarctions mass effect may result in clinical deterioration and death (see Chapter 5). Early signs of progressing oedema include decreased alertness and pupillary changes.[29] Treatment of elevated intracranial pressure following ischaemic stroke is difficult. Hyperventilation produces hypocapnia and vasoconstriction, with potential worsening of cerebral ischaemia.[30] Steroids are ineffective in ischaemic stroke.[31] We recommend mannitol at doses of 0.25–0.50 g/kg at 4–6-hour intervals, carefully managing electrolytes and maintaining serum osmolality below 300 mOsm.[32] In severe cases intravenous furosemide may be combined with mannitol.[33] Patients with cerebellar infarction developing brain stem compression may benefit from shunting and posterior fossa surgical decompression, an interesting but still unproved option in those with large hemispheric strokes.[34]

Swallowing, hydration and nutrition

Acute ischaemic stroke patients are at high risk of aspiration, a devastating complication in most instances. Oral fluids or food should not be given until a formal swallowing examination has been performed.[35] The risk of aspiration is particularly high in patients with absent gag reflex, coughing or choking when attempting to drink, dysarthria and in those who are obtunded.[36] For patients with swallowing difficulties, we recommend placement of a duodenal tube on the second day after the stroke as nasogastric tube feeding also carries the risk of aspiration. Duodenal tube fluid administration should be by continuous infusion to prevent regurgitation, acute gastric retention and osmotic diarrhoea. The head of the bed should be elevated at least 30 degrees at all times. The volume and caloric content can be increased gradually over the first 48–72 hours to meet daily requirements.

Glycaemic control

An association between elevated blood glucose levels and poor stroke outcome, perhaps due to the effect of lactic acidosis on infarcted brain, has been reported.[37] Some studies, however, have shown that there is no direct association between hyperglycaemia and stroke outcome.[38] Diabetic patients are best managed initially using a glucose sliding scale and corrections with regular insulin followed by diet and either oral hypoglycaemic agents or insulin depending on severity and requirements.

Pyrexia

Hyperthermia, even mild, is associated with increase of infarct size and higher morbidity and mortality.[39,40] Preceding or concomitant infection is common in ischaemic stroke patients.[41,42] Experimental studies in animals and humans have shown that moderate hypothermia might be beneficial in acute stroke.[43,44] Until the results of further trials of cooling are published it would be prudent to keep body temperature under control in these patients.

Pressure areas

Skin care and prevention of decubitus ulcers is achieved by the use of special mattresses and by mobilising the patient every 2 hours.[45]

Bladder management

Incontinence of urine is common in the first few days. Indwelling urinary catheters should be avoided if possible to prevent urinary tract infections.[46]

Venous thromboembolism prophylaxis

Deep vein thrombosis (DVT) is common in stroke patients[47] and even more so in patients with dense paralysis of the affected limb. Older subjects are at increased risk, particularly those with obesity, congestive heart failure, varicose veins, history of thromboembolism and hypercoagulable states.[47] However, clinically apparent DVT occurs in less than 10 per cent of subjects and pulmonary embolism in less than 2 per cent. Prophylactic measures for patients at risk include early mobilisation, external pneumatic compression, antiplatelet therapy and antithrombotic drug therapy using low dose subcutaneous heparin or low molecular weight heparinoids.[48–50]

Epileptic seizures

Seizures are frequent in patients with large infarctions especially during the first 48 hours.[51] Acute cerebrovascular events are the most common cause of seizures in subjects older than 65 years. The response to anticonvulsive therapy is usually satisfactory and there is no evidence to support the prophylactic use of antiepileptic drugs.

Rehabilitation

Physical and occupational therapy and assessment of speech difficulties should be initiated soon after admission. Rehabilitation programmes must be customised for each individual and should start as soon as the patient is clinically stable.

SPECIFIC TREATMENT

Stroke is a medical emergency with a narrow therapeutic window. Minimising the time interval between the onset of symptoms and the initiation of specific treatment is key to the patient's chances of a satisfactory recovery.[52]

Thrombolytic therapy

Multicentre, double blind, placebo controlled randomised trials in the USA and Europe have demonstrated the efficacy of early administration of activated recombinant tissue plasminogen activator (r-tPA) in patients with acute ischaemic stroke.[53–55] Nevertheless, the drug is underused in most centres in spite of the lack of alternative strategies because of delays in presentation to the emergency room, fears of haemorrhagic complications and the inadequacy of an infrastructure to manage stroke.

Intravenous r-tPA is effective at a dose of 0.9 mg/kg given intravenously over 60 minutes (10 per cent of dose as intravenous bolus over 1 minute; maximal dose 90 mg) when used within 3 hours of onset of symptoms in highly selected patients.[53,55] The number of patients who make an excellent recovery is significantly higher in those who receive r-tPA although there is no substantial difference in mortality and this is also true of ischaemic stroke subtypes. Studies using streptokinase in acute ischaemic stroke showed that it was unhelpful and ill advised.[56] The safety of using r-tPA continues to be a major concern, brain haemorrhage having been observed 10 times more frequently in patients receiving this treatment (6.4 v 0.6 per cent).

Criteria for r-tPA use are listed below. Strict adherence to these criteria is essential if catastrophic haemorrhagic complications are to be prevented. Inadequate control of blood pressure, stroke severity, and evidence of early signs of infarction on initial CT are important predisposing factors for haemorrhagic complications.

Criteria for treatment with r-tPA

- Stroke onset $\leqslant$ 3 hours
- Intensive care available for 24 hours post-treatment monitoring
- Patients already receiving antiplatelet agents prior to stroke are still eligible for r-tPA
- As the use of thrombolytic drugs carries a real risk of major bleeding, whenever possible the risks and potential benefits of r-tPA should be discussed with the patient and his or her family before treatment is initiated
- *Exclusion criteria*
  - Current use of oral anticoagulants or a prothrombin time greater than 15 seconds – international normalised ratio (INR) greater than 1.7
  - Use of heparin in the previous 48 hours and a prolonged partial thromboplastin time
  - A platelet count less than 100 000/mm^3
  - Another stroke or a serious head injury in the previous 3 months
  - Major surgery within the preceding 14 days
  - Pretreatment systolic blood pressure greater than 185 mmHg or diastolic blood pressure greater than 110 mmHg
  - Rapidly improving neurological signs
  - Caution is advised before giving r-tPA to persons with severe stroke (NIH Stroke Scale Score greater than 22)
  - Isolated, mild neurological deficits, such as ataxia alone, sensory loss alone, dysarthria alone or minimal weakness
  - Prior intracranial hemorrhage
  - Blood glucose less than 50 mg/dL or greater than 400 mg/dL
  - Seizure at the onset of stroke

- Gastrointestinal or urinary bleeding within the preceding 21 days
- Recent myocardial infarction
- r-tPA should be avoided in patients with evidence of mass effect or oedema on CT scan or early changes indicating involvement ≥ 1/3 of the middle cerebral artery territory. An expert must interpret the CT scan

Thrombolytic therapy is not recommended unless a physician with expertise in stroke management establishes the diagnosis aided by a CT of the brain. If the CT demonstrates early changes of recent major infarction such as sulcal effacement, mass effect, oedema or possibly haemorrhage, then thrombolytic therapy should be avoided. Exclusion criteria in the National Institute of Neurological Disorders and Stroke r-tPA Stroke Study (NINDS) must be considered to be contraindications for r-tPA use. Important measures in ancillary care, during and after administration of r-tPA are described below.

Ancillary care during and after administration of r–tPA

- Admission to a skilled care facility – intensive care unit or acute stroke care unit
- Careful management of arterial blood pressure, avoiding excessively high blood pressure and excessive lowering of blood pressure
- Central venous access and arterial punctures are restricted during the first 24 hours
- Placement of an indwelling bladder catheter should be avoided during drug infusion and for at least 30 minutes after infusion ends
- Insertion of a nasogastric tube should be avoided, if possible, during the first 24 hours after treatment

Intracranial and systemic bleeding are the most catastrophic complications after r-tPA use.[57] Thrombolytic therapy should not be used unless facilities to handle these bleeding complications are readily available. Bleeding should be presumed to be the cause of any neurological worsening after the use of a thrombolytic drug until confirmed by CT, which should be obtained immediately. The management of thrombolysis related bleeding depends on the location and size of the haematoma, the potential for controlling the bleeding mechanically, the neurological risk, the interval between administration of the drug and the onset of haemorrhage and the thrombolytic drug used. Appropriate measures are listed below.

Treatment of thrombolysis related bleeding

- Discontinue ongoing infusion of thrombolytic drug
- Obtain blood samples for coagulation tests
- Obtain surgical and haematological consultations
- Consider transfusion, cryoprecipitate and platelets

The Prolyse in Acute Cerebral Thromboembolism II (PROACT II) Study[58] showed that stroke patients treated with intra-arterial prourokinase within 6 hours of onset of symptoms were more likely to live independently after the stroke. The use of intra-arterial thrombolysis for patients with acute ischaemic stroke remains under continued review by the Food and Drug Administration (FDA) and has not yet been approved.

Ancrod, a potent fibrinogenolytic agent derived from snake venom, effective in the Stroke Treatment with Ancrod Trial (STAT) trial, is also awaiting FDA approval.[59]

Anticoagulation/antiaggregation

Anticoagulation started in the first day or two after stroke may reduce the risk of DVT and pulmonary embolism but there is no evidence of other short or long term neurological benefit.[60,61] There are a few exceptions to these criteria in which use of intravenous unfractionated heparin or subcutaneous low molecular weight heparins may be considered.[62,63]

Potential indications for anticoagulation in acute cerebrovascular disease

- Recent arterial dissection
- Cerebral venous thrombosis
- Frequent or imminent cardiac embolism
- Stroke-in-evolution specially in the posterior circulation
- Crescendo TIA
- High grade symptomatic stenosis specially in the posterior intracranial circulation

The efficacy of antiaggregants and anticoagulants in some acute stroke patients can probably be attributed to the prevention of early recurrence in subjects at risk.[64–66] Certain drugs such as warfarin and ticlopidine have latency effects limiting their use during the acute event. New agents such as clopidogrel at high doses of 300 mg, hirudin and antagonists of GPIIa/IIIb receptors have rapid antithrombotic effects and are being evaluated in clinical trials. In patients with acute ischaemic stroke and a proved cardioembolic source intravenous heparin followed by warfarin is recommended. This strategy is intended for acute secondary prevention and is unlikely to be beneficial for the already completed event. The timing for initiation of treatment is controversial. An acceptable approach would be to start anticoagulation 48–72 hours after the event in those cases in which the absolute contraindications of uncontrolled hypertension or haemorrhagic transformation in a follow-up CT do not apply. In patients with large infarcts anticoagulation is often delayed for 1–2 weeks. In patients with atrial fibrillation the risk of early recurrence is not very high and anticoagulation may be delayed for a few days.

Low to medium dose aspirin (160–300 mg) started in the acute phase of an ischaemic stroke slightly reduces morbidity and mortality probably because of the earlier initiation of secondary prevention of stroke and other thrombotic complications.[64,65]

Neuroprotective agents

Although over 100 compounds have been shown to diminish the extent of ischaemic damage in various laboratory models, none has yet been shown convincingly to benefit subjects with stroke.[67]

Treatment of haemorrhagic stroke

Medical management of increased intracranial pressure includes the use of osmotic agents such as mannitol, urea or glycerol as well as steroids and hyperventilation.[68] Occasionally, it is necessary to place an intraparenchymal or intraventricular catheter to directly measure intracranial pressure. Investigation and correction or reversal of any coagulation abnormality is mandatory especially when bleeding occurs after a surgical procedure.

Surgical evacuation of the haematoma is often considered although data from the literature are controversial.[68,69] It is possible that minimally invasive techniques such as stereotactic and endoscopic aspiration will allow early and safe removal of the clot. Large lobar and cerebellar haematomas are the most frequent indications for surgery.[70]

> ## Conclusions
>
> Acute stroke is common and carries a high morbidity and mortality rate. Recent advances in its treatment during the acute phase may help reduce its devastating consequences. The complexity of modern acute stroke care and the risks posed by the different strategies used have prompted the organisation of stroke services staffed by professionals with specialised training in the management of the disease and the potential complications of treatment. Specialised multidisciplinary stroke units may reduce morbidity and mortality for stroke patients.

> Acute stroke should be considered a medical emergency with a narrow therapeutic window. Fibrinolytic therapy is relatively safe and effective for patients with acute ischaemic stroke when administered early in the course of the disease and within very strict eligibility guidelines. Its use should be reserved for institutions with adequate infrastructure and experience in the management of the condition.

Key references

Adams H, Adams R, Del Zappo G, et al. Guidelines for the early management of patients with ischemic stroke. 2005 Guidelines update. A scientific statement from the Stroke Council of the American Heart Association/American Stroke Association. *Stroke* 2005; **36**: 916–21.

Adams HP Jr, Brott TG, Furlan AJ, et al. Guidelines for thrombolytic therapy for acute stroke: a supplement to the guidelines for the management of patients with acute ischemic stroke. *Circulation* 1996; **94**: 1167–74.

Adams HP, Bendixen BH, Kappelle LJ, et al. Classification of subtype of acute ischemic stroke. Definitions for use in a multicenter clinical trial. *Stroke* 1993; **24**: 35–41.

Brott T, Bogousslavsky J. Drug therapy: treatment of acute ischemic stroke. *N Engl J Med* 2000; **343**: 710–22.

The National Institute of Neurological Disorders and Stroke rt-PA Stroke Study Group. Tissue plasminogen activator for acute ischemic stroke. *N Engl J Med.* 1995; **333**: 1581–7.

REFERENCES

1 American Heart Association. *1991 Heart and Stroke Facts.* Dallas, TX: American Heart Association, 1991.

2 Alberts MJ, Perry A, Dawson DV, Bertels C. Effects of public and professional education on reducing the delay in presentation and referral of stroke patients. *Stroke* 1992; **23**: 352–6.

3 Foulkes MA, Wolf PA, Price TR, et al. The stroke data bank: design, methods, and baseline characteristics. *Stroke* 1988; **19**: 547–54.

4 Adams HP, Bendixen BH, Kappelle LJ, et al. Classification of subtype of acute ischemic stroke. Definitions for use in a multicenter clinical trial. *Stroke* 1993; **24**: 35–41.

5 Hart RG. Cardiogenic embolism to the brain. *Lancet* 1992; **339**: 589–94.

6 Amarenco P, Cohen A, Tzourio C, et al. Atherosclerotic disease of the aortic arch and the risk of ischemic stroke. *N Engl J Med* 1994; **331**: 1474–9.

7 Markus HS, Hambley H. Neurology and the blood: haematological abnormalities in ischaemic stroke. *J Neurol Neurosurg Psychiatry* 1998; **64**: 150–9.

8 Sandercock PA, Warlow CP, Jones LN, Starkey IR. Predisposing factors for cerebral infarction: the Oxfordshire community stroke project. *BMJ* 1989; **298**: 75–80.

9 Siesjo BK. Pathophysiology and treatment of focal cerebral ischemia. Part I: Pathophysiology. *J Neurosurg* 1992; **77**: 169–84.

10 Hossmann K-A. Viability thresholds and the penumbra of focal cerebral ischemia. *Ann Neurol* 1994; **36**: 557–65.

11 Pulsinelli WA. The therapeutic window in ischemic brain injury. *Curr Opin Neurol* 1995; **8**: 3–5.

12 Meyer JS, Shimazu K, Fukuuchi Y, *et al.* Impaired neurogenic cerebrovascular control and dysautoregulation after stroke. *Stroke* 1973; **4**: 169–86.

13 Fischberg GM, Lozano E, Rajamani K, *et al.* Stroke precipitated by moderate blood pressure reduction. *J Emerg Med* 2000; **19**: 339–46

14 Libman R, Wirowski E, Alvir J, Rao T. Conditions that mimic stroke in the emergency department. *Arch Neurol* 1995; **52**: 1119–22.

15 Fisher M, Prichard J, Warach S. New magnetic resonance techniques for acute ischemic stroke. *JAMA* 1995; **274**: 908–11.

16 Gautier JC. Stroke-in-progression. *Stroke* 1985; **16**: 729–33.

17 Brott T, Bogousslavsky J. Drug therapy: treatment of acute ischemic stroke. *N Engl J Med* 2000; **343**: 710–22.

18 Rout MW, Lane DJ, Wollner L. Prognosis in acute cerebrovascular accidents in relation to respiratory pattern and blood gas tensions. *BMJ* 1971; **3**: 7–9.

19 Potter JF. What should we do about blood pressure and stroke? *Q J Med* 1999; **92**: 63–6.

20 Wallace JD, Levy LL. Blood pressure after stroke. *JAMA* 1981; **246**: 2177–80.

21 Cole DJ, Matsumura JS, Drummond JC, Schell RM. Focal cerebral ischemia in rats: Effects of induced hypertension, during reperfusion, on CBF. *J Cereb Blood Flow Metab* 1992; 1264–9.

22 Jansen PAF, Schulte BPM, Meybook RHB, Gribnau FWJ. Antihypertensive treatment as a possible cause of stroke in the elderly. *Age Ageing* 1986; **15**: 129–38.

23 Ruff RL, Talman WT, Petito F. Transient ischemic attacks associated with hypotension in hypertensive patients with carotid artery stenosis. *Stroke* 1981; **12**: 353–5.

24 Paulson OB, Waldamer G, Schmidt JF, Strandgaard S. Cerebral circulation under normal and pathologic conditions. *Am J Cardiol* 1989; **63**: 2C–5C.

25 Yatsu FM, Zivin J. Hypertension in acute ischemic strokes. Not to treat. *Arch Neurol* 1985; **42**: 999–1000.

26 Bertel O, Conen D, Radu EW, *et al.* Nifedipine in hypertensive emergencies. *BMJ* 1983; **286**: 19–21.

27 Gonzalez ER, Peterson MA, Racht EM, *et al.* Dose response evaluation of oral labetalol in patients presenting to the emergency department with accelerated hypertension. *Ann Emerg Med* 1991; **20**: 333–8.

28 Garcia JH, Ho K-L, Pantoni L. Pathology. In: Barnett HJM, Mohr JP, Stein BM, Yatsu FM (eds). *Stroke. Pathophysiology, diagnosis, and management*. New York NY: Churchill Livingstone, 1998: 139–57.

29 Ropper AH, Shafran B. Brain edema after stroke. Clinical syndrome and intracranial pressure. *Arch Neurol* 1984; **41**: 26–29.

30 Raichle M, Plum F. Hyperventilation and cerebral blood flow. *Stroke* 1972; **3**: 566–75.

31 Norris JW, Hachinski VC. High dose steroid treatment in cerebral infarction. *BMJ* 1986; **292**: 21–3.

32 Schwarz S, Schwab S, Bertram M, *et al.* Effects of hypertonic saline hydroxyethyl starch solution and mannitol in patients with increased intracranial pressure after stroke. *Stroke* 1998; **29**: 1550–5.

33 Pollay M, Fullenwider C, Roberts A, Stevens A. Effect of mannitol and furosemide on blood-brain osmotic gradient and intracranial pressure. *J Neurosurg* 1983; **59**: 945–50.

34 Schwab S, Steiner T, Aschoff A, *et al.* Early hemicraniectomy in patients with complete middle cerebral artery infarction. *Stroke* 1998; **29**: 1888–93.

35 Gordon C, Hewer RL, Wade DT. Dysphagia in acute stroke. *BMJ* 1987; **295**: 411–14.

36 Horner J, Massey EW, Riski JE, *et al.* Aspiration following stroke: clinical correlates and outcome. *Neurology* 1988; **38**: 1359–62.

37 Pulsinelli WA, Levy DE, Sigsbee B, *et al.* Increased damage after ischemic stroke in patients with hyperglycemia with or without established diabetes mellitus. *Am J Med* 1983; **74**: 540–4.

38 Matchar DB, Divine GW, Heyman A, Feussner JR. The influence of hyperglycemia on outcome of cerebral infarction. *Ann Int Med* 1992; **117**: 449–56.

39 Chen H, Chopp M, Welch KM. Effect of mild hyperthermia on the ischemic infarct volume after middle cerebral artery occlusion in the rat. *Neurology* 1991; **41**: 1133–5.

40 Ginsberg MD, Busto R. Combating hyperthermia in acute stroke. A significant clinical concern. *Stroke* 1998; **29**: 529–34.

41 Ameriso SF, Wong VLY, Quismorio FP, Fisher M. Immunohematologic characteristics of infection-associated cerebral infarction. *Stroke* 1991; **22**: 1004–9.

42 Grau A, Buggle F, Heindl S, *et al.* Recent infection as a risk factor for cerebrovascular ischemia. *Stroke* 1995; **26**: 373–9.

43 Schwab S, Schwarz S, Spranger M, *et al.* Moderate hypothermia in the treatment of patients with severe middle cerebral artery infarction. *Stroke* 1998; **29**: 2461–6.

44 Yanamoto H, Nagata I, Niitsu Y, *et al.* Prolonged mild hypothermia therapy protects the brain against permanent focal ischemia. *Stroke* 2001; **32**: 232–9.

45 Nuffield Institute for Health. Effective health care. The prevention and treatment of pressure sores. *Effective Health Care* 1995; **2**: 1–16.

46 Nakayama H, Jorgensen HS, Pedersen PM, *et al.* Prevalence and risk factors of incontinence after stroke. The Copenhagen stroke study. *Stroke* 1997; **28**: 58–62.

47 Sioson ER. Deep vein thrombosis in stroke patients: an overview. *J Stroke Cerebrovasc Dis* 1992; **2**: 74–9.

48 Turpie A, Gallus A, Beattie WS, Hirsh J. Prevention of venous thrombosis in patients with intracranial disease by intermittent pneumatic compression of the calf. *Neurology* 1977; **27**: 435–8.

49 Antiplatelet Trialists' Collaboration. Collaborative overview of randomized trials of antiplatelet therapy. III: Reduction in venous thrombosis and pulmonary embolism by antiplatelet prophylaxis among surgical and medical patients. *BMJ* 1994; **308**: 235–46.

50 Turpie AG, Gent M, Cote R, *et al.* A low-molecular weight heparinoid compared with unfractionated heparin in the prevention of deep vein thrombosis in patients with acute ischemic stroke. *Ann Intern Med* 1992; **117**: 353–7.

51 Burn J, Dennis M, Bamford J, *et al.* Epileptic seizures after a first stroke: the Oxfordshire community stroke project. *BMJ* 1997; **315**: 1582–7.

52 Adams H, Adams R, Del Zappo G, *et al.* Guidelines for the early management of patients with ischemic stroke. 2005 Guidelines update. A scientific statement from the Stroke Council of the American Heart Association/American Stroke Association. *Stroke* 2005; **36**: 916–21.

53 The National Institute of Neurological Disorders and Stroke rt-PA Stroke Study Group. Tissue plasminogen activator for acute ischemic stroke. *N Engl J Med.* 1995; **333**: 1581–7.

54 Hacke W, Kaste M, Fieschi C, *et al.* Randomised double-blind placebo-controlled trial of thrombolytic therapy with

intravenous alteplase in acute ischaemic stroke (ECASS II). *Lancet* 1998; **352**: 1245–51.

55   Adams HP Jr, Brott TG, Furlan AJ, *et al.* Guidelines for thrombolytic therapy for acute stroke: a supplement to the guidelines for the management of patients with acute ischemic stroke. *Circulation* 1996; **94**: 1167–74.

56   Donnan GA, Davis SM, Chambers BR, *et al.* Trials of streptokinase in severe acute ischaemic stroke. *Lancet* 1995; **345**: 578–9.

57   The National Institute of Neurological Disorders and Stroke rt-PA Stroke Study Group. Intracerebral hemorrhage after intravenous t-PA therapy for ischemic stroke. *Stroke* 1997; **28**: 2109–18.

58   Furlan A, Higashida R, Wechsler L, *et al.* for the PROACT Investigators. Intra-arterial prourokinase for acute ischemic stroke: the PROACT II study: a randomized controlled trial. *JAMA* 1999; **282**: 2003–11.

59   Sherman DG, Atkinson RP, Chippendale T, *et al.* Intravenous ancrod for treatment of acute ischemic stroke: the STAT study: a randomized controlled trial. *JAMA* 2000; **282**: 2395–403.

60   Bousser MG. Aspirin or heparin immediately after a stroke? *Lancet* 1997; **349**: 1564–5.

61   The Publications Committee for the Trial of Org 10172 in Acute Stroke Treatment (TOAST) Investigators. Low molecular weight heparinoid, Org 10172 (danaparoid), and outcome after acute ischemic stroke: a randomized controlled trial. *JAMA* 1998; **279**: 1265–72.

62   Einhäupl KM, Villringer A, Meister W, *et al.* Heparin treatment in sinus venous thrombosis. *Lancet* 1991; **338**: 597–600.

63   Saver JL, Easton JD. Dissections and trauma of cervicocerebral arteries. In: Barnett HJM, Mohr JP, Stein BM, *et al.* (eds) Stroke: pathophysiology, diagnosis and management. New York: Churchill Livingstone, 1998: 769–86.

64   CAST (Chinese acute stroke trial) Collaborative Group. CAST: randomized placebo-controlled trial of early aspirin use in 20 000 patients with acute ischaemic stroke. *Lancet* 1997; **349**: 1641–9.

65   International Stroke Trial Collaborative Group. The International Stroke Trial (IST). A randomised trial of aspirin, subcutaneous heparin, both, or neither among 19,435 patients with acute ischaemic stroke. *Lancet* 1997; **349**: 1569–81.

66   Kay R, Wong KS, Yu YL, *et al.* Low molecular weight heparin for the treatment of acute ischemic stroke. *N Engl J Med* 1995; **333**: 1588–92.

67   Devuyst G, Bogousslavsky J. Clinical trial update: neuroprotection against acute ischaemic stroke. *Curr Opin Neurol* 1999; **12**: 73–9.

68   Qureshi AI, Tuhrim S, Broderick JP, *et al.* Medical progress: spontaneous intracerebral hemorrhage. *N Engl J Med* 2001; **344**: 1450–60.

69   Hankey GJ, Hon C. Surgery for primary intracerebral hemorrhage: is it safe and effective? A systematic review of case series and randomized trials. *Stroke* 1997; **28**: 2126–32.

70   Gerritsen van der Hoop R, Vermeulen M, Van Gijn J. Cerebellar hemorrhage: diagnosis and treatment. *Surg Neurol* 1988; **29**: 6–10.

12

Role of the Vascular Surgeon in Managing Stroke

JOHN P ROYLE, GEOFFREY A DONNAN, BRIAN CHAMBERS

THE PROBLEM

In 1954, Eastcott et al.[1] reported a successful carotid artery reconstruction in a patient with transient cerebral ischaemia. Following this report attention was focused on the carotid artery in the neck as a cause of stroke. It was realised that a stroke from carotid artery disease could occur due to a reduction in flow, or due to emboli, and transient ischaemic attacks (TIAs) could, similarly, arise from both of these causes.

There then developed a worldwide controversy over the place of carotid endarterectomy. With the results of two randomised trials of carotid artery surgery, the place of this operation was finally confirmed. In the European Carotid Surgery Trial (ECST)[2] and in the North American Symptomatic Carotid Endarterectomy Trial (NASCET),[3] it was firmly established that when a stenosis of 70–99 per cent was present in patients with symptomatic carotid disease, carotid artery surgery was clearly superior to best medical treatment. When the stenosis was 50–70 per cent, the results were, initially, unclear but it is now recognised that there is also some advantage of surgery over best medical therapy in this group of patients.[4]

More recently, carotid angioplasty and stenting has been used as an alternative to carotid endarterectomy, particularly in patients in whom there are relative contraindications to surgery. Routine deployment of a mesh funnel or other distal protection device reduces the risk of dislodging plaque material during the procedure, and stroke complications are now lower than when the technique was first used. Currently there are trials underway comparing carotid endarterectomy and carotid stenting. If stenting proves more efficacious than endarterectomy, most of the material presented in this chapter still applies.

SELECTION FOR URGENT SURGERY

The basis for urgent surgery follows the knowledge that a stroke may occur quickly after a TIA. A patient with an intact brain after a TIA has everything to save. Delay in surgery may result in a potentially preventable stroke. The 1977 study of Cartlidge et al. from the Mayo Clinic[5] showed that the risk of stroke was high in the first month after a TIA, and probably the greatest risk was in the first few days after the initial event.

The two most important aspects of selection of patients for surgery are diagnosis and timing. For this reason it is essential that neurologists and vascular surgeons work in close collaboration.

Wrong diagnosis

One of the most important aspects of selection of patients for carotid endarterectomy is to be certain that a carotid artery lesion is indeed responsible for the ischaemic deficit. An embolus may come from the heart, aortic valve, atheromatous aortic arch or carotid artery. There may occasionally be difficulty in distinguishing posterior from anterior circulation symptoms ipsilateral to a demonstrated carotid stenosis. Alternatively, although symptoms may relate to the anterior circulation, the pathology may be in small penetrating vessels quite unrelated to an ipsilateral carotid artery stenosis. The most common example of this is in a patient with lacunar TIA or minor stroke due to in situ single penetrator vessel disease and not caused by emboli from the heart or carotid artery. Lacunar TIAs may occasionally present in crescendo form with repeated bursts of hemiplegia, the so-called capsular warning syndrome.[6]

Cerebral haemorrhage

Where the initial TIA has in fact been due to a subdural haematoma, intracerebral tumour or cerebral haemorrhage, a carotid endarterectomy is strongly contraindicated. The relief of a tight stenosis will, by increasing the blood pressure at the site of the bleed, substantially increase the risk of further haemorrhage. A computed tomography (CT) scan performed early will exclude these entities.

Timing

There is anecdotal evidence that when an enhancing infarct is demonstrated on a CT scan there is an increased risk of converting a recent infarct into a haemorrhagic infarct. Therefore, operation is best delayed for at least 2–3 weeks after the stroke.

INVESTIGATIONS

A CT scan is required to determine whether there is any cerebral haemorrhage present and to determine whether there is any infarct present. However, when a CT scan is performed within 24 hours after an infarct, it may appear normal and an infarct may only be demonstrated on follow-up CT a few days later. When there is an established neurological deficit it is assumed that an infarct is present, even though the CT scan may not demonstrate it initially.

As magnetic resonance imaging (MRI) becomes more widely available in acute care hospitals, its superiority over CT in evaluation of acute stroke is appreciated more and more. Provided the scanning protocol includes a gradient echo sequence, cerebral haemorrhage is readily diagnosed. The main advantage over CT, however, is the use of diffusion-weighted imaging (DWI) to demonstrate acute brain infarction as early as 1 hour after the onset of symptoms. The sensitivity of MRI in detecting cerebral infarction is much greater than even delayed CT (see Chapter 13). Therefore MRI can identify those individuals in whom it may be better to delay carotid endarterectomy. In patients with infarction, the location of the infarct, e.g. anterior versus posterior circulation or cortical versus lacunar, helps determine whether or not carotid disease is implicated. Also, magnetic resonance angiography (MRA) of intracranial, and if necessary, extracranial vessels provides invaluable information concerning vascular pathology without injection of contrast media, and often, if performed within the first few hours after the onset of symptoms, embolic occlusion of the middle cerebral artery may be demonstrated.

Duplex scan versus angiography

A diagnosis of carotid stenosis used to be made by angiography, but with improvements of equipment and technique of duplex scanning, the latter is now the usual investigation employed in the demonstration of carotid stenosis. At our institution, we have found that transcranial Doppler gives valuable information about the status of the intracranial circulation and collaterals. Angiography is reserved for patients in whom a duplex scan presents technical difficulties, as sometimes occurs with heavily calcified lesions or when there is doubt about the result of a duplex scan. With experienced ultrasonographers, the percentage of patients in whom there will be a doubt is now very low. Gadolinium-enhanced MRI or CT angiography can be used instead of conventional angiography in selected cases.

MANAGEMENT

Current routine at the Austin and Repatriation Medical Centre (see Fig. 12.1)

Patients present to the emergency department in three ways:

- a local general practitioner has phoned the admitting officer regarding the patient
- the relatives have brought the patient directly to the emergency department without first attending a local doctor
- an ambulance has brought the patient following a 'collapse'.

When the admitting officer is forewarned of the patient's arrival, the patient will be shown directly to an assessment room, but when the patient comes unannounced, the triage sister will perform this task.

When a patient has a **neurological deficit** immediate admission is arranged. The emergency department medical staff make their initial assessment. A CT scan is usually arranged. Further assessment is done by a neurology registrar and/or neurologist concerning the need for a duplex scan. Patients with a gross deficit may have a duplex scan at a later time; as they will not be considered for surgery on an urgent basis there is no need for this to be expedited.

Patients **without a deficit**, or with a doubtful diagnosis, are usually assessed in the emergency department by the neurology registrar. If necessary, a CT scan and duplex study of carotid arteries may be performed immediately. An MRI scan may also be expedited. If these show a carotid stenosis, admission and surgery are expedited. If the duplex scan is doubtful, then angiography may be arranged, although this is not common nowadays. Some patients with no carotid pathology may be admitted for further detailed evaluation, looking for alternative sources of emboli. Others will be sent home either with or without aspirin and may have further evaluation on an outpatient basis.

In many instances, patients with **a minor neurological deficit** follow the same path as patients who have had a TIA and whose neurological signs have resolved completely,

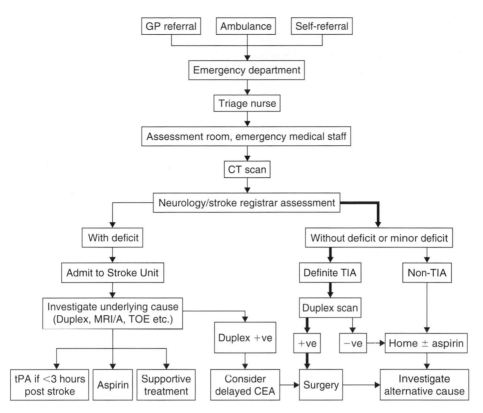

Figure 12.1 *Emergency management of patients with stroke at the Austin and Repatriation Medical Centre, Melbourne, Australia. CEA, carotid endarterectomy; CT, computed tomography; GP, general practitioner; MRI/A, magnetic resonance imaging/angiography; TIA, transient ischaemic attack; TOE, transoesophageal echocardiography; tPA, tissue plasminogen activator*

i.e. they have an urgent duplex scan, which, if it confirms a carotid stenosis, is then followed by an urgent operation. If the duplex scan is negative, there is no need for further consideration for carotid endarterectomy.

In difficult cases the CT scan is particularly important. It will exclude a haemorrhage, even a small one. In patients where CT scan is performed within 4 hours of the onset of an ischaemic deficit, only subtle changes of infarction are occasionally seen, but the majority of infarcts will show some changes within the first 48 hours. The use of MRI/MRA, when available, will usually demonstrate infarction even in early cases.

One area where a duplex scan may be in error is when the duplex scan shows complete occlusion when in fact 'trickle flow' may be present. An angiogram will demonstrate a 'carotid string sign'. This is a thin sliver of dye seen connecting the common carotid artery with an intracranial normal patent internal carotid artery. The appearance occurs when there is extremely low flow in the carotid artery and should not be confused with complete occlusion. In the stable patient, the risk of stroke is considered to be low as for complete occlusion, but there are patients with recurring or crescendo TIAs in whom carotid endarterectomy, which is not possible with complete occlusion, can be performed.

The management of **minor strokes** is more controversial. Usually, if a patient has had a mild cerebral deficit, carotid endarterectomy is delayed for a month unless a further TIA occurs. However, as mentioned earlier, if fluctuations of neurological deficit are occurring with almost complete resolution between, in spite of adequate medical therapy, consideration should be given to emergency endarterectomy. Such patients should be otherwise medically fit with a relatively minor neurological deficit between fluctuations.

The circle of Willis provides a theoretical collateral pathway for cerebral blood supply. In some patients this is congenitally incomplete. It has been shown that there is an added risk of stroke in patients with contralateral tight stenosis or occlusion,[7] associated intracranial disease,[8] or lack of intracranial collaterals.[9] In each of these situations, carotid endarterectomy improves the outcome.

Timing of urgent carotid endarterectomy

The 'emergency' operation is usually undertaken in the next operating session, rather than in the middle of the night. This obviates problems that may occur when non-regular staff are used to help. Similarly, when a patient, for whom a delay in surgery has been advised because of a mild deficit, sustains another TIA, operation is scheduled for the next available session. When the unit has an operating session on each day, as we do, there is little delay. However, in these circumstances, when an urgent operation is decided on a Friday, we prefer to do the operation on Saturday morning rather than leave the patient until the following Monday.

In situations where patients are having multiple TIAs, namely, those with so-called crescendo TIAs, a carotid endarterectomy is performed as a true emergency, if necessary in the middle of the night. In general, the mechanism of cerebral ischaemia in these patients is haemodynamic, secondary to a very tight carotid stenosis. Alternatively, an extensive haemorrhagic plaque repeatedly dislodging small emboli may be present. An angiogram may even show intraluminal clot on the surface of such plaques. In these cases intravenous heparin and/or plasma expanders have normally been commenced in order to reduce the risk of stroke. This therapy is ceased immediately prior to surgery. We do not use vasodilators, and hypertension is treated very cautiously indeed. We have seen three patients, each with a very tight stenosis, presenting with a TIA and marked hypertension, in whom the blood pressure had been reduced to 120 mmHg systolic, that promptly had a devastating stroke; the hypertension had been necessary to maintain flow past the tight stenosis.

TECHNICAL ISSUES

- When a non-specialist anaesthetist, inexperienced theatre staff or inexperienced assistants are used, the risks of operation rise.
- When there is a very tight stenosis, relief of the stenosis may result in loss of autoregulatory mechanisms, with resultant cerebral haemorrhage (so-called hyperperfusion syndrome – 1.3 per cent in our experience).
- When there is a haemorrhagic plaque with intraluminal thrombus which may be loose, that thrombus may be easily dislodged at the time of surgery.

This last group often contains those patients who are neurologically unstable. Even so, our experience would suggest that carefully performed endarterectomy is still associated with low morbidity and mortality. The emphasis is on 'carefully' performed endarterectomy.[10] When transcranial Doppler evaluation was first available we used it as a routine during carotid endarterectomy. This demonstrated that an increase in microembolic signals often occurred when the site of the plaque was dissected.

OPERATIVE TECHNIQUE (Fig. 12.2)

In patients that are unstable we prefer to perform the operation under local anaesthesia. However, this is inadvisable in the following: those who may not be able to understand the instructions because of language difficulties, those who

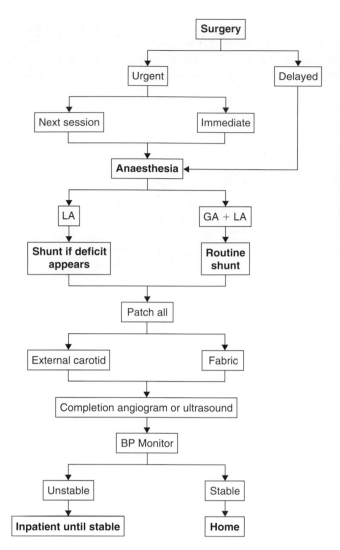

Figure 12.2 *Operative management and technique followed at the Austin and Repatriation Medical Centre, Melbourne, Australia. BP, blood pressure; L/GA, local/general anaesthesia*

are very anxious, those who have a short bull neck or those with a chronic cough.

When the operation is performed under local anaesthesia, there is no need to use a shunt routinely. However, the response to carotid clamping is quite variable. In some patients deficits or even loss of consciousness will occur within 10 seconds of clamping. On occasions the application of the clamp causes seizures; it may then be difficult to get the shunt in, and operation in these circumstances is certainly not for the inexperienced surgeon. When the operation is performed under general anaesthesia, a shunt is used as a routine and it is usually possible to get the shunt into position within one and a half minutes.

Monitoring

The blood pressure and electrocardiogram (ECG) of the patient are continually monitored. In particular, under general anaesthesia, great care has to be taken with induction of anaesthesia. An intra-arterial blood pressure line is required *before* induction of anaesthesia, as this is frequently when the most marked fall in blood pressure occurs. If hypotension occurs, it is routine for the anaesthetist to use vasopressor drugs such as metaraminol bitartrate (Aramine). The blood pressure should not be allowed to fall below 100 mmHg systolic during operation or below 120 mmHg systolic at the times of carotid clamping. If the blood pressure becomes very high before or during induction of anaesthesia, agents such as intravenous lidocaine (Xylocard) 1 mg/kg can be administered. The vocal cords are routinely sprayed with local anaesthetic (4 per cent lidocaine), and before closure of the neck wound at the end of the procedure the surgeon injects 0.5 per cent bupivacaine (Marcain) into the wound edges. The resulting analgesia reduces restlessness and thus helps to lessen rises in blood pressure which may occur at the end of the anaesthetic. It also avoids the need to give narcotic analgesia postoperatively.

The **induction of anaesthesia** is achieved by intravenous administration of 100 μg fentanyl and 2–3 mg midazolam while the patient breathes oxygen, followed by propofol (Diprivan). When Diprivan is given after fentanyl and midazolam, a lower dose is required than when Diprivan is used alone, and consequently the hypotensive effects of Diprivan are minimised.

Relaxant anaesthesia is used with nitrous oxide, oxygen isoflurane (Forthane) or seroflurane (Serorane). Dissection around the carotid sinus nerve or vagus nerve may induce a bradycardia that can be corrected with atropine before any effect on cardiac output occurs. If during the procedure hypertension occurs, increasing the dose of isoflurane or seroflurane, if either of these is being used to maintain anaesthesia, will bring the blood pressure down. Failing this, 5–10 mg hydralazine can be used. If tachycardia ensues, the β-blocker atenolol is used. Very rarely, sodium nitroprusside as a continuous infusion may be required. However, it is difficult to control swings of blood pressure with nitroprusside and we therefore reserve this for patients in whom other measures have failed. Postoperative hypertension similarly can be treated with hydralazine 4–40 mg, given in 5 mg increments with or without a β-blocker, or rarely, with sodium nitroprusside if elevation is otherwise uncontrolled.

Postoperative hypotension may be treated by elevation of the foot of the bed, and judicious use of intravenous fluids such as Haemacel. If these simple measures fail, we use 5 mL 0.5 per cent bupivacaine as an injection into the Redivac drain tube. Very occasionally, a dopamine infusion (2.5–5 μg/kg per minute) may be required.

Operation

It is important to check the position of the patient and the patient's head on the operating table before anaesthesia.

Sometimes rotation of the head and neck to the contralateral side, to provide optimal exposure at the time of operation, compromises the collateral circulation and will produce a neurological disturbance. Thus, *this should be checked before the patient is actually anaesthetised.*

The operative technique used by the author closely resembles that described by Lord.[10] There are, however, several points relevant to the urgent situation which should be stressed.

It is important to dissect the patient away from the artery. The artery must be handled as little as possible, particularly at the site of the plaque. If a haemorrhagic plaque with loose clots is present, some of the latter may easily become dislodged when pulling on the artery. If further dissection is required at this point, it is best done *after* application of the clamps. The effect of rough handling of a badly diseased carotid artery is very dramatically demonstrated by the use of a transcranial Doppler during surgery.

If a vessel loop is placed around the internal carotid artery, as is our routine, no clamp should be placed on the loop in case the weight of the clamp inadvertently pulls on the internal carotid artery and occludes it with its low pressure. The internal carotid artery pressure is not measured. If the operation is being undertaken under local anaesthesia, the patient acts as his or her own cerebral monitor. In patients undergoing carotid endarterectomy under general anaesthesia, a shunt is used routinely and placed in position as soon as possible.

It is important to anaesthetise the carotid sinus before application of clamps. Occasionally, the sinus is very sensitive to clamp application; a disturbance of blood pressure in these circumstances at this time can be disastrous. It is essential to have the shunt and shunt instruments readily available and to check these with the scrub nurse before the clamps are applied. There should be very little time gap between application of the clamp on the external carotid artery, the internal carotid artery and the common carotid artery, as the external carotid artery may well be providing major collateral blood flow.

Normally, if a patient presents with a TIA or minor stroke and angiography reveals complete occlusion of the internal carotid artery, no operation is performed. If complete occlusion is found at operation and the duplex scan or angiogram performed shortly before operation had shown a patent vessel, the vessel is opened. Gentle attempts to extract the clot are made, but if this is not successful, strenuous attempts are not made because of the risk of dislodging clot and subsequent cerebral embolism.

When closing, it is once again important not to have a long delay before flow is restored. A suture is commenced from each end. By this means, and by leaving a few loose sutures adjacent to the shunt on each side, it is possible to remove the shunt, flush out from the external carotid, internal carotid and common carotid arteries, wash the endarterectomy site with heparinised saline, complete the arteriotomy and restore flow, once again within about one and a half minutes. Flow is normally restored to the external carotid artery first, so that if there are any loose platelet aggregations inadvertently left at the reconstruction site, despite the saline washing, they will embolise to the external rather than the internal artery. It is our routine to perform a postoperative angiogram immediately after restoration of flow and before closure of the wound.

In the past we did not use a patch routinely but we do so now. If the external carotid artery runs parallel to the internal carotid artery, the external carotid artery is used as a patch following the technique described by Leather (see Bufo et al.[11]). Otherwise a fabric patch is used.

Dextran is a polysaccharide compound commonly used as a volume expander but it also has antiplatelet and rheologic properties. Although many vascular surgeons use dextran in the belief that it reduces perioperative stroke, no prospective randomised controlled trials have been performed. Our hospital has initiated such a trial. Patients randomized to dextran receive an intravenous bolus of 20 mL of dextran 1 (Promit) 2 minutes before skin incision to avoid anaphylaxis. This is followed by an intravenous infusion of 1000 mL of 10 per cent dextran 40 in normal saline commenced at the time of skin incision. The first 500 mL is administered over 4 hours (125 mL/hour) and the second 500 mL over the next 12 hours (42 mL/hour). Preliminary studies using transcranial Doppler monitoring have demonstrated that dextran reduces postoperative microemboli in the ipsilateral middle cerebral artery.[12] The Dextran in Carotid Endarterectomy (DICE) Trial continues in order to determine the effect of dextran on clinical outcome.

Postoperative surveillance

It is important that the patient's neurological status, and in particular the blood pressure, are carefully monitored postoperatively. Any hypertension should be promptly treated, as described earlier. Hypertension as a postoperative problem is usually evident very soon after surgery. Bourke and Crimmins have shown that in the absence of postoperative hypertension within 12 hours of surgery, it is safe to send the patient home on the next day.[13] All of our patients are followed for life by clinical surveillance and duplex scanning. Early restenosis, within two years of operation is usually due to fibrointimal hyperplasia, which occurs in 2 per cent of patients. The risk of later restenosis is very low and seldom requires reoperation, the risk of subsequent problems being very low.

Patients who have a small infarct have undergone operation without undue risk. However, when a small infarct is seen on CT or MRI, we still advocate a delay of 4–6 weeks before surgery.

Recent results

Of 412 consecutive carotid endarterectomies performed between January 1999 and November 2001, there were eight deaths (1.9 per cent) comprising seven strokes and one myocardial infarct. An independent audit showed that there were 22 (5.2 per cent) non-fatal strokes, a stroke being defined as a neurological deficit present for more than 24 hours. Thus stroke or death occurred in 7.1 per cent.

Conclusions

We showed previously that when there was a high grade contralateral carotid stenosis the procedure of carotid endarterectomy presented an increased risk. These patients of course have an increased risk of stroke anyway.[7] Patients with crescendo TIAs are clearly in a very high risk group. One has to accept, and explain to the patient and relatives, that whatever course of action is undertaken, be it conservative or operative, the patient's clinical condition is critical. We believe that, despite this, surgery produces a lower complication rate than nonoperative treatment.

Urgent carotid endarterectomy is one of the most satisfying operations in vascular surgery. However, to obtain good results, surgical technique must be impeccable, patient selection is vital and of utmost importance is the general organisation of hospital services. Patients who need such an operation require streamlined resources capable of recognising the urgency of the situation and treating it in appropriate and timely fashion.

Key references

Barnett HJM, Taylor DW, Eliasziw M, et al. Benefit of carotid endarterectomy in patients with symptomatic moderate or severe stenosis. N Engl J Med 1998; **339**: 1415–25.

Donnan GA, O'Malley H, Hurley S, et al. The capsular warning syndrome: pathogenesis and clinical features. Neurology 1993; **43**: 957–62.

European Carotid Surgery Trialists' Collaborative Group. MRC European Carotid Surgery Trial: interim results for symptomatic patients with severe (70–99%) or mild (0–29%) carotid stenosis. Lancet 1991; **337**: 1235–43.

Kappelle LJ, Eliasziw M, Fox AJ, et al. Importance of intracranial atherosclerotic disease in patients with symptomatic stenosis of the internal carotid artery. Stroke 1999; **30**: 282–6.

Levi CR, Stork JL, Chambers BR, et al. Dextran reduces embolic signals after carotid endarterectomy. Ann Neurol 2001; **50**: 544–7.

REFERENCES

1 Eastcott HHG, Pickering GW, Rob CG. Reconstruction of internal carotid artery in a patient with intermittent attacks of hemiplegia. Lancet 1954; **2**: 994–6.

2 European Carotid Surgery Trialists' Collaborative Group. MRC European Carotid Surgery Trial: interim results for symptomatic patients with severe (70–99%) or mild (0–29%) carotid stenosis. Lancet 1991; **337**: 1235–43.

3 North American Symptomatic Carotid Endarterectomy Trial Collaborators. Beneficial effect of carotid endarterectomy in symptomatic patients with high-grade carotid stenosis. *N Engl J Med* 1992; **325**: 445–53.

4 Barnett IIJM, Taylor DW, Eliasziw M, *et al.* Benefit of carotid endarterectomy in patients with symptomatic moderate or severe stenosis. *N Engl J Med* 1998; **339**: 1415–25.

5 Cartlidge NEF, Whisnant JPR, Elveback LR. Carotid and vertebral-basilar transient cerebral ischaemic attacks: a community study, Rochester, Minnesota. *Mayo Clin Proc* 1977; **52**: 117–20.

6 Donnan GA, O'Malley H, Hurley S, *et al.* The capsular warning syndrome: pathogenesis and clinical features. *Neurology* 1993; **43**: 957–62.

7 Gasecki AP, Ferguson GG, Barnett HJM. Long-term prognosis and effect of endarterectomy in patients with symptomatic severe carotid stenosis and contralateral carotid stenosis or occlusion: results from NASCET. *J Neurosurg* 1995; **83**: 778–82.

8 Kappelle LJ, Eliasziw M, Fox AJ, *et al.* Importance of intracranial atherosclerotic disease in patients with symptomatic stenosis of the internal carotid artery. *Stroke* 1999; **30**: 282–6.

9 Henderson RD, Eliasziw M, Fox AJ, *et al.* Angiographically defined collateral circulation and risk of stroke in patients with severe carotid artery stenosis. *Stroke* 2000; **31**: 128–32.

10 Lord RSA. *Surgery of occlusive cerebrovascular disease.* St Louis: CV Mosby, 1986.

11 Bufo AJ, Shaf DM, Chang BB, Leather RP. Carotid bifurcationplasty: an alternative to patching. *J Cardiovasc Surg* 1992; **33**: 308–10.

12 Levi CR, Stork JL, Chambers BR, *et al.* Dextran reduces embolic signals after carotid endarterectomy. *Ann Neurol* 2001; **50**: 544–7.

13 Bourke BM, Crimmins DC. Overnight hospital stay for carotid endarterectomy. *Med J Aust* 1998; **168**: 149–50.

Surgical Experience in Evolving Stroke Arising From the Carotid

R HUBER, RJ SEITZ, M SIEBLER, A AULICH, WILHELM SANDMANN

THE PROBLEM

The Joint Study of Extracranial Carotid Occlusion documented in 1969 the uselessness of emergency revascularisation in patients with acute stroke and carotid occlusion.[1,2] Only recently have neurologists accepted indications for urgent carotid surgery[3,4] based on new diagnostic techniques[5-8] and close clinical observation during care in the stroke unit.[9,10] Both the new and the old goals are prevention of recurrent or disabling stroke and prevention and reduction of the extent of brain infarction. For decades surgeons undertook carotid endarterectomy to remove the embolic source and to restore internal carotid artery (ICA) blood flow, but the indications for urgent reconstruction of the ICA were not defined precisely at that time. Since then the diagnostic armamentarium, the surgical safety measures and the drugs available to discourage thrombosis have changed substantially allowing new strategies to develop in dealing with these acute cases. Magnetic resonance imaging (MRI) can reveal structural damage by diffusion-weighted imaging (DWI) within 1 hour of onset of symptoms, and by comparing DWI and perfusion-weighted imaging (PWI) the size of the infarct as well as the tissue at risk can be determined at a very early stage.[6,7] By using this approach, patients who have a dangerous degree of ICA occlusive disease, but who also have a substantial amount of potentially rescuable brain tissue, in other words that forming the penumbra, can be identified.

MATERIAL AND METHODS

Selection based on clinical criteria

- Conscious patient
- Acute/recurrent stroke
- Recurrent/crescendo transient ischaemic attacks (TIAs)

Between 1 November 1997 and 31 December 2002 we prospectively monitored all patients diagnosed in the stroke unit at our centre and selected patients were transferred to our operating theatre for urgent carotid surgery. Neurologists, neuroradiologists and vascular surgeons had initially collaborated closely in arriving at a consensus on the criteria for patient selection: (i) radiologically, the presence of acute extracranial carotid occlusive disease, a patent intracranial component of the ICA, evidence of perfusion of the middle cerebral artery (MCA); and (ii) clinically, evidence of acute stroke, recurrent stroke or recent TIAs, possibly aggravated or crescendo in nature within the previous week. Unconscious patients who required ventilation were excluded.

Investigations: radiological/ultrasound

- Duplex scan
- Computed tomography (CT) scan of brain stem

- Magnetic resonance angiography (MRA)
- Intra-arterial digital subtraction arteriography (DSA)
- Transcranial Doppler sonography (TCD)
- Magnetic resonance imaging (MRI) (DWI/PWI)

Doppler and duplex sonography confirmed a diagnosis of stenosis or acute occlusion. In cases of multivessel involvement magnetic resonance arteriography and/or intra-arterial digital subtraction arteriography (DSA) was performed. Intracranial circulation and embolism were assessed by transcranial Doppler sonography (TCD) and high intensity transient signal (HITS) detection, respectively.[5] A patent middle cerebral artery (MCA) was documented by TCD, MRA or intra-arterial DSA.

Selection based on investigative findings

- Acute extracranial ICA disease
- Patent intracranial ICA
- Perfusing MCA
- HITS
- Evidence of penumbra

Magnetic resonance imaging procedures were used to assess acute reversible and irreversible ischaemic brain damage (see Chapter 12).[6–8] In order to evaluate actual brain tissue damage CT or whenever possible MRI with DWI and PWI was performed. The cerebral area of critical ischaemia was visualised by means of colour-coded PWI. As shown earlier, a time-to-peak delay in perfusion imaging of greater than 4 seconds compared with the contralateral hemisphere had to be considered 'tissue at risk'.[6,8] Because quantitative volumetry of the infarct, compared with the area of 'misery perfusion' or penumbra measured by DWI and PWI, is time consuming and not always available outside normal working hours, it was only performed in a small number of patients selected on precise clinical criteria.[11] Measurements were done before and 8 days after surgery. Impairment was assessed clinically using the Rankin impairment scale[12] and the Barthel index[13] before surgery, 8 days afterwards and during follow-up.

Objective clinical measurements

- Rankin impairment scale
- Barthel index

Surgery was performed under general anesthesia and was standardised with early clamping of the common carotid artery before dissection of the bifurcation and the distal ICA. Shunting was applied routinely after thrombectomy of the distal ICA on the basis of earlier studies in which a patient with a history of previous stroke or CT findings positive for stroke, regardless of the hemisphere involved, tended to have a better outcome with shunting.[14] Patients in the stroke unit were placed on heparin which was maintained during surgery and continued at a low dosage postoperatively, followed by aspirin 100 mg daily.

A total of 166 patients underwent 173 urgent carotid operations (seven bilateral under the same anaesthetic), representing 12.9 per cent of all carotid artery operations (n = 1285) performed during the period in question. These patients included 119 men (71.7 per cent) and 47 women (28.3 per cent), median age 64.7 years (range 31–86). Risk factors for both occlusive arterial disease and vascular surgery were: hypertension in 133 (80.1 per cent), smoking in 105 (63.3 per cent), cardiac disease in 84 (50.6 per cent), diabetes in 38 (22.9 per cent) and coagulation disorders in 7 (4.2 per cent).

All patients underwent preoperative Doppler and duplex sonography. Transcranial Doppler was performed in 104 patients (62.7 per cent) and in 46 (44.2 per cent) of these cases microemboli were detected. Intra-arterial DSA was performed in 83 of cases (50 per cent) and MRA in 91 cases (54.8 per cent). Preoperative vascular findings were ipsilateral carotid occlusion in 45 (27.1 per cent), tight stenosis in 111 (66.9 per cent) and pseudo-occlusion in 10 (6 per cent). Findings in the contralateral carotid artery were: normal in 116 (69.9 per cent), occluded in 27 (16.3 per cent), stenotic in 23 (13.8 per cent).

Preoperative clinical findings were stroke in 98 (59.1 per cent) and TIA in 67 (40.3 per cent); one patient (0.6 per cent) had an asymptomatic acute ICA occlusion, the progression from stenosis to carotid occlusion having been discovered accidentally on repeat duplex sonography within 12 hours. Clinical presentations were: stroke with a stable neurological deficit in 34 (20.5 per cent), stroke with stuttering symptoms in 27 (16.3 per cent), progressive stroke in 20 (12 per cent), stroke after TIA in 17 (10.2 per cent), crescendo TIA in 40 (24.1 per cent), TIA with positive microemboli detected in 11 (6.6 per cent), crescendo TIA with microemboli detected in 11 (6.6 per cent) and recent TIA in 5 (3 per cent). In these patients angiographic findings were critical: small mobile thrombus in one, subtotal carotid artery stenosis in two, bilateral high grade stenosis in two. None of the patients underwent surgery without a CT scan or MRI. Extended MRI evaluation by means of DWI and PWI was undertaken in 104 patients (62.6 per cent). Acute lesions with a large perfusion/diffusion mismatch were found in 47 cases (45.2 per cent) among which were 15 patients with TIA. Median time between onset of first symptoms and operation was 4.5 days (range 4 hours to 141 days).

Reconstructive techniques applied were conventional carotid endarterectomy with vein patch closure in 129 patients (77.7 per cent) and eversion endarterectomy[15] in 22 (13.3 per cent). In six cases (3.6 per cent) a vein interposition graft had to be inserted. Additional thrombectomies of the petrous portion of the ICA were necessary in 29 patients. In nine patients (5.4 per cent) the carotid artery could not be reconstructed because backflow after thrombectomy could not be achieved due to thrombosis extending into the siphon, and the wound was closed after thromboendarterectomy of the external carotid artery. In seven additional cases, the presence of bilateral subtotal occlusion led to contralateral ICA reconstruction under the same anaesthetic.

RESULTS

Subsequent to surgery 53 patients (31.9 per cent) remained free of symptoms. According to the Rankin scale[12] clinical disability improved in 63 (38 per cent) of the stroke patients. Thirty four stroke patients (20.5 per cent) remained stable, although 11 did so with severe disability (Rankin 4, 5). Sixteen patients (9.6 per cent) deteriorated: two had presented with TIAs and progressed to complete stroke and 14 (8.4 per cent) showed worsening of stroke symptoms. In the TIA group one stroke occurred intraoperatively in a patient with contralateral ICA occlusion having presented primarily with crescendo TIAs and highly positive detection of microemboli, and in a second patient a large DWI lesion present before surgery progressed during a hypertensive crisis 6 days after surgery. Nine patients experienced aggravation of MCA infarction symptoms, and one of them with contralateral occlusion died 2 days postoperatively. Three patients in whom flow through the ICA could not be restored developed brain oedema which resolved spontaneously in two of them. In the third patient a midline shift necessitated craniotomy. Another patient with contralateral occlusion developed secondary infarction with brain oedema 5 days postoperatively and died 24 days later. One patient sustained rupture of the carotid patch during gastroscopy 5 days postoperatively and died 12 days later. Of the 166 patients, only one suffered secondary intracerebral bleeding, detected on routine CT scanning, but without manifesting any new symptoms. The 30-day mortality was 2.4 per cent (4/166). Postoperative neurological morbidity was 9.6 per cent (n = 16), procedure related peripheral nerve lesions (n = 9) delayed wound healing (n = 6) and reoperation for haematoma (n = 6) was 12.6 per cent.

The volume of ischaemic brain lesions decreased in 17 patients until day eight as assessed by quantitative lesion volumetry[11] and was accompanied by improvement of the Barthel index[13] (Fig. 13.1). Early postoperative neurological assessment showed that 139 patients (83.7 per cent) benefitted from carotid surgery and 27 (16.2 per cent) patients remained severely disabled or deteriorated (Fig. 13.2).

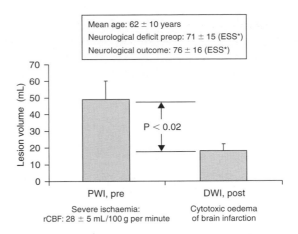

Mean age: 62 ± 10 years
Neurological deficit preop: 71 ± 15 (ESS*)
Neurological outcome: 76 ± 16 (ESS*)

Figure 13.1   *Rescue of 'tissue at risk' in acute symptomatic patients (emergent carotid endarterectomy). Patients were studied pre- and post-operatively with perfusion-weighted magnetic resonance imaging (PWI) (n = 17). *ESS, European Stroke Scale (0, severely abnormal; 100, normal). DWI, diffusion-weighted imaging*

Rankin (postoperative)

	0	1	2	3	4	5	6	Total
0	53			2				55
1	6	12						18
2	2	12	6	1				21
3	1	5	12	5	1	4	1	29
4	1	4	5	10	8	5		33
5			1		4	3	2	10
Total	63	33	24	18	13	12	3	

Rankin (preoperative)

Figure 13.2   *Outcome of carotid surgery in acute symptomatic patients (Black: stable (n = 34), free of symptoms (n = 53); red: improved and Rankin 0–3 (n = 63), blue: deteriorated and Rankin >3 (n = 16))*

Median follow-up until 31 December 2002 was 1.3 years and was complete for all but nine patients. During this time period all patients were on aspirin 100 mg/day. Ten patients died. The causes of death were: contralateral intracerebral bleeding with ventricular rupture (n = 1), cerebral infarction on the contralateral side (n = 1), myocardial infarction (n = 3), pulmonary embolism (n = 1) and cancer (n = 4). Survival after 1 year was 93.5 per cent and after 2 years 91.4 per cent (Fig. 13.3).

All surviving patients are living in their own homes, seven dependent on help from their families. No further strokes or TIAs occurred. Three patients developed grand mal seizures after stroke and remain on anticonvulsive medication. One patient was reoperated for asymptomatic recurrent stenosis and has remained asymptomatic.

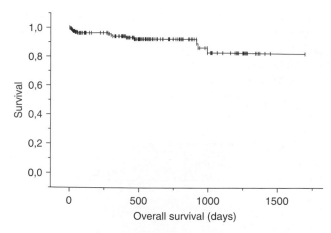

Figure 13.3 *Overall survival (Kaplan–Meier) after carotid endarterectomy in acute symptomatic patients (n = 166)*

DISCUSSION

We have come a long way since the days of condemnation of carotid artery reconstruction in patients presenting with symptoms of acute stroke[1] to the current recognition that restoration of carotid flow in the acute case is of value.[3,4] Although some surgeons have always insisted that surgery is indicated for this particular presentation, no clear guidelines and/or criteria defining the objectives of urgent carotid surgery have been spelt out. In earlier times however, clinicians were equipped with the patient's history, the results of a meticulous neurological examination, an arteriogram of reasonably acceptable quality, an echoencephalogram for imaging of brain oedema and finally, a surgeon willing to perform the operation.

The major concern with urgent surgery was the possibility of intracranial haemorrhage thought to result from rupture of the fragile capillaries in the infarction territory. It became evident from CT scanning, that localised oedema and small areas of bleeding can develop not only around ischaemic infarcts but also within the brain of patients suffering from TIAs, but this process would not necessarily progress to massive haemorrhage even though anticoagulation was being used more aggressively. It was felt that as long as the blood–brain barrier had not closed, reconstruction of the ICA was too dangerous an undertaking (see Chapter 5).[2] At our institution we began to disregard the phenomenon of the unclosed blood–brain barrier and our neurologists exhorted us to reconstitute carotid blood flow urgently. The indications were clinical instability in the presence of haemodynamic and/or angiographic evidence of deterioration of the occluding lesion and to our surprise intracranial haemorrhage did not occur. Today, with the availability of MRI derived assessment of structural and perfusion deficit, the decision to operate is made on the assessment of the volume of tissue at risk and the extent to which the patient might improve after eliminating the perfusion deficit. In our series intracranial

haemorrhage occurred in one patient only and even then no new symptoms had developed.

The results of the European Carotid Surgery Trial[16,17] and the North American Symptomatic Carotid Endarterectomy Trial[18,19] and the therapeutic demands made by stroke units[9,10,20] in the wake of new imaging techniques have changed attitudes to carotid surgery in acutely symptomatic patients. The results of these studies and our growing experience show that urgent surgery can be performed in carefully selected patients at risk of developing stroke, recurrent stroke and/or progression of stenosis to complete occlusion, if nothing other than anticoagulant therapy is given to alter the spontaneous course of the disease. We have to ask ourselves: Why have the results of urgent surgery improved? Although the reasons for intraoperative or postoperative deterioration are often a matter for speculation, they generally fall into three categories: (i) morphological abnormalities of the luminal surface of the ICA itself, (ii) extracranial and intracranial multivessel involvement and (iii) structural brain tissue lesions.

Specific morphological abnormalities of the ICA which test the technical skills of the surgeon include occlusive disease located near the base of the skull, siphon involvement, thrombus which is loose or not adherent to the vessel wall, continuous embolisation and even dissection. In those cases in our series in which deterioration followed attempts at carotid reconstruction, the ICA, contrary to preoperative angiographic appearances, was found at surgery to be occluded, the blockage extending intracranially. In those patients who deteriorated, embolisation during thrombectomy manoeuvres was the most probable cause. Nonetheless, in our opinion, an acute carotid artery occlusion should always be disobliterated if the probability of infarction or reinfarction is considered to be very high.[21,22]

Causes of perioperative deterioration

- Morphological abnormalities in the ICA
- Multisegmental vessel disease
- Brain tissue lesions

Other reasons for aggressive intervention are: first, the probability of spontaneous embolisation into an intracranial artery,[23,24] and second, the limitations of collateral circulation in acute infarction, either because of haemodynamic impairment within the territory of the exposed ICA, or, in the case of bilateral ICA occlusion, of the contralateral hemisphere as well. Furthermore, outcome studies of re-exploration have shown good long term results with the ICA remaining patent with a low risk of stroke recurrence.[25] In patients with contralateral ICA occlusion and multivessel involvement, clamping the common carotid artery can cause haemodynamic impairment even if a temporary shunt is used, unless unrestricted flow through the shunt can be ascertained. Placement of a shunt *per se* does not guarantee flow and therefore we recommend continuous shunt flow measurement and neuromonitoring using somatosensory evoked potentials. Additional stenosis or occlusion of the MCA, undiagnosed preoperatively, may present a further problem which we encountered only once: a patient with concomitant contralateral internal carotid occlusion, in whom shunting of a small calibre ICA was impossible, had a shunt inserted into the external carotid artery which probably helped to a degree in preventing perfusion ischaemia. The MCA was diseased in two cases of intraoperative embolisation in one of which evidence of embolism into the MCA was confirmed by comparing preoperative and intraoperative angiograms.

The key challenge presented by structural intracerebral lesions is estimating how much of the area recognised as malperfused is actually irreversibly damaged using modern imaging techniques. Magnetic resonance imaging reveals structural damage in DWI within 1–2 hours after onset of symptoms and is an early marker for brain infarction.[6,7] By means of parametric colour-coded PWI the cerebral area of critical ischaemia is visualised. As shown earlier, a time-to-peak delay in perfusion imaging of greater than four as compared with the contralateral hemisphere, has to be treated as 'tissue at risk'.[6,8] We worked on the basis that patients in whom the PWI area was significantly more extensive than the DWI lesion, reflecting the PWI/DWI area mismatch, were ideal candidates for urgent carotid artery reconstruction; this was because the volume mismatch of the two areas was anticipated to be the penumbra.[26,27]

In our series, clinical deterioration was observed either in patients with a large intracerebral structural deficit already present in DWI at the time of operation, or in patients with smaller structural deficits in DWI but a longer interval between onset of symptoms and surgery. The latter was the case in two patients in whom the interval was 8 days and 16 days. This leads to the critical issue of the optimal time interval between the onset of symptoms and the operation. A balanced approach is required in stabilising the patient in the stroke unit, gathering the complex morphological, haemodynamic and clinical data needed, and scheduling the patient for surgery. Our current experience suggests a period of 36 hours after onset of symptoms as the time frame within which the procedure should be undertaken.

Another important issue remains to be discussed: the new and sensitive MRI techniques of DWI and PWI have shown, even more clearly than CT, that clinical classification of brain ischaemia cannot be correlated reliably to brain tissue status. A patient thought to have a TIA clinically may easily be found to have a brain infarction as determined by MRI criteria. Two of our TIA patients deteriorated preoperatively and in both cases, just before operation, microembolism was detected and larger structural brain lesions were confirmed on MRI. In our opinion, this underlines the fact that embolisation renders carotid surgery even more urgent in TIA patients, especially when HITS are detected by TCD despite heparin therapy.

The results of surgery will always be classified clinically, but the influence of carotid flow in restoring the DWI/PWI deficit, thereby salvaging brain tissue at risk, is an equally important and challenging issue. In eight patients in whom we were able to obtain preoperative and postoperative MRIs, a decrease in the volume of the lesion and neurological improvement was evident using the Barthel score of daily activities.[13]

During the spontaneous course of the disease early reinfarction rates of 1.29 per cent,[28] as well as reinfarction rates of 12 per cent[29] and mortality rates of 19 per cent[30] within the first year of onset of symptoms have to be considered. In our patients, reinfarction within the former symptomatic hemisphere related to the reconstructed ICA did not occur, the one-year mortality was 6.5 per cent and two-year mortality 8.6 per cent. During follow-up restenosis was detected only in one asymptomatic patient who was reoperated and has remained asymptomatic ever since. Finally we pose this question: What might have happened to this subset of patients presenting with symptoms of acute stroke symptoms prior to having redefined the case for urgent carotid endarterectomy? Clearly, the spontaneous course would have been significantly worse, otherwise our neurology colleagues would not have considered those patients to be good candidates for carotid surgery.

Conclusions

On one hand, the traditional criteria for patient selection in urgent carotid surgery such as evidence of extracranial carotid artery disease, neurological deficit, loss of consciousness or not, will continue to be considered. On the other hand, the preservation of an open MCA, the status of embolisation, and PWI/DWI mismatch must also be taken into account. Although an expert stroke team should be able to acquire the necessary information within hours, the timeframe which obtains in practice, even in a university hospital, is still too long: at our centre a median of 4 days elapsed from onset of symptoms until surgery but recently that interval has shortened. A neurological morbidity rate of 9.6 per cent, a procedure related morbidity of 12.6 per cent as well as a 30-day mortality of 2.7 per cent still remain higher than that observed in the 2262 patients who underwent elective carotid surgery at our hospital from 1990 to 1999,[31] namely, morbidity 4.8 per cent, 30-day mortality 0.9 per cent. Nevertheless, these outcome figures no longer represent an objection to urgent carotid surgery, because the alternative course is much worse. The improvement in our series was achieved by detailed preoperative diagnosis and observing the indications for carotid surgery based on clinical assessment, Doppler and duplex sonography, TCD for microemboli detection, multimodal MRI and DSA.

Key references

Baird AE, Benfield A, Schlaug G, *et al*. Enlargement of human cerebral ischemic lesion volumes measured by diffusion weighted magnetic resonance imaging. *Ann Neurol* 1997; **41**: 581–9.

Futrell N, Millikan CH. Stroke is an emergency. *Dis Mon* 1996; **42**: 199–264.

Mahoney FI, Barthel DW. Functional evaluation: the Barthel index. *Md State Med J* 1965; **14**: 61–5.

Neumann-Haefelin T, Wittsack HJ, Wenserski F, *et al*. Diffusion- and perfusion weighted MRI. The DWI/PWI mismatch region in acute stroke. *Stroke* 1999; **30**: 1591–7.

Sandmann W, Willeke F, Kolvenbach R, *et al*. Shunting and neuromonitoring: A prospective randomized study. In: Greenhalgh RM (ed). *Surgery for stroke*. London: WB Saunders, 1993: 287–96.

REFERENCES

1   Blaisdell WF, Clauss RH, Galbraith, *et al*. Joint Study of Extracranial Carotid Occlusion IV. A review of surgical considerations. *JAMA* 1969; **209**: 1889–95.

2   Thompson JE, Austin DJ, Patman PD. Endarterectomy of the totally occluded internal carotid artery for stroke, results in 100 operations. *Arch Surg* 1967; **95**: 791–801.

3   Pritz MB. Timing of carotid endarterectomy after stroke. *Stroke* 1997; **28**: 2563–7.

4   Whittemore AD, Ruby ST, Couch NP, Mannick JA. Early carotid endarterectomy in patients with small, fixed neurologic deficit. *J Vasc Surg* 1984; **1**: 795–9.

5   Ringelstein EB, Droste DW, Babikian VL, *et al*. Consensus on microembolus detection by TCD. International Consensus Group on Microembolus Detection. *Stroke* 1998; **29**: 725–9.

6   Neumann-Haefelin T, Wittsack HJ, Wenserski F, *et al*. Diffusion- and perfusion weighted MRI. The DWI/PWI mismatch region in acute stroke. *Stroke* 1999; **30**: 1591–7.

7   Baird AE, Benfield A, Schlaug G, *et al*. Enlargement of human cerebral ischemic lesion volumes measured by diffusion weighted magnetic resonance imaging. *Ann Neurol* 1997; **41**: 581–9.

8   Neumann-Haefelin T, Wittsack HJ, Fink GR, *et al*. Diffusion- and perfusion weighted MRI. Influence of severe carotid artery stenosis on the DWI/PWI mismatch in acute stroke. *Stroke* 2000; **31**: 1311–17.

9   Bath P, Butterworth RJ, Soo J, Kerr JE. The King's College Hospital Acute Stroke Unit. *J R Coll Phys Lond* 1996; **30**: 13–17.

10   Futrell N, Millikan CH. Stroke is an emergency. *Dis Mon* 1996; **42**: 199–264.

11   Wittsack HJ, Ritzl A, Fink GR, *et al*. Magnetic resonance imaging in acute stroke: DWI and PWI. parameters predicting infarct size. *Radiology* 2002; **222**: 397–403.

12   Rankin J. Cerebral vascular accidents in patients over the age of 60. Prognosis. *Scottish Med J* 1957; **2**: 200–15.

13   Mahoney FI, Barthel DW. Functional evaluation: the Barthel index. *Md State Med J* 1965; **14**: 61–5.

14   Sandmann W, Willeke F, Kolvenbach R, *et al*. Shunting and neuromonitoring: A prospective randomized study. In: Greenhalgh RM (ed). *Surgery for Stroke*. London: WB Saunders, 1993: 287–96.

15   Raithel D. Carotid eversion endarterectomy: a better technique than the standard operation? *Cardiovasc Surg* 1999; **5**: 471–2.

16   European Carotid Surgery Trialists' Collaborative Group. Randomised trial of endarterectomy for recently symptomatic carotid stenosis: final results of the MRC European Carotid Surgery Trial (ECST). *Lancet* 1998; **351**: 1379–86.

17   European Carotid Surgery Trialists' Collaboratory Group. MRC European Carotid Surgery Trial: Interim results for symptomatic patients with severe (70–90%) or with mild (0–29%) carotid stenosis. *Lancet* 1991; **337**: 1235–43.

18   North American Symptomatic Carotid Endarterectomy Trial Collaborators Group. Beneficial effect of carotid endarterectomy in symptomatic patients with high-grade carotid stenosis. *N Engl J Med* 1991; **325**: 445–53.

19   Gasecki AP, Ferguson GG, Eliasziw M, *et al*. Early endarterectomy for severe carotid artery stenosis after nondisabling stroke: results from the North American Symptomatic Carotid Endarterectomy Trial. *J Vasc Surg* 1994; **27**: 288–95.

20   Hacke W, Kaste M, Olsen TS, *et al*. Acute treatment of ischemic stroke. *Cerebrovasc Dis* 2000; **10**(suppl 3): 22–33.

21   Hennerici M, Hulsbomer HB, Rautenberg W, Hefter H. Spontaneous history of asymptomatic internal carotid occlusion. *Stroke* 1986; **17**: 718–22.

22   Klijn CJM, Kappelle JK, van der Grond J, *et al*. Magnetic resonance techniques for the identification of patients with symptomatic carotidartery occlusion at high risk of cerebral ischemic events. *Stroke* 2000; **31**: 3001–7.

23   Barber PA, Davis SM, Darby DG, *et al*. Absent middle cerebral artery flow predicts the presence and evolution of the ischemic penumbra. *Neurology* 1999; **52**: 1125–32.

24   Kniemeyer HW, Aulich A, Schlachetzki F, *et al*. Pseudo- and segmental occlusion of the internal carotid artery: a new classification, surgical treatment and results. *Eur J Vasc Endovasc Surg* 1996; **12**: 310–20.

25   von Arbin M, Britton M, de Faire U. Mortality and recurrences during eight years following stroke. *J Intern Med* 1992; **231**: 43–8.

26   Astrup J, Siesjö BK, Symon L. Thresholds of cerebral ischemia: the ischemic penumbra. *Stroke* 1981; **12**: 723–5.

27   Lassen NA. Pathophysiology of brain ischemia as it relates to the therapy of acute ischemic stroke. *Clin Neuropharmacol* 1990; **13**: S1.

28   Sandercock P, Tangkanakul C. Very early prevention of stroke recurrence. *Cerebrovasc Dis* 1997; **7**(suppl 1): 10–15.

29   Easton DJ. Epidemiology of stroke recurrence. *Cerebrovasc Dis* 1997; **7**(suppl 1): 2–4.

30   Dennis MS, Burn JPS, Sandercock PAG, *et al*. Long term survival after first ever stroke: the oxfordshire community stroke project. *Stroke* 1993; **24**: 796–800.

31   Ommer A, Dziewanowski M, Pillny M, *et al*. Langzeitergebnisse nach Carotisrekonstruktion im Defektstadium der cerebrovaskulären Verschluβkrankheit. *Dtsch Med Wochenschr* 2002; **127**: 370–5.

14

Post-Carotid Endarterectomy Stroke

DAVID ROSENTHAL, ERIC D WELLONS

THE PROBLEM

After nearly half a century of carotid artery surgery, the pathogenesis and management of the postoperative neurological deficit remains controversial. Several reports[1-5] believe reperfusion injury or technical error resulting in thromboembolic events to be the cause, whereas others[6-8] attribute cerebral ischaemia during carotid occlusion to the pathogenesis of postoperative deficits. It is often difficult to determine the exact aetiology of a postoperative deficit, but each of these factors may play some role.

The purpose of this chapter is to discuss the most likely causes of early and late neurologic deficits after carotid endarterectomy (CEA) and to evaluate the safest and most efficient means of managing such patients in order to minimise permanent neurological impairment.

EARLY POSTOPERATIVE DEFICITS

Between 1980 and 1999, 1085 patients underwent 1238 CEAs. The indications for operation included hemispheric transient ischaemic attacks (TIAs) (n = 579), symptoms of vertebrobasilar insufficiency (n = 248), reversible ischaemic neurological deficit (RIND) or stroke (n = 165), prophylactic CEA (n = 111), amaurosis fugax (n = 108) and stroke in evolution (n = 27).

Based on the different operative techniques employed, the patients were categorised into three groups: (i) CEA performed with a shunt (n = 512); (ii) CEA without a shunt (n = 274); and (iii) CEA monitored by electroencephalogram (EEG) surveillance (n = 452). Of the 1085 patients, 705 (65 per cent) were men. The mean age was 66.5 years (range 40–86). A history consistent with coronary artery heart disease documented by electrocardiogram (ECG) was present in 716 (66 per cent), hypertension in 662 (61 per cent), diabetes mellitus in 391 (36 per cent) abnormal lipid profiles in 434 (40 per cent) and a history of cigarette smoking was elicited in 521 (48 per cent).

Postoperative neurological deficits were classified into three categories: (i) a focal episode of neurological dysfunction which resolved within 24 hours was defined as a TIA; (ii) a neurological deficit which lasted more than 24 hours, yet resolved completely within 3 weeks was designated a reversible ischaemic neurological deficit (RIND), whereas (iii) a fixed non-progressive neurological deficit lasting less than 24 hours and caused by cerebral infarction was characterised as a stroke.[9]

The incidence of postoperative neurological deficit was not significantly different if patients underwent CEA with routine shunting, routine non-shunting or selective shunting based on electroencephalogram (EEG) criteria. Of the patients who underwent CEA with a shunt (n = 512), a transient deficit occurred in 15 (2.9 per cent) and a permanent deficit in 11 (2.1 per cent). When CEA was performed without a shunt (n = 274), a transient deficit occurred in eight patients (2.9 per cent) and a permanent deficit occurred in nine (3.3 per cent). Transient deficit after CEA monitored by EEG surveillance (n = 452) occurred in 12 (2.7 per cent) and permanent deficit occurred in 11 patients (2.4 per cent). Overall, 35 patients experienced a transient postoperative deficit and 31 a permanent deficit. Although the incidence of postoperative stroke (3.3 per cent) was slightly higher in the routine non-shunting group, there was no significant statistical difference when the different methods of cerebral protection were compared (P > 6.25).

The preoperative arteriograms of all patients experiencing a postoperative neurological deficit were reviewed. Of 35 patients who experienced a transient postoperative deficit, 25 patients (72 per cent) had ulcerated plaque disease, as did 10 of 31 (32 per cent) who sustained a postoperative stroke. This suggests that embolisation from the ulcer bed may have been the cause of the postoperative deficit. Intracranial occlusive disease, namely, stenosis at the siphon or stenoses within the circle of Willis, was also noted in 29 patients.

The incidence of postoperative neurological complications was evaluated on the basis of indications for operation. It is of interest to note that patients with 'stable' preoperative symptoms such as TIAs, amaurosis fugax and vertebrobasilar insufficiency had nearly a *fourfold* increased incidence of transient and permanent deficits over patients whose neurological status was 'unstable', namely those presenting with stroke in evolution, RIND or stroke (Table 14.1), and these features have been observed by others.[10,11] After a RIND or stroke or during a stroke in evolution, a zone of ischaemic brain tissue is present which may be more vulnerable to diminished perfusion during carotid cross-clamping than normal brain tissue.[12,13] This ischaemic zone is supplied by highly resistant collateral vessels and a drop in perfusion pressure during carotid cross-clamping may cause further ischaemia. In order to diminish the potential for a postoperative neurological deficit in these neurologically 'unstable' patients, the wisest course of action is to shunt the carotids in order to avoid any drop in perfusion during CEA.

In the immediate postoperative period (<12 hours), 35 patients experienced a transient neurological deficit. Seventeen patients experienced a focal minor deficit, which resolved rapidly, and 18 patients experienced a more pronounced deficit such as contralateral sensory and motor changes of the face and extremities upon awakening from anaesthesia. Fifteen were reanaesthetised preparatory to immediate operative arteriography. Carotid re-exploration was necessary in four patients, and the others had normal arteriograms. Each of the 18 patients who experienced a more pronounced deficit had a computed tomography (CT) brain scan within 72 hours of operation: all scans were normal and all patients regained neurological function within 1 month of operation.

A total of 35 patients with immediate profound postoperative deficit and a suspected stroke required emergency operation. In 31 cases a deficit was identified upon awakening from anaesthesia and four deficits occurred in the recovery room within 3 hours of operation. A patent CEA site was identified in 15 patients and arteriography verified an intracranial embolic shower in 12, and three arteriograms were normal. In 20 patients a thrombosed carotid artery was found caused by technical errors: an intimal flap was identified in 11, a lateral tear in three and a residual plaque in two. Four other patients underwent thrombectomy of platelet–fibrin aggregates or 'white clot'. Despite arterial re-exploration and arteriography a cause could not be found and therefore it was assumed to be due to heparin induced thrombocytopenic thrombosis. After thrombectomy and correction of the technical error, a patch graft was constructed in 14 patients and in six the carotid bifurcation was replaced with saphenous vein. Of these 35 patients, three showed immediate return of neurological function, eight improved slowly, 20 were unchanged and four died of stroke related causes.

DISCUSSION

Early neurological deficits after CEA occur infrequently and both the causative factors and the management of these patients remains undefined. A comparison of the postoperative neurological deficit with the preoperative arteriograms reveals two findings of interest. First, most complications (72 per cent transient deficit, 32 per cent permanent deficit) occurred in patients who had ulcerative plaque disease identified at arteriography. It seems likely that patients with ulcerated plaque disease are more prone to embolic events during carotid artery mobilisation, where intraluminal cellular debris is not adherent to the ulcer bed, compared with patients who have calcific high grade obstructive lesions. Second, of the 65 patients who suffered a postoperative deficit, 29 had intracranial occlusive disease represented by stenoses within the siphon or circle of Willis. Severe intracranial arterial disease has been previously demonstrated to place patients at high risk of developing postoperative neurological complications, while neither recurrent stenosis nor contralateral occlusion appear to increase the stroke risk.[14–16] Extracranial arterial occlusive disease indicates the severity of cerebrovascular insufficiency present and the surgeon may selectively shunt this patient, but intracranial arterial occlusive disease is the limiting factor of cerebral ischaemia during carotid cross-clamping. In the absence of intraoperative EEG surveillance in the patient with severe intracranial arterial occlusive disease, the better part of surgical wisdom would be to use a shunt.

Table 14.1 *Postoperative deficit/indication for operation*

	Number	Transient Per cent (n)	Permanent Per cent (n)
Neurologically 'stable'			
TIA	579	2.0 (12)	2.2 (13)
VBI	248	2.8 (7)	2.3 (6)
Prophylactic	111	1.8 (2)	1.8 (2)
Amaurosis fugax	108	2.7 (3)	0.9 (1)
Total		2.3	1.8
Neurologically 'unstable'			
Stroke in evolution	27	48.8 (4)	11.0 (3)
RIND/stroke	165	4.2 (7)	3.6 (6)
Total		9.5	7.3

TIA, transient ischaemic attack; VBI, vertebrobasilar insufficiency; RIND, reversible ischaemic neurological deficit.

Since most surgeons have little experience with neurological deficit after endarterectomy, a succinct management schema is necessary (Fig. 14.1). When a focal, minor transient deficit or suspected TIA occurs and resolves within minutes, supportive non-operative treatment is most appropriate. This is the patient in whom urgent, carotid colour-flow duplex ultrasonography should be performed to evaluate the operative site. If, however, there is progression of the deficit, symptoms that wax and wane, the surgeon is unsure or the ultrasound examination is abnormal, then the safest and most expeditious means of managing the patient is prompt return to the operating room for neck exploration.

- A neurological deficit immediately after operation calls for emergency re-exploration

---

At re-exploration if a pulsatile artery is found, intraoperative arteriography is performed through a common carotid puncture proximal to the endarterectomy site. In this manner, the common carotid clamp site as well as the extracranial and intracranial internal carotid components can be visualised. If no defects are identified, the patient is simply kept under observation. If, however, there is evidence of intracranial embolism current wisdom would indicate the administration of local intra-arterial thrombolysis. Urokinase (1 MU (million units) in 100 mL saline over 1 hour) or tissue plasminogen activator (tPA) (10 mg in 100 mL saline over 1 hour) may be administered through a microcatheter inserted via the internal carotid artery intracranially up to middle cerebral artery level or via an indwelling shunt.[17–20] These reports are anecdotal, but offer encouraging results (Fig. 14.2). It must

be remembered, however, that postoperative neurological deficits caused by 'embolic showers' are likely to be made up of cholesterol–platelet–fibrin aggregates, and in this setting thrombolytic agents may have little benefit. Continued investigation of this therapeutic approach is, nevertheless, warranted.

When a pulseless, thrombosed endarterectomy site is found, the common and external carotid arteries are cross-clamped, the endarterectomy site is opened, and the internal carotid artery is allowed to back-bleed freely in the hope of washing out any thromboembolic material. If no back-bleeding occurs, thromboembolectomy using a no. 2 Fogarty catheter, and *very gently* executed to avoid cavernous sinus injury, is appropriate. Once back-bleeding is established, a temporary shunt is inserted to ensure restoration of cerebral blood flow. Technical errors should be corrected but, unfortunately, these may not always be found. The arteriotomy should be closed with a patch graft or the artery replaced with saphenous vein depending on the condition of the artery. A completion arteriogram is then mandatory.

As mentioned above, four endarterectomy sites were thrombosed by white clot composed of platelet–fibrin aggregates. This was probably heparin induced thrombocytopenic thrombosis caused by either heparin dependent platelet membrane antibodies, which induce platelet aggregation in the present of heparin,[21,22] or a disequilibrium in the balance of the prostaglandin systems (thromboxane A_2 and prostacyclin), affecting platelet proaggregation and disaggregation activity. Not a great deal of information exists on the 'white clot syndrome' after CEA, but faced with such a problem the wisest course of action may be systemic infusion of low molecular weight dextran, replacement of the endarterectomised segment with saphenous vein and adjunctive use of clopidogrel or ticlopidine.

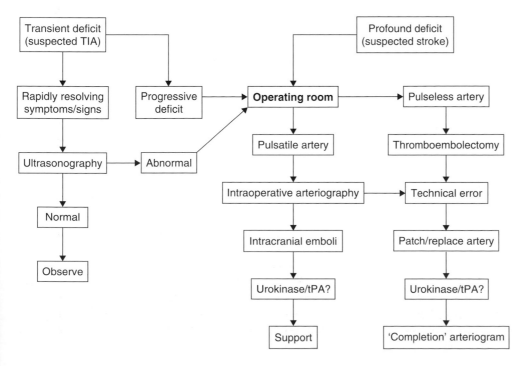

Figure 14.1 *Management schema in post-carotid endarterectomy stroke. TIA, transient ischaemic attack; tPA, tissue plasminogen activator*

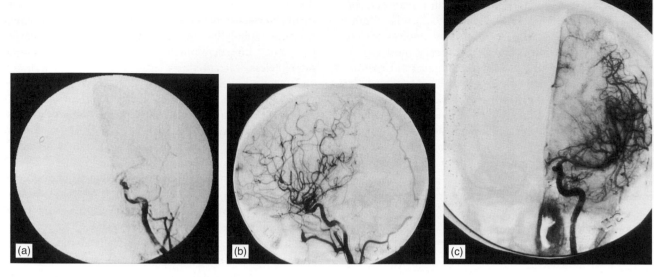

Figure 14.2   *(a) Thrombosed intracranial internal carotid artery (ICA) after left carotid endarterectomy; (b) ICA 20 minutes after tissue plasminogen activator (tPA) infusion; and (c) ICA 60 minutes after tPA infusion*

When a profound deficit in the form of a suspected stroke occurs upon 'awakening' from anaesthesia, the patient is immediately reanaesthetised and the wound reopened. If the deficit becomes apparent in the recovery room, the patient is immediately returned to the operating room and the steps shown in the algorithm in Fig. 14.1 are followed. The 'take home' message from the algorithm is that the safest and most expeditious step in managing these patients is immediate wound exploration in the operating room. Once in the operating room, arteriography, carotid exploration, thrombolytic therapy or any combination of these may be performed without delay.

> • Technical errors account for most postoperative strokes

In our experience the incidence of postoperative neurological deficits when CEA was performed with a shunt, without a shunt or under EEG surveillance has not been statistically different (see above). The concept of inadequate cerebral collateral flow during CEA, therefore, cannot be incriminated as the cause of the postoperative neurological complications. Technical errors causing carotid thrombosis or cerebral embolism rather than inadequate collateral cerebral flow, account for most cases of neurological deficit after CEA. When an early postoperative neurological deficit does occur, however, the most appropriate management is the immediate return of the patient to the operating room, which provides the opportunity to confirm the diagnosis and to take appropriate action. Although immediate reoperation is mandatory, the clinical outcome may not be significantly altered by this course of action.[23,24]

LATE NEUROLOGICAL DEFICITS

Late neurological deficit after CEA, which occurs in a very small percentage of patients, is represented by two pathological entities, namely, the cerebral hyperperfusion syndrome and intracerebral haemorrhage. Risk factors which place patients at risk of developing hyperperfusion syndromes are as follows: the relief of a high grade, preocclusive stenosis in the presence of a contralateral occlusion or contralateral high grade stenosis, recent (<3 months) contralateral CEA, a history of hypertension, postoperative use of systemic anticoagulants, an increase in cerebral blood flow of 100 per cent or more measured at the time of operation and patterns of cerebrovascular chronic hyperperfusion.[25,26] In areas of chronic cerebral ischaemia the 'autoregulatory mechanism' involving the intracerebral arterial system is known to be impaired. Brain tissue normally has the ability to resist changes in blood flow by the reflex contraction and relaxation of the intracerebral vessels as blood pressure increases. In the chronically ischaemic brain, this autoregulatory mechanism is lost and the arteriolar vessels tend to remain maximally dilated. With restoration of flow into a preocclusive internal carotid artery the delicate intracerebral small vasculature is suddenly exposed to an uncontrolled high pressure head.

> • The late development of a neurological deficit points to a diagnosis of cerebral hyperperfusion syndrome or intracerebral haemorrhage

The onset of symptoms associated with a hyperperfusion syndrome is heralded by a hemicranial vascular headache ipsilateral to the side of the endarterectomy. Additionally, the patient may experience uncontrollable hypertension, seizures and migrainous episodes associated with visual disturbances such as flashing lights or scotomata. The treatment for these symptoms is appropriate blood pressure control, possibly steroids to help stabilise the blood–brain barrier and antiseizure medication when indicated.[27] Considering the possible risk of intracerebral haemorrhage, it is safest to avoid any type of analgesic which has anticoagulant or antiplatelet effects.

> • Severe hemicranial headaches after CEA often herald the cerebral hyperfusion syndrome

Cerebral CT scan and EEG studies may be of benefit for establishing a diagnosis of the cerebral hyperperfusion syndrome. A postoperative CT scan may demonstrate patchy oedema, and an EEG demonstrates paroxysmal lateralising epileptiform discharges (PLEDs) ipsilateral to the side of endarterectomy, indicating a localised focus of irritability. A transient neurological deficit is occasionally seen with a hyperperfusion syndrome and is almost exclusively a postictal paresis.[27] Transcranial Doppler (TCD) and magnetic resonance imaging (MRI) may prove useful in establishing a definitive diagnosis of the hyperperfusion syndrome. Transcranial Doppler normally shows a return of velocities in the middle cerebral artery to the 40 mL/s range after a period of reactive hyperaemia. A greater than 100 per cent increase in peak velocity or pulsatility index of the middle cerebral artery compared with baseline values is consistent with the hyperperfusion syndrome.[28] Meticulous blood pressure control in these patients is essential.

> • A delayed neurological deficit should be evaluated systematically to establish cause: is it a technical error or an incorrigible event?

Intracerebral haemorrhage is the most feared sequela of the hyperperfusion syndrome. Risk factors associated with intracerebral haemorrhage are virtually identical to the hyperperfusion syndrome and include recent cerebral infarction, hypertension, relief of a high grade, preocclusive stenosis associated with drastic increases in cerebral blood flow and the use of anticoagulants. Presenting symptoms of intracerebral haemorrhage, which also occurs 3–7 days after endarterectomy are severe hemicranial headache, seizures, severe unremitting hypertension and a dilated unilateral pupil.[29,30]

Treatment is again symptomatic, but the most appropriate approach ought to be preventive, first, by recognising the symptoms and second, by controlling the patient's blood pressure effectively, because once haemorrhage occurs, herniation and death are all too common. The rate of incidence of intracerebral haemorrhage after CEA is less than 0.5 per cent.[31]

In summary, the symptom of severe hemicranial headache after CEA mandates swift evaluation and CT, MRI, TCD, anticoagulation profile and an EEG are appropriate. If the EEG reveals lateralising paroxysmal activity, the TCD demonstrates consistently elevated velocities or the CT/MRI shows patchy oedema, the patient may be started on anticonvulsants; any antiplatelet or anticoagulant medication is stopped and blood pressure is carefully controlled.

Conclusions

Stroke after CEA is a devastating event and a succinct, systematic management schema is necessary. A postoperative major deficit mandates immediate return to the operating room where arteriography, carotid exploration, thrombolytic therapy or a combination of these may be performed without delay. A minor or transient deficit, which resolves in minutes, necessitates urgent colour-flow duplex ultrasonography. If, however, there is any progression of the deficit, prompt return to the operating room is indicated. Late neurological events after CEA, which occur in a very small percentage of patients, are the cerebral hyperperfusion syndrome and intracerebral haemorrhage. These are generally heralded by hypertension and severe hemicranial headache ipsilateral to the side of CEA and are best managed medically.

Key references

Comerota AJ, Eze AR. Intraoperative high-dose regional urokinase infusion for cerebrovascular occlusion after carotid endarterectomy. *J Vasc Surg* 1996; **24**: 1008–16.

Pomposelli FB, Lamparello PJ, Riles TS, *et al.* Intracranial hemorrhage after carotid endarterectomy. *J Vasc Surg* 1988; **7**: 240–7.

Reigel MM, Hollier LH, Sundt TM Jr, *et al.* Cerebral hypoperfusion syndrome: a cause of neurologic dysfunction after carotid endarterectomy. *J Vasc Surg* 1987; **5**: 628–34.

Rockman CB, Jacobowitz GR, Lamparello PJ, *et al.* Immediate reexploration for the perioperative neurologic event after carotid endarterectomy: is it worthwhile? *J Vasc Surg* 2000; **32**: 1062–70.

Rosenthal D, Zeichner WD, Pano LA, Stanton PE Jr. Neurologic deficit after carotid endarterectomy; pathogenesis and management. *Surgery* 1983; **94**: 776–80.

REFERENCES

1 Riles TS, Imparato AM, Jacobowitz GR, *et al.* The cause of perioperative stroke after carotid endarterectomy. *J Vasc Surg* 1994; **19**: 206–16.

2   Rosenthal D, Zeichner WD, Pano LA, Stanton PE Jr. Neurologic deficit after carotid endarterectomy; pathogenesis and management. *Surgery* 1983; **94**: 776–80.

3   Hertzer NR, Beven EG, Greenstreet RL, Humphries AW. Internal carotid artery back pressure, intraoperative shunting, ulcerated atheromata, and the incidence of stroke during carotid endarterectomy. *Surgery* 1978; **83**: 306–12.

4   Hingorani A, Ascher E, Tsemekhim B, *et al.* Causes of early post carotid endarterectomy stroke in a recent series: the increasing importance of hyperperfusion syndrome. *Acta Chir Belg* 2002; **102**: 435–8.

5   Laman DM, Wieneke GH, van Duijin H, van Huffelen AC. High embolic rate early after carotid endarterectomy is associated with early cerebrovascular complications, especially in women. *J Vasc Surg* 2002; **36**: 278–84.

6   Frawley JE, Hicks RG, Beardon M, Woodey R. Hemodynamic ischemic stroke during carotid endarterectomy; an appraisal of risk and cerebral protection. *J Vasc Surg* 1997; **25**: 611–19.

7   Archie JP Jr. Technique and clinical results of carotid stump back pressure to determine selective shunting during carotid endarterectomy. *J Vasc Surg* 1991; **13**: 319–27.

8   Owens MC, Wilson SE. Prevention of neurologic complications of carotid endarterectomy. *Arch Surg* 1982; **117**: 551–5.

9   Moore WS, Barnett HJM, Beebe HG, *et al.* Guidelines for carotid endarterectomy; a multidisciplinary consensus statement from the ad hoc committee, American Heart Association. *Stroke* 1995; **26**: 188–201.

10 Whittemore AD, Ruby ST, Couch NP, *et al.* Early carotid endarterectomy in patients with small fixed neurologic deficits. *J Vasc Surg* 1984; **1**: 795–9.

11 Giodano JM, Trout HH, Kozloff L, DePalma RG. Timing Carotid Arterial Endarterectomy Surgery after Stroke. *J Vasc Surg* 1985; **2**: 250–5.

12 Pomposelli FB, Lamparello PJ, Riles TS, *et al.* Intracranial hemorrhage after carotid endarterectomy. *J Vasc Surg* 1988; **7**: 240–7.

13 Rothwell PM, Slattery J, Warlow CP. A systematic comparison of the risks of stroke and death due to carotid endarterectomy for symptomatic and asymptomatic stenosis. *Stroke* 1996; **27**: 266–9.

14 Thompson JE, Talkington CM. Carotid endarterectomy. *Adv Surg* 1993; **26**: 99–131.

15 Tu JV, Wang H, Bowyer B, *et al.* Risk factors for death or stroke after carotid endarterectomy. Observations from the Ontario Carotid Endarterectomy Registry. *Stroke* 2003; **34**: 2568–73 [epub ahead of print 2 October 2003].

16 Domenig C, Hamdan AD, Belfield AK, *et al.* Recurrent stenosis and contralateral occlusion: high-risk situations in carotid endarterectomy? *Ann Vasc Surg* 2003; **17**: 622–8 [epub ahead of print 23 October 2003].

17 Comerota AJ, Eze AR. Intraoperative high-dose regional urokinase infusion for cerebrovascular occlusion after carotid endarterectomy. *J Vasc Surg* 1996; **24**: 1008–16.

18 Barr JD, Harowitz MB, Mathis JM, *et al.* Intraoperative urokinase infusion for embolic stroke during carotid endarterectomy. *Neurosurgery* 1995; **36**: 606–11.

19 Del Zoppo GJ. Investigational use of tPA in acute stroke. *Ann Emerg Med* 1988; **11**: 1196–201.

20 Chalela JA, Katzan I, Liebskind DS, *et al.* Safety of intra-arterial thrombolysis in the postoperative stroke. *Stroke* 2001; **32**: 6:1365–9.

21 Kapsch D, Silver D. Heparin-induced thrombocytopenia and hemorrhage. *Arch Surg* 1981; **116**: 1423–9.

22 Adams JG, Humphrey LJ, Zhang X, Silver D. Do patients with heparin-induced thrombocytopenia syndrome have heparin specific antibodies? *J Vasc Surg* 1995; **21**: 247–54.

23 Stewart AH, McGrath CM, Cole SE, *et al.* Reoperation for neurological complications following carotid endarterectomy. *Br J Surg* 2003; **90**: 832–7.

24 Findlay JM, Marchak BE. Reoperation for acute hemispheric stroke after carotid endarterectomy: is there any value? *Neurosurgery* 2002; **50**: 486–92.

25 Waltz AG. Effect of blood pressure on blood flow in ischemic and in non-ischemic cerebral cortex. *Neurology* 1968; **18**: 613–21.

26 Ascher E, Markevich N, Schutzer RW, *et al.* Cerebral hyperperfusion syndrome after carotid endarterectomy: predictive factors and hemodynamic changes. *J Vasc Surg* 2003; **3**: 769–77.

27 Reigel MM, Hollier LH, Sundt TM Jr, *et al.* Cerebral hypoperfusion syndrome: a cause of neurologic dysfunction after carotid endarterectomy. *J Vasc Surg* 1987; **5**: 628–34.

28 Zanette EM, Fieschi C, Bozzao I, *et al.* Comparison of cerebral angiography and transcranial doppler sonography in acute stroke. *Stroke* 1989; **20**: 899–903.

29 Piepgras DG, Morgan MK, Sundt TF Jr, *et al.* Intracerebral hemorrhage after carotid endarterectomy. *J Neurosurg* 1988; **68**: 532–36.

30 Pomposelli FB, Lamparello PJ, Riles TS, *et al.* Intracranial hemorrhage after carotid endarterectomy. *J Vasc Surg* 1985; **51**: 114–15.

31 Rockman CB, Jacobowitz GR, Lamparello PJ, *et al.* Immediate reexploration for the perioperative neurologic event after carotid endarterectomy: is it worthwhile? *J Vasc Surg* 2000; **32**: 1062–70.

Acute Lower Limb Ischaemic States

15

Acute Limb Ischaemia: Surgical Options

CLIFFORD P SHEARMAN, MALCOLM H SIMMS

THE PROBLEM

Each year between 500 and 1000 per million of the population of northern Europe will suffer limb-threatening ischaemia due to atherosclerotic vascular disease.[1] The majority of these patients present with progressive deterioration in their condition and can be offered elective vascular reconstruction, resulting in limb salvage in up to 90 per cent.[2] Although demanding in terms of hospital resources, revascularisation currently offers the best therapeutic chance of the patient remaining ambulant and independent. Importantly, it is highly cost-effective when compared with amputation.[3,4]

Of the cohort of patients suffering severe limb ischaemia, a certain proportion, 20 per cent in most centres, present with a precipitate worsening of the condition requiring urgent or emergency intervention. When limb blood flow becomes insufficient to support resting tissue metabolism, a cascade of changes commences at the cellular level, which, if not reversed, will lead inevitably to tissue necrosis[5] (see Chapter 2). Early detection is therefore vital if revascularisation is to succeed. Acute limb-threatening ischaemia appears in a variety of guises and its recognition still remains a matter for clinical judgement rather than physiological measurement. In the classic presentation the patient reports that the limb has become painful, cold, immobile and numb, and the surgeon recognises that it is pale and pulseless. Pain, however, may not be reported if the patient is confused, demented or drugged. Similarly, physical signs may be obscured in a traumatised or oedematous limb. When acute deterioration occurs against a background of severe chronic ischaemia, the accompanying changes in symptoms and signs may be subtle and escape notice. While early recognition of impending gangrene is essential, it is just as important for the surgeon to recognise the onset of irreversible tissue death so that futile and potentially hazardous revascularisation procedures are avoided when amputation is the appropriate management.

Acute ischaemia and gangrene may be precipitated by spontaneous thromboembolism, acute deterioration in chronic ischaemia, failure of an established arterial bypass graft (see Chapter 2) or the consequences of either accidental, intentional or iatrogenic arterial trauma (see Chapters 38, 39 and 40). Arterial trauma is discussed elsewhere in this book (see Chapter 33). Intradermal ischaemia producing digital and cutaneous gangrene is characteristic of extensive arteriolar thrombosis secondary to diffuse endothelial injury, as seen in some forms of septicaemia, immune complex deposition, toxic injection and poorly controlled diabetes (see Chapter 19). Such cases of small vessel occlusion are not amenable to surgical intervention and treatment is supportive.

Aetiology of acute ischaemia

- Spontaneous thromboembolism
- Acute deterioration in chronic ischaemia
- Failure of arterial bypass graft
- Accidental/intentional trauma
- Iatrogenic trauma
- Diffuse endothelial injury – septicaemia, immune complex deposition, toxic injection, poorly controlled diabetes

It is important to note a shift in the spectrum of presentation of acute ischaemia. Recent decades have seen a decline in valvular heart disease, with its potential for dispatching emboli into a previously disease-free arterial bed. This decline has been offset by an increased prevalence of ischaemic heart disease that is frequently associated with peripheral vascular disease. Thus, even when the cause of the acute ischaemia is an embolus of cardiac origin, it is likely that this will lodge in an already diseased arterial tree, making simple measures such as balloon embolectomy ineffective.[6,7] Acute-on-chronic ischaemia is therefore an increasingly common mode of presentation, affecting an enlarging geriatric and diabetic population, while bypass graft related problems have become more frequent as reconstruction rather than primary amputation becomes the preferred treatment for critical limb ischaemia. The steady increase in the number and complexity of endovascular interventions undertaken in patients with advanced limb ischaemia has been accompanied inevitably by a proportion of complications that can lead to a precipitate worsening of ischaemia. The outcome for such patients presenting with acute and acute-on-chronic ischaemia is in general less favourable than in chronic ischaemia, and it is the management of this subgroup that we seek to address here.

DIAGNOSIS

The objectives of diagnosis are to ascertain the cause and severity of ischaemia, determine as far as possible the state of the arteries involved, and consider the patient's general medical condition, including the possible role of environmental factors. Obtaining a clear history followed by careful clinical examination provides most of the necessary information, and it is upon this that vital decisions regarding reconstruction or amputation are taken. In the context of impending gangrene, vascular imaging through ultrasound and angiography does not play its usual pivotal role. The reasons for this are twofold: first, the urgency of the situation may not allow sufficient time for vascular imaging to be performed, and second, a stagnant vascular bed does not facilitate the provision of satisfactory angiographic or ultrasonic images.

Clinical history

The aetiology of the ischaemic episode may be suggested by the clinical history.[8] Sudden, spontaneous and unheralded acute ischaemia favours a thromboembolic aetiology, whereas a prior history of claudication and rest pain suggests acute-on-chronic deterioration. Any history of previous vascular intervention warrants detailed interrogation and scrutiny of operative scars and medical records when available. Pain and sensory loss in the limb is usually the predominant symptom but may give way to loss of limb function as the effects of ischaemia progress.

Clinical examination

Patients should be examined supine and in a comfortable, warm environment. In assessing the severity of the peripheral perfusion deficit, it is important to take into consideration reversible systemic factors such as dehydration, anaemia, lung disease, heart failure and hypothermia.

Indicators for urgent revascularisation

- Peripheral neurosensory loss
- Inability to flex/extend ankle
- Loss of sensation distal to mid-calf

Examination of the affected limb, particularly in comparison with its pair, will help to determine the urgency of the situation. Peripheral neurosensory loss in an ischaemic limb implies that its viability is compromised and that revascularisation needs to be achieved without delay to prevent irreversible damage. In severe cases the patient is completely unable to flex or extend the ankle and there is no preservation of sensation distal to the mid-calf. Waxy pallor of the extremity which persists in full dependency of the limb and is accompanied by coldness, numbness and paralysis indicates a near complete loss of arterial perfusion, requiring urgent correction. Tenderness of the calf muscles suggests the onset of tissue damage whereas induration denotes irreversibility. Whenever there is evidence of muscle paralysis and tenderness, particularly if this is associated with pain on passive stretching, it is likely that cellular ischaemia is established and that muscle reperfusion will be followed by cellular swelling and interstitial oedema, resulting in raised pressure in vulnerable muscle compartments (see Chapter 2). In such cases revascularisation procedures should be followed by fasciotomy.

Extreme indicators for urgent revascularisation

- Fixed blotchy cyanosis of skin limited to forefoot and toes
- Waxy pallor persisting with full dependency of extremity
- Coldness, numbness and paralysis of calf muscles
- Tenderness of calf muscles

If in addition to these signs the muscles have a stiff and 'putty-like' consistency and the overlying and distal skin exhibits fixed cyanosis, the limb should be considered non-viable and amputation at the appropriate level should be offered. When the distribution of fixed blotchy staining of skin is limited to the forefoot and toes, such a finding in isolation should not deter attempted revascularisation.

Reperfusion of ischaemic skin and digits carries a low risk of systemic complications and superficial or peripheral necrosis of the foot is compatible with recovery. Varying degrees of distal necrosis or superficial ulceration may complicate diverse disorders such as chronic ischaemia, neuropathy, tissue trauma and venous disease and may be regarded as potentially reversible. Digital and cutaneous changes should therefore not influence the decision to revascularise unless they appear sufficiently extensive as to preclude functional rehabilitation.

Indicators of non-viability of leg

- Fixed cyanosis of overlying and distal skin
- Loss of movement
- Stiff and putty-like consistency of muscles

When placement of the ischaemic foot in a position of maximum dependency produces slow capillary return and there remains some active movement in the calf muscles, then, whether or not the foot remains anaesthetic, there is less immediate urgency to restore perfusion. Assuming facilities are available, there is time for angiography to be undertaken, with a view to evaluating the comparative merits of thrombolysis, angioplasty or reconstruction.

Some patients will present with a limb that already exhibits signs of established irreversible ischaemia. Loss of both movement and sensation, fixed cyanotic staining and tense muscle compartments indicate that the limb is beyond salvage. Attempts to revascularise such a limb are pointless and expose the patient to the systemic complications of reperfusion injury (see Chapter 4), notably pulmonary dysfunction and renal failure (Fig. 15.1) (see Chapter 4). Amputation is then the therapeutic option of choice.

Acute limb ischaemia may occur as an agonal event in some patients, especially in those with advanced malignancy or other severe debilitating disease. The decision to intervene with the limb then has to be balanced against the patient's overall prognosis and quality of life. We believe that if the patient has potential to use the limb and is likely to survive, even for only a few months, then revascularisation procedures should be considered. The worst scenario is for a patient to spend the last year of his or her life struggling not only with their primary disease but also with the challenge of rehabilitating from an amputation.

Assessment of the severity of limb ischaemia should be accompanied by thorough general examination to detect and evaluate comorbid conditions, particularly those likely to influence oxygen delivery such as shock, dehydration and cardiac or pulmonary insufficiency. Cardiovascular examination should concentrate on the identification of possible sources of embolism and on assessing the condition of the arteries by palpation, auscultation and Doppler insonation.

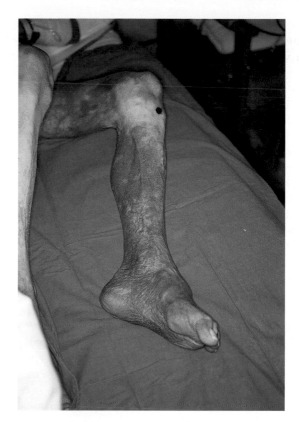

Figure 15.1 *Irreversibly ischaemic leg with fixed staining of the skin and a waxy, dough-like feeling of the calf muscles at which time the limb was painless*

Vigilance is required when assessing patients suffering from vasospastic and neurological disorders that affect the microvasculature of the extremities. Patients with paraplegia, stroke and poliomyelitis may exhibit changes in skin colour and temperature that bear a superficial resemblance to those of critical ischaemia. Careful assessment of ankle pulses and Doppler-derived ankle systolic pressure should prevent misdiagnosis. Similarly, chronic oedema can make assessment of peripheral arterial perfusion particularly difficult, especially when it is due to a combination of venous and arterial insufficiency.

Evaluation of arterial status

In patients exhibiting severe acute ischaemia, inspection of the limb with pulse palpation may provide all the necessary evidence to determine the cause and extent of the problem. Comparison of the affected and unaffected limbs is of particular value in distinguishing embolic events from the thrombotic complications of peripheral atherosclerosis. Palpation at the usual sites, i.e. abdomen, groins, knees, ankles and feet, should distinguish not only pulse volume but also note any evidence of mural calcification or aneurysmal dilatation. Palpation of the superficial femoral artery in the mid-thigh of a thin patient can occasionally localise the level of a femoropopliteal block. Detection of an arterial thrill or bruit can assist in the localisation of stenoses.

Portable Doppler ultrasound examination

With the patient in the supine position, insonation of the leg arteries with a handheld Doppler probe (8 MHz) can yield valuable information. In the groin the presence of a tapping signal is indicative of downstream occlusion in the common, superficial or profunda femoris arteries and the level of occlusion may be detected by insonation of the superficial femoral artery along the subsartorial canal and into the popliteal fossa. The presence of a palpable popliteal pulse with a 'pistol shot' Doppler signal is suggestive of a recent thromboembolic occlusion at the trifurcation of the popliteal artery (Fig. 15.2). Insonation of the tibial arteries is easiest at the malleolar level and allows calf sphygmomanometry to be employed to derive the ankle systolic blood pressure.

Ankle pressure values obtained by calf compression, however, can be elevated erroneously by loss of arterial wall compliance. This occurs most often in patients with diabetes or with chronic renal failure but it also occurs to some extent in all patients with peripheral vascular disease.[9] When calf derived ankle systolic blood pressure appears to be at variance with the clinical picture, the limb should be elevated (Fig. 15.3) while insonating one of the ankle arteries with the Doppler probe.[10] If the signal disappears reproducibly at a certain height of elevation above the heart, this indicates that the perfusion pressure at this level is equivalent to the height of elevation expressed as cm of water (1 mm pressure of mercury is equivalent to 1.36 cm water). In any limb the maximum recording of elevation pressure is limited by its length and therefore pressures exceeding around 50 mmHg are unrecordable.

In the presence of symptomatic ischaemia, more detailed information concerning the state of the infrapopliteal

arteries can be obtained by enlisting gravity in order to maximise distal perfusion pressure. The patient should be repositioned sitting up with both legs hanging in dependency over the edge of the bed. All three crural arteries should be insonated in the lower third of the calf, the peroneal artery being located by compressing the probe into the soft tissues posteromedial to the fibula. Under conditions of impending gangrene arterial signals may be so damped as to resemble venous signals. A distinction can be made, however, by continuing insonation while delivering a sharp squeeze to the foot. Augmentation of the signal suggests it is of venous origin and diminution arterial.

An understanding of the anatomy and interrelationships of the crural and pedal arteries is essential in the optimal surgical management of the ischaemic foot. This understanding is enhanced by habitual use of dependent Doppler insonation to map these arteries in both health and disease.

At the level of the ankle joint the dorsalis pedis artery lies immediately deep to the tendon of extensor hallucis longus but as it enters the foot the artery emerges lateral to this tendon to lie on the dorsal convexity of the foot. The

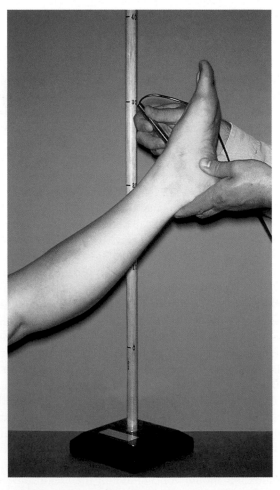

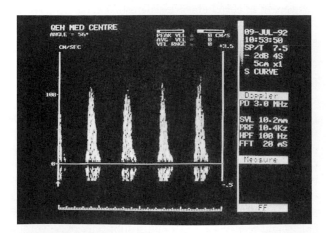

Figure 15.2 *Doppler waveform from a vessel proximal to an acute occlusion*

Figure 15.3 *Limb being elevated and ankle vessel being insonated with an ultrasound probe; the signal will disappear if the perfusion pressure is exceeded (the 'pole test')*

dorsalis pedis artery ends by entering the first metatarsal space to become the deep plantar artery.

The posterior tibial artery is insonated about 1 cm posterior to the tibial border and when patent can be traced under the medial malleolus into the foot. As it runs deep to the belly of adductor hallucis muscle it divides into its medial and lateral plantar branches, which are often difficult to trace.

The peroneal artery divides into its anterior and posterior communicating branches 2–3 cm proximal to the ankle joint. The anterior branch penetrates the interosseous membrane and runs distally onto the foot on the anterior surface of the lateral malleolus, where it is normally palpable. In the foot it communicates with the dorsalis pedis artery before anastomosing with the lateral end of the arcade that links the bases of the metatarsals. The posterior peroneal artery branch passes distally about 1 cm parallel to the posterior and inferior border of the lateral malleolus. It gives off a posterior communicating branch which passes between the back of the ankle joint and the tendo Achilles to join the posterior tibial artery before descending into the foot, where under normal conditions it may be palpated subcutaneously on the lateral aspect of the calcaneum. It then winds under the arch of the calcaneum to enter the foot where it terminates by anastomosing with branches of the lateral plantar artery in the sole of the foot.

The major component of the pedal arch is the deep plantar artery which links the dorsal and plantar metatarsal arcades through the first intermetatarsal space. This artery should be insonated with the probe placed over the base of the first intermetatarsal space. If an arterial flow signal is obtained, digital compression of the ankle arteries one by one should determine which is the dominant vessel supplying the pedal arch. When the dominant artery is compressed the pedal arch signal will disappear then return on release. Conversely, when the non-dominant artery is compressed the strength of the deep plantar signal may be enhanced. When neither the anterior nor the posterior tibial appears dominant the peroneal trunk should be occluded by digital compression posteromedial to the fibula. Whichever crural artery seems to provide dominant inflow to the deep plantar should be considered the best outflow when distal bypass is required.[11]

Unfortunately, in acute and severe ischaemia arterial Doppler signals are often unobtainable even with the limb dependent and the patient warm and hydrated. This situation provides a useful index of the severity of ischaemia but no clue as to run-off anatomy.

PATIENT AND TREATMENT SELECTION

Surgical intervention carries risk for the patient and is expensive in time and materials. The worst outcome for the patient and the least economical for the community is a failed bypass that results in amputation. For these reasons it is important to be realistic in selecting patients for surgery. In a one-year prospective audit in two centres we found that factors associated with a poor outcome were previous bypass surgery, absence of suitable vein for a bypass conduit, extensive ulceration of the foot and absence of an identifiable pedal arch with dependent Doppler. Diabetes mellitus was not associated with any worse outcome. A good outcome in terms of rehabilitation following either reconstruction or amputation could be predicted prior to intervention from the level of social support available, such as that from a partner living with the patient, and from the mental state of the patient.

The role of subintimal angioplasty (SIA) remains controversial. Most published reports fail to provide sufficient haemodynamic, anatomical or follow-up detail to enable valid comparisons to be made with surgical series. In units where access to both SIA and infrapopliteal bypass is unrestricted, selection of a preferred option can usually be made on the basis of clinical and angiographic criteria. In a significant proportion of patients presenting with acute ischaemia SIA is impracticable, for instance in multisegment iliofemoral occlusion, aneurysmal disease or severe acute ischaemia with fresh thrombus. When there is apparent equipoise in the potential application of the two techniques their relative merits have not yet been compared. This issue is now the subject of a randomised prospective study in the UK. Most reports seem to agree that failed SIA does not compromise subsequent attempts at bypass surgery so a rational policy when both alternatives are applicable would be either to randomise or to attempt SIA as the first line of treatment?

Questions in decision making

- Revascularisation or amputation?
- Will limb loss lead to patient's deterioration?
- Is effective treatment available to save the leg?
- Potential success/difficulty of chosen method of revascularisation?
- Fitness for anaesthesia either by GA or LA?

The decision on whether to proceed with any vascular intervention rests on the answers to two questions: first, whether the patient's overall situation will deteriorate if the limb is lost, and second, whether there is an effective treatment available. If the answer to either question is negative then the intervention should not be considered. If both answers are affirmative it still remains to weigh the difficulty and potential success of the intervention as well as its predictable mortality and morbidity. The alternatives of palliative therapy, percutaneous recanalisation, surgical bypass or primary amputation may all merit consideration. Of these, amputation remains the only irrevocable step although when it offers the patient the best prospect for recovery it should be adopted in a spirit of optimism. The concept of the 'unreconstructable leg' is flexible and open to biased interpretation and therefore it should legitimately be restricted to patients in whom arteriography has shown extensive infrapopliteal occlusion with good distal contrast filling but no axial arteries shown in the calf or the foot. Most patients in this category will be suffering from diabetes mellitus or Buerger's disease or thromboangiitis obliterans (see Chapter 42). Fitness for anaesthesia should not be used as an argument for amputation in preference to bypass; regional and local anaesthetic techniques are applicable to both. The limited life expectancy of the vascular patient has been deployed, with some justice, as an argument in favour of SIA, which often confers only short term benefit. Distal bypass is undoubtedly a more durable option but the potential for perioperative complication is greater.

The case for preintervention investigation

When initial clinical and Doppler assessment suggest that revascularisation is appropriate, further investigation should be considered with the objective of clarifying pathological anatomy and determining interventional strategy, whether thrombolysis, angioplasty or reconstruction. If, despite a normal femoral pulse, the foot remains cold and anaesthetic and ankle Doppler signals are unobtainable in dependency then the two points mentioned previously should be recalled: first, that there may be much less than a 12-hour window before the onset of muscle necrosis and second, that transfemoral arteriography is very unlikely to yield diagnostic images of the infrapopliteal arteries. In a significant proportion of patients presenting with impending gangrene, however, there is some evidence of continuing distal perfusion. In these cases vascular imaging is helpful in planning operative intervention and essential whenever percutaneous intervention is considered feasible.

Duplex ultrasonography

Colour flow duplex ultrasound scanning has been proved as a reliable means of determining the extent of femoropopliteal occlusive disease. It, therefore, has a major role in the non-invasive selection of cases that appear suitable for angioplasty. Claims have been made for the superiority of duplex over dependent Doppler for the evaluation of the infrapopliteal and pedal arteries. We remain unconvinced and continue to be swayed by the accessibility and simplicity of Doppler. Duplex ultrasound scanning requires special technical skills so may not be available out of hours.

Aneurysms of the femoral and popliteal arteries can be assessed with accuracy and the presence and extent of arterial and venous thrombus can be recorded. Duplex ultrasound is less reliable in the assessment of the aortoiliac segment, particularly in obese patients.

In all but the thinnest legs it is helpful to request ultrasound mapping of the long saphenous vein. This may

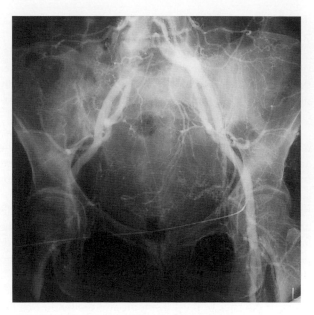

Figure 15.4 *Angiogram of a 68-year-old woman with a three-year history of intermittent claudication and sudden deterioration; despite clinical expectations she had a saddle embolus, which was removed by bilateral femoral balloon embolectomy*

facilitate vein harvesting and also aids strategy in those patients in whom the vein is absent or unsuitable and alternative sources of vein need to be identified.

Angiography

If time and the condition of the limb allows, angiography should be arranged. On the basis of the history and clinical examination it is often difficult to discern whether the patient has suffered an embolic or thrombotic event. If angiography reveals a simple embolus, the decision whether to proceed to catheter directed thrombolysis (CDT) or to surgical removal of clot will depend on clinical urgency (surgery is usually the quicker option), the relative availability of surgeon or radiologist and the presence or otherwise of contraindications to thrombolysis (see Chapter 16). Balloon embolectomy for acute limb ischaemia can be undertaken in most cases with reasonable expectation of a good result (Fig. 15.4). Conversely, if atherosclerotic occlusive disease is discovered, complex reconstruction may be required.

Investigation and assessment

- Doppler pressures/waveforms – simple and accessible
- Colour flow duplex scanning – not always available out of hours
- Ultrasound mapping of long saphenous vein
- Angiography – transfemoral (ipsilateral) orthograde ± CDT of embolus, (contralateral)

retrograde ± saddle embolectomy or inflow iliac percutaneous transluminal angioplasty (PTA), transbrachial, intravenous digital subtraction angiography (DSA)
- Magnetic resonance angiography
- Intraoperative angiography

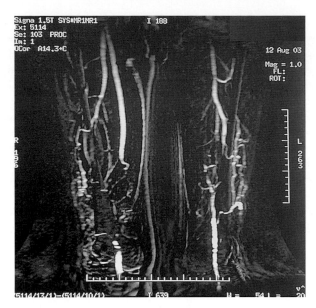

Figure 15.5 *Magnetic resonance angiogram of patient with femoropopliteal disease*

If the patient has a palpable femoral pulse on the side of the affected limb, ipsilateral orthograde transfemoral angiography should be undertaken, since its greater selectivity reduces contrast load and facilitates more detailed distal imaging. It is also the preferred point of access if percutaneous intervention is contemplated. Retrograde arteriography via the contralateral groin is an effective alternative. If neither femoral pulse is palpable, we favour brachial catheterisation and in over 250 cases have had only one episode of brachial artery injury. Intravenous DSA has in our experience not been particularly helpful in the emergency situation as unfit patients are seldom able to tolerate the large volumes of contrast necessary.

If the angiogram reveals underlying thrombus, a guidewire is passed into the thrombus, which is agitated, and a catheter is then passed along the guidewire. We currently use tissue plasminogen activator (tPA) delivered as a 5 mg bolus three times 30 minutes apart or as a low dose infusion (0.5 mg/hour). We found that the local complication rate became unacceptable after the catheter had been in place more than 24 hours and now no longer continue infusions beyond that period. If lysis reveals a lesion suitable to angioplasty, this is carried out at the same time. Often, however, the angiogram will reveal extensive distal disease that is only amenable to bypass surgery. These issues are dealt with in greater detail in Chapter 16.

Angioplasty for inflow occlusion

If a stenosis or short occlusion of the iliac artery is discovered in association with extensive distal disease, we favour angioplasty of the iliac lesion at the time of angiography, proceeding to distal surgery when necessary. If percutaneous access is difficult or the haemodynamic significance of the lesion is difficult to ascertain, peroperative angioplasty (PTA) can also be undertaken (see below). Extensive aortofemoral atheroma may warrant surgical treatment, either bypass or endarterectomy, as described below.

The choice between angioplasty and bypass has generated a shifting debate in recent years, although in the emergency situation the decision may be dictated by manpower logistics, reflecting the scarcity of skilled interventional radiologists in many centres. The planning of emergency revascularisation procedures involves matching the patient's condition, both arterial and general, to the resources, skills and experience of the vascular department, in order to achieve the best outcome for the individual.

Magnetic resonance angiography

With improvements in magnetic resonance technology we find this an increasingly useful tool, particularly for imaging the distal vessels (Fig. 15.5). It is ideal in patients with impaired renal function or those in whom arterial access is limited. The investigation can be disturbing to some elderly patients and access to the equipment may be difficult, especially in the emergency situation.

Peroperative angiography

In some patients with advanced ischaemia of the limb, time and haemodynamics do not favour a preoperative angiogram and in such cases intraoperative prebypass arteriography may be considered. In the presence of severe acute ischaemia distal perfusion may be so stagnant that direct intrafemoral injection of contrast fails to provide diagnostic images of the infrapopliteal segment. Under these circumstances it is preferable to clear femoral thrombus before embarking on angiography, or alternatively to choose a more distal injection point such as the below-knee popliteal artery. Fortunately, in most patients residual distal perfusion is sufficient to permit the distribution of contrast and so achieve satisfactory images via the common femoral artery. A 19 gauge butterfly needle is inserted into the artery, and 40 mL non-ionic X-ray contrast (Ultravist, Schering AG, Berlin, Germany) is injected by hand as rapidly as possible with the femoral artery cross-clamped above the needle. If an image intensifier is not available an X-ray plate is wrapped and placed beneath the calf and a single film obtained 5–10 seconds after injecting the contrast; the more severe and distal the ischaemia, the longer the delay. Some external rotation of the calf improves the perspective. This technique seldom fails to reveal the distal run-off vessels. Failure to obtain clear images implies either a technical failure with the contrast injection or an underestimate of the severity of distal ischaemia.

Intraoperative arteriography can be of value when a distal vessel has been explored but it is unclear whether the outflow bed is satisfactory. At the popliteal artery level, we use the same technique as for the femoral but reduce the X-ray contrast to 20 mL. Similarly, at the level of the calf and ankle, 10 mL of contrast is injected through a 21 gauge cannula (Venflon) via an arteriotomy. This technique is useful in seeking to confirm that the selected run-off vessel communicates with the pedal arch (Fig. 15.6).

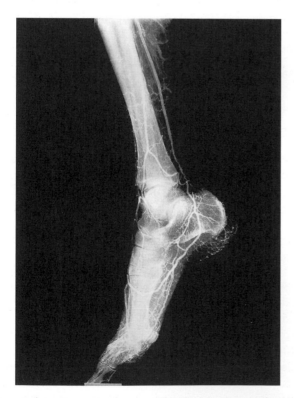

Figure 15.6 *Operative angiogram via proximal posterior tibial artery showing disease in the posterior tibial vessel at the ankle, which supplies the pedal arch and fills the peroneal artery via the posterior and anterior communicating branches; the dorsalis pedis artery is occluded; the proximal peroneal artery was used for distal run-off with a good result*

SURGICAL INTERVENTION

General supportive measures

The main concern should be to restore adequate blood supply to the limb as soon as possible. Most patients fortunately present with a cold painful foot in which there is some preservation of calf muscle function and only partial loss of sensation. This provides a window of a few hours for assessment and preparation during which time optimisation of the patient's general condition may be achieved. Marginal improvement may occur after admission to hospital with adequate analgesia and correction of any fluid depletion. Simple measures such as nursing the foot in dependency, intravenous dextran 40 (500 mL in normal saline over 4 hours) and inspired oxygen (28 per cent) may allow a well-developed collateral circulation to compensate. This may gain time for preintervention investigation of the patient.

Anaesthesia

Patients at imminent risk of limb gangrene are likely to be systemically unwell and are at increased risk of ischaemic heart disease, so that the early involvement of an experienced anaesthetist is advisable, both to help prepare the patient and to select the appropriate method of anaesthesia.

In our practice epidural anaesthesia is the favoured approach, particularly in patients with chronic obstructive airways disease. Spinal anaesthesia has the advantage of speed and simplicity and is useful for amputation procedures. Because its duration is limited to 2 hours it is generally unsuited to the uncertainties of revascularisation surgery. The ease of prolongation of epidural anaesthesia is a distinct advantage in lower limb vascular reconstruction and provides the option of maintaining good postoperative analgesia without suppressing respiratory function. When used in this way, bladder catheterisation and vigilant nursing care of pressure areas are essential. Epidural anaesthesia must be used with particular care in patients with ischaemic heart disease, in whom blood pressure must be rigorously controlled to avoid coronary hypoperfusion. Epidural anaesthesia also carries a small risk of spinal haematoma so should be avoided or used with caution whenever there is a possibility of impaired coagulation.

Inhalational anaesthesia is acceptable for many patients and can be used in combination with epidural anaesthesia, when analgesic requirements are reduced. There remains a difficult cohort of patients in whom neither neuraxial nor inhalational anaesthesia is safe or practicable. These include patients with myocardial instability, severe metabolic and renal dysfunction, coagulopathy and spinal deformity.

Fortunately, nearly all infrainguinal reconstructions can be carried out under local anaesthesia.[12] Expertise in carrying out percutaneous femoral, obturator and sciatic nerve block is useful but not essential and our favoured technique requires no special training or equipment. Prilocaine 0.5 per cent is used to infiltrate the skin and subcutaneous tissues in the groin; deeper infiltration lateral to the femoral pulse should block the medial and anterior sensory branches of the femoral nerve, so that it is rarely necessary to perform supplementary infiltration in order to expose the long saphenous vein in the thigh and calf. Next the skin and subcutaneous tissues of the distal medial thigh are infiltrated to allow a medial approach to the above-knee popliteal artery. Some additional infiltration of muscle fascia is usually required in order to dissect with a finger deep and posterior to the artery until the sciatic nerve is palpated, lying on the surface of the biceps femoris muscle. The nerve is then hooked round the forefinger and injected slowly and gently with about 10 mL of 0.5 per cent prilocaine so that the nerve trunk is felt to distend. This injection usually produces momentary discomfort but within a minute will induce complete distal anaesthesia for 2–4 hours, with no adverse neurological sequelae. Provided that this manoeuvre is performed sufficiently proximal to include the lateral popliteal nerve, as is nearly always the case, no further anaesthesia is required and it is notable that patients who have been suffering severe ischaemic pain will often relax and sleep. Adjunctive sedation is not necessary with this form of anaesthesia and may produce disinhibition and restlessness. By this means it should be possible to achieve sufficient anaesthesia for any infrainguinal reconstruction with around 80 mL of 0.5 per cent prilocaine.

When only infrapopliteal reconstruction is required the below-knee popliteal artery can be exposed using local infiltration of the skin, fat and fascia with 0.5 per cent prilocaine. The posterior tibial nerve will be sighted as it disappears under the soleus arch and it is there injected with 5–10 mL prilocaine to produce effective anaesthesia of the posteromedial aspect of the leg. Anaesthesia of the anterior tibial compartment will require separate percutaneous infiltration of the lateral popliteal nerve as it lies superficial to the neck of the fibula.

Occasionally revascularisation at ankle level only is required, usually as a result of distal thromboembolism complicating a more proximal surgical or endovascular intervention. Microtibial embolectomy can then be accomplished under formal ankle block or by simple subcutaneous infiltration over the malleolar portions of the anterior and posterior tibial arteries.[13]

Extra-anatomical procedures such as cross-femoral and axillofemoral bypass can be carried out with the help of local infiltration anaesthesia. However, the length of the subcutaneous tunnel in axillofemoral bypass is too great for local anaesthesia alone. Temporary supplementation using inhalational agents or ketamine will enable the tunnelling procedure to be covered.

Operation: general considerations

Systemic anticoagulant cover is not used routinely except in patients with suspected thromboembolic disease, when intravenous heparin is given by bolus and infusion to achieve perioperatively a partial thromboplastin ratio of around × 2 control. In general we favour the intraoperative use of a local flush comprising Hartmann's solution with heparin added at a concentration of 10 units/mL. Prophylactic antibiotic cover is administered routinely intravenously, commencing on induction of anaesthesia and continuing with two or more postoperative doses according to clinical circumstance. Our usual regimen is flucloxacillin 500 mg, metronidazole 400 mg and gentamicin 120 mg, unless the patient has renal impairment, but combination and dosage can vary.

The first step in most patients is exposure of the femoral artery and its branches, affording an opportunity for intraoperative arteriography when appropriate. If the femoral pulse is of normal volume, attention is directed towards distal reconstruction. If the common femoral pulse is inadequate due to local atheroma then local femoral endarterectomy should be planned.

Some patients may present with impending gangrene despite the presence of a palpable popliteal or superficial femoral pulse. In such cases, as well as those in whom the cause of ischaemia is known to be an aneurysm of the popliteal artery, the level of the initial exposure should be as dictated by the clinical picture. Whether at femoral or popliteal level, the object of the exposure should be to assess the condition of the artery wall, to gain all possible insight into the cause of ischaemia and to obtain sufficient control to facilitate all potential manoeuvres, whether diagnostic or therapeutic.

Care should be taken during arterial exposure to preserve the long saphenous vein and to consider the most appropriate orientation of the proposed arteriotomy, whether transverse, oblique or, as is usually the case, longitudinal. The use of transverse or oblique arteriotomy should be restricted to simple embolectomy procedures in arteries that appear free from atheroma. In this situation they have the advantage of easy closure without recourse to patching, and the use of interrupted suture technique will avoid any risk of stenosis.

Inflow procedures

If the external iliac pulse is weak and it is unclear whether downflow will prove sufficient to support a distal reconstruction, then femoral arterial pressure can be measured by direct cannulation with a 19 gauge needle connected to a pressure transducer. If this shows a normal arterial pressure compared with upper limb pressure, 30 mg papaverine is injected. A fall in pressure of greater than 30 mmHg is deemed an indication for an inflow procedure.

If adequate in-theatre imaging is available on-table angioplasty can be carried out. This can be difficult to achieve, especially if the femoral artery has been opened. In extreme situations a catheter may be passed up the iliac artery and withdrawn so as to measure the pressure gradient, permitting blind angioplasty to be performed at the site of pressure fall.

When an unexpectedly weak femoral pulse persists after local disobliteration of the common femoral artery and, if necessary, retrograde external iliac endarterectomy, the problem is most likely to involve the whole length of the external iliac artery and may extend into the common iliac. If the contralateral femoral pulse is of normal volume then cross-femoral bypass may be the best and safest operation. However when the patient is under a general or epidural anaesthetic and there is a satisfactory pulse at the aortic bifurcation the various options of iliofemoral revascularisation may be preferred. An ipsilateral oblique iliac incision provides good extraperitoneal exposure of the iliac bifurcation and palpation will convey a good impression of the density of atheroma and degree and extent of arterial calcification. In the majority of patients it will be possible to use external finger fracture to dissect and dislodge the core of atheroma from the external iliac artery and to squeeze it out through the open common femoral. If there is significant common iliac atheroma or thrombus this can be treated in similar fashion provided that the aortic bifurcation is judged to be compressible. The internal iliac artery should be clamped during the process of finger fracture to protect it from embolisation. The core of common iliac atheroma/thrombus will require fragmentation in order for it to be extruded down the external iliac. This process of pulsion endarterectomy should be continued until all luminal obstruction is eliminated and a uniformly soft, pulsatile segment can be palpated down to the common femoral. Proximal clamping should not be required, although intermittent distal clamping is required for haemostasis; the arterial pulse then aids extrusion of atheromatous fragments. In the presence of significant arterial calcification this technique is inappropriate and conventional iliofemoral bypass using a prosthetic graft is preferred. The advantage of pulsion endarterectomy is its speed and convenience through a limited exposure and the avoidance of prosthetic material, which carries increased potential for infective complications.

When clinical or angiographic assessment indicates that there is significant stenosis or occlusion at or proximal to the aortic bifurcation then iliofemoral or femoro-femoral procedures will be insufficient. Endovascular treatment is, at present, unlikely to be effective in these circumstances. Surgical options are likely to involve bypass reconstruction, obtaining inflow from the abdominal aortic or axillary artery level.

It is rare for removal of a saddle embolus from the aortic bifurcation to be achieved successfully by the retrograde transfemoral deployment of balloon embolectomy catheters.

Acute ischaemia associated with loss of both femoral pulses is much more likely to result from thrombotic occlusion of a grossly atheromatous aortoiliac segment. Recanalisation or bypass is usually required. Aortofemoral endarterectomy has the reputation of being bloody and unreliable whereas bypass procedures are tried and tested. The choice or aortic or axillary artery inflow will balance the better long term patency of aortofemoral reconstruction against the reduced anaesthetic requirements and lower mortality of axillofemoral bypass. When utilising aortic inflow, access to the infrarenal aorta may be either direct or retroperitoneal. The latter trades some limitation of access for a reduction in postoperative ileus and wound pain.

As with all suprainguinal inflow procedures, long term patency demands unimpeded outflow beyond the common femoral bifurcation. Achieving this may necessitate the addition of measures such as profundaplasty, the tacking of superficial femoral plaque or immediate sequential infrainguinal bypass.

Operation: inflow procedures

- On-table iliac angioplasty
- Retrograde iliac embolectomy/endarterectomy
- Iliofemoral bypass
- Femoro-femoral crossover bypass
- Aortofemoral endarterectomy
- Aortofemoral bypass
- Axillofemoral bypass

Staged *in situ* bypass

When revascularisation at femoral level is achieved, whether as a consequence of inflow reconstruction or following a femoral embolectomy, the adequacy of distal perfusion can be predicted from observation of the femoral outflow or from knowledge of the status of the distal vasculature. On rare occasions this prediction may be difficult and the surgeon is then faced with the dilemma as to whether or not it is necessary to proceed to immediate distal bypass in order to achieve limb salvage. A policy of 'wait and see' may lead to persisting distal ischaemia, which may in turn lead to compartment syndrome, tissue loss (see Chapter 2) or an untimely rush back to the operating theatre to reopen the groin incision and add a distal bypass.

A useful compromise in this situation is to mobilise the proximal end of the long saphenous vein and to use it to close the femoral arteriotomy, as for *in situ* bypass. Any accessible valves in the vein should be destroyed first by using scissors or by probing in order to procure some limited fistulous outflow. In this way the option of proceeding to distal bypass is reserved and can be implemented at any time, using local anaesthesia, without recourse to reopening the groin incision; downflow is achieved by retrograde deployment of a valvulotome into the pulsating proximal segment of long saphenous vein. If in the event no further bypass is found necessary, the persisting controlled saphenous vein fistula has no serious disadvantage and can be left alone or tied off as desired.

Distal procedures

Once satisfactory inflow to the femoral artery has been confirmed and distal bypass is judged essential, we prefer to use the long saphenous vein in a non-reversed configuration, ensuring that the widest and most proximal section of the vein is available for anastomosis to the common femoral arteriotomy. This may necessitate side-clamping the femoral vein in order to harvest the long saphenous vein flush with the common femoral vein, closing the resulting venotomy with a running suture. When a synchronous inflow procedure has been performed we employ a side-by-side technique for the junctional anastomosis, where the inflow graft and the proximal end of the distal bypass are anastomosed alongside one another on the common femoral arteriotomy. Any accessible valves in the proximal long saphenous vein should be incised with scissors before the proximal anastomosis is performed. On completion of the proximal anastomosis the femoral clamps are removed to restore flow into the profunda femoris. Palpating the pulsating proximal portion of the arterialised long saphenous vein provides some index of the quality of the inflow. Spontaneous thrombosis of this column of blood, which must remain stagnant until distal outflow is achieved, is rare and usually points to some thrombotic complication either proximally or in the vein itself.

It now remains to prepare the distal graft and the outflow artery prior to completion of the distal anastomosis; if two surgeons are collaborating these tasks can be undertaken synchronously. We no longer believe that it is important to leave the long saphenous vein undisturbed in its original bed, although every effort should be made to minimise its exposure to trauma and ischaemia. When, as is usually the case, the distal anastomosis is to lie below the knee joint, we mobilise the vein fully in order to re-route it through a deep anatomical tunnel, alongside the neurovascular bundle. In this position the graft is unlikely to be affected by cutaneous wound problems and should not be subject to abrupt angulation or tissue compression.

The artery selected for distal run-off is exposed, taking care to avoid damage to venous collaterals by the use of loupe magnification. Hopefully the artery will be disease free and compressible and if pricked gently with the point of a fine blade it will bleed briskly. When these ideals are knowingly compromised the surgeon should be satisfied that the artery selected is the best available. Occasionally, when arteriography and informed exploration fail to discover any artery capable of supporting a graft, an intraoperative

decision to abandon bypass in favour of primary amputation may have to be taken. Ideally such situations should be foreseen and the patient counselled and consented in advance. In general the prospect of salvaging the limb by bypass reconstruction should not be abandoned until the peroneal artery has been explored in the distal calf or the dorsalis pedis and lateral plantar arteries in the foot. When faced with a difficult intraoperative dilemma, the surgeon should keep in mind the basic principle that correction of critical ischaemia demands the restoration of pulsatile flow across two anatomical levels. Thus if the femoral pulse was palpable at the outset, the graft will have to cross the adductor hiatus and the popliteal trifurcation to perfuse a crural artery. If the popliteal pulse was still palpable, the bypass will have to cross the popliteal trifurcation and the malleolar anastomosis to reach a pedal artery.

Once the distal outflow site is selected, the vein graft can be cut to length and downflow established. When using the long saphenous in our favoured non-reversed configuration we proceed as follows: on completion of the proximal anastomosis a valvulotome (Hall, Cardial, Le Maitre, etc) is passed up the distal end of the vein to the femoral artery anastomosis and then withdrawn. Each time the valve cutter engages the valve cusp, its position on the skin is marked. When all valve cusps have been cut the vein graft is explored through short, discontinuous incisions at the sites of the valves. We have found that the majority of valve branches can be identified at these points and ligated. Following this a retrograde irrigation test or 'squirt' test is performed. The thumb and finger of the assistant occlude the vein graft through the incisions in the limb, and retrograde irrigation using heparinised Hartmann solution is carried out. If it is not possible to irrigate and the assistant feels transmitted pressure waves between the thumb and finger, it is assumed that no branches exist, and the assistant moves up to the next incision until the femoral anastomosis is reached.[14] We believe that the use of short, discontinuous incisions produces fewer wound complications, particularly in frail elderly patients with advanced ischaemia.

For crural and pedal anastomosis, haemostasis is best achieved with microvascular clamps or silastic slings and we have not found any advantage in the use of tourniquets. Usually 6-0 or 7-0 monofilament polypropylene material on an 8 mm curved atraumatic needle is suitable but 8-0 may be preferable for some delicate pedal anastomoses. Loupe magnification is desirable ($\times 2.5$ or $\times 3.5$) and a continuous suture line in a 'short parachute' configuration, commencing at the heel and completing in the middle of the second panel, is standard.

On release of the clamps some confirmation that graft flow is adequate and outflow resistance is low should be sought. Palpation of a distal pulse is reassuring, as is the detection below the anastomosis of a biphasic Doppler signal, with continuing flow in diastole. Graft flow in mL/min can be measured by various methods including electromagnetic flowmetry or controlled pressure infusion but the most widely used is the 'Op-Dop' ultrasound device (SciMed, Bristol, UK). If pressure in the bypass graft is measured using a cannula inserted through a side branch of the vein graft, peripheral resistance can be calculated. In grafts with a peripheral resistance of over 1.5 and flow rates below 80 mL/min, a bolus injection of 30 mg papaverine is given into the graft. If the flow and resistance do not improve, an angiogram is taken to determine the cause of this poor haemodynamic performance.

Alternatives to the long saphenous vein

In many patients the long saphenous vein will be found to be inadequate either in its entirety or over short segments, especially around the knee. In others the entire vein may be absent because of prior excision or grafting, in which case it is prudent to request duplex ultrasound scanning of the arms in advance. For short deficits, branches of long or short saphenous vein segments can be substituted. However, in order to avoid further incisions being made on the ischaemic limb we have a low threshold for utilising arm vein, which has been shown to yield results comparable with long saphenous vein grafts.[15] This may be harvested in a variety of configurations. The full length of the cephalic vein from wrist to shoulder will suffice for grafting to the proximal calf. Similar lengths can be obtained from the ulnar/basilic system or by figure of eight combinations of ulnar, cephalic and basilic vein linked by the antecubital vein. Another option is the upper arm loop, comprising cephalic, antecubital and basilic veins, although it should be remembered that in this configuration the valves are orientated in opposite directions in the two main sections of the graft.

In general, the more distal the arm vein the more robust is its wall but the more likely that it has been injured by previous cannulation. Although the proximal cephalic vein can seem alarmingly flimsy it usually improves in appearance with gentle dilatation and will withstand arterial pressures when implanted. The basilic vein in the medial upper arm is normally of good calibre but of limited length and in the interest of avoiding arm swelling is best not harvested proximal to its confluence with the axillary vein. In general there is minimal morbidity associated with arm vein harvest, with cutaneous neuropraxia and minor haematoma being the only problems we have experienced. Discontinuous skin incisions should be used over the elbow to avoid contractures. Harvest under local anaesthetic infiltration is acceptable and easily performed in patients undergoing neuraxial anaesthesia.

Veno-venous anastomoses may have to be constructed to obtain significant length. We have not found this to be a particular problem and it is not in our experience associated with an increased incidence of graft stenosis. The problem of the venous valves is little different from that encountered with the long saphenous except that with arm vein the calibre does not usually favour either a reversed or non-reversed configuration. In general we prefer to use the non-reversed configuration. The proximal anastomosis is performed first and the valves lysed with a valvulotome as usual so that the graft can be tunnelled while pulsating in order to reduce the risk of kinks, twists and compression. If using the reversed configuration we prefer to perform the distal anastomosis first in order to discourage the formation of intraluminal thrombus. In the event of graft occlusion, however, the residual valves tend to complicate thromboembolectomy procedures.

> ## Alternatives to ipsilateral long saphenous vein
>
> - Branches of long saphenous vein
> - Short saphenous vein
> - Arm vein – cephalic, ulnar/basilic, antecubital, figure of eight combinations of above, upper arm loop
> - Contralateral long saphenous vein

Arm vein is our first alternative to the ipsilateral long saphenous vein, the contralateral long saphenous vein is our second. The reasons for this order of priority are that donor site complications are more frequent and severe in the leg than in the arm and that there is a definite risk that the contralateral leg may develop occlusive disease in the future, requiring the vein for grafting.

If it proves impossible to obtain sufficient vein from any source to construct a femorodistal graft, other options may be considered. Grafts should never be made longer than necessary and if the femoropopliteal segment is patent then it should be used as the inflow site for the graft. Sometimes percutaneous angioplasty, either transluminal or subintimal, will recanalise the femoropopliteal sufficiently to support a popliteal to distal bypass. Similarly we have had occasional success with restoring popliteal inflow by semi-closed superficial femoral endarterectomy, using ring cutters to dissect and remove the core of atheroma. Unfortunately, as with angioplasty, there is a strong tendency towards restenosis. We have found it more reliable in this situation to use a thin-walled polytetrafluoroethylene (PTFE) graft, either 6 mm or 8 mm diameter, as a bypass from the common femoral to the above-knee popliteal artery. Ideally there should be angiographic evidence of an isolated patent popliteal segment but we have found when this is not the case that local endarterectomy can restore sufficient lumen to receive an anastomosis and may reopen previously occluded geniculate collaterals.[16] A vein jump graft is then taken from a composite anastomosis alongside the PTFE graft on the popliteal artery to the distal run-off

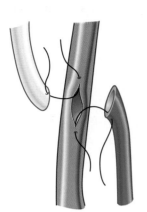
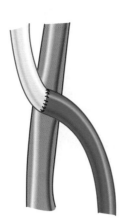
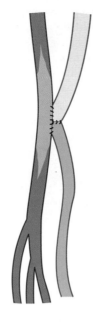

Figure 15.7 *Diagram illustrating composite sequential anastomosis: polytetrafluoroethylene (PTFE) bypass to blind popliteal segment with vein bypass to distal crural vessel; this technique can be used when there is insufficient vein for full length of bypass*

vessel, utilising a deep anatomical tunnel to traverse the knee joint. This technique of composite sequential grafting (Fig. 15.7) significantly reduces the amount of vein required and has provided results that are comparable with those of primary long saphenous vein bypass. We endorse the widely held consensus that regards prosthetic bypass to distal arteries as a last resort, with or without the addition of venous cuffs for the distal anastomosis. However, although patency rates for such grafts are consistently low, late failure, after healing of ischaemic lesions has taken place, may not necessarily precipitate recurrence of critical ischaemia. Thus each case must be considered individually.

Multiple outflow techniques

The aim of distal reconstruction is to achieve durable restoration of pulsatile flow to a healthy artery in the leg or foot which, through its direct or anastomotic communications, is capable of perfusing all previously ischaemic areas. In practice, this is usually an artery with direct access to the pedal arch. There are, however, a number of cases where identification of such an artery is not obvious. There may be two patent calf arteries below an occluded popliteal which appear to share equal access to the pedal arch, or an isolated popliteal segment may appear to be a more obvious recipient for a distal graft than a distal calf vessel, which seems to perfuse little more than the foot. In such cases it is possible to consider constructing a graft with two outflows, either in a bifurcated configuration (Fig 15.8a) or by utilising a single trunk with sequential anastomoses at two levels, the first side to side and the second end to side (Fig. 15.8b). We have taken an interest in bifurcated and sequential grafts over a number of years and have attempted to derive relevant data on flow and resistance where possible.

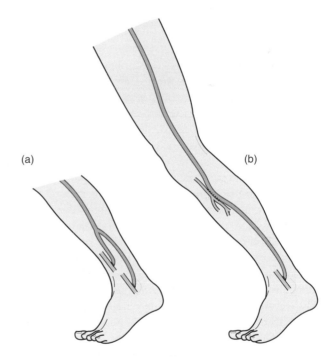

Figure 15.8 *Alternative configurations for multiple outflow in distal bypass: (a) bifurcated tibial outflow and (b) sequential popliteal-tibial outflow*

All that can be said as a consequence is that a second outflow will increase flow in the graft trunk by an average of 30–40 per cent and that there appears to be no increase in morbidity associated with the exercise (which is only undertaken when conditions are favourable). The fact that long term patency in this group appears better than would be expected with grafts having single artery outflow may be attributed to the fact that limbs with greater options for graft outflow constitute an intrinsically privileged subset.

Distal revascularisation procedures

- Staged *in situ* femorodistal bypass, preferably unreversed (valvulotomy) vein to popliteal (isolated?)/crural/pedal artery
- Femoral endarterectomy/percutaneous angiography (transluminal or subintimal) + popliteal-distal bypass
- PTFE femoropopliteal bypass ± popliteal endarterectomy
- Composite femorodistal bypass: PTFE to popliteal + vein jump graft to distal artery
- PTFE femoral/popliteal bypass to distal artery + vein cuff
- Multiple outflow bypass – dual bifurcated configuration/single sequential to distal arteries

SPECIFIC TECHNIQUES

Graft routing

We have already mentioned our preference for routing vein grafts across the knee in a deep anatomical tunnel alongside the popliteal neurovascular bundle, in the interests of avoiding kinking and compression and the potential consequences of wound failure. In distal bypass surgery, about 40 per cent of grafts are anastomosed to the anterior tibial or dorsalis pedis arteries and so have to cross from the popliteal fossa to the anterior tibial compartment. We prefer to make this tunnel through the upper third of the interosseous membrane, close to the route of the anterior tibial artery itself, running the vein graft distally alongside the anterior tibial vessels. A long curved clamp such as a Crafoord aortic clamp is suitable for this purpose but is too rigid to cross the ankle joint and pass under the extensor retinaculum into the foot. When bypassing to the dorsalis pedis we use a flexible tunnelling device such as the non-barbed head of the Cardial valvulotome or a stiffened balloon embolectomy catheter. This can be either used to pull down the graft directly or used to place a ligature with which the graft can be pulled through.

It is occasionally necessary to undertake a re-do bypass from the common femoral to the proximal anterior tibial artery using a free vein graft. For this purpose a lateral subcutaneous tunnel is more direct and avoids scarred tissue planes but it is important to cross the knee in the line of the lateral ligament in order to avoid traction during joint movement.

Microtibial embolectomy[9]

Occlusion of the arteries of the ankle and foot by thromboembolic material is a justifiably feared manifestation of acute lower limb ischaemia. It may be detected angiographically, sometimes as a complication of angioplasty or thrombolysis and is sometimes seen as a result of embolisation from aneurysms of the aorta or of the femoral or popliteal arteries. The term 'trash foot' implies distal microembolisation developing during aortic reconstructive procedures. The condition may also develop as a consequence of coagulopathy associated with malignancy or certain types of bacteraemia. The foot is observed to be persistently cold, blotchy and cyanotic despite the presence of an apparently satisfactory popliteal pulse. In these circumstances neither transpopliteal embolectomy nor systemic anticoagulation is effective and limb salvage depends on physical removal of the thrombotic material from the pedal arch. The anterior and posterior tibial arteries are exposed just above the ankle joint using local infiltration anaesthesia and proximal and distal embolectomy is performed through small transverse arteriotomies using a 2 Fr balloon catheter. It is necessary to partially deflate the balloon just prior to its emergence to avoid splitting the arteriotomy. Closure of the arteriotomies with interrupted 8-0 suture material avoids stenosis without recourse to patching. The liberal use of heparinised flushing solutions and of topical antispasmodics such as papaverine helps to prevent rethrombosis. Good results can be achieved when the cause of ischaemia is embolic but patients with spontaneous intravascular thrombosis secondary to malignancy or infection tend to do badly.

Fasciotomy

Successful revascularisation of the severely ischaemic limb will result inevitably in some degree of reactive tissue swelling. Influential variables, apart from the severity and duration of ischaemia, include the state of venous drainage, the position of the limb, the extent of operative trauma and blood loss and the presence of infection. Increases in tissue compartment pressure above 20 mmHg are abnormal, and above 40 mm Hg fasciotomy is mandatory. When calf muscles are found to be paralysed and tender prior to revascularisation, the likelihood of compartment syndrome developing is such as to justify prophylactic fasciotomy. In all other cases it is important to keep a careful watch on the limb in the first 12 hours after revascularisation. Swelling and induration of the calf muscles combined with the elicitation of calf muscle pain on passive stretching constitute grounds for intervention. Compartment pressure can be measured quickly at the bedside using very simple equipment if electronic manometry is not available (Fig. 15.9).

Although semiclosed fasciotomy can be used as a prophylactic measure, the correct treatment for elevated compartment pressure is open fasciotomy (Fig. 15.10), which will require a regional or general anaesthetic. In the recently operated calf the location of existing incisions may

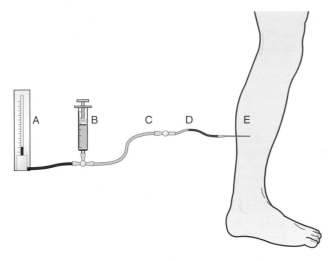

Figure 15.9 *A simple technique for measurement of compartment pressure: with all taps open the syringe is compressed slowly; the sphygmomanometer reading at the moment the meniscus of dyed saline moves towards the muscle is the compartment pressure. A, sphygmomanometer; B, air-filled syringe and three-way tap; C, drip tube and thumb clamp; D, dyed saline meniscus; E, no. 1 needle in muscle*

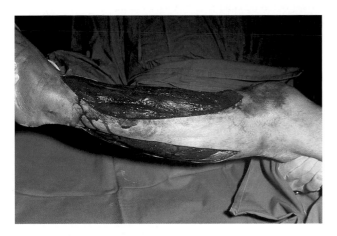

Figure 15.10 *Open fasciotomy*

influence the surgical approach. However in most cases a single lateral incision will decompress all four musculofascial compartments with minimal morbidity. With this approach the fascia between the peroneal muscles is incised to expose the full length of the fibula, taking care to protect the lateral popliteal nerve proximally. There is no need to excise the fibula, and the peroneal vessels which lie medially should not be exposed. Using scissor dissection, all tense fascial coverings over the anterior and posterior compartments are then split longitudinally until all muscle bundles are soft and bulging. This single lateral approach is simple and effective, incurs minimal morbidity and is

unlikely to expose vascular grafts. In addition it lends itself to delayed primary closure by means of a running polypropylene subcuticular suture, which serves initially to prevent excessive skin retraction and can then be closed by simple traction under analgesia once swelling has reduced sufficiently, usually in 4–5 days.

Reintervention

Early graft failure may be attributable to inappropriate operative strategy, technical error or systemic factors such as hypotension or hypercoagulability. Success in reintervention depends upon the cause of failure being identified, which in turn requires observation, deduction and experience. The correction of technical problems such as retained valve cusps, graft twists and residual intraluminal thrombus can often be undertaken under local anaesthesia with minimal morbidity and excellent outcome. More complex revisions and repeated failures call for careful risk/benefit review.

Wound management

Wounds should be planned to minimise trauma and ischaemia and should be closed in a way that will protect underlying structures, avoid fluid collections and promote tissue viability. Closed suction drainage is useful in selected cases. We favour discontinuous incisions for vein harvesting and find that in very obese patients the groin incision is best made along the skin crease. Closure of the groin wound in layers including a subcuticular skin stitch, using absorbable synthetic material throughout, has given the best results in our experience. In the thigh and proximal calf we leave fascia open and again use buried absorbable synthetics for the fat and skin. In the distal calf the absence of fat and the uncertain vascularity favours the use of interrupted monofilament material, the finer the better.

Because of the poor viability of the skin of the distal calf in patients with lower limb ischaemia we try to minimise dissection in this area. In popliteal to pedal bypass, the proximal portion of the long saphenous vein should be harvested and the vein transposed distally, rather than using a strict *in situ* technique. In some cases, arm vein segments can be used in preference to local vein. When parallel skin incisions in the lower leg are necessary, the incision overlying the graft and distal anastomosis should be closed and the other left to be covered with split skin.

Amputations

It is a general principle of vascular surgical management that prior to reconstruction, infection should be controlled by debridement and appropriate antibiotic therapy (see Chapters 18 and 33). Following reconstruction, definitive amputation should ideally be delayed until demarcation is established and the operative wounds have healed. In the context of acute or severe ischaemia, with imminent, progressive or established gangrene these principles may have to be adapted but they should not be ignored. Clearly, the priority is to restore arterial perfusion and prevent or halt ischaemic necrosis. Once this is achieved, however, steps must be taken to control infection and if this requires drainage of pus and/or excision of necrotic tissue then this should be undertaken at the time of reconstruction. It will hardly ever be appropriate to attempt primary closure after this type of surgery and the patient should be made aware of the possible need for further excision or amputation once demarcation is established.

Sadly, amputation remains a possible outcome after emergency surgery for severe lower limb ischaemia. Evidence that failed attempts at vascular reconstruction prejudice the level of subsequent amputation is contested. However, as far as is possible, incisions for infrainguinal reconstructive procedures should be placed so as to minimise interference with a potential below-knee amputation.

POSTOPERATIVE MANAGEMENT

We do not routinely anticoagulate these patients, who are often elderly and in whom the risk of anticoagulation may exceed any theoretical benefit. Unless contraindicated, they all receive 75 mg aspirin daily. Patients are followed up in the surveillance programme with duplex scanning of the graft at 6 weeks and then subsequently at 3-monthly intervals. Any patient who has a stenosis discovered in their graft with a more than 50 per cent velocity shift over 1 cm is referred for balloon angioplasty or, if this proves ineffective or of transient benefit, for patch angioplasty. Patients who are found to have failing grafts due to distal anastomotic stenosis or progression of disease in the native artery are treated with jump grafts. We have found percutaneous balloon angioplasty of some of the long grafts particularly difficult owing to the long length of catheter needed. In these patients the vein graft can be dissected and controlled proximal to the stenosis under local anaesthetic and an on-table balloon angioplasty carried out.

RESULTS

We adopted the above principles for the management of acute ischaemia of the lower limb over a 4-year period in two acute care hospitals. During that time 126 limbs were considered for surgical intervention. Fourteen patients were either too moribund for intervention or required primary amputation. Of the rest 42 were treated with embolectomy,

with a mortality rate of 28.6 per cent and a 30-day limb salvage/survival of 62 per cent. The remainder required surgical bypass, 22 per cent an inflow procedure, but the majority an infrainguinal reconstruction. The 30-day mortality rate for surgical bypass was 19.6 per cent and the overall limb salvage/survival rate 52 per cent.

Conclusions

The management of the acutely ischaemic leg remains a major challenge to the vascular surgeon. The key lies in good preintervention diagnostic information, which allows treatment to be undertaken with a reasonable expectation of a good outcome. In many cases this can be achieved by thrombolytic therapy or simple balloon embolectomy. In those patients in whom an advanced degree of ischaemia precludes thrombolysis, however, or in those patients with atheromatous vascular disease that makes embolectomy inappropriate, urgent surgical bypass will have to be undertaken. A number of simple manoeuvres can be performed which will aid the surgeon in undertaking these difficult procedures. Such techniques can produce acceptable limb salvage and survival in this challenging group of patients.

Key references

Hickey NC, Thomson IA, Shearman CP, Simms MH. Aggressive arterial reconstruction for critical lower limb ischaemia. *Br J Surg* 1991; **78**: 1476–8.

Mahmood A, Garnham A, Sintler M, *et al.* Composite sequential grafts for femorocrural bypass reconstruction: experience with a modified technique. *J Vasc Surg* 2002; **36**: 772–8.

McKay C, Razik WA, Simms MH. Local anaesthetic for lower limb revascularisation in high risk patients. *Br J Surg* 1997; **84**: 1096–8.

Second European consensus document on chronic critical leg ischaemia. *Eur J Vasc Surg* 1992: 6(A).

Shearman CP, Gwynn BR, Curran FT, *et al.* Non-invasive femoro-popliteal assessment: is that angiogram really necessary? *BMJ* 1986; **293**: 1086–9.

REFERENCES

1   Dormandy J (ed). *European Working Group on Critical Limb Ischaemia. European Consensus Document on Critical Limb Ischaemia.* Berlin: Springer Verlag, 1989.

2   Hickey NC, Thomson IA, Shearman CP, Simms MH. Aggressive arterial reconstruction for critical lower limb ischaemia. *Br J Surg* 1991; **78**: 1476–8.

3 Shearman CP, Ashley EMC, Gwynn BR, Simms MH. Rehabilitation of patients after vascular reconstruction for critical lower limb ischaemia. *Br J Surg* 1991; **77**: A346.

4 Cheshire NJ, Wolfe JHN, Noone MA, *et al*. The economics of femorocrural reconstruction for critical leg ischaemia with and without autologous vein. *J Vasc Surg* 1992; **15**: 167–75.

5 Second European consensus document on chronic critical leg ischaemia. *Eur J Vasc Surg* 1992: 6(A).

6 Fiorani P, Taurino M, Novelli G, *et al*. Acute occlusion of the lower limbs. In: Greenhalgh RM, Hollier LH (eds). *Emergency vascular surgery*. London: WB Saunders, 1992: 387–99.

7 Hight DW, Tilney NL, Couch NP. Changing clinical trends in patients with peripheral arterial emboli. *Surgery* 1976; **79**: 172–6.

8 Jivegard LE, Arfivdisson B, Holm J, Schersten T. Selective conservative and routine early operative treatment in acute lower limb ischaemia. *Br J Surg* 1987; **74**: 263–71.

9 Faris IB, Duncan HJ. The assessment of critical skin ischaemia. In: Greenhalgh RM, Jamieson CW, Nicolaides AN (eds). *Vascular Surgery: Issues in Current Practice*. London: Grune and Stratton, 1986: 91–6.

10 Smith FCT, Shearman CP, Simms MH, Gwynn BR. Falsely elevated ankle pressures in severe leg ischaemia: the pole test, an alternative approach. *Eur J Vasc Surg* 1994; **8**: 408–12.

11 Shearman CP, Gwynn BR, Curran FT, *et al*. Non-invasive femoro-popliteal assessment: is that angiogram really necessary? *BMJ* 1986; **293**: 1086–9.

12 McKay C, Razik WA, Simms MH. Local anaesthetic for lower limb revascularisation in high risk patients. *Br J Surg* 1997; **84**: 1096–8.

13 Mahmood A, Hardy R, Garnham A, *et al*. Microtibial embolectomy. *Eur J Vasc Endovasc Surg* 2003; **25**: 35–9.

14 Shearman CP, Gannon MX, Gwynn BR, Simms MH. A clinical method for the detection of arteriovenous fistulas during *in situ* great saphenous vein bypass. *J Vasc Surg* 1986; **4**: 578–81.

15 Andros G, Harris RW, Salles-Cunha SX. Arm veins for arterial revascularisation of the leg: arteriographic and clinical observations. *J Vasc Surg* 1986; **4**: 416.

16 Mahmood A, Garnham A, Sintler M, *et al*. Composite sequential grafts for femorocrural bypass reconstruction: experience with a modified technique. *J Vasc Surg* 2002; **36**: 772–8.

16

Acute Limb Ischaemia: Endovascular Options

BERNARD H NACHBUR, IRIS BAUMGARTNER, DO D DO, FELIX MAHLER, HANS–BEAT RIS

THE PROBLEM

Acute lower limb ischaemia poses a threat to both limb and life. Ischaemia of the upper limb is less frequent, and in the normal course of events more dangerous when associated with vascular trauma of the shoulder region than when caused by thromboembolic occlusion. Embolic occlusions of the axillary artery or around the elbow at the bifurcation of the cubital artery do not occur infrequently as a result of atrial fibrillation. The occluded native artery is practically always normal and surgical removal is so easy that endovascular options are unnecessary, disadvantageous and in fact impractical. This chapter will deal with the endovascular treatment options for ischaemia of the lower limb.

Acute ischaemia is by definition a sudden event which can therefore be timed quite exactly, most particularly so in the case of embolism into a previously normal arterial tree. Such emboli usually originate in the heart as a consequence of atrial fibrillation or mural thrombosis following myocardial infarction. They might occasionally originate from aortic ulcers or aneurysms, popliteal aneurysms being the most frequent source of arterio-arterial embolism. Mural thrombi from subclavian arteries exposed to repeated compression at the thoracic outlet produce similar effects (see Chapter 41).

Emboli have a certain given diameter and are swept distally to a point where the calibre of the vasculature prevents further migration. This is why embolic clots are usually found at the level of arterial bifurcations where they can be readily located either clinically, radiologically or by duplex ultrasonography. It is important to realise that they can also split into two or more fragments at a bifurcation and thus occlude more than just one artery. Therefore radiological visualisation is mandatory for the exact assessment of sites of occlusion. Figure 16.1 illustrates an example of such multiple splitting of an embolus. It shows the angiogram of a 17-year-old who collapsed on her way to school because of sudden paralysis of the lower limbs. The multiple occlusions of the iliac, femoral and distal vessels causing sudden muscular weakness had originated from a large myxoma of the left atrium and were removed surgically, followed by open heart surgery for removal of the myxoma. This emphasises the importance of harvesting material for histopathological examination.

More than 50 per cent of cases with acute lower limb ischaemia are probably not of embolic origin neither are they restricted to arterial bifurcations; they are caused by *in situ* thrombosis of a pre-existing atherosclerotic plaque, so-called acute-on-chronic ischaemia.[1] The arrest of arterial perfusion in the residual artery leads to propagation of thrombus distal to the occluding site. Angiographically, the difference between embolic occlusion and *in situ* thrombosis can be difficult but is possible in most cases. Duplex sonography can also be of help if the quality of the arterial wall can be defined. This is relevant because embolic occlusions at the level of the aortic, iliac or femoral bifurcation can readily be treated by a general surgeon who has sufficient

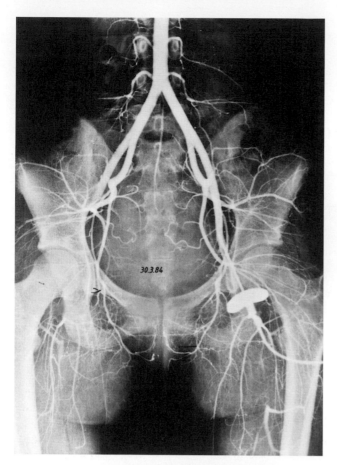

30.3.84

Figure 16.1   *A 17-year-old patient with multiple bilateral embolic occlusions of the external iliac and common femoral arteries and their branches*

Table. 16.1   *Predictive power of factors in favour of embolism versus thrombosis*

Factor	Predictive power
	+1 (embolism)
Atrial fibrillation/acute myocardial infarction	0.82
Duration of symptoms*	0.56
Age†	0.51
Diabetes	0.27
Systemic malignancy	−0.20
	−1 (thrombosis)

*The shorter the duration of symptoms, the greater the likelihood of embolism.
† The older the patient, the greater the likelihood of thrombosis.
Reproduced with permission from Goldstone J (ed). *Perspectives in vascular surgery*. Vol. 2. St Louis, MO: Quality Medical Publishing, 1989: 11–17.

knowledge, a special interest in vascular surgery and is conversant with modern techniques.[2] On the other hand, surgical thrombectomy in patients with acute-on-chronic occlusive disease can be hazardous and may actually worsen the degree of ischaemia if not dealt with optimally by an experienced vascular surgeon who has access to endovascular options and can call upon the support of ancillary investigators. The potential of these endovascular options has been subject to significant evolution in the past few years as a consequence of the discrete and diminishing role played by thrombolysis in the treatment of acute ischaemia. The examination of that potential is the objective of this chapter.

DIAGNOSIS

Some of the major factors and their discriminating power in the diagnosis of embolism and thrombosis are outlined in Table 16.1.[3] The degree of ischaemia in acute-on-chronic occlusive disease is usually less severe than in patients with sudden complete occlusion because of the

presence of pre-existing collaterals. A clear distinction between embolic occlusion and *in situ* thrombosis, or acute-on-chronic occlusive disease, cannot be made with sufficient reliability on clinical grounds alone; neither is the objective documentation of ischaemia using such investigations as Doppler ultrasound measurements or even duplex sonography decisive.

Imaging of the arterial tree is therefore of cardinal importance and for which, today, there are no contra-indications. The nephrotoxic effect of angiography with conventional contrast medium can be avoided by contrast-enhanced magnetic resonance imaging (MRI) using low osmolar gadolinium *as a viable alternative contrast agent* for angiographic investigation. Moreover, the *reduction in renal function* induced by radiographic contrast agents such as iopromide, a non-ionic, low osmolality contrast agent, can *now also be offset* by the prophylactic administration of the antioxidant acetylcysteine, along with hydration, in patients with chronic renal insufficiency.[4] Knowledge of the exact location of the occlusion as well as the extent of thrombosis will influence the tactical approach. It is relevant to note that in a prospective controlled study the serum creatinine concentration *decreased* significantly in the acetylcysteine group.[5] This is but one of the major recent developments. For practical purposes digital subtraction angiography (DSA) is the diagnostic test of choice and is a *prerequisite in the management of acute ischaemia*. It is also an indispensable method of *forewarning* the surgeon or physician in charge of the coexistence of chronic occlusive disease before surgical, lytic or other endovascular options are decided upon.

The non-opacification of peripheral run-off in an intra-arterial digital subtraction angiogram, however, can often be misleading. It has been shown that by applying pulse generated run-off techniques,[5] a significantly better functional picture can be obtained compared with conventional intra-arterial DSA alone. This can also be demonstrated by intraoperative angiography after exposure of the infragenicular popliteal artery. Non-opacification of the calf vessels by intra-arterial femoral DSA therefore does not preclude reconstructive procedures, be they surgical or endovascular. Endovascular techniques can be applied to the crural arteries intraoperatively following surgical exposure of a distal segment of the popliteal artery.[6–9]

Previous teaching has emphasised run-off as a significant discriminator between success and failure of reconstructive procedures in both acute and subacute occlusions.[10] The fallacy of this contention has been convincingly demonstrated by Do *et al.*[11] who point out both the advantages provided by pulse generated examination and intraoperative angiography of the peripheral arterial tree, and also the immense potential of intraoperative or catheter intraclot lysis.

SELECTION FOR TREATMENT[12]

The patient may present with a paralysed anaesthetic limb and the first signs of cutaneous mottling with, in a worst case scenario, rigor mortis. Further delay cannot be tolerated and immediate and decisive treatment is mandatory if amputation is to be avoided. When the condition is this serious there is no time for preoperative angiography. The situation might call for surgical intervention, but combined endovascular catheter treatment can now be considered to have equal potential. In general, however, it is the patient with acute-on-chronic occlusive disease who benefits most from endovascular treatment options. In some patients the collateral circulation opens up after initial treatment with analgesics and heparin and may even regain normal use of the extremity with little or no sign of anaesthesia. Indeed, pain may subside so as to justify a certain deferment of invasive action. Such an improvement allows time for decisions as to whether to treat with anticoagulants alone or to pursue either the surgical or endovascular option in a more leisurely fashion. Because of the need for ancillary diagnostic and therapeutic options (see Chapter 15), it is self-evident that treatment of acute-on-subacute ischaemia with impending gangrene should not be the business of a general surgeon with casual experience in the treatment of acute vascular occlusion. Referral to a specialist vascular unit, if that is possible, is important.[12]

DANGERS OF REVERSING ISCHAEMIA[13]

As with surgery it is important to identify those patients in whom reversal is contraindicated and life threatening. Thus on occasions the attending physician, who should be a vascular surgeon, will be confronted with an extremity in which acute and total ischaemia has led to a situation which is aptly described by the French expression of *ischémie dépassée*. The clinical picture is characterised by the grotesque mottled appearance of the skin of the involved extremity, total loss of sensitivity and motility of the foot and incipient or even well-developed rigor mortis of the muscles. Rigor mortis of the calf is easily diagnosed by examining passive motility of the toes and foot. If the knee joint has stiffened, occlusion has probably occurred at the level of the iliac arteries.

In this situation the ischaemic damage done to soft tissue is so extensive *that any attempts at revascularisation might endanger the life of the patient, whether the limb can be salvaged or not.* Following successful disobliteration in such patients, it is not unusual for them to die within a few hours, death usually being attributable to reperfusion injury (see Chapters 2 and 4). It is important to understand that, just as with surgical revascularisation, concepts such as rhabdomyolysis[11] and its associated metabolic disturbances, such as hyperkalaemia,[12,13] the closed compartment syndrome elevated serum phosphokinase, uraemia, hyperphosphataemia, hypocalcaemia and hypercalcaemia in association with anuria become critical parameters.[14] Indeed, because combined endovascular treatment options are so successful in the smaller arteries, such changes are likely to be more marked and acute. The *danger of revascularisation* must therefore be assessed by taking biochemical and individual clinical factors, such as renal insufficiency, into account.

WHAT IS *NEW* ABOUT ENDOVASCULAR OPTIONS FOR ACUTE LIMB ISCHAEMIA?

Percutaneous, catheter directed low dose infusion of thrombolytic agents has been used for many years since its introduction by Hans Hess *et al.* in 1982,[15] and has found widespread use as an alternative to open surgery for treatment of acute arterial occlusion of the legs.[16–26] The safety and efficacy of the procedure, however, continues to give rise to concern. For example, in the Thrombolysis Or Peripheral Artery Surgery (TOPAS) trial,[26] the latest most authoritarian prospective study comparing catheter directed thrombolysis with open surgery, serious bleeding problems as well as intracranial haemorrhage were associated with local thrombolysis requiring a considerable number of blood transfusions. Furthermore, in other studies reported hitherto, blood flow was restored more slowly than by immediate surgical revascularisation. Therefore, for endovascular techniques to be as efficient as the surgical treatment of acute limb-threatening ischaemia, the ideal catheter directed method must reduce haemorrhage and, if possible, reduce the time necessary for restoring arterial flow comparable to the duration of a surgical procedure. Ideally, catheter directed restoration of patency should be achieved within

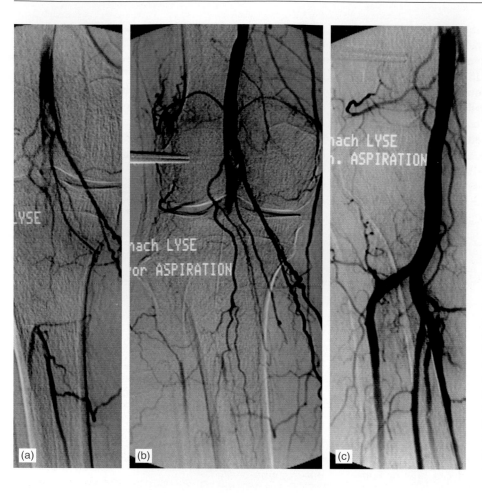

Figure 16.2 *Illustration of the efficacy of thrombus aspiration. (a) this patient had acute occlusion of the popliteal trifurcation with motor and sensory deficit of 20 hours duration. (b) following an intraclot instillation of 60 000 units of urokinase for 20 minutes there was only minor clot dissolution without clinical improvement. (c) following percutaneous catheter thrombus aspiration complete restoration of patency was achieved within 15 minutes*

the same time span as an open surgical procedure. That this is a viable option will be shown later in this chapter.

In the TOPAS trial reported by Ouriel *et al.* in 1998[26] it was shown that intra-arterial infusion of urokinase reduced the need for open surgical procedures with no significantly increased risk of amputation or death. Intra-arterial thrombolysis, however, was associated with a significantly higher number of major haemorrhages (12.5 per cent) than the surgery group (5.5 per cent; P = 0.005) and in both groups the amputation rate was surprisingly high. Moreover, of particular concern in the TOPAS study, are the four episodes of intracranial haemorrhage in the urokinase group (1.6 per cent), one of which was fatal. The development of these bleeding complications has been criticised by Porter.[27] In the surgical group there were, as expected, no episodes of intracranial haemorrhage. Therefore, although intra-arterial infusion of urokinase has significantly reduced the need for open surgical procedures, the safety of catheter thrombolysis necessitating the use of large amount of lytic agents has remained an awesome and serious threat to the patient. Furthermore, in the studies reported hitherto in the literature, blood flow was restored more slowly than by immediate surgical revascularisation, and tissue ischaemia may progress to necrosis before thrombolysis has taken effect; this is another reason for the reluctance to

accept catheter directed procedures, especially in the treatment of acute limb ischaemia.

It is now well established, however, that percutaneous catheter thrombus *extraction* can work, and by itself is capable of restoring patency following acute thrombotic or thromboembolic occlusion of the arteries of the leg.[28,29] The advantages and the potential which this regimen offers in terms of the significant reduction in the dosage of lytic agent used and in the duration of the procedure in restoring flow remains to be fully recognised. The important place of thrombus aspiration, in fact its superiority over lytic therapy alone, was recognised a number of years ago and is illustrated in Fig. 16.2.

It is the aim of this chapter, illustrated by a retrospective study, to demonstrate and to prove that by performing combined endovascular therapy either by percutaneous catheter aspiration alone or in association with thrombolysis and percutaneous transluminal angioplasty (PTA), high rates of primary success and limb preservation can be achieved both for acute and subacute ischaemia. In a majority of cases thrombus aspiration alone works and thrombolysis can be avoided altogether or reduced to harmless levels. Where necessary, thrombus infiltration with small doses of urokinase can loosen the thrombus and allow continuation of thrombus aspiration. In our study[30] in only one out of five cases was it necessary to apply a modest dose of intraclot urokinase. Thus the doses of urokinase are minimised and the duration of the intervention shortened substantially. If a culprit plaque is unmasked in the course of the intervention it can be treated by PTA. On balance then, the benefits of percutaneous catheter therapy should prevail over open surgical procedures. In fact amputation-free survival rates at 6 and 12 months are comparable to or better than those of open surgical procedures reported in the TOPAS trial and at no extra cost or risk of serious haemorrhage, death or secondary intervention.

In summary, the new achievements of endovascular treatment options areas follows:

1   By combining percutaneous clot aspiration with modest doses of thrombolytic agent only when necessary, and PTA of underlying stenotic plaques when unmasked, endovascular treatment can be shortened to periods of 35–160 minutes – comparable to the customary time spent in surgical interventions. This is achieved without serious bleeding risks and transfusions. For our unit endovascular options have become a valid and preferable option in managing cases of acute limb ischaemia including those with associated sensory and motor deficit.

2   Endovascular treatment implies repeated injection of small amounts of contrast medium. This can be hazardous in patients with chronic renal insufficiency. With prophylactic oral administration of the antioxidant acetylcysteine or the use of low osmolar gadodiamide for diagnostic and angiographic interventions, along with hydration, a fall in renal function induced by contrast medium can be offset entirely[4,5] and in patients with chronic renal insufficiency serum creatinine levels even improve.

During our preliminary experience we were impressed by the fact that with a minimal dose of lytic agent followed by percutaneous clot extraction, complete restoration of patency of an occluded popliteal trifurcation can be achieved within an hour (Fig. 16.2). With the passage of time and experience we eliminated the use of preliminary thrombolytic agents entirely and performed clot aspiration alone. In only one out of five cases was it necessary to apply small but safe doses of urokinase in order to loosen up residual clot and facilitate complete aspiration. In the presence of an underlying stenotic plaque identified as the cause of thrombotic or thromboembolic occlusion conventional PTA is performed immediately.

Given this experience it is our contention that the combined catheter approach as outlined above can be recommended as first line treatment for the group of patients with acute or subacute occlusions in infrainguinal arteries. The intervention proposed allows for clot aspiration, mild thrombolysis and PTA as an 'all-in-one' procedure and is performed under local anaesthesia. Only a minority of cases (20 per cent) will need modest amounts of lytic agent to obtain vascular patency. Hospital time is reduced and patient comfort considerably enhanced.

TECHNIQUE OF COMBINED ENDOVASCULAR CATHETER THERAPY[30]

Direct anterograde catheterisation of the common femoral artery is performed under local anaesthesia. Applying the Seldinger technique a 6–8 Fr sheath with a haemostatic valve and a side-port for flushing is introduced and a bolus of 5000 units of heparin is injected. In the presence of fresh thromboembolic material a thin walled 6–8 Fr catheter with an end-hole is positioned very closely to or barely into the proximal end of the thrombus, whereupon the clot is sucked and extracted with a 60 mL syringe. For extraction of larger pieces of clot, the haemostatic valve has to be removed. By repeated suction all the non-adherent material is removed, while residual thrombotic material adhering to the vessel wall is loosened with a wire loop[30] and subsequently also sucked away. In the crural arteries a 5 Fr aspiration catheter is used.

Should complete removal of the clot prove completely impossible, then local catheter thrombolysis is performed at the same session. To achieve that end a 0.035 inch (0.9 mm) guidewire is used to introduce a microporous balloon catheter down into the proximal part of the thrombus taking care not to pass beyond the clot so as to avoid peripheral embolism. Through the balloon catheter 10 000–20 000 units/cm of urokinase is infiltrated into the thrombus. Under fluoroscopic supervision the balloon catheter is advanced centimetre by centimetre until the distal end of the thrombus is reached. Clot material loosened by partial lysis is removed by repeated suction (Fig. 16.3). Angiography is performed at this time to confirm free peripheral outflow and underlying stenotic lesions are treated by PTA at the same session in keeping with the 'all-in-one' principle. Completion angiography is performed before removal of all instruments. The duration of the intervention and the total dose of the lytic agent are recorded.

VALIDATION OF THE COMBINED ENDOVASCULAR CATHETER TECHNIQUE[30]

Patient selection and immediate results

In the single centre study[30] performed by us between January 1995 and May 1997 there were 89 consecutive patients (42 men and 47 women; mean age 70.7 ± 14.9 years, range 29–100), 93 legs with acute or subacute thromboembolic occlusion of native femoropopliteal and crural arteries meeting the guidelines for reversible limb-threatening ischaemia. The indication and rationale for

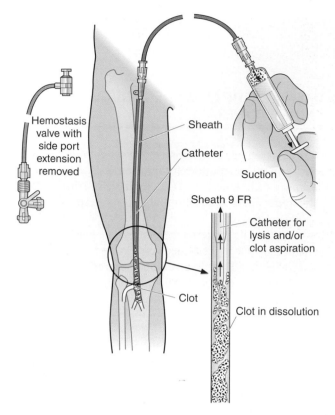

Figure 16.3 *The principle of clot extraction. The haemostatic valve with the side port extension (for heparinisation) has been removed and the radio-opaque sheath 8 or 9 Fr is left in place to protect the vessel wall from injury due to catheter manipulation. The catheter used for extraction is advanced into the clot which, in one out of five cases, has to be loosened up with modest doses of urokinase. The clots are readily aspirated. The wider the sheath, the larger the clots which can be extracted but by the same token the danger of intimal damage increases*

catheter therapy was critical ischaemia in all 69 patients presenting with rest pain and a further 20 patients with trophic lesions. The therapeutic decision was reached jointly by the vascular surgeon and the interventional angiologist. Percutaneous catheter directed treatment was restricted strictly to infrainguinal native arteries. Patients with occlusions of upper limb arteries, iliac arteries, the femoral bifurcation or bypass grafts were treated by open surgery. In the entire group of 89 patients with 93 treated legs, the minimum observation time was 12 months for all cases, but three patients were lost to follow-up after initial catheter therapy.

Catheter therapy had to be performed urgently on the same day or within 24 hours of onset of symptoms in 33 cases (37.5 per cent), whereas in 11 patients (12.5 per cent) the acute episode of occlusive disease was more than 14 days old (range 15–28 days). In the remaining 45 patients the acute onset of arterial occlusion was less than 14 days old. For the whole group the mean duration

Table 16.2 *Baseline patient characteristics*

Demographics	
Age (years ± SD)	70.7 (±14.9)
Number of patients	89
Gender	
Men	42
Women	47
Risk factors: n (per cent)	
History of smoking	39 (44)
Diabetes	14 (16)
Hypertension	49 (56)
Hypercholesterolaemia	17 (19)
Comorbidity: n (per cent)	
Cardiomyopathy	45 (50.5)
Coronary heart disease	41 (46.5)
Atrial fibrillation	19 (21.5)
Transient cerebral ischaemia or stroke	14 (16)
Chronic obstructive pulmonary disease	11 (12.5)
Pulmonary embolism	9 (10)
Multifocal arterial embolism	7 (8)
Renal insufficiency	9 (10)
Total number (per cent) of patients with polymorbidity	68 (76)

Table 16.3 *Clinical features and occlusion sites*

Clinical presentation	
Duration of symptoms (days)	6.2 (±7.3)
Pain at rest	89 (100 per cent)
Motor loss	7 (7.7 per cent)
Sensory loss	73 (81 per cent)
Embolism likely	55 (61.7 per cent)
Acute on chronic occlusive disease	40 (49 per cent)
Site of arterial occlusion	
Superficial and profunda femoral	24
Superficial femoral, popliteal, crurals	32
Crurals	26
Superficial and profunda femoral, popliteal	9
Profunda femoral	2
Superficial femoral	1

between onset of the acute occlusive episode and catheter therapy was 6.2 days (±7.3). A motor deficit was present in seven patients and a sensory deficit in 73; 20 legs presented with trophic lesions (21.5 per cent). Baseline patient characteristics (Table 16.2) and clinical presentation and sites of arterial occlusion (Table 16.3) were recorded.

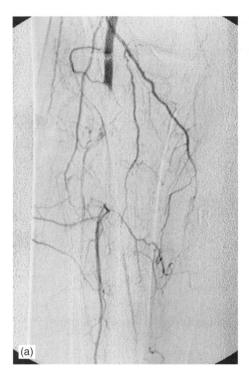
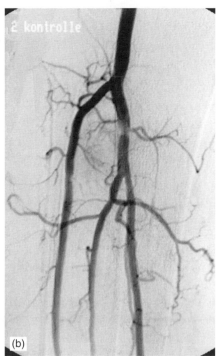

Figure 16.4 *(a) Acute occlusion, probably of embolic origin, of the popliteal trifurcation with non-opacification of the crural arteries presenting with motor and sensory deficit. (b) After clot aspiration, patency is achieved in all three crural arteries within 25 minutes*

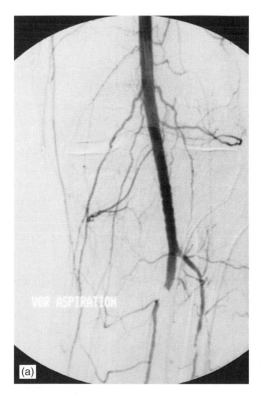
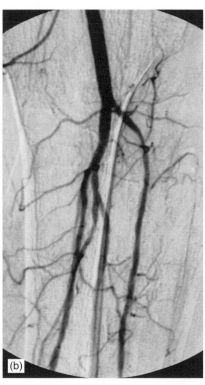

Figure 16.5 *(a) Acute-on-chronic occlusion of the infrapopliteal crural arteries with sensory deficit. (b) After thrombus aspiration combined with percutaneous angioplasty the infrapopliteal arteries are patent*

Procedures

Percutaneous thrombus aspiration was performed as a primary procedure in all patients and as the single therapeutic act in 30 legs (32.2 per cent). In 44 legs (47 per cent) thrombus aspiration was followed by balloon angioplasty of underlying atherosclerotic lesions. In only 20 patients/legs (21.4 per cent) was it necessary in the last resort to add a modest amount of urokinase to initiate thrombus dissolution and facilitate continuation of aspiration. In this last group all three therapeutic modalities were combined, namely, clot aspiration, thrombolysis and PTA (Figs 16.4 and 16.5). The duration of all percutaneous catheter interventions was between 35 and 160 minutes.

Outcome criteria

The primary endpoints of this study were mortality, amputation at 30 days, 6 and 12 months and amputation-free survival of the entire patient group at 6 and 12 months. Other endpoints were primary removal of occluding thrombus, i.e. primary success and patency rate achieved, and the number and percentage of secondary reinterventions necessary, whether open surgical or by catheter. Surgical reinterventions included femorodistal bypasses or thromboendarterectomy. Catheter reinterventions included repeat thrombus aspiration with and without adjuvant lytic therapy and PTA and the placement of a stent in one instance.

Secondary endpoints were the ankle systolic pressure index (ASPI) achieved by percutaneous thrombus aspiration with or without complementary PTA and thrombolysis and the occurrence of adverse effects of treatment. Special attention was given to bleeding complications including cerebral haemorrhage with or without associated mortality.

The extent of clot lysis attempted was based on completion arteriography immediately after catheter therapy in all patients. The ASPI was obtained during admission or from the referring hospital if treatment was ambulatory. Mortality was recorded at 30 days and 6 and 12 months; these outcome measures were obtained either from our own records or those of the referring hospitals and physicians. For a definition of episodes of major haemorrhage we adhered closely to the standards set in the TOPAS study. These were as follows: severe blood loss greater than 500 mL within 1 week after therapy (14 days in the TOPAS study), blood loss requiring surgery, transfusion or causing hypotension or intracranial haemorrhage. False aneurysms were also excluded.

The total dose of urokinase used for direct individual thrombus infiltration in the 21 patients treated with lytic agents was measured and considered in the light of possible bleeding complications.

Statistical analysis

Quantitative data were expressed as mean ± 1 SD. Times to events were analysed by Kaplan–Meier analysis (Stata, Release 5, Stata Corporation, College Station, TX, USA, 1997). Group differences were assessed with Student's t test and with the Mann–Whitney U test for non-parametric groups. A P value less than 0.05 was considered significant.

Clinical outcomes

The results are shown in Table 16.4. Primary success with complete dissolution and complete restoration of patency as proved by angiography was achieved in 84/93 legs

Table 16.4 *Results of combined endovascular catheter intervention*

	Number	Per cent
Procedures	93	100
Aspiration only	29	31
Thrombolysis	20	22
Percutaneous transluminal angioplasty	67	69
Primary success	84	90
Secondary procedures	28	30
Endovascular	14	
Surgical	16	
Amputation (6 months)	8	9
Below-knee	6	
Through-knee	1	
Above-knee	2	
Mortality		
30 days		8
6 months		16
12 months		19

(90.3 per cent), primary failure with ASPIs of 0.27 or less, immeasurable due to incomplete clot removal or re-occlusion in nine legs (9.7 per cent).

Eight patients underwent major amputation, two above-knee, five below-knee and one through-knee with an amputation-free survival of 82.5 per cent at 6 months and 77.9 per cent at 12 months (Fig. 16.6). The mean ASPI in 81 legs treated successfully and measured 1–7 days post intervention was 0.98 ± 0.23. The 30-day mortality was 7.8 per cent (seven patients). At 6 months 14 patients had died (mortality 15.7 per cent) and at 12 months, 17 patients (mortality 19 per cent). In 28 cases (30.1 per cent) a secondary intervention was required: in 14 cases this was an endovascular procedure (suction, lysis, PTA) and in 16 cases an open surgical procedure. Some patients had to undergo two reinterventions.

A total of 20 legs in 19 patients (21.5 per cent) did have thrombolytic therapy in the form of urokinase, not as the main line of treatment but as an adjunct to facilitate dissolution and aspiration; therefore, only modest doses were required, the lytic agent being sprayed within the clot. The individual doses were small and varied between 50 000 and 250 000 IU (mean: $112\,500 \pm 55\,901.7$ IU) thereby avoiding significant systemic fibrinolytic activity. Accordingly there were no major bleeding episodes and no haematomas at the puncture site with the exception of one case of false aneurysm which was treated successfully with local digital compression. No surgical interventions or blood transfusions were necessary and, of utmost importance, not a single case of intracranial haemorrhage occurrred.

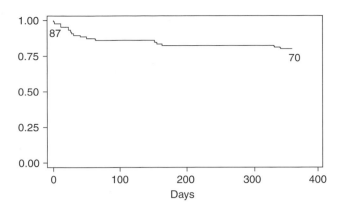

Figure 16.6 *Kaplan–Meier curve showing 12-month amputation-free survival in 77.9 per cent of patients*

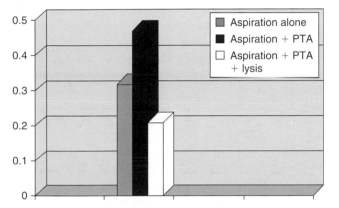

Figure 16.7 *Percutaneous catheter thrombus suction was performed in all patients in this series of 93 legs. It was the only form of therapy in 31 per cent of limbs, it was combined with percutaneous angioplasty (PTA) in 47 per cent and in only 22 per cent was it necessary to add modest doses of urokinase to produce clot disintegration to facilitate clot aspiration*

For the entire group of 89 patients the acute occlusive event had occurred within 6.2 ± 7.3 days. In the group of 19 patients (20 legs) requiring adjunctive thrombolysis to facilitate thrombus suction the process had taken longer (11.15 ± 9.8 days; $t = 2.56$; $P \approx 0.01$). In the 70 patients who did not need lytic therapy the duration of symptoms before treatment was shorter (4.7 ± 5.6 days; Mann–Whitney U test $P = 0.0045$).

Percutaneous catheter thrombus aspiration was performed in all patients in our series of 93 legs. It was the only form of therapy in 31 per cent and was combined with adjunctive PTA in 47 per cent (Fig. 16.7). In 22 per cent only was it necessary to add modest doses of urokinase to produce clot disintegration to facilitate clot aspiration.

DISCUSSION OF THE NEW EVIDENCE

The aim of our single centre retrospective study[30] comprising 93 legs in 89 patents was to show that by performing percutaneous catheter thrombus aspiration, thrombolysis

with its associated hazards is *unnecessary* in four out of five cases of acute limb ischaemia. Moreover, in those 20 legs (21.4 per cent) where urokinase was actually used the doses were small ($112\,500 \pm 55\,900$ IU) and not meant to dissolve the thrombus entirely but merely to loosen up the clot and to facilitate continued aspiration. The mean dose of urokinase in the TOPAS study[26] was, in contrast, 3.5 ± 1.8 million IU and the mean duration ($\pm$SE) of urokinase infusion 24.4 ± 14.2 hours. The mortality rates in our study and in those of the TOPAS study as well as the baseline patient characteristics indicate that the populations are comparable at least with respect to their comorbidity. In our study, the two mechanisms, minimal thrombolysis when necessary and clot suction in every case work in synergy. Small doses of lytic agents facilitate clot aspiration and conversely percutaneous clot removal decreases the need for urokinase. The result is a remarkable reduction of time necessary to obtain patency and certainly well within that taken for surgical intervention.

Eight patients (9 per cent) in our series underwent major amputation, six below-knee, two above-knee and one through-knee. In the TOPAS study the amputation-free survival rates in patients treated with urokinase were comparable to those achieved in the surgically treated group. Nevertheless, 58 major amputations were performed in the urokinase group (21 per cent), 33 below-knee and 25 above-knee. The percentage of amputees in the TOPAS study was therefore significantly greater than that in our series ($P < 0.05$); the proportion of above-knee amputations was also higher.

The 6-month and 12-month amputation-free survival rates in our retrospective study were 82.5 per cent and 77.5 per cent, respectively. In the first prospective randomised study by Ouriel *et al.*,[18] the Rochester trial, the amputation-free survival rates at 1 year were 75 per cent for the patients assigned to thrombolysis with urokinase and 52 per cent for those assigned to surgical treatment. While those figures are similar, both in the Rochester study and in our study there is a highly significant difference with respect to outcome and complications of catheter therapy. The Rochester study reported an 11 per cent rate of serious bleeding complications in patients receiving urokinase with one death due to haemorrhage.

The Surgery versus Thrombolysis for Ischaemia of the Lower Extremity (STILE) study[17] reported a 5.6 per cent rate of serious haemorrhage in patients receiving thrombolytic agents, with low fibrinogen values identified as a risk factor. In the recent report by Ouriel *et al.*[26] on the TOPAS study there was a 12.5 per cent incidence of major bleeding in the urokinase group, increasing when patients received heparin. In four cases these haemorrhages were intracranial and in one case fatal. The concomitant use of heparin had to be restricted and discontinued during the course of the study. Transfusions of more than 1 unit of packed red cells were necessary in 92 patients in the urokinase group of the TOPAS study (33.8 per cent). As stated earlier, there were no major haemorrhages at all in our single centre study, accordingly transfusions or surgical interventions for bleeding complications were unnecessary. These figures underline why it is so important to get away from using lytic agents and, if unavoidable, to minimise the dosage so as not to lower systemic fibrinogen levels by more than 5–10 per cent. This can be achieved by percutaneous clot suction. Before the introduction of suction therapy in a study combining short and long term catheter thrombolysis Do et al.[11] found that fibrinogen levels merely dropped from 2.6 ± 0.7 to 2.5 ± 1.2 g/L when urokinase was used.

In this study there were 28 patients (30.1 per cent) who needed a secondary intervention: in 14 cases endovascular, in 16 cases surgical. In contrast, in the TOPAS study urokinase group[26] the percentage of secondary interventions was 55 per cent, suggesting that routine primary catheter clot extraction, apart from avoiding major haemorrhage and shortening the procedure, has the added advantage of providing better patency results.

Although Dotter is credited with the recognition of the potential of selective clot lysis with low dose streptokinase, it was Hess et al.[15] who were most instrumental in confirming and establishing this procedure worldwide. Although Starck et al.,[28] Schneider and Hoffmann[29] and Mahler[31] repeatedly demonstrated that percutaneous catheter clot extraction was a valuable addition to the armamentarium of catheter therapy, its real potential was never fully recognised elsewhere. Reports on thrombolytic therapy proliferated with the sights constantly set on finding an ever better lytic agent. Once it was recognised that streptokinase had its drawbacks and limitations, especially with regard to duration of treatment, haemorrhagic complications and allergic reactions, attention turned to urokinase and then to recombinant tissue plasminogen activator (r-tPA)[32] in the hope of discovering a more powerful agent with less undesirable side effects. r-tPA has been shown to be faster acting and fibrinogen sparing and to have an improved safety record when compared with other agents, but for practical reasons it has not hitherto replaced urokinase.[31] Further improvement of local lytic treatment was sought by improving and altering the mode of local delivery either by means of pulsed delivery[33] or intraclot spray.[34]

Surprisingly however, the benefits of our regimen in limiting the dosage of, and in the majority of cases rendering superfluous, the lytic agent has not received the attention that it deserves. The shorter duration of aspiration, the adjunctive interventions and the limited exposure to thrombolytic agents when they become necessary are the factors we consider responsible for the lower rate of serious complications. As the procedure does not take more time than a surgical intervention we recommend it as first line treatment for acute or subacute infrainguinal arterial occlusions. It can be combined with PTA for the treatment of underlying stenotic lesions. Only in a minority of roughly 20 per cent of cases will a modest amount of lytic agent be necessary to facilitate clot disintegration and aspiration. Preoperative systemic heparinisation may preclude spinal anaesthesia if open surgery is considered, but it does not interfere with percutaneous clot aspiration, which is performed under local anaesthesia and offers extra benefit over open surgery by allowing for PTA and mild fibrinolysis – all in one. Hospital stay is reduced and patient comfort considerably enhanced.

WHEN SHOULD ENDOVASCULAR OPTIONS BE RECOMMENDED FOR ACUTE LIMB ISCHAEMIA?

Native arteries

Open surgical treatment for acute ischaemia requires either general or regional anaesthesia, the latter precluding prior administration of anticoagulant therapy which is an unfortunate requirement. Soft tissues are invariably injured at surgery and may delay wound healing. Surgical treatment involves the repeated use of Fogarty balloon catheters which can damage the intima, burst or break and occasionally perforate the vessel wall. The degree of patency achieved cannot be monitored during the process of disobliteration but can be assessed by completion angiography. Combined endovascular catheter therapy avoids all these drawbacks. Whereas surgical treatment is expeditious, straightforward and therefore preferable for embolic occlusions of the aorta, iliac and femoral bifurcations, it does require an inguinal incision and there is the additional likelihood of having to treat the ischaemia-reperfusion syndrome (see Chapter 2). Endovascular options should definitely be given preference in infrainguinal thromboembolic occlusions, which in practice means those distal to the level of Hunter's canal, and they are particularly relevant when the popliteal trifurcation is occluded.

The earlier caveats of lytic therapy and the absolute and relative contraindications of using large doses no longer play a decisive role when our combined treatment mode is employed. Nevertheless, these are listed here for those therapists still using lytic therapy alone with the inevitably large doses of urokinase or r-tPA. Despite intraclot instillation there can be leakage into the general vascular system causing episodes of internal bleeding. The following situations therefore represent absolute or relative contraindications: operative interventions upon the central nervous system, lumbar puncture, severe trauma, gastrointestinal and urogenital haemorrhages, uncontrolled hypertension (>200/100 mmHg), bleeding disorders, aortic aneurysms, severe hepatic and/or renal failure, pregnancy (before the third and after the seventh month), bacterial endocarditis, proliferative diabetic retinopathy and suspicion of thrombus in the left heart with its attendant danger of cerebral infarction. None of these contraindications, however, is a reason for not performing combined endovascular catheter therapy using only clot suction or extraction.

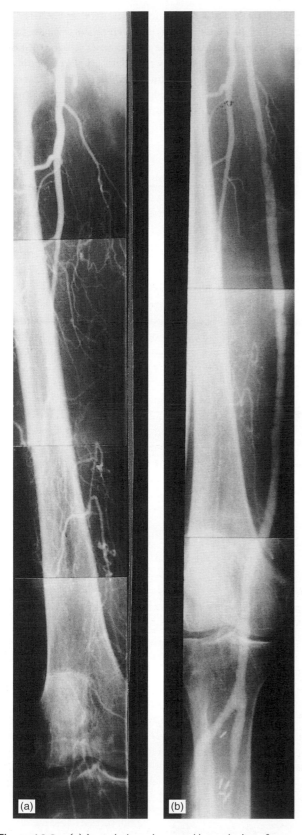

Our studies have shown that in those 70 legs where thrombolysis was not necessary the acute occlusive event was less than 4.7 ± 5.6 days old and significantly shorter than in those 20 legs in need of adjunctive thrombolysis (6.2 ± 7.3 days; Mann–Whitney U test, P = 0.0045). In other words the sooner acute limb ischaemia is treated the greater the chances that percutaneous clot aspiration alone will suffice.

Occluded synthetic grafts

Special awareness is justified when contemplating lysis of Dacron grafts as most lytic agents are capable of rendering such grafts porous. While positioning of catheters in thromboembolic occlusions of native arteries is successful in the vast majority of cases this is not always the case in autologous vein or synthetic bypass grafts. Catheter directed clot aspiration, however, is possible in some cases, as illustrated in Fig. 16.7. This is exemplified in Fig. 16.8 in which an occluded Dardik graft is disobliterated by percutaneous clot extraction. Figure 16.9 shows the thrombotic material sucked out of the graft. Occluded axillofemoral Dacron bypasses are readily amenable to surgical thrombectomy using a Fogarty balloon catheter, but the same procedure is not nearly as successful in graft bypasses in the infrainguinal position, usually because of intimal hyperplasia at the anastomotic site. Balloon dilatation of anastomotic stenosis does not have a lasting effect and revision surgery is usually envisaged in our experience. Comerota et al.[23] reported that in 39 per cent of patients randomised to lysis catheter placement failed and surgical treatment was required. Overall, a significantly better composite clinical outcome at 30 days and at 1 year was observed in the surgical group compared with lysis.

Autologous venous grafts

Here again the problems and difficulties are the same as those for synthetic grafts. In the case of acute ischaemia a re-do reconstruction is probably the best alternative.

Figure 16.8 *(a) Acute ischaemia caused by occlusion of an umbilical Dardik graft. (b) Patency restored after transcutaneous catheter clot extraction but the graft channel remains irregular (with kind permission of Prof J Largiadèr and Dr E Schneider, Zürich)*

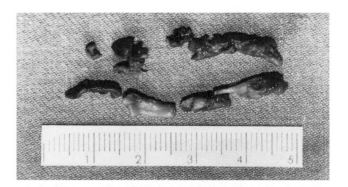

Figure 16.9 *Clots extracted percutaneously from occluded Dardik graft in Fig. 16.8 (with kind permission of Dr E Schneider, Zürich)*

Combined endovascular catheter directed treatment is not an easy option unless started immediately after graft occlusion.

Intraoperative intra-arterial local thrombolysis and clot aspiration

Since 1990 we have adopted a method of intra-arterial intraoperative lysis (IOL) adhering to the principles and experimental work of Quinones-Baldrich *et al.*[8] for those desperate cases in which viability of the limb is seriously threatened and the entire length of arterial vasculature cannot be opacified angiographically. Other authors have adopted a similar policy.[33–38] If, on exploration, the femoral, popliteal and all three crural arteries prove to be occluded, amputation is the usual outcome.

Rewarding results, however, can be obtained by bypassing the occluded femoropopliteal segment with a polytetrafluoroethylene (PTFE) graft and introducing catheters into all three crural arteries simultaneously (Fig. 16.10); up to 175 000 units of urokinase is injected into each vessel to a total dose of 500 000 units over a 25–30-minute period, with intermittent clot aspiration to hasten disobliteration and increase the efficacy of lysis. Simultaneously, another member of the operating team can prepare the femoral artery bifurcation for the upper anastomosis of a PTFE graft. In Fig. 16.11 a thrombolised distal artery offering the necessary run-off can be seen, a prerequisite for femoropopliteal bypass surgery. Figure 16.12 shows the result of IOL of the posterior tibial artery behind the medial malleolus.

This treatment protocol for IOL is similar to the University of California at Los Angeles (UCLA) protocol, which in turn is based on investigations of experimentally induced thrombosis:[8] the angiographic improvement following thrombectomy was 20 per cent reaching 80 per cent if thrombectomy was followed by IOL with streptokinase and heparin for 30 minutes. Our present protocol uses 250 000 units of urokinase dissolved in 100 mL 0.9 per cent sodium chloride with 1000 units of heparin administered into the clot for 30 minutes as described above. The results first published in 1993[9] are shown in Table 16.5, since

which time they have remained unchanged in practice. The impact and potential of IOL in lowering the dosage of lytic agent and in accelerating the restoration of blood flow has hitherto not been fully recognised and appreciated.[30,31,36–38] Further debate on advances in this area of management of acute lower limb ischaemia has been highlighted in the recent literature.[36–44]

WHAT DEVELOPMENTS DOES THE FUTURE HOLD?

The latest development in the treatment of acute and subacute thrombotic arterial occlusions has been the advent of

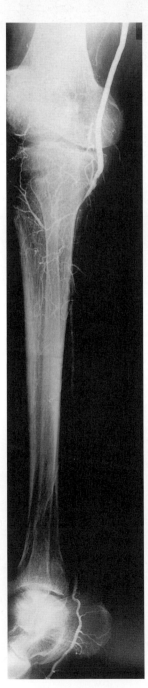

Figure 16.11 *Complete occlusion of the entire arterial vasculature from groin to foot. Local thrombectomy of the distal part of the popliteal artery has been performed for distal anastomosis to a polyfluorotetraethylene (PTFE) graft. From here on downwards intraoperative lysis using 500 000 units of urokinase for 25 minutes and clot suction of the crural arteries was performed reopening the previously occluded posterior tibial artery. There now is sufficient run-off to enable patency of the femoropopliteal bypass graft*

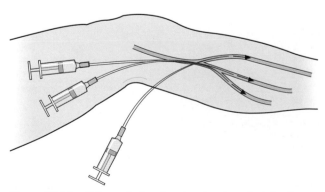

Figure 16.10 *Schematic drawing showing the principle of introducing three catheters from an infragenicular approach into the crural arteries for simultaneous intraoperative thrombolysis and clot suction*

a rotational thrombectomy device, the Stator Rotarex System (Straub Medical AG, Wangs, Switzerland; www.straubmedical.com) which has been clinically tested and improved over the past three years.[43,44] This Rotarex rotational thrombus debulking device is made of stainless steel fashioned into a wedge-shaped cutting head ground down to form a blunt rounded tip with a central opening for the guidewire over which the catheter passes. Two open slits

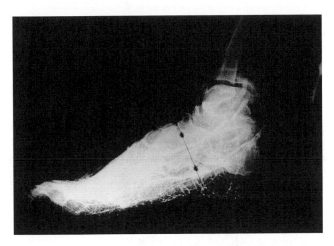

Figure 16.12 *A case of complete ischaemia of the right foot. Local fibrinolysis via the posterior tibial artery provides excellent visualisation of the pedal circulation*

Table 16.5 *Results of intraoperative clot lysis combined with clot suction for total ischaemia undertaken from 1 January 1990 to 31 July 1992*

Number of cases	34
Limb salvage rate	86 per cent
Patency rate	81 per cent
30-day mortality	14 per cent
Wound haematoma	4 per cent

5 mm from the tip rotate over two corresponding open slits in the internally placed stationary Stator. The Rotarex cutting head with its internally placed blades rotates around the Stator at 40 000 rotations per minute driven by a spiral which also has a transporting function; the thrombotic material is drawn by the suction force through the internally placed cutting edges and is broken down and removed through the middle of the catheter leaving no residual detached material in the lumen. The catheter follows the direction given by the guidewire in the blood vessel and allows controlled movements of the rotating head to be made.

This device has been designed for removing both fresh thrombus and organised thrombotic occlusions of up to 6 months but is not designed to deal with calcified plaque. When underlying plaques are uncovered they should be treated by balloon angioplasty. The diameter of the recanalised artery is approximately double that of the catheter used. The catheters presently available are 8 Fr antegrade, 8 Fr crossover and 6 Fr antegrade, all of which can be adapted to the motor unit. The aspiration capacity in fresh thrombus is 0.5–1 cm/s. For the sake of safety, mainly to avoid the danger of perforation, it is recommended that the Rotarex system not be used beyond the tibioperoneal trunk.

This mechanical 'four-in-one' device incorporates the combined functions of thrombus detachment, suction, cutting and transport of debris out of the vessel. It has enormous potential, acknowledging the aforementioned danger of perforation and the costs, one catheter currently priced at SF1500. Nevertheless, with commercially available devices such as this, the time spent in reopening occluded arteries is being significantly shortened and soon the use of thrombolytic agents may be dispensed with entirely.

The algorithm in Fig. 16.13 provides guidelines for the modern management of acute and subacute ischaemia of the lower limbs indicating optimal methods of dealing with occlusions at different levels of the arterial tree.

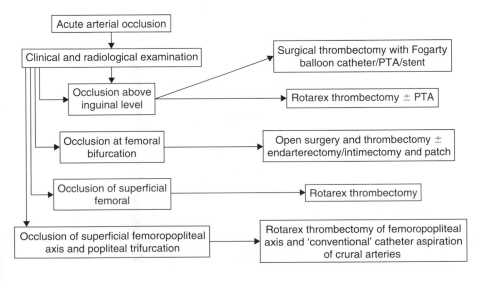

Figure 16.13 *Algorithm of the current treatment of acute and subacute ischaemia of the lower extremities. PTA, percutaneous angioplasty*

Conclusions

Acute and subacute thrombotic and embolic occlusions of the femoral, popliteal and infrapopliteal arteries are especially amenable to local endovascular catheter therapy. A new concept, combining clot aspiration with PTA whenever atherosclerotic plaques are uncovered, together with clot suction and modest doses of lytic agents when necessary, heralds a fresh era in the treatment of acute ischaemia of the limbs. The combined procedures shorten interventional disobliteration and at the same time avoid systemic thrombolysis with the inherent dangers of haemorrhage. We have shown that a 90 per cent primary patency rate and a 77 per cent amputation-free 12 month survival rate can be achieved with little risk of bleeding complications. Transfusions are unnecessary. This treatment modality works adequately with most degrees of acute ischaemia because of the rapidity of the procedure. It is therefore recommended as first line treatment for acute as well as subacute ischaemia caused by infrainguinal occlusions.

Currently, at the Vascular Department of the University of Berne, this approach is frequently being combined with Straub Rotarex catheter aspiration and significantly accelerating the reopening of occluded vessels. The success of this new technique has been such that thrombolytic agents are being dispensed with completely. It has already undergone extensive clinical trial and holds significant promise for the future.

Key references

Do DD, Mahler F, Triller J, Nachbur B. Combination of short and long-term catheter thrombolysis for peripheral arterial occlusion. *Eur J Radiol* 1987; **7**: 235–8.

Nachbur B. Treatment of acute ischaemia; every general surgeon's business? *Eur J Vasc Surg* 1988; **2**: 281–2.

Ouriel K, Veith FJ, Sasahara AA, for the TOPAS investigators. A comparison of recombinant urokinase with vascular surgery as initial treatment for acute arterial occlusions of the legs. *N Engl J Med* 1998; **338**: 1105–11.

Zehnder T, Birrer M, Do DD, *et al*. Percutaneous catheter thrombus aspiration for acute or subacute arterial occlusion of the legs: how much thrombolysis is needed? *Eur J Vasc Endovasc Surg* 2000; **20**: 41–6.

Zeller T, Frank U, Burgelin K, *et al*. Early experience with a rotational thrombectomy device for treatment of acute and subacute infra-aortic arterial occlusion. *J Endovasc Ther* 2003; **10**: 322–31.

REFERENCES

1 Jamieson CW. Is it important to differentiate between acute and acute on chronic ischaemia? In: Greenhalgh RM, Jamieson CW, Nicolaides AN (eds). *Limb Salvage and Amputation for Vascular Disease*. London: WB Saunders, 1988: 105–12.

2 Srinivasan R, Cooper G, Bell PRF. Popliteal embolectomy; does it still have a role? *Eur J Vasc Surg* 1992; **6**: 424–6.

3 Dinkel HP, Hoppe H, Baumgartner I, *et al*. Low-osmolar gadodiamide as alternative contrast agent for diagnostic angiography and angiographic interventions in patients with renal insufficiency. *Rofo Fortschr Geb Rontgenstr Neuen Bildgeb Verfahr* 2002; **174**: 56–61, (comment in *Rofo Fortschr Geb Rontgenstr Neuen Bildgeb Verfahr* 2003; **1**, author reply 571–2).

4 Tepel M, Van der Giet M, Schwarzfeld C, *et al*. Prevention of radiographic-contrast-agent induced reductions in renal function by acetylcysteine. *N Engl J Med* 2000; **343**: 180–4.

5 O'Brian RS, Thomas H, Crow A, Lamont PM. Calf vessel preservation in peripheral vascular disease – angiography versus pulse generated run-off. *Eur J Vasc Surg* 1993; **7**: 177–9.

6 Comerota AJ, White JV, Gosh JD. Intraoperative intra-arterial thrombolytic therapy for salvage of limbs in patients with distal arterial thrombosis. *Surg Gynecol Obstret* 1989; **169**: 283–9.

7 Alavaikka A. Local thrombolytic therapy as a support for catheter embolectomy in limb arterial occlusions. *Ann Chir Gynaecol* 1991; **80**: 357–62.

8 Quinones-Baldrich WJ, Baker JD, Busuttil RW, *et al*. Intraoperative infusion of lytic drugs for thrombotic complication of revascularization. *J Vasc Surg* 1989; **10**: 408–17.

9 Knaus J, Ris HB, Do D, Stirnemann P. Intraoperative thrombolysis as an adjunct to surgical revascularisation for infrainguinal limb-threatening ischemia. *Eur J Vasc Surg* 1993; **7**: 507–12.

10 Scott DJ, Wyatt MG, Wilson YG, *et al*. Intraarterial streptokinase infusion in acute lower limb ischaemia. *Br J Surg* 1991; **78**: 732–4.

11 Do DD, Mahler F, Triller J, Nachbur B. Combination of short and long-term catheter thrombolysis for peripheral arterial occlusion. *Eur J Radiol* 1987; **7**: 235–8.

12 Nachbur B. Treatment of acute ischaemia; every general surgeon's business? *Eur J Vasc Surg* 1988; **2**: 281–2.

13 Bywaters EGL, Beall C. Crush injuries with impairment of renal function. *BMJ* 1941; **1**: 427.

14 Nachbur B, Horber F, Sigrist S. Metabolic disorders in acute limb ischemia. In: Bergan JJ and Yao JS (eds). *Vascular Surgical Emergencies*. Orlando, FL: Grune and Stratton, 1987.

15 Hess H, Mietasch K, Rath H. Local low-dose thrombolytic therapy of peripheral arterial occlusions. *N Engl J Med* 1982; **307**: 1627–30.

16 Ouriel K. Comparison of surgical and thrombolytic treatment of peripheral arterial disease. *Rev Cardiovasc Med* 2002; **3**(suppl 2): S7–16.

17 Graor RA (Study Chairman). Results of a prospective randomized trial evaluating surgery *versus* thrombolysis for ischaemia of the lower extremity. The STILE trial. *Ann Surg* 1994; **220**: 251–68.

18 Ouriel K, Shortell CK, DeWeese JA, *et al*. A comparison of thrombolytic therapy with operative revascularization in the initial treatment of acute peripheral arterial ischemia. *J Vasc Surg* 1994; **19**: 1021–30.

19 Swischuk JL, Fox PF, Young K, *et al*. Transcatheter intraarterial infusion of rt-PA for acute lower limb ischemia: results and complications, *J Vasc Interv Radiol* 2001; **12**: 423–30.

20 Braithwaite BD, Petrik PV, Ritschie AWS, Earnshaw JJ. Computerized angiographic analysis of the outcome of peripheral thrombolysis. *Am J Surg* 1995; **170**: 131–5.

21 Braithwaite BD, Quinones-Baldrich WJ. Lower limb intraarterial thrombolysis as an adjunct to the management of arterial and graft occlusions. *World J Surg* 1996; **20**: 649–54.

22 Ouriel K, Veith FJ, Sasahara AA ,for the TOPAS investigators. Thrombolysis or peripheral arterial surgery: phase I results. *J Vasc Surg* 1996; **23**: 64–73.

23 Comerota AJ, Weaver FA, Hosking JD, *et al*. Results of a prospective, randomized trial of surgery versus thrombolysis for occluded lower extremity bypass grafts. *Am J Surg* 1996; **172**: 105–12.

24 Armon MP, Yusuf SC, Whitaker RH, *et al*. Results of 100 cases of pulse-spray thrombolysis for acute and subacute leg ischaemia. *Br J Surg* 1997; **84**: 47–50.

25 Davidian MM, Powell A, Benenati JF *et al*. Initial results of reteplasma in the treatment of acute lower extremity arterial occlusions. *J Vasc Interv Radiol* 2000; **11**: 289–94.

26 Ouriel K, Veith FJ, Sasahara AA, for the TOPAS investigators. A comparison of recombinant urokinase with vascular surgery as initial treatment for acute arterial occlusions of the legs. *N Engl J Med* 1998; **338**: 1105–11.

27 Porter JM. Thrombolysis for acute arterial occlusion of the legs [editorial]. *N Engl J Med* 1998; **338**: 1148–9.

28 Starck E, McDermott J, Crummy A, *et al*. Die perkutane Aspirations-Thromboembolektomie: eine weitere transluminale Angioplastiemethode. *Deutsche Med Wochenschr* 1986; **111**: 167–72.

29 Schneider E, Hoffmann U. Perkutane lokale Lysetherapie und Thrombenextraktion bei Verschlüssen der Extremitätenarterien. *Internist* 1996; **37**: 607–12.

30 Zehnder T, Birrer M, Do DD, *et al*. Percutaneous catheter thrombus aspiration for acute or subacute arterial occlusion of the legs: how much thrombolysis is needed? *Eur J Vasc Endovasc Surg* 2000; **20**: 41–6.

31 Mahler F. Lokale Katheterthrombolyse und Katheterthrombektomie. In: Mahler F (ed.) *Katheterinterventionen in der Angiologie.* Stuttgart: Thieme, 1990: 113–29.

32 Verstraete M, Hess H, Mahler F, *et al*. Femoro-popliteal artery thrombolysis with intra-arterial infusion of recombinant tissue-type plasminogen activator, report of a pilot trial. *Eur J Vasc Surg* 1988; **2**: 155–9.

33 Buckenham TM, George CD, Chester JF, *et al*. Accelerated thrombolysis using pulsed intra-thrombus recombinant human tissue type plasminogen activator (rt-PA). *Eur J Vasc Surg* 1992; **6**: 237–40.

34 Yusuf SW, Whitaker SC, Gregson HS, *et al*. Prospective randomised comparative study of pulse spray and conventional local thrombolysis. *Eur J Vasc Endovasc Surg* 1995; **10**: 136–41.

35 Parent FN, Piotrowski JJ, Bernhard VM, *et al*. Outcome of intraarterial urokinase for acute vascular occlusion. *J Cardiovasc Surg* 1991; **32**: 680–9.

36 Hopfner W, Bohndorf K, Vicol C, Loeprecht H. Percutaneous hydromechanical thrombectomy in acute and subacute lower limb ischemia. *Rofo Fortschr Geb Rontgenstr neuen Bildgeb Verfahr* 2001; **173**: 229–35.

37 Canova GR, Schneider E, Fischer L, *et al*. Long-term results of percutaneous thrombo-embolectomy in patients with infrainguinal embolic occlusions. *Int Angiol* 2001; **20**: 66–73.

38 Wang HJ, Kao HL, Liau CS, Lee YT. Export aspiration catheter thrombosuction before actual angioplasty in primary coronary intervention for acute myocardial infarction. *Katheter Cardiovasc Interv* 2002; **57**: 332–9.

39 Ouriel K. Comparison of surgical and thrombolytic treatment of peripheral arterial. *Rev Cardiovasc Med* 2002; Suppl 2: S7–S16.

40 Carlson GA, Hobollah JJ, Sharp WJ. Surgical thrombectomy: current role in thromboembolic occlusions. *Tech Vasc Interv Radiol* 2003; **6**: 14–21.

41 Kalinowski M, Wagner HJ. Adjunctive techniques in percutaenous mechanical thrombectomy. *Tech Vasc Interv Radiol* 2003; **6**: 6–13.

42 Henke PK. Approach to the patient with acute limb ischemia: diagnosis and therapeutic modalities. *Cardiol Clin* 2002; **20**: 513–20.

43 Zeller T, Frank U, Burgelin K, *et al*. Early experience with a rotational thrombectomy device for treatment of acute and subacute infra-aortic arterial occlusion. *J Endovasc Ther* 2003; **10**: 322–31.

44 Zeller T, Frank U, Burgelin K, *et al*. Treatment of acute embolic occlusions of the subclavian and axillary arteries using a rotational thrombectomy device. *Vasa* 2003; **32**: 11–16.

17

Graft Maintenance and Graft Failure

DAVID K BEATTIE, ALUN H DAVIES

THE PROBLEM OF GRAFT FAILURE

The advent of infrainguinal arterial reconstruction brought with it a new problem, that of graft stenosis and graft failure, irrespective of the conduit used for bypass. There has been no significant improvement in graft patency rates following such reconstructions since Szilagyi et al.[1] described the phenomena nearly 30 years ago, with most series reporting that 20–30 per cent of all grafts develop a stenosis or fail, usually within 1 year of surgery.[2–5]

The potential benefits of identifying a failing graft before it fails are clear. In one series 79 per cent of patients operated on for limb salvage were again at risk of limb loss following graft occlusion, and 91 per cent of claudicants were either worse or similar to their preoperative status.[6] Furthermore, the revision of surveillance detected graft stenoses using either surgical or endovascular techniques has been shown to give excellent primary assisted patency rates in excess of 80 per cent at 5 years[7–9] whereas revascularisation following graft occlusion yields poor long term limb salvage with secondary graft patency rates as low as 43 per cent at 5 years.[10–12] In the majority of cases it is technically easier to revise a graft before rather than after it fails.

This chapter addresses the question of both the detection and management of the 'at risk' graft and the management of the failed graft. However, it is important to stress that, where a graft has already failed, reintervention is only undertaken when there is renewed critical ischaemia or severe symptoms due to ischaemia.

GRAFT FAILURE: AETIOLOGY AND PATHOPHYSIOLOGY

Graft failure is conventionally described as occurring in one of three postoperative periods: **early** graft failure develops within 30 days of surgery, while the majority of failures occur during an **intermediate** period from 1 month to 1 year and **late** failures are those that come to light after 1 year.

Between 5 and 15 per cent of all infrainguinal grafts will fail within 1 month of surgery.[13] Continued early graft patency is dependent, given appropriate patient selection, upon technical factors and, where vein is used, vein quality. Technical problems occur in up to 15 per cent of femorodistal bypasses and identification of these is important to graft patency. Twisting and kinking of the vein graft are the usual causes of graft malfunction. The former is more common in reversed and fully mobilised grafts, though the latter is less common than in synthetic grafts.[14–16] Insertion of the graft under tension may also jeopardise flow.

While the use of an *in situ* technique decreases the risk of malalignment, the risk of persistent valves and tributaries is increased. The former may not always be immediately detectable, even with on-table arteriography, and failure to adequately disrupt the valves correlates with occlusion. There is evidence that, even in patients with reversed vein grafts, competent valves may create a pressure trap effect with segmental hypertension, flow stagnation and graft thickening, and stenosis.[17] Non-division of saphenous tributaries causes arteriovenous fistulae with shunting of blood to the

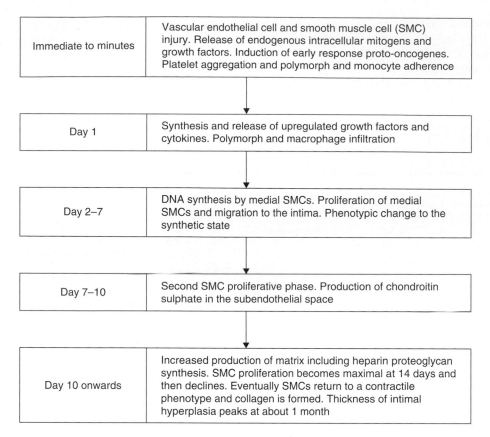

Immediate to minutes	Vascular endothelial cell and smooth muscle cell (SMC) injury. Release of endogenous intracellular mitogens and growth factors. Induction of early response proto-oncogenes. Platelet aggregation and polymorph and monocyte adherence
Day 1	Synthesis and release of upregulated growth factors and cytokines. Polymorph and macrophage infiltration
Day 2–7	DNA synthesis by medial SMCs. Proliferation of medial SMCs and migration to the intima. Phenotypic change to the synthetic state
Day 7–10	Second SMC proliferative phase. Production of chondroitin sulphate in the subendothelial space
Day 10 onwards	Increased production of matrix including heparin proteoglycan synthesis. SMC proliferation becomes maximal at 14 days and then declines. Eventually SMCs return to a contractile phenotype and collagen is formed. Thickness of intimal hyperplasia peaks at about 1 month

Figure 17.1   *The time course and events in the formation of intimal hyperplasia*

deep veins and a resultant decrease in distal graft flow;[18] this may occur in 20 per cent of *in situ* grafts. Occasionally fistulae enlarge causing graft failure.

Anastomoses are particularly prone to technical error, and the problem is magnified as the bypass becomes more distal and the recipient vessel therefore smaller. The most common problems are intimal dissection and luminal narrowing, and a number of techniques are used to prevent these complications. These include the use of fine sutures, passage of the suture from the intimal surface through to the adventitia, the fashioning of anastomoses over catheters and maintenance of an optimal ratio between cross-sectional area of the graft and artery. However, early graft patency is also substantially dependent on graft inflow and outflow. Poor cardiac output and proximal atherosclerotic disease are harbingers of a poor outcome. Nevertheless, a run-off deficiency is the most common cause of early graft failure and this is dependent upon graft site and the degree of preoperative ischaemia. For instance, it has been demonstrated that graft outcome correlates with tibial vessel patency[19] and that an intact pedal arch is important.

Up to 75 per cent of failures occur during the intermediate period, by far the most common cause being the development of neointimal hyperplasia with resultant, usually single, discrete stenoses, though valve cusp fibrosis and aneurysmal dilatation may also be responsible. Neointimal hyperplasia is a uniform vascular response to vessel injury,

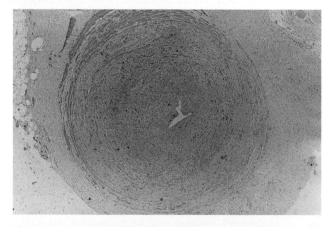

Figure 17.2   *Cross-section of a stenosed vein graft (alpha-actin stain × 40). Note the marked luminal narrowing secondary to the development of florid neointimal hyperplasia*

which can range from mild endothelial denudation to severe medial disruption. Histologically, medial smooth muscle cells alter phenotype, proliferate and migrate to the intima. In the intima a second phase of proliferation occurs and the cells become embedded in an extracellular matrix comprising mainly collagen.[20] Lesions develop quickly, often within 2 weeks of surgery; the time course of these events is shown in Fig. 17.1. A cross-section through a vein graft stenosis secondary to marked intimal hyperplasia can be seen in Fig. 17.2.

Late graft failure is significantly less common than intermediate or early failure. The primary cause is disease progression in the native inflow, or more commonly run-off, vessels compromising graft flow and leading to thrombosis which threatens survival of the limb (see Chapter 2). The act of grafting itself may increase the rate of progression of native vessel disease, though failure may also be due to the development of atheroma within the graft. Rarely vein grafts may fail due to other disease processes such as aneurysmal dilatation with subsequent thrombosis, embolism or rupture.

THE MAINTENANCE OF GRAFT PATENCY AND DIAGNOSIS OF THE FAILING GRAFT

The task of ensuring continued graft patency following infrainguinal reconstruction begins preoperatively. Preoperative assessment involves adequate assessment of both the arterial lesion and, if vein is to be used, the proposed donor vein. Traditionally, recourse to arteriography, preferably biplanar, has been necessary. Similarly, arteriography is used to assess outflow, particularly in the presence of distal disease, though it may fail to demonstrate patent distal vessels. Subtraction techniques may provide additional information. Duplex, however, has become the mainstay of non-invasive investigation, and Doppler insonation and pulse generated run-off are superior to arteriography in identifying patent distal vessels.[21]

The importance of assessing the donor vein prior to bypass is increasingly being recognised. Preoperatively, an assessment of vein anatomy, compliance and internal diameter is feasible. Previously, venography was the gold standard but in many units duplex Doppler is now the mainstay for preoperative venous assessment, providing information on vein wall morphology,[22] blood flow, calibre, varicosities and tributaries, as well as cusps.[23] Duplex accurately predicts vein location, size and quality[24] and is better than venography in assessing calf vein diameter.[25] In one series, duplex directly diagnosed pre-existing venous disease, with respect to wall thickness, calcification and occlusion, in 62 per cent of cases.[26] More recently, these pre-existing changes have been correlated with the development of vein graft stenosis.[27,28] Figure 17.3 shows a cross-section of a biopsy taken from the donor saphenous vein at the time of bypass surgery. Both preoperative internal vein diameter and compliance have been shown to correlate with graft survival.[5,29,30]

The importance of treating the patient medically as well as surgically at the time of operation, or well before it, is well documented, both to protect the graft and to limit the progression of native vessel disease. Issues to be addressed include the cessation of smoking, adequate treatment of hypertension and diabetes, the identification and treatment of hyperlipidaemias and hyperhomocysteinaemia and the institution of antiplatelet therapy where not contraindicated.

There are important peroperative steps to improve the immediate outcome of bypass surgery. Prior to arterial

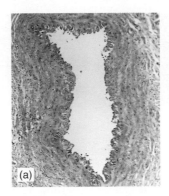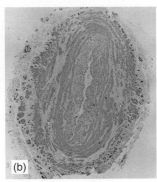

Figure 17.3 *Cross-section of a segment of saphenous vein taken at the time of bypass surgery. (a) Haematoxylin and eosin stained section of saphenous vein × 40. (b) Alpha-actin stain. Note the marked existing intimal hyperplasia present even before the vein has been arterialised*

clamping the patient should be heparinised. On completion of the bypass a check for patency and technical errors should be made. This may involve the use of intraoperative Doppler, on-table arteriography or angioscopy, though this has not found routine acceptance. A check on haemodynamic improvement should also be made prior to the patient leaving hospital. This should involve at least re-estimation of the ankle:brachial pressure index (ABPI), but preferably duplex examination.

DIAGNOSIS OF THE FAILING GRAFT

There is strong evidence that bypass graft surveillance increases the detection of flow limiting graft stenoses and that treatment of these prior to occlusion, i.e. when the graft is 'at risk' rather than 'failed' leads to improved long term graft patency.[31] The primary methods of graft surveillance include clinical examination, ABPI estimation, duplex imaging and arteriography. Of these, duplex scanning is increasingly recognised as the most valuable, though considerable debate surrounding its use and efficacy still exists.

Arteriography

Biplanar arteriography remains the gold standard in arterial assessment and is able to detect both native vessel and graft stenoses. It has advantages over non-invasive methods in that image resolution is not compromised proximal to the inguinal ligament, pressure gradients across iliac lesions can be measured and new techniques allow multiplanar imaging. However, as a means of surveillance it is unacceptable due to its invasive nature and the associated morbidity and mortality, the costs involved and the limited resource supply. Invasive arteriography no longer has a place in the routine surveillance of grafts postoperatively, but remains paramount in the confirmation of non-invasive findings and in planning revision procedures.

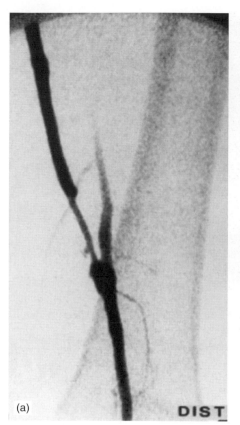

(a)   DIST

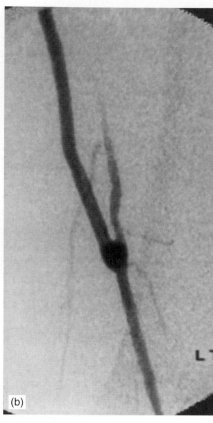

(b)   L T

Figure 17.4 *(a) Arteriogram showing intimal vein graft stenosis initially detected on duplex scanning. (b) Arteriogram after interposition grafting*

Figure 17.4 shows a vein graft stenosis initially detected on duplex scanning and here confirmed by arteriography at the time of balloon angioplasty.

Non-invasive surveillance

ANKLE:BRACHIAL PRESSURE INDICES

The use of resting ABPI estimation in the detection of graft stenoses has been accepted for some time. There are, however, considerable limitations to the technique. Ankle:brachial pressure index values may vary by as much as 0.1, without any change in the status of the patient. A fall of 0.15 in the ABPI is generally accepted as being significant, but such a fall requires the presence of a stenosis of at least 50 per cent. At this level graft occlusion is likely to be sudden and hence the opportunity to revise the graft before failure is lost. Several studies have shown that even a fall in the resting ABPI of at least 0.2 does not predict grafts that will fail.[32,33] Treadmill testing may however increase the sensitivity of ABPI measurements in the detection of stenosis, just as it has been shown to do for native vessel disease. A significant number of patients with stenosis and a stable resting ABPI have been shown to have a fall in the ABPI after exercise.[34] Ankle:brachial pressure index measurements may be of little use in diabetic patients due to vessel calcification.

DUPLEX GRAFT SURVEILLANCE

The rationale behind duplex graft surveillance is based upon the supposition that the detection and correction of graft stenoses, with consequent improvements in patency rates will result in improved limb survival. This, however, has never been proved in a large randomised trial. In fact, a large summation analysis of 6649 grafts comparing outcomes for grafts entered into a duplex surveillance programme with those where surveillance was not performed found that, while surveillance appeared to improve graft patency rates, there was no impact whatsoever upon limb salvage and amputation rates.[31] Furthermore, it has never been proved adequately that stenosis inevitably means either subsequent occlusion or potential limb loss. There are data, however, which suggest quite the opposite. Those from Bristol relating to 275 grafts showed that there was no difference in the 12-month cumulative patency rates between grafts with treated and those with untreated lesions.[35] In one study of 80 grafts followed angiographically, 22 grafts were shown to have a stenosis, five of which occluded, but four in the group of 58 with no stenosis also occluded.[36] Others have doubted that the non-invasive detection of graft stenoses identifies those grafts at risk of occlusion.[32,37,38] Even with the presumption that graft stenosis predisposes to graft occlusion and limb loss, a number of studies failed to find any benefit to duplex surveillance.

A randomised controlled Finnish study examining 185 vein grafts studied with either duplex surveillance or ABPI measurements failed to find any benefit of duplex surveillance.[39] Any differences in outcome were apparent during the first postoperative month, prior to the commencement of surveillance.

Another group looking at a mixture of 85 vein, polytetrafluoroethylene (PTFE) and composite grafts found no support for the efficacy of prophylactic graft revision for grafts identified as failing by currently accepted duplex criteria.[40] This perhaps reflects, at least in part, the increasingly accepted belief that duplex surveillance has a place in the surveillance of vein grafts but not prosthetic grafts. In a series of 69 prosthetic grafts from the Leicester group, for example, 14 failed after 30 days, 12 of which were not predicted by the surveillance programme.[41]

The results of an ongoing large randomised multicentre trial are awaited to provide direct evidence of the benefits of a duplex surveillance programme for vein grafts in terms of limb salvage, quality of life and cost benefit.[42]

The above evidence must call into question the place of duplex in graft surveillance but even if the concept of duplex graft surveillance is accepted there are problems. The generally accepted duplex criteria for the detection of a failing graft are shown in the box below, and Fig. 17.5 shows a duplex detected vein graft stenosis. A peak systolic velocity (PSV) greater than 150 cm/s implies a diameter reduction of at least 80 per cent.[43] The use of standardised criteria means that the precision and reproducibility of duplex in graft surveillance from laboratory to laboratory must be excellent. In a blinded trial of interobserver agreement in the duplex scanning of vein grafts the kappa statistic was just 0.69. This signifies 'good' agreement, but is it good enough?[44] The PSV criteria are open to question and there are doubts about the PSV ratio (PSVR) at which grafts should be revised. For example, there is evidence that graft stenoses with a PSVR of less than 3.0 can be safely left, provided that duplex surveillance is performed every 3 months.[45] This suggests that current duplex criteria for the detection of stenosis may be too sensitive, a viewpoint supported by a series of 46 grafts in which duplex detected abnormalities, as defined by a PSVR of more than 3.0, were followed up. Only 14 grafts were eventually revised, and only three occluded while being followed. All three showed a PSVR in excess of 7.0 prior to occlusion.[46] In the same group, and in a trial using the same criteria, a comparison of the outcome of failing grafts which underwent prophylactic revision with those in which no revision was performed, found that primary and secondary patency and limb salvage rates were not significantly different.[47] One suggestion, based on a study of 121 patients demonstrating that graft diameter and the location of the distal anastomosis significantly affect the flow velocity with the graft, is that currently established criteria for graft revision on the basis of velocity parameters may be improved if they can be modified to account for graft diameter and outflow.[48]

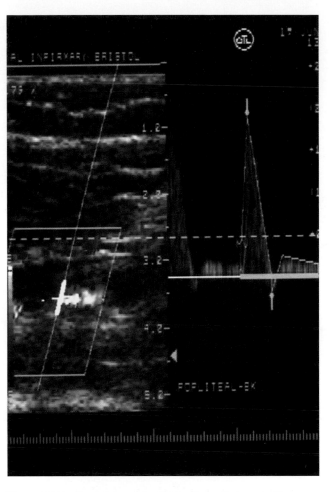

Figure 17.5 *Duplex scan of a tight vein graft stenosis. The duplex performed here demonstrates an elevated peak systolic velocity and hence stenosis*

Duplex criteria for the identification of the failing graft

- ABPI fall >0.2
- PSV <45 cm/s
- Increase in PSV to >150 cm/s
- PSVR across a stenosis >2.0

There is also ongoing controversy as to the ideal follow-up time for graft surveillance. On one hand there are the advocates of long term duplex surveillance. For example, Lundell *et al.* in their randomised trial of graft surveillance versus non-surveillance found that significant differences in patencies were found only by year 2.[49] This stance is shared by the Leicester group which feels that vein graft surveillance should be lifelong.[50] Mills *et al.*, however, found that of 91 grafts that were normal at 3 months only two subsequently developed *de novo* stenoses.[51] All grafts progressing to high grade stenosis had a duplex abnormality at

Table 17.1 *The Transatlantic inter-Society Consensus (TASC) guidelines for the surveillance of infrainguinal bypass grafts*

Recommended surveillance programme for vein bypass grafts

Patients undergoing vein bypass graft placement in the lower extremity for the treatment of claudication or limb-threatening ischaemia should be entered into a surveillance programme. This programme should consist of:

- Interval history (new symptoms)
- Vascular examination of the leg with palpation of inflow, graft and outflow pulses
- Periodic measurement of resting and, if possible, post-exercise ankle:brachial indices
- Duplex scanning of the entire length of the graft, with calculation of the peak systolic velocities and the velocity ratios across all identified lesions
- Surveillance should be performed in the immediate postoperative period and at regular intervals for at least 2 years

Recommended surveillance programme for prosthetic bypass grafts

Patients undergoing prosthetic femoropopliteal or femorotibial bypass for the treatment of claudication or limb-threatening ischaemia should be entered into a surveillance programme. This programme should consist of:

- Interval history (new symptoms)
- Vascular examination of the leg with palpation of inflow, graft and outflow pulses
- Periodic measurement of resting and, if possible, post-exercise ankle:brachial indices
- Surveillance should be performed in the immediate postoperative period and at regular intervals for at least 2 years

---

6 weeks. This suggests that grafts with a normal early scan need much less intensive surveillance. Similarly, in a prospective trial of 300 patients undergoing duplex surveillance after the first year of operation it was concluded that the duration of surveillance may be restricted to the first six months in those who have a normal bypass in that time.[52]

What is not disputed is the increased workload required to maintain vein graft patency consequent upon a graft surveillance programme, much of which is radiological.[53] Despite this, however, revision of a duplex identified stenosis has been shown to be significantly cheaper than revision after thrombosis has occurred. Similarly, limb salvage is more cost effective than amputation and, despite concern over the high frequency with which revisions have been required in some series, the expense of a duplex surveillance programme, together with the increased workload generated, appears to be justified.[54]

It is apparent that much controversy remains surrounding the use of duplex-based graft surveillance. Nevertheless, the TransAtlantic inter-Society Consensus[55] (TASC) Working Group on the Management of Peripheral Arterial Disease

has published surveillance guidelines as shown in Table 17.1. It is noted that there is a need for establishing the cost effectiveness and optimal duration for surveillance, but that surveillance should be for at least 2 years.

MANAGEMENT

An algorithm (Fig. 17.6) illustrates pathways of management, the treatment options available, the chances of bypass graft failure and surveillance to thwart that outcome.

The failing graft

Intervention in the failing graft has been shown to result in excellent primary assisted patency rates.[31] There is considerable inconsistency in the literature as to the level of stenosis, particularly with respect to vein grafts, at which intervention should be considered. It is generally agreed however that a rapidly progressive lesion, or a lesion deemed to be advanced on the basis of velocity criteria, should be revised. In our institution a PSVR in excess of 2.0, indicating a reduction in diameter of 50 per cent and a cross-sectional reduction of 70 per cent, is considered to be haemodynamically significant.

Many moderately severe lesions are detected on duplex scanning in the early postoperative period. Most will remain stable and will not require revision. Where intervention is deemed necessary options include percutaneous angioplasty, vein patch angioplasty and interposition or jump bypass grafting. Although some studies have shown equivalent results for surgery and balloon angioplasty for all stenoses,[56] in practice, short lesions such as isolated stenoses and webs tend to be addressed with balloon angioplasty, or increasingly, vein patch angioplasty, with more extensive graft revision being reserved for long lesions and grafts exhibiting multiple lesions.

Where a prosthetic graft is felt to be at risk by virtue of falling ABPIs, arteriography is usually required as duplex does not image the surface of the graft sufficiently, particularly where grafts are externally supported. Furthermore, a detailed assessment of the inflow and outflow vasculature is needed. Inflow and outflow lesions thus identified can be addressed by standard techniques. Where there is a lesion within the graft, the graft usually requires revision.[55] Restenosis at the site of a previous percutaneous or vein patch angioplasty usually requires resection and interposition grafting or jump grafting.

The failed graft – graft thrombosis

Despite the use of surveillance programmes, a significant number of grafts will not be identified as failing and will instead present as thrombosed grafts. A number of

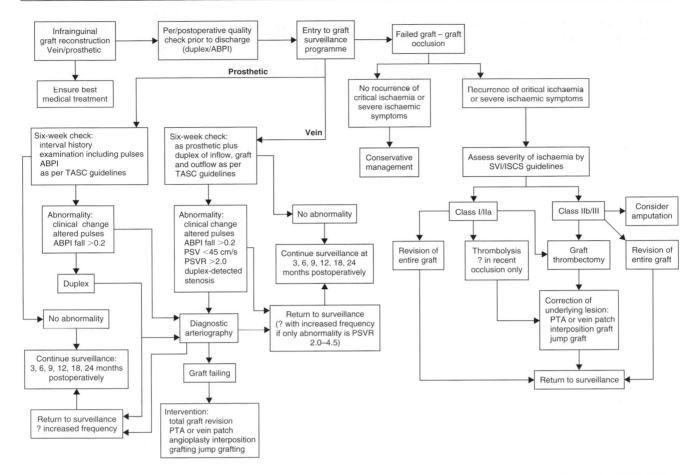

Figure 17.6 *Algorithm illustrating pathways of management. ABPI, ankle:brachial pressure index; PSV, peak systolic velocity; PSVR, PSV ratio; PTA, percutaneous transluminal angioplasty; SVI/ISCS, Society for Vascular Surgery/International Society of Cardiovascular Surgery; TASC, TransAtlantic inter-Society Consensus*

Table 17.2 *The Society for Vascular Surgery/International Society of Cardiovascular Surgery (SVS/ISCVS) grading system for limb ischaemia*

Class I	Viable. Not immediately threatened. Arterial Doppler signals audible, no sensory loss and no muscle weakness
Class IIa	Marginally threatened. Salvageable if promptly treated. Arterial Doppler signal often inaudible, minimal sensory loss and no muscle weakness
Class IIb	Immediately threatened. Salvageable with immediate revascularisation, arterial Doppler signal usually inaudible, sensory loss with rest pain in more than toes, mild to moderate muscle weakness
Class III	Irreversible. Major tissue loss or permanent nerve damage inevitable if there is significant delay before operation. Arterial and venous Doppler signal inaudible, profound limb anaesthesia and paralysis

considerations dictate the most appropriate management course. These include the nature of the symptoms exhibited by the patient, the severity of the ischaemia, the time from occlusion to presentation, and the time period since the original procedure.

Most patients presenting with an occluded bypass graft will require secondary intervention. A small number of grafts, however, do occlude asymptomatically due to the development of collaterals or healing of the tissue necrosis for which the original bypass was performed.[57] Such patients should not be subjected to further intervention. Furthermore, up to a quarter of patients who undergo surgery for critical limb ischaemia will have an effective functioning limb after occlusion, particularly if some time has elapsed since the original procedure.

Practically, where graft occlusion has occurred, the most vital initial assessment is that of the severity of ischaemia, and with it an assessment of the urgency of treatment (see Chapters 15 and 16). Although there is no substitute for experience in this situation, the Society for Vascular Surgery/International Society of Cardiovascular Surgery (SVS/ISCVS) grading system is accepted and is shown in Table 17.2.[58]

Those patients whose limbs exhibit Class II or worse ischaemia and hence require urgent intervention should be anticoagulated with heparin on presentation. The initial treatment options then rest between thrombolysis, usually with subsequent revision of any underlying lesion, and surgical revision.

Thrombolysis

It has been widely held that patients presenting with Class IIa ischaemia are suitable patients for thrombolysis; there is sufficient time to allow this, and a lesion may be unmasked which can be treated with limited intervention. The role of thrombolysis in the treatment of graft failure, however, requires closer scrutiny (see Chapter 16). Thrombolysis has a minimal role in graft occlusion[59] as it often unmasks a lesion requiring definitive treatment and hence merely delays an inevitable intervention.

At least four trials have failed to show any advantage to thrombolysis over surgery in the context of either acute lower limb ischaemia or an occluded bypass graft.[60–63] Thrombolysis however, has been shown to be more effective in terms of mortality and amputation where the occlusion is less than 14 days old.[60,63] The Surgery versus Thrombolysis for Ischemia of the Lower Extremity (STILE) trial[61] was a multicentre study randomising patients with acute lower limb ischaemia to treatment with surgery or one of two thrombolytic agents. Both vein and prosthetic bypass grafts were included. A disadvantage of the study was the use of a large number of clinical parameters to establish a primary endpoint. Overall there was a highly significant difference in favour of surgery, but subgroup analysis showed that, where the duration of ischaemia was less than 2 weeks, amputation rates were three times higher for surgery than for thrombolysis; after that period amputation rates were four times higher in the lytic group. STILE established surgery as a more effective and safer treatment than lytic therapy, and demonstrated that any benefit associated with thrombolysis is only gained if it is used within two weeks of the onset of symptoms.

The Thrombolysis Or Peripheral Arterial Surgery (TOPAS) study[60] demonstrated similar amputation and mortality rates at one year for thrombolysis and surgery. As with the STILE trial better results were claimed for graft occlusion than for native vessel occlusions. Furthermore, success was found to be predictable upon traversing the occlusion with a guidewire and lysis was more likely to be successful in prosthetic rather than vein grafts.

A recent four-centre study has questioned the justification for thrombolysis of occluded grafts having demonstrated a 20 per cent patency after thrombolysis.[64] Interestingly an additional procedure such as percutaneous or vein patch angioplasty appeared to make no difference to the patency rate. Table 17.3 shows guidelines with respect to thrombolysis in the presence of an occluded lower limb bypass graft.

Surgical intervention

Open surgical procedures form the basis for the traditional approach to graft occlusion. This tradition started in 1963 with the introduction of the Fogarty balloon embolectomy catheter and with it simple graft thrombectomy. It was

Table 17.3 *Guidelines for thrombolysis in the presence of an occluded lower limb bypass graft*

Thrombolysis may be considered as an option in those where bypass graft occlusion is a recent event, and where the limb is not immediately threatened

The intravenous route for the administration of high dose thrombolytic agents is associated with a high incidence of morbidity and mortality and should no longer be used

Where an intra-arterial infusion method is used there is still a significant morbidity and mortality

Adverse events include:

- Intracerebral bleeding (1.2–2.1 per cent in the STILE and TOPAS trials)
- Haematoma formation
- Distal embolisation
- Septicaemia
- Renal failure
- Pseudoaneurysm formation
- Angina
- Ulnar neuropathy

Where lysis is successful, adjuvant procedures are usually required to maintain patency. This may, however, be a lesser procedure than would otherwise be required

STILE, Surgery versus Thrombolysis for Ischaemia of the Lower Extremity;[61] TOPAS, Thrombolysis Or Peripheral Arterial Surgery.[60]

quickly realised however that this was usually unrewarding without the identification and correction of any underlying lesion.

Progression of native disease in either the inflow or outflow vessels is treated by angioplasty or bypass according to standard principles (see Chapter 16). Vein patch angioplasty was the initial favoured option where vein grafts develop discrete stenoses, but secondary patency rates below 25 per cent were reported[65,66] It is now accepted that secondary autogenous replacement of the graft gives the best results, with secondary patency rates in excess of 50 per cent reported.[67,68] Where localised problems are evident, such as a short discrete stenosis or a valve cusp stenosis, open repair is acceptable and yields better patency rates than dilatation.[9] Involvement of the distal anastomosis, or extension of native vessel disease, may require extension of the bypass graft. This is especially true where PTFE grafts develop distal anastomotic strictures as these lesions are less amenable to balloon dilatation. In treating graft failure, the recommendation of the TASC group should be considered, namely that, after the relief of acute limb ischaemia and the establishment of its aetiology, the choice of treatment of the underlying lesion should be similar to the treatment choice in the setting of chronic limb ischaemia and not linked to the method of clot removal.[55] It has certainly been shown that a pragmatic approach, where the revision strategy favours vein patch angioplasty for graft body lesions and jump grafts for distal anastomotic lesions, yields acceptable assisted primary patency rates.[69]

POSTOPERATIVE CARE

Immediate postoperative care does not differ substantively from those patients who are undergoing primary arterial reconstruction. Nevertheless, two points that have already been made are worth reiterating. First, all patients at the time of operation, and preferably considerably before, should be receiving best medical therapy to address smoking, hypertension, diabetes, hypercholesterolaemia, hyperhomocysteinaemia and cardiac failure and all should be receiving antiplatelet medication. Second, prior to discharge, all patients should undergo investigation to ensure that the haemodynamic integrity of the affected limb has been restored; ideally all patients should undergo postoperative duplex scanning, although in practice ABPI improvement may be considered sufficient.

The failed revascularisation

In many cases a failed attempt at graft salvage will lead inevitably to amputation (see Chapter 2). There is evidence, however, that a small number of patients with critical limb ischaemia following a failed revision will benefit from non-surgical treatments.

Iloprost, an extensively studied stable analogue of prostacyclin, has been shown to have beneficial effects on mortality and limb salvage at 3–6 months in three trials.[70–72] Its effects include prevention of platelet and leucocyte activation and vasodilatation, hence it works at a microcirculatory level. The administration regimens are all labour intensive and costly, requiring intravenous administration of iloprost for between 2 and 4 weeks. Patients receiving iloprost, however, were significantly more likely to be alive and to have avoided major amputation during the follow-up period than those having placebo, with a 16 per cent and 20 per cent risk reduction, respectively. Side effects may limit the efficacy of iloprost with flushing, headache, nausea, abdominal pain, hypotension and angina being reported. It does seem reasonable given the current evidence to consider the use of iloprost where surgery has failed or is not feasible, and the alternative would be amputation. Trials on a recently developed oral form of iloprost are awaited and, if successful, may have a profound effect upon the use of this therapy. A number of other agents have undergone trial in the treatment of critical ischaemia but are of little or no proven benefit. These include heparin, defibrinating agents, L-arginine, pentoxifylline and naftidrofuryl.

An exciting new approach to the problem is that of therapeutic angiogenesis which represents the clinical use of growth factors to enhance or promote the development of collateral blood vessels in ischaemic tissue.[73] Vascular endothelial growth factor (VEGF) is an angiogenic growth factor existing in four isoforms which vary in permeability and heparin binding properties.[74] It stimulates the growth, proliferation and migration of endothelial cells by binding to receptors; physiological effects include enhanced vascular permeability and vasodilatation. Growth factor and growth factor receptor expression is upregulated by hypoxia and ischaemia, thus allowing a targeted response and limiting pathological angiogenesis.

Recent studies have shown that recombinant angiogenic growth factors augment collateral development in animal models of hind limb ischaemia.[75] It has also been shown that VEGF can be used in an animal model to successfully modulate the disturbed endothelium dependent blood flow in the arterial circulation supplied by collateral vessels, thus implying a physiological as well as an anatomical advantage.[75] In a rabbit model of ischaemic hind limb the administration of VEGF caused a significant reduction in the haemodynamic deficit of the limb at 7 days and had positive effects upon both smooth muscle cell and endothelial cell proliferation.[76] This supports the concept that cellular augmentation contributes to enhanced collateral formation when therapeutic angiogenesis is employed.

Vascular endothelial growth factor is effective following direct gene transfer. In a rat model, ischaemia was induced followed by transfection of the plasmid encoding VEGF into the ischaemic limbs .[77] Gene transfer produced a significantly more extensive, though morphologically similar, pattern of collaterals to that seen in control limbs. A similar effect was seen when plasmid encoding each of the three main human VEGF isoforms was delivered on angioplasty balloons to the ischaemic hind legs of rabbits[78] and it thus appears that the transfer of naked DNA encoding a secreted cytokine is an alternative to the administration of recombinant protein in therapeutic angiogenesis. Striated muscle is capable of taking up and expressing foreign genes transferred in the form of naked plasmid DNA, albeit with low levels of gene expression. The efficacy of this technique when applied to VEGF augmented collateral development in the ischaemic limb has been shown[79] and intramuscular transfection of genes encoding angiogenic factors is an exciting prospect in those with peripheral vascular disease. Trials utilising this method of transfection have been performed with very small numbers of patients.[80] These appear to support the hypothesis that intramuscular injection of naked plasmid DNA leads to constitutive overexpression of VEGF sufficient to induce therapeutic angiogenesis in selected patients with critical limb ischaemia. Phase I trials with intravenous VEGF have been completed, but the results have not yet been published. Although it is notable that no pharmacological intervention shown to be successful in the laboratory or in animal models has subsequently been shown to be effective in humans, the recent dramatic increase in the number of trials of tissue angiogenesis reflects the success of the preclinical models and the favourable early clinical results.

The successful revascularisation

There is little available at present, besides that already mentioned, to augment a technically adequate revascularisation

Table 17.4   *Published primary, primary assisted and secondary patency rates following infrainguinal bypass surgery*

Authors	Year	Number of grafts	Nature of grafts	Follow-up (months)	Primary patency (per cent)	Primary assisted patency (per cent)	Secondary patency (per cent)	Limb salvage (per cent)
Shah *et al.*[91]	1995	2058	*In situ* vein	60			81	95
				120			70	90
Byrne *et al.*[92]	1999	165	Above-knee, popliteal – vein	48	62		64	
		150	Below-knee, popliteal – vein	48	77		81	
		94	Tibial – vein	48	86	82	90	
Eugster *et al.*[93]	2001	280	Infrainguinal non-reversed vein	60	63	85		
		107	Infrainguinal *in situ* vein	60	58	83		
Jamsen *et al.*[94]	2001	263	Femoropopliteal/distal	12	70	63		82
		263	Femoropopliteal/distal	60	52	65		77
Ihlberg *et al.*[39]	1998	185	Infrainguinal vein – duplex surveillance	12		74	71	81
			Infrainguinal vein – ABPI surveillance	12			84	88
Belkin *et al.*[95]	1996	189	Infrainguinal non-reversed vein	60	65		74	82
		568	Infrainguinal *in situ* vein	60	72		82	90

ABPI, ankle: brachial pressure index.

operation. Two very different interventions may however offer hope in future for improving graft patency where vein has been used.

It has been shown previously that the long term adaptation of vein to the arterial circulation can be modified by external stenting. Kohler *et al.*[81] postulated that wall stress regulates wall structure as vein graft thickening stops when the ratio of lumen radius to wall thickness equals that of a normal artery.[82] They found that, in rabbits, restrictive external support of vein grafts caused reduction of the wall area. Angelini *et al.*,[83] however, proposed that restrictive stenting, while reducing medial thickening, promoted neointimal thickening, thus leading to a reduction, not increase, in final luminal diameter. This may be due to reduced fluid flux around the graft, or vessel wall hypoxia due to adventitial disruption.[84] They therefore used a non-restrictive and porous external stent in a pig model of arteriovenous bypass grafting to reduce tangential wall stress, and found a dramatic decrease in both medial thickening and neointimal hyperplasia 4 weeks after implantation. The degree of oversize of the stent appears not to be important.[85] Subsequent work suggested a role for prostacyclin (PG12) and nitric oxide in promoting microangiogenesis in the adventitia of stented grafts, which may limit graft hypoxia.[86] Notably, stenting also seemed to result in a significant reduction in the expression of platelet derived growth factor (PDGF) by the graft .[87] Most recently, external stenting in a rat model has been shown to limit intimal hyperplasia and cellular proliferation, with the conclusion that external stenting will reduce atherosclerotic change in

arterialised vein and thus improve the patency of vein grafts.[88]

Finally, there may be a role for gene therapy in the reduction of intimal hyperplasia in bypass grafts. Vein grafts are well suited for gene therapy as there is direct access to the graft during vein preparation. Recent advances include adeno-associated and modifed adenovirus gene transfer, allowing prolonged expression *in vivo*. Targets for gene transfer have included tissue plasminogen activator, prostacyclin synthase and tissue inhibitors of metalloproteinases.[89] One example of such work has used an organ culture of human vein to demonstrate reduced intimal hyperplasia following adenovirus mediated transfer of nitric oxide synthase.[90]

RESULTS

Examples of published primary, primary assisted and secondary patency rates following infrainguinal arterial reconstruction are shown in Table 17.4, where available limb salvage rates are also shown.

Conclusions

The graft failure rate following infrainguinal reconstruction remains high and the consequences potentially serious both for the patient and financially. Graft revision surgery can be technically demanding. Prior to any intervention the most meticulous attention must be paid to both the overall condition of the patient and to the degree of ischaemia of the affected limb. Within the constraints of urgency, vigorous attempts to gain as much anatomical and haemodynamic information as possible must be made. Despite these measures, many revascularisations will fail. It remains to be seen whether the newer therapies currently in the experimental stage discussed above will lead to improved limb salvage rates, even when reintervention has not been successful.

Key references

Davies MG, Hagen PO. Pathobiology of intimal hyperplasia. *Br J Surg* 1994; **81**: 1254–69.

Ihlberg L, Luther M, Tierala E, Lapantalo M. The utility of duplex scanning in infrainguinal vein graft surveillance: results from a randomised controlled study. *Eur J Vasc Endovasc Surg* 1998; **16**: 19–27.

Ouriel K, Veith FJ, Sasahara AA. Thrombolysis or peripheral arterial surgery (TOPAS): Phase I results. TOPAS Investigators. *J Vasc Surg* 1996; **23**: 64–75.

Results of a prospective randomised trial evaluating surgery versus thrombolysis for ischemia of the lower extremity. The STILE trial. *Ann Surg* 1994; **220**: 251–68.

Szilagyi DE, Elliot JP, Hageman JH, *et al.* Biologic fate of autogenous vein implants as arterial substitutes – clinical, angiographic and histologic observations in femoro-popliteal operations for atherosclerosis. *Ann Surg* 1973; **178**: 232–46.

REFERENCES

1   Szilagyi DE, Elliot JP, Hageman JH, *et al.* Biologic fate of autogenous vein implants as arterial substitutes – clinical, angiographic and histologic observations in femoro-popliteal operations for atherosclerosis. *Ann Surg* 1973; **178**: 232–46.

2   Mamode N, Scott RN. Graft type for femoro-popliteal bypass surgery. *Cochrane Database Syst Rev* 2000; **2**: CD001487.

3   Englund R, Harris J, May J. Factors affecting the outcome of 463 femorotibial reconstructions. *Aust N Z J Surg* 1988; **58**: 279–83.

4   Luther M, Lepantalo M. Femorotibial reconstructions for chronic critical leg ischaemia: influence on outcome by diabetes, gender and age. *Eur J Vasc Endovasc Surg* 1997; **13**: 569–77.

5   Idu MM, Buth J, Hop WC, *et al.* Factors influencing the development of vein graft stenosis and their significance for clinical management. *Eur J Vasc Endovasc Surg* 1999; **17**: 15–21.

6   Brewster DC, Lasalle AJ, Robinson JG, *et al.* Femoropopliteal graft failures: Clinical consequences of success of secondary reconstructions. *Arch Surg* 1983; **118**: 1043–7.

7   Avino AJ, Bandyk DF, Gonsalves AJ, *et al.* Surgical and endovascular intervention for infrainguinal vein graft stenosis. *J Vasc Surg* 1999; **29**: 60–70.

8   Berkowitz HD, Fox AD, Deaton DH. Reversed vein graft stenosis: early diagnosis and management. *J Vasc Surg* 1992; **15**: 130–42.

9   Nehler MR, Moneta GL, Yeager RA, *et al.* Surgical treatment of threatened reversed infrainguinal vein grafts. *J Vasc Surg* 1994; **20**: 558–63.

10 Robinson KD, Sato DT, Gregory RT, *et al.* Long-term outcome after early infrainguinal graft failure. *J Vasc Surg* 1997; **26**: 425–37.

11 Bartlett ST, Olinde AJ, Flinn WR, *et al.* The reoperative potential of infrainguinal bypass: long-term limb and patient survival. *J Vasc Surg* 1997; **5**: 170–9.

12 Belkin M, Donaldson MC, Whittemore AD, *et al.* Observations on the use of thrombolytic agents for thrombotic occlusion of infrainguinal vein grafts. *J Vasc Surg* 1990; **11**: 289–94.

13 Budd JS, Brennan J, Beard JD, *et al.* Infra-inguinal bypass surgery; Factors determining late graft patency. *Br J Surg* 1990; **77**: 1382–7.

14 Taylor RS, McFarland RJ, Cox MI. An investigation into the causes of failure of PTFE grafts. *Eur J Vasc Surg* 1987; **1**: 335–43.

15 Stept LL, Flinn WR, McCarthy WJ, *et al.* Technical defects as a cause of early graft failure after femorodistal bypass surgery. *Arch Surg* 1987; **122**: 599–604.

16 Kehler M, Albrechtsson U, Alwmark A, *et al.* Intra-operative digital angiography as a control of the *in-situ* saphenous vein bypass graft. *Acta Radiol* 1988; **29**: 645–8.

17 Robicsek F, Thubrikar MJ, Fokin A, *et al.* Pressure traps in femoro-popliteal reversed vein grafts. Are valves culprits? *J Cardiovasc Surg (Torino)* 1999; **40**: 683–9.

18 Gannon MX, Goldman MD, Simms MH, *et al.* Peri-operative complications of *in-situ* vein bypass. *Ann R Coll Surg Engl* 1987; **74**: 252–5.

19 Szilagyi DE, Hageman JH, Smith RF, *et al.* Autogenous vein grafting in femoropopliteal atherosclerosis: the limit of its effectiveness. *Surgery* 1979; **86**: 836–51.

20 Davies MG, Hagen PO. Pathobiology of intimal hyperplasia. *Br J Surg* 1994; **81**: 1254–69.

21 Currie IC, Wilson YG, Davies AH, *et al.* Pulse generated run-off versus dependent Doppler ultrasonography for assessment of calf vessel patency. *Br J Surg* 1994; **81**: 1448–50.

22 Kupinsky AM, Evans JM, Khan AM, *et al.* Ultrasonic characteristics of the saphenous vein. *Cardiovasc Surg* 1993; **1**: 513–17.

23 Katz ML, Pilla TS, Comerota AJ. Technical aspects of venous duplex imaging. *J Vasc Technol* 1988; **12**: 100–2.

24 Seeger JM, Schmidt JH, Flynn TC. Preoperative saphenous and cephalic vein mapping as an adjunct to reconstructive arterial surgery. *Ann Surg* 1987; **205**: 733–9.

25 Leopold PW, Shandall AA, Corson JD, *et al.* Initial experience comparing B-mode imaging and venography of the saphenous vein before *in-situ* bypass. *Am J Surg* 1986; **152**: 206–10.

26 Panetta TF, Marin ML, Veith FJ, *et al.* Unsuspected pre-existing saphenous vein disease: an unrecognised cause of vein bypass failure. *J Vasc Surg* 1992; **15**: 102–12.

27 Davies AH. Vein factors that affect the outcome of femorodistal bypass. *Ann R Coll Surg Engl* 1995; **77**: 63–66.

28 Beattie DK, Sian M, Greenhalgh RM, Davies AH. Influence of systemic factors on pre-existing intimal hyperplasia and their effect on the outcome of infrainguinal arterial reconstruction with vein. *Br J Surg* 1999; **86**: 1441–7.

29 Davies AH, Magee TR, Baird RN, *et al.* Vein compliance: a pre-operative indicator of vein morphology and of veins at risk of vascular graft stenosis. *Br J Surg* 1992; **79**: 1019–21.

30 Davies AH, Magee TR, Sheffield E, *et al.* The aetiology of vein graft stenoses. *Eur J Vasc Surg* 1994; **8**: 389–94.

31 Golledge J, Beattie DK, Greenhalgh RM, Davies AH. Have the results of infrainguinal bypass improved with the widespread

utilisation of postoperative surveillance? *Eur J Vasc Endovasc Surg* 1996; **11**: 388–92.

32 Barnes RW, Thompson BW, MacDonald CM, *et al.* Serial non-invasive studies do not herald post-operative failure of femoropopliteal or femorotibial bypass grafts. *Ann Surg* 1989; **210**: 486–93.

33 Laborde AL, Synn AY, Worsey MJ, *et al.* A prospective comparison of ankle/brachial indices and colour duplex imaging in surveillance of the *in situ* saphenous vein bypass. *J Cardiovasc Surg* 1992; **33**: 420–5.

34 Tong Y, Somjen G, Teeuwsen W, Royle JP. Percutaneous transluminal angioplasty: follow-up with treadmill exercise testing. *Cardiovasc Surg* 1994: **2**: 503–7.

35 Wilson YG, Davies AH, Currie IC, *et al.* Vein graft stenosis; incidence and intervention. *Eur J Vasc Endovasc Surg* 1996; **11**: 164–9.

36 Moody P, DeCossart LM, Douglas HM, Harris PL. Asymptomatic strictures in femoropopliteal vein grafts. *Eur J Vasc Surg* 1989; **3**: 389–92.

37 Mattos MA, Van Bremmelen PS, Hodgson KJ, *et al.* Does correction of stenoses identified with colour duplex scanning improve infrainguinal graft patency? *J Vasc Surg* 1993; **17**: 54–66.

38 Ihlberg L, Luther M, Alback A, *et al.* Does a completely accomplished duplex-based surveillance programme prevent vein-graft failure? *Eur J Vasc Endovasc Surg* 1999; **18**: 395–400.

39 Ihlberg L, Luther M, Tierala E, Lapantalo M. The utility of duplex scanning in infrainguinal vein graft surveillance: results from a randomised controlled study. *Eur J Vasc Endovasc Surg* 1998; **16**: 19–27.

40 Dougherty MJ, Calligaro KD, DeLaurentis DA. Revision of failing lower extremity bypass grafts. *Am J Surg* 1998; **176**: 126–30.

41 Dunlop P, Sayers RD, Naylor AR, *et al.* The effect of a surveillance programme on the patency of synthetic infrainguinal bypass grafts. *Eur J Vasc Endovasc Surg* 1996; **11**: 441–5.

42 Kirby PL, Brady AR, Thompson SG, *et al.* The vein graft surveillance trial: rationale, design and methods. VGST participants. *Eur J Vasc Endovasc Surg* 1999; **18**: 469–74.

43 Buth J, Disselhoff B, Sommeling C, Stam L. Color-flow duplex criteria for grading stenosis in infrainguinal vein grafts. *J Vasc Surg* 1991; **14**: 716–28.

44 Ihlberg L, Alback A, Roth WD, *et al.* Interobserver agreement in duplex scanning for vein grafts. *Eur J Vasc Endovasc Surg* 2000; **19**: 504–8.

45 Olojugba DH, McCarthy MJ, Naylor AR, *et al.* At what peak velocity ratio should duplex-detected vein graft stenoses be revised? *Eur J Vasc Endovasc Surg* 1998; **15**: 258–60.

46 Dougherty MJ, Calligaro KD, DeLaurentis DA. The natural history of 'failing' arterial bypass grafts in a duplex surveillance protocol. *Ann Vasc Surg* 1998; **12**: 255–9.

47 Dougherty MJ, Calligaro KD, DeLaurentis DA. Revision of failing lower extremity bypass grafts. *Am J Surg* 1998; **176**: 126–30.

48 Treiman GS, Lawrence PF, Bhirangi K, Gazak CE. Effect of outflow level and maximum graft diameter on the velocity parameters of reversed vein bypass grafts. *J Vasc Surg* 1999; **30**: 16–25.

49 Lundell A, Lindblad B, Bergqvist D, Hansen F. Femoropopliteal-crural graft patency is improved by an intensive graft surveillance programme: a prospective randomised study. *J Vasc Surg* 1995; **21**: 26–34.

50 McCarthy MJ, Olojugba D, Loftus IM, *et al.* Lower limb surveillance following autologous vein bypass should be life long. *Br J Surg* 1998; **85**: 1369–72.

51 Mills JL, Bandyk DF, Gahtan V, Esses G. The origin of infrainguinal vein graft stenosis: a prospective randomised trial based on duplex surveillance. *J Vasc Surg* 1995; **21**: 16–25.

52 Idu MM, Buth J, Cuypers P, *et al.* Economising vein-graft surveillance programmes. *Eur J Vasc Endovasc Surg* 1998; **15**: 432–8.

53 Loftus IM, Reid A, Thompson MM, *et al.* The increasing workload required to maintain infra inguinal graft patency. *Eur J Vasc Endovasc Surg* 1998; **15**: 37–41.

54 Wixon CL, Mills JL, Westerband A, *et al.* An economic appraisal of lower extremity bypass graft maintenance. *J Vasc Surg* 2000; **32**: 1–12.

55 TASC Working Group. Management of peripheral arterial disease. TransAtlantic Inter-Society Consensus. *Eur J Vasc Endovasc Surg* 2000; **19**(suppl A): S217–218.

56 Tonnesen KH, Holstein P, Rordam L, *et al.* Early results of percutaneous transluminal angioplasty of failing below-knee bypass grafts. *Eur J Vasc Endovasc Surg* 1998; **15**: 51–6.

57 Brewster DC, Lasalle AJ, Robinson JG, *et al.* Femoropopliteal graft failures: clinical consequences of success of secondary reconstructions. *Arch Surg* 1983; **118**: 1043–7.

58 Rutherford RB, Baker JD, Ernst C, *et al.* Recommended standards for reports dealing with lower extremity ischaemia: revised version. *J Vasc Surg* 1997; **26**: 517–38.

59 Lacroix H, Suy R, Nevelsteen A, *et al.* Local thrombolysis for occluded arterial grafts: is the yield worth the effort? *J Cardiovasc Surg* 1994; **35**: 187–91.

60 Ouriel K, Veith FJ, Sasahara AA. Thrombolysis or peripheral arterial surgery (TOPAS): Phase I results. TOPAS Investigators. *J Vasc Surg* 1996; **23**: 64–75.

61 Results of a prospective randomised trial evaluating surgery versus thrombolysis for ischemia of the lower extremity. The STILE trial. *Ann Surg* 1994; **220**: 251–68.

62 Ouriel K, Shortell CK, DeWeese JA, *et al.* A comparison of thrombolytic therapy with operative revascularisation in the initial treatment of acute peripheral arterial ischaemia. *J Vasc Surg* 1994; **19**: 1021–30.

63 Comerota AJ, Weaver FA, Hosking JD, *et al.* Results of a prospective randomised trial of surgery versus thrombolysis for occluded lower extremity bypass grafts. *Am J Surg* 1996; **172**: 105–12.

64 Galland RB, Magee TR, Whitman B, *et al.* Patency following successful thrombolysis of occluded vascular grafts. *Eur J Vasc Endovasc Surg* 2001; **22**: 157–60.

65 Whittemore AD, Clowes AW, Couch NP, Mannick JA. Secondary femoropopliteal reconstruction. *Ann Surg* 1981; **193**: 35–42.

66 Cohen JR, Mannick JA, Couch NP, Whittemore AD. Recognition and management of impending vein graft failure. *Ann Surg* 1986; **121**: 758–9.

67 DeWeese JA, Leather R, Porter J. Practical guidelines: lower extremity revascularisation. *J Vasc Surg* 1993; **18**: 280–94.

68 Belkin M, Conte MS, Donaldson MC. Preferred strategies for secondary infrainguinal bypass: lessons learned from 300 consecutive operations. *J Vasc Surg* 1995; **21**: 282–95.

69 Sullivan TR, Welch HJ, Iafrati MD, *et al.* Clinical results of common strategies used to revise infrainguinal vein grafts. *J Vasc Surg* 1996; **24**: 909–17.

70 Norgren L, Alwmark A, Angqvist KA, *et al.* A stable prostacyclin analogue (iloprost) in the treatment of ischaemic ulcers of the

lower limb. A Scandinavian-Polish placebo controlled, randomised multicentre study. *Eur J Vasc Surg* 1990; **4**: 463–7.

71 UK Severe Limb ischaemia Study Group. Treatment of limb threatening ischaemia with intravenous iloprost: a randomised double blind placebo controlled study. *Eur J Vasc Surg* 1991; **5**: 511–16.

72 Guilmot JL, Diot E. Treatment of lower limb ischaemia due to atherosclerosis in diabetic and non -diabetic patients with iloprost, a stable analogue of prostacyclin. *Drug Invest* 1991; **3**: 351–9.

73 Henry TD. Therapeutic angiogenesis. *BMJ* 1999; **318**: 1536–9.

74 Ferrara N, Davis-Smyth T. The biology of vascular endothelial growth factor. *Endocri Rev* 1997; **18**: 1–22.

75 Bauters C, Asahara T, Zheng LP, *et al.* Recovery of disturbed endothelium-dependent flow in the collateral-perfused rabbit ischemic hindlimb after administration of vascular endothelial growth factor. *Circulation* 1995; **91**: 2802–9.

76 Takeshita S, Rossow ST, Kearney M, *et al.* Time course on increased cellular proliferation in collateral arteries after administration of vascular endothelial growth factor in a rabbit model of lower limb vascular insufficiency. *Am J Pathol* 1995; **147**: 1649–60.

77 Takeshita S, Isshiki T, Mori H, *et al.* Microangiographic assessment of collateral vessel formation following direct gene transfer of vascular endothelial growth factor in rats. *Cardiovasc Res* 1997; **35**: 547–52.

78 Takeshita S, Tsurumi Y, Couffinahl T, *et al.* Gene transfer of naked DNA encoding for three isoforms of vascular endothelial growth factor stimulates collateral development *in vivo. Lab Invest* 1996; **75**: 487–501.

79 Tsurumi Y, Takeshita S, Chen D, *et al.* Direct intramuscular gene transfer of naked DNA encoding vascular endothelial growth factor augments collateral development and tissue perfusion. *Circulation* 1996; **94**: 3281–90.

80 Baumgartner I, Pieczek A, Manor O, *et al.* Constitutive expression of phVEGF165 after intramuscular gene transfer promotes collateral vessel development in patients with critical limb ischaemia. *Circulation* 1998; **97**: 1114–23.

81 Kohler TR, Kirkman TR, Clowes AW. The effect of rigid external support on vein graft adaptation to the arterial circulation. *J Vasc Surg* 1989; **9**: 277–85.

82 Zwolak RM, Adams MC, Clowes AW. Kinetics of vein graft hyperplasia: association with tangential stress. *J Vasc Surg* 1987; **5**: 126–36.

83 Angelini GD, Izzat MB, Bryan AJ, Newby AC. External stenting reduces early medial and neointimal thickening in a pig model of arteriovenous bypass grafting. *J Thorac Cardiovasc Surg* 1996; **112**: 79–84.

84 Barker SGE, Talbert A, Cottam S, *et al.* Arterial intimal hyperplasia after occlusion of the adventitial vasa vasorum in the pig. *Arterioscler Thromb* 1993; **13**: 70–7.

85 Izzat MB, Mehta D, Bryan AJ, *et al.* Influence of external stent size on early medial and neointimal thickening in a pig model of saphenous vein bypass grafting. *Circulation* 1996; **94**: 1741–5.

86 Jeremy JY, Dashwood MR, Mehta D, *et al.* Nitric oxide, prostacyclin and cyclic nucleotide formation in externally stented porcine vein grafts. *Atherosclerosis* 1998; **141**: 297–305.

87 Mehta D, George SJ, Jeremy JY, *et al.* External stenting reduces long-term medial and neointimal thickening and platelet derived growth factor expression in a pig model of arteriovenous bypass grafting. *Nat Med* 1998; **4**: 235–9.

88 Meguro T, Nakashima H, Kawada S, *et al.* Effects of external stenting and systemic hypertension on intimal hyperplasia in vein grafts. *Neurosurgery* 2000; **46**: 963–9.

89 Newby AC, Baker AH. Targets for gene therapy of vein grafts. *Curr Opin Cardiol* 1999; **14**: 489–94.

90 Cable DG, Caccitolo JA, Caplice N, *et al.* The role of gene therapy for intimal hyperplasia of bypass grafts. *Circulation* 1999; **100**(19 suppl): II392–6.

91 Shah DM, Darling RC, Chang BB, *et al.* Long term results of *in situ* saphenous vein bypass. Analysis of 2058 cases. *Ann Surg* 1995; **222**: 438–46.

92 Byrne J, Darling RC, Chang BB, *et al.* Vascular surgical society of Great Britain and Ireland: review of 94 tibial bypasses for intermittent claudication. *Br J Surg* 1999; **86**: 706–7.

93 Eugster T, Stierli P, Aeberhard P. Infrainguinal arterial reconstruction with autogenous vein grafts: are the results for the *in situ* technique better than those of non-reversed bypass? A long-term follow-up study. *J Cardiovasc Surg (Torino)* 2001; **42**: 221–6.

94 Jamsen T, Tulla H, Manninen H, *et al.* Results of infrainguinal bypass surgery: an analysis of 263 consecutive operations. *Ann Chir Gynaecol* 2001; **90**: 92–9.

95 Belkin M, Knox J, Donaldson MC, *et al.* Infrainguinal arterial reconstruction with nonreversed greater saphenous vein. *J Vasc Surg* 1996; **24**: 957–62.

18

Acute Ischaemia Secondary to Occult Prosthetic Graft Infection

LINDA M REILLY

THE PROBLEM

The principles of treatment of prosthetic graft infection are straightforward: eliminate the infection while preserving perfusion to the vascular bed supplied by the infected graft. Two circumstances, however, pose significant challenges to successful treatment, namely, associated bleeding and associated ischaemia. In each case the urgency of the associated condition imposes an immediacy which may limit the options for evaluation, preparation and treatment, as well as have an adverse impact on outcome.

EPIDEMIOLOGY

While prosthetic vascular graft infection occurs in 2–4 per cent of patients[1–3] it is an uncommon cause of acute limb ischaemia. In our experience and that of others, less than 10 per cent of patients with graft infection present with graft or graft limb occlusion.[4,5] While the incidence of graft infection among all patients presenting with graft or graft limb occlusion is unknown, clearly most of these occlusions result from haemodynamic causes and not from underlying graft infection.

In most cases of graft occlusion and associated infection of the prosthesis, graft infection is occult and the ischaemia is not limb threatening. It is less likely for the infection to be evident or for the ischaemia to limb threatening. As the usual clinical setting is one of graft occlusion without any clinical evidence to suggest an infection, the vascular surgeon usually discovers the infection incidentally during treatment focused on relieving ischaemia. The challenge presented to the vascular surgeon, therefore, is the management of occult graft infection discovered during the treatment of graft or graft limb occlusion.

DIAGNOSIS

As mentioned, these patients usually lack the clinical signs and symptoms associated with vascular graft infection, namely, fever, malaise, persistent/recurrent wound fluid collection, cellulitis, drainage, chronic sinus tract or septicaemia.[6] The detected abnormalities, such as elevated white blood cell count and elevated sedimentation rate, are mild and quite reasonably attributed to the physiological effects of the ischaemia. The suspicion of a possible graft infection is first aroused by the intraoperative findings at exploration to treat the ischaemia. Typically, these include a lack of graft incorporation by the surrounding tissue, the presence of perigraft fluid, especially if within the perigraft capsule and white blood cells on Gram stain of that fluid. It is rare to see organisms on Gram stain of the fluid, but if found they are pathognomonic of graft infection. The standard approaches to the diagnosis of graft infection using imaging studies, nuclear medicine scans, aspiration of perigraft fluid or sinus tract injection will not have been applied in the setting of an occult graft infection.

BACTERIOLOGY

The absence of organisms on Gram stain and the common finding of no growth on subsequent cultures is consistent with the low virulence of the most common causative organism, *Staphylococcus epidermidis*.[7] Central to the pathogenesis of this organism is the production of a polysaccharide biofilm, commonly referred to as 'slime', which allows the *S. epidermidis* organisms to adhere to the surface and the interstices of the graft material in a protected environment which white cells, antibodies and antibiotics have difficulty penetrating effectively. The resultant tissue destruction is relatively confined to the perigraft area and produces a muted host response. It is this limited pathogenicity which allows the graft infection to remain occult, pursuing a chronic, indolent course over many months or years. Although there are no specific data regarding the bacteriology of occult graft infections presenting with graft or graft limb occlusion, in comparison to those in other manifestations of graft infection, infection is less likely to be occult when it results from more virulent organisms such as *Staphylococcus aureus* and Gram-negative organisms. The latter bacteria are more likely to cause significant tissue destruction resulting in a more obvious host response, manifesting itself as cellulitis, abscess, anastomotic disruption with either false aneurysm formation or actual bleeding.

MANAGEMENT

In general, the management of a patient with a graft infection requires evidence of that infection, definition of relevant arterial anatomy, determination of the extent of involvement of the graft by infection, and then selection of the best approach to treatment (Fig. 18.1). In the specific clinical situation where the patient presents with graft thrombosis, however, that approach will be determined by the severity of tissue ischaemia, the level of suspicion, if any, of an underlying graft infection, the infecting organism, once it has been identified, and the patient's associated comorbidities.

Factors determining approach

- Severity of tissue ischaemia
- Level of suspicion of infection
- Infecting organism
- Associated comorbidities

As the presenting feature in these patients is ischaemia, anticoagulation should be initiated promptly. In addition, antibiotics should be administered, not because of any suspicion of underlying graft infection, but in anticipation of invasive intervention. The antibiotic selected should have a spectrum of activity, which at the least, includes skin organisms. If tissue ischaemia is extensive, for example affecting both lower extremities or if it is advanced, i.e. present for some time, and especially with associated neuro-muscular deficit, then renal protection against myoglobin damage should be initiated by means of hydration and alkalinisation of the urine with a continuous infusion of bicarbonate. With extensive or advanced ischaemia the patient will also need volume resuscitation to correct the considerable sequestration of fluid accompanying this event. Renal protection is particularly important because administration of intravenous contrast will almost certainly be necessary at some point in evaluation and management of the patient. Electrolyte abnormalities should also be corrected. These basic elements of treatment must be accomplished expeditiously and should not delay rapid intervention to correct the ischaemia.

Initial management

- Anticoagulant treatment
- Antibiotic therapy
- Renal protection
  - hydration
  - alkalinisation of the urine
  - against intravenous contrast
- Volume resuscitation
- Correction of electrolyte abnormalities
- Intervention to correct ischaemia

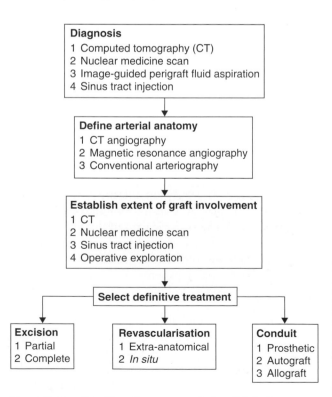

Figure 18.1 *Algorithm of management of graft infection*

Graft occlusion with occult infection

In the most common clinical setting, namely, graft occlusion with no clinical evidence or suspicion of graft infection, the vascular surgeon will be concentrating on treating the ischaemia. Therefore, the treatment chosen will be determined by the severity of the ischaemia (Fig. 18.2). If the patient has mild or moderate ischaemia, with no associated neuromuscular deficit, or at most a very mild sensory deficit, then either thrombolysis or thrombectomy are appropriate treatment options. The vascular anatomy can be defined by contrast arteriography performed just prior to initiating thrombolysis or performing thrombectomy, although complete definition of the anatomy may not be possible in the very poorly perfused ischaemic bed. Thrombolysis, if effective, has the potential benefit of averting an open procedure especially if extensive or even multiple procedures might have been necessary. Some consideration, however, should be given to the possibility that thrombolysis may increase the embolic potential of a pseudointima already destabilised by graft infection.[6] Embolisation of contents from an infected, occluded graft may create extensive soft tissue infection and destruction leading to limb loss. In those even rarer circumstances when the graft infection has presented with septic emboli at the time of occlusion, thrombolysis is contraindicated. Thrombolysis is obviously not advisable in the setting of advanced ischemia because of the associated delay in achieving reperfusion.

A particular risk of thrombolysis in this setting is the limited opportunity to diagnose graft infection. Occasionally, perigraft fluid will be detected during puncture of the graft to establish access for thrombolysis. If that does not occur, however, and if lysis is successful in restoring perfusion, and the lesion(s) responsible for the graft occlusion is(are) then managed endoluminally, it is likely that the graft infection will go undiagnosed. This is of particular concern if endoluminal treatment involves placing stents or stent-grafts through a graft in which infection is present but has not been recognised. The potential for contaminating the new endoprosthesis and for spreading the infection to other previously uninvolved areas of the graft or arterial tree is an alarming prospect. One approach, which would prevent such a missed diagnosis and would have no impact on the risk of spreading infection, is to define the arterial anatomy at the conclusion of successful thrombolysis and endoluminal treatment using fine-cut computed tomography (CT) with three-dimensional arterial reconstruction. This will demonstrate the perigraft soft tissue and detect any of the typical abnormalities associated with graft infection, i.e. perigraft fluid, air, indistinct tissue planes, abscess or false aneurysm. Artefacts from endoluminal prostheses, however, can make interpretation of the study difficult. If thrombolysis is unsuccessful or if treatment

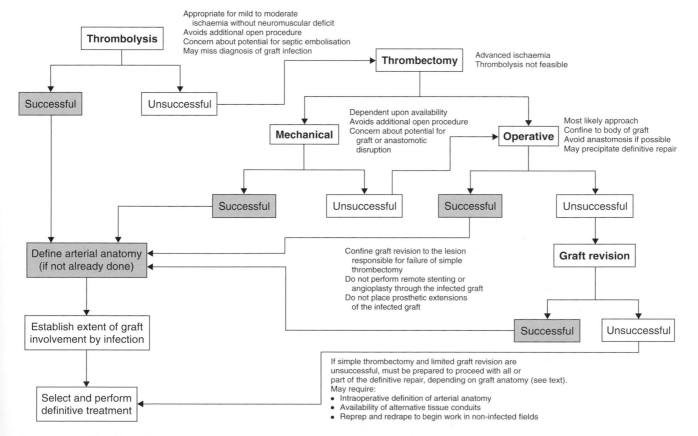

Figure 18.2 *Algorithm of management of graft occlusion with occult infection*

of the causative lesion requires open operation, then diagnosis of the occult graft infection will not be missed.

Thrombectomy is the treatment of choice in the setting of advanced or extensive ischaemia, or if thrombolysis is not safe or technically feasible. Thrombectomy may be performed using the percutaneous mechanical approach (see Chapter 16) or the standard open approach (see Chapter 15). Again, the percutaneous approach has the same advantages and disadvantages as thrombolysis, except that it can provide more rapid restoration of flow. Given that graft infection can result in structural weakening of the graft and its attachments, mechanical thrombectomy carries the potential for disrupting the conduit or the anastomoses, and that must be kept in mind. Finally, the use of mechanical thrombectomy is limited by the availability of the necessary devices.

Open thrombectomy is the most common approach in patients with extensive or advanced ischaemia, and will also be needed for a proportion of those in whom thrombolysis fails. When an occult graft infection is encountered at the time of graft exploration for thrombectomy several principles should be followed. An adequate sample of any perigraft fluid should be sent for immediate Gram staining as well as for culture and sensitivity. The goal of this operation should be to restore perfusion, allowing adequate time for appropriate assessment and planning for definitive treatment of the graft infection. Accordingly, the procedure should begin by transgraft thrombectomy avoiding exposure of any anastomosis. To do so increases the risk of disruption of an anastomosis already weakened by infection. Anastomotic disruption may precipitate immediate definitive treatment of the graft infection, which is most undesirable at this point because the extent of graft involvement is not known and the pertinent arterial anatomy may not be completely defined. The lack of such information may result in either an unnecessarily extensive or an inappropriately limited procedure, either of which can adversely affect outcome. Adequate drainage of the infection should be established, but extensive debridement of the soft tissue involved should not be performed at this time. If thrombectomy is successful in restoring flow, the procedure is then terminated. The patient should then undergo expeditious definition of the arterial anatomy and determination of the extent to which the graft is involved in the infection. With this information the surgeon can select an appropriate approach to definitive treatment.

If simple transgraft thrombectomy is not successful in restoring perfusion to the ischaemic bed, graft revision will be required. Careful consideration must be given to the technical aspects of this revision. Endoluminal angioplasty of stenoses limiting inflow or outflow can be utilised provided that access is through a non-infected site and does not involve traversing the infected graft. Placement of stents or stent-grafts to treat any flow-limiting, graft-threatening stenosis is not advisable in the setting of an infection, even if access is through a non-infected site and the planned deployment site is remote from the infected graft. Local anastomotic revision, for example, patch angioplasty to treat an anastomotic stenosis, should be limited to the shortest patch that will correct the stenosis. Prosthetic extensions of the infected graft such as proximal or distal jump-grafts are to be avoided, as they will certainly complicate the subsequent definitive treatment of the graft infection. In short, if graft revision is needed to ensure successful perfusion and reversal of ischaemia, it should be confined to the minimum that is needed and should be completed in a manner that does not make the subsequent definitive treatment of the graft infection any more complicated.

Occasionally, open thrombectomy will have the effect of precipitating immediate definitive treatment of the graft infection. The most common reasons for this are inability to re-establish adequate perfusion through the infected graft and/or bleeding as a result of disruption of an anastomosis or the conduit itself during attempts at thrombectomy or focal revision. The specific approach to the graft infection is individualised in each case but some examples will illustrate general principles.

Situations governing specific approaches to infection

- Occult infection of aortofemoral bypass graft limb
- Occult infection of femoropopliteal bypass graft
- Graft occlusion with suspected infection

Occult infection of aortofemoral graft limb

INADEQUATE OUTFLOW

If the patient presents with occlusion of one limb of an aortobifemoral bypass graft (AFBG) and occult infection is detected at open thrombectomy, the first step must be transgraft thrombectomy. If inflow is restored but there is a focal stenosis at the femoral anastomosis, the appropriate options would include prosthetic patch angioplasty or focal common femoral artery (CFA) endarterectomy (Fig. 18.3). The prosthetic patch angioplasty needs to be short and should not be extended for any distance onto either the superficial femoral artery (SFA) or the profunda femoris artery (PFA). Common femoral endarterectomy is only feasible if there is no suggestion of anastomotic weakening. Inappropriate options include prosthetic femoropopliteal bypass or a prosthetic extension graft from the AFBG limb to the SFA or PFA. If the SFA is occluded and the PFA does not provide sufficient outflow to maintain patency of the AFBG limb, a femoropopliteal bypass may be constructed using vein conduit only, with the graft originating from the PFA. Thereafter, subsequent resection of the infected AFBG limb and reconstruction, either extra-anatomical or in-line, can be undertaken without having to revise the proximal

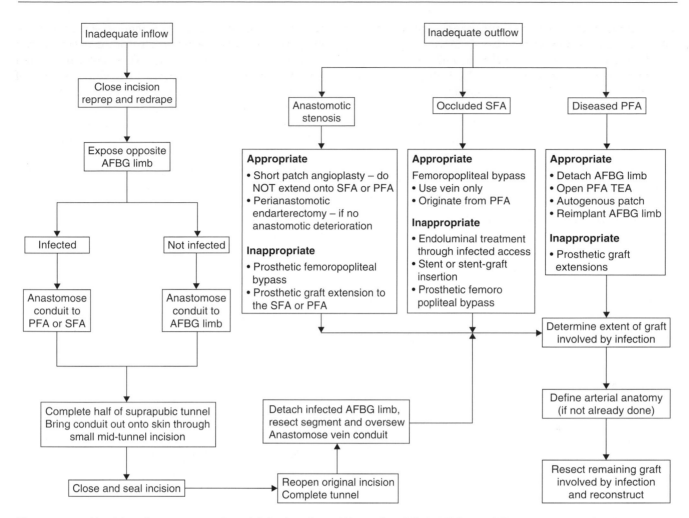

Figure 18.3 *Algorithm of management of occult infection of aortobifemoral graft limb. AFBG, aortobifemoral bypass graft; PFA, profundus femoris artery; SFA, superficial femoral artery; TEA, thromboendarterectomy*

anastomosis of the newly placed femoropopliteal graft. If the only outflow is the PFA and if that vessel has an extended lesion, then the appropriate technique is to detach the AFBG limb, extend the open arteriotomy down the PFA, perform an open endarterectomy, patch the arteriotomy with either vein or an endarterectomised segment of the occluded SFA and then re-anastomose the AFBG limb into the patch or into the CFA just proximal to the patch.

INADEQUATE INFLOW

If inflow is not restored by transgraft thrombectomy, then an alternative inflow source is needed (see Fig. 18.3). It will be necessary to close the incision used to explore the occluded, infected graft limb and begin again with a clean field and clean instruments. An incision is made exposing the contralateral patent, and presumably non-infected, AFBG limb. If that graft limb shows no evidence of infection, the perigraft space is swabbed and a Gram stain performed. If no white cells are seen on Gram stain, the AFBG limb can be used for inflow to the ischaemic limb. We do

not use another prosthetic conduit in this situation and prefer either the patient's superficial femoral vein harvested from the non-infected side, a cryopreserved superficial femoral vein or a cryopreserved arterial segment of appropriate size. The chosen conduit is anastomosed to the uninfected AFBG limb, tunnelled halfway across a suprapubic tunnel and, maintaining orientation within it, brought out through a short incision in the skin. The incision used to expose the non-infected AFBG limb and to perform that anastomosis is closed and sealed.

The original incision used to expose the infected graft limb is now re-opened and the vein conduit tunnelled the remainder of the way across the suprapubic region. The infected AFBG limb is now detached from the femoral artery and the vein conduit is anastomosed to the CFA. If necessary, the anastomosis of this vein conduit may be brought well down onto the PFA or SFA to treat any femoral anastomotic stenosis. The ample size of the conduit facilitates a lengthy anastomosis if it is needed. The infected AFBG limb is resected back to a point just proximal to the inguinal ligament and oversewn. After this procedure has successfully restored flow to the ischaemic limb, appropriate investigations can be undertaken to determine how much of the AFGB is involved by the infection. A second procedure will be needed to remove the remaining infected segments of the graft.

If there is any concern that the contralateral AFBG limb is involved by the infection, or that the body of the AFBG may be involved, then the vein conduit is *not* anastomosed to the contralateral AFBG limb. Instead the vein conduit is anastomosed either to the contralateral SFA or, if the SFA is occluded, to the PFA. If the entire AFBG subsequently proves to be involved by the infection, it can be removed without necessitating revision of the vein conduit anastomosis. If the entire AFBG requires removal, our preference is to perform in-line reconstruction, again using either the patient's superficial femoral vein or, more commonly, either cryopreserved superficial femoral vein or cryopreserved aortoiliac segments (see Chapter 25). The chosen conduit is anastomosed proximally to the infrarenal aorta and then distally to the recently placed cross-femoral vein conduit. The site of the distal anastomosis to the vein conduit is optional.

Occult infection femoropopliteal graft

INADEQUATE OUTFLOW

If the patient presents with occlusion of a femoropopliteal graft and at open thrombectomy an occult infection is detected, the first step is to proceed to transgraft thrombectomy (Fig. 18.4). If inflow is sufficient, but there is a distal anastomotic stenosis, focal balloon angioplasty may be performed through the graft, without risk of spreading infection because the graft is already involved. This may not be an appropriate intervention, however, if the graft infection seems localised, for example, confined to a segment of the body of the graft. Alternatively, a short focal patch angioplasty may be performed as long as it does not extend to any major tibial branch point. Inappropriate options would be prosthetic extension of the infected graft to a more distal segment of the popliteal artery or to a tibial artery.

If there is significant disease in the run-off arteries and adequate outflow can only be obtained by treating this disease or extending the graft to a more distal arterial segment, such as the below-knee popliteal artery or a tibial artery, the entire infected graft should be removed and replaced. In this situation, we would not place another prosthetic graft but choose instead the patient's greater saphenous vein if it is still available, the other choices being the lesser saphenous vein, an arm vein or a cryopreserved saphenous vein. An inappropriate option would be an angioplasty or stenting of the distal disease, there being no endoluminal approach to those lesions which does not involve traversing the infected graft. Excision of the infected graft without revascularisation is an acceptable option only if the patient has no symptoms of acute ischaemia, a clinical scenario not covered in this chapter.

INADEQUATE INFLOW

If inflow to femoral level is insufficient to maintain patency of the femoropopliteal graft, there are several other options

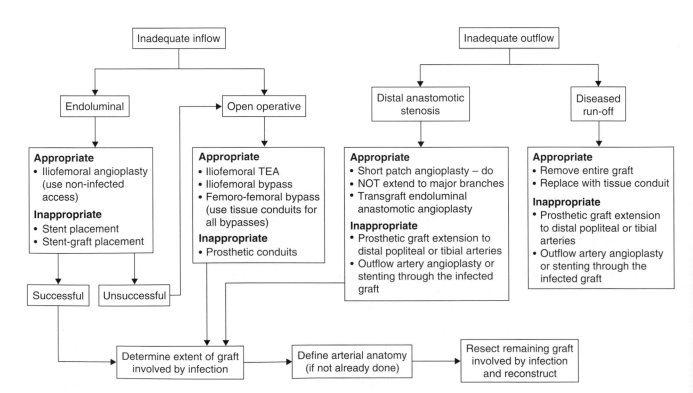

Figure 18.4   *Algorithm of management of occult infection of femoropopliteal graft. TEA, thromboendarterectomy*

(Fig. 18.4). Balloon angioplasty can be performed to treat any inflow lesion, provided that access is obtained through a non-infected site, for example via a contralateral retrograde femoral approach or an antegrade brachial approach. Stent placement should be avoided because of the risk of infection even though there is no direct continuity between the proximal stent and the infected femoropopliteal graft. Stent-graft placement should not be performed, even in a remote location. If ipsilateral inflow through the native iliofemoral arteries is insufficient and cannot be adequately improved by angioplasty, then an open approach to establish adequate inflow is needed. Appropriate options include ipsilateral iliofemoral endarterectomy, with or without patch angioplasty, ipsilateral iliofemoral bypass or cross-femoral bypass.

We would not use prosthetic material for any patch or another prosthetic conduit for the iliofemoral or cross-femoral bypass, instead preferring the patient's superficial femoral vein harvested from the uninfected leg, cryopreserved superficial femoral vein or cryopreserved arterial segments of an appropriate diameter. The patient's greater saphenous vein may be used if it is of adequate calibre, and we prefer to preserve this conduit and use it to replace the infected femoropopliteal graft. The distal anastomosis of the inflow iliofemoral bypass or cross-femoral bypass is to the native CFA or PFA and *not* to the infected femoropopliteal graft. Subsequent removal of the infected femoropopliteal conduit can then be performed without revising the distal anastomosis of the recently placed inflow graft.

Re-establishing perfusion to the ischaemic limb allows time for expeditious assessment of the extent of involvement of the graft by the infection, the relevant arterial anatomy and any associated comorbidities. Appropriate definitive treatment can then be selected. Occasionally an infection will involve only the body of a femoropopliteal graft, but more commonly the entire graft is infected. Although some investigators have recommended preservation or partial preservation of an infected lower extremity graft as the optimal treatment,[8–10] we prefer to remove the infected graft and replace it with a tissue conduit in the form of either the patient's vein (greater saphenous, lesser saphenous, or arm vein) or cryopreserved saphenous vein. We generally do not use cryopreserved arterial conduits for replacement of infected lower extremity grafts because the size is generally not well matched to the native arteries.

Graft occlusion with suspected infection

When graft occlusion occurs and graft infection is suspected, the severity of tissue ischaemia still determines the approach to treatment (Fig. 18.5). Thrombolysis, however,

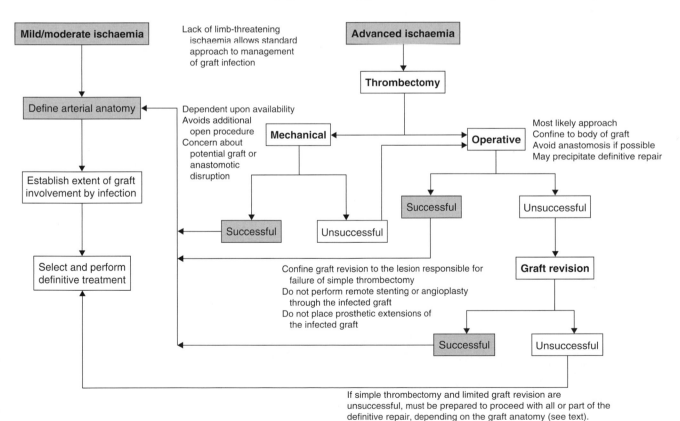

Figure 18.5 *Algorithm of management of graft occlusion with suspected infection*

is no longer an appropriate consideration. The inevitability of an open intervention eliminates the potential for total endoluminal management, the principal benefit of thrombolysis. Meanwhile, all of the potential disadvantages of thrombolysis remain, namely, delay in revascularisation, risk of bleeding and risk of septic embolisation. Therefore, patients with mild or moderate ischaemia will undergo expeditious assessment of the extent of infection, delineation of arterial anatomy and then definitive treatment of the infection. Patients with advanced ischaemia will most often undergo open thrombectomy. The approach to open thrombectomy and graft revision, if simple transgraft thrombectomy fails, is the same as that for totally occult graft infection discovered incidentally during treatment of graft occlusion. Again, the basic principles to be emphasised are to perform as minimal a procedure as possible which will successfully restore perfusion without further complicating subsequent definitive treatment of the graft infection. After restoration of flow and reversal of ischaemia, the patient will undergo routine assessment and management of the graft infection.

RESULTS

In general, patients who present with limb-threatening ischaemia of any aetiology have a higher rate of limb loss than patients who present with non-limb-threatening ischaemia. In addition mortality and morbidity rates are higher in this patient group, consistent with both the physiological effects and the need for an urgent, if not emergency, intervention. One would expect these observations also to apply to patients with acute ischaemia in the setting of occult or suspected graft infection. Although there are no outcome data specific to the clinical situation of occult graft infection

within the setting of acute graft or graft limb occlusion, one can use the available outcome data for generic prosthetic graft infection to establish a range of obtainable outcomes.

In general, the outcome of graft infection has improved as the principles of management have become better defined and the treatment options have expanded. Investigators usually acknowledge that the presence of the foreign body, i.e. the prosthetic graft, potentiates the infection. Therefore, complete removal of the infected prosthesis and avoidance of tissue planes by using extra-anatomical routes in any subsequent revascularisation procedure offers the best chance of eradicating the infection. Almost all investigators, however, also acknowledge that the parallel goal of maintenance of perfusion to the distal bed is not optimally achieved with extra-anatomical bypass. The standard approach to the management of infected grafts, i.e. complete graft excision with revascularisation through remote non-infected fields,[5,11–17] has been supplemented with *in situ* revascularisation utilising a variety of conduits including prostheses such as Dacron and expanded polytetrafluoroethylene (PTFE),[7,18–33] antibiotic (rifampin)-bonded prosthetic conduits,[34–38] autologous vein,[39–47] arterial allografts[48–60] and venous allografts.

The potential benefits of *in situ* revascularisation are that it is a simplified single operative procedure with lower amputation rates and possibly even lower mortality. The potential disadvantages are the risk of persistent or recurrent infection, particularly when another prosthetic conduit is placed in the tissue bed contaminated by graft infection. The use of autogenous deep venous conduits is associated with a risk of significant limb oedema and even the venous compartment syndrome.[39,45] Allograft use is associated with conduit failure either because of aneurysmal degeneration or stenosis/occlusion, possibly reflecting low grade chronic rejection.

Overall, the available results of these treatment approaches published during the past 15 years suggest that reasonable outcomes may be achieved (Table 18.1). Many of the

Table 18.1 *Outcome of prosthetic vascular graft infection: selected series 1990–2004*

Conduit	Number	Death (per cent)	Limb loss (per cent)	Conduit disruption (per cent)	Conduit failure (per cent)	Recurrent/ persistent infection (per cent)	Conduit dilation (per cent)
Venous autograft	62	10–33	0–20	0–33	0–17		
Arterial allograft	248	13–30	0–6	3–17	5–44	7–24	5–22
In situ prosthetic	72	0–50	0–40	0–7	0	10–60	
In situ prosthetic-antibiotic bonded	36	11–36	0	0–18	9–36	0–18	
Extra-anatomical bypass and infected graft removal – others	276	19	14		13–27	3–13	
Extra-anatomical bypass and infected graft removal – UCSF	55	24	15	0	25	5	
Venous allograft – UCSF	20	15	0	4	0	5	5

UCSF, University of California, San Francisco.

reported series, however, are small, the patients having been selected rather than taken consecutively, accumulated over long time intervals and during which there have been many changes in patient management. Outcome data beyond the perioperative interval are often limited or not available. Finally, most investigators triage their choice of the in-line conduit according to the clinical scenario; prosthetic in-line conduits tend to be used almost exclusively in the setting of aortoenteric fistula, whereas tissue in-line conduits tend to be used in the setting of chronic infection.

In general, *in situ* reconstruction is recommended for consideration in infections which are culture-negative or when there are no systemic signs of it. Such treatment is also appropriate when significant occlusive disease severely disadvantages the haemodynamic success of an extra-anatomical bypass, when the degree of occlusive disease itself demands treatment, and finally, and when major branches are involved in the infected graft, the last two situations being particularly relevant to infected aortic grafts.

In situ reconstruction

- Recommended
  - Culture-negative infections
  - No signs of systemic infection
  - Likely compromise of extra-anatomical bypass by significant occlusive disease
  - Significant disease in major (especially aortic) branches requiring treatment
  - Infection involving major (especially aortic) branches
- Not recommended
  - Abscess
  - Gross, virulent or invasive infection
  - Gram-negative, *S. aureus* or culture-positive infection
  - Systemic manifestations of infection

In general, *in situ* reconstruction is not recommended for consideration when there is an abscess or when infections are gross, culture-positive, caused by Gram-negative organisms, by *S. aureus*, particularly if methicillin sensitive or resistant (MRSA), and if there are systemic, virulent or invasive manifestations.

For the most part occult graft infection, manifesting as graft or graft limb occlusion, will not have any of the above features contraindicating *in situ* replacement of the infected graft, as almost all of them reflect an aggressive and invasive infection which is not likely to remain occult.

Conclusions

Acute ischaemia secondary to graft occlusion with an underlying occult graft infection is a rare occurrence. There are few specific data to guide treatment or establish expected outcomes. In general, the degree of ischemia will dictate the initial treatment approach. In the most common setting non-limb-threatening ischaemia, caused by the occluded graft, results in operative exploration and incidental discovery of graft infection. The principles guiding treatment are the relief of ischaemia using the simplest approach in restoring flow, avoiding any procedure which risks spreading infection or which makes subsequent definitive treatment of the graft infection more difficult.

Once ischaemia has been relieved expeditiously, the arterial anatomy is delineated, the extent of graft involved by the infection is established and definitive treatment is chosen and executed. *In situ* graft replacement is employed only for non-invasive, non-aggressive infections. The conduit chosen for *in situ* graft replacement is, in order of preference, vein autograft, vein allograft, arterial allograft, antibiotic-bonded prosthetic graft or a simple prosthesis. In following these guidelines the best possible combined outcome endpoints of patient survival, eradication of infection and limb salvage can be achieved.

Key references

Bandyk DF, Novotny ML, Back MR, *et al.* Expanded application of in situ replacement for prosthetic graft infection. *J Vasc Surg* 2001; **34**: 411–20.
Brown PM, Kim VB, Lalikos JF, *et al.* Autologous superficial femoral vein for aortic reconstruction in infected fields. *Ann Vasc Surg* 1999; **13**: 32–6.
Chiesa R, Astore D, Picolo G and the Italian Collaborative Vascular Homograft Group. Fresh and Cryopreserved arterial homographs in the treatment of prosthetic graft infections: experience of the Italian Collaborative Group. *Ann Vasc Surg* 1998; **12**: 457–62.
Hayes PD, Nasim A, London NJM, *et al.* In situ replacement of infected aortic grafts with rifampicin-bonded prostheses: The Leicester experience (1992–98). *J Vasc Surg* 1999; **30**: 92–8.
Seeger JM, Pretus HA, Welborn MB, *et al.* Long-term outcome after treatment of aortic graft infection with staged extra-anatomic bypass grafting and aortic graft removal. *J Vasc Surg* 2000; **32**: 451–61.

REFERENCES

1 Lorentzen JE, Nielsen OM, Arendup H, *et al.* Vascular graft infection: an analysis of sixty-two graft infections in 2411 consecutively implanted synthetic vascular grafts. *Surgery* 1985; **98**: 81–6.

2 Bunt TJ. Synthetic vascular graft infections. I: Graft infections. *Surgery* 1983; **93**: 733–46.

3 Seeger JM. Management of patients with prosthetic graft infection. *Am Surg* 2000; **66**: 166–77.

4 Reilly LM, Lusby RJ, Altman H, Kersh RA, *et al.* Late results following surgical management of vascular graft infection. *J Vasc Surg* 1984; **1**: 36–44.

5 Seeger JM, Back MR, Albright JL, *et al.* Influence of patient characteristics and treatment options on outcome of patients with prosthetic aortic graft infection. *Ann Vasc Surg* 1999; **13**: 413–20.

6 Wilson SE. New alternatives in management of the infected vascular prosthesis. *Surg Infect* 2001; **2**: 171–7.

7 Bandyk DF, Esses GE. Prosthetic graft infection. *Surg Clin North Am* 1994; **74**: 571–90.

8 Calligaro KD, Veith FJ, Yuan JG, *et al.* Intre-abdominal aortic graft infection: complete or partial graft preservation in patients at very high risk. *J Vasc Surg* 2003; **38**: 1199–205.

9 Calligaro KD, Veith FJ, Schwartz ML, *et al.* Selective preservation of infected prosthetic arterial grafts: analysis of a 20-year experience with 120 extracavitary infected grafts. *Ann Surg* 1994; **220**: 461–71.

10 Calligaro KD, Veith FJ, Schwartz ML, *et al.* Are Gram-negative bacteria a contraindication to selective preservation of infected prosthetic grafts. *J Vasc Surg* 1992; **16**: 337–46.

11 Reilly LM, Stoney RJ, Goldstone J, Ehrenfeld WK. Improved management of aortic graft infection: the influence of operation sequence and staging. *J Vasc Surg* 1987; **5**: 421–31.

12 Kuestner L, Reilly LM, Jicha D, *et al.* Secondary aortoenteric fistulas: Contemporary outcome using extra-anatomic bypass and graft excision. *J Vasc Surg* 1995; **21**: 184–96.

13 O'Hara PJ, Hertzer NR, Beven EG, Krajewski LP. Surgical management of infected abdominal aortic grafts: review of a 25-year experience. *J Vasc Surg* 1986; **3**: 725–31.

14 Schmitt DD, Seabrook GR, Bandyk DF, Towne JB. Graft excision and extra-anatomic revascularization: the treatment of choice for the septic aortic prosthesis. *J Cardiovasc Surg* 1990; **31**: 327–32.

15 Yeager RA, Taylor LM Jr, Moneta GL, *et al.* Improved results with conventional management of infrarenal aortic infection. *J Vasc Surg* 1999; **30**: 76–83.

16 Seeger JM, Pretus HA, Welborn MB, *et al.* Long-term outcome after treatment of aortic graft infection with staged extra-anatomic bypass grafting and aortic graft removal. *J Vasc Surg* 2000; **32**: 451–61.

17 Ricotta JJ, Faggioli GL, Stella A, *et al.* Total excision and extra-anatomic bypass for aortic graft infection. *Am J Surg* 1991; **162**: 145–9.

18 Robinson JA, Johansen K. Aortic sepsis: is there a role for *in situ* graft reconstruction? *J Vasc Surg* 1991; **13**: 677–84.

19 Bandyk DF, Novotny ML, Back MR, *et al.* Expanded application of in situ replacement for prosthetic graft infection. *J Vasc Surg* 2001; **34**: 411–20.

20 Menawat SS, Gloviczki P, Serry RD, *et al.* Management of aortic graft-enteric fistulae. *Eur J Vasc Endovasc Surg* 1997; **14**(suppl A): 74–81.

21 Towne JB, Seabrook GR, Bandyk D, *et al.* In situ replacement of arterial prosthesis infected by bacterial biofilms: long-term follow-up. *J Vasc Surg* 1994; **19**: 226–35.

22 Bandyk DF, Bergamini TM, Kinney EV, *et al.* In situ replacement of vascular prostheses infected by bacterial biofilms. *J Vasc Surg* 1991; **13**: 575–83.

23 Jensen LJ, Kimose HH. Prosthetic graft infections: a review of 720 arterial prosthetic reconstructions. *Thorac Cardiovasc Surgeon* 1985; **33**: 389–91.

24 Young RM, Cherry KJ Jr, Davis PM, *et al.* The results of *in situ* prosthetic replacement for infected aortic grafts. *Am J Surg* 1999; **178**: 136–40.

25 Fiorani P, Speziale F, Rizzo L, *et al.* Long-term follow-up after *in situ* graft replacement in patients with aortofemoral graft infections. *Eur J Vasc Endovasc Surg* 1997; **14**(suppl A): 111–14.

26 Miller JH. Partial replacement of an infected arterial graft by a new prosthetic polytetrafluoroethylene segment: a new therapeutic option. *J Vasc Surg* 1993; **17**: 546–48.

27 Henke PK, Bergamini TM, Rose SM, Richardson JD. Current options in prosthetic vascular graft infection. *Am Surg* 1998; **64**: 39–46.

28 Thomas WEG, Baird RN. Secondary aorto-enteric fistulae: Towards a more conservative approach. *Br J Surg* 1986; **73**: 875–8.

29 Jacobs MJHM, Reul GJ, Gregoric I, Cooley DA. In-situ replacement and extra-anatomic bypass for the treatment of infected abdominal aortic grafts. *Eur J Vasc Endovasc Surg* 1991; **5**: 83–6.

30 Vollmar JF, Kogel H. Aortoenteric fistulas as postoperative complication. *J Cardiovasc Surg* 1987; **28**: 479–84.

31 Higgins RSD, Steed DL, Julian TB, *et al.* The management of aortoenteric and paraprosthetic fistulae. *J Cardiovasc Surg* 1990; **31**: 81–6.

32 Sorensen S, Lorentzen JE. Case report: recurrent graft-enteric fistulae. *Eur J Vasc Endovasc Surg* 1989; **3**: 583–5.

33 Walker WE, Cooley DA, Duncan JM, *et al.* The management of aortoduodenal fistula by *in situ* replacement of the infected abdominal aortic graft. *Ann Surg* 1987; **205**: 727–32.

34 Nasim A, Hayes P, London N, *et al. In situ* replacement of infected aortic grafts with rifampicin-bonded prostheses. *Br J Surg* 1999; **86**: 695.

35 Hayes PD, Nasim A, London NJM, *et al. In situ* replacement of infected aortic grafts with rifampicin-bonded prostheses: the Leicester experience (1992–98). *J Vasc Surg* 1999; **30**: 92–8.

36 Torsello G, Sandmann W. Use of antibiotic-bonded grafts in vascular graft infection. *Eur J Vasc Endovasc Surg* 1997; **14**(suppl A): 84–87.

37 Naylor AR, Clark S, London NJM, *et al.* Treatment of major aortic graft infection: preliminary experience with total graft excision and *in situ* replacement with a rifampicin bonded-prosthesis. *Eur J Vasc Endovasc Surg* 1995; **9**: 252–6.

38 Batt M, Magne J-L, Alric P, *et al. In situ* revascularization with silver-coated polyester grafts to treat aortic infection: early and midterm results. *J Vasc Surg* 2003; **38**: 983–9.

39 Brown PM, Kim VB, Lalikos JF, *et al.* Autologous superficial femoral vein for aortic reconstruction in infected fields. *Ann Vasc Surg* 1999; **13**: 32–6.

40 Nevelsteen A, Suy R. Autogenous venous reconstruction in the treatment of aortobifemoral prosthetic infection. *J Cardiovasc Surg* 1988; **29**: 315–17.

41 Nevelsteen A, Lacroix H, Suy R. Autogenous reconstruction with the lower extremity deep veins: an alternative treatment of prosthetic infection after reconstructive surgery for aortoiliac disease. *J Vasc Surg* 1995; **22**: 129–34.

42 Franke S, Voit R. The superficial femoral vein as arterial substitute in infections of the aortoiliac region. *Ann Vasc Surg* 1997; **11**: 406–12.

43 Sicard GA, Reilly JM, Doblas M, *et al.* Autologous vein reconstruction in prosthetic graft infections. *Eur J Vasc Endovasc Surg* 1997; **14**(suppl A): 93–8.

44 Nevelsteen A, Lacroix H, Suy R. Infrarenal aortic graft infection: *in situ* aortoiliofemoral reconstruction with the lower extremity deep veins. *Eur J Vasc Endovasc Surg* 1997; **14**(suppl A): 88–92.

45 Benjamin ME, Cohn EJ Jr, Purtil WA, *et al.* Arterial reconstruction with deep leg veins for the treatment of mycotic aneurysms. *J Vasc Surg* 1999; **30**: 1004–15.

46 Clagett GP, Bowers BL, Lopez-Viego MA, *et al.* Creation of a neo-aortoiliac system from lower extremity deep and superficial veins. *Ann Surg* 1993; **218**: 239–49.

47 Clagett GP, Valentine RJ, Hagino RT. Autogenous aortoiliac/femoral reconstruction from superficial femoral-popliteal veins: feasibility and durability. *J Vasc Surg* 1997; **25**: 255–70.

48 Ruotolo C, Plissonnier D, Bahnini A, *et al. In situ* arterial allografts: a new treatment for aortic prosthetic infection. *Eur J Vasc Endovasc Surg* 1997; **14**(suppl A): 102–107.

49 Knosalla C, Goeau-Brissonniere O, Leflon V, *et al.* Treatment of vascular graft infection by *in situ* replacement with cryopreserved aortic allografts: an experimental study. *J Vasc Surg* 1998; **27**: 689–98.

50 Kieffer E, Bahnini A, Koskas F, *et al. In situ* allograft replacement of infected infrarenal aortic prosthetic grafts: results in forty-three patients. *J Vasc Surg* 1993; **17**: 349–56.

51 Bahnini A, Ruotolo C, Koskas F, Kieffer E. *In situ* fresh allograft replacement of an infected aortic prosthetic graft; eighteen months' follow-up. *J Vasc Surg* 1991; **14**: 98–102.

52 Chiesa R, Astore D, Piccolo G and the Italian Collaborative Vascular Homograft Group. Fresh and cryopreserved arterial homografts in the treatment of prosthetic graft infections: experience of the Italian Collaborative Vascular Homograft Group. *Ann Vasc Surg* 1998; **12**: 457–62.

53 Desgranges P, Beaujan F, Brunet S, *et al.* Cryopreserved arterial allografts used for the treatment of infected vascular grafts. *Ann Vasc Surg* 1998; **12**: 583–8.

54 Agrifoglio G, Bonalumi F, Scalamogna M, *et al.* Aortic allograft replacement: North Italy Transplant Programme (NITp). *Eur J Vasc Endovasc Surg* 1997; **14**(suppl A): 108–10.

55 Vogt PR, von Segesser LK, Goffin Y, *et al.* Eradication of aortic infection with the use of cryporeserved arterial allografts. *Ann Thorac Surg* 1996; **62**: 640–5.

56 Vogt PR, Brunner-La Rocca HP, Carrel T, *et al.* Cryopreserved arterial allografts in the treatment of major vascular infection: a comparison with conventional surgical techniques. *J Thorac Cardiovasc Surg* 1998; **116**: 965–72.

57 Lehalle B, Geschier C, Fieve G, Stolz JF. Early rupture and degeneration of cryopreserved arterial allografts. *J Vasc Surg* 1997; **25**: 751–2.

58 Kieffer E, Gomes D, Plissonnier D, *et al.* Current use of allografts for infrarenal aortic graft infection. In: Yao JSY, Pearce WH (eds). *Modern Vascular Surgery.* New York: McGraw Hill, 2000: 297–308.

59 Mestres CA, Mulet J, Pomar JL. Large-caliber cryopreserved arterial allografts in vascular reconstructive operations: early experience. *Ann Thorac Surg* 1995; **60**: S105–S107.

60 Verhelst R, Lacroix V, Vraux H, *et al.* Use of cryopreserved arterial homografts for management of infected prosthetic grafts: A multicentric study. *Ann Vasc Surg* 2000; **14**: 602–7.

19

The Acute Diabetic Foot

CAMERON M AKBARI, FRANK W LOGERFO

THE PROBLEM

With the rising incidence and prevalence of diabetes mellitus worldwide, there has been an even greater increase in the prevalence of diabetes related complications. Foot ulceration is one of the most common and formidable complications of diabetes, affecting almost 20 per cent of all diabetic patients during their lifetime. Despite advances in management, foot problems continue to be the most common reason for hospitalisation among these patients.[1] Diabetes remains the single strongest risk factor for limb loss, contributing to half of all lower extremity amputations in the USA. The relative risk for leg amputation is 40 times greater among diabetic patients. Moreover, up to 50 per cent of diabetic amputees will undergo a second leg amputation within 5 years of the first one.[2]

The spectrum of diabetic foot disease ranges from the asymptomatic patient, who may require only preventive foot care, to the unstable and critically ill patient in whom both loss of life and limb are imminent threats. Indeed, the variety of presentations of the diabetic foot often contributes to the clinical confusion and diagnostic and treatment delays which unfortunately lead to limb loss. It follows that the clinician needs to develop an orderly approach, grounded on firm pathophysiological principles, in order to prevent such disasters.

PATHOLOGY OF THE DIABETIC FOOT

The pathogenic mechanisms involved in diabetic foot disease include ischaemia, neuropathy and infection. Acting synergistically, they contribute to the sequence of tissue ulceration, necrosis and eventually gangrene. Prevention and treatment of diabetic foot problems should be tailored to these pathogenic factors, either solely or in combination.

Neuropathy

Peripheral neuropathy is a common complication of diabetes mellitus, affecting as many as 60 per cent of all patients in their lifetime and up to 80 per cent of those presenting with foot lesions.[3] Broadly classified as focal and diffuse, the latter is more common and includes both the autonomic neuropathy and chronic sensorimotor polyneuropathies implicated in foot ulceration.

Sensorimotor neuropathy initially involves the distal lower extremities; it progresses centrally and tends to be symmetrical. Sensory nerve fibre involvement leads to loss of the protective sensation of pain, while motor nerve fibre loss results in small muscle atrophy in the foot, flexion of the metatarsals and subsequent prominence of the metatarsal heads and clawing of the toes. This in turn results in the development of abnormal pressure points on the plantar bony prominence which lacks protective sensation culminating in ulceration at these pressure points. Loss of intrinsic muscle function also results in digital contractures, hammer toe and clawed toe deformities, pes cavus and ulceration. Because the motor neuropathy may affect the extensor musculature of the leg, deformities can also involve the ankle joint, with resultant so-called equinus deformity and abnormal bending forces.

Sensorimotor neuropathy

- Tends to be symmetrical
- Sensory – loss of protective sensation of pain
- Motor – small muscle atrophy, flexion contractures
- Deformities – callosities, hammer toe, clawed toes, pes cavus, equinus
- Necrosis and ulceration at pressure points

Autonomic denervation leads to loss of sympathetic tone and increased arteriovenous shunting in the foot with defective nutrient flow. Impaired autonomic regulation of the sweat glands leads to anhidrosis and cracking of dry skin, which creates a predisposition to skin breakdown and ulceration. Because of sympathetic innervation to the bone, autonomic neuropathy may also result in an increase in bone blood flow and subsequent osteopenia and 'bone washout'. This osteoarthropathy associated with diabetes is more commonly known as Charcot's foot, once historically associated with syphilitic tabes dorsalis, and now almost exclusively a complication of diabetes.

Autonomic neuropathy

- Loss of sympathetic tone
- Increased arteriovenous shunting – defective flow
- Anhidrosis – skin cracking and breakdown
- Increased bone blood flow – osteopenia or 'bone washout'

The aetiology of Charcot's foot deformity includes a combination of both sensorimotor and autonomic neuropathies. Continued walking on an insensate joint, combined with muscle imbalance and atrophy from motor neuropathy and limited joint mobility, leads to joint instability, loss of joint architecture and ultimately bone and joint destruction.[4] This destructive process leads to increased bone blood flow, concomitant resorption and softening of normal bone, which in turn leads to further bone destruction and ultimately fracture and Charcot's joint.

Pathology of Charcot's joint

- Aetiology – sensorimotor and autonomic neuropathy
- Insensate joint, muscle atrophy, contracture – reduced mobility
- Joint instability, loss of joint architecture
- Weight-bearing and walking – bone and joint destruction

Infection

The unique anatomy of the foot has implications for the presentation and treatment of infection. Most infections progress within the plantar aspect of the foot consisting of three compartments: medial, central and lateral.[5] The floor of each compartment is the rigid plantar fascia and the roof is composed of the metatarsal bones and interosseous fascia. A thick medial intermuscular septum, extending from the medial calcaneal tuberosity to the head of the first metatarsal, defines the medial and central compartments. The intrinsic muscles of the great toe are in the medial compartment whereas the central compartment is composed of the intrinsic muscles of the second, third and fourth toes as well as the extensor and flexor tendons of those toes, the medial and lateral plantar nerves, and the plantar vascular structures. The lateral intermuscular septum, from the calcaneus to the fifth metatarsal, delineates the lateral compartment, which contains the intrinsic muscles of the fifth toe.

Diabetic foot infection may result from a simple puncture wound, a neuropathic ulcer, the nail plate, or from the interdigital web space. Because the intrinsic muscles of each digit are essentially confined within the respective plantar compartment, untreated distal phalangeal infection may progress to a plantar abscess. Infection within these rigid anatomical compartments also creates high intra-compartmental pressures, which subsequently impairs capillary blood flow and leads to progressive tissue ischaemia and necrosis. Because the roof of each compartment is composed of bone and fascia, deep space infections show deceptively little abnormality on the dorsal foot. Left untreated, ongoing infection and cellulitis progresses to bacterial spread from one compartment to another through direct perforation of the medial or lateral intermuscular septum (Fig. 19.1), causing the development of

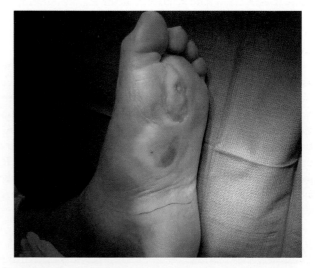

Figure 19.1   *Infection of the foot from a small plantar ulcer which has progressed from the central to medial compartments with proximal extension as well*

proximal foot and ankle abscesses at the calcaneal convergence of the septum and eventually leading to an unsalvageable foot.

The microbiology of the diabetic foot infection is dependent on the patient's environment, whether as outpatient or hospitalised, and the severity of the infection itself.[6] Mild localised and superficial ulcerations, particularly among outpatients, are usually caused by aerobic Gram-positive cocci such as *Staphylococcus aureus* or streptococci. In contrast, deeper ulcers and more generalised, limb-threatening infections are usually polymicrobial in content. In addition to Gram-positive cocci, the causative organisms in this latter group may include Gram-negative bacilli (*Escherichia coli*, *Klebsiella*, *Enterobacter aerogenes*, *Proteus mirabilis* and *Pseudomonas aeruginosa*) and anaerobes (*Bacteroides fragilis* and peptostreptococci). Enterococci may also be isolated from the wound, notably among hospitalised patients, and these, in the absence of other cultured virulent organisms, should probably be considered pathogenic.

Ischaemia – microvascular and macrovascular considerations

Two distinct types of vascular disease are seen in patients with diabetes.[7] The first is a non-occlusive microcirculatory impairment, characteristically involving the capillaries and arterioles of the kidneys (nephropathy), eye (retinopathy) and peripheral nerves (neuropathy) with significant effects in the diabetic foot. The second is a macroangiopathy, characterised by atherosclerotic lesions of the coronary and peripheral arterial circulation, which is morphologically and functionally similar in both non-diabetic and diabetic patients.

In the context of the diabetic foot and microvascular dysfunction, the so-called 'small vessel disease' of diabetes is an inaccurate term, since it suggests an untreatable occlusive lesion in the microcirculation. Prospective anatomical[8] and physiological studies have demonstrated that there is *no such microvascular occlusive disease*. Dispelling the notion of 'small vessel disease' is fundamental to the principles of limb salvage in patients with diabetes, since arterial reconstruction is almost always possible and successful in these patients.[9]

While there is no occlusive disease in the microcirculation, multiple structural and physiological abnormalities result in functional microvascular impairment.[10] Endothelial dysfunction and the response to nitric oxide is diminished in patients with diabetes, neuropathy and vascular disease.[11] Hyperglycaemia alone may lead to at least some of these abnormal responses.[12] Thickening of the capillary basement membrane is the dominant structural change in both neuropathy and retinopathy whereas alterations of the basement membrane are likely to contribute to albuminuria and the progression of diabetic nephropathy.[13] In the diabetic foot, capillary basement membrane thickening may theoretically impair the migration of leucocytes, and the hyperaemic

response following injury increases the susceptibility of the diabetic foot to infection.[14,15] These changes, however, do not lead to narrowing of the capillary lumen, and arteriolar blood flow may be normal or even increased despite these changes.[16]

A variety of other microvascular abnormalities may be demonstrated in the diabetic foot.[17] Both capillary blood flow and the maximal hyperaemic response to stimuli are reduced in the diabetic foot, suggesting that *functional* microvascular impairment is a major contributing factor in diabetic foot problems. Neurogenic vasodilatation is also impaired in the diabetic foot.[18] Normally, injury-mediated nociceptive C fibre stimulation results in adjacent neurogenic release of vasoactive peptides, which subsequently lead to vasodilation and increased blood flow to the area of injury. Absence of this axon reflex further reduces the inflammatory hyperaemic response to injury in the diabetic foot.

Microvascular functional impairment

- Endothelial dysfunction
- Thickening of the basement membrane
- Impairment of migration of leucocytes
- Impaired inflammatory hyperaemic response
- Susceptibility to sepsis
- Arterial flow may be normal or increased
- Neurogenic axon reflex mediated vasodilatation is impaired

As noted earlier, macrovascular lower extremity disease in the diabetic patient is morphologically similar to that in the non-diabetic patient. The major difference between these two populations of patients is the pattern and location of the occlusive lesions.[19] Whereas occlusive lesions of the superficial femoral and popliteal segment are commonly found in the non-diabetic patient with limb ischaemia, diabetic patients commonly have occlusive disease involving the infrageniculate, or tibial, arteries. However, the foot arteries are almost invariably patent, which allows for extreme distal arterial reconstruction despite extensive tibial or even proximal multisegmental disease. In addition, the popliteal, superficial femoral and more proximal arteries are less likely to be affected by atherosclerosis, which happily allows these vessels to serve as an inflow source for distal arterial bypass grafts.

Macrovascular disease

- Femoropopliteal system less affected by atherosclerosis
- Occlusive disease often in infrageniculate and tibial arteries
- Medial calcinosis of tibial arteries
- Foot arteries invariably patent

CLINICAL EVALUATION

As with all other disease processes, the initial evaluation of the patient with any diabetic foot problem begins with a complete history and careful physical examination. Broadly classified, this bedside assessment includes the healing potential of the foot, the details of the foot problem, e.g. ulcer, gangrene, infection, osteomyelitis, etc., the systemic consequences of diabetes, and any immediate threats to life and/or limb.[20]

History

The history of the foot problem itself can give valuable insight as to the potential for healing, the presence of coexisting infection or arterial occlusive disease and the need for further treatment. Any patient presenting with foot ulceration or gangrene should immediately arouse suspicion of underlying arterial insufficiency, even if neuropathy or infection is present. In the patient with diabetes and arterial insufficiency, the development of a non-healing foot ulcer may be a seemingly benign event such as cutting a toenail, soaking the foot in a warm bath or using a heating pad (Fig. 19.2).

The duration of ulceration also provides important clues to the extent that a long-standing, non-healing ulcer is

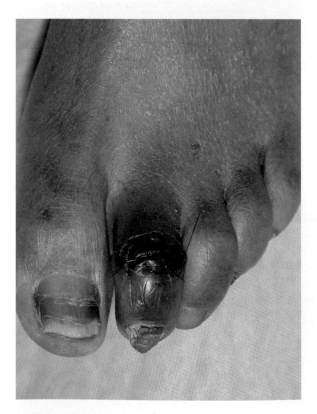

Figure 19.2 *Gangrene and non-healing following a 'simple' arthroplasty*

strongly suggestive of ischaemia. Certainly, an ulcer or gangrenous area which has been present for several months is unlikely to heal without some type of further additional treatment, whether it be off-loading of weight-bearing areas, treatment of infection, or, most commonly, the correction of arterial insufficiency. Had the present ulcer healed previously, and is the current episode a relapsing problem? A history of intermittent healing followed by relapse should raise suspicion of underlying untreated infection, such as recurrent osteomyelitis, or uncorrected architectural abnormality such as a bony pressure point or varus deformity.

It is helpful to consider past opinions and treatments, while still formulating an objective treatment plan based on presenting data. Many diabetic patients with correctable foot ulceration and limb ischaemia have been told that the only option is limb amputation, usually due to 'inherited pessimism' and inadequate knowledge of the advances made in limb and foot salvage. In these circumstances, when seeking an additional treatment opinion, it is best to 'start at the beginning' rather than blindly concur with previous actions.

The past history should be first directed to previous foot and limb problems. Recent ipsilateral ulceration or foot surgery, healed in timely fashion and with uncomplicated course, may suggest adequate arterial supply. When the history is more remote, such information becomes less useful. A history of previous leg revascularisation, including percutaneous therapies, also provides an important clue as to underlying arterial insufficiency. Other cardiovascular risk factors, such as cigarette smoking or hyperlipidaemia, should also be considered, as their presence increases the likelihood that ischaemia is contributing to the present foot problem.

Although claudication or rest pain has traditionally been associated with vascular disease, diabetic neuropathy may obscure those symptoms, and their absence in the diabetic patient certainly does not rule out ischaemia. Because even moderate ischaemia will preclude healing in the diabetic foot, the absence of rest pain is not a reliable indicator of adequate arterial blood supply; moreover, many patients may not walk a sufficient distance to develop true vasculogenic claudication. Conversely, some patients with true ischaemic rest pain are dismissed for years as having 'painful neuropathy'.

Because unrecognised infection in the diabetic patient may rapidly progress to a life-threatening condition, attention should be directed toward detecting the subtle manifestations of an infected foot ulcer. Worsening hyperglycaemia, recent erratic blood glucose control and higher insulin requirements all suggest untreated infection. Due to microvascular and neuropathic abnormalities in the diabetic foot, the classic symptoms of infection such as chills or pain are often absent, and hyperglycaemia is often the sole presenting symptom of undrained infection. As infection and hyperglycaemia progress, impending ketoacidosis or non-ketotic hyperglycaemic hyperosmolar coma may develop with symptoms of weakness, confusion and altered mental status.

The history should also include a comprehensive assessment of the patient's overall health, to help stratify perioperative risk should some type of operative intervention be needed. Knowledge of previous cardiac events, such as myocardial infarction or revascularisation, and present cardiac status, anginal severity and heart failure symptoms are all mandatory components of the history taking. Similarly, in the patient with suspected infection and ischaemia, a history of worsening renal function or impending need for haemodialysis will help determine the dose and choice of antibiotics and may alter plans for standard contrast arteriography. Functional status also becomes an important consideration at this point, and the history should carefully determine the ambulatory and rehabilitative potential of the patient, so that appropriate decisions may be made for limb salvage or amputation.

Physical examination

Initial evaluation of the diabetic foot ulcer should include a strong suspicion and thorough search for infection. In the patient with cellulitis, the entire foot, including the web spaces and nail beds, should be examined for any potential portals of entry, such as a puncture wound or an interdigital 'kissing' ulcer. Encrusted and heavily calloused areas over the ulceration should be deroofed, and the wound thoroughly inspected to determine the extent of involvement. An apparently benign dry gangrenous eschar can often hide an undrained infectious collection. Cultures should be taken from the base of the ulcer, avoiding superficial swabs which may only yield colonising organisms. Findings consistent with infection might include purulent drainage, crepitus, tenderness, mild erythema and sinus formation, although these findings may be entirely absent in the neuropathic foot. Close inspection of the ulcer and the use of a sterile probe may also confirm the presence of osteomyelitis, which occurs commonly even in benign appearing ulcers; if bone is detected with gentle probing, osteomyelitis is presumed to be present. Although not always present, fever and tachycardia are strongly suggestive of deep or undrained infection with impending or already established sepsis.

Because of its prevalence and causative role in diabetic foot problems neuropathy should be assessed in every diabetic patient, and appropriate preventive measures taken to ensure against foot ulceration in the high risk neuropathic foot. Protective sensation may be assessed with a Semmes–Weinstein 5.07 strength monofilament; inability to feel the monofilament when pressed to the skin correlates well with an increased risk of foot ulceration. Advanced sensorimotor neuropathy will lead to the presence of a 'claw' foot due to gradual atrophy of the intrinsic muscles. Charcot's deformity, with bone and joint destruction of the mid-foot, may also be seen.

Assessment of arterial perfusion in the diabetic foot is a fundamental consideration, since the diabetic foot needs maximal perfusion to heal. Inadequate or faulty assessment and treatment of underlying ischaemia will lead to failure of limb salvage in the patient with diabetic foot ulceration. Inspection of the leg and foot, including the ulcer itself will often provide suggestive clues. For example, distal ulceration at the tip of a digit, an ulcer unassociated with an exostosis or weight-bearing area, and the presence of gangrene, are all strongly consistent with underlying ischaemia. Multiple ulcers or gangrenous areas on the foot, the absence of granulation tissue or lack of bleeding with debridement of the ulcer should immediately raise concerns of underlying arterial insufficiency (Fig. 19.3). Other signs suggestive of ischaemia include pallor with elevation, fissures, particularly at the heel and absent hair growth. Although poor skin condition and hyperkeratosis may not always be good indicators of arterial disease, they should be noted, as they may help confirm initial clinical impressions.

Pulse examination, most notably the status of the foot pulses, is the single most important component of the physical exam, since, as has been emphasised, *ischaemia is always presumed to be present in the absence of a palpable foot pulse*. As such, special attention should be directed toward the foot pulses, which requires a knowledge of the usual location of the native arteries. The dorsalis pedis artery is located between the first and second metatarsal bones, just lateral to the extensor hallucis longus tendon, and its pulse is palpated

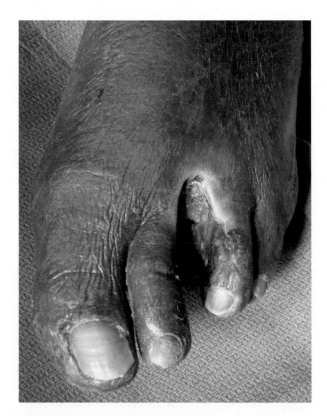

Figure 19.3 *Non-healing and lack of granulation tissue at the bed of a third toe open amputation site with extension of gangrene to the fourth toe*

by the pads of the fingers as the hand is partially wrapped around the foot. If the pulse cannot be palpated, the fingers may be moved a few millimetres in each direction, as the artery may occasionally have a slightly aberrant course. A common mistake is to place a single finger at one location on the dorsum of the foot. The posterior tibial artery is typically located in the hollow curve just behind the medial malleolus, approximately halfway between the malleolus and Achilles' tendon. The examiner's hand should be contralateral to the examined foot, i.e. the right hand should be used to palpate the left foot and vice versa, so as to allow the curvature of the hand to follow the ankle.

Non-invasive arterial evaluation

Non-invasive arterial testing has a limited role in the diabetic patient with foot ulceration, and should not be used in place of the bedside evaluation. In selected patients, and in conjunction with the clinical findings, non-invasive testing may provide useful information. Some examples might include the diabetic patient with absent foot pulses and a superficial ulcer showing evidence of healing and a previous history of a healed foot ulcer, or the patient without any foot lesions scheduled to undergo elective foot surgery. In the patient with poor healing or gangrene and absent foot pulses, however, non-invasive testing will add little additional information to the initial clinical evaluation and will serve only to further delay vascular reconstruction.

All the non-invasive arterial tests have limitations in the presence of diabetes.[21] Medial arterial calcinosis occurs frequently and unpredictably in patients with diabetes, and its presence renders the arteries non-compressible resulting in artificially elevated segmental systolic pressures and ankle:brachial indices (ABI). Therefore, a 'normal' ABI in a patient with diabetes should be interpreted with caution. Measurements may also be affected by the use of cuffs of inappropriate size. For example, too narrow a cuff will result in artefactually high pressures, and the so called 'narrow cuff artefact' is often associated with obese patients. Lower levels of calcification in the toe vessels support the use of toe systolic pressures as a surrogate measure of healing potential, but despite its advantages in the presence of calcified vessels, toe pressure measurements also have several limitations. The presence of a bandage or toe ulcer often precludes placement of the cuff. In addition, as a plethysmograph is used to detect the pressure at which volume increases, the quality of the tracing may be affected by any vasoconstricted states caused by cold weather such as a cold room, a nervous patient, etc. Finally, both the volume and photoplethysmographs require close calibration, and poor contact of the photocell with the skin will yield poor results.

Segmental Doppler waveforms and pulsed volume recordings are unaffected by medial calcification, but *evaluation of these waveforms is primarily qualitative and not quantitative*. Although a triphasic Doppler waveform suggests normal arterial perfusion at that level, in the occasional patient, the waveform may be triphasic at the ankle even though occlusive disease may be present more distally. In addition, the quality of the waveforms is affected by peripheral oedema and in that sense is technically dependent. Similarly, plethysmography and pulsed volume recordings have several shortcomings, primary among them being that it frequently underestimates the severity of proximal arterial disease mainly due to the presence of collateral vessels. As with segmental Doppler waveforms, the quality of the test is affected by several variables, including room temperature, since temperature differences in the air cuff can change the pressure measured by the air-filled plethysmograph; other factors are peripheral oedema and obesity. Finally, extensive casts or bandages preclude accurate waveform measurement.

Despite the invaluable role of duplex ultrasound in the diagnosis of carotid artery disease and in postoperative graft surveillance, multiple limitations apply to its use for the diagnosis of lower extremity arterial disease. A large variation in the range of 'normal' velocities for leg arteries may lead to a significant stenosis being misinterpreted. Although the femoral and popliteal vessels may be visualised relatively easily, the tibial vessels are more cumbersome to scan, and the velocities in the tibial arteries may be even more difficult to interpret. When one considers the usual pattern of diabetic vascular disease in diabetes, with a predilection toward atherosclerotic involvement of the tibial vessels, the limitations of duplex in the diagnosis of arterial insufficiency in the diabetic patient can be understood. Because the study depends on accurate sonographic localisation of the vessel, duplex is quite 'operator dependent'. Finally, multiple other variables can influence the quality of the image, including medial arterial calcification, which can cause artefactual shadowing, obesity and peripheral oedema, so compromising the imaging of tibial vessels.

Regional transcutaneous oximetry ($TcPO_2$) measurements are also unaffected by medial calcinosis, and some studies have noted its reliability in predicting healing of ulcers and amputation levels.[22] Because haemodynamics are not measured, the test is immune to many of the problems facing other non-invasive tests in the presence of diabetes, such as non-compressible vessels. Due to the unique considerations of the diabetic foot, however, *$TcPO_2$ measurements are not entirely reliable in the diabetic patient with foot ulceration*. Although values less than 20 and greater than 60 can be predictive, there is a large 'grey area' of intermediate values which are of little clinical use. Additionally, patients with diabetes develop foot ulceration at higher $TcPO_2$ values in comparison with the non-diabetic population and, due to the effects of arteriovenous shunting and microvascular dysfunction, a higher $TcPO_2$ value may not correlate with healing potential in the diabetic patient. Even in the patient with a 'normal' $TcPO_2$ value, the measurement may not accurately reflect healing potential at the target area. Because the probe is placed typically at the proximal dorsal foot, i.e. near the ankle, more distal ischaemia due to possible distal tibial and paramalleolar occlusive disease may not be identified. Technical problems, such as poor probe placement, lack of equipment standardisation and user variability and lack of familiarity, may also undermine the reliability of the study.

TREATMENT

Once the initial bedside history and physical evaluation has been completed, the astute clinician will have formulated a plan determining the type and urgency of subsequent treatment and diagnostic tests. Specifically, this timely assessment focuses on the presence and severity of infection, whether the limb is salvageable, which includes an assessment of the underlying medical condition of the patient, and the presence of ischaemia. These considerations are summarised in the algorithm in Fig. 19.4.

Infection

Evaluation and treatment of infection assumes first priority in the management of any diabetic foot problem.[23] Although radiographic tests may confirm initial clinical suspicions, the determination of the severity of infection is almost always made based on the clinical findings, and should be made without undue delay. Infection in the diabetic foot may range from a minimal superficial infection to fulminant sepsis with extensive necrosis and destruction of the foot. Accordingly, the assessment of infection and the subsequent treatment plan should consider the following: choice of antibiotic, which requires knowledge of the microbiology, the need for drainage, local or even guillotine amputation and the medical condition of the patient.

In the compliant patient with no evidence of deep space involvement or systemic infection, treatment may be performed as an outpatient, and consists of an oral antibiotic, pending culture results, and non-weight bearing of the involved extremity. Because most pathogens in this group of patients are either *Staphylococcus* or *Streptococcus*, an oral penicillin or first generation cephalosporin is usually adequate. The patient should be instructed on appropriate dressing changes to the wound, frequent follow-up and guidelines to recognise determining improvement or worsening.

Unfortunately, a more common presentation is the patient with ulceration or gangrene and a deep infection involving tendon or bone and possible systemic involvement. These patients require immediate hospitalisation,

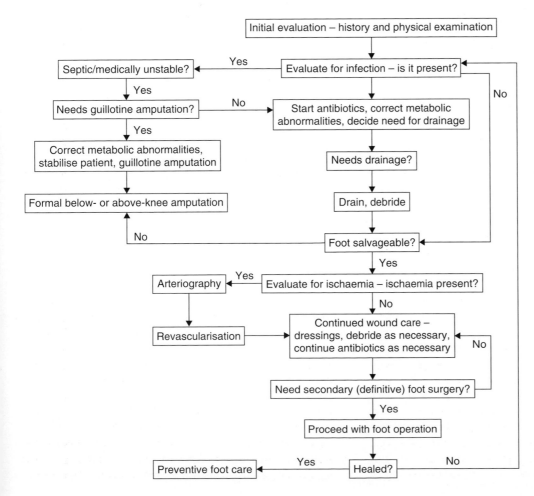

Figure 19.4 *Algorithm detailing evaluation and treatment of the diabetic foot*

bed rest with elevation of the infected foot, correction of any systemic abnormalities and broad spectrum intravenous antibiotics, the range of which is narrowed once culture results are complete. As noted earlier, the clinical findings of impending sepsis may be subtle, and therefore these patients should have a complete laboratory work-up to detect and correct electrolyte and acid–base imbalances.

Duration and choice of antibiotic therapy is dependent on the extent of infection. As noted earlier, deep or chronic, recurrent ulcers are typically polymicrobic, and appropriate empirical antibiotic choices for those infections which are not life-threatening might include the following: clindamycin plus a fluoroquinolone; clindamycin plus a third or fourth generation cephalosporin; an antipseudomonal penicillin. Subsequent culture results will then dictate any further antibiotic coverage. In the absence of osteomyelitis, antibiotics should be continued, typically 10–14 days, until the wound appears clean and all surrounding cellulitis has resolved. If osteomyelitis is present, treatment should include both surgical debridement and a prolonged course, say 4–6 weeks, of antibiotic therapy, though it may be abbreviated if the entire infected bone has been removed, as with digital or transmetatarsal amputation. Heel lesions will often present with some degree of calcaneal destruction, and the diagnosis of osteomyelitis may be made by either clinical examination alone or in conjunction with other radiographic tests such as plain X-rays or magnetic resonance imaging (MRI).

In the presence of an abscess or deep space infection, immediate drainage, of all infected tissue planes, is mandatory. Incisions should be chosen with consideration of the normal anatomy, including the compartments, of the foot and the need for subsequent secondary foot salvage procedures. These incisions should be placed to allow for dependent and complete drainage and all necrotic tissue must be debrided. If incision and drainage is adequate, placement of drains, for example of the Penrose type, is unnecessary, and reliance on such drains should be avoided. Repeat cultures, both aerobic and anaerobic, of the deep tissues should be obtained. Care is taken to avoid drainage incisions upwards to the dorsum of the foot. Abscesses in the medial, central or lateral compartments should be drained using longitudinal incisions in the direction of the neurovascular bundles and extending the entire length of the abscess. The medial and central compartments should be drained through a medial incision and the lateral compartment should be drained through a lateral incision, just above the plantar surface of the forefoot. Similarly, web space infections may be drained through the plantar aspect of the foot. In some instances, an open toe or transmetatarsal amputation may be necessary to allow complete drainage and resection of necrotic tissue. Strict adherence to textbook amputations may lead to unnecessary soft tissue removal and the possible need for a higher amputation in the future. Therefore all viable tissue should be conserved.

With continuing undrained infection, the patient may present with an unsalvageable foot and fulminant sepsis, haemodynamic instability, bacteraemia and severe acid–base and electrolyte abnormalities. Such a patient should undergo prompt open guillotine below-knee amputation. This type of amputation is usually performed at ankle level to remove the septic source and to allow for subsequent revision and closure at a later date. Intravenous antibiotics, correction of dehydration and electrolyte abnormalities and continuous cardiac monitoring are absolutely essential throughout the treatment process.

Once the infection has been drained and the tissues debrided, continued wound inspection and management is essential. Persistent necrosis should raise suspicion of undrained infection or untreated ischaemia and further debridement and treatments may be necessary. Wounds should be kept moist, avoiding caustic solutions, soaks or whirlpool therapy. Attention should also be focused on avoiding any weight-bearing on the affected foot, while also maximising nutrition and controlling hyperglycaemia.

Limb salvageability

While the infection is being treated and controlled, the surgeon should determine the chances and feasibility of limb salvage. Assessment should include the patient's functional status and the viability of the foot. For example, primary limb amputation may be considered in a non-ambulatory, bedridden patient or in a patient with severe Charcot destruction and degeneration and for whom no further reconstructive foot procedures are possible. *'Poor' medical condition is not necessarily an indication for primary limb amputation*, considering the higher perioperative morbidity associated with limb amputation. Moreover, in many patients, optimisation of the underling medical comorbidities may be accomplished during treatment of infection and while evaluating for ischaemia.

The assessment for limb salvage should be performed as the infection is being treated, as appropriate drainage and antibiotics can dramatically change the appearance and perceived viability of the foot. If, however, limb salvage is not deemed possible, the patient should undergo formal below-knee or above-knee amputation.

Ischaemia

The surgeon's initial evaluation, based on the history and physical examination, should offer a fairly accurate impression of the arterial circulation to the foot. That *assessment should be directed at the treatment goal, namely, the restoration of maximal, pulsatile arterial perfusion to the foot.* The limitations of non-invasive vascular testing in diabetic patients with foot ulceration emphasise the continued importance of thorough bedside evaluation and clinical judgement. To reiterate, the status of the foot pulses is the most important aspect of the physical examination and if impalpable, occlusive disease is present. As the restoration of pulsatile flow maximises the chances of healing in the diabetic foot, the absence of foot pulses must be an indication for contrast arteriography. This has particular relevance in the clinical setting of tissue loss, poor healing and gangrene, even if neuropathy may have been the antecedent cause of skin breakdown or ulceration. Arteriography is essential in determining and planning the type of arterial reconstruction likely to restore the foot pulses.

Concern about contrast induced renal dysfunction in the presence of diabetes should not contraindicate high quality arteriography of the entire distal circulation. Several prospective studies showing that the incidence of contrast induced nephropathy is no higher in the diabetic patient free from pre-existing renal disease, especially if it is undertaken with the judicious use of hydration and renal protective agents.[24] N-acetylcysteine in a 600 mg dose twice daily should be started the day before the arteriogram and continued for 48 hours,[25] and intravenous hydration with 0.45 per cent normal saline should be run at a rate of 1 mg/kg per hour, beginning 12 hours prior to the scheduled arteriogram. In selected patients, magnetic resonance angiography (MRA), carbon dioxide angiography or both may be used, either in conjunction with or in place of contrast arteriography.

Whatever preoperative imaging modality is chosen prior to arterial reconstruction, it is mandatory that consideration be given to the pattern of lower extremity vascular disease in patients with diabetes and that the complete infrapopliteal circulation be incorporated, including that of the foot vessels. It is essential that arteriograms should not end at mid-tibial level because foot vessels are often spared in the atherosclerotic occlusive process, even when tibial arteries are occluded.

PRINCIPLES OF ARTERIAL RECONSTRUCTION IN THE DIABETIC FOOT

The treatment of ischaemia in the diabetic foot is aimed at restoring maximal perfusion to the foot and ideally to restore a palpable foot pulse.[26] Possible approaches include the endovascular techniques of angioplasty and stenting, bypass grafting using autogenous or prosthetic grafts, or a combination of the two.[27] Ultimately, the choice of procedure should be tailored to the patient's anatomy, comorbidities and preoperative assessment, the goal being to provide the most durable procedure with the least risk. For example, angioplasty alone may be of benefit in the patient with an isolated iliac artery stenosis or a focal lesion in the superficial femoral artery, but it may also be used in combination with an infrainguinal bypass in the diabetic patient with multilevel disease.

In most patients, restoration of the foot pulse in the ischaemic diabetic foot is usually achieved by infrainguinal arterial bypass grafting to an outflow artery in direct continuity with the foot (see Chapter 15). Although proximal bypass to the popliteal or proximal tibioperoneal arteries may restore foot pulses, more distal revascularisation is often needed to achieve this goal, again owing to the pattern of occlusive disease in the diabetic patient. Similarly, although excellent results have been reported with peroneal artery bypass, this artery is not in continuity with the foot vessels and may not achieve the maximal flow required for healing, particularly at forefoot level. We therefore reserve peroneal artery bypass for those rare circumstances in which there is no dorsalis pedis or posterior tibial artery in continuity with the foot, or when limited venous conduit length mitigates against more distal bypass.

Autogenous vein grafting to the dorsalis pedis, distal posterior tibial and plantar arteries incorporates our knowledge of the anatomical pattern of diabetic vascular disease, satisfies the fundamental goal of restoration of the foot pulse and provides durable and effective limb salvage.[28] Indeed, extensive experience with arterial reconstruction to the pedal vessels has established the efficacy, durability and safety of these procedures and improved limb salvage rates in the diabetic patient may be directly attributed to the increasing use of pedal bypass.[29] The choice of outflow artery should be based on availability of conduit, the location of the foot ulcer and the quality of the outflow vessel.

The dorsalis pedis artery is exposed through a longitudinal incision 1 cm distal to an imaginary transverse line between the distal malleoli and 1 cm lateral to the extensor hallucis longus tendon. A continuous-wave Doppler probe may be used preoperatively to mark the location of the artery. Experience has shown that the artery is less likely to be calcified at the intermalleolar level. The incision is deepened through the fascia and the artery is found just beneath the inferior margin of the extensor retinaculum. The dorsalis pedis artery gives off a lateral tarsal branch proximally and then bifurcates into deep plantar and dorsal metatarsal arteries distally.

In the patient with an ischemic heel ulcer, first consideration should be given to the posterior tibial or plantar arteries if they are patent on preoperative imaging. The distal posterior tibial artery is found in the hollow just behind the medial malleolus, halfway between the bone and Achilles' tendon. Again, a Doppler probe may be used to mark its location preoperatively. A longitudinal incision is carried down through the fascia, upon which the artery may be visualised. If more distal dissection is required, such as for plantar artery exposure and bypass, the distal dense fascia and flexor retinaculum are divided. This exposes a trifurcation, with a medial calcaneal branch running directly posteriorly toward the heel, followed by the medial and lateral plantar arteries approximately 1 cm beyond the calcaneal branch. If further exposure of the plantar arteries is required, the muscle fibres of the abductor hallucis muscle may be divided.

The distal location of the dorsalis pedis and posterior tibial arteries theoretically necessitates a long venous conduit, which is often not attainable. By using the popliteal or distal superficial femoral artery as an inflow site, however, a shorter length of vein may be used, with excellent long term patency. This is particularly true in the diabetic patient, again due to the pattern of atherosclerotic disease. This avoids dissection in the groin and upper thigh, a common location for wound complications. In addition, the shorter length of saphenous vein obviates the need to extend the vein harvest incision into the foot, which is parallel to the one required to expose the paramalleolar and inframalleolar arteries; this avoids the resultant skin bridge which may occasionally become ischaemic from undue tension. If a skin bridge is created, as with an *in situ* bypass, care must be taken to create the subcutaneous graft tunnel proximal and not through the skin bridge.

The vein graft can be prepared as an *in situ*, reversed, or non-reversed graft, without any significant difference in outcome. We therefore advocate a flexible approach, taking advantage of the technical strategy best suited to individual vascular anatomy. The *in situ* technique minimises size mismatch between the graft and native arteries, eliminates the need to completely mobilise the vein and may prevent inadvertent twisting of the graft. We have used the *in situ* technique for most infrageniculate distal bypass grafts originating from the common femoral artery. Although the valves in the vein graft may be lysed blindly, we prefer to cut the valves under direct angioscopic guidance using a flexible valvulotome (Fig. 19.5) This also allows for assessment of the saphenous vein to detect intraluminal abnormalities and can help direct endoluminal interventions which upgrade the quality of the conduit and improve patency.

The *absence of an ipsilateral greater saphenous vein is not a contraindication for pedal bypass*, as comparable results may be attained using arm vein or lesser saphenous vein grafts. Prosthetic material should seldom, if ever, be used for extreme distal bypass grafting. When ipsilateral saphenous vein is not available, several alternatives exist for an autogenous conduit. Although the contralateral saphenous vein is

an obvious alternative, several considerations limit its use in the diabetic patient. A contralateral leg vein may not always be present in this population of patients who often require multiple cardiovascular interventions. More importantly, diabetes is a strong risk factor for subsequent contralateral limb bypass, and almost 60 per cent of patients require such a bypass at 3 years. Therefore, our approach has been to use arm vein grafts as the first alternative in the absence of ipsilateral saphenous vein.[30] The cephalic, basilic, or upper arm basilic-cephalic loop vein grafts may be harvested. Once the vein has been harvested, angioscopic evaluation is crucial, as many of these patients have undergone multiple venipunctures and cannulations with resultant scarring and web-like synechiae. Angioscopy allows for detection and correction of many of these areas, and allows for precise valve lysis within these thin-walled veins.[31]

Active infection in the foot is not a contraindication to dorsalis pedis bypass, as long as the infectious process is controlled.[32] Adequate control implies resolution of cellulitis, lymphangitis and oedema, especially in areas of proposed incisions required to expose the distal artery or saphenous vein. Occasionally, severe circumferential calcification of the distal artery may also be encountered. Strategies include the use of special intraluminal bulb-tipped vessel occluders or tourniquet occlusion, with or without attempts made at endarterectomy or 'cracking' the plaque. Results of bypasses to calcified vessels are comparable to non-calcified vessels.[33]

RESULTS

Several reports have summarised the results of the dorsalis pedis artery bypass, of which the most recent describes a decade-long experience of more than 1000 cases.[34] In that series, 5-year primary patency rate was 57 per cent with a

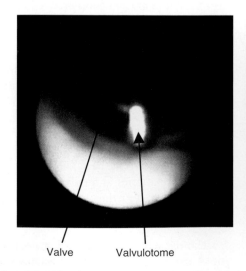
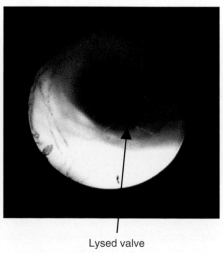

Valve   Valvulotome   Lysed valve

Figure 19.5 *Angioscopic evaluation allows for valve identification and precise lysis*

limb salvage rate of almost 80 per cent, confirming the efficacy and durability of these procedures. Additionally, concern regarding perioperative morbidity and long term outcome in diabetic patients has also been dispelled.[35,36]

Conclusions

These superior results are due the continued application of sound anatomical and pathological principles to a coordinated, systematic and aggressive approach in managing the diabetic foot. This, coupled with advances in technology and more sophisticated techniques in endovascular approaches, has undoubtedly led to even higher limb salvage rates among patients with diabetes.

Key references

Akbari CM, Macsata R, Smith BM, Sidawy AN. Overview of the diabetic foot. *Semin Vasc Surg* 2003; **16**: 3–11.

Akbari CM, LoGerfo FW. Distal bypasses in the diabetic patient. In: Yao JST, Pearce WH (eds). *Current Techniques in Vascular Surgery*. New York: McGraw-Hill, 2001: 285–96.

Akbari CM, LoGerfo FW. The diabetic foot. In: Wilmore DW, Souba WW, Fink MP, *et al.* (eds). *ACS Surgery: Principles and Practice*. New York: WebMD Professional Publishing, 2003: 1–11.

LoGerfo FW, Gibbons GW, Pomposelli FB Jr, *et al.* Trends in the care of the diabetic foot: Expanded role of arterial reconstruction. *Arch Surg* 1992; **127**: 617–21.

Pomposelli FB Jr, Kansal N, Hamdan AD, *et al.* A decade of experience with dorsalis pedis artery bypass: analysis of outcome in more than 1000 cases. *J Vasc Surg* 2003; **37**: 307–15.

REFERENCES

1 Reiber GE, Boyko EJ, Smith DG. Lower extremity foot ulcers and amputations in diabetes. In: *Diabetes in America*, 2nd edn, National Institute of Diabetes and Digestive Kidney Diseases NIH Publication No. 95–1468. National Diabetes Data Group. Bethesda, MD: National Institutes of Health, 1995, 409–28.

2 Nathan DM. Long-term complications of diabetes mellitus. *N Engl J Med* 1993; **328**: 1676–85.

3 Grunfeld C. Diabetic foot ulcers: etiology, treatment, and prevention. *Adv Intern Med* 1992; **37**: 103–32.

4 Frykberg RG, Kozak GP. The diabetic Charcot foot. In: Kozak GP, Campbell DR, Frykberg RG, Habershaw GM (eds). *Management of Diabetic Foot Problems*, 2nd edn. Philadelphia, PA: WB Saunders, 1995: 88–97.

5 Akbari CM, Macsata R, Smith BM, Sidawy AN. Overview of the diabetic foot. *Semin Vasc Surg* 2003; **16**: 3–11.

6 Joshi N, Caputo GM, Weitekamp MR, Karchmer AW. Infections in patients with diabetes mellitus. *N Engl J Med* 1999; **341**: 1906–12.

7 Akbari CM, LoGerfo FW. Diabetes and peripheral vascular disease. *J Vasc Surg* 1999; **30**: 373–84.

8 Strandness DE Jr, Priest RE, Gibbons GE. Combined clinical and pathologic study of diabetic and nondiabetic peripheral arterial disease. *Diabetes* 1964; **13**: 366–72.

9 LoGerfo FW, Coffman JD. Vascular and microvascular disease of the foot in diabetes. *N Engl J Med* 1984; **311**: 1615–19.

10 LoGerfo FW. Vascular disease, matrix abnormalities, and neuropathy: implications for limb salvage in diabetes mellitus. *J Vasc Surg* 1987; **5**: 793–6.

11 Veves A, Akbari CM, Primavera J, *et al.* Endothelial dysfunction and the expression of endothelial nitric oxide synthetase in diabetic neuropathy, vascular disease, and foot ulceration. *Diabetes* 1997; **47**: 457–63.

12 Akbari CM, Saouaf R, Barnhill DF, *et al.* Endothelium-dependent vasodilation is impaired in both micro- and macrocirculation during acute hyperglycemia. *J Vasc Surg* 1998; **28**: 687–94.

13 Morgensen CE, Schmitz A, Christensen CR. Comparative renal pathophysiology relevant to IDDM and NIDDM patients. *Diabetes Metab Rev* 1988; **4**: 453–83.

14 Flynn MD, Tooke JE. Aetiology of diabetic foot ulceration: A role for the microcirculation? *Diabet Med* 1992; **8**: 320–9.

15 Rayman G, Williams SA, Spencer PD, *et al.* Impaired microvascular hyperaemic response to minor skin trauma in Type I diabetes. *BMJ* 1986; **292**: 1295–8.

16 Parving HH, Viberti GC, Keen H, *et al.* Hemodynamic factors in the genesis of diabetic microangiopathy. *Metabolism* 1983; **32**: 943–9.

17 Akbari CM, LoGerfo FW. Microvascular changes in the diabetic foot. In: Veves A, Giurini JM, LoGerfo FW (eds). *The Diabetic Foot: Medical and Surgical Management*. Totowa, NJ: Humana Press, 2002: 99–112.

18 Parkhouse N, LeQueen PM. Impaired neurogenic vascular response in patients with diabetes and neuropathic foot lesions. *N Engl J Med* 1988; **318**: 1306–9.

19 Menzoian JO, LaMorte WW, Paniszyn CC, *et al.* Symptomatology and anatomic patterns of peripheral vascular disease: differing impact of smoking and diabetes. *Ann Vasc Surg* 1989; **3**: 224.

20 Akbari CM, LoGerfo FW. The diabetic foot. In: Wilmore DW, Souba WW, Fink MP, *et al.* (eds). *ACS Surgery: Principles and Practice*. New York: WebMD Professional Publishing, 2003: 1–11.

21 Akbari CM, LoGerfo FW. Peripheral vascular disease in the person with diabetes. In: Porte D, Sherwin RS, Baron AD (eds). *Ellenberg and Rifkin's Diabetes Mellitus*, 6th edn. New York: McGraw-Hill, 2003: 845–57.

22 Ballard JL, Eke CC, Bunt TJ, *et al.* A prospective evaluation of transcutaneous oxygen measurements in the management of diabetic foot problems. *J Vasc Surg* 1995; **22**: 485–92.

23 Akbari CM, Pomposelli FB Jr. Diabetes and diseases of the foot. *Intern Med* 2000; **21**: 10–17.

24 Solomon R, Werner C, Mann D, *et al.* Effects of saline, mannitol, and furosemide to prevent acute decreases in renal function induced by radiocontrast agents. *N Engl J Med* 1994; **331**: 1416–20.

25 Tepel M, van der Giet M, Schwarzfeld C, *et al.* Prevention of radiographic-contrast-agent-induced reductions in renal function by acetylcysteine. *N Engl J Med* 2000; **343**: 180–4.

26 Akbari CM, LoGerfo FW. Distal bypasses in the diabetic patient. In: Yao JST, Pearce WH (eds). *Current Techniques in Vascular Surgery*. New York: McGraw-Hill, 2001: 285–96.

27 Faries PL, Brophy D, LoGerfo FW, *et al.* Combined iliac angioplasty and infrainguinal revascularization surgery are

effective in diabetic patients with multilevel arterial disease. *Ann Vasc Surg* 2001; **15**: 67–72.

28 Akbari CM, LoGerfo FW. Saphenous vein bypass to pedal arteries in diabetic patients. In: Yao JST, Pearce WH (eds). *Techniques in Vascular and Endovascular Surgery*. Norwalk, CT: Appleton and Lange, 1998: 227–32.

29 LoGerfo FW, Gibbons GW, Pomposelli FB Jr, *et al*. Trends in the care of the diabetic foot: Expanded role of arterial reconstruction. *Arch Surg* 1992; **127**: 617–21.

30 Faries PL, Arora S, Pomposelli FB Jr, *et al*. The use of arm vein in lower-extremity revascularization: results of 520 procedures performed in eight years. *J Vasc Surg* 2000; **31**: 50–9.

31 Akbari CM, LoGerfo FW. Value of arm vein in femoral distal bypass. In: Yao JST, Pearce WH (eds). *Advances in Vascular Surgery*. New York: McGraw-Hill, 2001: 261–9.

32 Tannenbaum GA, Pomposelli FB Jr, Marcaccio EJ, *et al*. Safety of vein bypass grafting to the dorsal pedal artery in diabetic patients with foot infections. *J Vasc Surg* 1992; **15**: 982–90.

33 Misare BD, Pomposelli FB Jr, Gibbons GW, *et al*. Infrapopliteal bypasses to severely calcified outflow arteries: two year results. *J Vasc Surg* 1996; **24**: 6–16.

34 Pomposelli FB Jr, Kansal N, Hamdan AD, *et al*. A decade of experience with dorsalis pedis artery bypass: analysis of outcome in more than 1000 cases. *J Vasc Surg* 2003; **37**: 307–15.

35 Hamdan AD, Saltzberg SS, Sheahan M, *et al*. Lack of association of diabetes with increased postoperative mortality and cardiac morbidity. *Arch Surg* 2002; **137**: 417–21.

36 Akbari CM, Pomposelli FB Jr, Gibbons GW, *et al*. Lower extremity revascularization in diabetes: late observations. *Arch Surg* 2000; **135**: 452–6.

The Acutely Swollen Limb

20

Deep Vein Thrombosis

BO GH EKLOF, CURTIS B KAMIDA

THE PROBLEM

Deep vein thrombosis (DVT) and pulmonary embolism (PE) are major health hazards which have a great impact on healthcare costs. In the general population the rate of DVT is about 160 per 100 000 and the rate of fatal PE is 60 per 100 000. Pulmonary embolism is approximately half as common as myocardial infarction and about three times as common as cerebrovascular accident (see Chapter 21). About one-half to two-thirds of patients who die from PE do so within 1 hour of onset, too short a period of time to establish the diagnosis and institute specific treatment.[1] Prophylactic anticoagulant treatment might have prevented the development of DVT and some subsequent deaths. Therefore, primary prevention of DVT in defined risk groups is important. When DVT occurs, the secondary objectives are to prevent:

- extension of the thrombus and fatal PE
- progressive swelling of the leg and increased compartmental pressure, which can lead to phlegmasia caerulea dolens, venous gangrene and limb loss
- later development of severe post-thrombotic syndrome (PTS) by preservation of the venous outflow and valve function
- chronic pulmonary hypertension.

PREDISPOSING FACTORS

Rudolph Virchow presented his classical triad in 1856 for the aetiology of DVT: changes in the blood elements producing a **hypercoagulable state**, reduced blood flow velocity causing **stasis** and vein wall injury resulting in **endothelial damage**. An increased risk of thrombosis is demonstrated in association with an increase in procoagulant activity in the plasma, including increases in platelet count and adhesiveness, changes in the coagulation cascade and endogenous fibrinolytic activity. Additionally, deficiencies of antithrombin III, protein C, protein S and resistance to activated protein C, as well as the presence of a circulating lupus anticoagulant, indicate either primary or secondary hypercoagulable states. Stasis is generally accepted as a major factor causing DVT, and there is evidence that stasis occurs, for example, on the operating table. It is logical that reduced flow might prolong the contact time of activated platelets and clotting factors with the vein wall, thereby permitting thrombus formation. To date, no study has shown stasis alone to be causally related to DVT.[2] Virchow's third factor, endothelial damage, has now received more attention with experimental and clinical data.[3] The data show an intraoperative venodilatation that leads to endothelial damage and exposure of the subendothelial collagen, which is highly thrombogenic. The lesions were infiltrated with leucocytes and platelets, trapping the blood cells and stimulating fibrin deposition. It is postulated that the venodilatation is induced by products of tissue injury released at the operative site and which gain entry into the circulation.

RISK FACTORS

Surgical patients who sustain major trauma or undergo prolonged operative procedures are at risk of developing venous thromboembolic disease. The degree of risk is increased by age, obesity, malignancy, prior history of thromboembolism, varicose veins, recent operative procedures and thrombophilic states. These factors are further modified by general care, including duration of operation, type of anaesthesia, preoperative and postoperative immobility, level of hydration and presence of sepsis.[4] In medical patients the risk is increased after acute myocardial infarction and cerebrovascular accidents, and in immobile general medical patients.[4] Pulmonary embolism is the leading cause of death in cases following surgical procedures for gynaecological cancer and is a major contributor to maternal mortality. There is an increased risk of DVT in women taking oral contraceptives (OCPs) containing 50 μg or more of oestrogen. The third generation OCPs in combination with the hypercoagulable state (APC resistance) is reported to increase the risk of DVT 30–40 times. The same risk seems to involve women on hormone replacement therapy. With this knowledge and with the appearance of new risk factors for the hypercoagulable state, screening of larger groups of people at risk is increasingly favoured. In our own practice we perform hypercoagulation screening in all young patients with DVT and in all patients with recurrent DVT before we start treatment. Finally, all of the above factors may be compounded by long periods of immobility, such as in airline travel, to produce DVT.

PATHOPHYSIOLOGY OF DVT

The **development of a vein thrombus** is well described in a text on vein diseases.[5] The initial platelet cluster on the vessel wall is followed by coralline thrombus, which is produced, presumably in response to adenosine diphosphate or thromboxane release, by the deposition of more platelets. The thrombus then grows towards the centre of the vessel lumen, alternate layers of fibrin and red cells being trapped between layers consisting mainly of platelets. As the thrombus grows out into the blood stream, it bends in the direction of the flow and extends across the lumen. The flow beyond it becomes turbulent and gradually decreases. A red thrombus, a mixture of fibrin and red cells, extends in the direction of the flow and grows rapidly when flow falls to critical levels. When the vein becomes completely occluded the thrombus begins to adhere to the endothelium.

The process of **organisation**, namely, invasion with granulation tissue and replacement of the fibrin by fibrous tissue, occurs wherever the thrombus is adherent. Where the thrombus remains loose within the lumen, the polymerisation and maturation of the fibrin within the thrombus cause it to retract. Thrombus retraction and organisation eventually lead to **recanalisation and re-endothelialisation**. This process destroys all the valves in the affected segment of vein and is accompanied by enlargement of the collateral venous channels. There is a considerable **danger of embolism** until a non-adherent, non-occlusive thrombus begins to contract. Contraction usually occurs 5–10 days after thrombus formation. If a thrombus has not fragmented by this stage, it usually adheres to one side of the vein and organisation occurs as if the thrombus were fully adherent. In most cases DVT develops in the calf veins, extends proximally and can lead to secondary iliofemoral DVT. The soleal sinusoids and the valves of the calf veins are the common sites of origin of DVT. Primary iliofemoral DVT starts in the iliac vein, mainly owing to iliac vein compression, and extends distally.

New data on the inflammatory response to DVT are appearing. Downing *et al.* in Ann Arbor have shown that the leucocyte adhesion molecule P-selectin activates the leucocytes emigrating into the venous wall, creating inflammation which destroys the venous wall and the valves.[6] Using an experimental model See-Tho *et al.* in Stanford showed that if the thrombus were to be removed early then the inflammatory changes are reversible.[7] Caps *et al.* in Seattle had shown previously that the remaining thrombotic proximal occlusion in human leg veins will lead to progressive distal valvular incompetence.[8] The lesson from this new information is to *remove the thrombus as early and as quickly as possible.*

DIAGNOSIS

A patient, who, over a few hours, develops aching pain and swelling of one leg accompanied by pleuritic chest pain, shortness of breath and haemoptysis most certainly has DVT with PE.

This **clinical presentation**, however, is quite rare. In most cases the presentation is atypical and objective methods of diagnosis are necessary. In a patient with acute iliofemoral vein thrombosis (IFVT) and phlegmasia alba dolens, the clinical diagnosis is easy and usually correct. Given the abundance of differential diagnoses, clinical diagnosis in a patient with pain and swelling in the calf can be difficult. The Doppler ultrasound probe has high sensitivity and specificity for mainstem DVT but it is less accurate in calf DVT. The method of choice today is **duplex scanning**, particularly using colour flow imaging.[9] **Phlebography** is considered the gold standard for detection of DVT, but this position has been eroded for various reasons: high costs, painful and sometimes impossible access to foot veins, contrast induced phlebitis and allergic reactions.

The advantages of duplex scanning are several. It is non-invasive, easily repeated and permits imaging as well as flow studies. It is applicable to the venous system from the level of the inferior vena cava (IVC) down to the ankle. It distinguishes total from partial venous occlusion, estimates the age of the thrombus and can be used to follow the natural history and recanalisation of the thrombus.

Advantages of duplex scanning

- Non-invasive, easily repeated
- Images system from IVC down to ankle
- Gives data on both morphology and flow
- Distinguishes total from partial occlusion
- Estimates age of thrombus
- Allows monitoring of natural history of thrombosis and recanalisation

By the same token there are a number of disadvantages. Admittedly, duplex scanning equipment is expensive but as it replaces phlebography the investment argument is clearly valid. Nevertheless, it has to be acknowledged that duplex scanning remains a time consuming and operator dependent process. Technically, the quality of study is limited by gross oedema, the presence of plaster casts, etc. It is sometimes difficult to visualise the upper limits of the thrombus in the abdomen and pelvis and equally calf veins and duplicated vessels lower down. It is difficult, of course, to detect recurrent DVT in a chronically damaged vein.

Disadvantages of duplex scanning

- The equipment is expensive
- Studies are time consuming and operator dependent
- Technical limitations – gross oedema, plaster casts
- Difficulty visualising upper limit of thrombus, calf veins, duplicated vessels
- Difficult detecting recurrent DVT in chronically damaged vein

When DVT is suspected on the basis of history, clinical examination and Doppler ultrasonography, it is routine to proceed to duplex scanning using colour flow imaging. There are different protocols as to how a proper duplex scan in a patient with a suspected DVT should be performed. Many vascular laboratories only look at the common femoral and popliteal veins, disregarding the iliac and calf veins. There are studies showing that with such a protocol more than 30 per cent of clots will be missed in the iliac and calf veins. With improved technology and methodology using colour and power Doppler, not only the tibial and peroneal veins, but also the soleal and the gastrocnemial veins can be interrogated. In cases of extension of DVT into the iliac vein without visualisation of the upper end of the thrombus, a femoral phlebogram from the contralateral side is performed. This will show the IVC and localise the top of the thrombus in the involved iliac vein. With the advent of duplex scanning, indirect methods such as plethysmography and thermography have become obsolete and indications for isotope uptake tests are rare. The role of the D-dimer test for screening of DVT and PE is still controversial. A negative test may in the future reduce the need for duplex scans to eliminate the diagnosis of DVT and PE in patients in whom the diagnosis is suspected.

TREATMENT

Standard hospital treatment for patients with acute venous thromboembolism (VTE) in the USA is bedrest with leg elevation and anticoagulation using intravenous unfractionated heparin (UFH) for at least 5 days. Oral warfarin is started simultaneously and continued for 3 months. Heparin therapy is monitored by activated partial thromboplastin time (APTT) and the heparin infusion dose is adjusted to maintain the APTT ratio at 1.5–2.5 times control to minimise recurrent thrombotic events and risk of bleeding. The lower level should be reached within 24 hours. Warfarin therapy is monitored by the international normalised ratio (INR), the therapeutic range of which is defined by an INR of 2.0–3.0.

There are new actors on the scene and they will change our behaviour in the treatment of VTE: low molecular weight heparin (LMWH), catheter directed thrombolysis (CDT) with adjunctive angioplasty and stenting and venous thrombectomy (TE) with temporary arteriovenous fistula (AVF). Low molecular weight heparin has been used for several years in the treatment of VTE in Australia, Canada and Europe based on numerous level I clinical trials; in 1999 it was approved by the Food and Drug Administration (FDA) for treatment in the USA. Catheter directed thrombolysis is theoretically the method of choice for timely dissolution of the acute thrombus and preserving patency of the vein and competency of the valves, thereby preventing fatal PE (see Chapter 21) and the disabling PTS (for the use of CDT in acute *arterial* thromboembolic disease see Chapter 16). When there are contraindications to thrombolysis or when it fails, the combination of TE with AVF is a valid alternative.

CONSERVATIVE TREATMENT

The advent of LMWH has opened a new exciting chapter in the treatment of VTE. All LMWHs are easily absorbed from subcutaneous tissue and they have a much longer plasma half-life and better bioavailability at low doses than UFH as well as a more predictable dose–response relationship. These properties allow LMWHs to be administered once or twice daily without laboratory monitoring of coagulation factors. Although LMWHs seem to have less platelet interaction, the danger of heparin induced thrombocytopenia is still in the 1 per cent range, and therefore platelets should be monitored during therapy.

The results of 14 major randomised studies[10] have shown that LMWHs are highly effective in the initial treatment of established DVT and are superior to standard UFH in the following areas: superior or equal thrombolysis on repeat venography, fewer bleeding complications, reduced mortality at 90 days particularly in patients with cancer, reduced recurrence of DVT and no requirement for monitoring. Hence the potential for treatment in the outpatient setting. Partsch of Vienna[11] reported on 212 patients with IFVT treated with LMWH, compression bandage and ambulation: PE at admission was 45 per cent, new PE after 10 days was 7 per cent and one patient (0.2 per cent) suffered a fatal PE. The treatment recommended in an ambulatory patient with IFVT was LMWH given subcutaneously once a day based on body weight, starting warfarin therapy and continuing ambulation with a compression bandage.

A MEDLINE search showed that seven studies[12] have examined cost, and each found the efficacy of LMWHs and UFH to be comparable but the costs of the LMWHs to be less. Two studies involved home therapy and reported cost savings of up to US$1100 per patient over traditional in-hospital treatment. The drawbacks of LMWH treatment are that we cannot measure the effects on coagulation and that reversal of anticoagulation is more difficult. If one believes in the concept of early removal of the thrombus, particularly in extensive DVT, then it is a step backwards to treat all patients with LMWH given that there are no studies on the long term effect of LMWH on the development of the PTS.

Advantages of LMWH over UFH

- Longer plasma half-life and better bioavailability at low doses
- More predictable dose–response relationship
- Does not require laboratory monitoring – ideal for outpatient care
- Less platelet interaction, but it should be checked during treatment
- Highly effective thrombolysis at initial treatment of established DVT
- Fewer bleeding complications
- Lower mortality at 90 days, especially in cancer patients
- Lower recurrence rate of DVT

THE CONTROVERSY OF CALF VEIN THROMBOSIS

The clinical significance of calf vein thrombosis is controversial. Isolated calf vein DVT is estimated to be found in 5 per cent to 33 per cent of all cases of DVT diagnosed.[13,14] Reports on propagation in the absence of treatment vary from 8 to 28 per cent.[15] The direct relationship of isolated calf DVT and PE is controversial (see Chapter 21). In most series where calf DVT and PE were shown to have a high association, cases were selected by identifying those who presented with PE and were then subsequently scanned and found to have calf DVT. The question remains in these reports as to whether a larger, more proximal clot in the femoral or popliteal segment could have embolised before discovery of the calf clot. The development of the post-thrombotic sequelae is also controversial. Passman et al. reported a significant incidence of late onset abnormal venous haemodynamics, but only 5 per cent presented with swelling and 3 per cent with skin pigmentation and ulcer.[16] In our own study we found that the most common site for calf DVT was the peroneal vein (76 per cent) and there was no case of anterior tibial vein involvement. In the untreated group the incidence of propagation into proximal veins was 8 per cent with no case of clinical PE. At three-year follow-up 95 per cent were asymptomatic, 5 per cent had discoloration of the leg but no ulcers. Based on these results we recommended duplex scan surveillance for at least 2 weeks without treatment.[17] Passman et al. recommended for all patients treatment with LMWH followed by oral anticoagulants for 3 months.[16] At the discussion at the Third Pacific Vascular Symposium on Venous Disease in Hawaii in 1999 the compromise suggested was that most patients with calf vein thrombosis should be treated, while those at risk of complications from anticoagulation should be followed with duplex scans.

PERCUTANEOUS ENDOVASCULAR THERAPY

A variety of endovascular techniques can be used in the treatment of acute DVT, and most of them were initially developed for the treatment of limb ischaemia. They can be divided into procedures designed to remove obstructing thrombus and those which correct any underlying anatomical or structural abnormality. The procedures used to remove obstructing thrombus can be further divided into pharmacological and mechanical methods. In addition, the use of IVC filters will be discussed in this section.

Clot removal – catheter directed thrombolysis

Twenty years after Dotter et al.'s description of CDT in the treatment of arterial thromboembolism,[18] Semba and Dake published their experience in 22 patients with DVT treated with CDT.[19] The rationale for CDT is that by directly administering thrombolytic drug into an offending clot, the drug dosage needed would be lower than the amount used in systemic lytic therapy. This lower dose would still produce a drug concentration immediately adjacent to the clot higher than that achieved by intravenous systemic therapy (for details on CDT in acute arterial thromboembolism see Chapter 15). This method would lead to a decrease in drug cost, treatment time, and haemorrhagic complications while increasing treatment efficacy.

Until 1998, the drug of choice for thrombolytic therapy in the peripheral arterial and venous systems was urokinase (Abbokinase). Because of concerns regarding the risk of transmission of infectious disease inherent in the production of urokinase from human tissue, the FDA banned its sale in mid 1998.[20] Consequently, physicians in the USA turned to alteplase (recombinant tissue plasminogen activator (r-tPA)) and reteplase (r-PA), human plasminogen activators currently approved for intravenous use. The two drugs differ from urokinase and from each other in several respects, including half-life, fibrin specificity and clot penetration. Both drugs appear to be acceptable alternatives to urokinase, but no large clinical trials have been performed and extensive clinical experience has yet to be obtained.

The half-life of reteplase is between 13 and 16 minutes while the half-life of alteplase is much shorter, probably less than 5 minutes. The fibrin specificity of reteplase is less than that with alteplase. Theoretically, this may allow the molecule, less bound as it is with the fibrin on the surface of the clot, to penetrate deeper into the thrombus bring about faster clot lysis. This is because the fibrin-bound plasminogen inside the clot is better activated with r-PA, but this has not been demonstrated convincingly and remains unconfirmed. In the USA, r-tPA is probably the dominant agent used to replace urokinase although r-PA is being investigated and used in many centres, including ours. Until mid 2000, there were no published reports on the use of r-PA in catheter directed lytic therapy.

Most of the data discussed in the following sections were obtained using urokinase as the thrombolytic agent. We feel that the method of CDT therapy is more important than the actual drug used within a reasonable margin of safety, but obviously that has to be confirmed.

INDICATIONS AND CONTRAINDICATIONS

The rapid removal of clot in the acute phase of DVT will obviously reduce the risk of development of PE. In addition, phlegmasia and its symptoms can be alleviated by the removal of the offending thrombus obstructing venous blood return. The long term sequelae of venous insufficiency involve the inadequacy of valve function. Removing thrombus before the recanalisation process sets in leads to valve destruction and so thrombolytic therapy aids the maintenance of normal valve competence.[21]

Contraindications to the use of any thrombolytic drug include recent surgery, recent major trauma or biopsy, active or recent gastrointestinal bleeding, pregnancy, and recent stroke or the presence of intracranial neoplasm. Our own experience suggests that almost every other patient has a relative contraindication to thrombolysis. This reflects the underlying condition which predisposed the patient to developing thrombosis in the first place. Examples include DVT after joint replacement surgery and immobility subsequent to extensive trauma.

TECHNIQUE

Catheter directed thrombolysis involves the insertion of an angiographic catheter into the venous system, positioned immediately adjacent to the clot or embedded within the clot itself. The entry site for venous access does not seem to affect lytic success, as long as the catheter tip can be manipulated into the appropriate position.[22] We generally do not use additional mechanical methods such as pulse spray or injection of lytic agent via a power injector. Our concern is that the time advantage gained is outweighed by the risk of clot fragmentation, dislodgement and PE formation.

For iliofemoral thrombosis which does not involve the popliteal vein, the usual site of venepuncture and catheter insertion is the popliteal vein. The latter is approached using ultrasound guidance or fluoroscopic assistance while simultaneously injecting X-ray contrast into a pedal vein.[23] With this approach, however, the site for catheter entry is above the major popliteal vein valves and therefore these valves cannot be directly exposed to the lytic agent. To solve this problem without resorting to retrograde manipulation of a catheter through a valve cusp, Cragg has developed a technique for gaining access into the venous system below the popliteal vein.[24] This aspect of the technique is important because preservation of the integrity of the popliteal vein valves has been shown to be a major determinant in reducing the incidence of development of PTS.[25]

As mentioned previously, the most efficacious dose of the newer thrombolytic agents is still under investigation. Reteplase doses used currently range from 0.5 to 2.0 units per hour. We use 1.0 unit per hour with slight adjustment for patient size. A dose greater than 2.0 units per hour probably increases the rate of bleeding complications without improving the lytic effect to any significant degree.[26] Alteplase doses currently used are in the range of 0.5–1.0 mg per hour. Semba found that lysis tends to be faster and more complete when using alteplase compared with urokinase[23] but there is always a 'balancing act' between speed of lysis and haemorrhagic complications.

The use of heparin is controversial. Some fear that full heparinisation will lead to an increase in bleeding complications and consequently tend to use subtherapeutic doses or none at all.[23] A recent study with reteplase found that therapeutic levels of heparin do not seem to increase the rate of haemorrhagic complications[26] but the authors still advocate caution. Heparin should not be added directly to alteplase solutions because of the formation of precipitates and also because the degree of dilution seems to affect drug efficacy. Complete details and protocols have been published and are available for the interested reader.[27]

RESULTS

Recent small studies suggest that the efficacy of the newer thrombolytic agents will be similar to urokinase.[26] A clinically successful thrombolytic result should be expected in 80–90 per cent of patients[28] when using urokinase. Acute clot (<10 days) or patients with acute symptoms should respond to lysis faster and better than those with chronic disease or chronic disease with acute symptomatology.[22]

A health related quality of life survey was undertaken on patients who had lytic therapy as well as those treated with heparin alone. Improved quality of life scores were obtained in the lytic group when compared with those on anticoagulant treatment alone. Patients who failed to respond to lysis had outcomes similar to those treated with heparin alone. In addition, fewer post-thrombotic symptoms were elicited in those treated successfully with thrombolysis.[29] This reduction in post-thrombotic complications due to preservation of valve function has been seen in other large series where urokinase[30] was used.

Percutaneous endovascular therapies

- Clot removal – catheter directed therapy
- Clot removal – mechanical thrombectomy devices
- Adjunctive procedures – stents, AV fistulae
- IVC filter placement – permanent, temporary

Clot removal – mechanical thrombectomy devices

In those patients not eligible for thrombolytic therapy but who would benefit greatly from clot removal, a number of percutaneous mechanical devices have been developed which are of theoretical benefit.[31–33] We have not found any of them to be effective as a 'stand alone' method for venous clot removal but have used them in the treatment of small or persistent residual clot after lytic therapy. The lack of directional control, noted by others,[34] can sometimes be overcome by placing the device through a guiding catheter with an appropriate bend at the tip but this does necessitate placing a larger sheath than normally used. Anatomical and the histological integrity of vein valves does not seem to be compromised by the use of at least one of the more vigorous devices[35] but most of them have not been tested in this regard.

At the time of writing, none of the devices had FDA approval for the treatment of iliofemoral or native vein thrombosis. It should be re-emphasised that such approval is awaited for both reteplase and alteplase.

Adjunctive procedures

Once the acute clot has been removed, a large percentage of patients will require angioplasty or stenting of underlying anatomical or structural abnormalities. In the report of the National Venous Registry, 99 stent procedures were necessary to reestablish iliac venous outflow in 221 patients.[22] In particular, patients with strictures from radiation therapy, compression by pelvic malignancies and those sustained postoperatively will usually show better patency with metal stents than with angioplasty alone.[36]

One entity deserves special mention. The 'iliac vein compression syndrome', also known as the May–Thurner or Cockett–Thomas syndrome, is often encountered after successful thrombolytic therapy. It was first described in 1851 by Virchow who noted that thrombosis in the pelvic veins occurs more frequently on the left side than on the right.[37] He postulated that the right common iliac artery resting on the left common iliac vein leads to compression and venous obstruction. This prolonged extrinsic compression ultimately leads to intraluminal abnormalities within the left iliac vein, consisting of webs and synechiae which often do not respond to angioplasty alone and do require stent placement.[34]

The creation of an AVF to help patency after endovascular intervention is an option whose role is not clearly defined. Theoretically, an AVF helps to increase venous blood flow but in our practice we do not usually place a fistula when the lesion is short, has a reasonably large diameter, as in the case of an iliac vein, or when venous inflow is good. Nevertheless, we have created an AVF in patients with poor venous inflow is caused by multiple webs and synechiae found in a post-thrombotic superficial femoral vein.

Inferior vena caval filter

The indications for the placement of an inferior vena caval filter (VCF) include contraindications to or failure of anticoagulant therapy, the failure of a previous device to prevent PE by extension of thrombus through a filter, recurrent embolism and, in some instances, as a prophylactic measure.[38] Indications for prophylactic filter insertion include a free-floating caval thrombus, DVT with compromised cardiac or pulmonary function or an impending orthopaedic procedure.[39] In general, we do not place a permanent filter prior to CDT because of the low rate of complicating PE in patients undergoing this treatment.[22] The use of a temporary filter, however, might be reasonable in cases of a large clot burden. These filters are not currently approved by the FDA and are not widely available except in Europe. A recent multicentre registry of current practice of temporary VCF insertion has been published.[40] These filters can be left in place for up to 14 days. A total of 188 patients were described: in 53.1 per cent the indication was systemic, not catheter directed, lytic therapy; four patients died from PE but none died from filter induced complications.

Percutaneous techniques can be used to place any of the several permanent VCFs. Specific techniques differ according to the device and all of the manufacturers supply detailed instructions for placement. These can be placed from a femoral, jugular, or in the case of the Simon Nitinol filter (Nitinol Medical Technologies, Worburn, MA, USA), from an antecubital vein approach. There are currently five permanent devices available in the USA possessing relatively equivalent efficacy rates and long term outcomes.[41]

For the critically ill patient who cannot be safely transported from the intensive care unit to the angiography suite, a VCF can be placed using portable C-arm fluoroscopy.[42] Filter insertion using duplex ultrasonography alone is feasible and has been described.[43] This is highly operator dependent, patient size and the ability to visualise the IVC through bowel gas being complicating factors. Congenital anomalies such as a double IVC, a circumaortic or retroaortic left renal vein and a double renal vein may be extremely difficult to visualise with ultrasound. When possible, the filter should be inserted under direct and adequate fluoroscopic guidance with a cavogram performed prior to filter insertion because the diameter of the IVC will affect the choice of filter type. Currently, only the Bird's Nest device (Cook Group, Bloomington, IN, USA) can be placed in a large IVC or mega cava, i.e. with a diameter greater than 30 cm.

Indications for placement of VCFs

- Contraindications to anticoagulant therapy
- Failure of anticoagulant therapy
- Thrombus extension and PE through previously inserted device
- Recurrent PE
- Prophylactically
  - Free floating thrombus
  - DVT with compromised cardiac function
  - Impending orthopaedic procedure

Summary of endovascular techniques

Up until mid-1998, the mainstay of CDT had been the use of urokinase as the pharmacological agent. Since its withdrawal from the market, alteplase and reteplase have been used for the purpose of thrombolysis in acute DVT. The ideal dosing regimen and the use of additional heparin is still being investigated. Historical results obtained with urokinase may not strictly apply to the other thrombolytic agents but the method of drug delivery remains the same. Catheter directed thrombolysis and the use of adjunctive procedures such as stenting can relieve venous obstruction, preserve valve function and hopefully reduce the risk of PE (see Chapter 21).

THROMBECTOMY

Historical background

The history of TE in the USA is quite interesting. At the annual meeting of the New England Surgical Society in Poland Spring, ME, on 28 September 1940, John Homans[44] from Tufts-New England Medical Centre presented the paper, 'Exploration and division of the femoral and iliac veins in the treatment of thrombophlebitis of the leg'. Homans, who was an advocate for division of the femoral vein to prevent PE, made many suggestions and raised questions that are pertinent today: 'I believe that in the future, instead of at once dividing the various femoral veins, it might be permissible to repair the vein and institute for the next few days a vigorous heparinization. Such a procedure is probably, in skilled hands, less hazardous than non-operative treatment'. He also advocated division of the femoral or iliac veins to prevent reflux if these vessels were affected by previous thrombophlebitis. This 'will always do good, and never harm'. In this paper Homans discussed indications for TE with or without ligation of the femoral vein, the technique, the complications and the importance of preventing reflux.

The modern era of TE in the USA started with Howard Mahorner's paper,[45] 'New management for thrombosis of deep veins of extremities' in 1954 in which he advocated TE followed by restoration of vein lumen and regional heparinisation. He presented six patients, five of whom had an excellent result with rapid disappearance of leg swelling, very little late morbidity and minimal leg oedema. There was no instance of PE prior or subsequent to surgery. He claimed that this method restores vein function with preservation of the vein lumen and vein valves. In a paper in 1957[46] he reported 16 patients in whom TE had been performed on 14 legs and two arms with excellent results in 12, good in two and poor in two patients.

The wave of enthusiasm created by Mahorner's paper, boosted by the report by Haller and Abrams in 1963,[47] was effectively quelled by Lansing and Davis in 1968 presenting the results of a five-year follow-up of Haller and Abrams' patients.[48] Haller and Abrams had presented 45 patients with IFVT who underwent TE; of 34 patients with a short history (<10 days) excellent bidirectional flow was established in 31 patients (91 per cent). At follow-up after an average of 18 months, 26 out of these 31 patients (84 per cent) had normal legs and ascending venography permitted by 13 patients showed normal patency of the deep venous system in 11 (85 per cent). Lansing and Davis reported the five-year follow-up results of those 34 patients with a short history, and of 17 patients (50 per cent) interviewed 16 were found to have swelling of the leg requiring stockings; one patient had developed an ulcer. Ascending venography in the supine position in 15 patients showed patent veins in most patients but 'the involved area of the deep venous system was found to be incompetent in all cases and there were no functioning valves'. This study is flawed because they did not study the iliac vein to prove patency and their interpretation of incompetence of the valves in the femoral and popliteal veins cannot reliably be drawn from only an ascending venographic study in the supine patient.

Lansing and Davis' paper was presented at the annual meeting of the American Surgical Association in Boston on 18 April 1968, where Hanlon thought it was 'an important paper despite the rather melancholy message which it brings, reversing some previous optimistic reports' and requested the need 'to have a series of patients followed objectively with clinical and radiographic data over a long period of time after two treatment regimens, operative and non-operative'. At the annual meeting of the Southern Surgical Association at Hot Springs, VA, on 8–10 December 1969, Edwards et al.[49] presented a paper, 'Iliofemoral venous thrombosis: reappraisal of thrombectomy' where he argued with Lansing's results and concluded that: 'venous TE offers an effective and safe method of restoring flow in the deep venous system; when the thrombus is less than 10 days in duration and is of the iliofemoral segment, TE is recommended; venograms at operation to determine the patency of the deep venous system will aid in complete removal of the thrombus and give a basis for later comparison and evaluation of long-term patency'. In the discussion Lansing repeated his findings from the five-year follow-up and questioned the value of TE. Haller stated that he was never consulted about the follow-up report. At a recent visit to Louisville, he had studied 17 patients in whom total removal of the thrombus had been possible, none with any residual oedema. Despite some optimism for TE at this meeting, the impact of Lansing's report was striking, and few papers have since been published from the USA but they all showed very good clinical results above 75 per cent.

Two reports basically abolished TE in the USA: Karp and Wylie's[50] one-page short paper on 10 patients of whom eight had re-occlusion of the femoral vein before discharge, and Lansing and Davis'[48] skewed paper based on a third of the original material, using questionable methods to reach their verdict and arrived at without communicating with the original investigators. However, there seems to be renewed interest in TE judging by current American textbooks in vascular surgery. This revival is mainly based on positive reports from Europe.

Modern venous reconstructive surgery using valvuloplasty can give good long term results in primary venous disease with severe reflux while the results of vein segment transfer and autologous vein transplantation in secondary, or post-thrombotic, venous disease are much less promising.[51] It is, therefore, important to treat thrombosis of the leg early and successfully to avoid obstruction of the venous outflow tract and preserve valvular function in order to prevent the development of a severe PTS.

Surgical technique

The first thrombectomy for IFVT was performed by Lawen in Germany in 1937.[52] Surgery today is performed under intubation anaesthesia, 10 cm water positive end-expiratory pressure (PEEP) having been added during manipulation of the thrombus, to prevent perioperative PE. The involved leg and abdomen are prepared. A longitudinal incision is made in the groin to expose the long saphenous vein (LSV) to its confluence with the common femoral vein (CFV) dissected up to the inguinal ligament. The superficial femoral artery 3–4 cm below the femoral bifurcation is prepared for construction of the AVF. Further dissection depends upon the aetiology of the IFVT.

In **primary** IFVT with subsequent distal progression of the thrombus, a longitudinal venotomy is made in the CFV and a venous Fogarty thrombectomy catheter is passed through the thrombus into the IVC. The balloon is inflated and repeated exercises with the Fogarty catheter are performed until no more thrombotic material is extracted. With the balloon inflated in the common iliac vein a suction catheter is introduced to the level of the internal iliac vein to evacuate thrombus. Backflow is not a reliable sign of clearance as a proximal valve in the external iliac vein may be present in 25 per cent of cases preventing retrograde flow in a cleared vein. In contrast, backflow can be excellent from the internal iliac vein and its tributaries despite residual occlusion of the common iliac vein. An intraoperative completion venogram, therefore, is mandatory. Alternatively, an angioscope, which enables removal of residual thrombus, may be used under direct vision. The distal thrombus in the leg is removed by manual massage of the leg starting at the foot. The Fogarty catheter can sometimes be advanced gently in retrograde fashion, the aim being to remove all fresh thrombi from the leg.

In IFVT **secondary** to ascending thrombosis from the calf, the thrombus in the superficial femoral vein is often old and adherent to the venous wall, by which stage the battle of the valves has been lost. The objective is to restore patency and preserve valvular function. If iliac patency is established but the thrombus in the femoral vein is too old to be removed, ligation of the superficial femoral vein is preferable. Recanalisation will otherwise lead to valvular incompetence and subsequent reflux. In a 13-year follow-up after superficial femoral vein ligation Masuda et al.[53] found excellent clinical and physiological results without evidence of PTS. If normal flow cannot be re-established in the superficial femoral vein, we recommend extending the incision distally and exploring the orifices of the deep femoral branches where thrombus is usually isolated and venous flow can be restored with a small calibre Fogarty catheter. The superficial femoral vein is ligated. The venotomy is closed with continuous suture and an AVF is created using the long saphenous vein, anastomosing it end-to-side to the superficial femoral artery. An intraoperative venogram is performed through a catheter inserted in a branch of the AVF and, if satisfactory, the wound is closed in layers without drainage. If there are signs of iliac vein compression, which can occur in about 50 per cent of left-sided IFVT, we recommend intraoperative angioplasty and stenting.

If phlegmasia caerulea dolens or venous gangrene is present, we start the operation with fasciotomy of the calf compartments in order to release pressure and re-establish the circulation. If there is extension of the thrombus into the IVC, the cava is approached transperitoneally through a subcostal incision. The IVC is exposed by reflecting the ascending colon and duodenum medially (see Chapter 36). Depending upon the venographic findings relative to the upper end of the thrombus, the IVC is controlled, usually just below the renal veins. The IVC is opened and the thrombus is removed by massage, especially of the iliac venous system. If the iliofemoral segment is involved, the operation is continued into the groin as described above. When laparotomy is contraindicated in patients in poor condition, a caval filter of the Greenfield type can be introduced prior to TE in order to protect against fatal PE (see Chapter 21).

Heparin is continued at least 5 days postoperatively and warfarin, started on the first postoperative day, is continued routinely for 6 months. The patient is ambulant the day after the operation wearing a compression stocking and is usually discharged on the tenth postoperative day to return after 6 weeks for closure of the fistula. The objectives of a temporary AVF are to increase blood flow in the thrombectomised segment to prevent immediate re-thrombosis, to allow time for healing of the endothelium and to promote the development of collaterals in case of incomplete clearance or immediate re-thrombosis of the iliac segment. A new percutaneous technique for fistula closure was developed by Endrys et al. in Kuwait.[54] Through a puncture of the femoral artery on the opposite, surgically untouched, side a catheter is inserted and positioned at the level of the fistula. Prior to inflation and release of the balloon or coil, an arteriovenogram can be performed to evaluate the patency of the iliac and caval veins, a study which is also of prognostic value. Despite initial successful surgery more than 10 per cent of patients have been shown to have significant residual stenosis of the iliac vein. A transvenous percutaneous angioplasty and stenting can be performed under the protection of the AVF, which is then closed 4 weeks later after repeat arteriovenography.

Complications of surgical management

MORTALITY

One of the many reasons inducing surgeons to abandon TE in the 1960s was the high mortality. Surgery still bears a risk, but given the present perioperative precautions, results have improved. In our series of over 200 patients two died: one succumbed from acute respiratory failure due to chronic pulmonary fibrosis, the autopsy excluding fresh PE; an autopsy on the other patient showed preoperatively undetected cirrhosis of the liver and IVC extension of the thrombus, the patient dying in multiorgan failure on the 32nd postoperative day due to intra-abdominal haemorrhage and severe shock caused by over-anticoagulation.

PULMONARY EMBOLISM

In our experience there were no cases of fatal PE in the perioperative period. To avoid this problem it is of utmost importance to demand a preoperative venogram to exclude extension of thrombus into the IVC as it may fracture during manipulation with the Fogarty catheter. We do not use a separate balloon catheter to occlude the IVC but routinely ask the anaesthetist to apply PEEP during the procedure. In a prospective randomised study from Sweden,[55] we found positive perfusion scans at admission in 45 per cent of all patients; additional defects were seen after 1 and 4 weeks in the conservatively treated group in 11 per cent and 12 per cent, respectively, and in the thrombectomised group in 20 per cent and 0 per cent, respectively. Mavor and Galloway[56] demonstrated that incomplete clearance of the thrombus in the iliac vein increased the incidence of re-thrombosis and PE. In the Swedish series no additional perfusion defects developed after the first postoperative week following thrombectomy and AVF. Since the AVF effectively prevented re-thrombosis it is reasonable to assume that the fistula was one reason for the low incidence of postoperative PE.

Earlier reports of high mortality due to fatal PE have not been borne out in our experience. Several reasons may account for the decreased risk of developing significant symptomatic and fatal PE with the present technique: careful selection of patients; preoperative venographic demonstration of extension of thrombus and its upper limit, requiring an extended surgical approach if the IVC is involved; use of PEEP during surgery; intraoperative venography or venoscopy to prove clearance of the iliac vein; creation of an AVF.

EARLY MORBIDITY AFTER THROMBECTOMY

The rate of early re-thrombosis of the iliac vein varies. In a retrospective study from Hawaii[57] it was 34 per cent in primary IFVT (8/24) and 18 per cent in secondary IFVT (6/33) without the use of a temporary AVF. In a prospective randomised Swedish study[58] of TE using an AVF, 13 per cent developed early re-thrombosis of the iliac vein despite the temporary AVF. This re-thrombosis rate is corroborated in a series of 555 patients[59] in whom 12 per cent developed early re-thrombosis. This complication can be minimised by avoiding surgery in those patients with symptoms of iliac obstruction of more than 7 days. A Fogarty catheter to clear the external and the common iliac veins, giving special consideration to the internal iliac vein, and a direct caval approach when the IVC is involved is recommended. Intraoperative venography or venoscopy will confirm clearance of the iliac venous system. Early and liberal use of a temporary AVF and fasciotomy in patients with phlegmasia cerulea dolens are worthwhile adjunctive procedures. Early ambulation, compression stockings and carefully monitored postoperative anticoagulation are all very helpful measures.

Guidelines for reducing morbidity and mortality after TE

- Careful patient selection
- Avoiding thrombectomy when symptoms of iliac obstruction exceed 7 days
- Venographic demonstration of upper limit of thrombus (into IVC?)
- Direct caval approach when IVC involved
- Use of PEEP during surgery
- Venographic/venoscopic proof of clearance of iliac thrombus
- Early and liberal use of an AVF
- Carefully monitored postoperative anticoagulant therapy
- Compression stockings and early ambulation
- Evacuation of groin haematoma

Postoperative bleeding with haematoma formation in the groin was not uncommon despite drainage of the wound, as full anticoagulation with heparin was continued for 5 days after operation. Haematomas should be evacuated to avoid compression of the vein and the risk of thrombosis and infection.

Early re-thrombosis, previously common, is now down to 12 per cent with the use of a temporary AVF. In cases of immediate re-occlusion of the iliac vein, re-exploration followed by angioplasty and stenting or a femoro-femoral crossover bypass graft will help to prevent retrograde thrombosis and subsequent valve insufficiency.

Venous gangrene is very rare, in most cases caused by underlying malignancy and can be prevented in phlegmasia caerulea dolens by fasciotomy. Groin infection was very common until we improved preoperative hygiene and began using prophylactic antibiotics. We still see lymphatic leakage but it usually stops within 2–3 weeks. In two patients from the Swedish series the AVF caused high output cardiac failure, returning to normal immediately after the AVF was closed. Both operations had been performed in elderly patients with previously known compromised cardiac function; therefore, careful patient selection is essential. One objection to the AVF is the resulting rise in venous pressure and swelling of the lower limb. We did not observe any rise in iliac vein pressure when outflow was normal. Stenosis of the vein cephalad to the fistula produced higher pressures and stresses the importance of clearing the proximal vein.

'Late' results

There are few studies giving 'long term' results of TE with AVF. In eight studies comprising 521 patients, with more than two years' follow-up, 'clinical success' is claimed in 62 per cent.[59] In five studies of iliac vein patency involving 247 patients with more than two years' follow-up the figure was 82 per cent (range 77–88 per cent).[59] In five studies on femoro-popliteal valvular competence in 259 patients altogether, with more than two years' follow-up, competence was 60 per cent (range 36–84 per cent).[59]

In the prospective, randomised study from Sweden we found a highly significant difference in the number of asymptomatic patients after 6 months, 42 per cent in the surgical group and 7 per cent in the conservatively treated group.[58] At 5 years 37 per cent of the operated patients were asymptomatic compared with 18 per cent in the conservative group.[60] At 10 years 54 per cent in the surgical group were basically asymptomatic (class 0–2 using the CEAP classification) compared with 23 per cent in the conservative group, but the difference was not a significant.[61]

Iliac vein patency demonstrated by venography at 6 months was 76 per cent in the surgical group compared with 35 per cent in the conservative group,[58] a significant difference upheld at 5 years and 10 years with 77 per cent and 77 per cent patency, respectively, in the surgical group, and 30 per cent and 47 per cent, respectively, in the conservative group.[60,61] Femoro-popliteal valvular competence studied by descending venography using Valsalva at 6 months was 52 per cent in the surgical group compared with 26 per cent in the conservatively treated group, which is a significant difference.[58] After 5 years, the patients who underwent TE had significantly lower ambulatory venous pressures, improved venous emptying, as shown by plethysmography, and better calf pump function with less reflux, as measured by foot volumetry. Combining the results of all functional tests, 36 per cent of surgical patients had normal venous function compared with 11 per cent of the conservatively treated group but the differences were not statistically significant due to the loss of patients at follow-up.[60] At 10 years using duplex scanning, popliteal reflux was found in 32 per cent of the surgical group compared with 67 per cent of the conservative group. Six patients who had a successful TE 10 years previously, and in whom the iliac vein was not obstructed after surgery, were all asymptomatic with patent iliac veins, and 50 per cent of them had competent popliteal veins.[61] Successful TE seems to be beneficial in the long term.

CASE ILLUSTRATING OUR CURRENT APPROACH IN PROXIMAL DVT

A 13-year-old Chinese-American boy was admitted from another hospital with superficial thrombophlebitis involving the right long saphenous vein extending into the

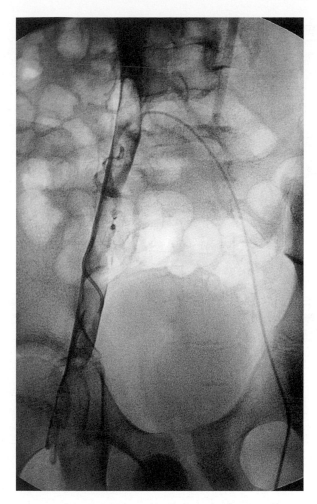

Figure 20.1 *Venogram via the left common femoral vein with the tip into the right external iliac vein shows thrombus partially occluding the common femoral, external and common iliac veins extending 2 cm into the inferior vena cava*

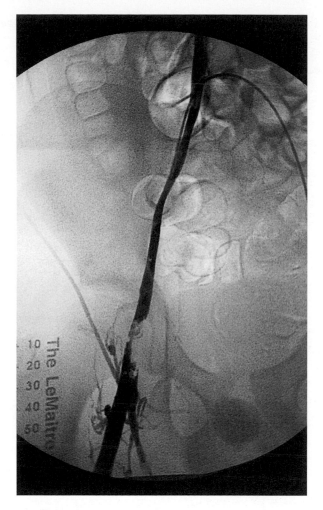

Figure 20.2 *Follow-up venogram 27 hours after catheter directed thrombolysis shows marked improvement, but with residual filling defect in the common femoral vein; attempts at percutaneous, mechanical destruction of the blood clot failed, and surgical thrombectomy with a temporary AVF was performed successfully*

common femoral vein, the iliac vein and protruding into the IVC. Five months before transfer, he was diagnosed with systemic lupus erythematosus (SLE) for which he was treated with steroids and hydroxychloroquine sulphate. For about 5 weeks before admission he had suffered from recurrent episodes of severe pain and swelling of the right lower leg. Duplex scanning of the leg at the onset of symptoms did not reveal any evidence of DVT. A repeat duplex scan from the groin to the knee 3 days before admission was still negative for DVT. The day before referral, however, a further scan revealed thrombus in the right common femoral vein. Upon admission there was slight swelling of the right calf and thigh, no chest symptoms or signs and the platelet count was 33 000. A repeat duplex scan showed thrombosis of the right common femoral vein occluding the long saphenous vein and extending up the iliac vein into the IVC but the deep veins of the leg were free from thrombus. A venogram via the left common femoral vein revealed no thrombus on the left side, but confirmed complete occlusion the right common femoral vein and iliac vein extending 2 cm into the IVC (Fig. 20.1).

Catheter directed thrombolysis with urokinase was started with an infusion of 100 000 IU/hour for 20 hours. A follow-up venogram showed marked improvement with a filling defect still present in the common femoral vein, which remained despite another 7 hours of treatment. Attempts were made to mechanically destroy and aspirate the clot attached to the vein wall (Fig. 20.2). Surgical exploration of the common femoral vein on the same day revealed organised thrombus, which was removed, the wall of the common femoral vein being severely inflamed and 1.5 mm thick. The long saphenous vein was also diseased with evidence of active thrombophlebitis. An AVF was created anastomosing the long saphenous vein end-to-side to the superficial femoral artery. An intraoperative venogram showed complete removal of the thrombus and a patent common femoral vein and iliac vein.

After some postoperative problems the patient rapidly improved and still remains on anticoagulation and other medication for his SLE. Three years later he has no swelling

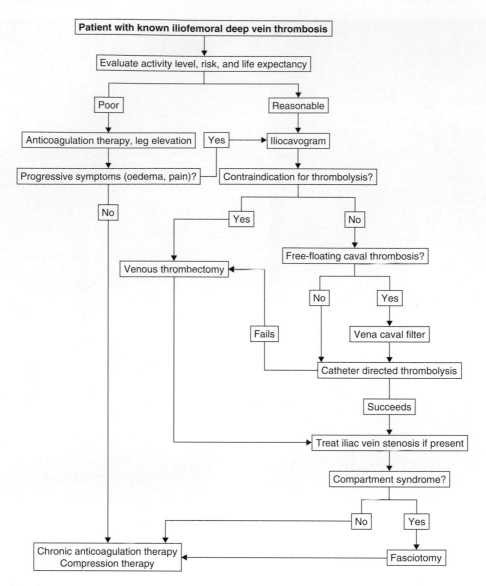

Figure 20.3   *Algorithm for managing patients with proved iliofemoral vein thrombosis (IFVT) (redrawn from Comerota AJ. Iliofemoral deep vein thrombosis. In: Cronenwett JL (ed). Decision Making in Vascular Surgery. Philadelphia: WB Saunders, 2001: 282–5)*

or pain in his leg. Repeated duplex scans have shown a patent deep venous system without any reflux. The AVF closed spontaneously after about 1 year. Three years after the extensive DVT he is fully active and playing basketball. The first line of treatment was CDT and although only partially successful, immediate TE with AVF resulted in a patent and competent deep venous system and, to date, had prevented the potential development of a severe PTS. An algorithm (Fig. 20.3) provides pathways of management of a patient with proved IFVT.

Conclusions

Early and quick removal of the thrombus is indicated to avoid the late PTS in active patients with acute iliofemoral DVT. The first line of treatment should be

CDT with or without adjunctive procedures such as angioplasty and stenting. When there are contraindications to thrombolysis or when it fails, TE with a temporary AVF is a valid alternative. Both interventions should be followed by anticoagulation. These aggressive interventions are not justified in chronically ill, bedridden, high risk or aged patients, or those with serious intercurrent disease and/or limited life expectancy. In this group of patients these interventions can only be justified for limb salvage in phlegmasia caerulea dolens, in which conservative treatment does not prevent the development of an acute compartment syndrome and venous gangrene. The role of LMWH in acute iliofemoral DVT in preventing the PTS should be tested in a prospective randomised trial comparing it with the interventional approach.

Key references

Eklof B, Kamida CB, Kistner RL, Masuda EM. Contemporary treatment of iliofemoral deep vein thrombosis. *Perspect Vasc Surg* 1999; **11**: 1–27.

Hull RD, Pineo GF. Prophylaxis of deep venous thrombosis and pulmonary embolism: current recommendations. *Med Clin North Am* 1998; **82**: 477–93.

Kalodiki E, Nicolaides AN. Low-molecular-weight heparin in the treatment of deep vein thrombosis. In: Pifarre R (ed). *New Anticoagulants for the Cardiovascular Patient.* Philadelphia: Hanley & Belfus, Inc, 1997: 609–19.

Mewissen MW, Seabrook GR, Meissner MN, *et al.* Catheter-directed thrombolysis for lower extremity deep venous thrombosis: Report of a national multi-center registry. *Radiology* 1999; **211**: 39–49.

Semba CP, Dake MD. Iliofemoral deep venous thrombosis: aggressive therapy with catheter directed thrombolysis. *Radiology* 1994; **191**: 487–94.

REFERENCES

1   Miller G. Pulmonary embolism. In: Browse NL, Burnand KG, Lea TM (eds). *Diseases of the Veins: Pathology, Diagnosis and Treatment.* London: Edward Arnold, 1988:558–80.

2   Comerota A. Causes of deep vein thrombosis. *Proceedings of the Straub Pacific Health Foundation* 1993; **57**: 2.

3   Comerota A, Stewart GJ. Operative venous dilation and its relation to postoperative deep venous thrombosis. In: Goldhaber SZ (ed). *Prevention of Venous Thromboembolism.* New York: Dekker 1993: 25–50.

4   Nicolaides AN, Arcelus J, Belcaro G, *et al.* Prevention of venous thromboembolism. European consensus statement, 1–5 November 1991, developed at Oakley Court Hotel, Windsor, UK. *Int Angiol* 1992; **11**: 151–9.

5   Browse NL, Burnand KG, Lea TM (eds). *Diseases of the Veins: Pathology, Diagnosis and Treatment.* London: Edward Arnold, 1988: 603–25.

6   Downing LJ, Wakefield TW, Strieter RM, *et al.* Anti-P-selectin antibody decreases inflammation and thrombus formation in venous thrombosis. *J Vasc Surg* 1997; **25**: 816–28.

7   See-Tho K, Harris EJJ. Thrombosis with outflow obstruction delays thrombolysis and results in chronic wall thickening of rat veins. *J Vasc Surg* 1998; **28**: 115–22.

8   Caps MT, Manzo RA, Bergelin RO, *et al.* Venous valvular reflux in veins not involved at the time of acute deep vein thrombosis. *J Vasc Surg* 1995; **22**: 524–31.

9   Douglas MG, Sumner DS. Duplex scanning for deep vein thrombosis: Has it replaced both phlebography and noninvasive testing? *Semin Vasc Surg* 1996; **9**: 3–12.

10 Kalodiki E, Nicolaides AN. Low-molecular-weight heparin in the treatment of deep vein thrombosis. In: Pifarre R (ed). *New Anticoagulants for the Cardiovascular Patient.* Philadelphia: Hanley & Belfus, Inc, 1997: 609–19.

11 Partsch H. Acute iliofemoral DVT: results of ambulatory treatment. *Vasc Surg* 1997; **31**: 307–9.

12 Leizorovicz A. Comparison of the efficacy and safety of low molecular weight heparins and unfractionated heparin in the initial treatment of deep venous thrombosis: an updated meta-analysis. *Drugs* 1996; **52**(suppl 7): 30–7.

13 Markel A, Manzo RA, Bergelin RO. Strandness DE. Pattern and distribution of thrombi in acute venous thrombosis. *Arch Surg* 1992; **127**: 305–9.

14 Mattos MA, Melendres G, Sumner DS, *et al.* Prevalence and distribution of calf vein thrombosis in patients with symptomatic deep venous thrombosis: a color-flow duplex study. *J Vasc Surg* 1996; **24**: 738–44.

15 Lohr JM, James KV, Deshmukh RM, Hasselfeld KA. Calf vein thrombi are not a benign finding. *Am J Surg* 1995; **170**: 86–90.

16 Passman MA, Moneta GL, Taylor LM, *et al.* Pulmonary embolism is associated with the combination of isolated calf vein thrombosis and respiratory symptoms. *J Vasc Surg* 1997; **25**: 39–45.

17 Masuda EM, Kessler DM, Kistner RL, *et al.* The natural history of calf vein thrombosis: lysis of thrombi and development of reflux. *J Vasc Surg* 1998; **28**: 67–74.

18 Dotter CJ, Rosch J, Seaqman AJ. Selective clot lysis with low-dose streptokinase. *Radiology* 1974; **111**: 31–7.

19 Semba CP, Dake MD. Iliofemoral deep venous thrombosis: Aggressive therapy with catheter directed thrombolysis. *Radiology* 1994; **191**: 487–94.

20 Hartnell GG, Gates J. The case of Abbokinase and the FDA: the events leading to the suspension of Abbokinase supplies in the United States. *J Vasc Interv Radiol* 2000; **11**: 841–7.

21 Eklof B, Kamida CB, Kistner RL, Masuda EM. Contemporary treatment of iliofemoral deep vein thrombosis. *Perspect Vasc Surg* 1999; **11**: 1–27.

22 Mewissen MW, Seabrook GR, Meissner MN, *et al.* Catheter-directed thrombolysis for lower extremity deep venous thrombosis: report of a national multi-center registry. *Radiology* 1999; **211**: 39–49.

23 Semba CP. Venous thrombolysis in the post-urokinase era. *Tech Vasc Interv Radiol* 2000; **3**: 2–11.

24 Cragg AH. Lower extremity deep venous thrombolysis: a new approach to obtaining access. *J Vasc Interv Radiol* 1996; **7**: 283–6.

25 Shull KC, Nicolaides AN, Fernandes E, *et al.* Significance of popliteal reflux in relation to ambulatory venous pressure and ulceration. *Arch Surg* 1979; **114**: 1304–6.

26 Ouriel K, Katzen B, Mewissen MW, *et al.* Reteplase in the treatment of peripheral arterial and venous occlusions. A pilot study. *J Vasc Interv Radiol* 2000; **11**: 849–54.

27 Valji K. Evolving strategies for thrombolytic therapy of peripheral vascular occlusion. *J Vasc Interv Radiol* 2000; **11**: 411–29.

28 Grossman C, McPherson S. Safety and efficacy of catheter-directed thrombolysis for iliofemoral venous thrombosis. *AJR Am J Radiol* 1999; **172**: 667–72.

29 Comerota AJ, Throm RC, Mathias SD, *et al.* Catheter-directed thrombolysis for iliofemoral deep venous thrombosis improves health-related quality of life. *J Vasc Surg* 2000; **32**: 130–7.

30 Bjarnason H, Kruse JR, Asinger DA, *et al.* Iliofemoral deep vein thrombosis: Safety and efficacy during five years of catheter directed thrombolytic therapy. *J Vasc Interv Radiol* 1997; **8**: 405–18.

31 Sharafuddin MJA, Hicks ME. Current status of percutaneous mechanical thrombectomy. Part I. General principles. *J Vasc Interv Radiol* 1997; **8**: 911–21.

32 Sharafuddin MJA, Hicks ME. Current status of percutaneous mechanical thrombectomy. Part II. Devices and mechanisms of action. *J Vasc Interv Radiol* 1998; **9**: 15–31.

33 Sharafuddin MJA, Hicks ME. Current status of percutaneous mechanical thrombectomy. Part III. Present and future applications. *J Vasc Interv Radiol* 1998; **9**: 209–34.

34 O'Sullivan GJ, Semba CP, Bittner CA, *et al.* Endovascular management of iliac vein compression (May-Thurner) syndrome. *J Vasc Interv Radiol* 2000; **11**: 823–36.

35 Sharafuddin MJA, Gu X, Urness M, Amplatz K. Lack of acute injury to venous valves by the Amplatz Thrombectomy Device during experimental antegrade venous thrombectomy. *J Vasc Interv Radiol* 1998; **9**(suppl): 203.

36 Nazarian GK, Bjarnason H, Dietz CA Jr, *et al.* Iliofemoral venous stenoses: Effectiveness of treatment with metallic endovascular stents. *Radiology* 1996; **200**: 193–9.

37 Virchow R. Uber die Erweiterung kleiner Gefasse. *Arch Path Anat* 1851; **3**: 427.

38 Greenfield LJ, Rutherford RB. Recommended reporting standards for vena caval filter placement and patient follow-up. *J Vasc Interv Radiol* 1999; **10**: 1013–19; Erratum in: *J Vasc Interv Radiol* 1999; **10**: 1270.

39 Hull RD, Pineo GF. Prophylaxis of deep venous thrombosis and pulmonary embolism: current recommendations. *Med Clin North Am* 1998; **82**: 477–93.

40 Lorch H, Welger D, Wagner V, *et al.* Current practice of temporary vena cava filter insertion: a multi-center registry. *J Vasc Interv Radiol* 2000; **11**: 83–8.

41 Athanasoulis C, Kaufman J, Halpern E, *et al.* Inferior vena caval filters: review of a 26-year, single-center clinical experience. *Radiology* 2000; **216**: 54–66.

42 Rose SC, Kinney TB, Valji K, Winchell RJ. Placement of inferior vena caval filters in the intensive care unit. *J Vasc Interv Radiol* 1997; **8**: 61–4.

43 Neuzil DF, Garrard CL, Berkman RA, *et al.* Duplex-directed vena caval filter placement: report of initial experience. *Surgery* 1998; **123**: 470–4.

44 Homans J. Exploration and division of the femoral and iliac veins in the treatment of thrombophlebitis of the leg. *JAMA* 1941; **224**: 179–86.

45 Mahorner H. New management for thrombosis of deep veins of extremities. *Am Surgeon* 1954; **20**: 487–98.

46 Mahorner H, Castleberry JW, Coleman WO. Attempts to restore function in major veins which are the site of massive thrombosis. *Ann Surg* 1957; **146**: 510–22.

47 Haller JAJ, Abrams BL. Use of thrombectomy in the treatment of acute iliofemoral venous thrombosis in forty-five patients. *Ann Surg* 1963; **158**: 561–9.

48 Lansing AM, Davis WM. Five-year follow-up study of iliofemoral venous thrombectomy. *Ann Surg* 1968; **168**: 620–8.

49 Edwards WH, Sawyers JL, Foster JH. Iliofemoral venous thrombosis: reappraisal of thrombectomy. *Ann Surg* 1970; **171**: 961–70.

50 Karp RB, Wylie EJ. Recurrent thrombosis after iliofemoral venous thrombectomy. *Surg Forum* 1966; **17**: 147.

51 Kistner RL. Valve repair and segment transposition in primary valvular insufficiency. In: Bergan JJ, Yao JST (eds). *Venous Disorders.* Philadelphia: WB Saunders, 1991: 261–72.

52 Lawen A. Uber Thrombektomie bei Venenthrombose und Arteriospamus. *Zentralbl Chir* 1937; **64**: 961–8.

53 Masuda EM, Kistner RL, Ferris EB. Long-term effects of superficial femoral vein ligation: thirteen-year follow-up. *J Vasc Surg* 1992; **16**: 741–9.

54 Endrys J, Eklof B, Neglen P, *et al.* Percutaneous balloon occlusion of surgical arteriovenous fistulae following venous thrombectomy. *Cardiovasc Intervent Radiol* 1989; **12**: 226–9.

55 Plate G, Ohlin P, Eklof B. Pulmonary embolism in acute iliofemoral venous thrombosis. *Br J Surg* 1985; **72**: 912–15.

56 Mavor GE, Galloway JMD. The iliofemoral venous segment as a source of pulmonary emboli. *Lancet* 1967; **i**: 871.

57 Kistner RL, Sparkuhl MD. Surgery in acute and chronic venous disease. *Surgery* 1979; **85**: 31–43.

58 Plate G, Einarsson E, Ohlin P, *et al.* Thrombectomy with temporary arteriovenous fistula: the treatment of choice in acute iliofemoral venous thrombosis. *J Vasc Surg* 1984; **1**: 867–76.

59 Eklof B, Kistner RL. Is there a role for thrombectomy in iliofemoral venous thrombosis? *Semin Vasc Surg* 1996; **9**: 34–45.

60 Plate G, Akesson H, Einarsson E, *et al.* Long-term results of venous thrombectomy combined with a temporary arterio-venous fistula. *Eur J Vasc Surg* 1990; **4**: 483–9.

61 Plate G, Eklof B, Norgren L, *et al.* Venous thrombectomy for iliofemoral vein thrombosis. 10-year results of a prospective randomized study. *Eur J Vasc Endovasc Surg* 1997; **14**: 367–74.

21

Pulmonary Embolism

ANH NGUYEN, ELAINE IMOTO, BO GH EKLOF

THE PROBLEM

Pulmonary embolism (PE) is a potentially fatal complication of deep venous thrombosis (DVT). While common, it remains underdiagnosed. The antemortem diagnosis of PE was made in only 30 per cent of patients confirmed as having had PE at autopsy.[1] Eighty per cent of patients with angio-proven PE had bilateral leg venography which showed evidence of DVT in 82 per cent, symptomatic in only 42 per cent.[2,3]

The astute physician must combine a high clinical suspicion for PE, based on presenting features and appropriate risk factors, with timely investigations and empirical therapy. The majority of PEs are caused by portions of thrombi originating in the upper leg and pelvic veins breaking off and travelling to the lungs. The focus of this chapter therefore will be the diagnosis and therapy of thombotic emboli. At all times less frequent causes of PE such as upper extremity thrombi, air, bone marrow, arthroplasty cement, amniotic fluid, talc, fat, septic and tumour emboli should be kept in mind.

CLINICAL PRESENTATION

The clinical presentation is quite diverse, depending on the size of the vessel occluded and the patient's cardiorespiratory reserve. A normal person may tolerate total occlusion of a unilateral pulmonary artery with minimal symptoms. A patient with pre-existing cardiopulmonary compromise may die from the same occlusion. Findings in PE can be understood in terms of the severity of PE as it increases from 'mild' with the pulmonary infarction syndrome, to 'moderate' with isolated dyspnoea syndrome and to 'severe' with circulatory collapse.[4] In assessing the patient with an acute presentation, the clinician must be able to distinguish between small and massive PE, as the latter is life threatening and must be diagnosed and treated promptly.[5]

Some or *none* of the following symptoms may be present in the patient with a submassive or massive PE presenting with circulatory collapse at risk of death in the next three hours:[4,6] dyspnoea, pleuritic pain, haemoptysis, wheeze, anterior chest pain, cough, and leg swelling and pain. The classic triad of symptoms of **dyspnoea**, **haemoptysis** and **pleuritic chest pain** occurred in only 28 per cent of the 160 patients in the Urokinase Pulmonary Embolism Trial (UPET) and in only 20 per cent of patients with massive embolism.[7] None of the five patients in the Prospective Investigation of Pulmonary Embolism Diagnosis (PIOPED) study with circulatory collapse from PE, loss of consciousness or blood pressure <80 mmHg, had haemoptysis, pleuritic pain, palpitations or angina-like pain.[4]

Symptoms of PE

- Dyspnoea, wheeze
- Pleuritic pain
- Cough, haemoptysis
- Leg swelling and pain

RISK FACTORS

As symptoms and signs vary between presentations, the presence of risk factor(s) will add to the suspicion of PE and

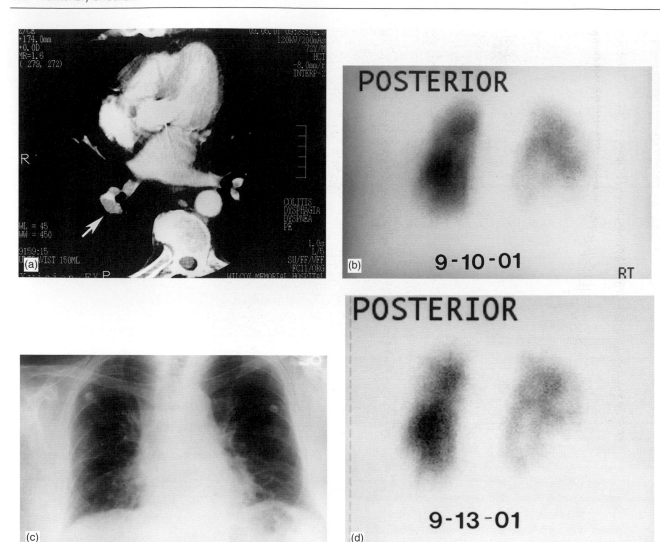

Figure 21.1 *A 72-year-old male developed pain and swelling of the right leg with shortness of breath 3 months after a lengthy flight from Africa. A duplex scan showed extensive deep vein thrombosis (DVT) in the right leg. (a) Computed tomography (CT) angiogram confirming right pulmonary artery embolism with the doughnut sign (arrow) despite having been on warfarin (Coumadin) treatment for an aortic valve prosthesis. After adding low molecular weight heparin an inferior vena cava (IVC) filter was placed below the renal veins. (b) A ventilation/perfusion (V/Q) scan 5 days later confirming pulmonary embolism (PE) of the right lung. He was discharged 2 days thereafter to continue on warfarin. (c) A chest radiograph on readmission following a syncopal attack and hypoxia on the day after discharge showing that the heart was not enlarged and pulmonary vascularity was normal. Several vague 'nodules' were seen projecting over the lung bases suspicious of metastatic disease. (d) A repeat V/Q scan showing increased embolism to the lungs. Lytic therapy in the form of tissue plasminogen activator (tPA) was commenced in the intensive care unit (ICU) but stopped in 24 hours because of gastrointestinal bleeding. He also developed severe swelling of the left leg and another duplex scan showed DVT in both legs extending from the tibial veins all the way up to the IVC filter. Following a fresh syncopal attack 2 days after readmission a further V/Q scan revealed more embolism to the right lung.*

help to decide whether further investigation is warranted.[8,9] They all revolve around the thrombotic triad elucidated by Virchow in 1856: local trauma to the vessel wall, hypercoagulability and stasis. Stasis and local augmentation of the coagulation process are the most important factors in thrombus formation making recognition of acquired risk factors (see Chapter 2) critical for therapy.[10] **Acquired risk factors** include recent major surgery or trauma, immobilisation, as for instance on long flights, advancing age, malignancy (Fig. 21.1), previous thrombosis, pregnancy and puerperium, use of contraceptives or hormone replacement

therapy (HRT), resistance to activated protein C, antiphospholipid antibodies and mild-to-moderate hyperhomocysteinaemia.[11] In the Nurses' Health Study,[12] nurses 60 years or older in the highest quintile of body mass index had the highest rate of PE. Heavy cigarette smoking and high blood pressure were identified as independent risk factors.

Genetic predisposition appears to explain one-fifth of cases of PE. The family history is critical if the patient is young and if there is a possibility of lifetime anticoagulation and avoidance of additional acquired risk factors.[11] The most common **inherited risk factors** are activated

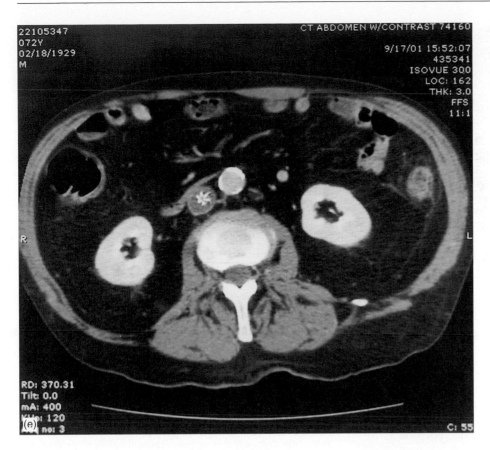

Figure 21.1 (*Continued*)
(*e*) *A CT angiogram 2 days later showing extension of IVC thrombus 2 cm above the filter ending about 1 cm below the renal vein. The IVC was ligated after removal of thrombus below the renal veins. He was discharged on warfarin, recovered and made it to the golf course. He died suddenly 3 months later with generalised metastatic cancer, the primary site still unknown*

protein C resistance due to a mutation in the factor V gene, namely, factor V Leiden, with a 5 per cent prevalence in the Caucasian population, G20210A mutation in the pro-thrombin (factor II) gene and homozygous C677T mutation in the methylene-tetrahydrofolate reductase gene.[13] Antithrombin, protein C and protein S deficiencies are rare while homozygous homocysteinuria is very rare.

Risk factors

- Acquired
  - Recent major surgery/trauma
  - Prolonged immobilisation
  - Advancing age
  - Malignancy
  - Previous thrombosis
  - Pregnancy/puerperium
  - Contraceptives/HRT
  - Antiphospholipid antibodies
- Inherited
  - Antithrombin deficiency
  - Protein C deficiency
  - Protein S deficiency
  - Factor V Leiden (Activated protein C resistance)
  - G20210A mutation prothrombin (F II) gene

- Homozygous C677T mutation in the methylene-tetrahydrofolate reductase gene
- Homozygous homocysteinuria

CLINICAL SIGNS

Signs of PE are often absent, and, even when present tend to be non-specific. The concurrent presence of DVT (30 per cent) must be investigated as supportive evidence for PE and as an indication for anticoagulation. The most common signs of PE[14,15] include cyanosis, tachypnoea, the use of accessory muscles of respiration, tachycardia, hypotension, elevated jugular venous pressure (JVP), left parasternal heave, chest wall tenderness, gallop rhythm on cardiac auscultation, pleural rub, crackles, thrombophlebitis, fever and sweating. Signs of right heart insufficiency should prompt early action. Elevated JVP, low blood pressure, gallop rhythm and cyanosis all suggest pulmonary hypertension as a result of massive PE.

Signs of PE

- Cyanosis, fever, sweating
- Tachypnoea, use of accessory muscles of respiration

- Tachycardia, hypotension, raised JVP
- Left parasternal heave, gallop rhythm
- Chest wall tenderness, pleural rub, crackles
- Thrombophlebitis

DIFFERENTIAL DIAGNOSIS

The signs and symptoms of PE are often non-specific but they should be considered in a differential diagnosis.[16] The possible diagnoses include acute myocardial infarction (MI), acute pulmonary oedema, pneumonia, asthma, pneumothorax, pleurisy, tachyarrhythmia, pericardial tamponade, musculoskeletal pain, rib fracture, lobar collapse, lung cancer, primary pulmonary hypertension, costochondritis, aortic dissection or anxiety. Overdiagnosis is as likely as underdiagnosis. A detailed history, whenever possible, physical examination and selective testing will improve diagnostic accuracy.

Differential diagnoses of PE

- Cardiovascular – acute MI, acute pulmonary oedema, tachyarrhythmia, pericardial tamponade, aortic dissection
- Pulmonary – pneumonia, asthma, pneumothorax, pleurisy, lobar collapse, lung cancer, primary pulmonary hypertension
- Chest wall – musculoskeletal pain, rib fracture, costochondritis
- Anxiety

INVESTIGATIONS

Laboratory tests for the diagnosis of PE should include an arterial blood gas (ABG), chest X-ray (CXR), electrocardiography (ECG) and D-dimer. Arterial blood gases are checked if the patient has hypoxia detected on pulse oximetry or if the patient is tachypnoeic. Increased minute ventilation is a sensitive indicator of larger PE. A respiratory alkalosis may be detected and hypoxaemia can be confirmed. In the case of a small embolus, however, these findings may not be present, so that the absence of findings on ABG does not exclude the possibility of an embolus.[5,17]

Frequently obtained, a CXR helps to exclude other diagnoses (Fig. 21.1c). Occasional, non-specific CXR findings in PE include an elevated hemidiaphragm, subsegmental atelectasis, small pleural effusions and patchy infiltrates due to associated oedema, haemorrhage or infarction. Large emboli can cause dilatation of a proximal pulmonary artery with oligaemia in the distant lung field known as the Westermark sign. More often than not, the CXR in PE is more likely to appear normal than to show the classic wedge-shaped defect or the Hampton hump. The most common X-ray finding is simple cardiomegaly.[18]

The ECG will help to exclude other diagnoses, especially acute MI and tachyarrhythmias. As with chest films, ECGs may suggest PE but they are usually not diagnostic.[19] The classic ECG changes of S1Q3T3 are present in only 25 per cent of patients with PE. The ECG will frequently reveal non-specific tachycardia or atrial fibrillation. Evidence of right ventricular insufficiency may exist in the form of right bundle branch block, P pulmonale, right axis deviation, and T wave inversion in leads V1–3.[5] These findings, however, are present only after significant obstruction ($\sim >50$ per cent) of the pulmonary vasculature has occurred in an otherwise healthy patient, but they are more pronounced in patients with previous cardiopulmonary disease.[20]

Plasma D–dimer

This is a sensitive but a non-specific test of venous thromboembolic disease.[21–23] D-dimers are crosslinks which are cleaved and then released into the circulation by the action of plasmin during fibrinolysis. This event occurs within one hour of thrombus formation. *D-dimer values $<500\,\mu g/mL$ reliably exclude PE in patients with intermediate and low probability lung scans.*[21,24,25] They do not, however, exclude PE in high probability scans. D-dimers also have no positive predictive value as a variety of reasons cause them to rise e.g. recent surgery, trauma, MI, congestive heart failure, pneumonia, cancer and sepsis. The D-dimer assay is useful in patients who present to the emergency department or physician's office without other systemic illnesses. If clinical likelihood is low, a D-dimer assay and duplex scan of the leg veins may be useful in ruling out PE/DVT. Because it is not 100 per cent sensitive, D-dimer cannot be used to rule out the diagnosis in patients in whom there is a high clinical suspicion of PE.[26,27]

Other laboratory tests are helpful in delineating disease processes such as elevated cardiac enzymes in MI and an elevated leucocyte count in infection. Leucocytosis, however, can also be present in a stressed state with lung infarction.

The decision to investigate further should be based on clinical suspicion as to whether a PE has occurred. The most common scenario is the patient with a risk factor who becomes breathless suddenly and has a normal CXR and perhaps mild hypoxia, without any obvious cause. Assessment of the patient allows the clinical probability of a diagnosis of PE to be expressed as high, intermediate, low or unlikely, depending on the predictive value ascribed to a particular presentation.[28]

Clinical probability of diagnosis of PE (per cent chance)

- High[*] (80–100 per cent)
  - Presence of a risk factor
  - CXR, ABG or D-dimer consistent finding; lack of evidence for another explanation

- Intermediate* (20–80 per cent)
  - Neither high nor low probability
- Low (1–19 per cent)
  - No risk factor
  - Clinical symptoms and signs explainable by other causes
  - ABG/CXR explainable by other causes
  - D-dimer positive
- Unlikely (<1 per cent)
  - Low clinical probability
  - D-dimer negative

*Further investigations should be undertaken in high and intermediate probability cases

FURTHER INVESTIGATIONS

Ventilation/perfusion lung scanning

This remains the first line investigation of possible PE when multidetector helical computed tomography (CT) scanning is unavailable.[25] The sensitivity and specificity of ventilation/perfusion (V/Q) scans has been investigated in the PIOPED multicentre trial. They can be performed rapidly with minimal risk to the patient (see Fig. 21.1b, d). The interpretation and use of V/Q scans seems most effective in conjunction with clinical probability assignment.[21,29–31] V/Q scan results should be interpreted as normal, or demonstrating low, intermediate or high probability for PE. A **normal** scan excludes PE with 96 per cent accuracy and a **high** probability scan with a risk factor is diagnostic of PE with 86–92 per cent accuracy. A **low** probability scan with no risk factors still requires further investigation to exclude PE but 8 per cent of patients with low probability lung scans and negative lower extremity Doppler ultrasound have PE.[32] Patients with **intermediate** scans and those with **incongruity** between the V/Q result and clinical suspicion require further investigation.[25,29]

Spiral CT of the lungs

Depending on radiological availability and cooperation at individual institutions, V/Q scans are not often performed until the day after presentation or after a weekend. This delay has prompted many clinicians to take advantage of spiral CT, if available, as the first line investigation, which it often is when a large PE is suspected and early diagnosis is needed (Fig. 21.1a) or when a patient has pre-existing cardiopulmonary disease which would limit interpretation of the V/Q scan results.[33–35]

The speed of spiral CT allows the pulmonary vasculature to be examined with the use of peripherally administered contrast during a single breath-hold. It is sensitive and specific for *central and segmental* vessels, but is not as good at detecting peripheral emboli, which may account for up to 20

per cent of PE.[35–38] Spiral CT and V/Q scans are comparable as first line testing for PE.[24] Multidetector CT (MDCT) provides the next step in diagnostic accuracy with the ability to obtain thin sections 2–3 mm at narrow intervals of 2–3 mm and yet perform the study within a 10–15 second breath-hold. Although no article with specific statistics has been published, the advantages are clear-cut for PE and have been addressed by studies on helical CT.[39] An additional advantage of MDCT is the ability to combine a CT venogram of the deep venous system with the CT pulmonary angiogram, two tests being performed together in a timely manner for diagnosis of PE with a good look at the inferior vena cava (IVC) and iliac veins when, in selected cases, consideration is given to inserting an IVC filter (Fig. 21.1e). This may be the single examination of choice when more institutions have MDCT installed.[40]

Further investigations

- V/Q lung scanning
- Spiral CT of the lungs
- Echocardiography
- Pulmonary angiography
- Duplex scanning of the legs

Echocardiography

V/Q scans have shown good results as seen in the PIOPED study,[31,41] PE being present in those scans indicating high probability. Unfortunately, only a small number of patients with PE have high probability scans.[41] Echocardiography has been looked at for its value in the diagnosis of PE.[21,42] It may be useful after a large PE in a haemodynamically compromised patient,[35] as it can reveal the presence of right heart dysfunction, the occasional intracardiac thrombus and increased pulmonary artery pressure readings with dilated pulmonary arteries. The presence and degree of right ventricular pressure overload can be important for diagnostic and prognostic purposes. These findings may be documented using either the transthoracic or transoesophageal approach. One limitation to consider is the presence of chronic obstructive pulmonary disease, which can make the differential diagnosis between acute PE and chronic cor pulmonale difficult.[43]

Pulmonary angiography

Pulmonary angiography remains the gold standard investigation for PE where MDCT is not available. It is invasive, expensive, not readily available, time consuming, and labour intensive.[5,25] It is most reliable if performed immediately after embolism has taken place and becomes less reliable with the passage of time because thrombolysis occurs rapidly within the pulmonary circulation. It should be considered if non-invasive tests are inconclusive, if there is a high clinical suspicion and if MDCT is not available. The mortality rate associated with pulmonary angiography in the PIOPED study was less than 1 per cent, major morbidity was 1 per cent and non-major complications 5 per cent.[41]

Duplex scanning of the legs

A positive duplex scan along with an intermediate probability lung scan provide strong evidence for PE.[5,29] Duplex scanning is a powerful adjunct to lung scanning and can be performed with minimal delay.

TREATMENT

The goals of therapy are to support and maintain life during the acute episode, to stop the spread of the thromboembolus, to foster spontaneous or induce fibrinolytic removal of the thromboembolus and to prevent recurrence. These goals can be further categorised as prevention, primary treatment and secondary prophylaxis, involving supportive care, anticoagulation, thrombolysis, and/or embolectomy. With early diagnosis and swift aggressive therapy many patients will survive PE with a low rate of recurrence.

Prevention

Identifying patients with risk factors is essential, as the incidence of venous thrombosis and PE can be reduced by limiting venous stasis or by administering drugs to inhibit coagulation.[44] Elastic stockings and pneumatic compression devices increase venous return, and the pneumatic pump may increase fibrinolytic activity with its rhythmic compressions. Prophylaxis with low molecular weight heparin (LMWH) by once-daily subcutaneous injection is simple and does not need monitoring as its effects are predictable and weight dependent. Perioperative use of low dose subcutaneous heparin can prevent about half of PEs and about two-thirds of DVTs, with a significant reduction in fatal episodes.[5]

Primary therapy

The response to pulmonary embolisation is determined by the size of the embolus and the patient's cardiopulmonary status. If the PE is *small* and the patient is reasonably well, then oxygen administration by mask or nasal prong may be all that is needed for supportive care.[5] Tracheal intubation and respiratory assistance may be necessary if the hypoxaemia is profound.

Specific treatment consists of intravenous heparin infusion following an initial bolus. When sufficient amounts of heparin are given to stabilise and stop the clotting process, the activated partial thromboplastin time (APTT) becomes about twice that of control. The APTT should be monitored 6 hours after initiation and 6 hours after any

change of dosage, then daily once the APTT level is stable with a target range of 1.5–2.5 times normal. Weight based nomograms may assist in rapid achievement of target APTT.[45] If clinical suspicion of PE is low, treatment does not have to be commenced until after pulmonary imaging. On the other hand, in the absence of specific contraindications such as an active bleed, patients with a moderate or high likelihood of PE should receive intensive anticoagulation while undergoing further investigation.[16] Heparin does not reduce acute mortality but significantly reduces further untoward events. Low molecular weight heparin is now first line treatment for DVT and is as effective as intravenous heparin in PE.[44,46–51] Figure 21.2 offers an algorithm on the management of patients with possible PE but who are haemodynamically stable.

With *massive* PE, the presentation may be quite dramatic, and immediate, aggressive institution of supportive care is crucial, consisting of attempts to increase venous return and maintaining filling pressures within the heart to ensure cardiac output. Approximately 10 per cent of patients with PE do not survive the initial embolic event.[52] Specific therapy consists of anticoagulation and lytic therapy. When there is cardiac compromise and a significantly unstable haemodynamic state, thrombolysis may be instituted.[48] Many patients die from massive PE because of right ventricular failure secondary to the sudden increase in pulmonary vascular resistance caused by embolism. Thrombolysis offers a theoretical advantage over heparin, achieving faster lysis and resolution of thrombus and resulting in a lowering of pulmonary hypertension and improvement in cardiac output. The long term outcomes, however, are similar.[50,53] In addition, thrombolysis has potentially devastating side effects and therefore its use is restricted to life-threatening cardiac compromise.

Faced with this severe situation and if thrombolysis has failed or if there are contraindications to this treatment, pulmonary embolectomy, either as suction catheter embolectomy or as open surgical embolectomy on cardiopulmonary bypass can be contemplated. This has an average perioperative morbidity rate of 26 per cent. Transfemoral removal of emboli was described by Greenfield in 1981 using a specially designed bell-mouthed suction catheter passed into the pulmonary artery under fluoroscopic control. In 1908 Trendelenburg had first described open pulmonary embolectomy, that today involves cardiopulmonary bypass and embolectomy using embolectomy catheters and manual compression of the affected lung. To avoid re-embolisation, an IVC filter may be placed concurrently with the procedure.[47,49,54,55] Figure 21.3 offers an algorithm for the management of patients with possible PE but who are haemodynamically unstable.

Secondary prophylaxis

Secondary treatment comprises oral anticoagulants in the form of subcutaneous heparin and insertion of an IVC

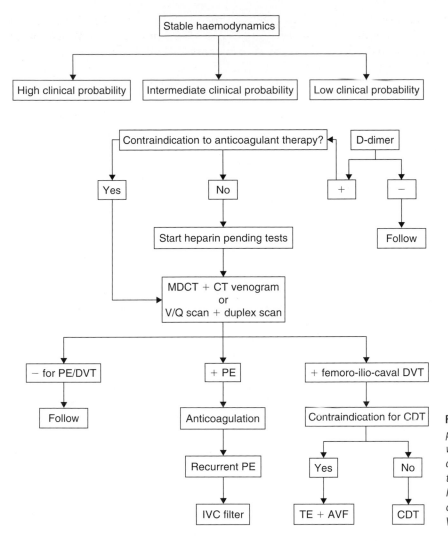

Figure 21.2 *Algorithm of management of patients with possible pulmonary embolism (PE) who are haemodynamically stable. AVF, arteriovenous fistula; CDT, catheter directed thrombolysis; DVT, deep vein thrombosis; IVC, inferior vena cava; MDCT, multidetector computed tomography; TE, thrombectomy; V/Q, ventilation/perfusion*

filter.[48] Warfarin is started in hospital and heparin continued until the prothrombin time is therapeutically elevated, with an international normalised ratio (INR) of two to three times normal.[47,49,50,56] This level must be maintained for 24 hours before heparin is discontinued, usually within 5–7 days. Warfarin can be started at the same time as heparin, as there is no advantage to prolonging heparin therapy beyond the few days needed to establish a goal INR with warfarin. Heparin is continued for a 24 hour overlap period with warfarin. Subcutaneous LMWH can be given in cases where warfarin is contraindicated, for example in pregnancy.

After the first episode of PE, treatment is recommended for at least 3 months.[47,49,57] With repeated episodes of PE, permanent anticoagulation is implemented unless there is an obvious reversible cause. Repeat duplex scans of the legs or repeat V/Q scans have been used to confirm complete resolution of thrombus before stopping anticoagulation. Elastic stockings and avoidance of positions of venous stasis are prescribed to reduce the incidence of recurrent embolism.

Patients with recurrent thromboembolic disease, and especially those in whom anticoagulant treatment is contraindicated or has been ineffective, are good candidates for IVC interruption to prevent fatal PE.[50] The IVC filters are inserted under radiological guidance via the femoral or jugular veins and are lodged below the renal veins. Complications of insertion are low but can be extremely significant, including events threatening life and limb. Transvenous insertion of a Greenfield titanium vena caval filter protects 97 per cent of patients from PE while maintaining patency of the IVC in 100 per cent of them.[55] In emergency situations, IVC filters can be placed under duplex ultrasound guidance. The rare complication of IVC filter failure may warrant ligation of the IVC.

Recurrent thromboembolic pulmonary disease

Recurrent pulmonary emboli, often occurring over many years, eventually lead to irreversible pulmonary hypertension with resultant right heart failure and cor pulmonale.[5] Dyspnoea is chronic and insidious, often with stepwise progression. Cyanosis and peripheral oedema is common. The JVP is elevated and S3, S4 heart sounds are often

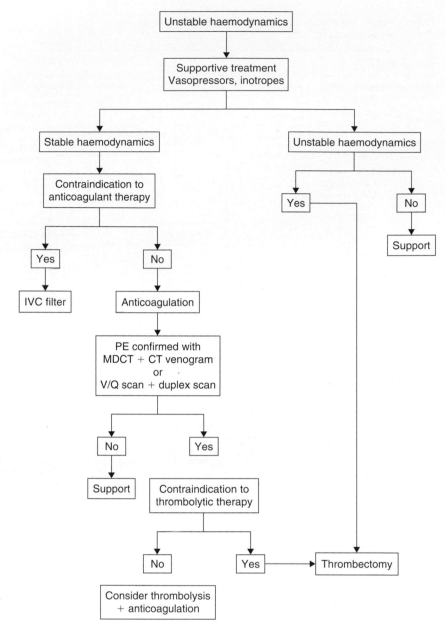

Figure 21.3 *Algorithm for management of patients with possible pulmonary embolism who are haemodynamically unstable. CT, computed tomography; IVC, inferior vena cava; V/Q, ventilation/perfusion*

present. The pulmonary component of S2 is loud. Systolic pulmonary artery pressure is often greater than 70 mmHg. Treatment is aimed at preventing further progression, but symptoms are unlikely to be reversed. Intervention consists of anticoagulation, domiciliary oxygen and treatment of peripheral oedema with diuretics, balanced with maintaining adequate filling pressures. Embolectomy evaluation should be done at specialised centres before considering heart–lung transplantation in appropriate patients.

Conclusions

Pulmonary embolism is a potentially fatal complication of DVT, in most cases originating in the upper leg and pelvic veins. While common, it remains underdiagnosed

as shown by autopsy studies: the diagnosis is established in only a third of patients. The astute physician must combine a high clinical suspicion for PE, based on presenting features and appropriate risk factors, with early diagnosis and swift, aggressive therapy involving supportive care, anticoagulation, thrombolysis, and/or embolectomy. Many patients will survive pulmonary embolism with a low incidence of morbidity and recurrence.

Key references

Anderson DR, Wells PS. Improvements in the diagnostic approach for patients with suspected deep vein thrombosis or pulmonary embolism. *Thromb Haemost* 1999; **82**: 878–86.

Bates S, Hirsch J. Treatment of venous thromboembolism. *Thromb Haemost* 1999; **82**: 870–7.

Gray HH, Firoozan S. Management of pulmonary embolism. *Thorax* 1992; **47**: 825–32.

Michiels JJ. Rational diagnosis of pulmonary embolism (RADIA PE) in symptomatic patients with suspected PE: an improved strategy to exclude or diagnose venous thromboembolism by the sequential use of a clinical model, rapid ELISA D-dimer test, perfusion lung scan, ultrasonography, spiral CT and pulmonary angiography. *Semin Thromb Hemost* 1998; **24**: 413–18.

PIOPED Investigators. Value of the ventilation/perfusion scan in acute pulmonary embolism: results of the Prospective Investigation of Pulmonary Embolism Diagnosis (PIOPED). *JAMA* 1990; **263**: 2753–9.

REFERENCES

1   Stein PD, Henry JW. Prevalence of acute pulmonary embolism among patients in a general hospital and at autopsy. *Chest* 1995; **108**: 978–81.

2   Girard P, Musset D, Parent F, *et al*. High prevalence of detectable deep venous thrombosis in patients with acute pulmonary embolism. *Chest* 1999; **116**: 903–8.

3   Lindblad B, Eriksson A, Bergqvist D. Autopsy-verified pulmonary embolism in a surgical department: analysis of the period from 1951 to 1988. *Br J Surg* 1991; **78**: 849–52.

4   Stein PD, Henry JW. Clinical characteristics of patients with acute pulmonary embolism stratified according to their presenting syndromes. *Chest* 1997; **112**: 974–9.

5   Gray HH, Firoozan S. Management of pulmonary embolism. *Thorax* 1992; **47**: 825–32.

6   Bell WR, Simon TL, Demets DL. The clinical features of submassive and massive pulmonary emboli. *Am J Med* 1977; **62**: 355.

7   Urokinase pulmonary embolism trial: Phase 1 results: a cooperative study. *JAMA* 1970; **214**: 2163.

8   Coon WW. Risk factors of pulmonary embolism. *Surg Gynecol Obstet* 1976; **143**: 385.

9   Goldhaber SZ. Optimizing anticoagulant therapy in the management of pulmonary embolism. *Semin Thromb Hemost* 1999; **25**(suppl 3): 129–33.

10 Dahl O. Mechanism of hypercoagulability. *Thromb Haemost* 1999; **82**: 902–6.

11 Seligsohn U, Lubetsky A. Genetic susceptibility to venous thrombosis. *N Engl J Med* 2001; **344**: 1222–31.

12 Goldhaber SZ, Grodstein F, Stampfer MJ, *et al*. A prospective study of risk factors for pulmonary embolism in women. *JAMA* 1997; **277**: 642–5.

13 De Stefano V, Chiusolo P, Piciaroni K, Leone G. Epidemiology of factor V Leiden: clinical implications. *Semin Thromb Hemost* 1998; **24**: 367–79.

14 Hull RD, Hirsch J, Carter CJ, *et al*. Pulmonary angiography, ventilation lung scanning and venography for clinically suspected pulmonary embolism with abnormal perfusion lung scan. *Ann Intern Med* 1983; **98**: 891–9.

15 Sasahara AA, Sharma GV, Barsamian EM, *et al*. Pulmonary Thromboembolism. *JAMA* 1983; **249**: 2945–50.

16 Goldhaber SZ. Pulmonary embolism. *N Engl J Med* 1998; **339**: 93–104.

17 Cvitanic O, Marino PL. Improved use of arterial blood gas analysis in suspected pulmonary embolism. *Chest* 1989; **95**: 48–51.

18 Elliot CG, Goldhaber SZ, Visani L, DeRosa M. Chest radiographs in acute pulmonary embolism. *Chest* 2000; **118**: 33–8.

19 Stein PD, Dalen JE, McIntyre KM, *et al*. The electrocardiogram in acute pulmonary embolism. *Prog Cardiovasc Dis* 1975; **17**: 247–57.

20 McIntyre KM, Sasahara AA, Littmann D. Relation of the electrocardiogram to hemodynamic alterations in pulmonary embolism. *Am J Cardiol* 1972; **30**: 205–10.

21 Anderson DR, Wells PS. Improvements in the diagnostic approach for patients with suspected deep vein thrombosis or pulmonary embolism. *Thromb Haemost* 1999; **82**: 878–86.

22 Ginsberg JS, Wells PS, Kearon C, *et al*. Sensitivity and specificity of a rapid whole-blood assay for D-dimer in the diagnosis of pulmonary embolism. *Ann Intern Med* 1998; **129**: 1006–11.

23 Perrrier A, Bounameaux H, Morabia A, *et al*. Contribution of D-dimer plasma measurements and lower-limb venous ultrasound to the diagnosis of pulmonary embolism: a decision analysis model. *Am Heart J* 1994; **127**: 624–35.

24 Indik J, Alpert J. Detection of pulmonary embolism by D-dimer assay, spiral computed tomography and magnetic resonance imaging. *Prog Cardiovasc Dis* 2000; **42**: 261–72.

25 Michiels JJ. Rational diagnosis of pulmonary embolism (RADIA PE) in symptomatic patients with suspected PE: an improved strategy to exclude or diagnose venous thromboembolism by the sequential use of a clinical model, rapid ELISA D-dimer test, perfusion lung scan, ultrasonography, spiral CT and pulmonary angiography. *Semin Thromb Hemost* 1998; **24**: 413–18.

26 Bounameaux H, de Moerloose P, Perrier A, Miron MJ. D-dimer testing in suspected venous thromboembolism: an update. *QJM* 1997; **90**: 437–42.

27 Kline JA, Johns KL, Colucciello SA, Israel EG. New diagnostic tests for pulmonary embolism. *Ann Emerg Med* 2000; **35**: 168–80.

28 Hyers T. Diagnosis of pulmonary embolism. *Thorax* 1995; **50**: 930.

29 Miniati M, Marini C, Allescia G, *et al*. Non-invasive diagnosis of pulmonary embolism. *Int J Cardiol* 1998; **65**(suppl 1): S83–6.

30 Wells PS, Ginsberg JS, Anderson DR, *et al*. Use of a clinical model for safe management of patients with suspected pulmonary embolism. *Ann Intern Med* 1998; **129**: 997–1005.

31 Worsley DF, Alavi A. Comprehensive analysis of the PIOPED study. *J Nucl Med* 1995; **36**: 2380–7.

32 Meyerovitz MF, Mannting F, Polak JF, Goldhaber SZ. Frequency of pulmonary embolism in patients with low-probability lung scan and negative lower extremity venous ultrasound. *Chest* 1999; **115**: 980–2.

33 Cross JJ, Kemp PM, Walsh CG, *et al*. A randomized trial of spiral CT and ventilation perfusion scintigraphy for the diagnosis of pulmonary embolism. *Clin Radiol* 1998; **53**: 177–82.

34 Kim KI, Muller NL, Mayo JR. Clinically suspected pulmonary embolism: utility of spiral CT. *Radiology* 1999; **210**: 693–7.

35 Torbicki A. Imaging venous thromboembolism with emphasis on ultrasound, chest CT, angiography and echocardiography. *Thromb Haemost* 1999; **82**: 907–12.

36 Grenier PA, Beigelman C. Sprial computed tomographic scanning and magnetic resonance angiography for the diagnosis of pulmonary embolism. *Thorax* 1998; **53**(suppl 2): S25–31.

37 de Monye W, van Strijen MJ, Huisman MV, *et al*. Suspected pulmonary embolism: prevalence and anatomic distribution in 487 consecutive patients. Advances in New Technologies Evaluating the Localization of Pulmonary Embolism (ANTELOPE) Group. *Radiology* 2000; **215**: 184–8.

38 Mullins MD, Becker DM, Hagspiel KD, Philbrick JT. The role of spiral volumetric computed tomography in the diagnosis of pulmonary embolism. *Arch Intern Med* 2000; **160**: 293–8.

39 Remy-Jardin M, Remy J, Deschildre F, *et al*. Diagnosis of pulmonary embolism with spiral CT: comparison with pulmonary angiography and scintigraphy. *Radiology* 1996; **200**: 699–706.

40 Cham MD, Yankelevitz DF, Shaham D, *et al*. Deep venous thrombosis: detection by using indirect CT venography. *Radiology* 2000; **261**: 744–51.

41 PIOPED Investigators. Value of the ventilation/perfusion scan in acute pulmonary embolism: results of the Prospective Investigation of Pulmonary Embolism Diagnosis (PIOPED). *JAMA* 1990; **263**: 2753–9.

42 Pavan D, Nicolosi GL, Antonini-Canterin F, Zanuttini D. Echocardiography in pulmonary embolism disease. *Int J Cardiol* 1998; **65**(suppl 1): S87–90.

43 Grifoni S, Olivotto I, Cecchini P, *et al*. Utility of an integrated clinical, echocardiographic, and venous ultrasonographic approach for triage of patients with suspected pulmonary embolism. *Am J Cardiol* 1998; **82**: 1230–5.

44 Goldhaber SZ. Venous thromboembolism prophylaxis in medical patients. *Thromb Haemost* 1999; **82**: 899–901.

45 Raschke RA, Reilly BM, Guidry JR, *et al*. The weight-based heparin dosing nomogram compared with a 'standard care' nomogram: a randomized controlled trial. *Ann Intern Med* 1993; **119**: 874–81.

46 Agnelli G, Sonaglia F. Anticoagulant agents in the management of pulmonary embolism. *Int J Cardiol* 1998; **65**(suppl 1): S95–8.

47 Bates S, Hirsch J. Treatment of venous thromboembolism. *Thromb Haemost* 1999; **82**: 870–7.

48 Goldhaber SZ. Contemporary pulmonary embolism thrombolysis. *Int J Cardiol* 1998; **65**(suppl 1): S91–3.

49 Hyers T, Hull R, Weg J. Antithrombotic therapy for venous thromboembolic disease. *Chest* 1995; **108**(suppl 4): S335–51.

50 Kearon C. Initial treatment of venous thromboembolism. *Thromb Haemost* 1999; **82**: 887–91.

51 Simonneau G, Sors H, Charbonnier B, *et al*. A comparison of low-molecular-weight heparin with unfractionated heparin for acute pulmonary embolism. The THESEE Study Group. *N Engl J Med* 1997; **337**: 663–9.

52 Matsumoto A, Tegtmeyer C. Contemporary diagnostic approaches to acute pulmonary emboli. *Radiol Clin North Am* 1995; **33**: 167–83.

53 Urokinase-streptokinase embolism trial: Phase 2 results: a cooperative study. *JAMA* 1974; **229**: 1606.

54 Doerge H, Schoendube FA, Voss M, *et al*. Surgical therapy of fulminant pulmonary embolism: early and late results. *Thorac Cardiovasc Surg* 1999; **47**: 9–13.

55 Greenfield LJ. Caval interruption procedures. In: Rutherford RB (ed). *Vascular Surgery*, 5th edn. Philadelphia: WB Saunders, 2000: 1968–78.

56 Prins MH, Hutten BA, Koopman MM, Buller HR. Long-term treatment of venous thromboembolic disease. *Thromb Haemost* 1999; **82**: 892–8.

57 British Thoracic Society Research Committee. Optimum duration of treatment for deep-vein thrombosis and pulmonary embolism. *Lancet* 1992; **340**: 873–6.

22

Upper Limb Vein Thrombosis

BENGT LT LINDBLAD, KRASSI IVANCEV, SIMON G DARKE

THE PROBLEM

Upper limb venous thrombosis (ULVT) is fairly uncommon. It is estimated to represent 1–3 per cent of recognised deep vein thromboses.[1-3] Cases of ULVT are divided into primary, when no certain explanation for development of the thrombosis of the axillary/subclavian vein is found, and secondary, when an obvious factor has caused the development.

Anticoagulation has been widely used and gives favourable results preventing re-thrombosis and pulmonary embolism (PE); it also lowers the frequency of patients having severe long term arm disability.[1-5] During the past decade many reports have been published suggesting more aggressive treatment with thrombolysis with or without thoracic outlet decompression, i.e. first rib resection, scalenectomy and venolysis.[6,7] Most of these reports concern primary thrombosis and the subgroup of young patients with so-called effort induced ULVT. As a result of the low incidence of ULVT, the experience of any one clinician is limited; this compounds the problems and the opportunities of finding an optimal therapeutic strategy. Furthermore, the disease fails to fall naturally into any particular medical specialty. This again dilutes experience and the expertise of any one individual or department and reduces the potential for prospective controlled trials of treatment options. This review includes a suggestion of treatment pathways depicted in an algorithm (Fig. 22.1), but it is essential to be aware that this is not based on solid evidence-based facts, but reflects the authors' opinion.

HISTORY

Perhaps the most exotic, dramatic and at the same time the first described case of probable ULVT was that of Henry of Navarre (1553–1610) who, as King Henry IV of France, led his army into the Battle of Ivry (1590). He used his sword arm to such excess that he could not move it for 6 weeks.[8] The first description of venous compromise of the upper extremity is credited to Sir James Paget in 1875. His perception, however, was that the underlying morphology was a type of 'gouty arthritis'.[9] The true venous cause was recognised nine years later by von Schroetter,[10] hence the eponymous term Paget–von Schroetter syndrome.

PATHOGENESIS, NOMENCLATURE AND CLASSIFICATION

Upper limb vein thrombosis has a multifactorial aetiology. The classification most used differentiates between primary and secondary axillary/subclavian vein thrombosis.[1-5] **Primary** thrombosis may occur spontaneously or following effort while **secondary** thrombosis may be iatrogenic or complicate malignancy and other miscellaneous causes. Before considering this in further detail it is of value to address the anatomy and the venographic appearances of these conditions.

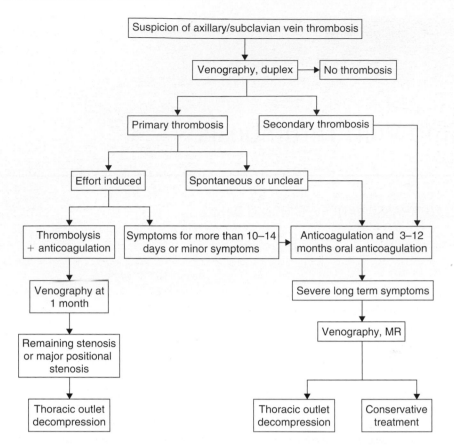

Figure 22.1   *An algorithm of the management of suspected axillary/subclavian vein thrombosis. MR, magnetic resonance (scan)*

ANATOMICAL CONSIDERATIONS

'Thoracic outlet syndrome' is a loose term which describes compression of the artery, vein or plexus of nerves as they pass through the neck to the upper extremity. In anatomical terms the problem seems to present in three distinct areas.[1,7,11] The first two of these, which do not in general concern us here, might be called 'axillo-pectoral compression' and 'the costo-scalene tunnel'. In axillo-pectoral compression intermittent compression of the axillary vein can be seen between the pectoral muscles and the rib cage. In the costo-scalene tunnel the artery or possibly the nerves become compressed between a cervical rib, a congenital fibrous band or the posterior surface of the scalenus anterior muscle. Removal of such constrictions (Fig. 22.2) decompresses the artery but normally not the vein.

In contrast, the vein is caught more medially in the costoclavicular tunnel. The axillary vein becomes the subclavian vein at the outer border of the first rib and passes through a potentially narrow space bounded inferiorly by the first rib and pleura. The vein is restricted, anteriorly, by the clavicle and subclavius muscle. Posteriorly, it is constrained by the anterior border of the scalenus anterior muscle and medially by the costoclavicular joint and ligament.[11] It is obvious, therefore, that cervical ribs, bands or associated structures have no relevance to subclavian venous problems.

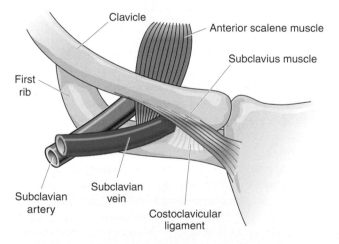

Figure 22.2   *Anatomy of the thoracic outlet. Note that the vein is most likely to be compressed by the subclavius muscle and costoclavicular ligament, and the artery by the anterior scalene muscle*

What then are the morphological features of apparently normal structures within this space which predispose to venous compression and thrombosis? There are two principal components and in most cases both contribute to a relatively greater or lesser extent. The first of these is that the gap quite simply is congenitally narrow[6] and can be detected at operation.[11] The second factor is related to physical activity.

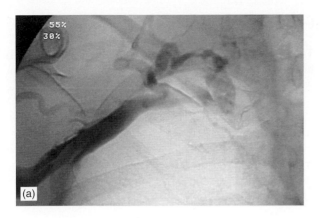

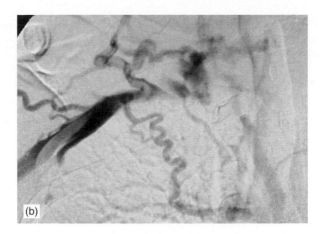

Figure 22.3   *(a, b) A short subclavian vein occlusion with collaterals which later fill central veins. During surgical venolysis some of these collaterals may be injured and occlude. Re-thrombosis may then give an even more symptomatic long term outcome*

This may be an acute and isolated episode of exceptional exertion, or it may be a consequence of prolonged activity such as training, sporting pursuits and similar avocations.[6,7,10,11] Here it is thought that the critically situated subclavius muscle becomes engorged or hypertrophied (see Fig. 22.2). Thrombosis, however, occurs clearly in only a few selected individuals who undertake these activities. It seems logical, therefore, that if the vein is to be harmed by physical activity, an element of anatomical narrowing referred to above must almost certainly coexist. It follows that in all cases of primary thrombosis this idiosyncratic anatomical narrowing is present.

Sites of thoracic outlet syndromes and vulnerable structures

- Axillo-pectoral compression – vein
- Costo-scalene tunnel – artery, nerve
- Costoclavicular tunnel – vein

VENOGRAPHIC AND HAEMODYNAMIC FINDINGS

A key issue in the strategy of treatment is the incidence of this anatomical narrowing, both in an unselected population and among those suffering from ULVT. There are a few venographic studies showing that 70 per cent of unselected individuals do have a degree of stenosis of the venous outflow, especially with the arm in hyperabduction.[12,13] Similarly, Stevenson and Parry reported that in patients with ULVT they could almost always document a compression abnormality of the vein in the contralateral arm in hyperabduction.[14] This has also been reported by others with a frequency ranging from 56 to 80 per cent.[6,15–17]

With the arm resting along the body compression of the axillary vein is not uncommon and best venographic filling is obtained with a 30 degree abduction. This compression is due to the closeness between the pectoral muscles and the rib cage.[18]

Venous arm pressure recordings also show that compression of the veins occurs in different positions of the arms. In the relaxed position, arm venous pressure is around 6–7 mmHg and is much the same when comparing healthy volunteers and patients with arm and shoulder disability with or without earlier ULVT.[19] In hyperabduction or the 'hurray position', and especially in a 'military position' with the shoulders drawn backwards, the pressure increases up to around 10 mmHg in normal individuals. In patients with chronic non-recanalised subclavians, venous pressure increased more prominently ($\approx$20 mmHg) in hyperabduction and especially in the 'military position'. Thus it appears that collaterals passing the narrow costoclavicular area are also affected by arm position.

In a number of studies evaluating haemodynamics using plethysmography, it has been shown that slightly reduced venous capacity and maximal venous outflow are observed in patients with chronic non-recanalised ULVT.[19] In venographic terms, two main patterns of ULVT are seen, namely, a short subclavian vein occlusion (Fig. 22.3) or a more extensive thrombotic process involving the axillary vein.[14,16–18]

CLASSIFICATION

Primary thrombosis, i.e. where no evidence is found to account for the development of axillary or subclavian vein thrombosis, is reported with very different frequencies in different reports (Table 22.1).[3,4,10,20–32] One reason for this is the manner in which population details are collected and another is whether they are representative of the population,[3,4 21,25] the other being that more severely symptomatic patients are referred.[6,7,26,27] In some patients a history of unusual upper limb activity precedes the development of ULVT, so-called effort induced thrombosis. This accounts for 5–10 per cent of patients in an unselected population.

A larger group of about 30 per cent are considered to be spontaneous cases of primary ULVT; in most cases the aetiology is multifactorial.

The number of cases of secondary thrombosis has now increased to approximately 60 per cent of those detected (Table 22.1).[3] This is due to an increased number of instances of iatrogenic thrombosis, such as those caused by central venous lines and pacemaker leads.

In an earlier series (1971–86) from Malmö University Hospital,[4] and representative of the population of the city, 61 per cent were considered to have primary thrombosis. The majority of these had no well-defined factors contributing to the development of thrombosis. Effort or physical activity related thrombosis was probably evident in only 6 per cent. A proved hypercoagulable state was seen in 9 per cent, to which should be added 17 per cent on contraceptive pills and those with previous thromboembolic episodes. In a recent analysis of the period 1987–2001 and within the same catchment area, only 3 per cent out of the total of 155 cases were effort induced while 30 per cent were probably cases of spontaneous ULVT.

Secondary thrombosis, in which a major contributory factor is found, comprised about 40 per cent of the patients with subclavian vein thrombosis in our series from 1971 to 1986.[4] In the recent series recorded from 1987 to 2001 the incidence of thrombosis has increased to 67 per cent: of these 44 per cent are due to central venous lines or pacemaker leads, 20 per cent to malignancy and another 3 per cent are considered to be miscellaneous cases. Just how many patients have undiagnosed secondary upper arm thrombosis may only be speculated upon.

Primary thrombosis

The term 'primary thrombosis' includes spontaneous, idiopathic, effort induced, positional, strain and Paget–von Schroetter syndrome. It even includes the term 'traumatic' when it has been used to describe probable anatomical abnormalities causing trauma to and compression of the subclavian vein.[2,6,7] It is obvious that the 'normal' narrowing of the costoclavicular space is a pathogenic factor in most of these patients; the problem is establishing how crucial this and the other factors are in causing the development of thrombosis.

Effort thrombosis

This presentation is an obviously recognisable and distinct entity.[2,3,6,7,10] It is of relevance not only because it can be defined as effort induced by the obvious sequence of events, but also because it relates to a possible long term outcome, a factor which must influence management strategy.

Effort induced thrombosis occurs as a result of excessive or prolonged physical activity in combination with the narrow space in the costoclavicular region through which the vein passes. A spectacular variety of provocative activities has been reported: throwing balls, playing handball or tennis, swimming, chopping wood, painting ceilings, pulling a propeller, rowing a boat, washing walls, starting an outboard motor, lifting weights, carrying a suitcase, wearing a figure-of-eight splint, falling asleep with one's arm over the back of the chair and windsurfing.[1–7,10]

Table 22.1 *Classification of upper extremity deep venous thrombosis*

Authors	Primary (per cent)				Secondary (per cent)		
	Year	No.	Effort	Spontaneous	Iatrogenic	Malignant	Others
Hughes[10]	1949	320	49	34	0	0	17
Adams et al.[20]	1965	25	52	32	0	0	16
Coon and Willis[21]	1967	60	23	5	38	10	24
Tilney et al.[22]	1970	48	21	21	17	6	35
Donayre et al.[23]	1986	41	22	5	51	12	10
Lindblad et al.[4]	1988	120	6	55	25	11	3
Hauptli et al.[25]	1989	96	3	24	34	28	10
Horattas et al.[24]	1988	33	6	12	40	24	18
AbuRahma et al.[26]	1991	23	100	0	0	0	0
Malcynski et al.[27]	1993	23	52	0	35	9	4
Martin and Brors[28]	1995	91	13	39	13	9	26
Adelman et al.[29]	1997	38	16	20	[.................................64.................................]		
Beygui et al.[30]	1997	32	42	6	29	29	
Hingorani et al.[3*]	1997	170	1	21	65	37	11
Marie et al.[31]	1998	49	10	14	22	33	21
Sakakibara et al.[32]	1999	12	9	9	67	17	0
Zell et al.[33]	2001	82	34	4	[.................................62.................................]		
Malmö University Hospital	2001	155	3	30	44	20	3

*33 per cent of the patients had multiple risk factors.

A variant of this category occurs when thrombosis follows excessive long term activities. These include excessive weight training, javelin throwing and occupations such as window cleaning.[11] In these cases contralateral venography often reveals a bilateral abnormality and previously undetected and asymptomatic thrombosis on the opposite side.[11]

Classification of ULVT

- Primary
  - Spontaneous, idiopathic
  - Effort, positional, strain (Paget–von Schroetter syndrome)
- Secondary
  - Iatrogenic
  - Malignancy
  - Miscellaneous

Hypercoagulable states

Many reports have reported different coagulation and fibrinolytic defects in patients developing ULVT. [4,34–37] In some reports 9–42 per cent of patients had a hypercoagulable state (also see Chapters 2 and 20). Heron and coworkers analysed 51 patients with primary thrombosis: comparing the spontaneous thrombosis group (n = 31) with the effort induced thrombosis group (n = 20) there was a higher frequency of a family history of DVT, 42 per cent and 15 per cent, respectively, and at least one coagulation abnormality, 42 per cent and 15 per cent, respectively.[35] Leebeek and associates found a 27 per cent frequency of antiphospholipid antibodies.[36] In an analysis of 60 patients collected from our hospital in Malmö during the 1970s, a decreased fibrinolytic defence mechanism was seen in 49 per cent, F VIII:C activity was increased in 48 per cent and F VIII:R Ag was elevated in 20 per cent.[34] Activated protein C resistance, polymorphism in prothrombin fragments 1 and 2, antithrombin, protein C and protein S deficiency were coagulation defects seen in just a small percentage of patients.[37]

Reports relating thrombosis to ingestion of the oestrogen containing contraceptive pill may well be coincidental. However, within some larger series there are a small number of patients in whom this appears to be a contributory factor.[4,6,22–24,26,38]

Secondary thrombosis

A large and increasing proportion of patients are diagnosed with secondary upper arm thrombosis. In this group of patients anatomical narrowing in the costoclavicular space is not a major cause but local trauma or compression from malignancy is of major aetiological importance.

Iatrogenic thrombosis

Iatrogenic thrombosis may account for up to two-thirds of cases of ULVT nowadays.[3] A large proportion of these are subclinical and undetected and therefore not treated.

CENTRAL VENOUS CATHETERS

The incidence of clinical symptomatic thrombosis caused by indwelling central venous lines is low at 1–6 per cent (Table 22.2).[39–55] If carefully investigated, however, a large proportion of, if not all, catheters will have a fibrin sleeve as a coating over the foreign material (Table 22.3).[39,42,43,48,49,56–59] Mural or occlusive thrombosis is not uncommon and is found in 12–68 per cent of patients undergoing prospective venographic examination (Table 22.2). Many patients with central venous cannula induced thrombosis remain undiagnosed.

The stiffness of the catheter, the lumen size, the length of the catheter and the length of catheterisation required are all reflected in the frequency of thrombosis.[40,55,56] The type of infusion given, i.c. total parenteral nutrition, hyperosmolarity solutions or chemotherapy and the reason for the use of a central venous line, e.g. malignancy, are likewise important. Normally short catheterisation periods will not induce significant thrombosis.[41]

Studies of the long term use of central venous catheters and prevention of induced thrombosis confirm the efficacy

Table 22.2 *Central venous catheters: mural and occlusive thrombosis*

Authors	Year	No.	Frequency (per cent)	Diagnostic method
Hoshal et al.[39]	1971	55	4	PM
Ryan et al.[40]	1974	34	24	PM
Lindblad et al.[41]	1981	28	32	PM
Ahmed[42]	1976	63	20	POP
Bennegård et al.[43]	1982	22	68	POP
Braun et al.[44]	1970	50	23	CP
Fassolt and Braun[45]	1978	50	12	CP
Ladefoged et al.[46]	1979	32	49	CP
Lindblad et al.[41]	1981	95	12	CP
Magalhaes et al.[47]	1986	51	23	CP
Balestreri et al.[48]	1995	57	46	CP
Martin et al.[49]	1999	60	12	CP
Allen et al.[50]	2000	137	24	CP
Male et al.[51]	2003	85	34	CP + Duplex + MRI
Frank et al.[52]	2000	319	35	RNP
Wu et al.[53]	1999	81	25	Duplex
Soto-Velasco et al.[54]	1984	1311	0.8	Clinical
Schwarz et al.[55]	2000	791	6.5	Clinical

PM, postmortem; POP, pull-out phlebography; CP, conventional phlebography; MRI, magnetic resonance imaging; RNP, radionuclide phlebography.

of standard heparin, low molecular weight heparin (LMWH) and low dose warfarin therapy.[60–64] The number of studies available is not sufficient for evidence-based recommendations, but they warrant further analysis. If possible, such prevention ought to be used more frequently than most centres do today. Prevention will not only reduce the risk of thrombosis but also that of pulmonary embolism, a not too infrequent sequela to secondary ULVT.

PACEMAKER LEADS

In spite of improved pacemaker lines during the last decade, more complex implants such as double-lead pacemakers and defibrillators have been developed. Clinically symptomatic thrombosis is not as common,[65] but routine

Table 22.3 *Central venous catheters: fibrin sleeve formation*

Authors	Year	No.	Frequency (per cent)	Diagnostic method
Scholz and Loewe[55]	1969	60	55	PM
Hoshal et al.[39]	1971	55	100	PM
Hoshal et al.[39]	1971	31	100	POP
Ahmed[42]	1976	63	75	POP
Brismar et al.[57]	1980	35	66	POP
Andersson et al.[58]	1981	60	85	POP
Bennegård et al.[43]	1982	22	100	POP
Starkhammar et al.[59]	1992	16	100	POP
Balestreri et al.[48]	1995	57	78	CP
Martin et al.[49]	1999	60	58	CP

PM, postmortem; POP, pull-out phlebography; CP, conventional phlebography.

venography reveals a 30–50 per cent incidence.[66,67] The discrepancy between clinically documented and prospectively recorded thrombosis is significant, with most asymptomatic cases going undetected.

Iatrogenic causes of ULVT

- Central venous catheters, type of infusate
- Pacemaker and defibrillator leads – single/double
- Haemodialysis catheters, arteriovenous (AV) fistula and late central vein stenosis

---

HAEMODIALYSIS CATHETERS

These are large, often double lumen, catheters that pose a high risk for thrombosis (11–40 per cent).[68] Later, when patients are evaluated for angio-access, occluded or stenotic central veins are often found[68–71] (see Chapter 7B). Few of these patients have any symptoms in their arms and many centres routinely perform venography before an angio-access operation if the patient has had a haemodialysis catheter on that side.[69] A stenosis or an occlusion in the venous outflow will reduce patency of peripherally constructed AV fistulae. Central vein stenosis can develop several months after an AV fistula operation resulting in higher resistance to venous return. Angioplasty has shown acceptable results at 6 months, primary patency being 31–42 per cent and secondary patency 71–80 per cent, but restenosis often develops requiring repeated dilatations.[68,70] Stenting of such veins has been used and seems a reasonable alternative (Fig. 22.4 a, b),[68,72] but repeated endovascular procedures are needed at approximately 3-month intervals and if considerable

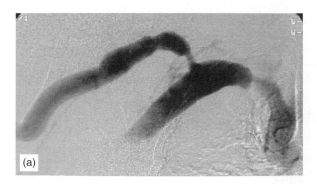
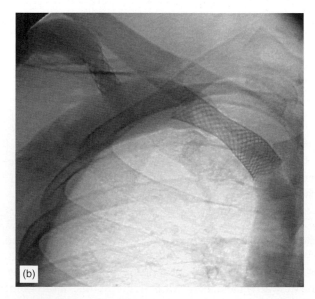

Figure 22.4 *(a, b) An enlarged cephalic vein resulting from a distal arteriovenous fistula with stenosis of the most proximal portion of the cephalic vein as well as of the subclavian vein, both of which were stented. Restenosis made repeated dilatations necessary about every third month and patency was maintained for over 4 years*

narrowing in the costoclavicular tunnel is noted, the risk of stent breakage must be considered.[73]

Malignant disease

In the majority of these cases the cause is direct pressure by tumour mass. They account for 10–30 per cent of ULVT.[4,25,33] Less frequently the thrombosis is ascribable to a hypercoagulable state adding to the other risk factors.[3] Local radiotherapy may also be a contributory factor in the development of thrombosis (see Chapter 33).

Miscellaneous causes

Other causes that have been reported are congestive heart failure, myocardial infarction, congenital anomaly, vascular malformations, drug abuse (see Chapter 44) and trauma.[1–5,31] There are even case reports of patients with vasculitis and vasospasm. In some cases severe illness, for example sepsis, ulcerative colitis, filariasis, otitis media, etc., is associated with ULVT and these are considered secondary occurrences, but the main causative factor may be difficult to identify.

Congenital webs are known to cause thrombosis at other sites as in the iliac vein web and Budd–Chiari syndrome but there must be doubt as to whether this occurs in the axillary/subclavian vein. Thus, an intraluminal 'web' is likely to be a secondary phenomenon due to incomplete recanalisation after previous thrombosis or a function of local trauma.

Miscellaneous causes of ULVT

- Congestive heart failure, myocardial infarction
- Congenital venous anomalies – webs, malformations
- Vasculitides
- Drug abuse
- Trauma
- Sepsis – focal or systemic

CLINICAL PRESENTATION

The characteristic findings are swelling of the affected arm, distension of superficial veins, especially in the shoulder region, mild cyanosis, and pain.[1–5,10,38] In our earlier reported series[4] oedema was seen in 97 per cent, pain in 50 per cent, distended collateral veins in 35 per cent, acrocyanosis in 10 per cent and erythema in 10 per cent. Few had altered skin temperature and only 4 per cent had fever. Importantly, about half of the patients with symptoms and suspicion of ULVT had normal venograms.[4]

Normally, patients present with a history of 2–3 days of symptoms, but a delay of up to several months is not unusual.[3,4,10,25,30] In many reports a male preponderance has been reported.[10,21,26] In the Malmö series[4] and others[38] no such difference was observed between the sexes; neither was there any predominant involvement of the right upper limb compared with the left. Venous gangrene is a rare finding and underlying malignancy should be considered.

INVESTIGATIONS

Normally, a conventional arm venogram will establish the diagnosis of ULVT. Alternative techniques are duplex, ultrasound, spiral computed tomography (CT) and magnetic resonance angiography (MRA).[1–5,53] Each of these techniques has limitations and needs to be evaluated based on the experience of the examiner. With the arm held by the side of the body it is not unusual for the axillary vein to be compressed by surrounding muscles.[18] If the contrast is not injected mainly into the basilic vein, the venogram will be of poor quality[16] as precise timing is required in assessing the central veins.[17] Duplex ultrasound has the advantage of being non-invasive, but a large collateral cannot be easily distinguished from the axillary/subclavian veins. New imaging techniques such as spiral CT and MR imaging are most promising.[51]

Routine laboratory testing should be performed and in cases of primary thrombosis a coagulation screen is recommended. A chest X-ray will rule out osteal malformation of the clavicle or an unknown pulmonary malignancy.

COMPLICATIONS

Pulmonary embolism

Pulmonary embolism (PE) is considered first because it threatens the patient's life (see Chapter 21). Table 22.4 documents the frequency of selected series reporting on non-fatal and fatal pulmonary embolism.[3,4,6,7,10,20–22,24,25,27,29,31,32,38,51,74–85] For patients with ULVT classified as primary, a 1 per cent (10/1017) incidence of non-fatal PE has been reported. A 7 per cent incidence of PE, 10 fatal and 49 non-fatal, has been documented followed secondary ULVT among 807 patients. In this group, major associated aetiological factors were taken into account in many of the patients who developed PE. In a prospective study Monreal and co-workers[79] followed 86 patients with central venous cannula induced upper extremity thrombosis. Anticoagulant treatment was started and perfusion/ventilation scintigraphy revealed pulmonary embolism in 15 per cent of patients, of whom two died of recurrent pulmonary embolism in spite of prophylactic anticoagulant therapy.

Table 22.4 *Fatal and non-fatal Pulmonary embolism*

Authors	Primary			Secondary		
	Year	No.	NFPE	No.	NFPE	FPE
Hughes[10]	1949	269	1	51	2	
Adams et al.[20]	1965	21	3	4		1
Coon and Willis[21]	1967	17	0	43	3	
Swinton et al.[744]	1968	23	1			
Tilney et al.[22]	1970	17	0	31	0	
Campbell et al.[75]	1977	9	0	10		2
Harley et al.[76]	1984	3	1	11	4	
Horattas et al.[24]	1988	4	0	29	4	
Lindblad et al.[4]	1988	73	0	47	2	3
Hauptli et al.[25]	1989	26	0	70	1	
Reed et al.[77]	1992			5	0	
Thompson et al.[78]	1992	6	0			
Malcynski et al.[27]	1993	12	0	11	0	
Monrcal et al.[79]	1994			86	11	2
Machleder[6]	1993	50	0			
Molina[80]	1995	18	0			
Adelman et al.[29]	1997	14	0	24	0	
Hingorani et al.[3]	1997	2	0	168	10	2
Azakie et al.[81]	1998	33	2			
Marie et al.[31]	1998	12	1	37	5	
Sakakibara et al.[32]	1999	2	0	10	0	
Urschel and Razzuk[7]	2000	294	0			
Angle et al.[82]	2001	18	0			
Feugier et al.[83]	2001	10	0			
Kreienberg et al.[85]	2001	23	0			
Lokanathan et al.[85]	2001	28	1			
Sabeti et al.[38]	2002	33	0	85	7	
Male et al.[51]	2003			85	0	
Total		1017	10	807	49	10

FPE, fatal pulmonary embolism; NFPE, non-fatal pulmonary embolism.

Complications of ULVT

- Pulmonary embolism
- Residual vein thrombosis
- Recurrent vein thrombosis
- Chronic vein stenosis
- Disabilities of restricted venous outflow

Long term symptoms

Although less dramatic than PE, long term symptoms are the crucial area, in practical terms, on which management is based. The widening of existing collaterals and/or recanalisation is normally seen during the first six months after axillary/subclavian vein thrombosis. Collaterals can be seen from the arm/shoulder extending to the chest wall, the anterior/posterior neck veins and contralateral neck veins as well. Many of these collaterals also pass through the costoclavicular space, and if there is an anatomical narrowing, these collaterals may also be dependent on arm position. This narrowing is usually visible on venography with the arm in different positions[16–19] and is also verifiable with pressure recordings.[19]

It is not possible to predict long term sequelae on the basis of presenting symptomatology.[4,10,19] Even in patients whose occluded veins recanalise, normally possible in 10–20 per cent, a clear reduction in long term disability is not consistently found.[2,4,26,38] Of those referred from outside the normal recruitment area of our university department, there is a preponderance of young patients with primary thrombosis and severe symptomatology. Often the time from onset of symptoms until referral is more than 7–14 days. Each aetiological group must be considered separately because, inherently, the outcome may be different.

Primary subclavian thrombosis

Long term symptoms are difficult to quantify and evaluate objectively. Protagonists of more aggressive surgery such as first rib resection are likely to take a pessimistic view of the unoperated outcome. An element of bias can easily cloud the issue. Thus, in the literature different opinions exist on the frequency of long term disability, especially after primary ULVT (20–82 per cent),[1–7,10,38] this difference is also due to differences in the selection of patients reported upon. Most authors report that a proportion of patients will have mild symptoms with occasional swelling, increased superficial networks of veins over the shoulder and pain, but few patients develop more severe disability requiring, for example, a change of occupation.[1,2,4,25,28,31] Patients usually complain of difficulties working for long periods with the arm in an elevated position.

The analysis from Malmö[4] covering the entire population and the outcome of all symptomatic cases, comes as close as it is possible to get an accurate estimate of the long term outcome. An attempt was made to quantify the severity of the outcome. 'Mild' sequelae were defined as occasional pain and some restrictions in arm capacity, 'moderate' as symptoms limiting certain activities and 'severe' as daily symptoms with severe limitation, often leading to a change of occupation. Of the 73 patients with primary thrombosis 15 (21 per cent) had mild long term symptoms and in a further three (4 per cent) they were moderate after a median of 6 years of follow-up.

The small group of patients with effort induced ULVT seems to have more frequent long term disability,[6,7,26,27,29,30,80–85] but other reports show lower frequencies of long term sequelae.[2–5,34,38,86] Many reports, especially from North American centres, seem to include cases of spontaneous primary thrombosis. In those patients with what can be clearly classified as effort induced thrombosis, up to 50 per cent complain of moderate long term sequelae, and in 25 per cent this leads to working disability.[6,7,26]

Secondary subclavian thrombosis

In many patients any disability arising from ULVT will be hidden by other serious diseases.[2–4] Most authors agree that the frequency of long term sequelae is low, that severe and even moderate symptoms are unusual and that mild symptoms occur in 30–74 per cent.[2–4,25,31] In iatrogenic ULVT late problems are uncommon and the majority may remain totally symptom free.[41,54] In the Malmö series, 47 patients had secondary thrombosis, 14 (30 per cent) had mild and two (4 per cent) had moderate long term sequelae.[4] If one analyses different treatment modalities in our series, the outcome was worse in the more aggressively treated patients, but these presented with more severe symptoms. What then is the evidence that treatment influences long term disability? In a retrospective review by Hicken and Ameli[2] persistent symptoms were reported in 52 per cent of conservatively treated patients, in 32 per cent of those anticoagulated and in 26 per cent of those treated by thrombolysis.

TREATMENT ALTERNATIVES

Many patients with ULVT were treated conservatively using arm elevation and rest with favorable outcomes.[10] More modern alternatives employed were anticoagulation and thrombolysis with or without thoracic outlet decompression. An algorithm (see Fig. 22.1, page 262) provides treatment options for ULVT. The plethora of published algorithms and surgical approaches in achieving decompression of the thoracic outlet underlines our limited understanding of the aetiology of ULVT.

Anticoagulation

In many reports and reviews the beneficial effect of anticoagulation has been advocated,[1–5,20,23,25,28,31,38] but there are no comparative studies of non-medical conservative treatment[10] and anticoagulation. Extrapolating from studies on deep venous thrombosis in the lower extremity, the value of anticoagulation in ULVT has also been established. Intravenous heparin or LMWH[1–5,79,86,87] combined with 3–12 months of oral anticoagulation is safe and reliable and that has been evaluated reasonably scientifically. This view is further endorsed by the circumstantial evidence that anticoagulation prevents occlusion of collaterals and may favourably influence the potential for long term symptoms. There are a few reviews compiling data on the effectiveness of anticoagulant treatment and which record a low frequency of treatment complications.[1,2,5,30] Pulmonary embolism has also been reported, but there have been no fatal cases.[2,5–7,21,26] Early re-thrombosis is infrequent, and more often seen after anticoagulation ceases.[2,5–7,21,26]

For patients with secondary ULVT, anticoagulation in the form of heparin or LMWH for 5–7 days should be the first treatment alternative.[2] The risk of PE speaks in favour of oral anticoagulation for 3–12 months. In patients with catheter induced thrombosis, it may be wiser not to withdraw the cannulae immediately after diagnosis. One can speculate as to whether anticoagulant treatment should be initiated and whether the thrombus should be a little more organised so as to minimise the risk of PE at removal of the catheter.

Thrombolysis

Although thrombolytic therapy is of no proven benefit in the lower limb, there is increasing interest in its employment in axillary/subclavian vein thrombosis and many reports, together including 569 patients, have been published, especially during the last decade.[6,7,26,27,29,30,77–86,88–91] Most reports on thrombolysis have used catheter directed low dose therapy, and in general, treatment has been required for 1–2 days. Three or four non-fatal cases of PE have been reported during treatment.[2,38] The success of initial recanalisation is reported to be high (40–100 per cent), the results seeming better if the treatment time span from the onset of signs of thrombosis to the commencement of thrombolysis is less than 14 days.[7,26,81]

The re-occlusion frequency is high (34 per cent),[6,7,26,38] but it has been reduced by endovascular and surgical measures aimed at decompression of the costoclavicular narrowing. The majority of patients treated with thrombolysis are young patients with effort induced thrombosis,[6,7] but many reports also include patients with spontaneous primary thrombosis. In a retrospective comparison of systemic thrombolysis and anticoagulation more veins remained open after thrombolysis and long term problems in the arm were infrequent, there being no difference between the groups.[38] The effectiveness of thrombolysis in cases of thrombosis of central venous cannulae has also been reported.[30,31]

Most reports have used urokinase in treatment but streptokinase and tissue plasminogen activator (tPA) are reported to be as effective.[6,7,77–79,81,83–86,88,89] Currently, in selected cases, we use catheter directed low dose thrombolysis into the thrombus with repeated venography and adjustment of the catheter position every 12 hours. We normally use tissue plasminogen activators at a dose of 1–2 mg/hour. Most centres today use this form of local thrombolytic therapy but the risk of potentially dangerous bleeding complications must be considered, and it should only be advocated in selected cases. In our selected series of over 550 patients receiving thrombolytic therapy, however, no major bleeding complications were reported although bleeding and pericatheter thrombosis at the access site were observed. Our patients are selected on non-evidence-based criteria, such as the probable factors responsible for the development of thrombosis, the magnitude of presenting symptoms and the collateral pattern on diagnostic venography prior to recommending specific therapy. All these factors, of course, are biased by the authors' judgement of each individual case. Currently, about 10 per cent of patients with ULVT would be recommended for thrombolysis.

Normally in secondary axillary/subclavian thrombosis the long term outcome of thrombolysis is less disabling but more risky than anticoagulation and therefore should be carefully evaluated before being recommended. A few patients will have disabling long term arm symptoms having failed to develop collaterals wide enough for acceptable venous outflow, but it is impossible to select them at the outset.

Treatment options

- Anticoagulant therapy – intravenous heparin, LMWH, oral (longer term)
- Catheter directed thrombolysis – urokinase, tPA, streptokinase
- Angioplasty ± stenting
- Thoracic outlet decompression – first rib resection, scalenectomy
- Venolysis – excision medial clavicle/subclavius/costoclavicular ligament
- Jugular vein transposition or saphenous vein bypass ± AV fistula

---

Angioplasty and stenting

One advantage of thrombolytic therapy is that completion venography will show residual stenosis, compression or fibrosis. These lesions might indicate a risk of subsequent re-thrombosis and a less favourable long term outcome. Based on this, further intervention may be proposed. In primary axillary/subclavian vein thrombosis angioplasty is often used after thrombolysis.[6,84,85] Other centres are more restrictive in their use of angioplasty.[7,82,86] The restenosis and re-thrombosis rate is high if not combined with surgical thoracic outlet decompression.[6] Supplementary stenting should not be undertaken as many reports have shown that the narrow anatomical space in the costoclavicular region will frequently cause stent fracture, distortion and re-thrombosis.[91] Currently, angioplasty can be used in primary thrombosis of the axillary/subclavian vein, but the benefits of such a procedure are restricted to short remaining lesions. Stenting should not be employed except in association with decompression of the thoracic outlet,[84] although we have seen stents break despite decompression.

Recanalisation of chronically stenosed or occluded segments could be an alternative if secondary thrombosis has not been caused by narrowing of the costoclavicular space.[80] In patients with previously inserted haemodialysis catheters, a high number of central vein abnormalities is often seen.[68] These stenoses or occlusions are caused by indwelling large lumen catheters and could be treated by angioplasty or stenting. The likelihood of restenosis seems to be high, certainly higher than normally reported.[68–71]

Surgical thoracic outlet decompression

Several reports, especially from North America, recommend thoracic outlet decompression including first rib resection, scalenectomy, thrombectomy, venolysis and even medial claviculectomy to reduce long term disability, especially in the subgroup of patients with effort induced thrombosis.[6,7,26,78] Using more aggressive surgical decompression treatment in acute cases, i.e. those with a history of less than 14 days, only 25 per cent are reported to suffer from chronic arm disabilities.[6,7,26,28,81,84] The case series described, however, differ and not only include patients with effort induced thrombosis but also what we would classify as spontaneous primary thrombosis. The anatomical narrowing, justifying thoracic outlet decompression, often also exists in the contralateral arm. Nevertheless, development of bilateral thrombosis is only seen in a small subset of patients (6 per cent).[7] The decision to decompress is often based on venographic evidence of narrowing after thrombolysis, representing the phlebitic reaction around the vein in which thrombus had been dissolved. Initial symptoms, or a venographically existing stenosis, are not useful pointers in predicting long term arm disability.

In performing a first rib resection care should be given to excise its most medial part for optimal vein decompression.[7,81,84] Medial claviculectomy may be an effective way of thoracic decompression, especially if more medial components, such as the subclavius muscle, costoclavicular ligament and the most medial part of the first rib are responsible.[92] Transaxillary resection of the first rib, because it approaches the problem from below, carries the advantage of minimising the risk of interfering with existing collateral veins.

First rib resection has been advocated after a suitable period subsequent to thrombolysis, if symptoms or morphological evidence of residual subclavian vein stenosis persists (Fig. 22.5).[6,78,83,85,89] Equally, many recommend decompression at the time of initial presentation after thrombolysis.[7,80,82,84,90] Both policies appear to give durable symptomatic relief, and few complications have been reported in both early and more selective decompression later.[7,80] Advocates of immediate exploration feel that to delay runs a risk of re-thrombosis and missing the window of opportunity to achieve patency and a durable outcome. On the other hand, a delayed operation is more selective: patients with effort induced thrombosis who benefit from thrombolysis and have no residual stenosis at follow-up, do not require surgery as compression is not a major causative factor.

The value of venolysis, normally requiring a supraclavicular approach, is apparent in some studies but is not utilised routinely by other experts.[6,7,28,78,81] Such an approach may jeopardise the collaterals. It is important to be aware, however, that most recommendations of aggressive treatment

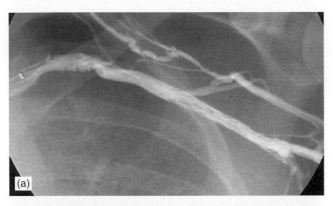

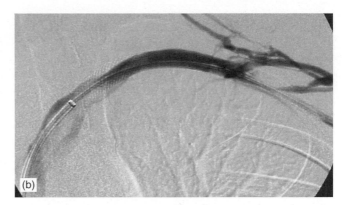

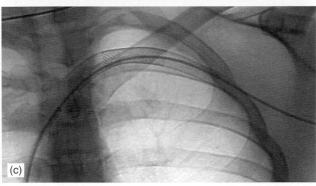

Figure 22.5 *(a–c) A 20-year-old man working as a butcher, who, 12 months after developing a probable effort induced thrombosis, had remaining severe arm symptoms in spite of recanalisation of the axillary/subclavian vein. Note the fibrous trabeculae. After first rib resection the vein was stented but symptoms were only partly alleviated*

modalities are based on uncontrolled case series. Some studies, however, are based on the subgroup of young patients with effort induced thrombosis in whom late arm sequelae are reduced by more aggressive therapy and therefore, such an approach is to be advocated.[6,7,80,82,90] Nevertheless, it is difficult to base one's treatment strategy on these reports. The frequent venographic finding of stenosis of the subclavian vein in 'normal' individuals as well as in the contralateral arm of patients with axillary/subclavian thrombosis but no higher incidence of bilateral upper arm thrombosis,[7] argues strongly against thoracic outlet compression being the major cause of primary subclavian thrombosis. Thoracic decompression can be a valuable tool, but the role of anticoagulation must not be forgotten.

Chronic occlusion

Venous reconstruction has been attempted in extreme circumstances where distressing symptoms persist.[80,83,90] The use of the ipsilateral internal jugular vein, which is divided high in the neck and anastomosed to the distal and unoccluded subclavian vein, seems to have been technically successful.[93] This procedure may be combined with an AV fistula and/or excision of the clavicle. Bypasses using the saphenous vein have had mixed results.

In some severe chronic cases, often referred from other centres to our specialised unit in Malmö, thoracic outlet decompression combined with venous recanalisation and stenting has given relief of symptoms but it has not become standard treatment. Other series have shown that those with chronic symptoms can be relieved by aggressive decompression and an endovascular treatment modality in about 50 per cent of cases.[7,80]

Conclusions

Optimal management of subclavian/axillary vein thrombosis remains contentious. There are numerous underlying causes and multiple treatment options but no comparative trials. The aetiology falls naturally into two categories: primary, due to 'effort' or 'spontaneous' thrombosis, and secondary, due to catheter/pacemaker placement, malignancy or drug abuse. Recent experience has seen a relative increase in the secondary type. Swelling is present in nearly all cases at presentation. Pain and superficial vein dilatation occur in up to half of the cases. Pulmonary embolism occurs in both primary (2 per cent), and more frequently, secondary thrombosis (7 per cent). It may be fatal. Long term symptoms, following primary or secondary thrombosis, occur in about a quarter of the patients, and a small but definite proportion is significantly incapacitated. This is probably more frequent among patients with effort induced thrombosis.

Anticoagulants should be given in the form of heparin or low molecular weight heparin and then oral anticoagulation to address the risks of PE. They may also improve the long term symptomatic outcome. Local thrombolysis has been shown to have a high technical success rate. Overall the justification for more aggressive primary treatment such as thrombectomy, thrombolysis, stenting, first rib resection and venolysis remains controversial. Only a prospective randomised trial, however, will determine whether its routine use in preference or in addition to anticoagulants is justified. First rib resection may be employed in the few seriously incapacitated symptomatic patients with effort induced thrombosis. The essential dilemma is that there remains no way of knowing which patient would be one of the few to be left with truly persisting debilitating symptoms if treated with anticoagulation alone. The use of surgical thoracic decompression as a primary procedure at the time of presentation, inevitably means unnecessary operations in the majority. Surgical bypass procedures, angioplasty and stenting have been reported with mixed results; they should be reserved for the rare and exceptional case.

Key references

Hicken GJ, Ameli FM. Management of subclavian-axillary vein thrombosis: a review. *Can J Surg* 1998; **41**: 13–25.

Hingorani A, Ascher E, Lorenson E, *et al*. Upper extremity deep venous thrombosis and its impact on morbidity and mortality rates in a hospital-based population. *J Vasc Surg* 1997; **26**: 853–60.

Lindblad B, Tengborn L, Bergqvist D. Deep vein thrombosis of the axillary–subclavian veins: epidemiologic data, effects of different types of treatment and late sequelae. *Eur J Vasc Surg* 1988; **2**: 161–5.

Monreal M, Alastrue A, Rull M, *et al*. Upper extremity deep venous thrombosis in cancer patients with venous access devices-prophylaxis with a low molecular weight heparin (Fragmin). *Thromb Haemost* 1996; **75**: 251–3.

Thompson RW, Schneider PA, Nelken NA, *et al*. Circumferential venolysis and paraclavicular thoracic outlet decompression for 'effort thrombosis' of the subclavian vein. *J Vasc Surg* 1992; **16**: 723–32.

REFERENCES

1 Becker DM, Philbrick JT, Walker FBT. Axillary and subclavian venous thrombosis. Prognosis and treatment. *Arch Intern Med* 1991; **151**: 1934–43.

2 Hicken GJ, Ameli FM. Management of subclavian-axillary vein thrombosis: a review. *Can J Surg* 1998; **41**: 13–25.

3 Hingorani A, Ascher E, Lorenson E, *et al*. Upper extremity deep venous thrombosis and its impact on morbidity and mortality rates in a hospital-based population. *J Vasc Surg* 1997; **26**: 853–60.

4 Lindblad B, Tengborn L, Bergqvist D. Deep vein thrombosis of the axillary–subclavian veins: epidemiologic data, effects of different types of treatment and late sequelae. *Eur J Vasc Surg* 1988; **2**: 161–5.

5 Prandoni P, Bernardi E. Upper extremity deep vein thrombosis. *Curr Opin Pulm Med* 1999; **5**: 222–6.

6 Machleder HI. Evaluation of a new treatment strategy for Paget-Schroetter syndrome: spontaneous thrombosis of the axillary-subclavian vein. *J Vasc Surg* 1993; **17**: 305–15; discussion 316–17.

7 Urschel HC Jr, Razzuk MA. Paget-Schroetter syndrome: what is the best management? *Ann Thorac Surg* 2000; **69**: 1663–8; discussion 1668–9.

8 Bailey H, Love M. King Henry IV of France – Battle of Ivry in 1590. In: Rains AJ, Ritchie HD (eds). *Bailey & Love's Short Practice of Surgery*. London: Lewis, HK, 1981: 175–84.

9 Paget J. *Clinical Lectures and Essays*. London: Longman's Green, 1875.

10 Hughes ESR. Venous obstruction in the upper extremity (Paget-Schroetter's syndrome). A review of 320 cases. *Int Abs Surg* 1949; **88**: 89–127.

11 Pittam MR, Darke SG. The place of first rib resection in the management of axillary-subclavian vein thrombosis. *Eur J Vasc Surg* 1987; **1**: 5–10.

12 Dunant JH. Subclavian vein obstruction in thoracic outlet syndrome. *Int Angiol* 1984; **3**: 157–9.

13 Broome A, Eklof B, Gothlin J, Hallbook T. [Phlebography and plethysmography in venous obstruction of the arm]. *Radiology* 1971; **11**: 155–61.

14 Stevenson IM, Parry EW. Radiological study of the aetiological factors in venous obstruction of the upper limb. *J Cardiovasc Surg (Torino)* 1975; **16**: 580–5.

15 Galea MH, Berridge DC, Gregson RHS, *et al*. Axillary/subclavian vein thrombosis: a clinical and radiological evaluation of conservative management. *Phlebology* 1990; **5**: 193–9.

16 Barker NW, Nygaard KK, Watters W. Statistical study of postoperative venous thrombosis and pulmonary embolism. Location of thrombosis. Relation of thrombosis and embolism. *Proc Mayo Clin* 1941; **16**: 33–7.

17 Kunkel JM, Machleder HI. Treatment of Paget-Schroetter syndrome. A staged, multidisciplinary approach. *Arch Surg* 1989; **124**: 1153–7; discussion 1157–8.

18 Kerr TM, Lutter KS, Moeller DM, *et al*. Upper extremity venous thrombosis diagnosed by duplex scanning. *Am J Surg* 1990; **160**: 202–6.

19 Lindblad B, Bornmyr S, Kullendorff B, Bergqvist D. Venous haemodynamics of the upper extremity after subclavian vein thrombosis. *Vasa* 1990; **19**: 218–22.

20 Adams JT, McEvoy RK, DeWeese JA. Primary deep venous thrombosis of upper extremity. *Arch Surg* 1965; **91**: 29–42.

21 Coon WW, Willis PW 3rd. Thrombosis of axillary and subclavian veins. *Arch Surg* 1967; **94**: 657–63.

22 Tilney NL, Griffiths HJG, Edwards EA. Natural history of major venous thrombosis of the upper extremity. *Arch Surg* 1970; **101**: 792–6.

23 Donayre CE, White GH, Mehringer SM, Wilson SE. Pathogenesis determines late morbidity of axillosubclavian vein thrombosis. *Am J Surg* 1986; **152**: 179–84.

24 Horattas MC, Wright DJ, Fenton AH, *et al*. Changing concepts of deep venous thrombosis of the upper extremity – report of a series and review of the literature. *Surgery* 1988; **104**: 561–7.

25 Hauptli W, Schmitt HE, Huber P, *et al*. [Etiology and long-term course of subclavian vein thrombosis with reference to acute therapy]. *Schweiz Med Wochenschr* 1989; **119**: 647–52.

26 AbuRahma AF, Sadler D, Stuart P, *et al*. Conventional versus thrombolytic therapy in spontaneous (effort) axillary-subclavian vein thrombosis. *Am J Surg* 1991; **161**: 459–65.

27   Malcynski J, O'Donnell TF Jr, Mackey WC, Millan VA. Long-term results of treatment for axillary subclavian vein thrombosis. *Can J Surg* 1993; **36**: 365–71.

28   Martin M, Brors G. [Subclavian vein thrombosis: epidemiologic data of the PHLEKO (phlebothrombosis conservative treatment) Study]. *Vasa* 1995; **24**: 120–5.

29   Adelman MA, Stone DH, Riles TS, *et al.* A multidisciplinary approach to the treatment of Paget-Schroetter syndrome. *Ann Vasc Surg* 1997; **11**: 149–54.

30   Beygui RE, Olcott Ct, Dalman RL. Subclavian vein thrombosis: outcome analysis based on etiology and modality of treatment. *Ann Vasc Surg* 1997; **11**: 247–55.

31   Marie I, Levesque H, Cailleux N, *et al.* [Deep venous thrombosis of the upper limbs. Apropos of 49 cases]. *Rev Med Interne* 1998; **19**: 399–408.

32   Sakakibara Y, Shigeta O, Ishikawa S, *et al.* Upper extremity vein thrombosis: etiologic categories, precipitating causes, and management. *Angiology* 1999; **50**: 547–53.

33   Zell L, Scheffler P, Heger M, *et al.* The Paget-Schroetter syndrome: work accident and occupational disease. *Ann Acad Med Singapore* 2001; **30**: 481–4.

34   Sundqvist SB, Hedner U, Kullenberg HK, Bergentz SE. Deep venous thrombosis of the arm: a study of coagulation and fibrinolysis. *BMJ (Clin Res Ed)* 1981; **283**: 265–7.

35   Heron E, Lozinguez O, Alhenc-Gelas M, *et al.* Hypercoagulable states in primary upper-extremity deep vein thrombosis. *Arch Intern Med* 2000; **160**: 382–6.

36   Leebcck FW, Stadhouders NA, van Stein D, *et al.* Hypercoagulability states in upper-extremity deep venous thrombosis. *Am J Hematol* 2001; **67**: 15–19.

37   Fijnheer R, Paijmans B, Verdonck LF, *et al.* Factor V Leiden in central venous catheter-associated thrombosis. *Br J Haematol* 2002; **118**: 267–70.

38   Sabeti S, Schillinger M, Mlekusch W, Haumer M, *et al.* Treatment of subclavian-axillary vein thrombosis: long-term outcome of anticoagulation versus systemic thrombolysis. *Thromb Res* 2002; **108**: 279–85.

39   Hoshal VL Jr, Ause RG, Hoskins PA. Fibrin sleeve formation on indwelling subclavian central venous catheters. *Arch Surg* 1971; **102**: 253–8.

40   Ryan JA Jr, Abel RM, Abbott WM, *et al.* Catheter complications in total parenteral nutrition. A prospective study of 200 consecutive patients. *N Engl J Med* 1974; **290**: 757–61.

41   Lindblad B, Efsing HO, Mark J, Wolff T. Central venous catheters and thromboembolic complications. A comparison of three different materials. *Thromb Haemost* 1981; **46**: 318.

42   Ahmed N. Thrombosis after central venous cannulation. *Med J Aust* 1976; **1**: 217–20.

43   Bennegård K, Curelaru I, Gustavsson B, *et al.* Material thrombogenicity in central venous catheterization. I. A comparison between uncoated and heparin-coated, long antebrachial, polyethylene catheters. *Acta Anaesthesiol Scand* 1982; **26**: 112–20.

44   Braun U, Fassolt A, Teske HJ. [Phlebographic studies on foreign body induced thrombosis caused by infraclavicular subclavian catheterization]. *Anaesthesist* 1970; **19**: 432–7.

45   Fassolt A, Braun U. [The prophylaxis of thrombosis due to central venous catheter with low-dose-heparin (author's transl)]. *Schweiz Rundsch Med Prax* 1978; **67**: 57–60.

46   Ladefoged K, Davidsen HG, Efsen F, *et al.* [Complications of prolonged parenteral nutrition. Experiences from an 11-year period]. *Ugeskr Laeger* 1979; **141**: 3356–60.

47   Magalhaes P, Humair L, Jacot C, de Torrente A. [Venous thrombosis in central venous catheterization: incidence and promoting factors]. *Schweiz Med Wochenschr* 1986; **116**: 579–82.

48   Balestreri L, De Cicco M, Matovic M, *et al.* Central venous catheter-related thrombosis in clinically asymptomatic oncologic patients: a phlebographic study. *Eur J Radiol* 1995; **20**: 108–11.

49   Martin C, Viviand X, Saux P, Gouin F. Upper-extremity deep vein thrombosis after central venous catheterization via the axillary vein. *Crit Care Med* 1999; **27**: 2626–9.

50   Allen AW, Megargell JL, Brown DB, *et al.* Venous thrombosis associated with the placement of peripherally inserted central catheters. *J Vasc Interv Radiol* 2000; **11**: 1309–14.

51   Male C, Chait P, Andrew M, Hanna K, Julian J, Mitchell L, for the PARKAA investigators. Central venous line-related thrombosis in children: association with central venous line location and insertion technique. *Blood* 2003; **101**: 4273–8.

52   Frank DA, Meuse J, Hirsch D, *et al.* The treatment and outcome of cancer patients with thromboses on central venous catheters. *J Thromb Thrombolysis* 2000; **10**: 271–5.

53   Wu X, Studer W, Skarvan K, Seeberger MD. High incidence of intravenous thrombi after short-term central venous catheterization of the internal jugular vein. *J Clin Anesth* 1999; **11**: 482–5.

54   Soto-Velasco JM, Steiger E, Rombeau JL, *et al.* Subclavian vein thrombophlebitis: complication of total parenteral nutrition (TPN). *Cleve Clin Q* 1984; **51**: 159–66.

55   Schwarz RE, Coit DG, Groeger JS. Transcutaneously tunneled central venous lines in cancer patients: an analysis of device-related morbidity factors based on prospective data collection. *Ann Surg Oncol* 2000; **7**: 441–9.

56   Scholz G, Loewe KR. [Puncture of the subclavian vein and its complications from the pathological and anatomical viewpoint]. *Med Welt* 1969; **41**: 2248–51.

57   Brismar B, Hardstedt C, Malmborg AS. Bacteriology and phlebography in catheterization for parenteral nutrition. A prospective study. *Acta Chir Scand* 1980; **146**: 115–19.

58   Andersson T, Brodin M, Lindberg E, Wickbom G. Frequency of thrombosis in patients with central venous catheter. *Svensk Kirurgi* 1981; **36**: 189.

59   Starkhammar H, Bengtsson M, Morales O. Fibrin sleeve formation after long term brachial catheterisation with an implantable port device. A prospective venographic study. *Eur J Surg* 1992; **158**: 481–4.

60   Cobos E, Dixon S, Keung YK. Prevention and management of central venous catheter thrombosis. *Curr Opin Hematol* 1998; **5**: 355–9.

61   Randolph AG, Cook DJ, Gonzales CA, Andrew M. Benefit of heparin in central venous and pulmonary artery catheters: a meta-analysis of randomized controlled trials. *Chest* 1998; **113**: 165–71.

62   Boraks P, Seale J, Price J, *et al.* Prevention of central venous catheter associated thrombosis using minidose warfarin in patients with haematological malignancies. *Br J Haematol* 1998; **101**: 483–6.

63   Bern MM, Bothe A Jr, Bistrian B, *et al.* Prophylaxis against central vein thrombosis with low-dose warfarin. *Surgery* 1986; **99**: 216–21.

64 Bern MM, Lokich JJ, Wallach SR, *et al.* Very low doses of warfarin can prevent thrombosis in central venous catheters. A randomized prospective trial. *Ann Intern Med* 1990; **112**: 423–8.

65 Kar AK, Ghosh S, Majumdar A, *et al.* Venous obstruction after permanent pacing. *Indian Heart J* 2000; **52**: 431–3.

66 Sticherling C, Chough SP, Baker RL, *et al.* Prevalence of central venous occlusion in patients with chronic defibrillator leads. *Am Heart J* 2001; **141**: 813–16.

67 Stoney WS, Addlestone RB, Alford WC Jr, *et al.* The incidence of venous thrombosis following long-term transvenous pacing. *Ann Thorac Surg* 1976; **22**: 166–70.

68 Quinn SF, Schuman ES, Demlow TA, *et al.* Percutaneous transluminal angioplasty versus endovascular stent placement in the treatment of venous stenoses in patients undergoing hemodialysis: intermediate results. *Vasc Interv Radiol* 1995; **6**: 851–5.

69 Surratt RS, Picus D, Hicks ME, *et al.* The importance of preoperative evaluation of the subclavian vein in dialysis access planning. *Am J Roentgenol* 1991; **156**: 623–5.

70 Lumsden AB, MacDonald MJ, Isiklar H, *et al.* Central venous stenosis in the hemodialysis patient: incidence and efficacy of endovascular treatment. *Cardiovasc Surg* 1997; **5**: 504–9.

71 Jean G, Vanel T, Chazot C, *et al.* Prevalence of stenosis and thrombosis of central veins in hemodialysis after a tunneled jugular catheter. *Nephrologie* 2001; **22**: 501–4.

72 Gray RJ, Horton KM, Dolmatch BL, *et al.* Use of Wallstents for hemodialysis access-related venous stenoses and occlusions untreatable with balloon angioplasty. *Radiology* 1995; **195**: 479–84.

73 Verstandig AG, Bloom AI, Sasson T, *et al.* Shortening and migration of Wallstents after stenting of central venous stenosis in hemodialysis patients. *Cardiovasc Intervent Radiol* 2003; **26**: 58–64.

74 Swinton NW, Edgett JW, Hall RJ. Primary subclavian-axillary vein thrombosis. *Circulation* 1968; **38**: 737–45.

75 Campbell CB, Chandler JG, Tegtmeyer CJ, Bernstein EF. Axillary, subclavian and brachiocephalic vein obstruction. *Surgery* 1977; **82**: 816–26.

76 Harley DP, White RA, Nelson RJ. Pulmonary embolism secondary to thrombosis of the arm. *Am J Surg* 1984; **141**: 221–4.

77 Reed JD, Harman JT, Harris V. Regional fibrinolytic therapy for iatrogenic subclavian vein thrombosis. *Semin Interv Radiol* 1992; **9**: 183–9.

78 Thompson RW, Schneider PA, Nelken NA, *et al.* Circumferential venolysis and paraclavicular thoracic outlet decompression for 'effort thrombosis' of the subclavian vein. *J Vasc Surg* 1992; **16**: 723–32.

79 Monreal M, Alastrue A, Rull M, *et al.* Upper extremity deep venous thrombosis in cancer patients with venous access devices – prophylaxis with a low molecular weight heparin (Fragmin). *Thromb Haemost* 1996; **75**: 251–3.

80 Molina JE. Need for emergency treatment in subclavian vein effort thrombosis. *J Am Coll Surg* 1995; **181**: 414–20.

81 Azakie A, McElhinney DB, Thompson RW, *et al.* Surgical management of subclavian-vein effort thrombosis as a result of thoracic outlet compression. *J Vasc Surg* 1998; **28**: 777–86.

82 Angle N, Gelabert HA, Farooq MM, *et al.* Safety and efficacy of early surgical decompression of the thoracic outlet for Paget-Schroetter syndrome. *Ann Vasc Surg* 2001; **15**: 37–42.

83 Feugier P, Aleksic I, Salari R, *et al.* Long-term results of venous revascularization for Paget-Schroetter syndrome in athletes. *Ann Vasc Surg* 2001; **15**: 212–18.

84 Kreienberg PB, Chang BB, Darling RC, *et al.* Long-term results in patients treated with thrombolysis, thoracic inlet decompression, and subclavian vein stenting for Paget-Schroetter syndrome. *J Vasc Surg* 2001; **33**: S100–5.

85 Lokanathan R, Salvian AJ, Chen JC, *et al.* Outcome after thrombolysis and selective thoracic outlet decompression for primary axillary vein thrombosis. *J Vasc Surg* 2001; **33**: 783–8.

86 Lee WA, Hill BB, Harris EJ Jr, *et al.* Surgical intervention is not required for all patients with subclavian vein thrombosis. *J Vasc Surg* 2000; **32**: 57–67.

87 Savage KJ, Wells PS, Schulz V, *et al.* Outpatient use of low molecular weight heparin (Dalteparin) for the treatment of deep vein thrombosis of the upper extremity. *Thromb Haemost* 1999; **82**: 1008–10.

88 Theiss W, Wirtzfeld A. [Fibrinolytic treatment of acute and subacute thromboses of the deep veins of the shoulder girdle.] *Dtsch Med Wochenschr* 1982; **107**: 933–6.

89 Strange-Vognsen HH, Hauch O, Andersen J, Struckmann J. Resection of the first rib, following deep arm vein thrombolysis in patients with thoracic outlet syndrome. *J Cardiovasc Surg* 1989; **30**: 430–3.

90 Lee MC, Grassi CJ, Belkin M, *et al.* Early operative intervention after thrombolytic therapy for primary subclavian vein thrombosis: an effective treatment approach. *J Vasc Surg* 1998; **27**: 1101–8.

91 Meier GH, Pollak JS, Rosenblatt M, *et al.* Initial experience with venous stents in exertional axillary-subclavian vein thrombosis. *J Vasc Surg* 1996; **24**: 974–83.

92 Green RM, Waldman D, Ouriel K, *et al.* Claviculectomy for subclavian venous repair: long-term functional results. *J Vasc Surg* 2000; **32**: 315–21.

93 De Weese JA. Results of surgical treatment of axillary subclavian venous thrombosis. In: Bergan JJ, Yao JST (eds). *Venous Disorders.* London: Saunders WB, 1991: 421–33.

Thoracoabdominal Catastrophes

23

The Emergency Aortic Aneurysm

JONATHAN REFSON, JOHN HN WOLFE

THE PROBLEM

Emergency aneurysms pose a difficult healthcare problem, as health resources are currently unable to provide the necessary expertise to all patients at the point of presentation. Therefore, diagnosis of this problem needs to be accurate with rapid passage of the patient from admitting unit to operating theatre, whether in the same hospital or after transfer. The diagnosis, management and common problems of this condition are discussed.

The ratio of planned aneurysm surgery to urgent and emergency aneurysms has remained remarkably constant at roughly 2:1 over the past 30 years.[1,2] Emergency aneurysms can present with a history of back, loin or abdominal pain associated with an episode of circulatory collapse or persistent hypotension; approximately 70 per cent will not be known to have an abdominal aortic aneurysm (AAA).[3] The level of urgency dictates the management of the 'emergency aneurysm'; has the aneurysm ruptured or is the rupture impending? In order to make the discussion of the subject easier, we have drawn a distinction between **urgent** and **emergency** aneurysms. Urgent aneurysms are those where the aneurysm has obviously become symptomatic but has not caused the patient to be hypotensive.

DIAGNOSIS

The history of sudden back or abdominal pain with cardiovascular collapse in a middle aged or elderly patient should alert the clinician to the possibility of a ruptured AAA, particularly where the patient is known to have such an aneurysm. On examination, the patient may be obviously shocked, pale, cold, clammy and agitated. Abdominal examination may reveal a pulsatile mass, but it may be difficult to palpate, particularly in an obese individual; it is also important to feel the peripheral pulses. The investigations of these patients should be kept to a minimum and an electrocardiogram (ECG) is really all that is required to rule out possible myocardial infarction, which may be a differential diagnosis. In the haemodynamically challenged patient radiological investigation is contraindicated, in particular computed tomography (CT) scanning, as it will only delay the patient's transfer to the operating theatre for definitive treatment.

Resuscitation should be simple and minimal; if the patient is talking sensibly there is enough blood pressure to perfuse the vital organs. High flow oxygen should be delivered by facemask, venous access should be achieved with two large bore cannulae (see Chapter 7B) and no fluid need be given. If fluid is administered to restore the patient's blood pressure to normality, further bleeding may occur with catastrophic consequences. Blood should be taken for baseline investigations, namely blood count, clotting studies, typing and crossmatching 10 units of blood and renal function. It is advisable to ensure that fresh frozen plasma and platelets are also available, as the coagulopathy associated with both haemorrhage and massive transfusion causes troublesome and life-threatening bleeding. No further intervention is required in the emergency department and the patient should be transferred directly to the operating theatre.

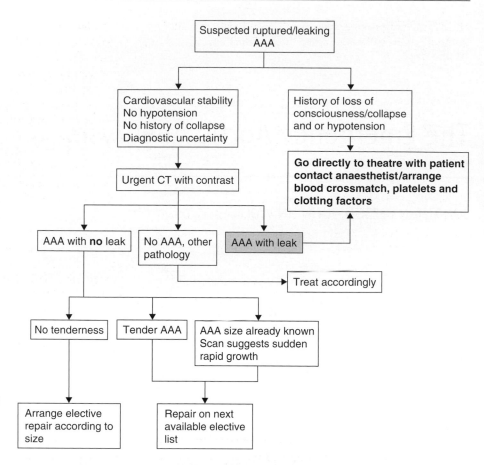

Figure 23.1 *Algorithm of management of suspected ruptured abdominal aortic aneurysms (AAAs). CT, computed tomography*

In the scenario of the **urgent** aneurysm, the patient may complain of pain or tenderness *but hypotension will not have been documented.* Therefore, it is acceptable to perform an urgent CT scan to assess the extent of the aneurysm and to establish whether or not it has leaked. It will also identify small leaks that have not caused circulatory collapse and some thoracoabdominal aneurysms that should be transferred to a specialist centre. This time window allows a more indepth assessment of the patient's overall fitness for surgery, but in the event that a leak is diagnosed on CT scanning, surgery should not be delayed. Where there has been hypotension, however, time is of the essence in getting the patient to theatre for surgery. An algorithm (Fig. 23.1) provides pathways of care in managing patients with suspected AAA rupture.

DIFFERENTIAL DIAGNOSIS

Age is important in distinguishing patients with aneurysmal disease. As this is a problem occurring almost invariably in the over-fifties, a patient under this age is unlikely to have leaked or ruptured an aneurysm. There is, however, an important rare group of exceptions to this rule including such conditions as Marfan's and Ehlers Danlos syndromes. Congenital connective tissue disorders are the pathological basis of these conditions and patients develop aneurysms in their late teens and early twenties. Other conditions that can be difficult to distinguish from the ruptured AAA are myocardial infarction, pancreatitis and renal stone disease, but a quick and careful history, examination and simple investigations should help to establish the diagnosis. It is important to note that renal stones rarely present for the first time in the over-fifties.

PATIENT SELECTION

An untreated leaking aneurysm has a mortality approaching 100 per cent.[4] Not to operate will, therefore, almost certainly result in the patient's demise. In these circumstances the patient and relatives should be advised that *if no surgery* were to be undertaken then the patient would die, but also that operative intervention carries a 50/50 chance of survival. Unless the patient flatly refuses surgery, or has an extensive thoracoabdominal (type II) aneurysm, we offer surgery to all-comers. Even if patients have such serious comorbidity that they have been turned down for an elective procedure it is appropriate, now that the AAA has ruptured, to offer intervention. This approach is reinforced by aggressive initial support in the intensive care unit during the first 24–48 hours, but unless there are clear signs of recovery that support may then be withdrawn. This is because preoperative assessment is very difficult in the absence of prior knowledge about the patient, indeed some surgeons will not operate on anuric patients with low blood pressure.[5]

Contraindications to surgery

- Patient alert but flatly refuses
- Extensive thoracoabdominal (type II) aneurysm

In the urgent scenario certain risk factors strongly influence outcome for both elective and urgent aneurysm surgery. Age seems to be the strongest predictor with patients over the age of 70 having a mortality rate between five and seven times that of those under the age of 70.[6,7]

Renal function also relates to outcome; patients with elevated creatinine beyond the normal range, i.e. over 50 per cent loss of nephron mass, have a mortality rate two to three times normal creatinine values.

Poor respiratory function, especially in the form of chronic obstructive airways disease (COAD), is another predictor of poor outcome.[8] Many patients with aneurysmal disease are smokers and, as such, will have a chronic respiratory problem. This does not pose an immediate threat, but makes the postoperative management and weaning from ventilation much more difficult and predisposes the patient to hospital acquired pneumonia. Serious consideration should be given to early tracheostomy to aid bronchial toilet and in weaning the patient off the ventilator and avoiding the deleterious effects of sedation. Placing an epidural catheter for analgesia postoperatively may aid respiratory function and, provided that the patient's clotting function is not deranged, should be done as early as possible.

Predictors of poor outcome in ruptured AAAs

- Raised creatinine levels, >50 per cent loss of nephron mass – mortality × 2–3 times normal
- Chronic respiratory failure (COAD) carries a high mortality rate
- Advancing age – beyond 70 years – mortality × 5–7 times normal

---

PATIENT TRANSFER

In hospitals fully equipped to look after ruptured aneurysms there should be no delay in making the transfer from the accident and emergency department to the operating theatre once the diagnosis is made. The vascular surgical team must ensure that all the relevant teams are contacted: operating theatre staff, anaesthetists, transfusion technicians and the intensive care unit.

So far, we have dealt with a scenario where the expertise needed to manage the patient is available in the hospital to which the patient has been admitted. Not infrequently, however, an aneurysm presents to a team without the necessary expertise to deal with the patient's problem. If this is the case the patient needs to be transferred to a unit able to perform the surgery, with the necessary intensive postoperative support. The logistical problems surrounding this exercise are beyond the scope of this chapter, but ideally the patient should be stable for transfer and the receiving hospital should have a vascular surgeon and an intensive care bed available. In the ambulance the patient should have a nurse and medical escort. In the scenario where the patient remains unstable, and in spite of the potential dangers, it is probably preferable to transfer rather than to attempt repair.[9]

This situation of insufficient cover is being addressed and some hospital groups have developed collaborative networks to provide full vascular cover 24 hours a day, 7 days a week (see Chapters 1A–1C). In this situation hospitals provide a collective on-call rota and one surgeon covers all the hospitals. The surgeon, therefore, may have to travel to the patient rather than the other way round. This ensures that patients need not be exposed to a risky transfer.

CONSENT

If the patient is fully conscious it is important to explain the nature of the procedure in simple terms, stressing the urgent need for surgery. In the circumstances, a detailed discussion of all the possible complications is less relevant. If family members are present it is important that they understand the situation and they should be included in any discussion. If the patient is not able to give his/her own consent the procedure can continue on the basis that it is in the patient's best interests. With the advent of living wills, however, it is prudent to enquire whether the patient has expressed an objection to surgery.

OPERATIVE TECHNIQUE

The patient is placed supine on the operating table with the arms abducted. This allows the anaesthetist access for insertion of arterial and venous cannulae. Two wide bore cannulae should be inserted for rapid transfusion access (see Chapter 7B). The patient is prepared and draped awake and the anaesthetist should only induce anaesthesia when the surgeon is ready to make the incision. This is because the abdominal wall musculature provides tamponade, and paralysis of the muscles is often followed by a precipitous fall in blood pressure.

Ideally, three surgeons should be available for the procedure, and in our case the principal surgeon stands on the left of the patient with the scrub nurse opposite. The first assistant stands opposite the surgeon and the other provides retraction to his or her right. This can be difficult with the arm abducted. A long midline incision is made from the xiphisternum to a point halfway between umbilicus and pubic symphysis allowing good exposure to the abdominal cavity. In the event of a retroperitoneal rupture there will be blood-stained fluid in the peritoneal cavity and a retroperitoneal haematoma.

The mobilisation of the aortic neck should continue as for an elective or unruptured case, with evisceration of the transverse colon and omentum cranially and the small bowel to the patient's right. It is tempting to rush the mobilisation of the aorta, but a few extra minutes spent carefully dissecting around the neck of the aneurysm will save much time later trying to control venous bleeding from the inferior mesenteric vein, left gonadal vein and renal vein. It is often venous bleeding that leads to exsanguination, not arterial. In fact, the retroperitoneal haematoma often facilitates dissection by lifting the peritoneal layers off the front of the aorta. Having incised the peritoneum over the aneurysm the sac is easily found and should be followed cranially to the left of the duodenum until the neck is found and a suitable clamp can then be applied anteroposteriorly on the aorta. The practice of fully mobilising the back of the aorta and clamping transversely is not necessary and may cause avulsion of a lumbar artery.

Whether the patient is rapidly exsanguinating or if the leak is contained, iliac artery control is necessary. This is usually straightforward as the ectatic and elongated arteries tend to be looped forward facilitating clamping. Extending the peritoneal incision caudally and dissecting along the surface of the aneurysm sac exposes the common iliac arteries. No attempt should be made to dissect around and sling the iliac arteries, as they are densely adherent to the iliac veins, which are easily damaged. If the common iliac arteries are aneurysmal then the external iliac artery should be mobilised and clamps should be applied at this level. If mobilisation is difficult, for example, because it is an inflammatory aneurysm, then balloons can be inserted to occlude flow, rather than resorting to the use of clamps.

Having isolated the aneurysm proximally and distally, the sac should be opened along its right anterolateral aspect and thrombus removed. At this point bleeding from the lumbar arteries is usually encountered. This can be controlled by direct suture with 3-0 Prolene. The inferior mesenteric artery (IMA) may back-bleed and this vessel, too, can be controlled with sutures from within the sac.

Colonic ischaemia is a potential problem, particularly in emergency aneurysm repair. This may be due to a number of reasons. First, clumsy manhandling of the sac may lead to 'trash' embolisation of the colon as well as more distal tissues. Second, ligation of the IMA through the haematoma may cause damage to the colonic arteries, particularly the ascending colic artery. Third, the aneurysmal process may compromise the internal iliac arteries and if both of these are occluded, as well as the IMA, then sigmoid and pelvic ischaemia may ensue. Fourth, mobilisation of the iliac artery bifurcation lateral to the sigmoid colon mesentery may also damage sigmoid arteries.

These points must be taken into consideration when performing the emergency procedure and if the IMA is patent with poor back bleeding the surgeon should be alerted to the possible need for IMA reimplantation. This reimplantation may also be necessary if one internal iliac artery is aneurysmal and therefore has to be ligated, particularly if the orifice of the other is compromised, in which case the surgeon cannot predict continuing internal iliac artery flow with confidence.

On opening the sac and removing the thrombus sac dark venous blood may well up copiously; this is usually due to the presence of an aortocaval fistula. In these circumstances, external compression by the assistant should allow the surgeon to oversew the defect from within the aortic sac using large bites with 2-0 Prolene. At this stage haemostasis is of more importance than the potential for narrowing the inferior vena cava. No attempt should be made to mobilise the cava and delay only leads to further dramatic blood loss. At this point haemostasis should have been achieved and the anaesthetist should have corrected the hypovolaemia. The next step is to suture in the graft. It should be noted that heparin is not given in cases of rupture as it may further aggravate a coagulopathy.

An appropriately sized graft is chosen. A 120 cm 3-0 Prolene suture is ideal for the proximal anastomosis. If the anastomosis is sound, except for a single bleeding point, then a carefully placed 4-0 suture should suffice. If, on the other hand, entire segments of the back wall appear to have torn away then the anastomosis should be fully revised without further delay. Wasting time on a number of poorly placed sutures that also tear out could lead to disastrous further haemorrhage. Occasionally a Teflon felt patch can be used to buttress the proximal anastomosis, and equally a 2 mm button of Teflon can be extremely useful in ensuring that a single stitch to a solitary bleeding point in a friable aortic wall does not tear through.

Once the proximal anastomosis is secure the surgeon can concentrate on the distal anastomosis; the latter can also be performed using 3-0 Prolene and slightly dilated iliac arteries should not deter the surgeon from using a tube graft as this will expedite the procedure. It is advisable to release the clamped iliac arteries at this point and check for back flow. As no heparin has been given it is quite likely that clot will have been formed. Provided that back flow is good a 50 mL bladder syringe charged with heparinised saline should be flushed down each iliac artery and the vessels reclamped. If back flow is poor and if femoral pulses were present preoperatively a suction catheter should be gently inserted into the iliac artery and clot aspirated until good back flow has been restored; if not, balloon thrombectomy

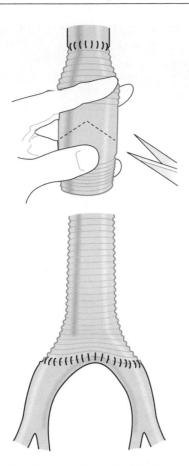

Figure 23.2 *Creating a 'swallow tail' at the lower end of a tube graft to facilitate iliac anastomosis*

is indicated. The artery should then be flushed with heparinised saline as described above. Prior to completion of the distal anastomosis back flow should be rechecked. It should also be ensured that there is good forward flow in the graft and that it has been flushed free of any clot.

Cutting the graft into a 'swallow tail' (Fig. 23.2) ensures that there is sufficient width to splay across the orifices of the aneurysmal aorta.[10] Without this technique the distal Dacron may be too narrow for the separated, dilated orifices and attempts to pull the orifices together with the anastomotic stitch may result in stenosis of the origins of the arteries.

At this point the anaesthetist should be warned that the surgeon is about to release the distal clamp and reperfuse the legs, and that should be done slowly. A drop in systolic blood pressure will indicate that the legs are being reperfused, as will a rise in end tidal carbon dioxide, as the accumulated ischaemic metabolites are cleared from the leg (see Chapter 2). There is often further bleeding from lumbar arteries as they are reperfused from the iliac circulation and they should be underrun with a 3-0 Prolene suture. It is important to check that a femoral pulse is palpable on both sides.

Patience is now required to ensure good haemostasis and this may require the administration of clotting factors,

such as pooled platelets and fresh frozen plasma. While haemostasis is being ensured the feet should be inspected to assess perfusion. The foot pulses may not be present but the feet should be pink and blanch on pressure, with reasonably brisk capillary refill.

Once this has been achieved the remaining aneurysm sac can be closed over the graft with an absorbable suture. The sac should be plicated to avoid dead space, which then fills with haematoma. It is important to ensure that the duodenum is not in contact with the graft as this may lead to erosion through the duodenum and a subsequent aortoenteric fistula. Closing retroperitoneal fat behind the duodenum using a tongue of omentum helps to avoid this complication. Care should be taken that the duodenum is not tethered down anterior to the graft. Any clots should now be evacuated from the abdominal cavity and a brief laparotomy performed as in most cases there is no time to do so prior to aneurysm repair. Care is taken to ensure that the nasogastric tube is correctly placed. The abdominal musculature can now be closed with a continuous mass closure, using a monofilament suture such as nylon.

In the case of **free peritoneal rupture** exsanguination occurs rapidly and therefore the technique has to be modified. On opening the abdomen the supracoeliac aorta can be compressed manually by an assistant while the surgeon places their left hand in the open aneurysm sac and plugs the neck of the aneurysm with the thumb. The aorta can then be cannulated through the site of rupture with a spigoted 24 Fr Foley catheter and a 50 mL syringe connected to the balloon. This is advanced to the suprarenal aorta and the balloon inflated, so gaining proximal control. Alternatively, the thumb allows the right hand to rapidly perform quite accurate blunt dissection around the neck of the aorta. Once this is exposed a clamp can be placed. It is also possible to temporarily clamp the aorta at the diaphragm: the lesser omentum is divided as is the left crus of the diaphragm, and by pushing the oesophagus to the left, the aorta is approached and then clamped. Whatever technique is employed, the aim should be to dissect out the neck as quickly and as safely as possible. If the clamp cannot be applied below the renal arteries then using either the Foley catheter or a suprarenal clamp the proximal anastomosis is carried out. Once complete, the clamp is moved down to the graft, reinstating renal flow.

SPECIAL PREOPERATIVE PROBLEMS

Aortocaval fistula

An aortocaval fistula can be diagnosed preoperatively if one or more of the following signs are found: a loud machinery murmur over the aneurysm, pulsatile leg veins or high central venous pressure in the presence of hypotension. At operation a small volume of arterial blood should come out of the sac but if venous blood continues to well

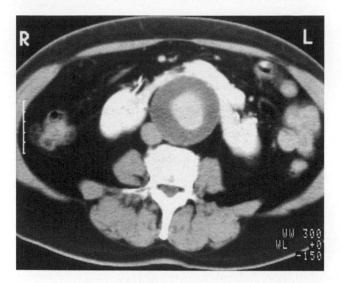

Figure 23.3   *Computed tomography scan demonstrating a horseshoe kidney*

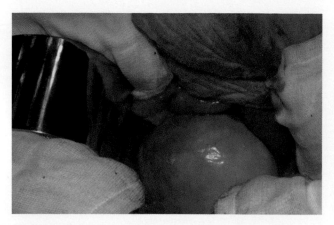

Figure 23.4   *Pearly white appearance of an inflammatory aneurysm*

out from it then a fistula is almost certainly present. This loss can be controlled by pressure on the vena cava having warned the anaesthetist that there will be a fall in venous return. Repair of the fistula is best effected by suturing it from within the aorta with large bites of a large suture which is remarkably easy. No attempt should be made to disconnect the fistula or repair the cava directly.

Horseshoe kidney

A horseshoe kidney is extremely rare. If a CT scan (Fig. 23.3) has been performed then the diagnosis will be clear-cut allowing a retroperitoneal operative approach to be used and the kidney is not involved in the operation. In most cases the surgeon faced with the unexpected anatomy associated with this condition. Once the proximal neck has been controlled the upper sac is opened and the proximal anastomosis is performed. The graft is then tunnelled through the unopened sac to the iliac arteries. Access to bleeding lumbar arteries within the sac can be difficult.[11]

Inflammatory aneurysms

These account for about 5 per cent of all AAAs. If diagnosed preoperatively they can be repaired using a retroperitoneal approach. At operation they can be recognised by the glistening white, pearly carapace involving the aortic wall (Fig. 23.4).

When confronted with the situation in an emergency the safest approach is to expose the supracoeliac aorta, which is rarely involved in the process. This can be done through the lesser sac by cutting the right crus of the diaphragm. There is a significant amount of muscle at this

level, but once it has been swept aside the plane and areolar tissue around the aorta can be cleared rapidly and a clamp applied. Having done this the sac can be opened to the left of the densely adherent duodenum and the proximal anastomosis can be done. Once the latter has been completed the clamp may be moved on to the graft, thus reperfusing the visceral and renal arteries. It is neither safe nor sensible to attempt to dissect the duodenum off the aortic wall unless the inflammatory process is in its very early stages and a plane is readily identified.

Special problems discovered at operation

- Aortocaval fistula
- Horseshoe kidney
- Inflammatory aneurysm
- Thoracoabdominal aneurysm
- Other abdominal pathology – gallstones, malignancy

Thoracoabdominal aneurysm

In an unstable patient with a ruptured aneurysm there will be little opportunity to diagnose a thoracoabdominal aneurysm. Fortunately, the most common site for rupture of these aneurysms is in the abdominal element (Fig. 23.5). Under these very difficult circumstances an attempt should be made to control the aneurysm at a narrow point, either in the pararenal area or the supracoeliac aorta through the lesser sac. Once control has been achieved the proximal anastomosis will have to be performed to a baggy aorta, and this is best achieved by plicating the arterial wall into a large diameter graft. If this anastomosis holds the situation can be salvaged and the operation completed.

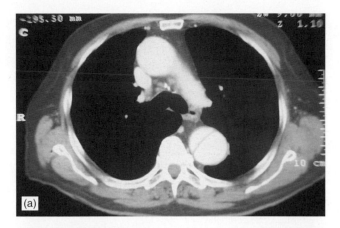

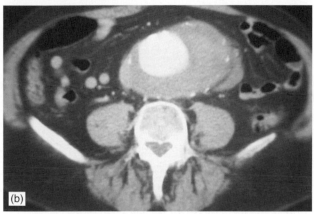

Figure 23.5 *(a) Type B aortic dissection, (b) the aneurysmal abdominal component of which had leaked, necessitating a type IV thoracoabdominal aneurysm repair*

In the postoperative phase the full extent of the aneurysm can be assessed and a judgement made as to whether further surgery is appropriate. Fortunately, a significant number of these aneurysms become symptomatic and the surgeon is in a position to investigate the aneurysm prior to surgery. If a thoracoabdominal aneurysm is diagnosed under these circumstances then referral to an appropriate specialist unit is sensible. That unit will then perform further appropriate investigations, including cardiac, respiratory and renal assessment, prior to elective repair using standard techniques.

Associated abdominal pathology

Other coexisting pathological conditions are encountered in about 5 per cent of patients undergoing aneurysm surgery.[12] With the exception of gallstone disease synchronous procedures should be avoided because of the risk of graft sepsis. In the scenario of the ruptured aneurysm the priority is haemostasis and restoration of circulation and all secondary procedures should be left to a later date, even if malignancy is found.

POSTOPERATIVE CARE

The majority of patients coming to surgery survive the operative procedure but many of these elderly patients then succumb to the multiorgan failure precipitated by massive blood loss and transfusion (see Chapters 4 and 7A). Meticulous attention to postoperative patient care is crucial if survival is to be improved. The systemic problems frequently encountered following emergency surgery are renal failure requiring support in the form of haemofiltration and respiratory failure requiring ventilatory support. An intensive care facility is essential with good cooperation between surgeon and intensivist. If an elderly patient with extensive comorbidity survives initial emergency surgery, but is obviously not thriving, then the clinical team must take stock.

During the first 48 hours intensive support should be given to the patient and discussions should take place with the family so that they are fully aware of the situation. Within this period it will become apparent that some of these patients are most unlikely to survive. Under these circumstances the surgeon, intensivist and nursing staff should discuss among themselves, and then with the family, whether escalating support should be withdrawn.

RECENT ADVANCES

Screening

Recent advances in the fields of screening and surveillance of small aneurysms have refined our knowledge as to whether to offer surgery to patients with abdominal aortic aneurysms. The Small Aneurysm Study demonstrated that it was safe to pursue a policy of surveillance of aneurysms up to 5.5 cm in diameter.[13] Some screening studies have suggested that surveillance may be safe in an aneurysm of up to 6 cm diameter.[14] Screening has also demonstrated a 50–60 per cent reduction in the incidence of ruptured AAAs in a screened population.[15,16] Currently in the UK 33 per cent of all aneurysm surgery is undertaken on an emergency basis,[1,17] which is nearly double the European average.[17]

Stenting

Recent reports have demonstrated that endovascular techniques can be successfully employed in managing emergency AAAs. Others[18–20] have demonstrated a 92 per cent success rate in managing leaking aneurysms in cases where the anatomy of the aorta was suitable for endovascular repair. These results compare favourably with open repair. The endovascular technique is currently available to only a small minority of centres and should be used by units which regularly perform elective aneurysm stenting.

Conclusions

Death from abdominal aortic aneurysmal disease is the tenth commonest cause of death in the UK and accounts for 1 per cent of all male deaths.[21] The rate of ruptured aneurysms across Europe varies from 12 to over 55 per cent of all aneurysm repairs.[17] The reasons for this disparity are not clear, but may relate to healthcare funding. The survival of all operated ruptures, however, is remarkably constant across both Europe and the USA at 35–60 per cent.[23,24] Dramatic improvements in surgical and anaesthetic techniques, as well as intensive care support, have had little impact.

The distinction between urgent and emergency aneurysms has been set out in terms of the level of urgency of definitive care necessary, and hypotension is employed as the discriminating factor. This parameter has been shown to determine outcome with 'urgent' aneurysms having a morality rate of 10–20 per cent, while emergency repair has a mortality rate of 35–60 per cent. The risk of elective infrarenal AAA repair is approximately 5 per cent, whereas the mortality rate of operations for ruptured aneurysms remains stubbornly at 35–60 per cent.[23] The true mortality rate of a ruptured aneurysm is in fact 80–90 per cent since many of the patients do not reach hospital.[25]

The increasing enthusiasm for screening programmes may, in the future, reduce the need for emergency aneurysm repair in the same way as advances in the management of peptic ulcers have reduced the need for repair of perforated peptic ulcers.

There is much discussion about the use of stents for elective infrarenal aneurysm repair as reintervention rates are high. If, however, the technique is successful in occluding the rupture and maintaining flow to organs and limbs, then it has an important role in the emergency situation. Once the patient has survived emergency surgery further investigations can be undertaken electively, with considerably reduced attendant risks.

Key references

Bown MJ, Sutton AJ, Bell PR, Sayers RD. A meta-analysis of 50 years of ruptured abdominal aortic aneurysm repair [review]. Br J Surg 2002; **89**: 714–30.
Brady AR, Fowkes FG, Greenhalgh RM, et al. Risk factors for postoperative death following elective surgical repair of abdominal aortic aneurysm: results from the UK Small Aneurysm Trial. On behalf of the UK Small Aneurysm Trial participants. Br J Surg 2000; **87**: 742–9.
Hewin DF, Campbell WB. Ruptured aortic aneurysm: the decision not to operate. Ann R Coll Surg Engl 1998; **80**: 221–5.

Scott RA, Ashton HA, Lamparelli MJ, et al. A 14-year experience with 6 cm as a criterion for surgical treatment of abdominal aortic aneurysm. Br J Surg 1999; **86**: 1317–21.
Wilmink AB, Quick CR, Hubbard CS, Day NE. Effectiveness and cost of screening for abdominal aortic aneurysm: results of a population screening program. J Vasc Surg 2003; **38**: 72–7.

REFERENCES

1 Castleden WM, Mercer JC. Abdominal aortic aneurysms in Western Australia: descriptive epidemiology and patterns of rupture. Br J Surg 1985; **72**: 109–12.
2 Samy AK, MacBain G. Abdominal aortic aneurysm: ten years' hospital population study in the city of Glasgow. Eur J Vasc Surg 1993; **7**: 561–6
3 Sterpetti AV, Cavallari N, Allegrucci P, et al. Seasonal variation in the incidence of ruptured abdominal aortic aneurysm. J R Coll Surg Edinb 1995; **40**: 14–15.
4 Walker EM, Hopkinson BR, Makin GS. Unoperated abdominal aortic aneurysm: presentation and natural history. Ann R Coll Surg Engl 1983; **65**: 311–13.
5 Hewin DF, Campbell WB. Ruptured aortic aneurysm: the decision not to operate. Ann R Coll Surg Engl 1998; **80**: 221–5.
6 Refson JS, Wilmink A, Kerle M, et al. Age, renal dysfunction and aneurysm outcome. Br J Surg 2001; **88**: 611.
7 Bayly PJ, Matthews JN, Dobson PM, et al. In-hospital mortality from abdominal aortic surgery in Great Britain and Ireland: Vascular Anaesthesia Society audit. Br J Surg 2001; **88**: 687–92.
8 Brady AR, Fowkes FG, Greenhalgh RM, et al. Risk factors for postoperative death following elective surgical repair of abdominal aortic aneurysm: results from the UK Small Aneurysm Trial. On behalf of the UK Small Aneurysm Trial participants. Br J Surg 2000; **87**: 742–9.
9 Adam DJ, Mohan IV, Stuart WP, et al. Community and hospital outcome from ruptured abdominal aortic aneurysm within the catchment area of a regional vascular surgical service. J Vasc Surg 1999; **30**: 922–8.
10 Gilling-Smith GL, Wolfe JH. The tailed aortic graft: a technique for widening the distal orifice of an aortic tube graft. Br J Surg 1986; **73**: 208
11 Stroosma OB, Kootstra G, Schurink GW. Management of aortic aneurysm in the presence of a horseshoe kidney. Br J Surg 2001; **88**: 500–9
12 Szilagyi DE, Elliott JP, Berguer R. Coincidental malignancy and abdominal aortic aneurysm. Problems of management. Arch Surg 1967; **95**: 402–12.
13 Mortality results for randomised controlled trial of early elective surgery or ultrasonographic surveillance for small abdominal aortic aneurysms. The UK Small Aneurysm Trial Participants. Lancet 1998; **352**: 1649–55.
14 Scott RA, Ashton HA, Lamparelli MJ, et al. A 14-year experience with 6 cm as a criterion for surgical treatment of abdominal aortic aneurysm. Br J Surg 1999; **86**: 1317–21.
15 Wilmink AB, Quick CR, Hubbard CS, Day NE. Effectiveness and cost of screening for abdominal aortic aneurysm: results of a population screening program. J Vasc Surg 2003; **38**: 72–7.

16 Lindholt JS, Juul S, Fasting H, Henneberg EW. Hospital costs and benefits of screening for abdominal aortic aneurysms. Results from a randomised population screening trial. *Eur J Vasc Endovasc Surg* 2002; **23**: 55–60.

17 Emergency AAA. Vascular news. 2001; 1.

18 Veith FJ, Ohki T. Endovascular approaches to ruptured infrarenal aorto-iliac aneurysms. *J Cardiovasc Surg (Torino)* 2002; **43**: 369–78.

19 Hinchliffe RJ, Braithwaite BD, Hopkinson BR. The endovascular management of ruptured abdominal aortic aneurysms. *Eur J Vasc Endovasc Surg* 2003; **25**: 191–201.

20 Peppelenbosch N, Yilmaz N, van Marrewijk C, *et al.* Emergency treatment of acute symptomatic or ruptured abdominal aortic aneurysm. Outcome of a prospective intent-to-treat by EVAR protocol. *Eur J Vasc Endovasc Surg* 2003; **26**: 303–10.

21 Office of National Statistics. *Mortality Statistics. Cause 1993.* London: HMSO, 1995.

22 Neary WD, Crow P, Foy C, *et al.* Comparison of POSSUM scoring and the Hardman Index in selection of patients for repair of ruptured abdominal aortic aneurysm. *Br J Surg* 2003; **90**: 421–5.

23 Bown MJ, Sutton AJ, Bell PR, Sayers RD. A meta-analysis of 50 years of ruptured abdominal aortic aneurysm repair [review]. *Br J Surg* 2002; **89**: 714–30.

24 Podlaha J, Gregor Z, Roubal P, *et al.* Ruptured abdominal aortic aneurysm – outcomes in the last ten years. *Bratisl Lek Listy* 2000; **101**: 191–3.

25 Buskens FG. Incidence, risk and operability of abdominal aortic aneurysm in the elderly patient [in Dutch]. *Tijdschr Gerontol Geriatr* 1990; **21**: 169–71.

24

Stenting in Acute Aortic Dissection

MICHAEL D DAKE

THE PROBLEM

Acute dissection is the most frequent catastrophe affecting the aorta. The mean age of patients at the time of diagnosis of acute aortic dissection is 60 years, a decade younger than that observed in other thoracic aortic diseases such as aneurysm, penetrating aortic ulcer or aortic intramural haematoma. Although hypertension is clearly recognised as a *sine qua non* for its occurrence, a number of other clinical factors are associated with its aetiology.

PATHOPHYSIOLOGY

Aortic dissection occurs when blood enters the aortic wall through a disruption of the intimal lining. The tear in the intima allows flowing blood to cleave a plane within the medial layer of the wall. The intimal entry is associated with intramural extension of blood which creates a longitudinal delamination of the aortic wall. The dissecting blood or thrombus may progress from the entry tear in a proximal and/or distal direction. As the process extends, a dissection flap or septum, consisting of the cleaved lamellar layer of intima and partial thickness of media is formed separating the original 'true' lumen lined by intima from the newly formed 'false' intramural channel. The trajectory of flap progression results in dissection with a distinct morphological features in each case of dissection. The anatomical relationships between the flap, true lumen, and false lumen and importantly, the aortic branch vessels they engage, are idiosyncratic to the individual concerned.

CLASSIFICATION AND RATIONALE

The process of aortic dissection is traditionally categorised by the extent of disease. The most widely adopted classification schemes rely on the ability to diagnose ascending aortic dissection and distinguish it from isolated involvement of the aortic arch and/or descending aorta. The rationale for this critical distinction is based on well-established prognostic implications and, consequently, therapeutic considerations associated with dissection of the ascending aorta. Presently, without immediate surgical intervention, the prognosis for aortic dissection of the ascending aorta managed with medical therapy alone is extremely grave, and the risk of aortic rupture, pericardial tamponade or cardiac death from proximal extension into the coronary arteries is considerable. Thus, standard therapy for this pattern of disease is open surgical repair of the ascending aorta. The most commonly used classification scheme is the Stanford categorisation. This straightforward system is predicated on the determination as to whether there is involvement of the ascending aorta irrespective of the distal extent of the dissection or location of the entry tear. If the ascending aorta is involved the dissection is defined as type A; exclusive dissection distal to the ascending aorta is type B.

MANAGEMENT

Currently, conventional therapeutic strategies for type B disease are **medical** management with pharmacological β-blockade and antihypertensive agents for uncomplicated cases; **surgical** repair is reserved for dissection complicated by ischaemic abdominal aortic branch vessel compromise or aortic rupture. In this regard, a new alternative for managing complicated acute type B aortic dissection has recently emerged. **Endovascular stent-grafts** combine self-expanding stent technology, originally designed to treat patients with arterial occlusive disease, with vascular graft materials used in vascular bypass or replacement surgery. Initially, these devices were used to repair abdominal aortic aneurysms and subsequently, thoracic aortic and peripheral arterial aneurysms. Recently, the spectrum of applications for this technology has expanded to include peripheral arterial occlusive disease, failing haemodialysis access conduits, venous and arterial traumatic injuries, transjugular intrahepatic portal-systemic stent shunts (TIPSS), and malignant biliary, oesophageal and tracheo-bronchial lesions.

ENDOVASCULAR STENT-GRAFT REPAIR

The concept of endovascular stent-graft repair of aortic dissection is predicated on successful placement of the device over the intimal entry tear in order to obliterate blood flow into the false lumen. The intent is to mimic the effect of successful operative repair of dissection with isolation of the false lumen from the circulation and redirection of blood flow into the true lumen. This endovascular surrogate for open surgery is capable of reversing ischaemic branch vessel involvement, thrombosing the aortic false lumen, and holds the attractive potential of reducing the frequency of thoracic false lumen aneurysm formation. In this regard, the false lumen in type B dissection has the propensity to become aneurysmal in patients who are treated medically. The frequency of this complication ranges from 30 to 40 per cent at 3 years after the initial diagnosis. It is important to note that the management of chronic dissection with false lumen aneurysm formation continues to represent a formidable surgical challenge.

Clinical evaluation of stent-grafts, for complicated or uncomplicated acute type B dissection, selected patterns of type A dissection as well as chronic dissection with false lumen aneurysm formation, is in progress at a growing number of institutions around the world. This chapter will focus on treatment considerations and early results related to stent-graft management of acute aortic dissection.

The particular manifestations of dissection which constitute imperatives for intervention in the setting of acute type B disease require an evaluation of many clinical symptoms, physiological effects and the findings of imaging studies. After weighing these considerations, however, and discarding many of them, it is possible to narrow the criteria down to three distinctive reasons for intervention. These include: early aortic expansion within 30 days of the initial onset of symptoms, associated with persistent pain or other findings suggestive of impending rupture (Fig. 24.1); aortic rupture, free or contained (Figs 24.2 and 24.3); and peripheral branch vessel involvement with correlative

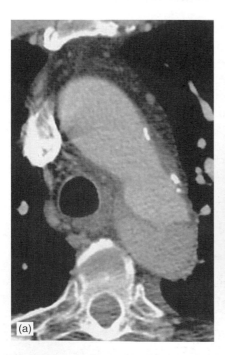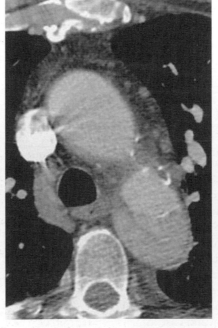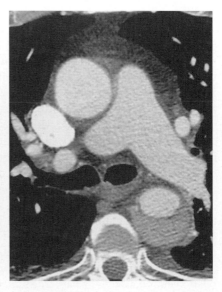

Figure 24.1 *Early dilatation of false lumen in type B dissection in a 68-year-old man with acute back pain. (a) Computed tomography (CT) scan shows type B aortic dissection.*

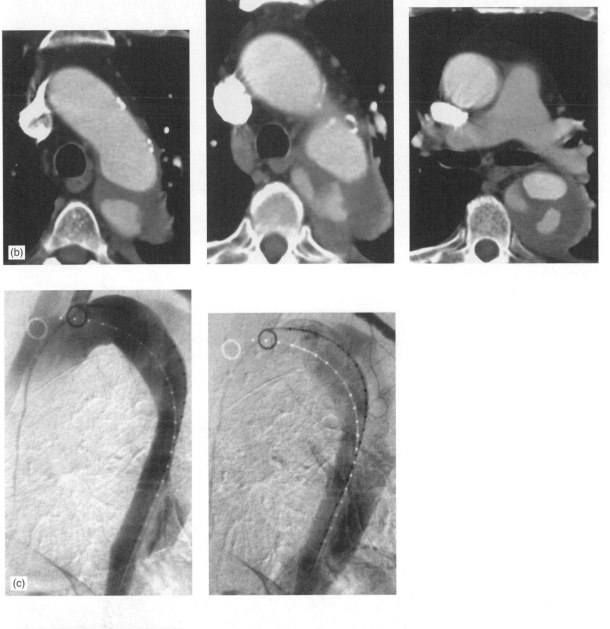

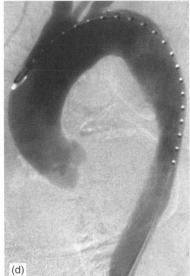

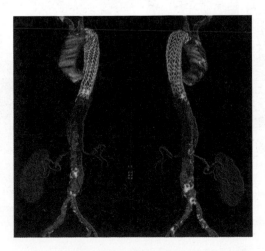

Figure 24.1 *(b) Follow-up CT 5 weeks after previous scan shows marked increase in diameter of descending aorta at the axial level of the pulmonary arteries associated with development of partial thrombosis of the false lumen. (c) Thoracic aortogram shows multiple communications between true and false lumens through tears in the flap located in the proximal and mid-descending aorta. (d) Aortogram and three-dimensional CT angiogram after stent-graft placement show obliteration of the tears and thrombosis of the thoracic aortic false lumen over the length of the stent-graft*

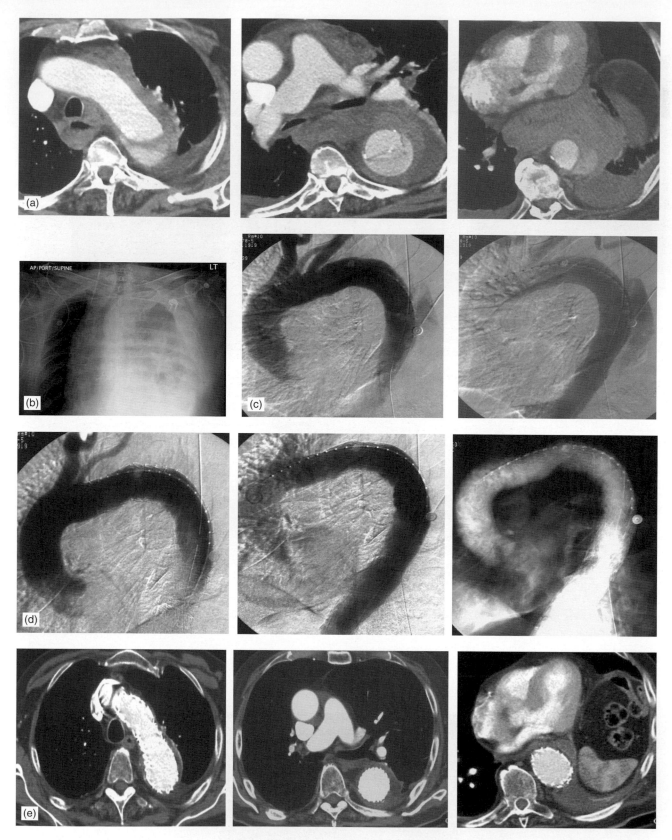

Figure 24.2 *Acute type B aortic dissection and rupture in an 84-year-old man with acute back pain and shock. (a) Computed tomography (CT) scan done elsewhere at 6 pm shows type B dissection with substantial mediastinal haemorrhage. (b) After helicopter transfer, chest X-ray at 8:14 pm shows complete opacification of left hemithorax with marked displacement of the trachea. (c) Initial aortogram demonstrates entry tear and false lumen filling but no evidence of the exact site of rupture. (d) Endovascular placement of a 20 cm stent-graft centred on the entry tear and aortogram at 8:43 pm shows no false lumen, opacification or evidence or extravascular contrast medium. (e) Follow-up CT scan 6 weeks after stent-graft placement shows only true lumen filling, with marked reduction in the volumes of the false lumen and mediastinal haematoma*

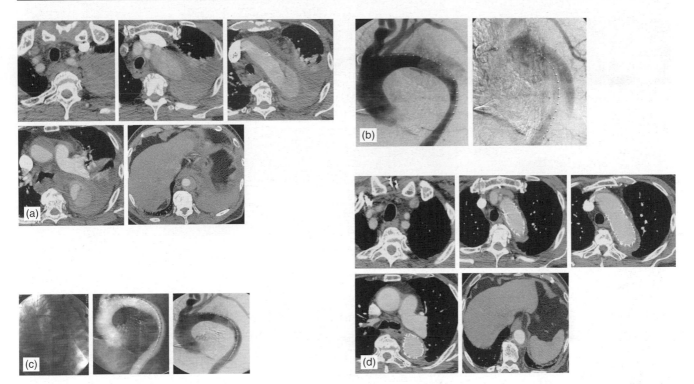

Figure 24.3 *Acute type A dissection with rupture and entry tear distal to left subclavian artery in a 74-year-old man with acute back pain and shock. (a) Computed tomography (CT) scan shows aortic rupture associated with type A dissection. (b) Aortography outlines entry tear in the proximal descending aorta. (c) Aortography shows stent-graft placement covering entry tear with no flow in the false lumen and no extravascular flow. (d) Follow-up CT scan 5 weeks after stenting shows marked resolution of the mediastinal haematoma and reduction in size of the thrombosed aortic false lumen*

evidence of end organ or tissue ischaemia (Fig. 24.4). In any of these clinical settings, the mortality and morbidity associated with open surgical intervention are high and dramatically greater than similar results for elective thoracic aneurysm repair. Consequently, the universally acknowledged high risk diagnostic group of complicated acute type B aortic dissection, represents both a challenge and an opportunity for stent-grafts to prove they are better, less invasive alternatives to the current default strategy of open repair.

Acute type B dissection – interventional imperatives

- Early aortic expansion or evidence of impending rupture
- Aortic rupture (free or contained)
- Symptomatic aortic branch vessel involvement

Initial results from published reports of experience with stent-graft technology in treating patients with aortic dissection are encouraging. Unfortunately, however, it is often difficult to determine from these publications the precise characteristics of the treatment group, in terms of the age of

dissection (acute *v* chronic), extent of aortic disease (type A *v* type B), indications for intervention (uncomplicated *v* complicated), patient symptoms and involvement of branch vessels. Nonetheless, valuable lessons from this early experience have served to fuel progress in our understanding of the disease process as well as its management by less invasive means.

DEVICES

Currently, there are three commercially manufactured thoracic stent-grafts that are widely available and marketed outside the USA. The TAG (WL Gore & Associates, Flagstaff, AZ, USA), the Talent device (AVE/Medtronic Inc., Santa Rosa, CA, USA), and the TX2 (Cook, Inc., Bloomington, IN, USA) are the most commonly implanted thoracic prostheses with a worldwide aggregate experience approaching 5000 patients. At the present time, however, not a single thoracic endograft has been approved by the Food and Drug Administration (FDA) for general clinical use in the USA. Nevertheless, all three devices mentioned above are currently undergoing phase II patient trials.

Published reports are also available of experiences with less widely distributed devices and of expectations with

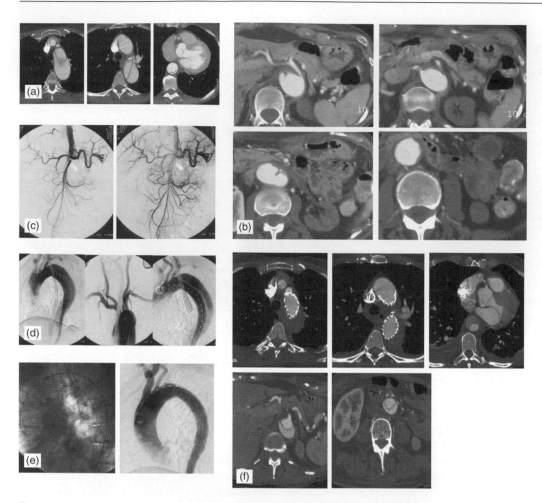

Figure 24.4   *Acute type B dissection with mesenteric ischaemia associated with dynamic branch vessel involvement and aortic true lumen collapse in a 75-year-old woman with abdominal pain. (a) Chest computed tomography (CT) scan shows type B dissection. (b) Abdominal CT scan reveals near obliteration of anteriorly positioned aortic true lumen. (c) Aortography shows marked compression of aortic true lumen distal to coeliac trunk. (d) Arch aortogram outlines type B dissection. (e) Aortogram after stent-graft deployment shows incremental true lumen size and no evidence of false lumen flow. (f) CT evaluation at discharge from hospital demonstrates thrombosed thoracic aortic false lumen with retained patency of abdominal false lumen and marked increase in diameter of aortic true lumen*

several newly developed endografts specifically targeting the challenges presented by thoracic aortic diseases. In all cases, however, the condition most commonly treated is descending thoracic aortic aneurysm rather than aortic dissection.

Detailed discussion of the various first generation home-made devices is only of modest historical interest. Suffice to say, most of these prostheses prototypes were self-expanding and based on a combination of a polyester graft with a modified type of Gianturco Z stent. Most delivery systems were large (24–27 Fr), relatively rigid, and depending upon the anatomy, as well as the length and diameter of the device, difficult to target and deploy due to marked frictional resistance encountered during withdrawal of the outer device containing sheath. Detailed descriptions of individual systems, components, fabrication processes and deployment techniques are provided elsewhere.

The current designs of the three most frequently used stent-grafts represent the second generation of each device

and feature considerable improvements over those of the previous generation. The individual benefits of these new products are detailed below, but in general, manufacturers are focused on improved durability, deliverability and reliability.

The **Gore TAG** is composed of a self-expanding nitinol stent lined with polytetrafluoroethylene (PTFE) graft material. Previously, the first generation of this device, the TAG Excluder, was lined with ultra-thin wall PTFE graft with a 30 µ internodal distance similar to the pore size of conventional PTFE vascular grafts. The new TAG uses a different proprietary multilayer composition which, in preclinical *in vitro* comparison tests, was found to be more durable and scratch resistant than the graft material previously used.

The ends of the device have a scalloped contour to enhance graft contact with the aortic wall over a wide range of aortic tortuosities and angulations. The scalloped projections are covered with PTFE and their length is directly proportional to the diameter of the graft. The device is very flexible radially and longitudinally. The new TAG does not have the S-shaped stabilisation wires that were anchored 180 degrees apart and spanning the length of its previous counterparts. Worryingly, fracture(s) of these longitudinally oriented wires has been observed after implantation in a number of patients. This complication occurred in 10–30 per cent of the implants and appeared to be related to the length of time since implantation, tortuosity of the device once implanted and, perhaps, the presence of overlapping endografts. Fortunately, no deaths related to this complication were reported to or observed by the independent core laboratory monitoring the follow-up of US clinical trials. There were, however, five untoward events caused by spine fractures. Two patients in the USA developed a type 3 endoleak through the graft material, presumably via a puncture hole created by an end of the fractured spine: one was managed successfully by adding another TAG device to line the damaged prosthesis while the second led to a rupture of the aneurysm necessitating surgical conversion and explantation of the device. The other three serious events occurred in Europe: in two cases, the type 3 endoleak was managed endovascularly by placement of an additional device, while in the third, elective surgical conversion with removal of the device was performed.

In view of the potential for clinical sequelae, Gore voluntarily suspended enrolment in its phase II US trial, withdrew the product from the global market and suspended sales in 2001. In the current newly redesigned TAG, the graft material is engineered to perform the same function as that provided by the former longitudinal wires, that is, to stabilise the implant and prevent any longitudinal compression during deployment. The graft is axially compressed onto the end of the delivery catheter and constrained by a PTFE corset laced with PTFE suture. The suture runs down the length of the catheter and is attached to a deployment knob at the opposite end. Grafts are available in a range of diameters between 26 and 40 mm, and a selection of lengths between 7.5 and 40 cm. The sizes of the delivery system and compatible introducer sheaths vary according to the diameter of the device and scale over a range of 20–24 Fr.

After preliminary arteriography studies have defined the preferred proximal and distal stent-graft 'landing zones', and these targets have been confirmed by transoesophageal ultrasound, a suitably sized 30 cm long introducer sheath is advanced over a guidewire to the infrarenal aorta. Alternatively, in certain situations, the catheter delivery system may be introduced over the guidewire without the use of a sheath. In either case, the device catheter is tracked over the wire until it reaches the selected target in a manner that bridges the entry tear.

After final positioning of the device has been achieved, deployment is effected by pulling the knob adjacent to the hub of the catheter. As the knob is smoothly retracted, the attached suture is withdrawn and opening of the corset occurs initially in the middle and then proceeds towards both ends. An instantaneous release of the underlying, self-expanding stent-graft occurs. After deployment, the delivery catheter is removed. The procedure is complete if the desired position of the graft is achieved without arteriographic or transoesophageal ultrasound imaging evidence of inadequate obliteration of the entry tear with persisting flow through it into the false lumen. If, however, the device is poorly positioned or not fully expanded and there is a perigraft leak, supplemental manoeuvres including placement of additional stent-graft(s) or gentle balloon expansion over the segment proximal to the entry opening, where the leak is suspected, may prove beneficial. As a general rule, if no false lumen filling is noted via the entry tear during post-placement aortography, balloon expansion of the device is discouraged in order to avoid the creation of secondary tears in the dissection septum. Resumption of the sales of the new TAG device by Gore began in March 2004 and the results of treatment of patients with a variety of thoracic aortic diseases are anxiously awaited.

The second device currently available for treatment of patients with descending thoracic aortic aneurysm is the **Talent endoprosthesis**. The design of this product has evolved since its introduction into clinical practice. The current version has a lower profile and more flexible delivery catheter than the original system. The prosthesis is composed of sinusoidal nitinol stent elements sandwiched between thin layers of polyester graft material. The individual stent forms are secured in place with oversewn sutures to prevent migration, but they are not connected to one another and there are segments of unsupported graft interposed between stents. This design allows independent stent motion and confers a degree of longitudinal flexibility. As with the earlier generation of the TAG Excluder device, the Talent utilises two longitudinal wires to provide stabilisation and prevent longitudinal compression.

A unique aspect of the device is its proximal margin with broad-based nitinol wire scallops. The wide, uncovered interstices may be placed across the origin of the left subclavian artery in cases where there is a short proximal neck of between 10 and 20 mm. In this setting, placement of the uncovered stent across the left subclavian artery helps to orient the graft optimally, stabilise its position and during deployment, secure precise targeting of the graft material at the distal subclavian margin.

The stent-grafts are available in a wide range of diameters and lengths. In addition, custom fabrication of a prosthesis based upon an individual patient's anatomy is possible within 3 weeks. The delivery profile for Talent is between 22 and 27 Fr depending on the diameter and length of the device. The delivery catheter has a flexible, conical tip. Set back from the tip is an integrated balloon used for smoothing the graft material and promoting adequate stent expansion following deployment of the self-expanding device. The prosthesis is collapsed over the distal segment of the delivery catheter and maintained in this packed configuration by an overlying transparent sheath. Proximal to the loaded stent-graft is a blunt metal stopper functioning as a brace to maintain the device position as the constraining sheath is withdrawn.

Once the stent-graft is properly positioned, usually 1–3 cm proximal to the optimal landing zone to mitigate against inadvertent downstream drift during deployment, the overlying sheath is slowly withdrawn. As the initial uncovered stent elements cantilever open, gentle retraction of the device is applied until the exact desired position of the proximal graft margin is contained. After the device is fully deployed, the balloon may be withdrawn and, if necessary, expanded within the proximal segments to fully expand the prosthesis. Subsequently, the final result is documented angiographically and the arteriotomy repaired surgically.

In an analysis of the relative merits of the devices, it is important to note that both devices described so far have established records of technical and clinical successes. In certain cases, however, the particular disease process and anatomy may recommend one device over the other. The marked flexibility of the Excluder device and its delivery system, as well as its smaller introduction profile, make it better suited for patients with severely angled aortic anatomy or those with small, calcified, or tortuous iliofemoral conduits. In aortic dissection cases, with short (<15 mm) proximal necks where the primary entry tear is very close to the left subclavian artery, the Talent device may be preferred because of its leading segment of uncovered stent. In terms of ease of use, the Excluder has some advantages. The maximum graft length available is 20 cm compared with 13 cm for an individual, non-custom Talent device. This, in combination with its simple and straight forward deployment, make it more efficient in extending the treatment zone. In aortic dissection, the relative radial force exerted by the prosthesis may be a consideration. In the acute setting, the lower hoop strength of the Excluder may allow adequate coverage of the entry site without causing an iatrogenic secondary tear in the thin, fragile dissection flap. In this regard, there are reports that the relatively rigid leading bare metal proximal segment of the Talent device can injure the aortic wall adjacent to the entry tear and create a retrograde type A dissection. On the other hand, the greater radial force of the Talent may be beneficial in cases of chronic dissection to displace a thick and resistant dissection septum and thus enhance the true lumen diameter.

The third device, the **Cook TX2 thoracic endograft** is made up of two components and is currently undergoing FDA phase II clinical trial in the USA. The predecessor of this device, the TX1, was a single piece device sold exclusively outside the USA. The current modular device and the uni-body former version both incorporate a distal uncovered stent-body, in conjunction with graft material extending to the proximal margin of the endograft. In both cases, fixation barbs are employed around the proximal aspect (pointing distally) and distal extent (pointing proximally).

The modular design of the TX2 endograft requires that two components, proximal and distal pieces, be placed, in each case, irrespective of the length of diseased aorta to be treated. The intent behind this concept is to confer increased flexibility upon the endograft and to allow for optimal accommodation within potential changes that may be likely to occur in the long term. At the time of writing this chapter, the use of the TX2 in the management of patients with aortic dissection is limited.

STENT–GRAFT PLACEMENT AND EFFECTS

There is growing worldwide experience with endovascular stent-graft placement in treating acute type B dissections as well as chronic dissections with coexisting descending aortic false lumen aneurysm.[1–5]

In both pathologies, successful management is predicated on the obliteration of the primary entry tear of the dissection by placement of the prosthesis within the true lumen across the entry tear. Stent-graft coverage of the entry site closes the primary communication to the false lumen and its flow is markedly reduced or choked off completely. In acute type B dissection, the true lumen immediately increases in diameter without a corresponding incremental change in the overall aortic diameter. Downstream, any dynamic compromise of the branch arteries of the abdominal aorta by the dissection process is expeditiously reversed within seconds of stent-graft placement.

In cases of both acute and chronic dissection, stagnant blood in the false lumen of the thoracic aorta will clot. In the majority of patients, progressive thrombosis of the false lumen proceeds from the point of proximal involvement of the thoracic aorta distally, irrespective of the location of the primary tear. The tempo of this process varies and is influenced by certain factors: the size of the false lumen, abdominal branch vessel distribution off the aortic lumens, the amount of residual flow through the false lumen via uncovered additional tears in the dissection flap, retrograde false lumen branch vessel flow via collaterals, retrograde perfusion from the abdominal aortic false lumen, etc.

Acute type B dissection – branch vessel involvement

- Static – direct extension of flap into aortic branch with or without distal re-entry tear
- Dynamic – true lumen collapse or obliteration with prolapse of aortic septum over ostia of abdominal branches with true lumen origin
- Both – co-existing static and dynamic processes affecting an individual branch

It is expected that isolated sections of the abdominal aortic false lumen will be kept patent via natural fenestrations in the dissection flap at levels corresponding to the abdominal branches coming off the false lumen. This phenomenon permits sufficient perfusion of the false lumen branches via true lumen trans-septal flow after stent-graft obliteration of the primary communication to the thoracic aortic false lumen. In cases of acute dissection, if thrombosis occurs in the false lumen after stent-graft placement, progressive false lumen resolution may occur with a corresponding gradual enlargement of the true lumen. In this regard, follow-up imaging at 1 year has shown apparent 'healing' of the dissection in a number of cases, there being no computed tomography (CT) evidence of a residual thoracic aortic false lumen or dissection flap.[1,2]

RESULTS

Early results from clinical series of stent-graft management in limited numbers of patients with acute type B and acute type A aortic dissection, where the primary tear is identified distal to the left subclavian artery, are encouraging.[1,5–9] Obliteration of flow through the entry tear into the false lumen was achieved in greater than 90 per cent of cases, with associated complete thrombosis of the proximal thoracic aortic false lumen segment apparent in 80–100 per cent and distal thoracic segment thrombosis noted less frequently. Progressive false lumen shrinkage at 1, 6, and 12 months follow-up imaging was observed in most cases. Complications, including paraplegia, rupture and iatrogenic extension of the dissection into the ascending aorta, have been reported anecdotally in the early experience with stent-graft placement in acute dissection.[6–9]

TECHNICAL CHALLENGES

In terms of the procedure, some technical challenges related to a specific set of morphological manifestations of aortic dissection are often discussed when stent-graft therapy is considered. A common issue for consideration is the optimal method of selecting the diameter and the length of the prosthesis. As the diameter of the true thoracic aortic lumen represents a fraction of that of the overall vessel trunk, and is rarely cylindrical in shape, choosing the 'right' device dimensions is a unique logistical dilemma. Most practitioners base their selection on more than one measurement. Perhaps, the most compelling is the diameter of the non-dissected aorta immediately proximal to the entry tear. This is a good estimate of the original size of the proximal involved segment prior to dissection. This measurement, plus an oversize factor of 20 per cent to ensure secure anchoring and a tight circumferential seal, is

the approximate size of the device most frequently used in current practice. Obviously, if there is retrograde proximal extension of the dissection from the entry site, other planning steps must be taken. These include calculation of the mean true lumen diameter from measurements of the maximum and minimum true lumen dimensions, selections of an arbitrary diameter corresponding to a value larger than the true lumen but smaller than the overall aortic diameter, etc.

In terms of the device length, most investigators implant devices which are clearly longer than the entry tear and usually in the range of 10–15 cm. After implantation this added length confers a more normal anatomical appearance to the aortic morphology, especially in the arch, than that observed following placement of a short device focally over the entry tear. In addition, the longer device promotes accelerated thrombosis within the proximal thoracic aortic false lumen. Further extension of the overall length of the device into the distal third of the descending thoracic aorta, however, should be avoided in this setting because of an associated increased risk of spinal cord ischaemia.

In those cases of aortic dissection in which the primary entry site is located classically at the isthmus, the tear may be within 10 mm of the left subclavian artery. In this situation, a device with a proximal segment consisting of a bare stent can be placed across the left subclavian artery effectively maximising the length of graft contact with the aortic wall cephalad to the tear. When retrograde proximal extension of the dissection occurs from the tear, however, it may be necessary to place the graft over the origin of the subclavian artery with its leading margin between the left carotid and subclavian arteries. In addition to carefully monitoring the patient post procedure for ischaemic symptoms in the left arm caused by a 'covered' left subclavian, it is important to image the thoracic aorta carefully to exclude persistent perfusion of the false lumen via retrograde subclavian flow around the device into the arch.

As with acute type B dissection, experience is mounting in treating patients with chronic aortic dissection and false lumen aneurysm using endografts as an alternative to open surgical repair. In this regard, multiple studies record rates of aneurysm thrombosis and subsequent false lumen shrinkage mirroring those in reported series of acute dissection.[2–11] One controlled investigation comparing stent-graft therapy with open surgery in matched groups of patients with chronic type B dissection reported improved survival and decreased neurological complications with the less invasive procedure.[2]

The therapeutic options available in managing type A or type B acute aortic dissections, depending on the entry tear location of the former and the status of involvement of the latter, taking into account the level of acceptability as well as the risk attached to each of those choices, are illustrated in the algorithm provided (Fig. 24.5).

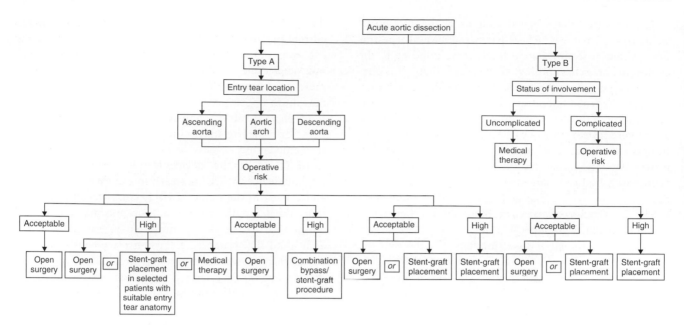

Figure 24.5 *Algorithm of therapeutic options available in managing acute aortic dissection: the degree of acceptability and the level of risk attached to choices made in treating type A dissections with different entry tear locations, and in dealing with complicated or uncomplicated type B dissections, are shown*

Conclusions

The recent development of endovascular stent-graft technology and its application as an alternative management strategy to medical therapy or open surgical treatment of patients with aortic dissection is an exciting and potentially valuable advance. The next major challenge that interventionists are facing is the important task of objectively elucidating the 'real' benefits, risks and complication of thoracic stent-grafts through rigorous, prospective controlled investigations of each possible anatomical and clinical manifestation of dissection. Only after this type of scientific scrutiny is performed can clinicians confidently counsel patients with accurate information regarding their therapeutic options.

Key references

Czermak BV, Waldenberger P, Fraedrich G, *et al.* Treatment of Stanford type B aortic dissection with stent-grafts: preliminary results. *Radiology* 2000; **217**: 544–50.

Dake MD, Kato N, Mitchell RS, *et al.* Endovascular stent-graft placement for the treatment of acute aortic dissection. *N Engl J Med* 1999; **340**: 1546–52.

Kato N, Hirano T, Shimono T, *et al.* Treatment of chronic type B aortic dissection with endovascular stent-graft placement. *Cardiovasc Intervent Radiol* 2000; 23: 60–2.

Nienaber CA, Fattori R, Lund G, *et al.* Non-surgical reconstruction of thoracic aortic dissection by stent-graft placement. *N Engl J Med* 1999; **340**: 1539–45.

Sakai T, Dake MD, Semba CP, *et al.* Descending thoracic aortic aneurysm: thoracic CT findings after endovascular stent-graft placement. *Radiology* 1999; **212**: 169–74.

REFERENCES

1 Dake MD, Kato N, Mitchell RS, *et al.* Endovascular stent-graft placement for the treatment of acute aortic dissection. *N Engl J Med* 1999; **340**: 1546–52.

2 Nienaber CA, Fattori R, Lund G, *et al.* Non-surgical reconstruction of thoracic aortic dissection by stent-graft placement. *N Engl J Med* 1999; **340**: 1539–45.

3 Sakai T, Dake MD, Semba CP, *et al.* Descending thoracic aortic aneurysm: thoracic CT findings after endovascular stent-graft placement. *Radiology* 1999; **212**: 169–74.

4 Kato N, Hirano T, Shimono T, *et al.* Treatment of chronic type B aortic dissection with endovascular stent-graft placement. *Cardiovasc Intervent Radiol* 2000; 23: 60–2.

5 Czermak BV, Waldenberger P, Fraedrich G, *et al.* Treatment of Stanford type B aortic dissection with stent-grafts: preliminary results. *Radiology* 2000; **217**: 544–50.

6 Ehrlich MP. Thoracic aorta endografting: the Austrian experience. The First International Summit on Thoracic Aorta Endografting, Tokyo, Japan, 2001.

7 Fattori R. Endovascular treatment of the thoracic aorta. The First International Summit on Thoracic Aorta Endografting, Tokyo, Japan, 2001.

8 Ishimaru S. Thoracic aorta grafting; the reliable treatment option. The First International Summit on Thoracic Aorta Endografting, Tokyo, Japan, 2001.

9 Lauterjung L. Endovascular stent-grafting for the thoracic aorta. The First International Summit on Thoracic Aorta Endografting, Tokyo, Japan 2001.

10 Dake MD. The advent of thoracic aortic endografting. The First International Summit on Thoracic Aorta Endografting, Tokyo, Japan, 2001.

11 Iwase T. Endovascular repair for chronic aortic dissection by Inoue stent-graft system. The First International Summit on Thoracic Aorta Endografting, Tokyo, Japan, 2001.

25

Prosthetic Aortic Graft Infection

CHARLES W BOUCH, JAMES M SEEGER

THE PROBLEM

Management of patients with infected prosthetic aortic grafts is one of the most difficult challenges faced by the vascular surgeon. Patients often present with non-specific symptoms and confirmation of the diagnosis of an aortic graft infection can be difficult. Delay in treatment of an infected aortic graft, however, can lead to life-threatening sepsis and/or haemorrhage. Patients with infected aortic grafts are also elderly and have multiple medical problems so that sepsis, haemorrhage and major surgical reconstructive procedures are associated with significant morbidity and mortality. Furthermore, the infected aortic graft is in the most favourable anatomical position for revascularisation, making maintenance of adequate lower extremity perfusion after graft removal difficult. Because of all of these factors, elimination of the infection, preservation of limb perfusion and long term survival are achieved in at most 70–80 per cent of patients presenting with prosthetic aortic graft infection.

This chapter will discuss diagnosis and treatment of patients with prosthetic aortic graft infection, emphasising the basic principles necessary for successful management of this complex problem. Essential information about the incidence, aetiology and bacteriology of such vascular graft infections will also be reviewed briefly. The pros and cons of the various treatments of aortic graft infection and the factors that lead to selection of a particular type of treatment for an individual patient will also be discussed as one form of treatment is not applicable to all patients with this difficult problem.

INCIDENCE, AETIOLOGY AND BACTERIOLOGY

Fortunately, infection of prosthetic aortic grafts is very uncommon. Although prospective series assessing the precise risk of aortic graft infections are not available, retrospective review of patients followed for at least 5 years after graft implantation suggests that the incidence of prosthetic vascular graft infection is between 0.5 and 2.5 per cent.[1] The risk of infection varies with the position of the graft, with the incidence of infection for aortic grafts confined to the abdomen being 0.5 to 1 per cent, and for aortofemoral grafts being 1.5 to 2.5 per cent. The incidence of infection in thoracic and thoracoabdominal grafts is less well known, but it appears to be similar to that of prosthetic aortic grafts limited to the abdomen.

Although it has not been definitively established, it is likely that infection occurs in most cases at the time of graft implantation, at the time of a subsequent procedure which involves the graft, e.g. revision or repair of a graft, arteriography through an aortofemoral graft or an infrainguinal bypass originating from it, or from involvement of the graft by an adjacent infection. Late infection from bacteraemia, although uncommon, is also a possible cause. The risk of development of aortic graft infection increases when there is a break in sterile technique, when leg infection is present at the time of graft placement or when a postoperative wound infection develops, even if it appears to be only superficial. In addition, the thrombus within an aortic aneurysm sac contains bacteria in approximately 13 per cent of cases[2] and the atherosclerotic plaque in the arterial wall at the graft–artery anastomosis has been shown to harbour bacteria in up to 40 per cent of cases.[2]

Factors influencing prosthetic aortic graft infection

- Break in sterile technique at time of graft implantation
- Leg infection present at time of graft placement
- Intra-aneurysmal thrombus containing bacteria (approximately 13 per cent)
- Plaque at the graft–artery anastomosis harbouring bacteria (up to 40 per cent)
- Postoperative wound infection
- Revision or repair of graft
- Arteriography through aortofemoral graft or linked infrainguinal bypass
- Late infection from bacteraemia

Natural history of prosthetic aortic graft infection

- Low grade sepsis
- 'Dis-incorporation' of graft
- Systemic sepsis
- Erosion into adjacent structures
- Graft occlusion
- Anastomotic disruption/life-threatening haemorrhage

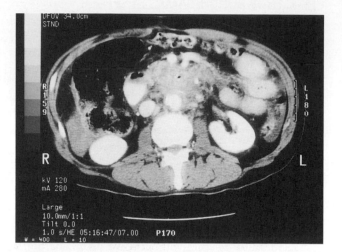

Figure 25.1 *Computed tomography (CT) scan of a patient showing obvious infection surrounding an aortic graft used to repair an abdominal aortic aneurysm 6 months previously. Extensive perigraft inflammation containing air can be seen in the midline adjacent to and above the aortic graft*

Organisms responsible for prosthetic graft infections include *Staphylococcus aureus*, *Staphylococcus epidermidis* and *Escherichia coli* in approximately 60 per cent of cases, with *Pseudomonas*, *Klebsiella*, *Proteus*, *Enterobacter*, *Bacteroides*, *Enterococcus* or other non-haemolytic streptococci and occasionally yeast accounting for most of the remainder.[2,3] Two or more organisms may be isolated from 10–37 per cent of infected aortic grafts, particularly in cases of graft-enteric erosion[4–6] and an alarming rise in the frequency of graft infection by methicillin resistant *S. aureus* (MRSA) has been observed over the past decade. Use of perioperative antibiotics reduces the risk of prosthetic vascular graft infection: prophylaxis against *S. aureus* in most cases and prophylaxis against MRSA in recently hospitalised patients. In addition, small anecdotal reports suggest that omental coverage of the graft may reduce the risk of late infection, although the superiority of this approach over peritoneal coverage alone has not been documented.

Identification of the organisms responsible for the infection is important in selecting appropriate antibiotic therapy and, at times, in deciding on appropriate treatment of the infected vascular graft, e.g. *in situ* graft replacement versus graft removal. No organisms, however, can be cultured from up to a quarter of patients with an obviously infected prosthetic vascular graft, unless special methods for recovering *S. epidermidis* from the graft material are used. In such instances, so called 'dis-incorporation' of the prosthetic vascular graft can be used to describe infection of the vascular graft as over 70 per cent of these grafts will have positive bacterial cultures using advanced culture techniques.[7] Furthermore, the natural history of a disincorporated, culture negative prosthetic vascular graft is the same as for one that is culture positive. This can range from initially low grade sepsis if the site can drain and if an anastomosis is not involved in the long term to systemic sepsis, erosion into adjacent structures, graft occlusion and/or anastomotic disruption with life-threatening haemorrhage.

DIAGNOSIS

When an aortofemoral bypass graft limb is seen in an infected groin wound, visualised on computed tomography (CT) or magnetic resonance imaging (MRI) or clearly outlined by a sinogram, the diagnosis of vascular graft infection is obvious. In Fig. 25.1 an aortic prosthesis is seen within an abscess. In all other circumstances, some degree of diagnostic uncertainty exists until the graft is explored surgically and/or cultured. This is because most signs and symptoms of prosthetic aortic graft infection are non-specific: malaise, low grade fever, unexplained weight loss and anorexia. On investigation, the findings associated with prosthetic vascular graft infection tend to be subtle. As previously noted, a history of leg sepsis prior to graft implantation, postoperative groin wound infection or systemic sepsis, a recent invasive procedure involving the graft or an episode of septicaemia, increases the likelihood of vascular graft infection. These historical findings, however, are far from definitive. Similarly, the systemic signs of sepsis, namely, fever, elevated white blood cell count, elevated sedimentation rate, without specific local signs of graft infection such as an abscess adjacent to the prosthetic graft, a pseudoaneurysm, inflammatory groin mass, etc., suggest vascular graft infection only when more common causes of sepsis have been excluded. This is particularly true in the early postoperative period after graft implantation when aortic graft infection is a rare cause of systemic signs of sepsis.

In contrast, localised sepsis adjacent to a prosthetic aortic graft such as a late groin abscess or purulent drainage from a previously healed groin wound must be assumed to be related to infection of the aortic graft unless it can be definitively proved otherwise. This assumption is strengthened significantly when what initially appears to be a superficial cellulitis in the groin fails to resolve with antibiotic therapy or recurs immediately after it has been discontinued. Early postoperative groin erythema following aortofemoral bypass, however, may simply represent the presence of a groin haematoma or seroma and early re-exploration provides diagnostic certainty, evacuation and treatment of the haematoma/seroma and groin closure. Similarly, the presence of multiple anastomotic pseudoaneurysms strongly suggests the presence of aortic graft infection while a single anastomotic pseudoaneurysm is usually not associated with infection but should prompt speedy evaluation of the other vascular graft anastomoses. Aortofemoral limb thrombosis is also usually due to progressive infrainguinal arterial occlusive disease but aortic graft thrombosis may be associated with infection in up to 25 per cent of cases.[8] Patients with infected prosthetic aortic grafts can also present with symptoms of obstruction of surrounding structures such as the ureter (Fig. 25.2) and such obstruction occurring late after aortic graft implantation should be considered to be caused by aortic graft infection until proved otherwise. Haemoptysis and haematemesis are signs also warranting graft evaluation in patients with thoracic or thoracoabdominal grafts and may be due to aortobronchial or aorto-oesophageal erosions. In rare instances, patients may present with septic emboli or hypertrophic osteoarthropathy, each of which strongly suggests the presence of vascular graft infection.

Gastrointestinal haemorrhage in a patient with a prosthetic aortic graft is of special concern; although patients who require aortic grafts are usually elderly and, therefore, at risk of more common causes of gastrointestinal bleeding, including diverticulosis, peptic ulcer disease, arteriovenous malformation, malignancy, portal hypertension and varices, etc. Gastrointestinal haemorrhage due to graft-enteric erosion, particularly involving a suture line, is such a catastrophic event that it is a possibility which must be excluded when gastrointestinal bleeding occurs in any patient with a prosthetic aortic graft. Bleeding can be slow and intermittent when the graft-enteric erosion does not involve an anastomosis, or it may be massive when anastomotic disruption from infection has occurred. Bleeding, in conjunction with other signs of sepsis or graft infection,

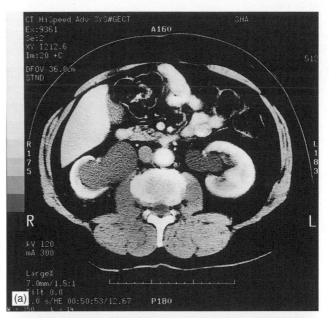

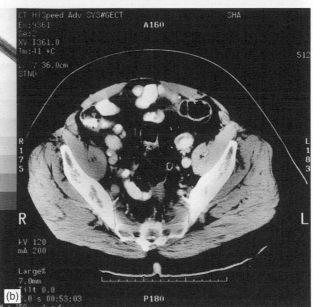

Figure 25.2 *Computed tomography (CT) scan of a patient showing (a) bilateral ureteric obstruction and (b) an infected aortobifemoral prosthetic graft, surrounding both limbs of which fluid can be seen. These findings were confirmed at surgical exploration, when the graft was removed followed by* in situ *graft replacement constructed from superficial femoral vein*

increases the likelihood of graft-enteric erosion being the cause. In the absence of other signs of graft infection, however, when a patient with gastrointestinal bleeding, manifested as haematemesis, melaena or haematochezia, has a history of implantation of a thoracic or intra-abdominal vascular graft, all efforts must be made to establish the cause of the bleeding and/or prove that an infected vascular graft and a graft-enteric erosion do not exist.

Clinical diagnosis of prosthetic aortic graft infection

- Non-specific symptoms and signs of sepsis
- Inflammatory groin mass, seroma, cellulitis, abscess, discharge
- Graft visible within groin abscess
- Haematemesis, melaena, haemoptysis/shock
- Pseudoaneurysm at femoral anastomosis
- Septic embolism/hypertrophic osteoarthropathy
- Aortofemoral limb thrombosis

Diagnostic studies can usually confirm or exclude aortic graft infection and/or graft-enteric fistula. At times, however, the diagnosis can only be made by surgical exploration of either a groin abscess to determine the presence and extent of a vascular graft infection or of an aortic graft to confirm or exclude graft-enteric erosion. Initially, the aortic graft should be imaged using either CT or MRI. Findings suggestive of vascular graft infection include perigraft fluid, ectopic gas, swelling of soft tissue adjacent to the graft and pseudoaneurysm formation (Fig. 25.3). Computed tomography imaging may also be used to guide aspiration of perigraft fluid for culture to help establish the diagnosis of vascular graft infection, although this is seldom necessary in our experience. The sensitivity and specificity of CT scanning in the diagnosis of vascular graft infection has been reported to be approximately 90 per cent in experienced hands,[9] and that has certainly been our experience at the University of Florida. Findings of vascular graft infection on CT scanning, however, can be very subtle, especially when minimal fluid is present around the graft such as is seen with infection by *S. epidermidis* and therefore the graft must be clearly visualised and normal throughout its course if aortic graft infection to be excluded. Computed tomography scanning is also of limited value in the diagnosis of vascular graft infection during the early postoperative period because the normal perigraft changes seen on CT scanning during the first three months after graft implantation are similar to the findings associated with vascular graft infection.[10] Magnetic resonance imaging has been reported to be potentially superior to CT in detecting small amounts of fluid and limited inflammatory changes surrounding an infected vascular graft, as would be seen in a patient with *S. epidermidis* infection. Experience with MRI scanning in patients with vascular graft infections, however, is limited at present. In addition, MRI imaging cannot differentiate between sterile and infected fluid or between the normal early inflammatory changes associated with graft implantation and those due to infection.[11]

Radionuclide imaging studies have been extensively used in the diagnosis of infected prosthetic aortic vascular grafts. The overall accuracy of indium-111 white blood cell scans has been reported to be 83–88 per cent[12,13] and the specificity

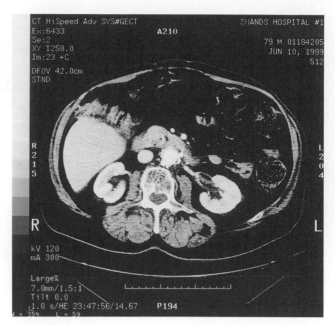

Figure 25.3   *Computed tomography (CT) scan of a patient with upper gastrointestinal haemorrhage showing a previously inserted aortic graft. The inflammatory changes and air adjacent to the area of the proximal anastomosis of the aortic graft were strongly suggestive of an aortoenteric fistula, which was confirmed at surgical exploration*

of gallium-67 scanning (Fig. 25.4) to be 94 per cent which is superior to that of CT scanning.[14] Nevertheless, both techniques are time consuming, can produce false positive studies due to cross-labelling of platelets or inflammation from other causes and can also be made falsely negative by antibiotic therapy. This is particularly true early after graft implantation and in patients with minimal evidence of infection by CT or MRI scanning. Technetium-99m exametazime has been used more recently to label leucocytes with repeatedly improved results and a small study with surgical/bacteriological confirmation of findings demonstrated 100 per cent sensitivity, 94 per cent specificity, 90 per cent positive predictive value and 100 per cent negative predictive value.[15] Regardless, at least in our experience, these radionuclide studies add little to CT or MRI scanning in the evaluation of patients suspected of having vascular graft infection and the exclusion of infection, in patients in whom CT and MRI studies are inconclusive, remains difficult.

Diagnosis of aortic prosthetic infection on investigation

- Fluid collection in groin for culture
- Positive sinogram of groin
- CT/MRI findings indicative of infection of body of graft and perigraft tissues, ureteric obstruction (? bilateral)

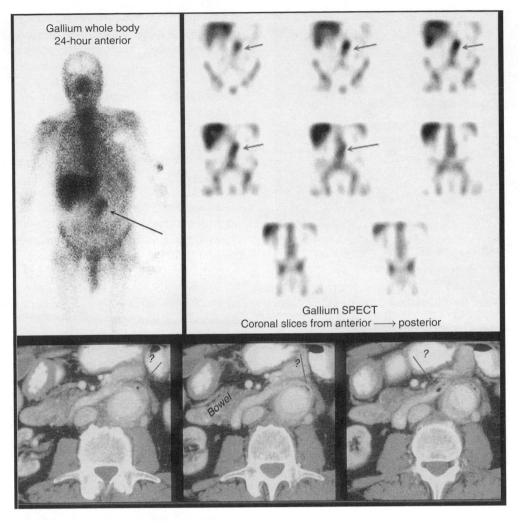

Figure 25.4 *Whole-body gallium and selected computed tomography (CT) scan images of a patient with an infected aortic graft. Uptake in the body of the graft (arrows) can be seen on the 24-hour gallium single photon emission computed tomography (SPECT) images. Selected CT images (lower three) from the same area show inflammatory changes and air adjacent to the graft (reproduced with permission from Drane WE (ed).* Nuclear Medicine: The basic, the advanced and the controversial. *Gainesville, FL: NMNF, Inc)*

- CT-guided aspiration of aortic perigraft fluid for culture
- Angiographic evidence of pseudoaneurysm (multiple) at aortic/femoral anastomosis, graft limb thrombosis
- Radionuclide imaging using Tc-99m hexametazime, gallium-67 or indium-111, but they add little to CT/MRI findings
- Upper gastrointestinal endoscopy – negative study unreliable
- Surgical exploration and culture of biofilm

The appropriate use of diagnostic studies in a patient suspected of having an aortic graft-enteric erosion depends on the degree of the gastrointestinal haemorrhage and the haemodynamic stability of the patient. When the bleeding is slow and intermittent the patient should undergo imaging of the graft as described above to determine the presence of signs of infection of the aortic graft. Demonstration of an anastomotic pseudoaneurysm, particularly at the proximal aortic anastomosis, is pathognomonic and any evidence of aortic graft infection also essentially confirms the diagnosis (Fig. 25.5). In the absence of evidence of vascular graft infection on the imaging studies, upper and lower gastrointestinal endoscopy should be done to search for other causes of the bleeding. Upper gastrointestinal endoscopy should also be done in a patient who is bleeding more rapidly, haemodynamic stability permitting, to exclude other causes such as peptic ulcer disease or oesophageal varices. Furthermore, a normal study except for bleeding from the third or fourth portion of the duodenum essentially establishes the diagnosis of aortic graft-enteric erosions in such patients. In contrast, a normal study without evidence of bleeding does not exclude the diagnosis of graft-enteric erosion as anastomotic fistulous connections can occur to the stomach,

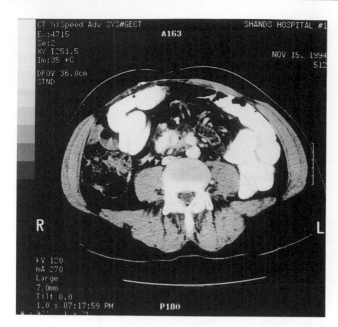

Figure 25.5 *Computed tomography (CT) scan of patient with an aortic graft infection subsequently found to have a graft-enteric erosion into the small bowel. Although the air seen adjacent to the graft is suggestive of graft-enteric erosion, infection by a gas producing organism may also be responsible*

small bowel or colon. Because of this, in the face of persistent, intermittent bleeding or massive bleeding without a definitive cause, surgical exploration is mandatory, graft-enteric erosion being excluded only when the bowel is completely freed from the retroperitoneum. Complete graft incorporation in this setting effectively rules out erosion or infection.

PREOPERATIVE MANAGEMENT

As previously noted, patients with infected prosthetic aortic grafts are usually elderly and have multiple medical problems. In addition, they may be debilitated by chronic sepsis and at times by acute or chronic blood loss. Treatment of these problems is therefore essential in reducing morbidity and mortality associated with management of the infected vascular graft. Fortunately, time for possible correction or improvement of such problems and preparing the patient for surgical treatment, is usually available, as most procedures are urgent rather than emergent in nature. Specific preparation for treatment of vascular graft infection includes bilateral non-invasive vascular testing to assess limb haemodynamics and arteriography of both lower and upper extremities, including the aortic arch when appropriate. This defines the anatomy of arteries adjacent to the infected vascular graft and identifies potential extra-anatomical bypass inflow sites. Venous duplex ultrasound should also be done to assess potential venous conduits, including deep leg veins, available for arterial reconstruction.

Antibiotic therapy should be initiated based on graft and/or wound cultures, if available, or on the pathogens most likely to be present, depending on the location and timing of the graft infection. Plans should also be made for the administration of intravenous antibiotics for 4–6 weeks after graft removal and possibly oral antibiotics for an additional 6–12 weeks. Importantly, operative records of implantation of the prosthetic graft now infected should be reviewed to determine the precise anatomy of the infected vascular graft so that graft removal and reconstruction can be planned appropriately.

Clearly, in this serious situation, the patient and family members must be counselled preoperatively regarding the extreme gravity of the situation in order to avoid false expectations. Taken overall, postoperative mortality ranges from 10 to 30 per cent, amputation from 0 to 15 per cent, reinfection post reconstruction 0 to 20 per cent and 5-year survival averages 50 per cent. Furthermore, multiple surgical procedures are frequently required to preserve lower extremity perfusion.

SURGICAL TREATMENT

Infection of a prosthetic aortic graft is a grave problem. In our experience, only 58 per cent of patients with this serious problem are alive and still have their limbs at 30 months after treatment though this varies with the original indication for placement of the infected aortic graft: 48 per cent in patients whose grafts were placed for occlusive disease, 65 per cent for patients whose grafts were placed for aneurysmal disease.[16] Types of treatment currently used in patients with prosthetic aortic graft infection include first, staged graft excision and extra-anatomical bypass and second, simultaneous graft excision and *in situ* graft replacement using a variety of types of graft, namely a new prosthetic graft, an autogenous graft constructed from deep vein or a homograft. Graft preservation may also be attempted in selected patients with presumed graft contamination rather than obvious infection and in those with evidence of low grade infection and severe life-limiting medical comorbidities. Each of these approaches has advantages and disadvantages and no one type of therapy is applicable to all patients. Therefore, in the individual patient with an aortic graft infection, many things must be considered to determine the treatment most likely to achieve eradication of the infection and long term limb salvage with the lowest risk (Fig. 25.6).

Aims of treatment
• Control bleeding and save life
• Restore flow
• Eradicate infection
• Prevent amputation(s)

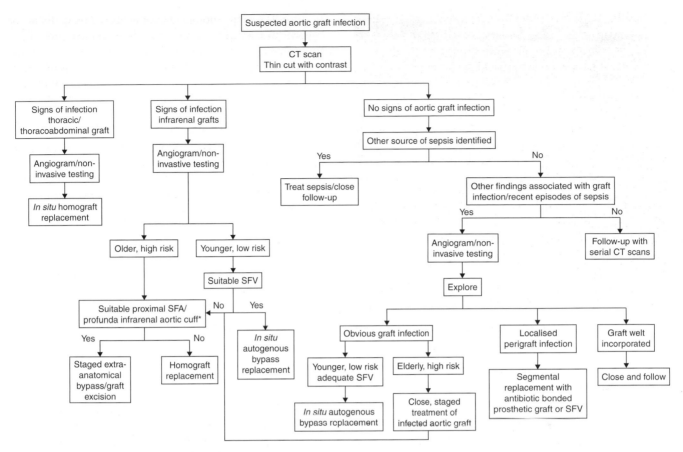

Figure 25.6 *Algorithm for the diagnosis and management of aortic graft infections. *Adequate length of infrarenal aorta for secure stump closure, patent SFA or profunda with adequate run-off. SFA, superficial femoral artery; SFV, superior femoral vein*

Infection can occur in prosthetic vascular grafts in any portion of the aorta. Fortunately, most infected aortic grafts encountered by the vascular surgeon are in the infrarenal aorta while infected suprarenal and thoracic aortic grafts are very uncommon. Graft excision and *in situ* prosthetic graft or homograft replacement is the usual treatment for infected thoracic and suprarenal aortic grafts as graft excision and extra-anatomical bypass is generally not possible. Only limited reports of this approach in patients with this exceedingly complex problem are available, but average mortality rates of 10–36 per cent, and of complication rates such as <5 per cent for amputation and approximately 20 per cent for early graft failure/infection, appear acceptable.

In situ graft replacement has also been used in the management of selected patients with infrarenal prosthetic aortic graft infection. Kieffer *et al.*[17] used aortic allografts to replace infected infrarenal prosthetic grafts in 43 patients, including 36 with aortic graft infections, with a mortality of 12 per cent and no early amputations. There were, however, early allograft complications in two patients and late allograft complications in nine patients, i.e. 26 per cent overall, including one death thought to be due to allograft graft rupture. Verhelst *et al.*[18] reported results from a multicentre trial of the use of cryopreserved homografts in 90 patients with vascular graft infections, including 41 with infected aortic grafts. Thirty-day mortality was 6.8 per cent for patients without aortoenteric fistulae (AEF) and 65 per cent for patients with AEF. Again, there were significant allograft complications in almost one-third of the patients: allograft rupture in 10, thrombosis in 9, dilatation in 7 and stenosis in 4. The mortality rate as a direct result of early and late homograft failure was 21 per cent.

Hayes *et al.*[3] used new rifampicin-bonded polyester grafts to replace infected prosthetic aortic grafts in 11 patients with a mortality of 18.2 per cent and no early amputations. Unfortunately, once again late catastrophic complications were common with two patients dying of recurrent graft infections within 30 months. Finally, Bandyk *et al.*[19] treated 40 patients with prosthetic vascular grafts infected by biofilms caused by *Staphylococcus* spp., including 25 with infected aortic grafts, by graft excision and *in situ* graft replacement using rifampin-bonded polyester and polytetrafluoroethylene (PTFE) grafts with a 2.5 per cent 30-day mortality and no limb loss. No late graft failures were seen at an average follow-up of 18 months but 10 per cent developed recurrent graft infection. Early reinfection due to rapid development of rifampin-resistant *S. epidermidis* has also been reported by Bandyk *et al.*[20] It seems likely that rifampin has limited efficacy against Gram negative and MRSA organisms *in vivo*. Because of these findings, we limit the use of *in situ* replacement of infected prosthetic aortic grafts, using either allografts or rifampin-bonded polyester grafts, to patients with suprarenal or thoracic aortic infections, a select group of patients with AEF, as will be discussed later, and those few patients not appropriate for treatment with either of the two main options.

Excision and extra-anatomical bypass using a prosthetic graft has been the most commonly used treatment of infrarenal aortic graft infection and results of treatment of aortic infection using this approach have gradually improved since it was introduced by Blaisdell *et al.* in 1970.[21] This was particularly true following the observation by Reilly *et al.*[22] that staged extra-anatomical bypass followed by graft excision was associated with lower mortality and improved initial limb salvage. Postoperative mortality and amputation rates after treatment of an aortic graft infection with this approach now average 10–12 per cent and 0–10 per cent, respectively, and Yeager *et al.*[23] recently reported a 73 per cent primary and 92 per cent secondary extra-anatomical bypass graft patency at 5 years in 50 patients treated for aortic graft infection in this manner. They also demonstrated that late aortic stump disruption, which previously had been a common cause of late death, was now uncommon. Seeger *et al.*[24] reported similar results in 36 patients with 64 per cent primary and 100 per cent secondary patency at 5 years with one case of aortic stump disruption. Thus, modern results of this approach to treatment of aortic graft infection appear acceptable. The long term patency of extra-anatomical bypass after aortic graft excision, however, remains problematic and this has led to the investigation of *in situ* replacement of infected aortic grafts with a new prosthetic graft or a homograft, as discussed above, or a graft constructed of infection-resistant autogenous tissue.

Ehrenfeld *et al.*[25] and Seeger *et al.*[26] used grafts constructed of endarterectomised aortoiliac and superficial artery segments combined with portions of saphenous vein to replace 15 and 10 infected aortobifemoral grafts, with early mortalities of 20 per cent and 9 per cent and early amputation rates of 7 per cent and 9 per cent, respectively. Unfortunately, long term graft failure, due primarily to stenosis of the saphenous vein portion of the autogenous graft, occurred in two-thirds of the patients in the report by Seeger *et al.*[26] More recently, Clagett *et al.*[4] and Nevelsteen *et al.*[27] reported the results of the use of autogenous grafts constructed using deep femoral veins to treat patients with infected aortic grafts. Postoperative mortality rates in these studies were 10 per cent and 7 per cent, and early amputation rates 5 per cent and 7 per cent, respectively. Furthermore, in the Clagett study, primary graft patency at 5 years was 83 per cent, secondary graft patency 100 per cent and significant lower extremity oedema was uncommon. However, major morbidity occurred in 49 per cent of the patients in Clagett's series, including compartment syndrome in 12 per cent and limb paralysis in 7.5 per cent. More recently, these two complications appear to have been reduced by the liberal use of prophylactic fasciotomies, but

in situ aortic graft replacement using one constructed from superficial femoral vein remains a demanding procedure for both patient and surgeon.

At present, we use both staged extra-anatomical bypass with graft excision, and *in situ* graft replacement using a graft constructed from superficial femoral vein, in the treatment of aortic graft infection. The treatment used in an individual patient is selected based on the location of the infected graft, the degree of occlusive disease present and the patient's age and other medical problems. If the infected aortic graft is confined to the abdomen, staged axillofemoral bypass to the common femoral artery followed by graft excision appears to be the simplest method of managing a patient with this problem. The procedure is staged because such an approach clearly limits the physiologic stress compared with simultaneous extra-anatomical bypass and graft removal and, surprisingly, the staged approach is also associated with a lower rate of graft failure, amputation and infection of the extra-anatomical bypass.[22]

Operative approaches

- Staged graft excision and extra-anatomical bypass using axillofemoral, obturator foramen bypass or autogenous vein iliofemoral or femoro-femoral bypass
- Simultaneous graft excision and *in situ* graft replacement using new prosthetic graft (rifampicin-bonded polyester or PTFE), autogenous graft constructed from deep vein and/or endarterectomised aortoiliac and superficial artery segments, homograft
- Graft preservation
- Other procedures – closure of bowel, fasciotomies, amputation(s)
- Endovascular option – stent-graft to arrest bleeding plus one of the above approaches

---

Similarly, if the infection appears to be limited to the distal portion of one limb of an aortobifemoral bypass graft, we use staged extra-anatomical bypass, i.e. axillary to profunda femoris artery bypass or axillary to superficial femoral artery bypass (Fig. 25.7), and excision of the infected portion of the graft. If the ipsilateral profunda femoris and superficial femoral arteries are unsuitable as distal targets for an extra-anatomical bypass in this setting, an obturator foramen bypass or an autogenous graft iliofemoral or femoro-femoral may be used to provide lower extremity perfusion after the infected graft limb has been excised. The above knee popliteal artery, however, must be patent for an obturator foramen bypass to be successful, the use of an *in situ* autogenous graft replacement risks spread of infection to the non-infected portion of the graft through the autogenous graft tunnel. Axillopopliteal bypass is not used because of extremely poor patency of this type of bypass in this setting,

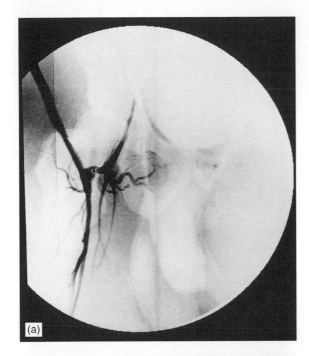

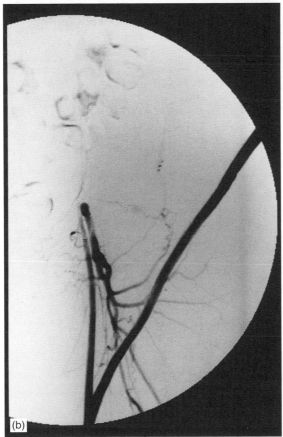

Figure 25.7 *Arteriogram showing the distal anastomoses in a patient treated for aortic graft infection by staged bilateral axillofemoral bypasses and graft excision. (a) The right bypass is to the profunda femoris artery, the right superficial femoral artery having occluded, and (b) the left bypass is to the proximal superficial femoral artery, the left profunda femoris branching early and being of relatively small calibre*

secondary patency being 33 per cent at 12 months.[16] Alternatively, if a localised biofilm infection is present, graft excision and *in situ* prosthetic PTFE graft replacement is reported to have equivalent results to either graft excision and extra-anatomical bypass or *in situ* graft replacement with deep vein, although published results concerning this approach are limited.

When the infection involves the body or both limbs of a prosthetic aortobifemoral bypass graft, thus involving both common femoral arteries with infection, the choice of treatments is between extra-anatomical bypass followed by graft excision and simultaneous graft excision and *in situ* replacement with an autogenous graft constructed from superficial femoral vein. As noted previously, reported postoperative mortality and early risk of amputation are essentially the same after these two procedures. Nevertheless, the incidence of major postoperative morbidity after *in situ* replacement of an infected aortobifemoral graft with an autogenous graft made of superficial femoral vein was as high as 49 per cent in early reports[4] while the long term risk of graft failure and subsequent graft infection is lower than after extra-anatomical bypass and aortic graft excision. Based on these results, we choose graft excision and autogenous graft replacement for younger, healthier patients who would benefit from a more definitive procedure and those patients whose profunda femoris and proximal superficial femoral arteries are unsuitable as distal targets for extra-anatomical bypasses (Fig. 25.8). In contrast, we use staged extra-anatomical bypass and graft excision in patients with infected aortobifemoral bypass prostheses.

MANAGEMENT OF PROSTHETIC GRAFT EROSIONS/FISTULAE

Patients with slow intermittent gastrointestinal bleeding from prosthetic graft-enteric erosions but who are haemodynamically stable can be managed in a manner similar to those with such infections but no evidence of gastrointestinal bleeding (Fig. 25.9). In fact, such patients are usually thought to have graft infection alone and the graft-enteric erosion is found incidentally at the time of removal of the infected graft. In a patient who is actively bleeding with a known or strongly suspected aortoenteric fistula, the traditional approach has been control of the fistula and removal of the aortic graft followed by extra-anatomical bypass for lower limb revascularisation. Alternatively, fistula repair and *in situ* graft replacement with a new prosthetic graft has been described by Walker *et al.*[28] and repair of the fistula alone has been reported by Eastcott.[29] Reported mortality rates for AEF using the traditional approach to treatment are up to 40 per cent with an early amputation rate of up to 10 per cent. In contrast, mortality after fistula repair and *in situ* prosthetic graft replacement was reported to be 22 per cent with an amputation rate of 0 per cent; after

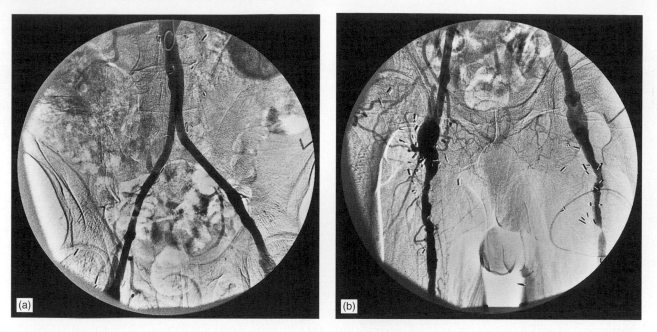

Figure 25.8 *Arteriogram of a patient previously treated for aortic graft infection with graft removal and in situ graft replacement constructed from superficial femoral vein showing (a) the proximal aortic anastomosis and body of the graft and (b) the distal anastomoses. This approach was chosen because first, both profunda femoris arteries were occluded and second, there was severe superficial femoral artery occlusive disease*

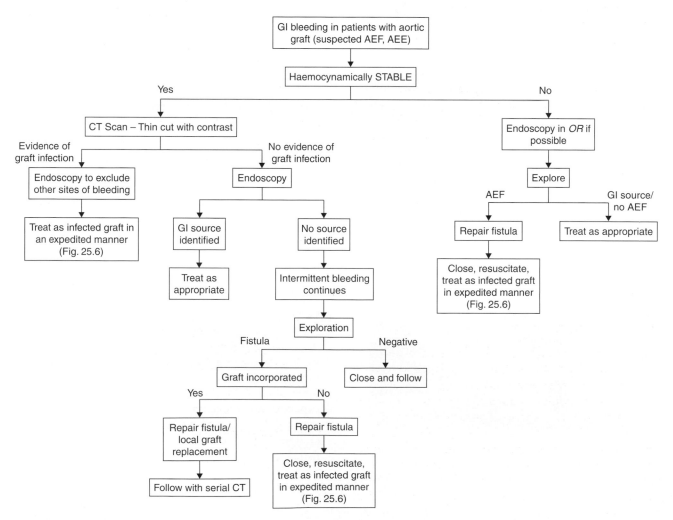

Figure 25.9 *Algorithm for the diagnosis and management of aortoenteric fistulae or erosions. AEE, aortoenteric erosion; AEF, aortoenteric fistula; CT, computed tomography; GI, gastrointestinal; OR, operating room*

fistula repair alone mortality was 0 per cent with an amputation rate of 0 per cent. After fistula repair and *in situ* prosthetic graft replacement, three patients (17 per cent) had recurrent graft infection and rupture of the proximal anastomosis, causing death in two, while after fistula repair alone, four patients (40 per cent) had evidence of recurrent infection, all of whom subsequently underwent graft excision and extra-anatomical bypass.

Based on the results of these studies, we have recently adopted a modified approach to treating the patient with an actively bleeding AEF, similar to that suggested by Stoney:[30] the patient is rapidly explored, the bleeding is controlled, the fistula is identified and the bowel is closed. If the majority of the aortic graft is well incorporated, the graft is cultured, the proximal portion of the graft is replaced with a PTFE graft, the patient is treated with 6 weeks of antibiotics and is then followed carefully with serial CT scanning. Alternatively, if the graft is obviously infected, the bowel and fistula are repaired, the abdomen is closed and the patient is allowed to recover for a few days after which the aortic graft infection is dealt with in a less urgent setting. Our experience with this modified protocol for the treatment of AEF is limited and the follow-up brief but the results have been good: 0 per cent mortality, 0 per cent amputation rate.

A novel, endovascular approach to the management of AEF has also been recently described in three case reports.[31–33] In each case, the infrarenal aortic graft had eroded into the duodenum resulting in haemorrhage, and deployment of a covered aortic stent-graft within the old graft successfully arrested the bleeding. In one case, further erosion occurred during follow-up requiring subsequent staged extra-anatomical bypass and graft excision.[32] Nevertheless, these reports suggest a possible role for an aortic stent-graft as a method of controlling active bleeding in patients with AEF, potentially with less physiological stress. More experience with these new approaches will be required to characterise their role in the management of AEF and only a larger experience and longer follow-up will determine whether the change in our approach to these patients is of value.

LATE COMPLICATIONS

Patients must be carefully followed up, essentially for life, after initially successful treatment of an infected aortic graft. Depending on the type of treatment used, they are at risk of developing complications associated with extra-anatomical or *in situ* bypass graft stenosis/failure, aortic stump disruption, recurrent infection of new *in situ* prosthetic grafts or extra-anatomical bypass grafts and degeneration/rupture of homograft or autogenous grafts. Extra-anatomical bypass graft failure occurs in approximately 25 per cent of patients[23] and can be treated with either repair of the failed graft or re-do aortic grafting as long as 6–12 months have passed after removal of the infected aortic graft, as described by Dimuzio *et al.*[34]

Late complications

- Stenosis/failure of extra-anatomical or *in situ* bypass
- Degeneration/rupture of graft
- Aortic stump disruption

Aortic stump disruption, although uncommon, does occur and, in our experience, patients who require repositioning of the renal arteries, and sometimes of the superior mesenteric artery to allow adequate aortic debridement, are at high risk. Homograft degeneration occurs in at least 25 per cent of patients, commonly resulting in graft rupture if left untreated. Durability of autogenous grafts constructed from superficial femoral vein appears good at present but follow-up has been limited and graft or anastomotic stenosis has been reported.[4] Because of all of these factors, we follow patients after successful treatment of infected prosthetic vascular grafts at 3, 6, 12, 18 and 24 months and yearly thereafter for haemodynamic testing and CT imaging at each visit. Long term suppressive antibiotics, beyond the previously described 3–4 months after graft removal, are not used as there is no evidence to support the value of such an approach. Only to those patients in whom an attempt is made to preserve the infected aortic graft are suppressive antibiotics given.

Conclusions

Treatment of infected prosthetic vascular grafts remains challenging. Familiarity with multiple types of treatment, experience with complex surgical reconstructions and careful long term follow-up is necessary to achieve optimal results in patients presenting with this grave problem. Fortunately, prosthetic vascular graft infection is uncommon but by the same token significant experience in the management of patients with this problem is also comparatively rare. For this reason, it is important that patients with prosthetic vascular graft infection are referred to centres with significant experience in this area. With appropriate application of the techniques currently available for treatment of prosthetic aortic graft infection, long term elimination of infection and limb preservation is possible and can be achieved in the great majority of patients.

Key references

Bandyk DF, Novotney ML, Back MR, *et al.* Expanded application of *in situ* replacement for prosthetic graft infection. *J Vasc Surg* 2001; **34**: 411–20.

Clagett GP, Valentine RJ, Hagino RT. Autogenous aortoiliac/femoral reconstruction from superficial femoral-popliteal veins: feasibility and durability. *J Vasc Surg* 1997; **25**: 255–70.

Low RN, Wall SD, Jeffery RB Jr, *et al.* Aortic enteric fistula and perigraft infection; evaluation by CT. *Radiology* 1990; **175**: 157–62.

Seeger JM, Pretus HA, Welborn MB, *et al.* Long term outcome after treatment of aortic graft infection with staged extra-anatomic bypass grafting and aortic graft removal. *J Vasc Surg* 2000; **32**: 451–61.

Verhelst R, Lacroix V, Varaux H, *et al.* Use of cryopreserved arterial homografts for management of infected prosthetic grafts: a multicentric study. *Ann Vasc Surg* 2000; **14**: 602–7.

REFERENCES

1 Liekweg WG Jr, Greenfield LJ. Vascular prosthetic infections: collected results of treatment. *Surgery* 1977; **81**: 335–42.

2 Yeager RA, Porter JM. Arterial and prosthetic graft infection. *Ann Vasc Surg* 1992; **6**: 485–91.

3 Hayes PD, Nasim A, London NJM, *et al. in situ* replacement of infected aortic grafts with rifampicin-bonded prostheses: the Leicester experience (1992 to 1998). *J Vasc Surg* 1999; **30**: 92–8.

4 Clagett GP, Valentine RJ, Hagino RT. Autogenous aortoiliac/femoral reconstruction from superficial femoral-popliteal veins: feasibility and durability. *J Vasc Surg* 1997; **25**: 255–70.

5 Vogt PR, Brunner-La Rocca HP, Carrel T, *et al.* Cryopreserved arterial allografts in the treatment of major vascular infection: a comparison with conventional surgical techniques. *J Thorac Cardiovasc Surg* 1998; **116**: 965–72.

6 Chiesa R, Astore D, Piccolo G, *et al.* Fresh and cryopreserved arterial homografts in the treatment of prosthetic graft infections: experience of the Italian Collaborative Vascular Homograft Group. *Ann Vasc Surg* 1998; **12**: 457–62.

7 Padberg FT, Smith SM, Eng RHK. Accuracy of disincorporation for identification of vascular graft infection. *Arch Surg* 1995; **130**: 183–7.

8 Southern FN, Eidt JF, Barnes RW, Moursi MM. Thrombosis and infection in aorta femoral bypass grafts. Presented at the 23rd Annual Meeting of the Southern Association for Vascular Surgery, January 1999.

9 Low RN, Wall SD, Jeffery RB Jr, *et al.* Aortic enteric fistula and perigraft infection; evaluation by CT. *Radiology* 1990; **175**: 157–62.

10 Qvarfortdt PG, Reilly LM, Mark AS, *et al.* Computerized tomographic assessment of graft incorporation after aortic reconstruction. *Am J Surg* 1985; **150**: 227–31.

11 Spartera C, Morettini G, Petrassi C, *et al.* Role of magnetic resonance imaging in the evaluation of aortic graft healing, perigraft fluid collection and graft infection. *Eur J Vasc Surg* 1990; **4**: 69–73.

12 Brunner MC, Mitchell RS, Baldwin JC, *et al.* prosthetic graft infection: limitations of indium white cell scanning. *J Vasc Surg* 1986; **3**: 42–8.

13 Reilly DP, Grigg MJ, Cunningham DA, *et al.* Vascular graft infection: the role of indium scanning. *Eur J Vasc Surg* 1989; **3**: 393–7.

14 Johnson KK, Russ PD, Bair JH, Friefeld GD. Diagnosis of synthetic vascular graft infection: comparison of CT and gallium scans. *Am J Roentgenol* 1990; **154**: 405–9.

15 Fiorani P, Speziale F, Rizzo L, *et al.* Detection of aortic graft infection with leukocytes labeled with technetium 99m-hexametazime. *J Vasc Surg* 1993; **17**: 87–95.

16 Seeger JM, Back MR, Albright JL, *et al.* Influence of patient characteristics and treatment options on outcome of patients with prosthetic aortic graft infection. *Ann Vasc Surg* 1999; **13**: 413–20.

17 Kieffer E, Bahnini A, Koskas F, *et al. in situ* allograft replacement of infected infrarenal aortic prosthetic grafts: results in forty-three patients. *J Vasc Surg* 1993; **17**: 349–56.

18 Verhelst R, Lacroix V, Varaux H, *et al.* Use of cryopreserved arterial homografts for management of infected prosthetic grafts: a multicentric study. *Ann Vasc Surg* 2000; **14**: 602–7.

19 Bandyk DF, Novotney ML, Back MR, *et al.* Expanded application of *in situ* replacement for prosthetic graft infection. *J Vasc Surg* 2001; **34**: 411–20.

20 Bandyk DF, Novotney ML, Johnson BL, *et al.* Use of rifampin-soaked gelatin-sealed polyester grafts for *in situ* treatment of primary aortic and vascular prosthetic infections. *J Surg Res* 2001; **95**: 44–9.

21 Blaisdell FW, Hall AD, Lim RC Jr, Moore WC. Aorto-iliac arterial substitution utilizing subcutaneous grafts. *Ann Surg* 1970; **172**: 775–80.

22 Reilly LM, Stoney RJ, Goldstone J, Ehrenfeld WK. Improved management of aortic graft infection: the influence of operation sequence and staging. *J Vasc Surg* 1987; **5**: 421–31.

23 Yeager RA, Taylor LM, Moneta GL, *et al.* Improved results with conventional management of infrarenal aortic infection. *J Vasc Surg* 1990; **30**: 76–83.

24 Seeger JM, Pretus HA, Welborn MB, *et al.* Long term outcome after treatment of aortic graft infection with staged extra-anatomic bypass grafting and aortic graft removal. *J Vasc Surg* 2000; **32**: 451–61.

25 Ehrenfeld WK, Wilbur BG, Olcott CN IV, Stoney RJ. Autogenous tissue reconstruction in the management of infected prosthetic grafts. *Surgery* 1979; **85**: 82–92.

26 Seeger JM, Wheeler JR, Gregory RT, *et al.* Autogenous graft replacement of infected prosthetic grafts in the femoral position. *Surgery* 1983; **93**: 39–45.

27 Nevelsteen A, Lacroix H, Suy R. Autogenous reconstruction with the lower extremity deep veins: an alternative treatment of prosthetic infection after reconstruction surgery for aortoiliac disease. *J Vasc Surg* 1995; **22**: 129–34.

28 Walker WE, Cooley DA, Duncan JM, *et al.* The management of aortoduodenal fistula by *in situ* replacement of the infected abdominal aortic graft. *Ann Surg* 1987; **205**: 727–32.

29 Eastcott HHG. Aortoenteric fistula. possibilities for direct repair. In: Greenhalgh RM, ed. *Extra-anatomic and Secondary Arterial Reconstruction.* London: Pitman, 1982: 58.

30 Stoney RJ. Discussion of Peck JJ, Eidemiller LR: Aortoenteric Fistula. *Arch Surg* 1992; **127**: 1191–4.

31 Deshpande A, Lovelock M, Mossop P, *et al.* Endovascular repair of an aortoenteric fistula in a high risk patient. *J Endovasc Surg* 1999; **6**: 379–84.

32 Chuter TA, Lukaszewicz GC, Reilly LM, *et al.* endovascular repair of a presumed aortoenteric fistula: late failure due to recurrent infection. *J Endovasc Ther* 2000; **7**: 240–4.

33 Grabs AJ, Irvine CD, Lusby RJ. Stent-graft treatment for bleeding from a presumed aortoenteric fistula. *J Endovasc Ther* 2000; **7**: 236–9.

34 Dimuzio PJ, Reilly LM, Stoney RJ. Redo aortic grafting after treatment of aortic graft infection. *J Vasc Surg* 1996; **24**: 328–37.

26

The Acutely Compromised Renal Artery

MICHAEL P JENKINS, GEORGE HAMILTON

THE PROBLEM

A kidney is in imminent danger once its blood supply is interrupted for whatever reason. A previously healthy kidney without prior vascular compromise will survive for only 40–50 minutes without a blood supply. In the presence of chronic renal artery stenosis (RAS) the kidney is preconditioned to ischaemia, thereby allowing it to survive without a blood supply for up to 60 minutes and sometimes even 90 minutes before irreversible damage occurs. This time between interruption of arterial supply and renal infarction is known as the **warm ischaemia time** during which it is mandatory to achieve reperfusion or employ renal cooling if kidney survival is to be ensured.

Renal blood flow may be compromised either by rupture or occlusion of the main renal artery and these scenarios will be considered in turn. Trauma and iatrogenic injury are the commonest causes of acute injury, but in the latter situation, pre-existing atherosclerotic or fibromuscular disease is common. Increasing use of catheter-based diagnostic and therapeutic interventions result in manipulation in the region of the renal ostia. These procedures may jeopardise renal perfusion even without selective catheterisation or renal artery intervention *per se*.

In this chapter the more commonly encountered causes of renal artery compromise will be documented, the therapeutic options available discussed and authors' preferential treatment modality highlighted. Individual experience of such situations is unlikely to be great and the often unique set of circumstances involved and need for urgency, exclude any hope of meaningful trials contributing to our current knowledge. Thus, much of the advice within this chapter is based on data from reported case series, first principles and personal experience.

IATROGENIC INJURY IN RENAL ARTERY INTERVENTIONS

Thrombosis

Despite the advent of computed tomography (CT) and magnetic resonance (MR)-based diagnostic imaging, any renal artery intervention will, as a prerequisite, involve selective catheterisation. Even prior to attempted balloon angioplasty or stent placement, catheter manipulation can lead to plaque disruption or dissection, both of which can progress to renal artery thrombosis. Although primary stenting is increasingly used for treatment of ostial atherosclerotic stenoses, more distal lesions and those secondary to fibromuscular dysplasia are more likely to be treated by angioplasty without stenting. At present there is no good evidence to suggest that renal artery stenting has any long term beneficial effect in terms of hypertension control or preservation of renal function over angioplasty alone.[1]

In non-ostial stenoses there is therefore a place for keeping stent placement in reserve to treat extensive dissection or occlusion, albeit accepting that such complications are less likely to occur away from the ostium. The most comprehensive review of thrombotic complications in percutaneous renal artery interventions (as seen in Fig. 26.1) suggests an incidence of 2.3 per cent.[2]

If possible, an acute dissection or thrombosis secondary to plaque rupture should be treated immediately with the placement of a stent. If successful, this is obviously an

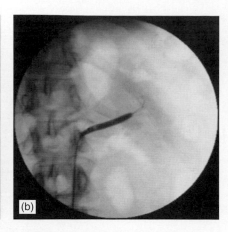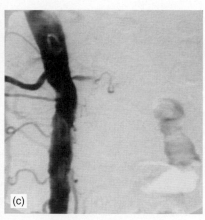

Figure 26.1   *Angiogram showing thrombosis of the left renal artery following balloon angioplasty prior to the use of stents. (a) Preintervention, (b) during balloon inflation and (c) post angioplasty. Today, this situation may be averted by primary stenting or rescued by the introduction of a stent post angioplasty*

attractive proposition as it maintains the minimally invasive nature of the procedure and obviates the time delay involved in transferring a patient to theatre for open surgery. Under such conditions, secondary stenting for angioplasty failure or complications thereof has been reported to offer equivalent outcome results to primary angioplasty, but at a cost of a 9.1–21.0 per cent major complication rate.[3,4] If unable to place a stent or in the face of a more distal thrombosis, urgent surgery is the treatment of choice, although in some cases there may be a role either for thrombolysis or for doing nothing, both of which will be discussed later.

In our unit, there is prearranged surgical cover for every renal angioplasty. Notwithstanding the aforementioned warm ischaemia times, a chronically stenosed renal artery has often promoted collateralisation, allowing a window of several hours in which to salvage a kidney even if the main renal artery occludes. Wong *et al.* have reported a series of 51 consecutive patients salvaged operatively following failed renal artery angioplasty.[5] Although this included a mixed bag of indications for initial and emergency intervention, among the atherosclerotic cases, surgical revascularisation was performed with a mortality of 9.4 per cent. In the presence of an on-table renal artery thrombosis, the operative decision is based on anatomical criteria, i.e. the total blood supply of the kidney and whether any segmental branches remain patent in addition to preintervention physiological factors. These include the overall renal function, differential function of the contralateral kidney, angioplasty indication and the fitness of the patient. Surgical options for revascularisation then depend on the condition of the infrarenal aorta, whether it is aneurysmal or not, and the presence or absence of disease within the coeliac trunk.

If the aorta is aneurysmal or contains a large amount of atheromatous plaque, then it should be replaced in the usual way and a 6–8 mm side branch sutured end-to-end to the renal artery. Obviously, such an approach will extend the renal ischaemia time and if there is concern regarding renal viability, the kidney should be cooled with topical ice and the renal artery perfused with ice-cold perfusate. Ideally such a patient would have been better treated by surgery in the first place as extensive aortic occlusive or aneurysmal disease is a relative contraindication to a percutaneous approach.

If the aorta is in good condition a Dacron or polytetrafluoroethylene (PTFE) bypass could be taken directly from the infrarenal aorta. This is probably the fastest approach in an acutely ischaemic kidney. It also has the attraction of not requiring a complete aortic cross-clamp in a patient who may not have had full preoperative preparation.

In the presence of an unattractive infrarenal aorta, the supracoeliac portion often remains soft and well preserved despite extensive atheroma elsewhere. Access to this segment is achieved via the lesser sac between the crura and again controlled with a side-biting clamp obviating complete aortic cross clamping. A prosthetic bypass can then be fashioned to one or both kidneys with good long term results, the latest reported series suggesting a 96 per cent secondary patency rate at 5 years.[6]

Other options include a splenorenal bypass to the left renal artery or a hepatorenal to the right using either the gastroduodenal artery or a reversed saphenous vein bypass from the common hepatic artery (see Fig. 26.2). Both these options require a healthy coeliac trunk and the dissection involved would be a relative contraindication in the acute situation.

Thrombolysis has been used to retrieve an iatrogenically thrombosed renal artery but there are few reports in the literature, although Salem *et al.* have described a small series[7] and there are many anecdotal reports of success. It would seem prudent to employ the fastest lysis technique available and at present this would involve using a high dose 'pulse spray' technique. This may buy time to allow a further endovascular approach, with or without stent placement,

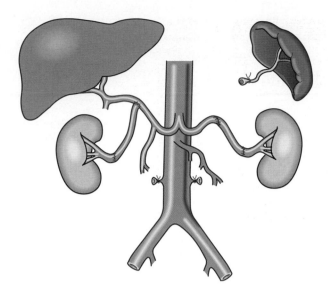

Figure 26.2 *Diagrammatic illustration of extra-anatomic bypass procedure either to revascularise the right kidney from the common hepatic artery (in approximately 40% of cases via the gastroduodenal branch) or to the left kidney using the splenic artery (the spleen remains* in situ *receiving blood from splenic collaterals and the short gastric arteries). Alternatively, in either case, a vein graft may be used.*

or allow the opportunity to arrange a formal surgical reconstruction. Thrombolysis should not be commenced as a 'knee-jerk' reaction to an angiographic occlusion and it is important to weigh up the estimated time to clot dissolution against renal ischaemia time.

If the contralateral kidney contributes the majority of overall renal function and the indication for angioplasty is hypertension, then, in the presence of an on-table occlusion, there is no mandate for insisting on revascularisation especially in an unfit patient. Leaving the renal artery occluded will remove the renin drive to uncontrolled hypertension without greatly affecting overall renal function.

- Before embarking on renal angioplasty, ensure the availability of an appropriate stent and surgical cover. Stent placement should be attempted as the first response to on-table thrombosis
- Despite predicted ischaemia times, surgical revascularisation can be worthwhile even after a few hours. If the situation is not salvageable radiologically, it remains the preferred option
- Only attempt revascularisation if the kidney contributes significantly to overall renal function

---

Occlusion during endovascular aortic repair

In endovascular aortic aneurysm repair (EVAR), accurate sizing and placement should allow a stent-graft to be deployed sufficiently distal to the renal ostia to allow adequate

perfusion of both kidneys. With a short neck, asymmetrical renal take-off or a distal separate lower pole artery, compromises are sometimes made. A catheter should be retained in the juxtarenal aorta to allow an angiogram after partial deployment in order that the final position with respect to the renal arteries can be checked prior to complete deployment.

The incidence of renal occlusion by the covered portion of the stent-graft during EVAR is largely unknown, but in Hopkinson's series (Kalliafas *et al.*[8]) of 204 patients over 4 years, five (including one bilateral) renal artery occlusions were reported. Although efforts should be made to reposition the graft, in reality this is often unsuccessful and the situation is often managed expectantly. It is therefore vital to know as much as possible about renal size and differential function preoperatively in order that a measured decision can be made at a time of crisis.

Contemporary issues surrounding EVAR and renal perfusion involve the 'short proximal neck problem' and long term renal artery patency with different stent-graft types. One novel method of ensuring adequate proximal stent fixation, in a neck of inadequate length, is to perform an iliorenal bypass prior to stent deployment over the renal ostium.[9] A more elegant approach uses the newly available fenestrated stent-grafts, allowing suprarenal deployment with precision alignment to allow flow through the fenestrations into the renal artery. This would allow many more patients with difficult or short necks to be treated by EVAR.

Current stent-grafts effectively fall into two main types with respect to proximal fixation technology: those with uncovered suprarenal segments and those without. Although the message from the RETA and EUROSTAR registries is unclear, anecdotal evidence would suggest that migration problems are reduced in the former, but at the expense of an incidence of renal artery thrombosis during long term follow up. At present it is unclear how common this is[10,11] (see Chapter 31).

Renal artery perforation

A perforation during catheter manipulation or more commonly balloon dilatation is easily detected by the presence of extra-arterial contrast. Although dramatic, bleeding can often be stopped by a 10–15 minute period of balloon tamponade and heparinisation reversed with protamine while blood is being cross-matched. If a longer period of occlusion is required, distal perfusion with ice-cold saline can be employed. If this fails, a covered stent may be deployed to seal the perforation and it is advisable to keep appropriately sized stents on the shelf for just this purpose. Once haemorrhage has been arrested the patient should be observed closely and re-imaged to exclude an expanding retroperitoneal haematoma.

If endovascular measures fail, surgical exploration is mandatory and during transport to theatre the angioplasty balloon should remain deployed to reduce blood loss.

- Attempt catheter balloon occlusion and arrange for availability of cross-matched blood
- Appropriately sized covered stents can be used very effectively if available
- If surgery becomes necessary, do not remove the balloon catheter as this can provide essential tamponade during operative exposure

EMBOLISM AND ATHEROEMBOLISM

In the majority of cases renal emboli emanate from the heart and unlike the situation in occlusion following a long period of RAS, acute occlusion of a previously normal renal artery supplying a kidney without a collateral circulation rapidly lead to irreversible ischaemic damage. The insult may be silent or manifest itself late with signs of infarction: loin pain and haematuria. Either way it is a difficult condition to diagnose early and time is of the essence.

Once suspected, urgent angiography is the investigation of choice as it allows catheter placement for thrombolysis. A number of reports in the literature suggest promising results from local intra-arterial lysis, some with clot lysis achieved even after a 7-day period of thrombosis.[12] However, immediate radiological success does not necessarily translate into preservation of renal function and longer term scintigraphy studies have shown lack of recovery in many examples of complete occlusion despite apparent complete lysis. This is probably explained by the existence of irreversible nephron ischaemia or reperfusion injury (see Chapters 2 and 4).

In view of the time required to achieve complete lysis and the known renal warm ischaemia time, one could make a case for urgent surgery. However, such patients are often very poorly, with a high incidence of ischaemic heart disease, and often a recent myocardial infarct as the aetiology behind the embolus, so it is not surprising that surgical revascularisation carries a mortality of up to 25 per cent.[13,14]

In the presence of a high burden of atherosclerotic soft plaque commonly seen in this area of the aorta, athero-embolism is a very real risk. Indeed significant athero-embolism leading to acute renal failure has a universally poor prognosis. Cholesterol embolisation occurs acutely at the time of catheterisation, but the resulting damage manifests itself insidiously over the next few weeks. In one of the largest reviews of histologically proven cholesterol embolisation, Fine et al. reported that 17 per cent of 221 cases had undergone recent angiography.[15]

The mainstay of treatment is supportive. Heparinisation is instituted, but there is no evidence for any additional benefit from thrombolysis. Haemofiltration is required in the face of the development of acid–base, electrolyte and fluid overload complications as in any other cause of acute renal failure, but as stated above, the prognosis for renal recovery under these circumstances is poor.

TRAUMA

Traumatic disruption of the renal pedicle is usually associated with high velocity and deceleration injuries typically seen in road traffic accidents (see Chapter 36). They are thus rarely seen in isolation and often occur in patients with significant multiple injuries. The emphasis in management is therefore skewed towards arrest of haemorrhage and preservation of life rather than renal reperfusion.

Here, more than in any other circumstance, each case must be treated based on its individual merit, but some principles will be outlined below. The first decision to make depends on the stability of the patient. In the face of an unstable patient with a haemoperitoneum, urgent laparotomy is required. If a torn renal pedicle is encountered, it should be ligated and the kidney sacrificed as the priority lies with stabilising the patient and transferring him or her to the intensive care unit or dealing with the other injuries. Assuming that a patient can be stabilised, imaging can be used to confirm the presence of a functioning contralateral kidney and whether there is any ongoing haemorrhage. A decision can then be made to manage a retroperitoneal hematoma conservatively or to embolise a kidney in the presence of ongoing active bleeding. In a cold multiply injured patient with a coagulopathy this approach has many attractions compared with open surgery.

Revascularisation via an operative approach may be used in more isolated injuries associated with stabbing or low velocity ballistic injuries (see Chapter 36). Any of the revascularisation methods described above may be employed with the proviso that in a contaminated wound, a prosthetic conduit should be avoided.

In the patient with a less severe initial injury managed conservatively, false aneurysm formation is not an uncommon sequela. If involving the main stem renal artery, these can often be treated with a covered stent, but more distal lesions are problematic. A recent report[16] suggests that microembolisation techniques can be very successful in excluding the false aneurysm cavity without adversely affecting renal perfusion or function.

- The patient should be resuscitated and initial management prioritised along Advanced Trauma Life Support (ATLS) principles
- Urgent laparotomy is required in an unstable patient with a haemoperitoneum
- A conservative approach plus or minus endovascular intervention is recommended in patients without life-threatening haemorrhage, especially in the presence of other injuries

PROBLEMS DURING AORTIC SURGERY

It cannot be stressed enough that the majority of aortic aneurysm/renal artery configurations can be anticipated from a good quality spiral CT and therefore a strategy for renal protection or revascularisation should be worked out in advance. However, this is not always possible in the case of a very angulated or tortuous neck where it can be difficult to define the exact morphology and, of course, in the majority of ruptured aneurysms imaging is not available. The following scenarios can cause problems:

- **Large lower pole renal artery:** It is not uncommon for multiple renal arteries to be present, but the majority are close together and proximal to the aneurysm neck. Less commonly, there is a large separate lower polar artery which contributes significantly to renal perfusion (Fig. 26.3) or even a low single renal artery (Fig. 26.4). These should always be implanted expeditiously using a Carrel patch technique. If the proximal aortic anastomosis is predicted to be difficult and time consuming, cooling can again be employed.
- **Insufficient aortic neck:** Clamp placement has to ensure a sufficient segment of aortic neck below the renal arteries to fashion an anastomosis. If the neck is too short for this, the clamp can be placed above one or both renal arteries and under such circumstances it is prudent to commence dopamine and mannitol. Such a situation should be predictable from a preoperative CT scan (as seen in Fig. 26.5). If the left renal vein is fully mobilised and slung, it is often possible to avoid ligating and dividing it. However, if division is essential to allow access, it should be performed as there is no good evidence to suggest it has any deleterious effect on renal function.[17] The suprarenal aorta can then be inspected to assess a suitable site for cross-clamping avoiding heavy calcification and extensive

atherosclerosis. If this area is unattractive or difficult to access safely, a supracoeliac clamp position is employed to perform the proximal anastomosis and the clamp moved down to the graft once the

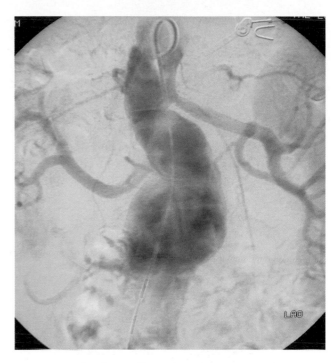

Figure 26.4 *Arteriogram illustrating asymmetrical renal artery take-off. The right renal artery was reimplanted into the Dacron graft*

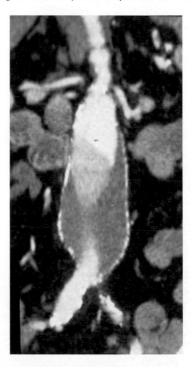

Figure 26.5 *Computed tomography reconstruction from which it should be anticipated that aortic cross-clamping at renal artery level would be difficult. In this case the aorta was clamped just below the diaphragm and the clamp moved down once the proximal anastomosis had been completed*

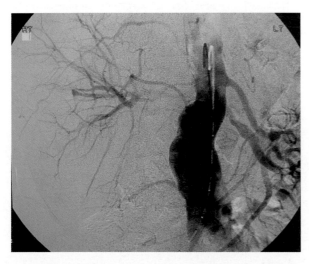

Figure 26.3 *Angiogram illustrating a significant lower pole left renal artery which was reimplanted at the time of surgery*

anastomosis is complete. The supracoeliac aorta is best approached through the lesser sac, dividing the crura if necessary, where it often remains relatively soft even in the presence of disease above and below it.

In a very diseased aorta, clamp placement abutting the renal arteries can risk plaque disruption leading to renal artery occlusion. In such situations, the renal arteries should be exposed and slung to allow an assessment of renal blood flow on clamp removal. This can be done with digital palpation but is best done with a Doppler probe. If there is doubt regarding the adequacy of perfusion a direct puncture with a 21 gauge needle attached to a pressure manometer will reveal any gradient with respect to the aortic pressure. Renal artery endarterectomy with patch closure would be the intervention of choice if necessary.

Conclusions

Although the situations described above represent diverse scenarios, some basic principles can be applied universally.

1 The viability of the renal parenchyma should be assessed prior to making any therapeutic decisions.
2 The renal arterial anatomy must be defined radiologically. The presence of multiple renal arteries, stenoses, low accessory lower pole arteries and the configuration of the neck of the aneurysm, if present, must be clarified before intervention is planned.
3 Surgical cover is mandatory for all endovascular renal artery procedures.
4 Endovascular complications should ideally be rescued by immediate further endovascular intervention.
5 During operative approaches, flexibility is crucial and the many sources of possible inflow remembered, while not forgetting the option of nephrectomy if appropriate.

Key references

Dyet JF, Ettles DF, Nicholson AA, Wilson SE. *Textbook of Endovascular Procedures.* Philadelphia, PA: Churchill Livingstone, 2000: 151–73.
Earnshaw JJ, Murie JA. *The Evidence for Vascular Surgery.* Cheltenham: TFM Publishing Ltd, 1999: 165–72.
Novick A, Scoble J, Hamilton G. *Renal Vascular Disease.* London: WB Saunders, 1996.
Textor SC, Wilcox CS. Renal artery stenosis: a common treatable cause of renal failure? *Annu Rev Med* 2001; **52**: 421–42.

REFERENCES

1 van de Venn PJ, Kaatee R, Beutler JJ, *et al.* Arterial stenting and balloon angioplasty in ostial atherosclerotic renovascular disease: a randomised trial. *Lancet* 1999; **353**: 282–6.
2 Bergentz S-E, Bergqvist D. *Iatrogenic Vascular Injuries.* Berlin: Springer Verlag, 1989.
3 Bush RL, Najibi S, MacDonald J, *et al.* Endovascular revascularization of renal artery stenosis: technical and clinical results. *J Vasc Surg* 2001; **33**: 1041–9.
4 Boisclair C, Therasse E, Oliva VL, *et al.* Treatment of renal angioplasty failure by percutaneous renal artery stenting with Palmaz stents: midterm technical and clinical results. *Am J Roentgenol* 1997; **168**: 245–51.
5 Wong JM, Hansen KJ, Oskin TC, *et al.* Surgery after failed percutaneous renal artery angioplasty. *J Vasc Surg* 1999; **30**: 468–82.
6 Paty PSK, Darling RC, Lee D, *et al.* Is prosthetic renal artery reconstruction a durable procedure? An analysis of 489 bypass grafts. *J Vasc Surg* 2001; **34**: 127–32.
7 Salem TA, Lumsden AB, Martin LG. Local infusion of fibrinolytic agents for renal artery thromboembolism: report of ten cases. *Ann Vasc Surg* 1993; **7**: 21–6.
8 Kalliafas S, Albertini JN, Macierewicz J, *et al.* Incidence and treatment of intra-operative problems during endovascular repair of complex abdominal aortic aneurysms. *J Vasc Surg* 2000; **31**: 1185–92.
9 Lin PH, Madsen K, Bush RL, *et al.* Iliorenal artery bypass grafting to facilitate endovascular abdominal aortic aneurysm repair. *J Vasc Surg* 2003; **38**: 183–5.
10 Lau LL, Hakaim AG, Oldenburg WA, *et al.* Effect of suprarenal versus infrarenal aortic fixation on renal function and renal artery patency: a comparative study with intermediate follow up. *J Vasc Surg* 2003; **37**: 1162–8.
11 Bove PG, Long GW, Shanley CJ, *et al.* Transrenal fixation of endovascular stent-grafts for infrarenal aortic aneurysm repair: mid-term results. *J Vasc Surg* 2003; **37**: 938–42.
12 Fischer P, Konnak JW, Cho KJ, *et al.* Renal artery embolism: therapy with intra-arterial streptokinase infusion. *J Urol* 1981; **125**: 402–4.
13 Lacombe M. Surgical versus medical treatment of renal artery embolism. *J Cardiovasc Surg* 1977; **18**: 281–90.
14 Nicholas GC, De Muth WE. Treatment of renal artery embolism. *Arch Surg* 1984; **119**: 278–81.
15 Fine MJ, Kapoor W, Falanga V. Cholesterol crystal embolization: a review of 221 cases in the English literature. *Angiology* 1987; **38**: 769–84.
16 Cantasdemir M, Adaletli I, Kantarci F, *et al.* Emergency endovascular embolization of traumatic intrarenal arterial pseudoaneurysms with *N*-butyl cyanoacrylate. *Clin Radiol* 2003; **58**: 560–5.
17 Elsharawy MA, Cheatle TR, Clarke JM, *et al.* Effect of left renal vein division during aortic surgery on renal function. *Ann R Coll Surg Engl* 2000; **82**: 417–20.

27

Renal Artery Aneurysms

JAMES C STANLEY, PETER K HENKE

THE PROBLEM

Aneurysms of the renal artery are an uncommon vascular disease, the clinical importance of which is a matter of controversy.[1–13] The emergency surgical treatment of renal artery aneurysms represents an ill-defined practice, with most reported experiences being anecdotal. The two most common complications leading to emergency operations are aneurysm rupture and thrombosis with peripheral embolism. Occurrences of these complications are often overestimated in that most published reports describe operative rather than population-based experiences. These emergency scenarios require careful clinical judgement and skilled surgical intervention if optimal care is to be achieved. The two most relevant renal artery macroaneurysms, namely, true aneurysms and those associated with dissections, deserve individual discussion.

TRUE RENAL ARTERY ANEURYSMS

The prevalence of true renal artery aneurysms in the general population approaches 0.09 per cent.[12] The group of patients being studied bears greatly on the reported frequency of these lesions. Macroaneurysms were identified in 0.7 per cent of arteriographic studies performed in patients suspected of renal disease,[14] 2.5 per cent of those studies having been undertaken for suspected renovascular hypertension,[12] and 9.2 per cent of studies performed in hypertensive adults with renal artery fibrodysplasia.[15]

Clinical manifestations

Rupture is the most serious complication attending renal artery aneurysms. Exsanguinating haemorrhage with aneurysm rupture is fatal in 10 per cent of cases, reflecting the seriousness of this complication. This mortality rate is less than suggested in earlier reports.[4,8,16,17] Nevertheless, loss of the involved kidney continues to be a nearly universal outcome of renal artery aneurysm rupture.[12,17]

In the largest reported experience with renal artery aneurysms, overt extraparenchymal rupture (Figs 27.1 and 27.2) occurred in 1.8 per cent of patients harbouring these lesions, and covert rupture (Fig. 27.3) caused renal arteriovenous fistulae in an additional 1.2 per cent.[5] The combined 3 per cent frequency of overt and covert rupture in the latter review is higher than that reported in non-surgical series.[7,13] The rate of rupture of renal artery aneurysms during pregnancy is unknown, but the sequelae are often catastrophic, causing foetal death in nearly 85 per cent of cases and maternal death in over half of them.[18–21]

Increased risks of renal artery aneurysm rupture have been attributed to large size, absence of calcification and elevated blood pressure, but these factors are not always relevant. In fact, overt rupture often occurs in normotensive patients as well as in patients with calcific aneurysms.[12] When rupture does occur it usually involves the base of the aneurysm and not the aneurysmal dome as might be expected. A large aneurysm, in contrast to a small one, has an inconsistent but relatively greater potential for rupture. Aneurysm rupture during pregnancy does not appear to be related to age or number of prior pregnancies.[18]

Overt renal artery aneurysm rupture usually causes unremitting costovertebral, flank and abdominal pain of varying intensity. In addition to pain, perirenal bleeding into the retroperitoneal space is usually associated with an ileus and abdominal distension. Nausea and vomiting are common in this setting. Most patients develop microhaematuria in association with rupture. Loss of retroperitoneal containment with free bleeding into the peritoneal cavity may result in life-threatening shock.

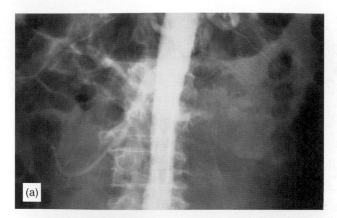

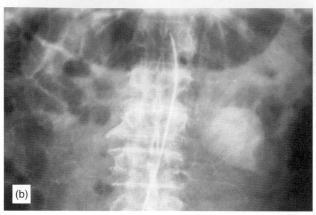

Figure 27.1 *Overt renal artery aneurysm rupture. (a) Aortographic demonstration of renal artery aneurysm rupture with no evidence of distal parenchymal vessels. (b) Later peripelvic collection of contrast medium (from Stanley JC, Whitehouse WM Jr. Renal artery macroaneurysms. In: Bergan JJ, Yao JST (eds). Aneurysms. Orlando, FL: WB Saunders, 1982: 417–31)*

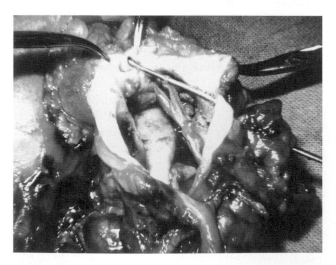

Figure 27.2 *Gross specimen of ruptured renal artery aneurysm depicted in arteriographic study in Fig. 27.1 (from Stanley JC, Whitehouse WM Jr. Renal artery macroaneurysms. In: Bergan JJ, Yao JST (eds). Aneurysms. Orlando, FL: WB Saunders, 1982: 417–31)*

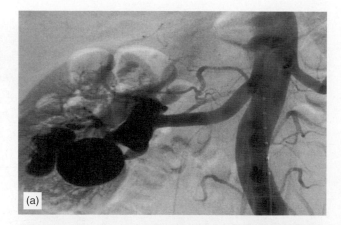

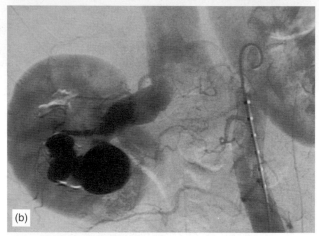

Figure 27.3 *Covert renal artery aneurysm rupture. (a) Arterial phase digital subtraction arteriography demonstrating large inferior pole arterial aneurysm communication with an adjacent vein. (b) Venous phase demonstrating rapid filling of the inferior vena cava with contrast (from Henke PK, Cardneau JD, Welling TH III, et al. Renal artery aneurysms: A 35-year clinical experience with 252 aneurysms in 168 patients. Ann Surg 2001; 234: 454–63)*

A renal artery aneurysm may rupture covertly into an adjacent renal vein producing an arteriovenous fistula (see Fig. 27.3). These patients may initially experience vague flank pain, but more often than not they are asymptomatic. As these fistulae expand in size, nearly half of them become associated with hypertension and chronic microhaematuria. It is uncommon for an arteriovenous fistula of the renal vessels to present as a surgical emergency.

Thromboembolism of dislodged material originating in an aneurysm results in renal ischaemia and infarction. Atheromatous plaque rupture and ulceration within large aneurysmal sacs may predispose to these embolic complications (Fig. 27.4). Small aneurysms without calcific atherosclerosis may also be the source of embolic renal arterial occlusion (Fig. 27.5). In a study reported from our institution, embolism was a clear complication of renal artery aneurysms in only three of 118 patients.[12] This complication, manifested by hypertension alone, is not considered a surgical emergency.

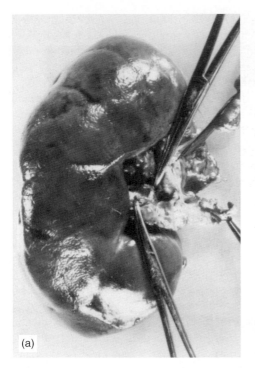
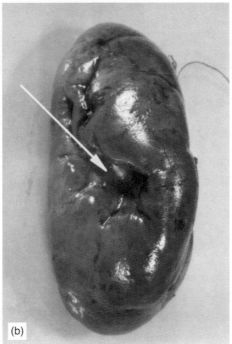

Figure 27.4   *(a) Large arteriosclerotic renal artery aneurysm containing thrombus. (b) Deep cortical infarct (arrow) secondary to thromboembolism from the hilar aneurysm (from Stanley JC, Whitehouse WM Jr. Renal artery macroaneurysms. In: Bergan JJ, Yao JST (eds). Aneurysms. Orlando, FL: WB Saunders, 1982: 417–31)*

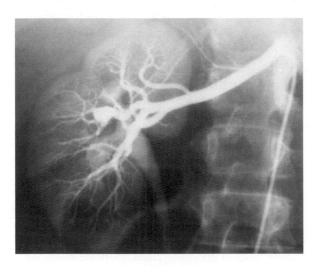

Figure 27.5   *Small non-atherosclerotic intraparenchymal aneurysm associated with segmental thromboembolic renal ischaemia and cortical infarct (from Stanley JC, Whitehouse WM Jr. Renal artery macroaneurysms. In: Bergan JJ, Yao JST (eds). Aneurysms. Orlando, FL: WB Saunders, 1982: 417–31)*

Aneurysm related thromboembolism may present with vague flank discomfort caused by an inflammatory perinephritis in the case of a small renal infarct, or with severe back, flank and abdominal pain following a large renal infarct. This is an uncommon but recognised presentation as a surgical emergency. The patient is usually febrile, exhibits a leucocytosis and develops haematuria and albuminuria. Severe hypertension, lasting for a few days, may accompany acute renal infarction. It is often attributed to pain experienced, but is more likely to be renin mediated provoked by profoundly ischaemic renal tissue. Eventually, with scarring and the loss of the affected kidney parenchyma, the blood pressure usually returns to normal. A small number of individuals will have such severe discomfort with renal infarction that urgent operative intervention will be required. Similarly, in rare instances, the infarcted segment will rupture into the renal pelvis causing massive haematuria. These patients require emergency nephrectomy.

Renal infarction usually results in a rise in the concentrations of a number of serum enzymes. Although somewhat non-specific, these elevations may be useful in supporting a diagnosis of renal infarction. Immediate increases in alanine aminotransferase are often observed followed 1 or 2 days later by peak levels of lactose dehydrogenase. Later, 3–5 days after infarction, peak elevations in alkaline phosphatase will be noted.

Compression of a renal artery aneurysm or kinking of an adjacent segment causing renal ischaemia and consequent severe uncontrolled renovascular hypertension has been documented in the literature.[22,23] Unless the patient develops malignant hypertension, which is unlikely, this complication is not considered a surgical emergency. A patient presenting with marked blood pressure elevations usually has coexisting renal artery stenotic disease in the vicinity of the aneurysm accounting for the secondary hypertension.

Aetiology

Renal artery aneurysms usually arise as a result of a congenital elastic tissue defect or medial degenerative process. Fragmentation of the internal elastic lamina and in the media a paucity of elastic tissue and loss of recognisable smooth muscle are characteristic features of these aneurysms. The well-known discontinuity of internal elastic lamina at the bifurcation of all muscular arteries further compromises the structural integrity of the renal artery and, together with the elevated blood pressure observed in 40–80 per cent of these patients, contributes to the development of an aneurysm.

Complicated atherosclerotic manifestations such as calcium deposition, collections of cholesterol, necrotic debris, haemorrhage and a matrix of fibrous tissue are often present in the walls of larger aneurysms. These changes are considered part of a secondary rather than a primary aetiological event. The observation that atherosclerotic changes are present in some, but not all, aneurysms in a patient with multiple aneurysms, supports the tenet that a non-atherosclerotic cause is responsible for most renal artery aneurysms.[12] Nevertheless, secondary atherosclerosis contributes to further vessel wall weakness.

> ## True renal artery aneurysms: presentation and manifestations
>
> - Rare – less than 1 in 1000 individuals
> - Aneurysms are usually discovered incidentally, often in association with hypertension
> - Risk of aneurysm rupture – not solely dependent on size, significantly higher during pregnancy
> - Renal infarction may result from thromboembolism

Diagnosis

The clinical manifestations of renal artery aneurysm rupture or acute thromboembolism are quite protean. The diagnosis is usually not immediately clear, the differential diagnoses including other vascular emergencies such as ruptured or expanding aortic or splanchnic artery aneurysms. Acute renal colic with the passage of kidney stones may also mimic the complications of certain aneurysms. Inflammatory processes such as diverticulitis with abscess formation, pancreatitis and acute biliary tract diseases may lead to urgent surgical intervention at which point a ruptured renal artery aneurysm may be discovered.

Imaging studies in some of the settings noted above may reveal renal artery aneurysm calcification, and distortion of the kidney substance and collecting system by the aneurysm or a haematoma if rupture has occurred. If a renal artery aneurysm is suspected in a haemodynamically stable patient based on the history, physical examination or non-specific imaging studies, then arteriography becomes an essential diagnostic study.[5,12]

Arteriographic documentation of renal arterial anatomy in the region of an aneurysm is especially necessary in planning emergency operative intervention if salvage of the kidney with a revascularisation procedure is intended. Gadolinium-enhanced magnetic resonance arteriography[24] and three-dimensional reconstructed computed tomography (CT) scanning[25] have a potential but unproved role in the anatomical delineation of these aneurysms.

Intraoperative diagnosis of a ruptured aneurysm should be entertained when a large retroperitoneal haematoma surrounding the kidney is noted during an emergency operation for pain or suspected haemorrhage. In this setting, the exact diagnosis is usually evident upon examination of the excised kidney. On rare occasions, lesser degrees of bleeding or thromboembolism may facilitate dissection and exposure of the aneurysm followed by revascularisation of the kidney.

Management

The objective of surgical therapy is to eliminate the renal artery aneurysm without removing the kidney or compromising its function.[5,12,26–29] This objective is rarely met in emergency procedures. Nephrectomy is the usual outcome in managing most ruptured aneurysms or extensive thromboembolic complications of these aneurysms. As far as overall health of the patient is concerned, nephrectomy may be well tolerated. In a recent report on the management of renal artery aneurysms with a follow-up of nearly a decade, planned nephrectomy, and in a few instances unplanned nephrectomy, did not result in renal failure.[5] Nevertheless, arterial reconstruction should be considered whenever the kidney does not appear to have been irreparably injured from ischaemia.

In attempting to salvage a kidney after an aneurysm has ruptured, it is important to recognise that renal function is impaired after blood flow has been interrupted for 40 minutes. After 60 minutes of warm ischaemia, retrieval of renal function becomes unlikely. If prolonged renal ischaemia is anticipated during a reconstructive procedure, renal hypothermia using cold (4 °C) hypertonic electrolyte solution infusions should be undertaken to protect the kidney. Longer periods of interruption of renal blood flow may be tolerated in those patients with pre-existing stenotic disease and the presence of collateral vessels to the kidney.

Partial nephrectomy may be possible when aneurysmal erosion has occurred into an adjacent vein causing an arteriovenous fistula or when thromboembolism has caused a limited area of segmental infarctions. Acute arteriovenous fistulae may be treated occasionally by endovascular means, namely, with transcatheter instillation of absolute alcohol to eliminate diseased tissue or embolisation of particulate matter or coils to obliterate the fistula, selectively infarcting small areas of the kidney.

Most renal artery aneurysms are best approached via a transabdominal, extraperitoneal exposure of the renal vasculature, displacing the overlying colon and foregut viscera medially. In the situation of active bleeding from a ruptured aneurysm, the renal artery is compressed or clamped proximally near its aortic origin before attempting to dissect distal tissue around the aneurysm. The patient's overall haemodynamic state and estimated renal ischaemia time will dictate whether a simple nephrectomy is performed or an arterial repair and renal salvage is attempted.

Large aneurysms affecting the main renal artery bifurcation can usually be excised with a simple angioplastic closure. Excision of smaller aneurysms may require arterial closure with a vein patch. More extensive renal artery reconstructions using autogenous saphenous vein or internal iliac artery as aortorenal grafts are favoured for those aneurysms associated with functionally important stenoses of the renal artery.[5,12,29] Aneurysmectomy with reimplantation of the involved vessel or vessels into a normal adjacent or proximal renal artery is appropriate for treating many first and second order branch aneurysms. These procedures are usually undertaken *in situ*, although *ex vivo* reconstructions may be preferred in certain cases,[30–32] especially with coexistent segmental renal artery stenotic disease. These arterial reconstructive procedures are often lengthy and are usually only undertaken for treatment of symptomatic intact aneurysms. Extensive tissue disruption and blood staining associated with aneurysm rupture may preclude completion of a complex renal artery reconstruction.

Renal artery aneurysms are not usually amenable to endovascular intervention and are even less so when they present as emergencies. Bleeding aneurysms may be an exception. Certainly if life-threatening haemorrhage is evident at angiography, coil or balloon occlusion of the renal artery may be quite acceptable and appropriate. In anecdotal reports, aneurysms of the main renal artery in a non-emergency setting have been successfully excluded by stent graft placement and branch aneurysms successfully embolised.[33–36] Embolisation of intact intraparenchymal aneurysms is a reasonable alternative to partial nephrectomy in selected symptomatic patients. Endovascular treatment of renal artery aneurysms may become more common as the technology improves in the future.

True renal artery aneurysms: diagnosis and management

- Non-specific abdominal complaints uncommon with intact aneurysms, most are asymptomatic
- Ruptured aneurysms are associated with severe flank pain, ileus and haemodynamic instability
- Confirmed rupture in unstable patients justifies emergency operation, usually nephrectomy
- Suspected rupture in haemodynamically stable patients warrants urgent arteriography and an operative attempt to salvage the kidney
- Consider endovascular embolisation for rupture of a segmental renal artery branch aneurysm in haemodynamically stable patients

DISSECTING RENAL ARTERY ANEURYSMS

Isolated renal artery dissection causing an aneurysm is rare.[37–40] Dissections are usually classified into two types: the first type is due to blunt abdominal trauma or intraluminal catheter induced injury and the second occurs spontaneously.

Clinical manifestations

Flank and back pain, haematuria, ileus and hypertension frequently accompany acute dissections regardless of the cause.[38,41,42] Acute dissections often present as emergencies with excruciating pain, associated nausea and vomiting suggestive of an acute abdomen. It is uncommon for renal artery dissection to result in vascular disruption and uncontrolled haemorrhage. Chronic renal artery dissection, when clinically relevant, is usually associated with renovascular hypertension or impaired renal function but it does not immediately threaten life or the kidney concerned, very rarely presenting as a surgical emergency.

Aetiology

Dissection of the renal artery affects men nearly 10 times more often than women,[43] indeed men have a greater likelihood of developing trauma induced dissections. Although an overall predilection for right renal artery involvement exists, trauma related dissection more commonly affects the left renal artery.

Blunt trauma contributes to renal artery dissection by two specific mechanisms. The first mechanism is violent displacement of the kidney, causing the renal artery to stretch, fracturing the intima and resulting in a subintimal dissection; this happens most frequently in deceleration injuries (see Chapters 26 and 36). The second relates to traumatic compression of the renal artery against the vertebra, causing haemorrhage within the deeper media, false aneurysm formation and vessel wall disruption. Both forms of trauma are most commonly associated with motor vehicle accidents.

Iatrogenic catheter related injury during diagnostic arteriography is an uncommon cause of renal artery dissection (Fig. 27.6). In an earlier series from our institution, only four catheter related renal artery dissections were encountered in more than 11 000 abdominal diagnostic arteriographic examinations, including more than 2200 selective renal arteriograms.[38] Iatrogenic dissections of this type usually occur within the inner media or subintimal tissues of the renal artery. Dissections accompanying therapeutic balloon angioplasty are very common, although only a few cause critical narrowing or occlusion of the renal artery.[44] In those instances of critical stenoses, stent placement

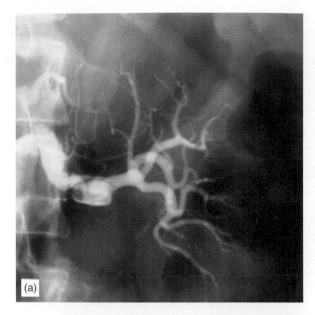

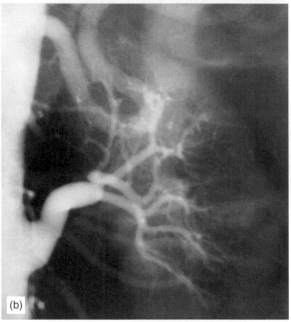

Figure 27.6 *(a) Catheter induced dissecting renal artery aneurysm. (b) Postoperative appearance following aneurysmectomy and arterial reconstruction with an aortorenal bypass (from Gewertz BL, Stanley JC, Fry WJ. Renal artery dissections. Arch Surg 1977; 112: 409–14)*

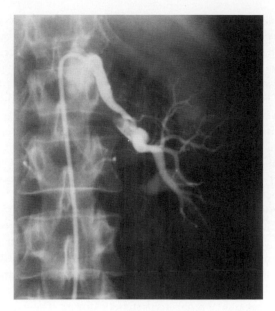

Figure 27.7 *Spontaneous saccular dissecting renal artery aneurysm in a patient with coexisting fibrodysplasia (from Gewertz BL, Stanley JC, Fry WJ. Renal artery dissections. Arch Surg 1977; 112: 409–14)*

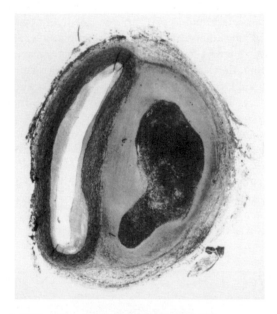

Figure 27.8 *Dissection exhibiting deep mural haematoma and compression of adjacent lumen (haematoxylin eosin stain, original magnification ×60) (from Stanley JC. Pathologic basis of macrovascular renal artery disease. In: Stanley JC, Ernst CB, Fry WJ (eds). Renovascular Hypertension. Philadelphia, PA: WB Saunders, 1984: 46–74)*

at the moment when the dissection is recognised will usually restore the renal artery lumen.[45]

Spontaneous dissection causing a pseudoaneurysm affects the renal arteries more than any other peripheral artery. Most of these lesions are associated with coexisting atherosclerotic or fibrodysplastic renovascular disease (Fig. 27.7). These dissections usually occur within the outer media adjacent to the external elastic lamina (Fig. 27.8). Spontaneous renal artery dissection most often affects the proximal vessel and terminates at its branching.

Diagnosis

A correct initial clinical diagnosis of a renal artery dissection is uncommon, occurring in less than half of these patients.[42] Intravenous pyelography has been advocated in evaluating serious renal hilar injuries, including dissecting aneurysms, but in view of the high incidence of false negative and false positive studies, such examination should be deferred in favour of arteriography.

Arteriography is necessary to diagnose as well as define the extent of a renal artery dissection and is essential in planning operative therapy. The features of dissection include:

- luminal irregularities with fusiform aneurysmal dilatation or saccular outpouchings associated with segmental stenoses
- extension of the dissection to the first renal artery branching
- cuffing at branchings
- variable degrees of reversibility documented on serial studies.

In the case of renal artery occlusion with infarction of the kidney, increases occur in the levels of the same array of enzymes previously described when true aneurysms are complicated by thromboembolism.

Dissecting renal artery aneurysms: presentation and diagnosis

- Often present with severe abdominal and back pain and nausea
- Blunt trauma is a more common cause than spontaneous dissection and a more common cause than catheter related dissecting aneurysm
- Arteriography will reveal the diagnosis

Management

Emergency arterial reconstruction of trauma induced dissection is vital in haemodynamically significant narrowing of the main renal artery or a major segmental branch.[38,39] Spontaneous dissecting aneurysms, when acute, are technically easier to treat than traumatic lesions and once diagnosed most should be dealt with urgently.

Operative intervention is indicated in chronic trauma related and spontaneous dissections associated with severe renovascular hypertension, and in some instances deteriorating renal function (see Chapter 26); these latter circumstances, however, do not often constitute surgical emergencies. Endovascular stent graft placement may be an appropriate alternative for short proximal renal artery dissections with a defined distal endpoint, but there is little in the literature pertaining to the long term durability of such treatment.

Kidney preservation must be the paramount concern when treating renal artery dissection, particularly as contralateral renal artery dissection occurs in a third of cases, and in addition the contralateral kidney may be diseased in half of the patients sustaining blunt abdominal trauma.[38] Nephrectomy, under such circumstances, should be avoided.

Local angioplastic procedures, often undertaken in the treatment of true renal artery aneurysms, are inappropriate in the treatment of dissections, regardless of the cause. In this situation the affected arterial segment usually demands replacement or bypass with a graft. Renal artery dissections with preserved renal blood flow allow time for a repair to be planned and executed in a semi-elective fashion. Standard arterial reconstruction in the form of an aortorenal bypass using autogenous saphenous vein or hypogastric artery (see Fig. 27.6), and *ex vivo* repairs in selected cases, provide reasonable kidney salvage rates.[38,39]

Conclusions

A patient with a renal artery aneurysm, regardless of aetiology, may present as an emergency, if the aneurysm ruptures causing severe haemorrhage and shock or if thromboembolism results in segmental infarction of the kidney. In both circumstances, and given the commoner acute abdominal conditions which mimic those two scenarios, the clinical diagnosis may not become immediately apparent. Arteriography is the investigation of choice in establishing the diagnosis. Ideally, the objectives of surgical treatment are to eliminate the aneurysm, reconstruct the artery and salvage the kidney. In reality, nephrectomy is often the outcome, as it is when endovascular techniques are used to occlude the renal artery as a life-saving measure. A patient with acute dissection of the renal artery, and the possible (pseudo)aneurysms complicating it, whether caused by blunt trauma, balloon angioplasty or if it occurs spontaneously, is also likely to be hypertensive. In such a case, operative replacement or bypass of the renal artery should remedy the problem while also preserving the kidney.

Key references

Cohen JR, Shamash FS. Ruptured renal artery aneurysms during pregnancy. *J Vasc Surg* 1987; **6**: 51–9. Comprehensive review of renal artery aneurysm rupture during pregnancy.

Henke PK, Cardneau JD, Welling TH III, *et al.* Renal artery aneurysms: a 35-year clinical experience with 252 aneurysms in 168 patients. *Ann Surg* 2001; **234**: 454–63. Largest reported series of renal artery aneurysms, from a surgical perspective.

Reilly LM, Cuningham CG, Maggisano R, *et al.* The role of arterial reconstruction in spontaneous renal artery dissection. *J Vasc Surg* 1991; **14**: 468–77. Comprehensive review of non-iatrogenic, spontaneous renal artery dissections.

Schorn B, Falk V, Dalichau H, Mohr FW. Kidney salvage in a case of ruptured renal artery aneurysm: case report and literature review. *Cardiovasc Surg* 1997; **5**: 134–6. Brief review of patient survival and kidney salvage after renal artery aneurysm rupture.

Stanley JC, Messina LM, Wakefield TW, Zelenock GB. Renal artery reconstruction. In: Bergan JJ, Yao JST (eds). *Techniques in Arterial Surgery.* Philadelphia, PA: WB Saunders, 1990: 247–63. Depiction of various techniques available for the surgical treatment of renal artery aneurysms.

REFERENCES

1 Bastounis W, Pikoulis E, Georgopoulos S, *et al.* Surgery for renal artery aneurysms: A combined series of two large centers. *Eur Urol* 1998; **33**: 22–7.

2 Bulbul MA, Farrow GA. Renal artery aneurysms. *Urology* 1992; **40**: 124–6.

3 Dzsinich C, Gloviczki P, McKusick MA, *et al.* Surgical management of renal artery aneurysm. *Cardiovasc Surg* 1993; **3**: 243–7.

4 Hageman JH, Smith RF, Szilagyi DE, Elliott JP. Aneurysms of the renal artery: problems of prognosis and surgical management. *Surgery* 1978; **84**: 563–72.

5 Henke PK, Cardneau JD, Welling TH III, *et al.* Renal artery aneurysms: A 35-year clinical experience with 252 aneurysms in 168 patients. *Ann Surg* 2001; **234**: 454–63.

6 Henriksson C, Bjorkerud S, Nilson AE, Pettersson S. Natural history of renal artery aneurysm elucidated by repeated angiography and pathoanatomical studies. *Eur Urol* 1985; **11**: 244–8.

7 Henriksson C, Lukes P, Nilson AE, Pettersson S. Angiographically discovered, non-operated renal artery aneurysms. *Scand J Urol Nephrol* 1984; **18**: 59–62.

8 Hubert JP Jr, Pairolero PC, Kazmier FJ. Solitary renal artery aneurysm. *Surgery* 1980; **88**: 557–65.

9 Lumsden AB, Salam TA, Walton KG. Renal artery aneurysm: a report of 28 cases. *Cardiovasc Surg* 1996; **4**: 185–9.

10 Martin RS III, Meacham PW, Ditesheim JA, *et al.* Renal artery aneurysm: selective treatment for hypertension and prevention of rupture. *J Vasc Surg* 1989; **9**: 26–34.

11 Soussou ID, Starr DS, Lawrie GM, Morris GC. Renal artery aneurysm: long-term relief of renovascular hypertension by *in situ* operative correction. *Arch Surg* 1979; **114**: 1410–15.

12 Stanley JC, Rhodes EL, Gewertz BL, *et al.* Renal artery aneurysms: significance of macroaneurysms exclusive of dissections and fibrodysplastic mural dilations. *Arch Surg* 1975; **110**: 1327–333.

13 Tham G, Ekelund L, Herrlin K, *et al.* Renal artery aneurysms: natural history and prognosis. *Ann Surg* 1983; **197**: 348–52.

14 Edsman G. Angiography and suprarenal angiography. *Acta Radiol* 1965; Suppl 155: 104.

15 Stanley JC, Gewertz BL, Bove EL, *et al.* Arterial fibrodysplasia: histopathologic character and current etiologic concepts. *Arch Surg* 1975; **110**: 561–6.

16 Hidai H, Kinoshita Y, Murayama T, *et al.* Rupture of renal artery aneurysm. *Eur Urol* 1985; **11**: 249–53.

17 Schorn B, Falk V, Dalichau H, Mohr FW. Kidney salvage in a case of ruptured renal artery aneurysm: case report and literature review. *Cardiovasc Surg* 1997; **5**: 134–6.

18 Cohen JR, Shamash FS. Ruptured renal artery aneurysms during pregnancy. *J Vasc Surg* 1987; **6**: 51–9.

19 Lacroix H, Bernaerts P, Nevelsteen A, Hanssens M. Ruptured renal artery aneurysm during pregnancy: Successful *ex situ* repair and autotransplantation. *J Vasc Surg* 2001; **33**: 188–90.

20 Love WK, Robinette MA, Vernon CP. Renal artery aneurysm rupture in pregnancy. *J Urol* 1981; **126**: 809–11.

21 Rijbroek A, van Dijk HA, Roex AJM. Rupture of renal artery aneurysm during pregnancy. *Eur J Vasc Surg* 1994; **8**: 375–6.

22 Reiher L, Grabitz K, Sandmann W. Reconstruction for renal artery aneurysm and its effect on hypertension. *Eur J Endovasc Surg* 2000;20;454–6.

23 Youkey JR, Collins GJ, Orecchia PM, *et al.* Saccular renal artery aneurysm as a cause of hypertension. *Surgery* 1985; **97**: 498–501.

24 Prince MR, Narasimham DL, Stanley JC, *et al.* Breath-hold gadolinium-enhanced MR angiography of the abdominal aorta and its major branches. *Radiology* 1995; **197**: 785–92.

25 Cikrit DF, Harris VJ, Hemmer CG, *et al.* Comparison of spiral CT scan and arteriography for evaluation of renal and visceral arteries. *Ann Vasc Surg* 1996; **10**: 109–16.

26 Forbes TL, Abraham CZ, Pudupakkam S. Repair of ruptured giant renal artery aneurysm with kidney salvage. *Eur J Vasc Endovasc Surg* 2001; **22**: 278–9.

27 Hupp, T, Allenberg JR, Post K, *et al.* Renal artery aneurysms: surgical indications and results. *Eur J Vasc Surg* 1992; **6**: 477–86.

28 Mercier C, Piquet P, Piligian F, Ferdani M. Aneurysms of the renal artery and its branches. *Ann Vasc Surg* 1986; **1**: 321–7.

29 Stanley JC, Messina LM, Wakefield TW, Zelenock GB. Renal artery reconstruction. In: Bergan JJ, Yao JST (eds). *Techniques in Arterial Surgery.* Philadelphia, PA: WB Saunders, 1990:247–63.

30 Belzer FO, Raczkowski A. *Ex vivo* renal artery reconstruction with autotransplantation. *Surgery* 1982; **92**: 642–5.

31 Bugge-Asperheim B, Sdal G, Flatmark A. Renal artery aneurysm: ex vivo repair and autotransplantation. *Scand J Urol Nephrol* 1984; **18**: 63–6.

32 Dubernard JM, Martin X, Gelet A, Mongin D. Aneurysms of the renal artery: surgical management with special reference to extracorporeal surgery and autotransplantation. *Eur Urol* 1985; **11**: 26–30.

33 Bui BT, Oliva VL, Leclerc G, *et al.* Renal artery aneurysm: Treatment with percutaneous placement of a stent-graft. *Radiology* 1995; **195**: 181–2.

34 Centenera LV, Hirsch JA, Choi IS, *et al.* Wide-necked saccular renal artery aneurysm: endovascular embolization with the Guglielmi detachable coil and temporary balloon occlusion of the aneurysm neck. *J Vasc Interv Radiol* 1998; **9**: 513–516.

35 Karkos CD, D'Souza SP, Thompson GJ, *et al.* Renal artery aneurysm: endovascular treatment by coil embolization with preservation of renal blood flow. *Eur J Vasc Endovasc Surg* 2000; **19**: 214–16.

36 Tateno T, Kubota Y, Sasagawa I, *et al.* Successful embolization of a renal artery aneurysm with preservation of renal blood flow. *Int Urol Nephrol* 1996; **28**: 283–7.

37 Edwards BS, Stanson AW, Holley KE, Sheps SG. Isolated renal artery dissection: presentation, evaluation, management and pathology. *Mayo Clin Proc* 1982; **57**: 564–71.

38 Gewertz BL, Stanley JC, Fry WJ. Renal artery dissections. *Arch Surg* 1977; **112**:409–14.

39 Reilly LM, Cuningham CG, Maggisano R, *et al.* The role of arterial reconstruction in spontaneous renal artery dissection. *J Vasc Surg* 1991; **14**: 468–77.

40 Smith BM, Holcomb GW 3rd, Richie RE, Dean RH. Renal artery dissection. *Ann Surg* 1984; **200**: 134–46.

41 Hare WS, Kincaid-Smith P. Dissecting aneurysm of the renal artery. *Radiology* 1970; **97**: 255–63.

42 Rao CN, Blaivas JG. Primary renal artery dissecting aneurysm: a review. *J Urol* 1977; **118**: 716–19.

43 Bakir AA, Patel K, Schwartz MM, Lewis EJ. Isolated dissecting aneurysm of the renal artery. *Am Heart J* 1978; **96**: 92–6.

44 Stanley JC. Surgery of failed percutaneous transluminal renal artery angioplasty. In: Bergan JJ, Yao JST (eds). *Reoperative Arterial Surgery*. Orlando, FL: Grune & Stratton, 1986: 441–54.

45 Mali WP, Geyskes GG, Thalman R. Dissecting renal artery aneurysm: Treatment with an endovascular stent. *Am J Radiol* 1989; **153**: 623–4.

28

Visceral Artery Aneurysms

SANDRA C CARR, WILLIAM D TURNIPSEED

THE PROBLEM

Aneurysms of the visceral arteries (VAAs) represent an uncommon but potentially lethal form of vascular disease. These lesions are rare, with an incidence of 0.01–0.2 per cent in routine autopsies.[1] The most commonly involved vessels include the splenic, hepatic, superior mesenteric (SMA) and coeliac arteries. The gastric-gastroepiploic, jejunal-ilieal-colic, pancreaticoduodenal-pancreatic, gastroduodenal and inferior mesenteric arteries are less often involved.

In the past, most VAAs were discovered at autopsy, rupture often being the cause of death. With the widespread use of computed tomography (CT) and angiography many asymptomatic aneurysms are now discovered. Despite this many of these patients still present acutely with rupture. Recent literature documents mortality ranging from 21 per cent to nearly 100 per cent,[2] depending upon the vessel involved. As these aneurysms frequently present as life-threatening clinical emergencies, it is essential that vascular surgeons know how to diagnose and treat VAAs.

PRESENTING SYMPTOMS AND SIGNS

Making the correct diagnosis requires an appropriate index of suspicion and knowledge of various associated conditions. Visceral pseudoaneurysms result from inflammation and/or trauma to the artery. Splenic aneurysms are commonly associated with pancreatitis and/or pseudocyst. Similarly, aneurysms of the pancreaticoduodenal, pancreatic, gastroduodenal, gastric and gastroepiploic arteries often result from pancreatic inflammation. Blunt or penetrating liver trauma is the most common cause of intrahepatic pseudoaneurysms. True aneurysms of the splenic artery are found in multiparous women and in patients with portal hypertension and splenomegaly. Mycotic aneurysms most commonly occur in the coeliac and superior mesenteric arteries and are associated with subacute bacterial endocarditis, *Salmonella* infection or syphilis. Patients with fibromuscular dysplasia, connective tissue disorders such as Ehlers–Danlos syndrome, and inflammatory conditions such as polyarteritis nodosa, systemic lupus erythematosus, Behçet's disease and Takayasu's disease are also at increased risk of developing visceral aneurysms.

The clinical findings associated with VAAs vary depending upon the artery involved. Splenic artery aneurysms (SAAs) are more common in women (78 per cent) than in men (21 per cent)[3,4] (Fig. 28.1). More than 90 per cent of SAAs are asymptomatic having been discovered in plain films, CT scan or magnetic resonance imaging (MRI) performed for other reasons.[4] Multiple SAAs are found in 5 per cent of patients.[4] Only 4.5 per cent present with rupture. Patients taking β-blockade medication may be at decreased risk of rupture.[4] The most common symptoms are abdominal pain, epigastric or left upper quadrant or back pain.[2] Patients with ruptured aneurysms may present with shock or gastrointestinal haemorrhage. Bleeding may be confined initially to the lesser sac but continued haemorrhage therefrom through the foramen of Winslow into the peritoneal cavity results in haemorrhagic shock; this is known as the 'double rupture phenomenon'.[5]

Unlike SAAs, those of the hepatic artery (HAAs) occur more frequently in men.[2] The routine use of abdominal CT scan for blunt liver trauma and the increasing numbers of percutaneous biliary procedures has led to an increase in

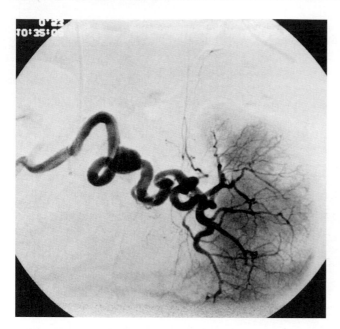

Figure 28.1 *Multiple splenic artery aneurysms in a 52-year-old multiparous woman. This patient was treated with splenectomy and resection of the aneurysms*

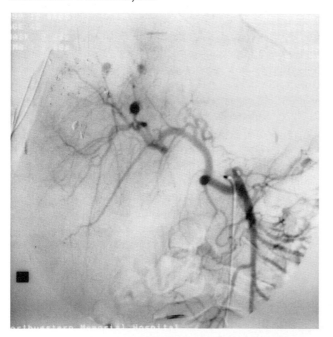

Figure 28.2 *Multiple intrahepatic artery aneurysms in a young male patient following blunt liver trauma*

the discovery of HAAs. Intrahepatic pseudoaneurysms may be associated with percutaneous biliary procedures, biopsy, abdominal trauma or pancreatitis[2] (Fig. 28.2). Aneurysms of the hepatic artery have been discovered recently in patients who had previously undergone previous liver transplantation.[6] In a current series by Abbas *et al.*, 78 per cent of the HAAs were extrahepatic and 25 per cent of the HAAs were symptomatic, including 14 per cent presenting with rupture.[7] The most common symptoms are right upper quadrant pain, radiating to the back and unrelated to meals. Rupture may

occur into the peritoneal cavity, retroperitoneum, common bile duct, gallbladder, duodenum or portal vein. Erosion into the bile duct may cause haemobilia, and erosion into the duodenum will result in gastrointestinal haemorrhage.[5] About half of the symptomatic patients will have abdominal pain and half will present with gastrointestinal haemorrhage or haemobilia. Biliary colic and jaundice may occur in up to 10 per cent of patients because of extrinsic compression of the bile duct by the aneurysm.[2] The 'classic triad' of pain, haemobilia and obstructive jaundice is seen in less than 30 per cent of patients. Less commonly, patients may present with a right upper quadrant mass.

The majority of patients with SMA or coeliac artery aneurysms are symptomatic at the time of presentation, 38 per cent of them having ruptured aneurysms with a resulting mortality of 30–40 per cent.[2,8] As with SAAs, there may be a decreased risk of rupture of SMA aneurysms in patients taking β-blockade medication.[4] Most patients have abdominal pain which may be postprandial and mimic the symptoms of chronic mesenteric occlusive disease. Other signs and symptoms include a palpable abdominal mass, nausea, vomiting, jaundice or anaemia.[3] Rupture may result in gastrointestinal haemorrhage, haematemesis, shock or bowel infarction. Approximately 5 per cent of SMA aneurysms are mycotic, associated with systemic infection or subacute bacterial endocarditis.[4]

Aneurysms of the gastroduodenal, pancreatoduodenal and pancreatic arteries are often associated with pancreatitis and its complications. Up to 68 per cent of these aneurysms present with rupture and mortality as high as 50 per cent.[3] More than 80 per cent of these aneurysms are symptomatic causing abdominal pain at the time of diagnosis. Rupture at the time of diagnosis has been observed in 56 per cent of gastroduodenal aneurysms and 68 per cent of pancreatoduodenal aneurysms. Aneurysms may erode into an adjacent portion of the gastrointestinal tract, causing gastrointestinal haemorrhage or may rupture into the peritoneal cavity. Gastrointestinal haemorrhage or haemobilia occurs in approximately 50 per cent of patients. Jaundice occurs in an additional 14–31 per cent.[2,9]

Gastric and gastroepiploic aneurysms are rare, comprising only 4 per cent of all VAAs. The vast majority (90 per cent) of these aneurysms present as emergencies with rupture and gastrointestinal or intraperitoneal haemorrhage. Visceral aneurysms may also occur in the jejunal, ileal, colic or inferior mesenteric arteries. In a report by Tessier *et al.*, rupture occurred in 25 per cent of the mesenteric branch artery aneurysms and all were in colic arteries.[10] These patients may present with abdominal pain or haemorrhagic shock and a haematoma in the mesentery.[10]

DIAGNOSTIC STUDIES

With the increasing use of CT and angiography, more asymptomatic visceral artery aneurysms are being discovered.

Many VAAs contain calcification in the wall appearing as a curvilinear or signet ring shaped density on plain abdominal film or intravenous pyelogram (IVP). Characteristic 'egg shell' patterns of calcification may be seen in the epigastrium or upper abdominal quadrants.

Ultrasound or CT scans can be used to size these aneurysms accurately. Typical ultrasound findings include cystic or solid masses with sonolucent or mixed echo signals but ultrasound is very technician dependent. Contrast-enhanced CT is more appropriate in delineating and establishing the patency of the artery from which the visceral aneurysm arises. Non-contrast CT scans may reveal a low attenuation mass with or without peripheral rim calcification, haematomas around the porta hepatis, liver or in the retroperitoneal space. A haematoma in the lesser sac is often associated with a ruptured SAA. Contrast-enhanced CT scans will increase diagnostic accuracy. Visceral artery aneurysms will appear as a brightly enhanced lesion with a variable amount of luminal thrombus. Spiral CT angiography is an additional technique which can be of value in identifying VAAs and their arteries or origin.[8]

Magnetic resonance imaging is another imaging modality that can be used to evaluate visceral artery aneurysms. Non-iodinated contrast agents such as gadolinium used in MR angiography (MRA) are not nephrotoxic. Magnetic resonance angiography can define the vessels of origin and provide information on collateral flow. Despite advances in spiral CT angiography and MRA, conventional digital subtraction angiography is still the most commonly used diagnostic test. Contrast angiography provides accurate preoperative information and can also be used for therapeutic embolisation.

TREATMENT OPTIONS: SURGICAL AND ENDOVASCULAR

Most visceral aneurysms, excluding coeliac and SMA lesions, can be treated with surgical ligation. Endovascular methods of thromboembolisation are appropriate for treating selected visceral aneurysms.[11]

Splenic artery aneurysms

The risk of rupture of SAAs, in cases not associated with pregnancy, is low at only 2–5 per cent. However, the mortality associated with rupture is high, being approximately 30–40 per cent.[4] Splenic artery aneurysms can be especially dangerous in the pregnant patient, the majority of which rupture during the last trimester. Rupture during pregnancy is associated with a maternal mortality of 70 per cent and a foetal death rate of 95 per cent.[12,13] Therefore, women of childbearing age, even with small aneurysms, should be treated when diagnosed. Pseudoaneurysms associated with inflammation or trauma are fragile and likely to rupture,

and therefore should be treated urgently. Treatment is also indicated in patients with symptomatic or enlarging aneurysms.[5,14] Conversely, small asymptomatic aneurysms, less than 2–3 cm in diameter, can be safely observed, especially in older women.[4,15]

Operative treatment most frequently consists of splenectomy and removal of that portion of the splenic artery containing the aneurysm. Surgical exposure is obtained though the lesser sac where the splenic artery can be easily controlled. Proximal aneurysms can be excised or ligated, often with preservation of the spleen,[4,15] whereas those in the midportion of the vessel can be excluded with proximal and distal ligation or reconstructed with an end-to-end anastomosis.[16] Inflammatory aneurysms associated with pancreatitis are more difficult to treat, as the aneurysm may be embedded within the pancreas. Pseudoaneurysms associated with pancreatitis are most safely treated by direct ligation from within the aneurysm sac. Distal SAAs may necessitate partial pancreatectomy along with resection of the aneurysm.[15] Laparoscopic ligation of the splenic artery proximal and distal to the aneurysm provides a minimally invasive treatment option.[17]

Many patients with SAAs have acute or chronic medical conditions, such as pancreatitis, which put them at high risk for open surgical intervention.[18] Advances in guidewire techniques and microvascular instruments have encouraged the development of percutaneous embolisation as an alternative treatment of SAAs and other VAAs. Although most SAAs are treated surgically, transcatheter embolisation (TCE) is becoming a more commonly used form of treatment.[18,19] Selective catheterisation of the splenic artery or the aneurysm sac is followed by the introduction of coils, Gelfoam particles, or detachable balloons into the vessel. In the case of a saccular aneurysm, it is possible to fill the aneurysm sac with coils, also known as the 'packing' method, while maintaining flow within the splenic artery and thus preserving the spleen. A possible complication of this form of therapy is embolic ischaemia of the spleen, infarction and even abscess formation[19] (Fig. 28.3). Other complications include pain, fever, embolisation to other visceral arteries, incomplete occlusion and recanalisation.[20] The postembolisation syndrome, consisting of abdominal pain, fever, slowed transit and elevation of pancreatic enzymes, can occur in up to 30 per cent of cases and generally resolves over 3–5 days.[18] Staged TCE, inducing arterial occlusion over a few days, may reduce the risk of splenic infarction. Recently, stent grafts, such as the Wallgraft endoprosthesis and the Jostent stent graft have been used to treat large visceral aneurysms and preserve splenic flow.[21]

Hepatic artery aneurysms

About 34 per cent of HAAs are intrahepatic, many of them small and multiple, making surgical exposure difficult.

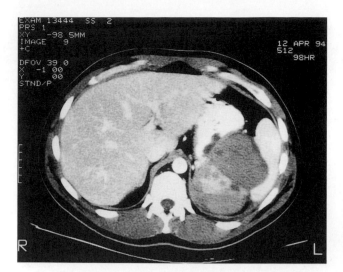

Figure 28.3 *A splenic artery aneurysm was successfully thrombosed with percutaneous transcatheter embolisation. The patient developed ischaemic infarction of the spleen with abscess formation*

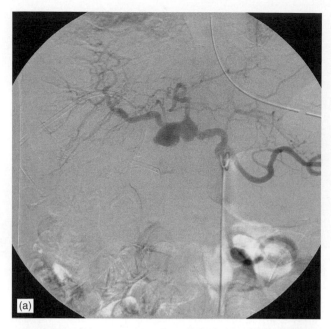

(a)

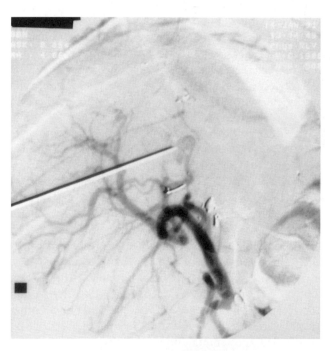

Figure 28.4 *Recurrence of this hepatic artery aneurysm occurred after embolisation of the right hepatic artery. Successful thrombosis was obtained using a combined percutaneous transhepatic and transarterial approach. Note the needle approaching the aneurysm for direct puncture and occlusion*

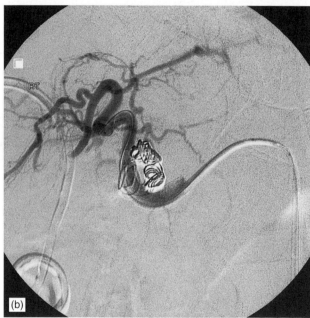

(b)

Figure 28.5 *(a) A 56-year-old man developed haemobilia following common bile duct resection and placement of a transhepatic biliary catheter. Arteriography demonstrated a pseudoaneurysm originating from the right hepatic artery. (b) The aneurysm was treated with coil embolisation followed by the placement of a Viabond stent graft (Gore)*

Although partial liver resection is a therapeutic option, this operation is performed for HAA much less commonly today. Most of these intrahepatic aneurysms are treated with TCE.[3] Selective catheterisation of the hepatic artery and its branches allows for TCE and thrombosis of the aneurysm sac. The feeding vessel should be embolised as distally as possible because occlusion of a more proximal vessel may result in incomplete thrombosis and recurrence.[22] Recanalisation or incomplete thrombosis can occur and therefore it is necessary to obtain follow-up angiography. Often a staged approach is required to achieve complete thrombosis. Transcatheter embolisation can be combined with direct percutaneous puncture of the HAA in some cases[15] (Fig. 28.4). As with SAAs, stent grafts may be used in the common hepatic artery or its proximal branches[21] (Fig. 28.5).

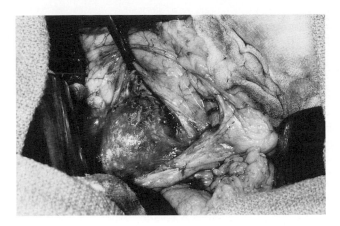

Figure 28.6 *Intraoperative photograph of an aneurysm of the common hepatic artery. The aneurysm was treated with excision and revascularisation using autogenous saphenous vein*

Larger, extrahepatic aneurysms usually require surgical ligation with or without revascularisation (Fig 28.6). Aneurysms proximal to the gastroduodenal artery can be treated by excision or exclusion without reconstruction because of collateral flow from the SMA via the gastroduodenal artery. In cases where collateral flow is insufficient or if the gastroduodenal artery is involved arterial reconstruction is required. Surgical options for vascular reconstruction include interposition graft, aorto-hepatic artery bypass or spleno-hepatic bypass using saphenous vein or hypogastric artery.[3,14] Non-operative management may be appropriate in the following situations: patients at high operative risk, those with a life expectancy less than 2 years, when HAAs are asymptomatic and of less than 2 cm diameter. Careful observation with serial radiological examinations is recommended.[7]

Superior mesenteric and coeliac artery aneurysms

The potential for SMA and coeliac aneurysms to produce life-threatening haemorrhage or bowel ischaemia makes intervention with ligation or resection of the aneurysm entirely appropriate. For proximally located aneurysms, vascular reconstruction using aorto-mesenteric bypass or reimplantation is required.[16] Aneurysms of the midportion of the SMA may be treated with excision or ligation and an interposition graft[3,19,23] (Fig. 28.7).

Similarly, patients with coeliac artery aneurysms are most often treated with excision and vascular reconstruction. Exposure of the coeliac artery is obtained through a transabdominal incision with medial rotation of the viscera or directly through the lesser sac (also see Chapter 36). In a life-threatening emergency, simple ligation of the coeliac artery aneurysm may be indicated. Ligation, however, may result in hepatic necrosis in patients with insufficient collateral flow and should be used with caution in those with pre-existing liver disease.[24]

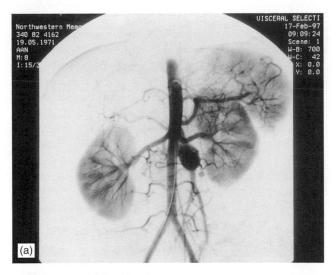

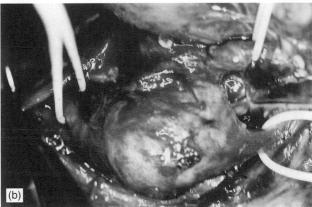

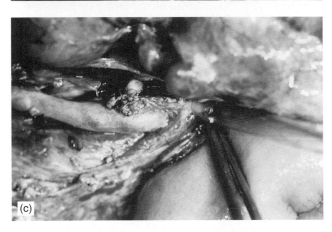

Figure 28.7 *A large superior mesenteric artery aneurysm was discovered in a 32-year-old woman who presented with intermittent abdominal pain in the postpartum period. (a) Visceral arteriogram demonstrating the superior mesenteric artery (SMA) aneurysm. (b) Intraoperative view of the aneurysm. (c) Interposition autogenous saphenous vein graft replacing the excised SMA aneurysm*

In high risk patients, TCE may be a useful alternative to open surgery.[23] This may be particularly useful for saccular aneurysms arising from the side of the SMA and for some pseudoaneurysms. Aneurysms of the first branch of the

SMA with sufficient collaterals may also be treated with TCE.[25] Slow growing aneurysms with enlarged collateral vessels present may be successfully occluded without vascular reconstruction. Embolisation, however, is not recommended for fusiform aneurysms of the SMA trunk. Because of the risk of intestinal infarction, TCE should be reserved for high risk patients with favourable anatomy and adequate collateral flow. Embolisation of the coeliac artery is a potential treatment option, but little has been published regarding this form of therapy. Aneurysms may also occur in the coeliac axis for which resection of the aneurysm and revascularisation will be necessary.[26,27]

Gastroduodenal, pancreaticoduodenal and pancreatic artery aneurysms

Surgery for aneurysms of the gastroduodenal, pancreatico-duodenal and pancreatic arteries involves ligation and may also necessitate treatment of associated pancreatitis or pseudocyst.[28,29] Aneurysms in the middle or distal region of the pancreas call for distal pancreatic resection. These aneurysms often have multiple communicating vessels making simple ligation difficult. Endoaneurysmectomy and suture ligation of the feeding vessels from within the sac will prevent recurrence.

Open surgery in patients with these aneurysms can be especially dangerous with mortality of 13 per cent or higher. Percutaneous treatment with TCE has become more popular and is becoming the preferred treatment for most gastroduodenal, pancreaticoduodenal and pancreatic artery aneurysms [28,30] The availability of wires and catheters for super-selective catheterisation of small feeding vessels permits the precise localisation and treatment of these difficult aneurysms. The collateral circulation between the coeliac artery and SMA ensures that satisfactory blood flow remains even after embolisation of the parent artery in both the distal and proximal portion of the aneurysm.[31,32] These aneurysms, and especially pseudoaneurysms, can be very fragile and embolisation may result in secondary rupture.[30,32]

There have been several case reports of aneurysms of the GDA or the pancreaticoduodenal artery associated with coeliac artery occlusive disease. The increased blood flow in these enlarged collateral vessels is thought to be the causative factor. Coeliac artery occlusive disease may result from atherosclerosis or from compression by the median arcuate ligament. Transcatheter embolisation of these aneurysms via the SMA can be especially useful in the treatment of a bleeding aneurysm.[33] Most ruptured aneurysms are still treated surgically with mesenteric revascularisation of the coeliac artery and ligation or resection of the aneurysm[34] (Fig. 28.8).

Gastric and gastroepiploic artery aneurysms

Gastric and gastroepiploic artery aneurysms occurring in an extragastric location may be treated with ligation or

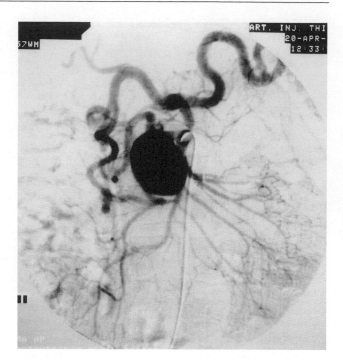

Figure 28.8   *Visceral arteriogram demonstrating an aneurysm of the pancreaticoduodenal artery (PDA) in a patient with arterial occlusive disease of the coeliac and superior mesenteric arteries. The PDA aneurysm developed in an important collateral vessel. The patient was treated with aorto-coeliac and aorta-to-superior mesenteric artery bypass, using autogenous saphenous vein, followed by ligation of the aneurysm*

excision of the aneurysm. In these situations TCE represents a good treatment option and is being increasingly employed.[24]

Mesenteric branch artery aneurysms

Surgical treatment of aneurysms of the jejunal, ileal and colic arteries usually involves ligation or resection of the aneurysm, sometimes along with a portion of the bowel which it supplies.[14] Super-selective catheterisation of the aneurysm with the injection of embolic material has been reported as a possible option[10,25] (Fig. 28.9). Transcatheter embolisation must be used with caution in these lesions because of the risk of infarcting the segment of bowel supplied by the parent artery.[24]

MANAGEMENT STRATEGIES AND RECOMMENDATIONS

The various types of VAAs differ somewhat in their natural history and treatment options. The surgeon must decide whether or not to treat an aneurysm based on their knowledge of the natural history of the disease and the risks associated with a particular intervention. Unlike abdominal aortic aneurysms, the natural history of visceral artery

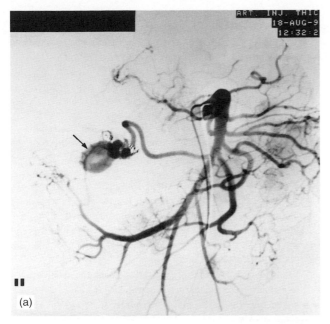

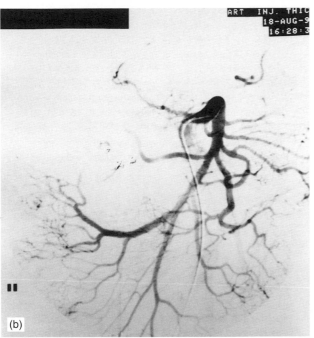

Figure 28.9 *An aneurysm of a branch of the superior mesenteric artery in a high risk patient with a 'hostile abdomen' successfully treated using transcatheter embolisation. (a) The aneurysm (arrowed) originating from a branch of the superior mesenteric artery. (b) Successful thrombosis with coils*

aneurysms is mostly unknown. At our institution, 42 per cent of the VAAs that were diagnosed presented with rupture. In this series the mortality rate from rupture was 25 per cent.[19] Although ruptured VAAs must be treated, controversy surrounds management when they are found incidentally and remain asymptomatic. Unlike aortic aneurysms, the relation between VAA aneurysm size and risk of rupture is not clear. There may be several appropriate

treatment options for a particular type of VAA. The understandable lack of a large patient series precludes consensus on best practice but recommendations can be made based upon published literature and current experience.

The CT scan is the best test for detecting a VAA. As multiple VAAs are often seen, all patients with known VAAs should undergo contrast arteriography. Haemodynamically unstable patients are best taken directly to the operating room for emergency exploration and ligation of the bleeding vessel.[35,36] If the patient is stable enough to undergo arteriography, information obtained radiologically will assist in planning an operative procedure or in considering treatment either by TCE or the insertion of a stent graft.

Most SAAs which present with rupture are at least 2 cm in diameter. Patients with enlarging or symptomatic aneurysms should be treated. The tendency for these aneurysms to expand and rupture during pregnancy requires that women of childbearing age should have them treated electively. Aneurysms found during pregnancy should be dealt with before the third trimester. Patients with portal hypertension or those who have a portocaval shunt are also at increased risk of rupture. These aneurysms may rupture following liver transplantation and therefore aneurysm repair at the time of transplantation, or in a staged approach, should be considered.[37] Although SAAs in young patients should be treated, smaller aneurysms in elderly or high risk patients may be safely observed.[15] Open surgery is the preferred treatment for ruptured SAAs. Although in the elective setting preservation of the spleen is preferred in order to avoid postsplenectomy sepsis, in the case of rupture, splenectomy and resection of the aneurysm is necessary. In patients presenting with pancreatitis or portal hypertension the operative mortality for open surgery can be quite high. Transcatheter embolisation or stent graft treatment may be a better option for patients who are not good surgical candidates. Percutaneous therapy is especially attractive for aneurysms associated with pancreatic inflammation or the 'hostile abdomen'.[19,36]

The optimal size at which HAAs should be treated has not been clearly established. There is evidence to suggest that some small aneurysms of less than 2 cm diameter may be safely observed.[7] Although more HAAs are being discovered in asymptomatic patients, many still present with rupture. The known mortality rate from rupture of approximately 30 per cent supports an aggressive approach to incidentally discovered lesions in the patient with a low risk for surgical intervention.[7] Risk factors for rupture include multiple HAAs and those of non-atherosclerotic origin, in particular aneurysms associated with polyarteritis nodosa.[7] Pseudoaneurysms may also be at increased risk of rupture. Intrahepatic artery aneurysms are most commonly treated with transarterial or TCE techniques. Aneurysms of the common hepatic artery should be treated by open surgery and arterial reconstruction.[15,24] Endovascular stent graft placement offers another option for aneurysms of the common hepatic artery in patients at high risk for surgery.[10]

Many SMA and coeliac artery aneurysms are symptomatic at the time of diagnosis. The dangers of bowel ischaemia or life-threatening haemorrhage are persuasive reasons for treating them, except for small asymptomatic aneurysms in the high risk patient. Ligation or resection of the aneurysm with arterial revascularisation is the treatment of choice.

Faced with aneurysms of the gastroepiploic, pancreaticoduodenal or pancreatic arteries the best treatment is TCE.[38,39] Open surgery is indicated when a pseudocyst or other intra-abdominal pathology is present, when percutaneous treatment fails or in the low risk patient.[40] Bleeding aneurysms of the gastric and gastroepiploic arteries are best treated with TCE. As at least 90 per cent of these aneurysms present with rupture, incidentally discovered gastric or gastroepiploic artery aneurysms should be treated electively with TCE. Mesenteric branch artery aneurysms are best treated with ligation of the aneurysm and resection of the adjacent portion of the bowel.[10]

Conclusion

An aggressive approach is indicated in the treatment of most VAAs. In our experience, these aneurysms usually tend to expand, produce symptoms and rupture, sometimes with fatal results. Once rupture occurs, ligation of the bleeding vessel is most often sufficient, but revascularisation is sometimes indicated because of lack of adequate collateral flow. Endovascular interventional choices for VAAs should take into account the location of the aneurysm, the perceived risk of rupture and the anticipated morbidity and mortality of the intended treatment.

Key references

Abbas MH, Fowl RJ, Stone WM, et al. Hepatic artery aneurysm factors that predict complications. J Vasc Surg 2003; **38**: 41–5.

Abbas MH, Stone WM, Fowl RJ, et al. Splenic artery aneurysm: two decades experience at Mayo Clinic. Ann Vasc Surg 2002; **16**: 442–9.

Carr SC, Pearce WH. Management of visceral artery aneurysms. Practical Vasc Surg 1999: 241–58.

Shanley CJ, Shah NL, Messina BS, Messina LM. Common splanchnic artery aneurysms: splenic, hepatic, and celiac. Ann Vasc Surg 1996; **10**: 315–22.

Tessier DJ, Abbas MH, Flowl RJ, et al. Management of rare mesenteric arterial branch aneurysms. Ann Vasc Surg 2002; **16**: 586–90.

REFERENCES

1 Rokko S, Amundsen S, Bjerke-Larssen T, et al. The diagnosis and management of splanchnic artery aneurysms. Scan J Gastroenterol 1996; **31**: 737–42.

2 Shanley CJ, Shah NL, Messina BS, Messina LM. Common splanchnic artery aneurysms: splenic, hepatic, and celiac. Ann Vasc Surg 1996; **10**: 315–22.

3 Messina LM, Shanley CJ. Mesenteric ischemia. Surg Clin North Am 1997; **77**: 425–43.

4 Abbas MH, Stone WM, Fowl RJ, et al. Splenic artery aneurysm: two decades experience at Mayo Clinic. Ann Vasc Surg 2002; **16**: 442–9.

5 Rokko S, Amundsen S, Bjerke-Larssen T, Jensen D. Review: the diagnosis and management of splanchnic artery aneurysms. Scand J Gastroenterol 1996; **31**: 737–43.

6 Leelaudomlipi S, Bramhall SR, Gunson BK, et al. Hepatic-artery aneurysm in adult transplantation. Transpl Int 2003; **16**: 257–61.

7 Abbas MH, Fowl RJ, Stone WM, et al. Hepatic artery aneurysm factors that predict complications. J Vasc Surg 2003; **38**: 41–5.

8 Stone WM, Abbas M, Cherry KJ, et al. Superior mesenteric artery aneurysm: is presence an indication for intervention? J Vasc Surg 2002; **36**: 234–7.

9 Shanley CJ, Shah NL, Messina BS, Messina LM. Uncommon splanchnic artery aneurysms: pancreaticoduodenal, gastroduodenal, superior mesenteric, inferior mesenteric, and colic. Ann Vasc Surg 1996; **10**: 506–15.

10 Tessier DJ, Abbas MH, Flowl RJ, et al. Management of rare mesenteric arterial branch aneurysms. Ann Vasc Surg 2002; **16**: 586–90.

11 Hossain A, Reis ED, Dave SP, et al. Visceral artery aneurysms: experience in a tertiary-care center. Am Surgeon 2001; **67**: 432–7.

12 Asokan S, Chew EK, Ng KY, et al. Post partum splenic artery aneurysm rupture. J Obstet Gynecol Res 2000; **26**: 199–201.

13 Herbeck M, Horbach T, Putzenlechner C, et al. Ruptured splenic artery aneurysm during pregnancy: a rare case with both maternal and fetal survival. Am J Obstet Gynecol 1999; **181**: 763–4.

14 de Perrot M, Buhler L, Deleaval J, et al. Management of true aneurysms of the splenic artery. Am J Surg 1998; **175**: 466–8.

15 Carr SC, Pearce WH, Vogelzang RL, et al. Current management of visceral artery aneurysms. Surgery 1996; **120**: 627–33.

16 Grego FG, Lepidi S, Ragazzi R, et al. Visceral artery aneurysms: a single center experience. Cardiovasc Surg 2003; **1**: 19–25.

17 Arca MJ, Gagner M, Hentford BT, et al. Splenic artery aneurysms: methods of laparoscopic repair. J Vasc Surg 1999 **30**: 184–8.

18 Guillon R, Garcier JM, Abergel A, et al. Management of splenic artery aneurysms and false aneurysms with endovascular treatment in 12 patients. Cardiovasc Intervent Radiol 2003; **26**: 256–60.

19 Carr SC, Mahvi DM, Hoch JR, et al. Visceral artery aneurysm rupture. J Vasc Surg 2001; **33**: 806–11.

20 Melissano G, Chlesa R. Successful surgical treatment of visceral artery aneurysms after failure of percutaneous treatment. Tex Heart Inst J 1998; **25**: 75–8.

21 Larson RA, Solomon J, Carpenter JP. Stent graft repair of visceral artery aneurysms. J Vasc Surg 2002; **36**: 1260–3.

22 Tarazov PG, Ryzhkov VK, Polysavov VN, et al. Extraorganic hepatic artery aneurysm: failure of transcatheter embolization. HPB Surg 1998; **11**: 55–60.

23 Zimmerman-Klima PM, Wixon CL, Bogey WM Jr, et al. Considerations in the management of aneurysms of the superior mesenteric artery. Ann Vasc Surg 2000; **14**: 410–14.

24 Carr SC, Pearce WH. Management of visceral artery aneurysms. Practical Vasc Surg 1999: 241–58.

25 Lorelli DR, Cambria RA, Seabrook GR, Towne JB. Diagnosis and management of aneurysms involving the superior mesenteric artery and its branches. A report of four cases. *Vasc Endovasc Surg* 2003; **37**: 59–66.

26 Veraldi GF, Dorrucci V, deManzoni G, *et al.* Aneurysm of the celiac trunk: diagnosis with US-color-doppler. Presentation of a new case and review of the literature. *Hepatogastroenterology* 1999; **46**: 781–3.

27 Detroux M, Anidjar S, Nottin R, Robinson LP. Aneurysm of a common celiomesenteric trunk. *Ann Vasc Surg* 1998; **12**: 78–82.

28 Coll DP, Ierardi R, Kerstein MD, *et al.* Aneurysms of the pancreaticoduodenal arteries: a change in management. *Ann Vasc Surg* 1998; **12**: 286–91.

29 Konstantakos AK, Coogan S, Husni EA, Raaf JH. Aneurysm of the gastroduodenal artery: an unusual cause of obstructive jaundice. *Am Surgeon* 2000; **66**: 695–8.

30 Yamagami T, Arai Y, Sueyoshi S, *et al.* Letter to editor re: embolization of ruptured pancreaticoduodenal artery aneurysm: report of two cases. *Cardiovasc Intervent Radiol* 1999; **22**: 440–2.

31 Kasirajan K, Greenberg RK, Clair D, Ouriel K. Endovascular management of visceral artery aneurysm. *J Endovasc Ther* 2001; **8**: 150–5.

32 de Perrot M, Berney T, Deleaval J, *et al.* Management of true aneurysm of the pancreaticoduodenal arteries. *Ann Surg* 1999; **229**: 416–20.

33 Kobayashi S, Yamaguchi A, Isogai M, *et al.* Successful transcatheter embolization of a pancreaticoduodenal artery aneurysm in association with celiac axis occlusion: a case report. *Hepatogastroenterology* 1999; **46**: 2991–4.

34 Suzuki K, Kashimura H, Sato M, *et al.* Pancreaticoduodenal artery aneurysms associated with celiac axis stenosis due to compression by median arcuate ligament and celiac plexus. *J Gastreoenterol* 1998; **33**: 434–8.

35 Wagner WH, Allins AD, Treiman RL, *et al.* Ruptured visceral artery aneurysms. *Ann Vasc Surg* 1997; **11**: 342–7.

36 Carmeci C, McClenathan J. Visceral artery aneurysms as seen in a community hospital. *Am J Surg* 2000; **179**: 486–9.

37 Jovine E, Mazziotti A, Grazi GL, *et al.* Rupture of splenic artery aneurysm after liver transplantation. *Clin Transplantation* 1996; **10**: 451–4.

38 deWeerth A, Buggisch P, Nicolas V, Maas R. Pancreaticoduodenal artery aneurysm – a life-threatening cause of gastrointestinal hemorrhage: case report and review of the literature. *Hepatogastroenterology* 1998; **45**: 1651–4.

39 Neschis DG, Safford SD, Golden MA. Management of pancreaticoduodenal artery aneurysms presenting as catastrophic intraabdominal bleeding. *Surgery* 1998; **123**: 8–12.

40 Yeh TS, Jan YY, Jeng LB, *et al.* Massive extra-enteric gastrointestinal hemorrhage secondary to splanchnic artery aneurysms. *Hepatogastroenterology* 1997; **44**: 1152–6.

29

Mesenteric Ischaemia

DARYLL M BAKER, JANICE TSUI, AVERIL O MANSFIELD

THE PROBLEM

Mesenteric ischaemia can be classified into acute and chronic disease, which present very differently clinically and require different management approaches. Here, the focus will be on acute mesenteric ischaemia, which presents as a catastrophic surgical emergency with high morbidity and mortality. It represents 0.1 per cent of hospital admissions[1] with reported mortality rates of 60–100 per cent.[1–4]

Prompt diagnosis and aggressive management are required. Correct diagnosis in the early stages, however, is often difficult due to the non-specific nature of symptoms resulting in delay in diagnosis.[5]

AETIOLOGY

The commonest causes of mesenteric ischaemia are mesenteric arterial occlusion due to thrombus or embolus, mesenteric venous occlusion and non-occlusive mesenteric ischaemia.[1] Rare causes include mechanical causes, haematological, vasculitic and endocrine conditions and drug induced events. The relative frequencies of these causes are shown in Table 29.1.

PATHOPHYSIOLOGY

Acute insufficiency of the blood supply to the small bowel and/or right colon causes hypoxic insult to the gut. At cellular

Table 29.1 *Aetiology of acute mesenteric ischaemia*

Causes	Frequency (per cent)[6]
Acute mesenteric arterial embolus	50
Acute mesenteric arterial thrombosis	25
Non-occlusive mesenteric ischaemia	20
Acute mesenteric venous thrombosis	5
Miscellaneous causes	Rare

level, high energy phosphates such as adenosine 5′ triphosphate (ATP) are depleted, with a build-up of catabolic products and lactate.[7] Mucosal permeability increases and tissue injury, which is initially reversible, occurs (see Chapter 3). The severity of the injury depends on the duration and severity of ischaemia, and ranges from mucosal infarction where the lesion does not extend deeper than the muscularis mucosae, to mural infarction involving the mucosa and submucosa and to transmural infarction where all visceral layers are affected[8] (Fig. 29.1).

Subsequent reperfusion may lead to ischaemia-reperfusion injury resulting in further tissue damage, which is in part due to free radical production via the xanthine oxidase pathway[9] (see Chapter 2). Further tissue necrosis occurs, with increased capillary permeability, protein leak into the gut lumen and translocation of bacteria, endotoxin and gut enzymes into the portal circulation,[10] and systemic complications.[11] This could lead to the development of multiple organ dysfunction syndrome with its associated high mortality[12] (see Chapter 4).

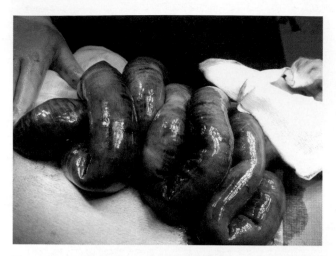

Figure 29.1 *Mesenteric infarction*

Acute mesenteric arterial embolism

The usual sources of emboli are left atrial or ventricular mural thrombi or cardiac valvular lesions.[1] The majority of emboli impact on the superior mesenteric artery (SMA) just distal to the origin of the middle colic artery. Reactive mesenteric vasoconstriction may also occur, reducing collateral flow and exacerbating ischaemic injury.

Acute mesenteric arterial thrombosis

Thrombosis of the SMA or coeliac axis usually occurs at regions of pre-existing atherosclerotic plaques. This usually occurs at the origin of the vessel.[1]

Non-occlusive mesenteric ischaemia

Low mesenteric flow may result in mesenteric ischaemia in the absence of anatomical arterial or venous obstruction. Causes of low-flow states include cardiogenic shock, sepsis and administration of vasoconstrictors such as digoxin or α-adrenergic agents. Excessive sympathetic activity is stimulated during these conditions in an attempt to maintain cardiac and cerebral perfusion, and may cause mesenteric vasospasm.[13] Underlying atherosclerotic arterial disease is usually also present.

Acute mesenteric venous thrombosis

Conditions predisposing to acute mesenteric venous thrombosis include hypercoagulability, cirrhosis, splenomegaly, malignancy, infection, trauma, pancreatitis and diverticular disease.[14] Bowel wall oedema, increased outflow resistance and increased blood viscosity impede arterial flow resulting in bowel infarction.[1] Massive fluid influx into the bowel wall and lumen can occur, resulting in hypovolaemia and haemoconcentration.

DIAGNOSIS

Clinical presentation

Patients present with severe abdominal pain which is frequently out of proportion to the physical findings.[6] This may be accompanied by sudden gut emptying, by vomiting and/or defaecation. Symptoms may occur suddenly and progress within a few hours, usually due to acute mesenteric ischaemia secondary to embolisation, but may also present more insidiously with progression of symptoms over a few days.

On physical examination, few signs are present in the early phases. The abdomen may be distended but bowel sounds are present. As bowel ischaemia progresses to infarction, peritoneal signs develop. The abdomen becomes severely tender and grossly distended with absent bowel sounds.

Investigations

Investigations should not lead to unnecessary delays in revascularisation. Laboratory investigations are non-specific and abnormal findings tend to develop late. They include a rise in the haemoglobin and haematocrit consistent with haemoconcentration, leucocytosis with left shift, elevated liver enzymes, serum amylase and lactic dehydrogenase, and metabolic acidosis.[6]

Plain abdominal X-rays are useful in excluding other causes of abdominal pain such as bowel obstruction and perforation. An ileus or bowel wall thickening due to submucosal oedema or haemorrhage may be seen in mesenteric ischaemia, but in 25 per cent of these patients completely normal plain abdominal X-rays have been reported.[15] In the late stages, pneumatosis of the bowel wall may be detected and portal vein gas indicates an extremely poor prognosis.[1]

Duplex ultrasonography is a simple, non-invasive test which can help in assessing the patency of the mesenteric vessels.[16] However, technical expertise is required and the presence of dilated loops of bowel in many patients makes it impossible to image the coeliac axis and the SMA.

Abdominal computed tomography (CT) scan may show bowel wall thickening in subacute mesenteric ischaemia. In mesenteric vein thrombosis, thrombus or lack of opacification of the mesenteric veins with intravenous contrast may be observed,[17] whereas non-enhancement of the mesenteric arteries following timed intravenous contrast injections may identify mesenteric arterial thrombosis or embolisation. Pneumatosis and portal vein gas can also be visualised.

Mesenteric angiography remains the definitive diagnostic test. It is performed via a transfemoral approach and both anteroposterior and lateral views are required for adequate assessment of the vessels. Angiography not only enables visualisation of the mesenteric vessels with identification of the cause of ischaemia, but also detects any underlying atherosclerotic disease, which is important in the planning of revascularisation procedures. Intra-arterial infusion of vasodilators can be also commenced and endovascular procedures carried out if appropriate (see below).

ANGIOGRAPHIC FINDINGS

Superior mesenteric artery emboli appear as sharp rounded filling defects on the angiogram but they may also occlude the origin of the SMA and be mistaken for thrombosis. Distal vessels are poorly visualised due to poor collateral flow and intense vasospasm but minimal atherosclerotic changes are usually seen in other vessels. Acute SMA thrombosis appears as an abrupt cut-off of the vessel at or within 2 cm of the origin. Atherosclerotic narrowing of other vessels and vasospasm are often seen. Large collaterals from the coeliac axis or inferior mesentery artery suggest underlying chronic mesenteric ischaemia.

In non-occlusive mesenteric ischaemia, SMA occlusion is not seen but narrowing of the SMA branch origins and irregularities and impaired filling of vessels indicative of vasospasm are observed. Partial occlusion or non-opacification of the superior mesenteric and portal veins occurs in mesenteric vein thrombosis. Delayed arterial emptying and vasospasm may also be seen.

TREATMENT

General principles

The patient should be resuscitated aggressively, intravenous anticoagulation commenced to prevent thrombus propagation and angiography performed promptly if acute mesenteric ischaemia is suspected. Endovascular procedures may be suitable in selected patients with no peritoneal signs, proceeding to surgery if symptoms deteriorate or success is not evident within 4 hours. Surgical management involves revascularisation and resection of necrotic bowel. Frankly necrotic bowel should be resected and the extent of bowel resection minimised by planning a second look laparotomy in 12–24 hours to reassess bowel viability and for further resection if necessary. Bowel continuity can be restored primarily or stomas exteriorised and anastomosed at a later stage.

Initial resuscitation

Resuscitation should be commenced immediately under adequate monitoring with a urinary catheter, central venous access or pulmonary artery catheter where necessary. Admission to the intensive care unit may be required. Volume deficit and metabolic disturbances should be corrected with intravenous crystalloids and blood products where necessary. Causative factors such as cardiac failure should be treated. Intravenous heparin should be commenced to prevent further thrombus propagation. Antibiotics effective against bowel flora should be administered. Nasogastric decompression should be instituted to avoid aspiration.

Endovascular procedures

SELECTIVE INTRA-ARTERIAL VASODILATOR INFUSIONS

At the time of angiography, selective SMA catheter infusion of vasodilating agents such as papaverine can be administered. This is the primary therapy for non-occlusive mesenteric ischaemia, but is also useful in reducing visceral vasoconstriction present in all forms of acute mesenteric ischaemia. Heparin is also administered to prevent thrombosis in the cannulated vessel but must be infused through a separate line to avoid precipitation when mixed with papaverine. Other vasodilators such as phenoxybenzamine and prostaglandin E_1 have also been used in this way but with less success than papaverine. Local complications of intra-arterial vasodilator infusions include pericatheter thrombosis and puncture site haematoma and haemorrhage. Systemic hypotension is rare unless the catheter becomes dislodged from the SMA.[18]

THROMBOLYSIS AND ANGIOPLASTY

In highly selected patients with an early diagnosis of SMA embolus with no signs of peritonism, intra-arterial thrombolytic therapy delivered at the time of angiography may be used in specialised units.[19,20] During therapy, patients must be closely monitored and development of any peritoneal signs or failure of lysis within 4 hours are indications for immediate surgical exploration.[1] Percutaneous angioplasty of atherosclerotic plaques at the SMA origin unmasked by thrombolysis has also been reported.[21,22] However, this is technically difficult and restenosis rates of 25–50 per cent have been reported.

Surgery

Most patients with acute mesenteric ischaemia require surgical exploration when the diagnosis is confirmed, other pathologies excluded, the bowel revascularised and infarcted bowel removed. The operating room should be kept as warm as possible to prevent further vasoconstriction. A midline incision is used and the abdomen fully explored. The extent of bowel ischaemia and necrosis is assessed (see below). Revascularisation is carried out before resecting necrotic bowel, but if the extent of bowel necrosis is very extensive, endarterectomy or palliative treatment are the only options.

SURGICAL EXPOSURE OF THE SMA

The proximal SMA is exposed by first retracting the transverse colon superiorly and the small bowel inferiorly and

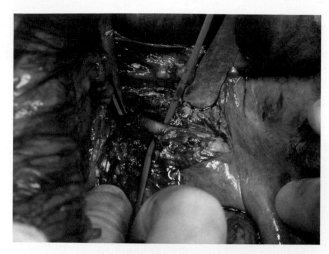

Figure 29.2 *Superior mesenteric artery exposed*

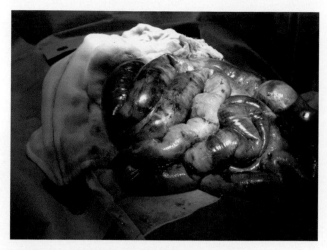

Figure 29.3 *Rationale for 'second look': a segment of bowel had undergone resection but at the 'second look' exploration there are further areas of necrosis requiring further resection*

to the right. The small bowel mesentery is incised at a point in the root of the transverse mesocolon where the middle colic artery ascends, and the proximal SMA is dissected free between the pancreas and the fourth part of the duodenum. To expose both the SMA and the coeliac axis, the lesser sac is opened lateral to the oesophagus. The supracoeliac aorta is exposed by dividing the median arcuate ligament and carefully dissected caudally until the coeliac axis is reached. The SMA is then exposed under the upper border of the pancreas (Fig. 29.2).

ASSESSMENT OF BOWEL ISCHAEMIA

Necrotic bowel must be resected to prevent perforation and sepsis. It is important, however, to preserve as much viable bowel as possible to avert the complications of the short bowel syndrome.

Intraoperatively, bowel viability is assessed visually according to its colour, sheen, peristaltic activity and presence of pulses, where dark, dull bowel with no visible peristalsis and absent pulses indicate non-viable bowel. These signs, however, are not always reliable. Doppler ultrasonography can be used to aid in the assessment of bowel viability by detecting arterial and venous flow in the mesentery. This is a simple, inexpensive method but it requires experience to obtain reliable results.

An alternative or additional method is the administration of intravenous fluorescein followed by illumination with Wood's ultraviolet light to confirm bowel perfusion. Normal bowel shows a homogeneous yellow-green pattern while patchy fluorescence or areas of non-fluorescence are not viable. Other techniques have been investigated, but Doppler ultrasonography and fluorescein dye remain the most useful although limited in their sensitivity and specificity.[23]

MANAGEMENT OF BOWEL ISCHAEMIA

The management of infarcted bowel depends on the degree and extent of tissue necrosis. A single short segment of non-viable bowel can be resected and a primary anastomosis

performed. More commonly, several regions of the bowel are affected and the degree of ischaemia is unclear. Obviously necrotic areas are resected and bowel ends are exteriorised as stomas. A 'second-look' laparotomy is undertaken 12–24 hours later to assess bowel of questionable viability (Fig. 29.3) when non-viable bowel is resected and the ends may be anastomosed.[24] This allows a conservative approach to bowel resection at the initial laparotomy preserving as much bowel as possible. Once the decision to perform a 'second look' laparotomy has been made, it should be carried out regardless of the patient's clinical condition because a significant proportion of patients not showing signs of clinical deterioration at this time do require further bowel resection.[5]

Where there is extensive small bowel infarction, the patient's prognosis is extremely poor, and the decision to carry out extensive bowel resection or to manage the patient palliatively has to be made. The premorbid medical condition of the patient is important because those with other atherosclerotic manifestations such as severe ischaemic heart disease and previous debilitating cerebrovascular episodes are poor candidates for massive bowel resection. Bowel perforations, sepsis and multiple organ dysfunction syndrome are indicators of high mortality (see Chapters 3 and 4). Where extensive small bowel resection is carried out, lifelong total parenteral nutrition will be required in surviving patients. An algorithm (Fig. 29.4) provides a pathway of care in suspected acute mesenteric ischaemia.

Definitive operative treatment

Operative procedures are designed to meet specific manifestations of acute mesenteric ischaemia.

ACUTE MESENTERIC ARTERIAL EMBOLISM

The site and extent of the embolus can be determined by direct palpation of the SMA, where the proximal pulse is

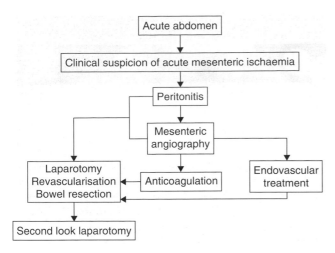

Figure 29.4 *Algorithm providing a pathway of care for patients with suspected acute mesenteric infarction*

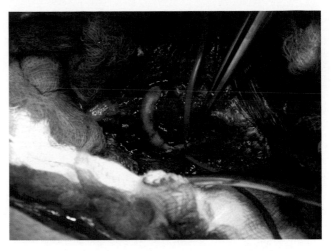

Figure 29.5 *Saphenous vein bypass onto the superior mesenteric artery*

usually palpable. The SMA is then mobilised at or just distal to the level of the obstruction. Vascular loops are used for proximal and distal control. Heparin should have been administered by this stage. A small transverse or a longitudinal arteriotomy is made. The embolus is removed and a balloon embolectomy catheter passed proximally and distally in the artery to retrieve residual embolus. Once adequate inflow and back-bleeding have been established, the vessel is flushed with heparin saline. Transverse arteriotomies are closed primarily in a transverse fashion and longitudinal arteriotomies are closed with a vein patch to prevent narrowing of the vessel.

ACUTE MESENTERIC ARTERIAL THROMBOSIS

The site of thrombosis is most commonly in the proximal 1–3 cm of the SMA and therefore the proximal pulse is not palpable. Thrombosis usually occurs at the site of atherosclerotic narrowing. Revascularisation is usually required as thrombectomy and endarterectomy is technically difficult, requiring exposure of the supracoeliac aorta and the proximal mesenteric vessels[25] and early re-occlusion rates are high.[18]

Retrograde or antegrade bypasses can be used. A short side-to-side bypass graft from the aorta to the SMA distal to the obstruction is the simplest procedure.[18] However, extensive aortic atherosclerosis may preclude its use and a retrograde iliac to SMA bypass may be more suitable. Alternatively, an antegrade bypass from the supracoeliac aorta to both the SMA and the coeliac axis can be performed if both vessels are diseased. A temporary arterial shunt may be inserted to allow restoration of blood flow during bypass grafting.[25] An autologous conduit, most commonly the reversed long saphenous vein, should be used in the presence of abdominal contamination from necrotic bowel[6] (Fig. 29.5). If no suitable vein is available, polytetrafluoroethylene (PTFE) or Dacron grafts may be used.

> **Operative procedures for acute mesenteric ischaemia**
>
> - SMA embolism – embolectomy
> - SMA thrombosis – aorta or iliac artery to SMA bypass using vein, Dacron or PTFE, supracoeliac aorta to SMA
> - Coeliac axis/SMA thrombosis: bifurcated graft bypass
> - Ischaemic bowel: resection and planned 'second look'

NON-OCCLUSIVE MESENTERIC ISCHAEMIA

As mentioned above, selective arterial administration of papaverine is the primary therapy in non-occlusive mesenteric ischaemia. In addition, the underlying cause should be treated and any vasoconstricting agents such as α-agonists stopped. Surgical exploration is limited to patients with peritonitis indicating bowel necrosis and the need for bowel resection.

MESENTERIC VEIN THROMBOSIS

Patients with no signs of peritonitis or any other evidence of bowel necrosis are managed conservatively with anticoagulation. Intravenous heparin should be started at the time of diagnosis and patients should be maintained on lifelong therapy with warfarin to reduce the chances of recurrence. Surgical treatment is limited to resection of necrotic bowel as venous thrombectomy is difficult and rarely successful.

POSTOPERATIVE CARE

Patients should be managed on an intensive care unit with close monitoring and support to prevent and manage multiple organ failure (see Chapter 4). Fluid balance and serum electrolytes must be monitored carefully and corrected. Intravenous heparin should be continued. Broad spectrum antibiotics commenced preoperatively should also be continued until culture results are available and adjusted accordingly.

Alimentation should be introduced as soon as possible, the exact timing and type given depending on the procedure untaken. Parental nutrition is often required until normal oral intake is resumed. Long term parenteral nutrition should be managed by specialist teams. Further investigations into any underlying causes of acute mesenteric ischaemia should be carried out, e.g. in patients sustaining mesenteric embolism, cardiac echocardiography is required.

Anticoagulation should be continued in the postoperative period in all patients unless there are contraindications. Patients with mesenteric venous thrombosis, arterial embolism and proved haematological disorders should be commenced on warfarin, whereas those with mesenteric arterial thrombosis and non-occlusive disease should be treated with antiplatelet agents.[2] The decision for lifelong anticoagulation must be made after balancing the low risk of recurrent mesenteric ischaemia with the risk of haemorrhage. In patients where the risks of anticoagulation are low, therapy should probably be continued.

COMPLICATIONS

Multiple organ failure is an important and common complication following acute mesenteric ischaemia and must be treated aggressively (see Chapter 4). Other early specific complications include **thrombosis** at arteriotomy sites or of bypass grafts. This results in early recurrence of symptoms and requires angiography and re-exploration. **Haemorrhage** may also occur from the arteriotomy or graft anastomosis site and is often due to infection. Later, **persistent diarrhoea** is a problem in many patients, even in those without short bowel syndrome. **Gastrointestinal bleeding** may occur due to ulceration or rarely from a SMA intestinal fistula. Late **arterial strictures** may occur at arteriotomy or anastomotic sites with recurrence of symptoms.

RESULTS

Despite increased awareness and better understanding of the pathophysiology of acute mesenteric ischaemia, morbidity and mortality have remained high over the past 30 years. Overall mortality rates of 60–100 per cent have been reported.[1–4] There is evidence that mesenteric arterial occlusion and non-occlusive mesenteric ischaemia carry a worse prognosis, with mortality rates of 70–90 per cent,[2] whereas patients with mesenteric vein thrombosis have a better chance of survival, with mortality rates of 20–70 per cent.[26,27]

The average hospital stay for patients who survive surgery is 2 months. Most patients return to their premorbid level of independent life[18] but many will suffer from gastrointestinal symptoms such as weight loss, loss of appetite, abdominal pain, diarrhoea, constipation, nausea and vomiting. Most of these symptoms, however, will be mild.[2] The reported incidence of clinically apparent chronic short bowel syndrome ranges from 20 per cent to 60 per cent.[2]

Recurrent arterial mesenteric ischaemia is rare, with a higher (5 per cent) incidence of recurrent mesenteric vein thrombosis which increases to 25 per cent if the patient is not anticoagulated.[18] Despite the low incidence of recurrent mesenteric ischaemia, the life expectancy of these patients is low. In a retrospective study of the outcome of 31 patients discharged following surgery for acute mesenteric ischaemia, the 2-year survival rate was less than 70 per cent and the 5-year survival rate was 50 per cent.[2] This was mainly due to cardiovascular comorbidity, in particular myocardial infarction and cerebrovascular events, and malignancies.

Conclusions

Acute mesenteric ischaemia is a rare but catastrophic acute surgical emergency. It represents a diagnostic challenge and therefore a high index of suspicion is required as patients often present without obvious physical signs. Angiography should be carried out promptly if it is suspected, but revascularisation should not be delayed by investigations. Aggressive resuscitation, intraoperative and postoperative management are all important.

Key references

Baker DM, Mansfield AO. Acute mesenteric ischaemia. In: Monson JM, Duthie G, O'Malley K (eds). *Surgical Emergencies.* Oxford: Blackwell Science, 1999: 305–15.

Endean ED, Barnes SL, Kwolek CJ, *et al.* Surgical management of thrombotic acute intestinal ischemia. *Ann Surg* 2001; **233**: 801–8.

Klempnauer J, Grothues F, Bektas H, Pichlmayr R. Long-term results after surgery for acute mesenteric ischemia. *Surgery* 1997; **121**: 239–43.

Mansour MA. Management of acute mesenteric ischemia. *Arch Surg* 1999; **134**: 328–30.

McKinsey JF, Gewertz BL. Acute mesenteric ischemia. *Surg Clin North Am* 1997; **77**: 307–18.

REFERENCES

1 McKinsey JF, Gewertz BL. Acute mesenteric ischemia. *Surg Clin North Am* 1997; **77**: 307–18.

2 Klempnauer J, Grothues F, Bektas H, Pichlmayr R. Long-term results after surgery for acute mesenteric ischemia. *Surgery* 1997; **121**: 239–43.

3   Montgomery RA, Venbrux AC, Bulkley GB. Mesenteric vascular insufficiency. *Curr Probl Surg* 1997; **34**: 941–1025.

4   Stoney RJ, Cunningham CG. Acute mesenteric ischemia. *Surgery* 1993; **114**: 489–90.

5   Endean ED, Barnes SL, Kwolek CJ, *et al.* Surgical management of thrombotic acute intestinal ischemia. *Ann Surg* 2001; **233**: 801–8.

6   Mansour MA. Management of acute mesenteric ischemia. *Arch Surg* 1999; **134**: 328–30.

7   Parums DV. The pathology of ischaemic-reperfusion injury. In: Grace PA, Mathie RT (eds). *Ischaemia-Reperfusion Injury*. Oxford Blackwell Science, 1999: 3–19.

8   Crawford JM. The oral cavity and gastrointestinal tract. In: Kumar V, Contran RS, Robbins SL (eds). *Basic Pathology*. Philadelphia, PA: Saunders, 1997: 470–515.

9   Parks DA, Granger DN. Contributions of ischemia and reperfusion to mucosal lesion formation. *Am J Physiol* 1986; **250**: G749–53.

10 Stahl GL, Pan HL, Longhurst JC. Activation of ischemia- and reperfusion-sensitive abdominal visceral C fiber afferents. Role of hydrogen peroxide and hydroxyl radicals. *Circ Res* 1993; **72**: 1266–75.

11 Haglund U, Osterberg J. Local consequences of reperfusion in the gut. In: Grace PA, Mathie RT (eds). *Ischaemia-Reperfusion Injury*. Oxford: Blackwell Science, 1999: 65–70.

12 Deitch EA. Multiple organ failure. Pathophysiology and potential future therapy. *Ann Surg* 1992; **216**: 117–34.

13 Bassiouny HS. Nonocclusive mesenteric ischemia. *Surg Clin North Am* 1997; **77**: 319–26.

14 Rhee RY, Gloviczki P. Mesenteric venous thrombosis. *Surg Clin North Am* 1997; **77**: 327–38.

15 Smerud MJ, Johnson CD, Stephens DH. Diagnosis of bowel infarction: a comparison of plain films and CT scans in 23 cases. *AJR Am J Roentgenol* 1990; **154**: 99–103.

16 Nicoloff AD, Williamson WK, Moneta GL, *et al.* Duplex ultrasonography in evaluation of splanchnic artery stenosis. *Surg Clin North Am* 1997; **77**: 339–55.

17 Rosen A, Korobkin M, Silverman PM, *et al.* Mesenteric vein thrombosis: CT identification. *AJR Am J Roentgenol* 1984; **143**: 83–6.

18 Baker DM, Mansfield AO. Acute mesenteric ischaemia. In: Monson JM, Duthie G, O'Malley K (eds). *Surgical Emergencies*. Oxford: Blackwell Science, 1999: 305–15.

19 McBride KD, Gaines PA. Thrombolysis of a partially occluding superior mesenteric artery thromboembolus by infusion of streptokinase. *Cardiovasc Intervent Radiol* 1994; **17**: 164–6.

20 Rivitz SM, Geller SC, Hahn C, Waltman AC. Treatment of acute mesenteric venous thrombosis with transjugular intramesenteric urokinase infusion. *J Vasc Intervent Radiol* 1995; **6**: 219–23.

21 Hallisey MJ, Deschaine J, Illescas FF, *et al.* Angioplasty for the treatment of visceral ischemia. *J Vasc Intervent Radiol* 1995; **6**: 785–91.

22 VanDeinse WH, Zawacki JK, Phillips D. Treatment of acute mesenteric ischemia by percutaneous transluminal angioplasty. *Gastroenterology* 1986; **91**: 475–8.

23 Ballard JL, Stone WM, Hallett JW, *et al.* A critical analysis of adjuvant techniques used to assess bowel viability in acute mesenteric ischemia. *Am Surg* 1993; **59**: 309–11.

24 Levy PJ, Krausz MM, Manny J. Acute mesenteric ischemia: improved results – a retrospective analysis of ninety-two patients. *Surgery* 1990; **107**: 372–80.

25 Whitehill T, Rutherford R. Acute mesenteric ischaemia caused by arterial occlusions: optimal management to improve survival. *Semin Vasc Surg* 1990; **3**: 149–55.

26 Anane-Sefah JC, Blair E, Reckler S. Primary mesenteric venous occlusive disease. *Surg Gynecol Obstet* 1975; **141**: 740–2.

27 Gertsch P, Matthews J, Lerut J, *et al.* Acute thrombosis of the splanchnic veins. *Arch Surg* 1993; **128**: 341–5.

Acute Complications of Endovascular Aortic Repair (EVAR)

30

Endoleak Complicating EVAR

ROBERT J HINCHLIFFE, BRIAN R HOPKINSON

THE PROBLEM

The feasibility of endovascular repair of infrarenal abdominal aortic aneurysm (EVAR) was demonstrated over a decade ago by Parodi, Volodos and coworkers.[1,2] The technology associated with EVAR has evolved at a rapid pace in parallel with recognition of the factors required for successful endovascular aneurysm exclusion. Enthusiasm for this technique has, however, been tempered by reports of significant device and non-device related complications. These complications have included aneurysm rupture, prevention of which is the basis of treatment.[3] In fact, a cumulative risk of 1 per cent per year has been reported by the European collaborators on Stent-graft Techniques for abdominal aortic Aneurysm Repair (EUROSTAR) using first and second generation endovascular grafts.[4]

Of all possible complications the one that has attracted most attention has been endoleak, which is peculiar to EVAR. The term 'endoleak' was coined by White et al.: 'a condition associated with endoluminal vascular grafts, defined by the presence of blood flow outside the lumen of the endoluminal graft, but within an aneurysm sac or an adjacent vascular segment being treated by the graft'.[5] Although all endoleaks share a common feature of blood flow outside the stent-graft it soon became apparent that a variety of types of endoleak with differing aetiology and natural history existed.

The importance of endoleak is its ability to predict success or failure of endografting and, crucially, whether it predisposes to aneurysm rupture. Early reports that endoleak may act as a reliable indicator of outcome were encouraging.[6] Recent evidence with longer follow-up has

been unable to confirm this report. The absence of endoleak does not reliably predict treatment success.[7–9]

INCIDENCE

The incidence of endoleak from the literature varies tremendously from values as high as 44 per cent to 10 per cent or less.[10–12] Critical analysis of these figures serves to illustrate the multifactorial aetiology of endoleak following endografting. As will be discussed later, the presence of endoleak depends upon patient selection criteria, endovascular graft (EVG) type, operator experience, imaging modality, classification, timing of investigation and duration of patient follow-up.

The incidence of primary endoleak differs from the secondary rate. Primary endoleak occurs in the perioperative period (within 30 days of the EVAR), whereas secondary endoleak manifests later. The Sidney experience discovered 12 per cent of cases with secondary endoleak requiring intervention.[12] The secondary endoleak prevalence is likely to increase in time. It is interesting to note that the intervention rate for endoleak in the Sydney experience was double the quantity of interventions required for other complications. These figures clearly show the scale of the problem.

AETIOLOGY/PATHOPHYSIOLOGY

Endoleak is an important consideration when talking about the success of EVAR. Endoleaks may transmit pressure to

Table 30.1 *Classification of endoleaks*

Type	Cause
1	Attachment sites (or occluder in aorto-uni-iliac endovascular graft)
2	Retrograde sac filling by patent aortic side branches
3	Graft tear, disintegration or modular limb dislocation
4	Angiographic 'blush' experienced on completion angiography with certain thin walled devices. ? Self-limiting
'5'	'Endotension'. Evidence of raised intrasac pressure (usually aneurysm sac expansion) in the absence of radiological evidence of endoleak

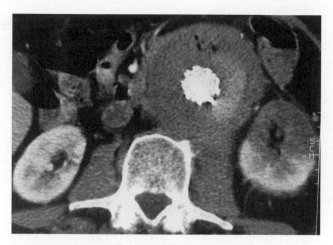

Figure 30.2 *Type 1 endoleak (proximal)*

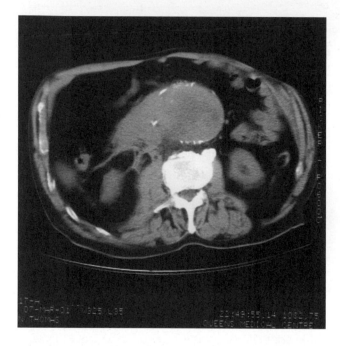

Figure 30.1 *'Endotension': rupture of a thrombosed abdominal aortic aneurysm in a patient who had endovascular repair five years previously; he subsequently developed graft migration, kinking and occlusion and was eventually admitted with aneurysm rupture*

thrombus has been well recognised in open surgery for a number of years (Fig. 30.1). Endoleaks may be present singly or multiply and each may act as an inflow or outflow channel with respect to the aneurysm sac.

Type 1 endoleak

Type 1 endoleak[15] (Fig. 30.2) is due to inadequate seal at the interface between stent-graft and arterial wall at the attachment zones. It occurs in up to 10 per cent of patients undergoing EVAR. Early type 1 endoleak (occurring within 30 days of operation) has two major causative factors. The first factor, 'bad planning', is related to patient selection criteria. Accurate preoperative imaging of aneurysm morphology is mandatory and a prerequisite of successful aneurysm exclusion. The proximal aneurysmal neck is a particularly important consideration to ensure a good seal.[16] Consideration of the aneurysm neck must take into account its length, diameter, angulation, shape and wall constitution. Essentially all these factors simply relate to the amount of covered stent providing a seal with the aortic wall. Unfortunately, there is insufficient evidence to implicate all these factors in type 1 endoleak. Indeed, controversially, a recent study of 100 patients found no statistically significant association between any of the above factors and the subsequent development of type 1 endoleak.[17] Experimental aneurysm flow models have, however, found significantly increased proximal perigraft endoleak flow for proximal neck angulation ≥ 30 degrees.[18] *In vivo* studies have also confirmed the importance of neck angulation and to a lesser degree the width of the aortic neck in the causation of type 1 endoleak.[19] The concept of stent-graft oversizing is now widely believed to be a relevant factor in stent-graft planning. Oversizing of 10–20 per cent of the original aortic diameter has been found to significantly reduce the incidence of endoleak.[20]

the aneurysm sac and therefore predispose to aneurysm rupture. Four types of endoleak (1–4) have been described (Table 30.1). The classification is further dependent upon anatomical site (a, b, c) and the presence of an outflow channel. Subclassification of the four types of endoleak is not generally undertaken in everyday practice, instead an anatomical description is preferred to prevent confusion.

Before describing endoleak in detail two factors must be considered. Pressure transmitted by an endoleak channel is not related to the size of the endoleak (diameter or length).[13] Thrombosis of the endoleak channel may not abolish pressure transmission.[14] Pressure transmission via

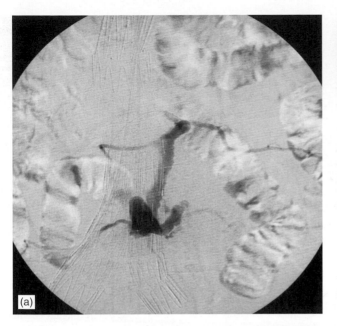 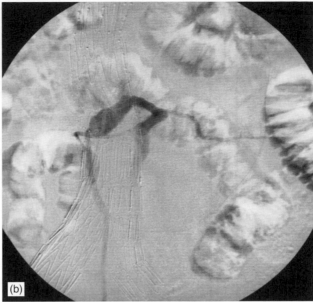

Figure 30.3   *Type 2 endoleak at angiogram: (a) lumbar vessels providing aneurysm inflow, (b) inferior mesenteric artery outflow*

The second factor in the development of primary type 1 endoeak is 'bad deployment'. Operator error, deploying the graft too low in the aortic neck or even in the aneurysm sac will result in endoleak. A particular hazard encountered in angulated necks is a parallax error which results in maldeployment.

In general there has been a reduction in the development of early type 1 endoleak brought about by improvements in preoperative imaging, an awareness of aneurysm morphology required for successful EVAR, the necessity of oversizing and increased technical expertise.

Finally, it is important to appreciate the differences among commercially available stent-grafts. Each graft has different deployment characteristics and sizes, making some aneurysms suitable for one stent-graft but unsuitable for another. The differences are most marked in the accommodation of neck morphology, particularly width.

Secondary development of type 1 endoleak has a different pattern from its early counterpart. Of course, if the aneurysm is excluded from the circulation via a tenuous seal due to 'bad planning' or 'bad deployment' then a leak may be expected. Unsurprisingly EVGs suffer from the same lack of incorporation into the aortic tissues as an open graft.[21] They are also subject to the forces exerted on it by aortic blood flow and elastic recoil. The pattern of endoleak which emerges in medium and long term follow-up is related to changing aneurysm morphology and graft migration. Significant graft migration is most commonly seen 2–3 years post implantation (see Chapter 31). There are intimate relations between migration and changing morphology. The fate of the proximal aneurysm neck following EVAR, like its open counterpart is controversial, with reports of both stability and expansion.[22–24] There appears to be a subgroup of patients prone to neck

expansion. Identifying this group of patients preoperatively is not yet possible.

Type 2 endoleak

Type 2 endoleak arises from retrograde flow in patent aortic side branches.[15] The most commonly involved vessels are the inferior mesenteric artery (IMA) and one or more lumbar arteries, although other vessels such as the gonadal or accessory renal vessels may be responsible (Fig. 30.3). Accepted type 2 endoleak rates are in the order of 10–25 per cent.[5,25] There appear to be no reliable factors, which predispose to the subsequent development of type 2 endoleak,[26,27] although Armon *et al.*'s results suggested patterns of thrombus distribution may be able to predict patients at risk from persistent endoleak via lumbar vessels.[28] Only a quarter of patent IMAs will subsequently perfuse the aneurysm sac. And there is little evidence to suggest that graft design has any bearing on the incidence of type 2 endoleak. Approximately two-thirds of side branch endoleaks seen on completion angiography will spontaneously thrombose in the early postoperative period.[29] A small proportion will persist.

One technique that has been found to be a useful indicator of subsequent development of type 2 endoleak is the intra-operative 'sacogram' (Fig. 30.4). This technique involves injection of contrast into the aneurysm sac alongside the deployed EVG. In a series of patients in Nottingham undergoing EVAR a negative sacogram was found to predict a group in whom the subsequent risk of development of type 2 endoleak was low.[30]

The natural history of type 2 endoleak remains undetermined. Early work on type 2 endoleak discovered a rather benign course.[31] Indeed, the EUROSTAR database, the largest accumulation of data currently available, revealed no relation between type 2 endoleak and sac rupture, this being in contrast to types 1 and 3 endoleak. More recently there have been worrying reports of aneurysm sac expansion (Fig. 30.5) and even rupture.[32,33] It is not surprising that type 2 endoleak is associated with adverse outcome in some patients. In patients with aneurysms treated by surgical ligation and bypass a 2 per cent aneurysm sac patency via 'type 2 endoleaks' was recorded despite intraoperative ligation of collateral vessels. Almost a quarter of the patients with persistent collaterals subsequently presented with sac rupture.[34]

In vivo pressure manometry in patients with type 2 endoleak has recorded systemic pressures and pulsatile waveforms.[35] We cannot reliably identify which type 2 endoleaks result in aneurysm expansion or rupture; suffice to say the reports of type 2 rupture have all been predictable events.

Type 3 endoleak

Type 3 endoleak[36] is primarily a device related complication. It has a well documented association with aneurysm rupture. It encompasses any form of graft disruption leading to leak of blood in to the aneurysm sac and includes graft tears and iliac limb disconnection (modular EVGs). Many of these problems have been attributed to first and second generation EVGs. The underlying problems have been investigated and corrected. Two particular EVGs have been implicated in type 3 endoleak, the Stentor (Mintec, LaCiotat, France) and the Vanguard (Boston Scientific, Natick, MA, USA). The former experienced endoleak due to seam defects and the latter due to metallic wear of the fabric.

An interesting observation has been made by the Liverpool group in patients with successful aneurysm exclusion. They noted a number of graft kinks, precipitating type 3 endoleak in modular grafts, which they were unable to attribute to graft migration (see Chapter 31). They attributed this complication to longitudinal shrinkage of the aneurysm sac. This observation highlights the requirement for ongoing graft surveillance to ensure patency of the graft.[37] Of course graft migration without longitudinal sac shrinkage may precipitate either type 1 or

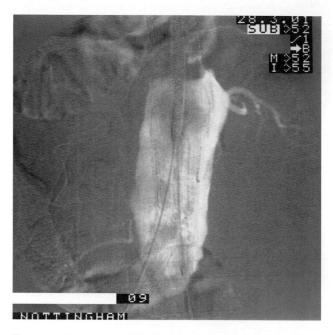

Figure 30.4 *Intraoperative sacogram revealing patent aortic side branch, a previously unrecognised left accessory renal artery*

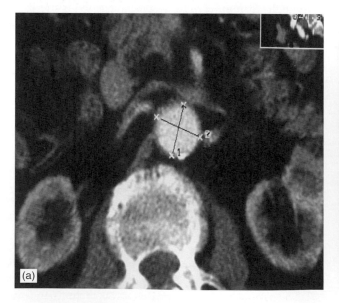

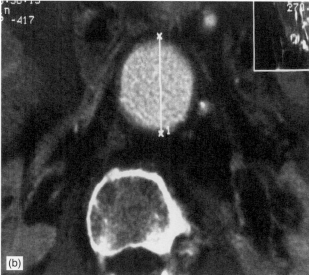

Figure 30.5 *Neck of aneurysm: (a) at time of EVAR, and (b) showing dilation post endografting*

type 3 endoleak. Modular grafts clearly remain at higher risk of developing type 3 endoleak when compared with their unitary counterparts.

Type 4 endoleak

Type 4 endoleak[36] is seen as an 'angiographic blush' on completion angiography. The placement of ultrathin endovascular grafts, in part conceived to reduce sheath diameter and employ a percutaneous introduction, were associated with this observation. The AneuRx graft allowed leakage of contrast at suture holes and from fabric interstices. The leaks have all been reported to be sealed at 1 month. Type 4 endoleak appears to be a self-limiting leak with, as yet, no recorded adverse sequelae.[38] The long term durability of thin walled porous grafts remains undetermined.

Type 5 (endotension)

Type 5 (endotension) was first introduced as a concept because a number of aneurysm sacs were undergoing expansion without evidence of endoleak.[39,40] In essence pressure is transmitted to the aneurysm sac in the absence of detectable blood flow. There has been no clear explanation for this phenomenon, however, it is thought that intermittent endoleak,[41] missed endoleak[42] or thrombosed endoleak are responsible either singly or in combination.

Recent evidence that thrombus may transmit pressure has been presented in a variety of both experimental[43] and clinical reports.[44] This property of thrombus has been recognised in open surgery for many years (see Fig. 30.1 showing rupture of a thrombosed abdominal aortic aneurysm).

Experimental data have, however, explained why type 1 endoleaks remain dangerous even when thrombosed whereas a thrombosed type 2 endoleak rarely causes problems. Pressure transmission is greater by short thrombosed endoleak channels with a large cross-sectional area than it is by long ones with a smaller cross-sectional area,[45] whereas the pressure transmission of a patent endoleak channel is unaffected by either cross-sectional area or length.[13] These results may explain why coil embolisation of endoleak channels does not always effectively reduce pressure transmission despite successful thrombosis.[14]

Three grades of endotension

- Grade 1 – high flow
- Grade 2 – low flow
- Grade 3 – 'no flow – no detectable' endoleak

Endotension may also be due to an endoleak with no outflow where the blood is allowed in during systole and then will oscillate in the endoleak channel at the point where the mean arterial pressure in the sac equals that in the body. This oscillation of blood can be identified on duplex scanning with a good 'window' but is missed by computed tomographic angiography (CTA).

In general the importance of endoleak has moved away from flow and concentrated on pressure. This has resulted from the realisation that thrombus may transmit pressure just as well as blood.

DIAGNOSIS

Clinical

Endoleak is invariably asymptomatic. Patients experience symptoms only when the endoleak is associated with sudden aneurysm expansion or rupture. As endoleak was first described and essentially remains a radiological diagnosis, little work has been done to assess its relation with clinical examination. Clinical examination hinges upon the detection of pulsatile wall motion of the sac, the absence of which, it is hoped, indicates successful aneurysm exclusion. Greenberg and Green have incorporated physical examination in their EVAR follow-up protocol.[45] Convincing evidence of its usefulness in the diagnosis and management of patients with endoleak is awaited.

Investigations

The purpose of any investigation with respect to endoleak is to:

- identify the presence of an endoleak
- classify the endoleak (1–4)
- identify the anatomical site of the endoleak
- identify endotension/identify successful aneurysm exclusion (shrinking of aneurysm sac, intrasac pressure reduction, reduced pulsatile wall motion).

Management of endoleak is dependent upon answers to these investigations. Unfortunately, no single currently available investigation has the ability to fulfil all these criteria.

Plain abdominal X-ray (AXR) has little place in the armamentarium for investigation of endoleak. It is a useful tool for the detection of stent fracture, disruption or migration (see Chapter 31). These signs may infer the presence of an endoleak. The detection of migration with AXR is probably less accurate than computed tomography (CT) due to the problems of parallax error. Lateral films help to reduce this problem.

Spiral CTA (SCTA) remains the gold standard for detection of endoleak. It is minimally invasive but, importantly, is limited by its inability to reliably distinguish the type of endoleak. The use of delayed acquisition scans may increase the identification of endoleak by up to 11 per cent.[46] The optimum technique of SCTA to diagnose endoleak has yet to be determined. Current problems with SCTA are related to blood flow. Low flow endoleaks or thrombi are not detected on current imaging but, significantly, maintain the ability to transmit pressure.[47] The use of 'blood pool' contrast agents and platelets labelled with radioisotope may offer further assistance in the detection of low flow endoleak or fresh thrombus transmitting pressure to the sac.

Worries over the invasiveness, cost and dose of radiation during follow-up with angiography and CT have increased the demands for other techniques. Ultrasound is a technique gaining popularity for its use in EVG surveillance. Duplex ultrasonography is observer dependent and may be technically difficult, especially in the early postoperative period where the aorta is often obscured by bowel gas. The technique is able to identify the anatomical site of endoleak but critically requires flow to determine the presence of an endoleak. Its use as a diagnostic tool may be enhanced with intravascular ultrasound contrast agents.[48]

Digital subtraction angiography (DSA) is frequently used to identify the type and anatomical site of an endoleak. It is usually a second line investigation due to its invasive nature. Selective views allow assessment of a variety of anatomical sites including the lumbar and inferior mesenteric arteries. The technique can differentiate inflow and outflow tracts and may permit therapeutic procedures such as embolisation. Digital subtraction angiography is frequently used intraoperatively at completion of endograft deployment, i.e. completion angiography, where it remains a useful tool in identifying primary endoleak. Detection of patent side branches can be facilitated by waiting for delayed filling or by using a 'sacogram' achieved by injecting contrast into the aneurysm sac post deployment.

Magnetic resonance angiography has proved effective as a sole imaging modality for the assessment of the suitability of the aorta for endografting. Its role in the investigation of endoleak appears attractive but is restricted to stent-grafts containing non-ferrous metals.

The detection of endotension usefully predicts those patients who will require intervention to prevent abdominal aortic aneurysm rupture. Endoleak may remain undetected despite the presence of endotension. Signs of endotension include an increasing sac diameter or volume, pulsatile wall motion and raised intrasac pressure. Both duplex and CTA are able to reproduce aneurysm sac diameter. More recently, however, sac volume has been found to be a more accurate predictor of successful aneurysm exclusion.[49] Unfortunately, this technique remains rather cumbersome for everyday practice.

The effect of endoleak on the aneurysm wall can be investigated in a dynamic fashion by ultrasound. Ultrasound tracking documents aneurysm wall motion. Malina et al. found the absence of pulsatile wall motion to be an indicator of successful aneurysm exclusion.[50] Interestingly, in Resnikoff et al.'s experience of open aneurysm exclusion and bypass, all aneurysms which subsequently ruptured exhibited pulsatile wall motion on echo-tracking ultrasound.[34]

Measurement of long term intrasac pressure appears to be the holy grail of successful endovascular aneurysm exclusion. One-off and short duration postoperative manometry has demonstrated quite clearly that successful EVAR is associated with a significant reduction of intrasac pressure.[51] The presence of endoleak has been associated with raised intrasac pressure.[35] Permanent intrasac manometry appears desirable and in itself will raise many questions. These are likely to include the relevance of the site of pressure readings from within the sac (there is evidence that an aneurysm sac may be compartmentalised so that a decrease in pressure in one part of the sac does not necessarily equal complete depressurisation of the entire sac[42]), the absolute level of pressure reduction required to prevent rupture and the significance of the pressure waveform and the level of pressure transmitted from the endoleak channel to the wall of the aneurysm. Importantly, the pressure readings will not tell us which sacs are going to rupture because all sacs are not the same. Experience from the management of abdominal aortic aneurysms has revealed that some will rupture at 5 cm whereas others will not do so until they reach 9 cm. More confusingly still, Baum et al. measured systemic pressures which were transmitted to the wall of the sac in a number of type 2 endoleaks.[35] Despite this evidence the majority of type 2 endoleaks generally follow a benign course. The development of a chronic intrasac pressure transducer is awaited.

Current methods of imaging are severely limited by the time delay between scans. Interval ruptures may be preventable if an early warning sign is available to allow timely intervention of endoleak. Intrasac manometry with readily available or continuous pressure recordings is certainly an attractive proposition.

MANAGEMENT

Management strategies are outlined in Table 30.2. It is generally accepted that type 1 and 3 endoleak require intervention to prevent rupture. The same cannot be said of type 2 endoleak. It is not yet clear which type 2 endoleaks require intervention to prevent rupture. Consequently, the EUROSTAR database found type 2 endoleak a risk factor for secondary intervention but not rupture.[52]

Table 30.2 *Management strategies for endoleaks*

Type 1	Urgent treatment
Type 2	Observation unless associated with aneurysm expansion
Type 3	Urgent treatment
Type 4	Conservative
Type 5	Try to identify cause. If no cause found consider open conversion

Prevention of endoleak

Primary, type 1, 3 and 4 endoleaks can be prevented by appropriate case selection, graft oversizing and accurate deployment. The endoleak rate increases markedly when operating on patients with adverse aneurysm morphology.[53] Uncovered suprarenal stent fixation and grafts with increased columnar strength may prevent migration and subsequent endoleak but the evidence for their efficacy is awaited in the long term (Fig. 30.6).

Some institutions elect to embolise patent aortic side branches preoperatively. Embolisation is usually performed at the preoperative angiogram with insertion of metallic coils to induce vessel thrombosis and subsequent fibrosis. As already alluded to, there really is no evidence to support this manoeuvre and it is not performed in our unit.[54] The procedure of intraoperative filling of the aneurysm sac with thrombogenic sponge, as it is performed in our unit, may be undertaken in all cases (Fig. 30.7). It is preferable, however, to apply it on a more selective basis where the sacogram reveals patent side branches. A negative sacogram has been found to be a useful predictor. Type 2 endoleak development is unlikely in patients who have had a negative sacogram.[30]

Treatment of endoleak

Management of endoleak requires a full medical assessment of the patient. A medically high risk, frail patient may be better served by non-operative management. That said, the majority of interventions can be performed by the less invasive endovascular route, open treatment being reserved for cases refractory to endovascular methods.[55]

Intraoperative management of type 1 endoleak is widely believed to be necessary to prevent early complications, including rupture[56] (Table 30.3). A number of the commercially available self-expanding stent-grafts are supplied with a low pressure balloon in order to 'mould' the graft to the wall and allow it to conform to the aorta. If the low pressure balloon fails then an angioplasty balloon may offer some benefit.

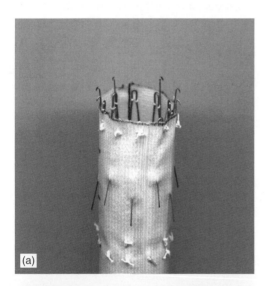

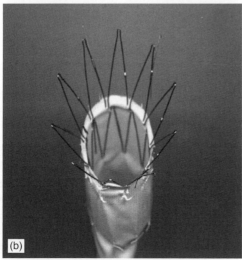

Figure 30.6 *(a) Suprarenal and (b) infrarenal stent fixation*

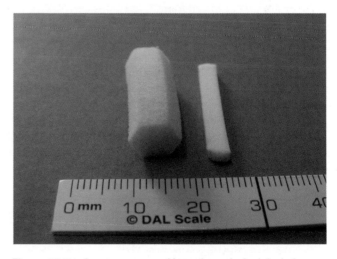

Figure 30.7 *Aneurysm sac packing using polyvinylalcohol sponge (Netcell, Skipton, UK) for the prevention of type 2 endoleak*

Table 30.3 *Management of type 1 endoleak*

Cause	Endovascular/open treatment
EVG landed too low/migration	Extension piece
Poor EVG/aortic wall interface	Balloon angioplasty/Palmaz stent
Angulated neck	Palmaz stent (straighten aortic neck)
Dilated neck	Periaortic ligature

EVG, endovascular graft.

Table 30.4 *Management of type 2 endoleaks*

Preoperative	Coil embolisation, laparoscopic ligation
Intraoperative	Aneurysm sac packing (thrombogenic sponge), coil embolisation, laparoscopic ligation
Postoperative	Coil embolisation, laparoscopic ligation, open ligation or conversion

A stent deployed too low in the proximal aortic neck is rectified by the insertion of a covered extension graft. Deployment as close to the renals as possible is desirable. For patients with difficult aortic necks, especially those that are angulated, the giant Palmaz stent is an ideal adjunct. These stainless steel balloon expandable stents straighten out angulated aortic necks and improve the seal at the stent-graft/aortic wall interface. Failure of the Palmaz stent to eliminate an endoleak requires the placement of periaortic ligatures.[57] The periaortic ligatures are applied at mini-laparotomy or laparoscopy following dissection of the aortic neck. Placement of the periaortic ligatures is facilitated by the Palmaz stent. The rigid stent provides a firm structure on which to 'snug' the nylon periaortic tapes, in so doing preventing stenosis or occlusion of the aorta or kinking of the endograft.

A variety of methods have been used for the treatment of type 2 endoleak (Table 30.4). Endovascular embolisation with metallic coils or other embolic agents including liquids has been described.[58] There are concerns about the use of liquid embolic agents, especially when treating lumbar arteries because of their proximity to the spinal circulation. Embolisation of endoleak channels has also been performed via a direct translumbar approach and in some cases has been combined with embolisation of the aneurysm sac itself. There have even been suggestions to fill the aneurysm sac with a non-absorbable medium, creating a permanent solid sac. The direct approach is useful where endovascular access is difficult or there are fears regarding the disturbance of an endograft iliac limb with wires or catheters. Opponents of 'open' techniques warn of the dangers of introducing infection and the potential bleeding complications subsequent to creating a hole in an aneurysm sac which may be under systemic pulsatile pressure.

Laparoscopic ligation of vessels is an attractive method of treating type 2 endoleak. The aorta may be approached either by the transperitoneal or the retroperitoneal route. It is an intervention best undertaken at the same sitting as EVAR or in the early postoperative period. The inflammatory reaction which tends to develop in the perioperative period often makes periaortic dissection and identification of feeding vessel difficult.[59]

Endoleak from the iliac limbs or occluding devices in the case of aorto-uni-iliac prostheses, is usually managed best by open methods via an extraperitoneal approach. Extension cuffs can, of course, be used if the iliac limb has landed short or if there is a type 3 endoleak in a modular graft. If an occluding device fails the best policy is to ligate the common iliac artery or the external and internal iliac arteries separately.

Open transperitoneal procedures for the treatment of endoleak vary from ligation of side branch vessels to conversion to traditional aneurysmorrhaphy.[52] They have a role, particularly where less invasive techniques have failed. In the case of endovascular embolisation procedures this is usually due to access failure or the presence of multiple endoleak channels. Although an open ligation of side branch endoleak appears particularly invasive it is not nearly so stressful for the patient as a conventional open repair, the latter requiring prolonged clamping of the aorta with its attendant sequelae. In some patients with type 2 endoleak open methods are reassuring in their exclusion of other causes of endoleak, for example, a proximal type 1 endoleak providing inflow to the aneurysmal sac and a type 2 endoleak the outflow channel.

The techniques for open conversion have been reviewed thoroughly by May *et al.*[60] Patients in whom the device has migrated entirely into the aneurysm sac may be treated by conventional aneurysm repair. In patients who have had the device deployed suboptimally, the technique required is a modified conventional repair suturing the top of the graft to the aneurysm neck. In addition to proximal and distal clamping the graft is clamped in order to reduce blood loss and facilitate removal of proximal and distal stents from the infrarenal aorta and iliac arteries, respectively. Surprisingly little damage is encountered in these vessels post-endografting.

Patients who have had a suprarenal endograft that needs to be removed, usually require supracoeliac clamping or the use of a large (30 mm) angioplasty occlusion balloon placed in the aorta above the renal arteries. At secondary conversion the metal suprarenal frame is usually left *in situ* because it is frequently well incorporated. The suprarenal component is incorporated into the anastomosis.

Treatment of complications of endoleak (rupture)

Aneurysm rupture is *the* complication of endoleak. The feasibility of endovascular repair of ruptured abdominal aortic aneurysm has been demonstrated in a number of institutions. Endovascular repair of rupture post endografting is possible but clearly depends upon the cause of the rupture and the patient's fitness and stability to tolerate a preoperative delay for investigations. A great many of the ruptures experienced in the early years of endografting required open repair. Frequently no endoleak could be identified at laparotomy. A number of risk factors have been identified for rupture. If the cause of the leak/rupture can be identified preoperatively then endovascular treatment may salvage the situation. If the anatomical site of the leak cannot be identified then open repair is required.

POSTOPERATIVE CARE

The majority of secondary endovascular procedures can be performed under local anaesthesia. Where instrumentation of the iliac arteries or aorta is required and large sheaths are used then edpidural or spinal anaesthesia with sedation or general anaesthesia is more comfortable for the patient and reduces movement artefact. The recovery time for elective cases is short and major complications are rare.

RESULTS

Endovascular aneurysm surgery is in its infancy and therefore there are very few long term follow-up results. Many of the early endoleaks occurred when the requirements for successful endografting were not understood and the devices were first and second generation.

It was initially suggested by May *et al.* that a stent-graft may confer some benefit to the patient if sac rupture occurs,[61] an effect presumed to be due to the attenuated haemodynamic disturbance. A more recent and contradictory report from a larger experience compiled by the EUROSTAR database found the mortality to be 50 per cent (similar to that of open repair of *de novo* rupture).[62] Open conversion carries an 18 per cent mortality when performed primarily and 27 per cent at secondary conversion. Primary conversion is usually performed for access failure or device migration. Secondary conversion is generally required for rupture or persistent endoleak.[52] These high mortality rates highlight the importance of endoleak prevention and early endovascular intervention to prevent open conversion.

The use of Palmaz stents and periaortic ligatures has been confined to experimental models, case reports and small series with relatively short duration of follow-up.[63,64] They are certainly feasible techniques and appear efficacious in the short term although their effect on device durability is unknown.

It has been claimed that coil embolisation of endoleak channels may not effectively seal lower intra-aneurysmal pressure,[14] whereas as others have reported successful occlusion of aortic aneurysms using this technique. One of these reports has claimed to reduce the pressure to zero with coils before tying the iliacs and doing an extra-anatomical bypass for high risk aneurysms.[65] This is not an original approach having been first performed by Moore in the

1800s and published by Peacock and Brown in 1968.[66] Many are sceptical of the efficacy of this technique. Similarly, embolisation for type 1 and type 3 endoleak has proved disappointing. An analysis of experimental data shows why type 1 and 3 endoleaks do not appear to be successfully treated using embolisation techniques, whereas their type 2 counterparts do.[43] Both type 1 and 3 endoleaks tend to be of large cross-sectional area and short length, and therefore even when thrombosed, either naturally or induced by embolic material, they may be expected to transmit a significant level of pressure. Type 2 endoleaks are usually longer and of smaller cross-sectional area and consequently dampen pressure transmission.

Conclusions

Types 1 and 3 endoleak should be regarded as dangerous and accordingly managed with a degree of urgency. If these lesions are recognised intraoperatively then they are best treated at the same sitting. The outcome of type 2 endoleaks is generally benign although some are associated with aneurysm expansion. There is insufficient evidence to suggest that treatment of type 2 endoleaks is required to prevent rupture. Those endoleaks resulting in aneurysm expansion require intervention. Further investigation is required to predict the type 2 endoleaks which will result in aneurysm expansion.

Early endoleak can be prevented by accurate assessment of aneurysm morphology, appropriate patient selection and precise endograft deployment. Whereas early endoleak is now largely avoidable, the problems of late endoleak remain. Late endoleak occurs as a result of a previously unrecognised or missed endoleak, graft failure, changing aneurysm morphology and endograft migration. Improved graft durability will hopefully reduce the incidence of type 3 endoleak and improved graft design, including more secure fixation, may prevent graft migration and type 1 endoleak. Changing aneurysm morphology, and neck dilatation in particular, is likely to require alternative techniques to ensure adequate seal and fixation of the proximal endograft. New technology such as an endovascular staple is in development.

Our ability to detect endoleaks is largely dependent upon significant blood flow. Low flow endoleaks and the pressure transmitted by thrombus are more difficult to detect. Current methods of investigation can only reliably detect the secondary effects of raised pressure on the sac, i.e. an expanding aneurysm sac or pulsatile wall motion. The introduction of long term pressure telemetry and more sophisticated imaging techniques offer some promise in the detection of these types of endoleak. It is hoped that these techniques will allow a more rational approach in the follow-up of EVAR and act as early warning signs of aneurysm exclusion failure.

Most endoleaks can be treated successfully by endovascular methods. Open methods may be used but are less favourable. A good proportion of the first and second generation grafts have developed endoleaks. Many of these endoleaks will require secondary interventions. To reduce endoleaks and the number of secondary interventions in future there must be an improvement in EVG design, a greater understanding of the principles required for successful aneurysm exclusion and a heightened awareness of the natural history of individual endoleaks.

Key references

Gilling-Smith GL, Brennan J, Harris P, *et al.* Endotension after endovascular aneurysm repair: definition, classification, and strategies for surveillance and intervention. *J Endovasc Surg* 1999; **6**: 305–7.

Mohan IV, Laheij RJ, Harris PL. EUROSTAR collaborators. Risk factors for endoleak and the evidence for stent-graft oversizing when undergoing endovascular aneurysm repair. *Eur J Vasc Endovasc Surg* 2001; **21**: 344–9.

Schurink GW, Aarts NJ, Van Baalen JM, *et al.* Experimental study of the influence of endoleak size on pressure in the aneurysm sac and the consequences of thrombosis. *Br J Surg* 2000; **87**: 71–8.

White GH, May J, Petrasek P, *et al.* Endotension: an explanation for continued AAA growth after successful endoluminal repair. *J Endovasc Surg* 1999; **6**: 308–15.

White GH, May J, Waugh RC, *et al.* Type 3 and Type 4 endoleak: toward a complete definition of blood flow in the sac after endoluminal AAA repair. *J Endovasc Surg* 1998; **5**: 305–9.

REFERENCES

1   Parodi JC, Palmaz JC, Barone HD. Transfemoral intraluminal graft implantation for abdominal aortic aneurysms. *Ann Vasc Surg* 1991; **5**: 491–6.

2   Volodos NL, Karpovich IP, Troyan VL, *et al.* Clinical experience of the use of self-fixing prostheses for remote endoprosthetics of the thoracic and abdominal aorta and iliac arteries through the femoral artery and as intraoperative endoprosthesis for aorta reconstruction. *Vasa Suppl* 1991; **33**: 93–5.

3   Torsello GB, Klenck E, Kasprzak B, Umscheid T. Rupture of abdominal aortic aneurysm previously treated by endovascular stent-graft. *J Vasc Surg* 1998; **28**: 184.

4   Laheij RJF, Buth J, Harris PL, *et al.* Need for secondary interventions after endovascular repair of abdominal aortic aneurysms. Intermediate-term follow-up results of a European collaborative registry (EUROSTAR). *Br J Surg* 2000; **87**: 1666–73.

5   White GH, Yu W, May J, *et al.* Endoleak as a complication of endoluminal grafting of abdominal aortic aneurysms. *J Endovasc Surg* 1997; **4**: 152.

6   Matsumara JS, Moore WS. Clinical consequences of periprosthetic leak after endovascular repair of abdominal aortic aneurysm. *J Vasc Surg* 1998; **27**: 606–13.

7   Gilling-Smith GL, Martin J, Sudhindran S, *et al.* Freedom from endoleak after endovascular aneurysm repair does not equal treatment success. *Eur J Vasc Endovasc Surg* 2000; **19**: 621–5.

8   Lee WA, Yehuda GW, Fogarty TJ, *et al.* Does complete aneurysm exclusion ensure long-term success after endovascular repair? *J Endovasc Ther* 2000; **7**: 494–500.

9   Rhee RY, Eskandari MK, Zajko AB, *et al.* Long-term fate of the aneurysmal sac after endoluminal exclusion of abdominal aortic aneurysms. *J Vasc Surg* 2000; **32**: 689–96.

10   Moore WS, Rutherford RB, for the EVT investigators. Transfemoral endovascular repair of abdominal aortic aneurysm: results of the North American phase I trial. *J Vasc Surg* 1996; **23**: 543–53.

11   Yusuf SW, Whitaker SC, Chuter TA, *et al.* Early results of endovascular aortic aneurysm surgery with aortouniiliac graft, contralateral iliac occlusion and femoro-femoral bypass. *J Vasc Surg* 1997; **25**: 165–72.

12   Blum U, Voshage G, Lammer J, *et al.* Endoluminal stent-grafts for infrarenal abdominal aortic aneurysms. *N Engl J Med* 1997; **336**: 13–20.

13   Schurink GW, Aarts NJ, Van Baalen JM, *et al.* Experimental study of the influence of endoleak size on pressure in the aneurysm sac and the consequences of thrombosis. *Br J Surg* 2000; **87**: 71–8.

14   Marty B, Sanchez LA, Ohki T, *et al.* Endoleak after endovascular graft repair of experimental aneurysms: does coil embolization with angiographic 'seal' lower intraaneurysmal pressure? *J Vasc Surg* 1998; **27**: 454–61.

15   White GH, May J, Waugh RC, *et al.* Type 1 and type 2 endoleaks: a more useful classification for reporting results of endoluminal AAA repair [letter]. *J Endovasc Surg.* 1998; **5**: 189–91.

16   May J, White GH, Yu W, *et al.* Focus on the proximal neck: the key to durability of endoluminal AAA repair. *J Endovasc Surg* 1997; **4**: 1–27.

17   Petrik P, Moore WS. Endoleaks following endovascular repair of abdominal aortic aneurysm: the predictive value of preoperative anatomic factors – a review of 100 cases. *J Vasc Surg* 2001; **33**: 739–44.

18   Albertini JN, Macierewicz JA, Yusuf SW, *et al.* Pathophysiology of proximal perigraft endoleak following endovascular repair of abdominal aortic aneurysms: a study using a flow model. *Eur J Vasc Endovasc Surg* 2001; **22**: 53–6.

19   Albertini J, Kalliafas S, Travis, *et al.* Anatomical risk factors for proximal perigraft endoleak and graft migration following endovascular repair of abdominal aortic aneurysms. *Eur J Vasc Endovasc Surg* 2000; **19**: 308–12.

20   Mohan IV, Laheij RJ, Harris PL, EUROSTAR collaborators. Risk factors for endoleak and the evidence for stent-graft oversizing when undergoing endovascular aneurysm repair. *Eur J Vasc Endovasc Surg* 2001; **21**: 344–9.

21   McArthur C, Teodorescu V, Eisen L, *et al.* Histopathologic analysis of endovascular stent grafts from patients with aortic aneurysms: Does healing occur ? *J Vasc Surg* 2001; **33**: 733–8.

22   Walker SR, Macierewicz J, Elmarasy NM, *et al.* A prospective study to assess changes in proximal aortic neck dimensions after endovascular repair of abdominal aortic aneurysms. *J Vasc Surg* 1999; **29**: 625–30.

23   Matsumara JS, Chaikof EL. Continued expansion of aortic necks after endovascular repair of abdominal aortic aneurysms. *J Vasc Surg* 1998; **28**: 422–31.

24 Illig KA, Green RM, Ouriel K, *et al.* Fate of the proximal aortic cuff: implications for endovascular aneurysm repair. *J Vasc Surg* 1998; **28**: 184–7.

25 Jacobowitz GR, Rosen RJ, Riles TS. The significance and management of the leaking endograft. *Semin Vasc Surg* 1999; **12**: 199–206.

26 Walker SR, Halliday K, Yusuf SW, *et al.* A study on the patency of the inferior mesenteric and lumbar arteries in the incidence of endoleak following endovascular repair of infrarenal aortic aneurysms. *Clin Radiol* 1998; **53**: 593–5.

27 Velazquez OC, Baum RA, Carpenter JP, *et al.* Relationship between preoperative patency of the inferior mesenteric artery and subsequent occurrence of type 2 endoleak in patients undergoing endovascular repair of abdominal aortic aneurysms. *J Vasc Surg* 2000; **32**: 777–88.

28 Armon MP, Yusuf SW, Whitaker SC, *et al.* Thrombus distribution and changes in aneurysm size following endovascular aortic aneurysm repair. *Eur J Vasc Endovasc Surg* 1998; **16**: 472–6.

29 Kato N, Semba CP, Dake MD. Embolization of perigraft leaks after endovascular stent-graft treatment of aortic aneurysms. *J Vasc Intervent Radiol* 1996; **7**: 805–11.

30 Lehmann JM, Macierewicz JA, Davidson IR, *et al.* Prevention of side branch endoleaks with thrombogenic sponge: one year follow-up. *J Endovasc Ther* 2000; **7**: 431–3.

31 Resch T, Ivancev K, Lindh M, *et al.* Persistent collateral perfusion of abdominal aortic aneurysm after endovascular repair does not lead to progressive change in aneurysm diameter. *J Vasc Surg* 1998; **28**: 242–9.

32 Arko FR, Rubin GD, Johnson BL, *et al.* Type 2 endoleaks following endovascular repair: preoperative predictors and long-term effects. International Congress 14 on Endovascular Interventions, New York, 2000.

33 Hinchliffe RJ, Singh-Ranger R, Davidson I, Hopkinson BR. Rupture of an abdominal aortic aneurysm sac secondary to type II endoleak. *Eur J Vasc Endovasc Surg* (in press).

34 Resnikoff M, Darling RC 3rd, Chang BB, *et al.* Fate of the excluded abdominal aortic aneurysm sac: long-term follow-up of 831 patients. *J Vasc Surg.* 1996; **24**: 851–5.

35 Baum RA, Carpenter JP, Cope C, *et al.* Aneurysm sac pressure measurements after endovascular repair of abdominal aortic aneurysms. *J Vasc Surg* 2000; **33**: 32–40.

36 White GH, May J, Waugh RC, *et al.* Type 3 and Type 4 Endoleak: Toward a complete definition of blood flow in the sac after endoluminal AAA repair. *J Endovasc Surg* 1998; **5**: 305–9.

37 Harris PL, Brennan J, Martin J, *et al.* Longitudinal shrinkage following endovascular aneurysm repair: a source of intermediate and late complications. *J Endovasc Surg* 1999; **6**: 4.

38 Zarins CK, White RA, Schwarten DE, *et al.* AneuRx stent-graft versus open repair of abdominal aortic aneurysms: multicentre prospective clinical trial. *J Vasc Surg* 1999; **29**: 292–308.

39 White GH, May J, Petrasek P, *et al.* Endotension: an explanation for continued AAA growth after successful endoluminal repair. *J Endovasc Surg* 1999; **6**: 308–15.

40 Torsello GB, Klenck E, Kasprzak B, Umscheid T. Rupture of abdominal aortic aneurysm previously treated by endovascular stent-graft. *J Vasc Surg* 1998; **28**: 184.

41 Gilling-Smith GL, Brennan J, Harris P, *et al.* Endotension after endovascular aneurysm repair: definition, classification, and strategies for surveillance and intervention. *J Endovasc Surg* 1999; **6**: 305–7.

42 Wever JJ, Blankensteijn JD, Eikelboom BC. Secondary endoleak or missed endoleak? *Eur J Vasc Surg* 1999; **18**: 458–60.

43 Mehta M, Ohki T, Veith FJ, Lipsitz EC. All sealed endoleaks are not the same: a treatment strategy based on analysis. *Eur J Vasc Endovasc Surg* 2001; **21**: 541–4 .

44 Ruurda JP, Rijbroek A, Vermeulen EGJ. Continuing expansion of internal iliac artery aneurysms after surgical exclusion of the inflow. *J Cardiovasc Surg* 2001; **42**: 389–92.

45 Greenberg R, Green R. A clinical perspective on the management of endoleaks after abdominal aortic aneurysm repair. *J Vasc Surg* 2000; **31**: 836–7.

46 Golzarian J, Dussaussois L, Abada HT, *et al.* Helical CT of the aorta after endoluminal stent-graft therapy: value of biphasic acquisition. *Am J Roentgenol* 1998; **171**: 329–31.

47 Schurink GWH, Aarts NJM, Wilde J, *et al.* Endoleakage after stent-graft treatment of abdominal aortic aneurysm: Implications on pressure and imaging – an *in vitro* study. *J Vasc Surg* 1998; **28**: 234.

48 McWilliams R, Martin J, Gould D, *et al.* Levovist-enhanced ultrasound as the primary follow-up investigation after endovascular aneurysm repair. *J Intervent Radiol* 1998; **13**: 146–7.

49 Singh-Ranger R, McArthur T, Della Corte M, *et al.* The abdominal aortic aneurysm sac after endoluminal exclusion: a medium-term morphologic follow up based on volumetric technology. *J Vasc Surg* 2000; **31**: 490–500.

50 Malina M, Lanne T, Ivancev K, *et al.* Reduced pulsatile wall motion of abdominal aortic aneurysms after endovascular repair. *J Vasc Surg* 1998; **27**: 624–31.

51 Treharne GD, Loftus IM, Thompson MM, *et al.* Quality control during endovascular aneurysm repair: Monitoring aneurismal sac pressure and superficial femoral artery flow velocity. *J Endovasc Surg* 1999; **6**: 239–45.

52 Harris PL, Vallabhameni SR, Desgranges P. Incidence and risk factors of late rupture, conversion, and death after endovascular repair of infrarenal aortic aneurysms: the EUROSTAR experience. European Collaborators on Stent-graft Techniques for aortic Aneurysm Repair. *J Vasc Surg* 2000; **32**: 739–49.

53 Lawrence-Brown MMD, Semmens JB, Hartley DE. The Zenith endoluminal stent-graft system: suprarenal fixation, safety features, modular components, fenestration and custom crafting. In: Greenhalgh RM, Becquemin J-P, Davies A *et al.* (eds). *Vascular and Endovascular Surgical Techniques*, 4th edn. London: WB Saunders, 2001: 219–23.

54 Walker SR, Macierewicz JA, Hopkinson BR. Endovascular AAA repair: prevention of side branch endoleaks with thrombogenic sponge. *J Endovasc Surg* 1999; **6**: 350–3.

55 May J, White G, Yu W, *et al.* Endovascular grafting for abdominal aortic aneurysms: Changing incidence and indications for conversion to open operation. *Cardiovasc Surg* 1998; **6**: 194–7.

56 Harris PL. Management of endoleak and endotension. In: Greenhalgh RM, Becquemin J-P, Davies A *et al.* (eds). *Vascular and Endovascular Surgical Techniques*, 4th edn. London: WB Saunders, 2001: 265–70.

57 Kalliafas S, Albertini JN, Macierewicz J, *et al.* Incidence and treatment of intraoperative technical problems during endovascular repair of complex abdominal aortic aneurysms. *J Vasc Surg* 2000; **31**: 1185–92.

58 Marin ML, Dolmatch BL, Fry PD, *et al.* Treatment of type II endoleaks with onyx. *J Vasc Intervent Radiol* 2001; **12**: 629–32.

59 Edoga JK. Laparoscopic treatment for endoleak resolution following endoprosthesis exclusion of AAA. Presented to the International Workshop 'New Technologies in Vascular Surgery', Rome, 27 June 2001.

60 May J, White GH, Harris JP. Techniques for surgical conversion of aortic endoprosthesis. *Eur J Vasc Endovasc Surg* 1999; **18**: 284–9.

61 May J, White GH, Waugh R, *et al.* Rupture of abdominal aortic aneurysms: a concurrent comparison of outcome of those occurring after endoluminal repair versus those occurring *de novo. Eur J Vasc Endovasc Surg* 1999; **18**: 344–8.

62 Cuypers PWM, Laheij RJF, Buth J, on behalf of the EUROSTAR collaborators. Which factors increase the risk of conversion to open surgery following endovascular abdominal aortic aneurysm repair ? *Eur J Vasc Endovasc Surg* 2000; **20**: 183–9.

63 Sonesson B, Montgomery A, Invancev K, Lindblad B. Fixation of infra-renal aortic stent-grafts using laparoscopic banding – an experimental study. *Eur J Vasc Endovasc Surg* 2001; **21**: 40–5.

64 Hopkinson BR. Methods for dealing with difficult aortic necks: short, wide, conical or angulated. The 27th Global Symposium. Vascular and Endovascular Issues, Techniques and Horizons. New York, 17 November 2000.

65 Huber KL, Joseph A, Mukherjee D. Extra-anatomic arterial reconstruction of common iliac arteries and embolization of the aneurysm sac for the treatment of abdominal aortic aneurysms in high risk patients. *J Vasc Surg* 2001; **33**: 745–51.

66 Peacock JH, Brown GJ. Wiring of abdominal aortic aneurysms. *Br J Surg* 1968; **55**: 344–6.

31

Graft Breakdown and Migration Complicating EVAR

S RAO VALLABHANENI, PETER L HARRIS

INTRODUCTION

Endovascular aneurysm repair (EVAR) using stent-graft systems that could be deployed through femoral arteries was introduced in 1991. Although the early results were encouraging, late follow-up has been characterised by a high rate of secondary intervention, reaching a cumulative annual incidence of nearly 10 per cent for any intervention and approximately 3 per cent for late conversion.[1,2] Despite close surveillance and such high rates of secondary intervention, late rupture has been observed at an annual rate of 1 per cent.[2] Although correction of an endoleak, most often type 2, has been the commonest indication for a secondary intervention, a recent EUROSTAR analysis revealed no significant association between isolated type 2 endoleak and late rupture.[2,3] The important and significant risk factors leading to late rupture were migration of stent-graft leading to a type I endoleak and device disintegration leading to a type 3 endoleak, both signifying device failure.[3] Therefore the surveillance and secondary interventions should be aimed at ensuring stent-graft stability and integrity. Endoleak, as a consequence of device failure (secondary type 1 and type 3), is a potentially serious finding and is a late event (see Chapter 30).

Although the durability of endovascular devices is invariably subjected to rigorous testing prior to release for clinical use, some of the mechanisms of EVAR failure have come to light only with long term follow-up of early recipients. It is possible that some potential mechanisms for device failure remain as yet unrecognised. This chapter addresses the clinical issues associated with device migration and disintegration related to endovascular aneurysm repair.

AETIOLOGY/PATHOPHYSIOLOGY

Mechanism of stent-graft function

Devices which can be delivered by a transfemoral route to exclude aortic aneurysms, avoiding all transabdominal manoeuvres, call for design features that differ radically from a simple fabric tube fixed by conventional sutured anastomosis at open repair.[4] A brief overview of the stent-graft design and function relevant to stent migration and disintegration is presented here to facilitate understanding of these modes of failure. Stent-grafts require not only a fabric tube to isolate the aneurysm sac from the blood flow but also some form of frame or stent to effect a 'seal' and fix the device in place. Sutures have been used to attach the stent rings to each other and to the fabric in early devices. More recent models incorporate the metal rings within the layers of fabric. In addition, a system of radio-opaque markers is required to facilitate visualisation and orientation of the device during deployment and at follow-up. The entire device is crimped into a delivery mechanism which is narrow and flexible enough to traverse the iliofemoral segment. Thin Dacron has been used to facilitate smaller profile construction but it is more susceptible to wear than standard thickness fabric. Polytetrafluoroethylene (PTFE), the other fabric used in stent-graft construction, appears to be more resistant to wear.

Adequate apposition between stent fabric and native vessel wall, at the neck of aneurysm and in iliac segments, is necessary to seal these junctions or 'anastomoses' against type 1 endoleak. This is largely dependent on radial forces exerted by the stent. Such radial forces are brought into action by balloon expansion (e.g. Lifepath, Edwards Life Sciences, Irvine, CA, USA) or spring-expansion (e.g. Zenith, Cook, Bloomington, IN, USA) or as a mechanical function of 'memory' alloys from which the stent is constructed (e.g. Talent, World Medical Corp).

Once deployed, the columnar strength of the device assists the radial forces in stabilising the stent-graft in its position and resists its movement. In some devices, fixation may be enhanced by the addition of hooks and barbs to the proximal or distal stent-graft enabling it to anchor on to the neck of aneurysm or iliac arteries.[5] Natural healing does not contribute significantly to fixation and stent-grafts therefore rely permanently upon their mechanical properties for their stability and integrity.[6] A section of uncovered metal stent on the top end of the device may assist fixation by increasing the frictional forces. One device (Zenith, Cook) incorporates a proximal uncovered stent with hooks intended to cross the renal artery ostia and engage into the relatively healthy suprarenal aorta for additional fixation.

The columnar strength of a device depends on its construction. Some devices (e.g. AneuRx, Medtronic, Minneapolis, MN, USA) comprise metal rings which articulate with each other throughout its height providing high columnar strength. Devices with stents at fixation sites only, with the fabric tube unsupported in the middle, have negligible columnar strength and depend entirely on radial forces and hooks for fixation. Other devices contain partially articulating struts or vertical wire frames to provide columnar strength of intermediate and variable degree.

Most devices are bifurcated but straight tube designs intended for endoluminal aorto-uni-iliac use are available. Bifurcated design is preferred since aorto-uni-iliac repair requires an additional femoro-femoral bypass. Some bifurcated models are available as a single piece. The more frequently used modular construction allows customisation of the device to utilise the anatomy fully, to extend applicability of EVAR to a wider range of aneurysms and in some cases to facilitate accurate deployment. Modular systems are made up of two or three components which can be docked and deployed to construct a bifurcated device *in vivo*. A major disadvantage of modular devices is the potential for disjunction of the modular parts.

Device failure

Materials that are known to be safe for implantation into humans have been adopted for the fabrication of stent-grafts. The physiological conditions within an aortic aneurysm, however, such as the constant pulsation, the haemodynamic forces, host reaction, etc., have proved to be detrimental to the structural integrity of the device, upon which the state of the aneurysm repair depends.[7] Additionally, the morphology of the aneurysm sac changes following implantation of an endograft, with potential adverse impact upon both the fixation and structure of the endograft.[8]

Stent–graft disintegration

The approximately 30 000 000 pulsations a year to which the devices are subjected increase the risk of stress fracture of the suture material bonding the stent frames together or to the fabric. Suture breakage may result in wire frame separation and dislocation, which, in turn, may lead to distortion. Consequently the columnar strength is compromised and in severe cases the basic integrity of the device may be lost.

Nitinol from which the wire frames of some devices are constructed has been shown to be susceptible to corrosion by a host reaction leading to weakening and fracture of stents.[9] It is probable that other alloys are similarly vulnerable. Wire frames are also susceptible to stress fracture. This not only compromises the strength of the device but the sharp ends of broken wire can also come into contact with the fabric. Pulsatile movement can then result in erosion of fabric resulting in holes or tears with a risk of sudden reperfusion of the aneurysm sac (type 3 endoleak). Integrity of the flow channel of the stent-graft depends on adequate fixation between the modular components. Loss of structural integrity and distortion may cause dislocation of the contralateral limb from the main stent-graft precipitating sudden reperfusion of the aneurysm sac.

An aneurysm that has been excluded successfully shrinks in size not only in its anteroposterior (AP) and lateral diameters but also longitudinally. This may lead to kinking and buckling of the stent-graft which could lead to dislocation of limb engagement or modular separation.[10] In addition, stent-graft distortion alters the spatial relationship between the components of the device. This, in turn, may exaggerate movement between them causing tears in the fabric, suture breakage or fracture of stent struts.[7]

Stent migration

The infrarenal neck of some aortic aneurysms increases in diameter at the landing zone of the stent-graft at a rate approximating 1 mm per year following stent-graft implantation.[11,12] It is usual to 'oversize' the diameter of the device relative to that of aneurysm neck by at least 10 per cent or 3–4 mm. Therefore, one may expect to see compromise of proximal fixation and seal resulting in proximal type 1 endoleaks and stent migration 3–4 years after implantation.[12] Aneurysmal changes in common iliac arteries resulting in widening and shortening could result in the loss of distal fixation (Irfan Raza, unpublished data).

The physiological haemodynamic forces of the aorta generate vectors due to flow channel geometry.[13,14] The cephalo-caudal narrowing of the flow channel leads to a 'wind sock effect', the force attempting to cause distal migration of the entire device. The curvature in the stent-graft elicits a 'hose pipe effect' (the force that causes an open fire hose to move vigorously side to side like a snake), which encourages proximal dislocation of the iliac limb engagement and distal

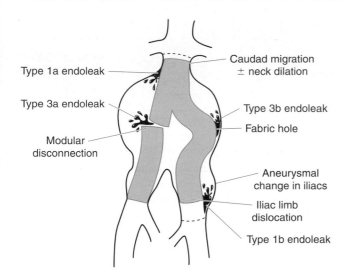

Figure 31.1 *Schematic diagram of some possible modes of stent-graft failure*

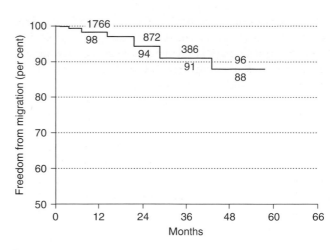

Figure 31.2 *Kaplan–Meier graph of freedom from stent-graft migration. The numbers above line are patients at risk and those below the line are the percentage free from migration*

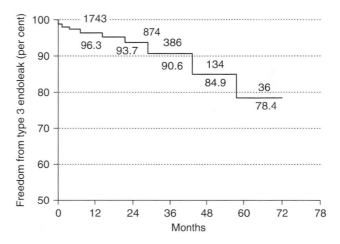

Figure 31.3 *Kaplan–Meier graph of freedom from secondary type 3 endoleak. The numbers above line are patients at risk and those below the line are the percentage free from migration*

migration of the proximal engagement at the neck. The haemodynamic forces are of significant magnitude and are exaggerated by curvature, angulation or kinking of the device, all of which may worsen with aneurysm shrinkage and play an important role in promoting device migration.

Figure 31.1 is a diagrammatic representation of some modes of failure of endoaortic stent-grafts. The design of these devices is under constant review and later generations of devices incorporate features intended to address these modes of failure.

THE PROBLEMS AND THEIR INCIDENCE

Stent-graft migration and disintegration are observed throughout the follow-up. The Kaplan–Meier curve of the incidence of migration in Figure 31.2 is derived from an analysis of 3264 patients from EUROSTAR with a mean and median follow-up of approximately 1 year. The incidence of stent-graft migration can be noted to be persistent without signs of reaching a plateau at 4 years and by then affecting nearly 12 per cent of the cohort. The mean time after EVAR to the diagnosis of migration is approximately 20 months.[13]

Stent-graft disintegration is a progressive phenomenon with its effects once again noted throughout the late follow-up of all models. Suture breakage, detected on plain X-rays as alteration in the alignment of stent struts, is a common and universally noted finding affecting the earliest, now withdrawn, models. Fracture of metal struts is also a common finding. Secondary mid-graft endoleaks due to stent-graft disintegration (fabric hole or modular component dissociation), a finding that can be used as a surrogate measure of

serious disintegration, shows a steady incidence affecting 21.6 per cent of the cohort by 5 years (Figure 31.3).

Consequences of device failure

Stent migration or disintegration may not show any immediate effects and may lead to complacency in dealing with these failures in their early stages. Haemodynamic isolation of the aneurysm sac, which is the aim of stent-graft repair, should aim at isolating the sac not only from blood flow but also from systemic blood pressure. Endotension, the phenomenon of pressurisation of the stent-grafted aneurysm sac, denotes a risk of rupture. Pressure can be transmitted through thrombus[15] and through fixation sites with inadequate overlap in the absence of a detectable endoleak. In general, a 10 mm overlap is considered the essential minimum for an adequate seal. The consequences of 'silent' pressurisation of the sac may not be detectable straight away by the routine means of surveillance but may only appear as an enlarging sac over time.[16,17] An enlarging aneurysm sac with a migrating stent-graft and inadequate seal is at risk of precipitous graft related endoleak and ensuing rupture. Even an aneurysm that has been shown to be shrinking, however, may be at risk if there is evidence of increasing distortion of the stent-graft and compromise of the seal due to stent-graft disintegration or migration.[18] Endoleak due to migration or disintegration is a late finding and indicates that the ideal time for intervention has already been missed. Poor fixation, catastrophic migration and disintegration of the stent-graft have been incriminated in reports of late ruptures.[19] An aneurysm sac may undergo atrophy following successful exclusion and a sudden reperfusion may render it more liable to rupture than it might have been prior to exclusion. Current surveillance methods are limited by their inability to demonstrate directly the presence or absence of endotension. The time interval between the surveillance scans, according to current schedules, also means that an adverse development could go undetected for as long as nearly a year and, more significantly, may lead to a catastrophe before it can be detected. Patients with subtle or early changes of stent migration or disintegration are at higher risk of such an event and call for the adoption of flexible surveillance schedules permitting more frequent investigation in selected patients.

Since the mechanisms of device failure related to material fatigue and the morphological changes in the aneurysm sac take time to evolve, inevitably, it also takes time to evaluate each new device or malfunction of that device. For this reason it is essential that all patients treated with aortic endografts for repair of an aneurysm are subjected to lifelong surveillance.

Risk factors

Analysis of EUROSTAR data has revealed a number of statistically significant risk factors associated with migration.[13,20] The association may not be causal for each factor and the mechanisms by which the risk factors could possibly be associated with device failure are not discussed here.

> ### Risk factors for the development of migration[6,20]
>
> - Patient factors
>   - Smoking
>   - Hypertension
>   - Higher ASA (Amercan Society of Anesthesiologists) class
> - Graft related feature
>   - Higher proximal diameter

> - Anatomical factors
>   - Aortic neck angulation
>   - Angulation of iliac artery
>   - Higher maximal aneurysm diameter
>   - Higher terminal aortic transverse diameter

DIAGNOSIS

Diagnosis of device failure in its early stages is dependent upon an adequate programme of postoperative surveillance.

Clinical manifestations

Migration and stent-graft disintegration occur insidiously and, initially, may not be associated with any symptoms or signs until rupture ensues.[21] The majority of stent-graft failures are detected on routine surveillance imaging. Absence of symptoms or signs does not signify adequacy of stent-graft function or integrity.

Investigations

PLAIN RADIOGRAPHY

Plain X-rays may demonstrate evidence of suture breakage by showing misalignment of metal struts of adjacent stent rings. Breakages and dislocations of metal struts and fractures of hooks and barbs may also be seen well on plain X-rays. The anatomical relationship of the stent-graft to bony landmarks serves as a guide in evaluating changes in stent-graft position over time. Plain radiographs should be performed in four planes: AP, lateral and oblique views from both directions. A methodical assessment of all sets of plain radiographs taken since implantation is necessary in order to discern the subtle changes. Lateral views reconstructed from computed tomography (CT) images eliminate inconsistencies due to variable centring and projection. Good understanding of the radiological appearances of stent disintegration and migration is crucial to utilising the plain X-rays to the fullest. Subtle findings can easily go unnoticed.

COMPUTED TOMOGRAPHY

Dual-phase CT scan provides detailed information regarding the morphology of the aneurysm and the presence or absence of an endoleak and is currently the mainstay of surveillance. The position of the stent-graft can be determined accurately in relation to anatomical landmarks such as the ostia of visceral arteries in order to diagnose migration. The extent and adequacy of overlap at the landing zones can be assessed precisely to establish the quality of seal. Three-dimensional reconstruction of images using a workstation provides useful information in specific circumstances.

Migration of subtle degree between each interval can add up to significant levels over time. Therefore, a review of all previous imaging is necessary at each evaluation rather than simply comparing the most recent CTs to the immediately preceding set.

ANGIOGRAPHY

Angiography is not an appropriate tool for routine surveillance. The indications for diagnostic angiography should be considered for each patient on the merits of the situation. Examples of such indications include the enlarging aneurysm where there is plain X-ray evidence of borderline fixation or structural deformation and deterioration of a stent-graft sufficient to suspect that a fabric hole might have occurred but remained undetected on CT.

ULTRASOUND SCAN

Duplex ultrasound scan, enhanced with microbubble contrast media can provide useful information regarding the presence or absence of endoleak.[22] Being an operator dependent investigation, however, it is not specific or sensitive enough to replace CT even in the diagnosis of endoleak. The major limitation remains the poor quality of information obtained regarding changing sac and stent-graft morphology and migration.

MAGNETIC RESONANCE IMAGING

Magnetic resonance imaging (MRI) is free from ionising radiation and is performed with or without intravenous contrast and functional measurements such as renal perfusion can also be made. A major proportion of patients will be unsuitable due to the magnetic properties of the device used, the presence of metal implants such as cardiac pacemakers or in cases of claustrophobia. The anatomical detail obtained is also limited. For these reasons, MRI is not used as a tool of routine surveillance and has a limited role in investigation.

MANAGEMENT

General principles

Complications of stent-graft migration and disintegration may be detected on routine surveillance in apparently asymptomatic patients. Since the consequences of delayed diagnosis are potentially serious, even fatal, there is a need for a methodical and organised surveillance system. A failsafe arrangement to ensure patient compliance with surveillance protocol and prompt review of results is therefore essential.

Minor structural failures such as suture or strut breakage are very common. While not compromising the overall repair on their own, they may be harbingers of further and more serious failure later. Severe disruption of stent-graft integrity may lead to rupture of the aneurysm by causing graft related endoleak either directly or through stent-graft migration. It is important to recognise that any degree of migration is a significant finding and points to a compromise in fixation even if an 'adequate seal' is maintained at the time of examination. Migration may not progress at a uniform rate, and the possibility that a minor degree of migration may appear as a forerunner of precipitous loss of fixation, should be considered when management plans are made.

The risk of unintended conversion to open repair due to complications during a secondary intervention needs to be assessed in each patient and preoperative assessment performed accordingly.

Selection and timing of secondary intervention

Late ruptures continue to occur despite a high incidence of secondary interventions.[2,19] Evidence pointing to the importance of stent-graft migration and disintegration is clear and growing stronger.[3,19,21] This suggests that currently accepted indications and timing of secondary intervention are inappropriate or require modification. The hitherto conventional focus on endoleaks should be shifted towards ensuring stent-graft integrity and stability so that earlier and more selective secondary interventions could be undertaken before secondary type 1 or type 3 endoleaks appear. Such early remedy could be expected to reduce the incidence of catastrophic device failure. Some factors to be considered when deciding secondary interventions in the absence of an associated endoleak are listed in below and in the algorithm in Figure 31.4.

> ### Considerations in endograft failure when not associated with consequent endoleak
>
> - Suture breakage without severe or multiple metal ring dislocations is unlikely to compromise integrity of the system
> - Multiple metal ring breaks or dislocations can threaten the structural integrity
> - 'Landing zones' shorter than 10 mm are prone to dislocation and consequent endoleak or development of endotension
> - Risk is worsened in all the above if associated with stent-graft angulation or kinking
> - Loss of proximal or mid-graft seal can be more serious than loss of distal seal
> - Any migration is significant and may be followed by precipitous loss of fixation

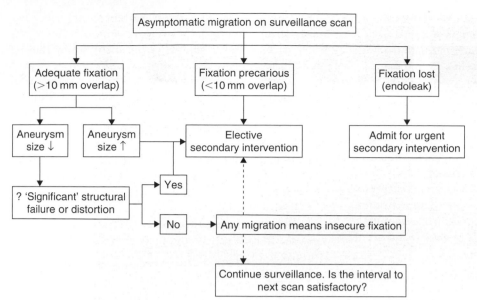

Figure 31.4 *Algorithm of management of stent-graft migration*

Late conversion has been reported to be associated with considerable postoperative morbidity and mortality. That, combined with the fact that the majority of secondary interventions are feasible via the transfemoral route, meant that late conversion has been considered to be the last resort and undertaken only when no other means of intervention is possible. In the EUROSTAR and other series, however, mortality following late conversion was confined to patients having emergency operations for rupture[2,21,23] and elective conversion was associated with very low risk of death. When transfemoral intervention only serves as a temporary measure to 'shore-up' the integrity of a disintegrating stent-graft, elective conversion is likely to be the preferred option.

Stent-graft migration or disintegration may present as an acute emergency having already caused a rupture of the aneurysm and this situation requires to be dealt with along the same lines as a ruptured aortic aneurysm. Acute situations in which the aneurysm sac may be exposed to systemic blood pressure require to be treated urgently, i.e. as soon as possible, even if there are no symptoms. Modular dislocation endoleaks, perigraft endoleak and graft-hole endoleak are examples of this.

ENDOVASCULAR SECONDARY INTERVENTIONS

Technical considerations

Most secondary interventions can be accomplished via the transfemoral route but they can be challenging and frequently call for a very high degree of expertise, dexterity and catheter skills. The aim is to deploy a covered stent to restore stent-graft integrity and haemodynamic 'seal'. A gap between dissociated modular components or a gap

between stent-graft and native vessel may be bridged with a covered stent (Figure 31.5). Similarly, fabric holes can be covered and 'landing zones' of fixation sites extended with stent extensions. Deployment of a new complete stent-graft system within a failing stent-graft has also been undertaken on rare occasions. Conversion of a bifurcated into an aorto-uni-iliac reconstruction is also a useful approach in some circumstances, e.g. a modular disconnection that could not be repaired directly. Knowledge about the device *in situ* and current anatomy, forward planning of access and route of deployment are essential. A vast array of catheters, guidewires and techniques could be drawn from but a comprehensive account of their technical details is not within the scope of this chapter.

Practical considerations

The requirement for sophisticated imaging with a digital subtraction facility, access to a wide array of disposables used for catheter techniques, aseptic conditions and facilities for anaesthesia demand a highly sophisticated environment for these procedures. The exact location of such facilities depends on the hospital. It is common for short percutaneous transfemoral procedures such as iliac limb extensions to be performed in the interventional radiology suite under local anaesthetic. Longer or complex procedures, those that require surgical exposure of access vessels, interventions requiring regional or general anaesthesia and those with some risk of conversion are best undertaken in operating theatres with imaging facilities.

Conversion to conventional repair

Conversion is indicated for late rupture and also when other forms of secondary intervention are not feasible. All

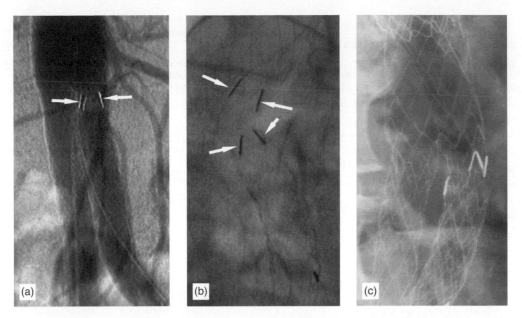

Figure 31.5   *Modular disconnection. (a) Arrows point to the radio-opaque markers of stent-graft system well aligned initially. (b) Later separation of these markers due to modular disconnection. (c) Treatment of the problem by a bridging stent*

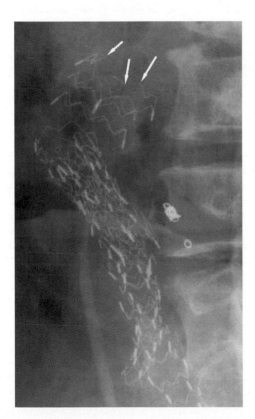

Figure 31.6   *Severe stent-graft disintegration. The metal struts not only show misalignment but also breakage (arrows)*

fit patients with severe structural failure or migration of stent-graft, where other forms of secondary intervention may serve only as a temporary measure (Figure 31.6), should be considered for an elective conversion to conventional repair.

Assessment of fitness for such major surgery should include objective assessment of cardiorespiratory status in addition to baseline blood tests and electrocardiography. Spirometry for respiratory function and echocardiography or multiple gated acquisition scan (MUGA) scan for estimation of left ventricular ejection fraction ought to be carried out. Arterial blood gases, echocardiography, creatinine clearance, etc., could be considered depending on individual circumstances.

The aorta at and above the upper limit of the stent-graft needs to be evaluated carefully by preoperative imaging to ascertain the level of aortic cross-clamping. A suprarenal aortic clamp is frequently required and on occasions, a supracoeliac clamp. The risk of renal failure and the need for dialysis is relatively high. Technical difficulties in the removal of the stent-graft, as a result of incorporation of the uncovered stent-graft into native vessels and the effects of fixation barbs or hooks, should be expected. Wire cutters should be available for cutting the struts.

Conclusions

Until completely durable devices become available, EVAR patients will remain at a lifelong risk of device failure with migration and disintegration, leading to secondary endoleak and late rupture. With the conventional primary focus on endoleaks, the diagnosis of subtle but incremental development of migration or deterioration of graft integrity is often overlooked and the consequences may be disastrous. There is a need to re-examine the indications and timing of secondary interventions to eliminate the risk of late rupture. Transfemoral interventions are adequate in extending the seal or in bridging defects and are usually feasible in the majority of patients. Although late conversion is technically challenging, it should be considered in all patients with severe stent-graft disintegration or migration, where endoluminal interventions may only be able to offer a temporary solution. Actual or imminent loss of seal requires urgent intervention. Long term solutions lie in alterations in the stent-graft design and construction to impart stronger fixation and resistance to structural deterioration.

ACKNOWLEDGEMENT

We wish to acknowledge Gillian Rycroft, Medical Illustrator, for assistance with Figure 31.1.

EUROSTAR (European collaborators on Stent-Graft Techniques for Aneurysm Repair) a Europe-wide project launched in 1996 to scientifically evaluate endovascular aneurysm repair, was adopted by the European Society for Vascular and Endovascular Surgery in September 2001. By September 2001, collaborators from 107 centres had enrolled in excess of 4000 patients into the Eurostar database. Comprehensive data regarding preoperative, intraoperative and follow-up details are collected prospectively and periodically analysed. The follow-up is structured and uniform. See the website at www.esvs.org/start/index.asp (accessed 21 December 2004).

Key references

Albertini J, Kalliafas S, Travis S, *et al.* Anatomical risk factors for proximal perigraft endoleak and graft migration following endovascular repair of abdominal aortic aneurysms. *Eur J Vasc Endovasc Surg* 2000; **19**: 308–12.

Beebe HG, Cronenwett JL, Katzen BT, *et al.* Vanguard Endograft Trial Investigators. Results of an aortic endograft trial: impact of device failure beyond 12 months. *J Vasc Surg* 2001; **33**(suppl 2): S55–63.

Broeders IA, Blankensteijn JD, Wever JJ, Eikelboom BC. Mid-term fixation stability of the EndoVascular Technologies endograft. EVT Investigators. *Eur J Vasc Endovasc Surg* 1999; **18**: 300–7.

Jacobowitz GR, Lee AM, Riles TS. Immediate and late explantation of endovascular aortic grafts: the endovascular technologies experience. *J Vasc Surg* 1999; **29**: 309–16.

Vallabhaneni SR, Harris PL. Lessons learnt from the EUROSTAR registry on endovascular repair of abdominal aortic aneurysm repair. *Eur J Radiol* 2001; **39**: 34–41.

REFERENCES

1   Laheij RJ, Buth J, Harris PL, *et al.* Need for secondary interventions after endovascular repair of abdominal aortic aneurysms. Intermediate-term follow-up results of a European collaborative registry (EUROSTAR). *Br J Surg* 2000; **87**: 1666–73.

2   Harris PL, Vallabhaneni SR, Desgranges P, *et al.* Incidence and risk factors of late rupture, conversion, and death after endovascular repair of infrarenal aortic aneurysms: the EUROSTAR experience. European Collaborators on Stent/graft techniques for aortic aneurysm repair. *J Vasc Surg* 2000; **32**: 739–49.

3   Vallabhaneni SR, Harris PL. Lessons learnt from the EUROSTAR registry on endovascular repair of abdominal aortic aneurysm repair. *Eur J Radiol* 2001; **39**: 34–41.

4   Veith FJ, Abbott WM, Yao JST, *et al.* Guidelines for development and use of transluminally placed endovascular prosthetic grafts in the arterial system. *J Vasc Surg* 1995; **21**: 670–85 and *J Vasc Interv Radiol* 1995; **6**: 477–92.

5   Broeders IA, Blankensteijn JD, Wever JJ, Eikelboom BC. Mid-term fixation stability of the EndoVascular Technologies endograft. EVT Investigators. *Eur J Vasc Endovasc Surg* 1999; **18**: 300–7.

6   Malina M, Brunkwall J, Ivancev K, *et al.* Endovascular healing is inadequate for fixation of Dacron stent-grafts in human aortoiliac vessels. *Eur J Vasc Endovasc Surg* 2000; **19**: 5–11.

7   Guidoin R, Marois Y, Douville Y, *et al.* First-generation aortic endografts: analysis of explanted Stentor devices from the EUROSTAR Registry. *J Endovasc Ther* 2000; **7**: 105–22.

8   Resch T, Ivancev K, Brunkwall J, *et al.* Midterm changes in aortic aneurysm morphology after endovascular repair. *J Endovasc Ther* 2000; **7**: 279–85.

9   Heintz C, Riepe G, Birken L, *et al.* Corroded nitinol wires in explanted aortic endografts: an important mechanism of failure? *J Endovasc Ther* 2001; **8**: 248–53.

10 Harris P, Brennan J, Martin J, *et al.* Longitudinal aneurysm shrinkage following endovascular aortic aneurysm repair: a source of intermediate and late complications. *J Endovasc Surg* 1999; **6**: 11–16.

11 Wever JJ, de Nie AJ, Blankensteijn JD, *et al.* Dilatation of the proximal neck of infrarenal aortic aneurysms after endovascular AAA repair. *Eur J Vasc Endovasc Surg* 2000; **19**: 197–201.

12 Prinssen M, Wever JJ, Mali WP, *et al.* Concerns for the durability of the proximal abdominal aortic aneurysm endograft fixation from a 2-year and 3-year longitudinal computed tomography angiography study. *J Vasc Surg* 2001; **33**(suppl 2): S64–9.

13 Mohan IV, van Marriewijk, Harris PL, *et al.* Factors and forces influencing stent-graft migration after endovascular aortic aneurysm. *J Endovasc Ther* 2002; **9**: 748–55.

14 Liffman K, Lawrence-Brown MM, Semmens JB, *et al.* Analytical modeling and numerical simulation of forces in an endoluminal graft. *J Endovasc Ther* 2001; **8**: 358–71.

15 Marty B, Sanchez LA, Ohki T, *et al.* Endoleak after endovascular graft repair of experimental aortic aneurysms: does coil embolization with angiographic "seal" lower intraaneurysmal pressure? *J Vasc Surg* 1998; **27**: 454–61; discussion 462.

16 Gilling-Smith G, Brennan J, Harris P, *et al.* Endotension after endovascular aneurysm repair: definition, classification, and strategies for surveillance and intervention [review]. *J Endovasc Surg* 1999; **6**: 305–7.

17 White GH, May J, Petrasek P, *et al.* Endotension: an explanation for continued AAA growth after successful endoluminal repair. *J Endovasc Surg* 1999; **6**: 308–15.

18 Alimi YS, Chakfe N, Rivoal E, *et al.* Rupture of an abdominal aortic aneurysm after endovascular graft placement and aneurysm size reduction. *J Vasc Surg* 1998; **28**: 178–83.

19 Zarins CK, White RA, Fogarty TJ. Aneurysm rupture after endovascular repair using the AneuRx stent graft. *J Vasc Surg* 2000; **31**: 960–70.

20 Albertini J, Kalliafas S, Travis S, *et al.* Anatomical risk factors for proximal perigraft endoleak and graft migration following endovascular repair of abdominal aortic aneurysms. *Eur J Vasc Endovasc Surg* 2000; **19**: 308–12.

21 Beebe HG, Cronenwett JL, Katzen BT, *et al.* Vanguard Endograft Trial Investigators. Results of an aortic endograft trial: impact of device failure beyond 12 months. *J Vasc Surg* 2001; **33**(suppl 2): S55–63.

22 McWilliams RG, Martin J, White D, *et al.* Detection of endoleak with enhanced ultrasound imaging: comparison with biphasic computed tomography. *J Endovasc Ther* 2002; **9**: 170–9.

23 Jacobowitz GR, Lee AM, Riles TS. Immediate and late explantation of endovascular aortic grafts: the endovascular technologies experience. *J Vasc Surg* 1999; **29**: 309–16.

32

Atheroembolism Complicating EVAR

JUAN C PARODI, LUIS M FERREIRA

THE PROBLEM

Atheroembolism results from the release of cholesterol rich atheromatous debris from an ulcerated aorta or an abdominal aortic aneurysm (AAA) into the systemic arterial circulation.[1-2] Atheroembolism is a rare condition, but it is becoming more common with the growing indications for endovascular procedures and increasing numbers of candidates undergoing them. At the same time, an ageing population represents a rising incidence of atheromatous 'shaggy' aortas and aneurysms warranting treatment. The technical feasibility of endovascular aneurysm repair (EVAR) has been conclusively established, with many centres reporting the successful exclusion of AAAs by endoprostheses.[3-5] The surgical community has also enthusiastically embraced this new technology because it offers potentially significant advantages over conventional aneurysm repair in that it avoids transperitoneal or retroperitoneal interventions, general anaesthesia and prolonged aortic clamping while also ensuring rapid recovery.

In spite of the potential advantages of EVAR, early reports documented a high incidence of perioperative complications and mortality in excess of 5 per cent. Parodi et al.,[6] Gitlitz et al.[7] and Thompson et al.[8] reported cases of massive microembolism as a significant complication of this technique with an incidence of 4–17 per cent, all invariably fatal cases. In contrast, however, several other representative series failed to document evidence of peripheral microembolism which suggests that this complication may be related either to technique or the device used. The fact that even those who reported such incidents did so in the early

stages of their experience, and were no longer experiencing them, shows that it was at least partly to do with a learning curve or perhaps better patient selection. The aim of this chapter is to discuss our experience of treating patients who suffered atheroembolism and offer our approach in averting this serious complication in endovascular procedures.

AETIOLOGY/PATHOPHYSIOLOGY

Atheroembolism consists of cholesterol crystal microemboli which generally occlude arterioles of 200–900 μm calibre, often leading to the development of the typical blue toe syndrome (Fig. 32.1), in which arterial occlusions are located at the level of the digital arteries of the feet.[1-2] This atheromatous embolism syndrome is a frequently misdiagnosed, and sometimes unrecognised, condition the true incidence and consequences of which are unknown, and although often clinically silent, associated with significant morbidity and mortality. Clinically it may present in a variety of ways. Atheroembolism may be spontaneous but it sometimes occurs after lifting weights, coughing or tenesmus, although it is definitely more frequently observed during or after open aortic interventions, endovascular procedures and anticoagulant or thrombolytic therapy. During the latter, the blue toe syndrome may occur at any time but, typically, it does so within 4–12 weeks of having been started. The mechanism of embolism is presumed to be due to unsuccessful fibrin apposition and loosening of fresh thrombus at ulcerated plaques, but it may also be precipitated by sudden haemorrhage into plaques, leading to

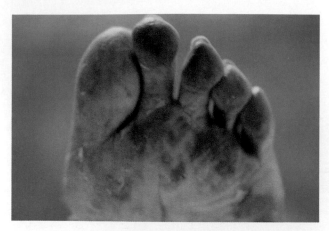

Figure 32.1 *Embolisation to the dermal vessels with areas of focal ischaemia, purplish discoloration of the skin and surrounding petechial haemorrhages (blue toe syndrome)*

their disruption. Data suggesting that anticoagulant therapy causes embolism, however, are not overwhelmingly convincing.

Atheroembolism can be a serious complication associated with procedures undertaken for diagnostic or therapeutic purposes. In a retrospective study of autopsy findings of patients who died soon after coronary angiography, almost 30 per cent were found to have evidence of atheroembolism.[1] In contrast, in 70 age-matched patients with diffuse atherosclerotic disease, but no history of having undergone endoluminal procedures, the incidence of atheroembolism was only 4.3 per cent.[1]

Thromboembolic complications are relatively uncommon after surgical AAA repair but they have been reported in many series of endoluminal treatment. While perioperative mortality in patients undergoing conventional AAA repair is primarily cardiac, in those subjected to the endoluminal approach it is mainly associated with local or vascular complications. One of them, namely, massive microembolim, is a devastating complication and proved to be fatal in over 90 per cent of affected patients. In some initial series, including ours, one of the most important causes of perioperative death was related to diffuse embolism during endograft deployment.[9–13]

MECHANISMS

The mechanism of thromboembolism is probably related to intrasac manipulation by large and rigid devices dislodging laminated thrombus lining the sac of the aneurysm. Most endovascular teams witnessed massive microembolism during their early experience of inserting endografts. With bilateral distal clamping, the debris loosened by guidewires and catheters is rapidly dispersed in retrograde fashion upwards into the visceral and renal artery with devastating results. When we reviewed our cases of atheroembolism it became clear that large and tortuous aneurysms have a potentially higher likelihood of causing this problem. First, that is probably because in advancing the guidewire from the femoral artery into the aorta and then into the proximal neck, the operator is negotiating the device through a tortuous chamber often lined with friable material which can become dislodged by those manoeuvres. In large aneurysms especially, therefore, it is advisable to insert the guidewire percutaneously via the brachial artery or, better still, a floating balloon mounted on a wire, as will be discussed later. A second possible cause of atheroembolism applies to large aneurysms which create the necessity of adding extensions to lengthen the device or to cover any type of endoleak. In short, the more intravascular manipulations performed, the greater the risk for dislodgement of material and embolism.

A new generation of endografts has evolved of greater flexibility and of slimmer profile compared with initial models. These changes in design are also probably responsible for the lower incidence of atheroembolism in more recently reported series.

CLINICAL MANIFESTATIONS

A variety of clinical manifestations are observed in atheroembolism, most commonly involving the lower limbs. The condition may be heralded by hypertension, pain and a livedo reticularis pattern on the abdomen and lower extremities, cyanosis, discoloration, blue toes, gangrene, and later, ulceration. These features of embolism to dermal vessels generally appear on the buttocks, thighs, legs and feet (see Fig. 32.1). They are painful lesions caused by focal ischaemia, recognisable by their purplish discoloration and surrounding petechial haemorrhages, and present in spite of palpable foot pulses. If left untreated, the natural history of microembolism of the extremities is one of repetitive such events; more than 50 per cent of patients develop further complications and nearly 40 per cent experience some degree of tissue loss. Long term follow-up shows that up to 20 per cent of these patients will die within a year of the initial event.

The most common clinical manifestation of visceral atheroembolism is diffuse abdominal pain, distension, paralytic ileus and bleeding. In cases of renal atheroembolism the clinical picture is one of hypertension, fever, eosinophilia and acute renal failure.

The diagnosis of atheroembolism is made having first anticipated that possibility, recognising the symptoms and signs and confirming the source of embolism by appropriate imaging. In most cases, colour duplex scans, transoesophageal echocardiography and computed tomography (CT) scans are of value in defining the territory responsible.

Keen and Yao describe the following CT findings in patients who suffered spontaneous atheroembolism from an AAA: irregular luminal surface, multiple lumens, heterogeneity of thrombus, calcification within the thrombus, fissures extending from the lumen into the thrombus and non-contiguous areas of intraluminal thrombus.[14]

MANAGEMENT

Treatment should be directed towards three goals: removal of the source of atheromatous debris, symptomatic care of the end organ wherein the emboli are located and risk factor modification to prevent re-embolism and progression of the disease.

Medical management described in the literature includes the use of heparin, dextran, papaverine, urokinase and vasodilators, among other agents. Unfortunately, the results have not been uniformly satisfactory. Atheroembolism often produces tissue loss and even death. Since 1985, in our institution, we have treated patients with severe lower extremity microembolism by means of intra-arterial prostaglandin E1 (PGE_1) infusion.[15] The encouraging results achieved with PGE_1 in Buerger's disease (see Chapter 42) induced us to try the drug in cases of severe atheroembolism.

Kurzock and Lieb discovered prostaglandins in 1930. Von Euler in 1934 coined the term prostaglandin because he mistook the substance for the secretory product of the prostate. Prostaglandin E1 has several biological properties which make it a suitable drug for maintaining patency of the microcirculation. Prostanoids have been used extensively in Europe for the treatment of peripheral arterial disease (prostacyclin PGI2, PGE_1, and the chemically stable prostacyclin analogue, iloprost). PGI2 is chemically unstable and needs to be administered at high pH, which also has the potential of causing vascular damage. Prostaglandin E1 is used intra-arterially because one passage through the lung inactivates almost 70–90 per cent of the drug.

The treatment of microembolism itself should be considered if the effects are severe enough to cause tissue loss or uncontrollable pain, but attention should also be given to eliminating the cause. A trial, started in 1985, using intra-arterial PGE_1 in 29 patients admitted to our clinic with the diagnosis of blue toe syndrome caused by severe atheroembolism, has been reported.[15] All the following criteria had to be satisfied for inclusion in that trial: persistent pain resistant to medication, severe ischaemia with risk of tissue loss but with distal pulses or a positive Doppler signal present. Patients with asymptomatic or mild symptoms of microembolism were not included in the series and treatment was directed solely at dealing with its source. In 19 patients the source of microembolism was an AAA, occurring spontaneously in nine, during open repair in four, secondary to endoluminal treatment in five and due to diagnostic instrumentation in one. In six of these patients the emboli had come from an atherosclerotic 'shaggy' aorta, and in another from a limited ulcer which was activated by anticoagulant therapy. In addition to this cohort, three other patients who developed atheroembolism were treated: one from poststenotic dilatation of the subclavian artery as a component of the thoracic outlet syndrome, another from a popliteal artery aneurysm and one from iliac stenosis.

The source of microembolism was defined by contrast-enhanced CT scan or angiography. Pathological studies of skin and muscle were carried out in only two patients. Clinical presentation included all or some of the following features: severe limb pain, livedo reticularis and lesions with serpiginous edges, elevated serum levels of creatinine phosphokinase (CPK), abdominal pain, uncontrolled hypertension, renal failure requiring dialysis, weight loss and paraparesis.

Once the decision to treat the patient was made, a 3 Fr multiperforated catheter was placed in the popliteal artery, most frequently inserted via the contralateral femoral artery. That allowed us to combine a urokinase infusion (bolus 300 000 U at an infusion rate of 60 000–100 000 U per hour) with 250 µg of alprostadil (Prolisina VR 0.5 mg/mL, Upjohn, Pururs, Belgium) diluted in 250 mL of normal saline solution administered as a continuous infusion over a period of 2–4 hours, the rate adjusted to the patient's tolerance of vasodilator effects of the latter in terms of discomfort and even pain. The infusion was repeated depending on the response, either on the same day or on subsequent days. In the series of patients presented here the total dose varied between 500 and 8000 µg of PGE_1.

RESULTS

Twenty-nine patients, men of average age 71 years (58–78), were treated as follows: by AAA conventional repair (n = 6), AAA endoluminal treatment (n = 6), aortobifemoral bypass (n = 9), resection of cervical rib (n = 1), resection of popliteal aneurysm (n = 1), iliac stenting (n = 1) and axillo-bifemoral bypass (n = 2). The remaining three high risk patients were treated only medically. Treatment with PGE_1 preceded that of the source of embolism by several days (4–18 days).

In three of the cases of massive microembolism caused by endoluminal treatment of AAAs, the intra-arterial injection of PGE_1 only provided temporary and partial improvement in skin perfusion. Two patients died of multiorgan failure (see Chapters 2 and 4), and one of them suffered spinal cord injury with paraparesis. Primitive endovascular devices were inserted in three of the patients with AAA. Neither visceral nor renal embolism was recorded with the new generation of devices, all of which were of a slimmer profile and much more flexible and only three patients who received them developed distal embolism.

One AAA patient with recurrent lower limb and renal microembolism, receiving dialysis for anuria, was successfully treated with a stent-graft after the distal ischaemia had been relieved by PGE_1. Immediately after excluding the aneurysm, urine production recommenced, but unfortunately he suffered massive fatal pulmonary embolism a few days later. In this group 30-day mortality was 25 per cent. The side effects and complications of treatment were minimal.

Recovery from renal failure occurring immediately after aneurysm exclusion was achieved in two patients, one having been treated endoluminally and the other by conventional open repair, the inference being that microembolism is an important factor in renal failure. Equally, interruption of the continuous showers of microemboli improves renal function.

All other patients showed improvement in peripheral ischaemia and either had minor loss or no loss of tissue. Long term follow-up data were available for 10 patients and all had favourable outcomes.

Prostaglandin E1 is a potent vasodilator which activates fibrinolysis and inhibits leucocyte migration and activation, release of leucotrienes, oxygen free radicals and proteolytic enzymes. Prostaglandin E1 provokes platelet disaggregation and inhibits platelet release of thromboxane and 5-hydroxytryptamine. It increases deformability of red blood cells and has an antiproliferative action on vascular smooth muscle cells. In our experience of patients whose distal pulses are present despite peripheral ischaemia and tissue loss, the intra-arterial infusion of PGE_1 reversed pregangrenous changes in the toes and relieved pain. Capillary filling and pain relief are evident almost immediately after the injection of PGE_1. Unfortunately, there have not been any controlled trials demonstrating its efficacy.

ENDOVASCULAR APPROACH

In most instances, direct aortic reconstruction may be the treatment of choice in the presence of peripheral atheroembolism from an ulcerated lesion in a 'shaggy' or dilated aorta. Nevertheless, comorbidities, severe pulmonary disease and limited life expectancy weigh heavily against conventional aortic bypass and in favour of an alternative procedure such as EVAR. We believe that avoidance of general anaesthesia contributed to the lower rate of complications in this type of patient in whom successful postoperative weaning from mechanical ventilation might have been very difficult. In high risk patients with non-aneurysmal aortic disease conventional extra-anatomical procedures such as axillo-bifemoral bypass are acceptable alternatives.

The relation between the use of stent-grafts and microembolism deserves special comment. Atheroembolism is the most dreaded complication associated with stent-grafting and, paradoxically, endoluminal exclusion of an AAA is a rapidly emerging therapeutic tool in treating that complication. While the rigidity and the broader profile of the older devices played a significant role in atheroembolism, the most important factor determining who will or will not develop emboli is probably the severity of atherosclerotic disease in the aorta. Thompson et al., using an ultrasound based method of detecting lower limb atheroembolism, demonstrated a higher incidence of particle embolisation during endovascular repair compared with conventional aneurysm surgery.[16] In addition, bilateral iliac artery occlusion generates turbulent flow and a net movement of those particles into the suprarenal aorta. As Lipsitz et al.[17] demonstrated in an animal model, initial distal clamping minimises distal embolisation, but renal and/or visceral embolisation may follow. However, if outflow into one iliac artery is being maintained, embolism into that extremity is more likely to occur.

Based on these findings, we have designed our own device (Parodi Antiembolism System or PAESreg; ArteriA, San Francisco Science, San Francisco, CA, USA) using a new concept which ensures protection from distal embolisation. It had been designed originally for use in the carotid territory to ensure reversal of flow during carotid angioplasty and stenting.[18] It consists of a 7–8 Fr guiding catheter with an inverted pear-shaped balloon at the tip to occlude the common iliac artery (CIA) through which antegrade iliac flow is permitted. Flow through the CIA is achieved by an iliac-to-femoral arterio-arterial shunt connecting the guiding catheter to the distal superficial femoral artery introducer at the time the endovascular device is introduced and deployed.

To avoid dislodgement of fragments of thrombus, no wires were advanced via a femoral approach retrogradely into the aneurysm. Instead, a catheter was inserted into the aorta via the left brachial artery. Once the catheter had reached the descending aorta, a **Percusurge** (Percusurge Inc, Sunnyvale, CA, USA) balloon guidewire (0.014 and 0.018 inches) was inserted through the catheter and allowed to navigate freely with aortic flow down into the aneurysm. As one iliac artery had its flow interrupted by the PAES device, the catheter was directed into the chosen iliac artery; when the wire and the catheter mounted on it were felt within the exposed common femoral artery on the latter side, they were exteriorised through an arteriotomy and an extra-stiff guidewire used to replace the navigator wire. The stiff wire was finally passed up to the brachial artery introducer and gently held, creating in this way a 'through and through' guidewire. Applying tension on the wire, we introduced the endograft without angulation and so prevented disruption of thrombus. Further, to avoid intra-aortic manipulation in relation to contralateral stump cannulation, we prefer an aorto-uni-iliac device for this application.

In cases in which thrombus was situated at the level of the renal arteries, the **Angioguard** device (Angioguard Inc, Plymouth, MN, USA) was placed occluding the ostia of the superior mesenteric and renal arteries. It consists of a low

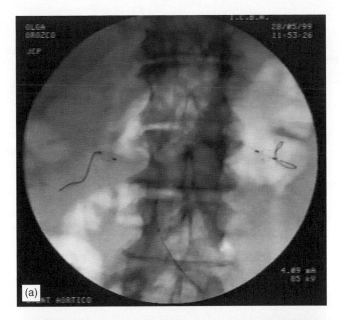

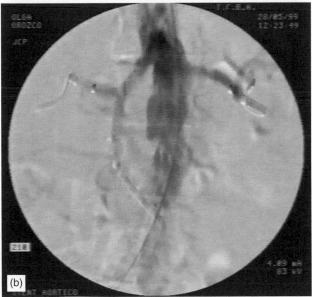

Figure 32.2   *Angioguard device seen on angiography (a) positioned within the renal arteries and (b) within both renal and superior mesenteric arteries*

profile guidewire based, 4 Fr filter-type device which was placed in the arterial ostium, capturing and removing embolic debris while maintaining distal perfusion (Fig. 32.2).

Conclusions

Intra-arterial infusion of PGE$_1$ appears to be an effective treatment of severe atheroembolism when all other treatment has failed. Surgical or endoluminal treatment of the primary source of atheromatous embolism is indicated to prevent recurrence. This serious complication can be prevented by the judicious use of endoluminal

diagnostic and therapeutic methods when needed. We describe two approaches for patients with distal atheroembolism in whom endoluminal exclusion of the aortic source of emboli is attempted using three different devices. In each case, the stent-graft was positioned within the infrarenal aorta preventing visceral and distal embolisation. The dilated segment of the aorta was thereby safely excluded from the circulation.

Key references

Kauffman JL, Shah DM, Leather RP. Atheroembolism and microembolism syndrome. (Blue toe syndrome and disseminated atheroembolism). In: Rutherford RB (ed). *Vascular Surgery*. Philadelphia, PA: WB Saunders Company, 1995: 669–77.

Lipsitz EC, Veith FJ, Ohki T, Quintos RT. Should initial clamping for abdominal aortic aneurysm repair be proximal or distal to minimise embolisation? *Eur J Vasc Endovasc Surg* 1999; **17**: 413–18.

Messina LM. Peripheral arterial embolism. In: Greenfield LJ (ed). *Surgery, Scientific Principles and Practice*. Philadelphia, PA: JB Lippincott Company, 1993: 1478–92.

Parodi JC. Treatment of blue toe syndrome with intra-arterial injection of Prostaglandin E1. In: Yao JST, Pearce WH (eds). *Aneurysms: New Findings and Treatment*. Norwalk, CT: Appleton & Lange, 1994: 325–31.

Thompson MM, Smith J, Naylor AR, *et al*. Microembolization during endovascular and conventional aneurysm repair. *J Vasc Surg* 1997; **25**: 179–86.

REFERENCES

1   Messina LM. Peripheral arterial embolism. In: Greenfield LJ (ed). *Surgery, Scientific Principles and Practice*. Philadelphia, PA: JB Lippincott Company, 1993: 1478–92.

2   Kauffman JL, Shah DM, Leather RP. Atheroembolism and microembolism syndrome. (Blue toe syndrome and disseminated atheroembolism). In: Rutherford RB (ed). *Vascular Surgery*. Philadelphia, PA: WB Saunders Company, 1995: 669–77.

3   May J, White GH, Waugh R, *et al*. Improved survival after endoluminal repair with second-generation prostheses compared with open repair in the treatment of abdominal aortic aneurysms: a 5-year concurrent comparison using life table method. *J Vasc Surg* 2001; **33**: S21–6.

4   Beebe HG, Cronenwett JL, Katzen BT, *et al*. Results of an aortic endograft trial: impact of device failure beyond 12 months. *J Vasc Surg* 2001; **33**: S55–63.

5   Bush RL, Lumsden AB, Dodson TF, *et al*. Mid-term results after endovascular repair of the abdominal aortic aneurysm *J Vasc Surg* 2001; **33**: S70–6.

6   Parodi JC, Criado FJ, Barone HD, *et al*. Endoluminal aortic aneurysm repair using a balloon-expandable stent-graft device: a progress report. *Ann Vasc Surg* 1994; **8**: 523–9.

7 Gitlitz DB, Ramaswami G, Kaplan D, *et al.* Endovascular stent grafting in the presence of aortic neck filling defects: early clinical experience. *J Vasc Surg* 2001; **33**: 340–4.

8 Thompson MM, Smith J, Naylor AR, *et al.* Microembolization during endovascular and conventional aneurysm repair. *J Vasc Surg* 1997; **25**: 179–86.

9 Jaeger HJ, Mathias KD, Gissler HM, *et al.* Rectum and sigmoid colon necrosis due to cholesterol embolization after implantation of an aortic stent-graft. *J Vasc Interv Radiol* 1999; **10**: 751–5.

10 Sandison AJ, Edmondson RA, Panayiotopoulos YP, *et al.* Fatal colonic ischaemia after stent graft for aortic aneurysm. *Eur J Vasc Endovasc Surg* 1997; **13**: 219–20.

11 Lindholt JS, Sandermann J, Bruun-Petersen J, *et al.* Fatal late multiple emboli after endovascular treatment of abdominal aortic aneurysm. Case report. *Int Angiol* 1998; **17**: 241–3.

12 Zempo N, Sakano H, Ikenaga S, *et al.* Fatal diffuse atheromatous embolization following endovascular grafting for an abdominal aortic aneurysm: report of a case. *Surg Today* 2001; **31**: 269–73.

13 Thompson MM, Smith JL, Bell PR. Thromboembolic complications during endovascular aneurysm repair. *Semin Vasc Surg* 1999; **12**: 215–19.

14 Keen RR, Yao JST. Aneurysm and embolization: detection and management In: Yao JST, Pearce WH (eds). *Aneurysms: New Findings and Treatment.* Norwalk, CT: Appleton & Lange, 1994: 305–14.

15 Parodi JC. Treatment of blue toe syndrome with intra-arterial injection of Prostaglandin E1. In: Yao JST, Pearce WH (eds). *Aneurysms: New Findings and Treatment.* Norwalk, CT: Appleton & Lange, 1994: 325–31.

16 Thompson MM, Smith J, Naylor AR, *et al.* Ultrasound-based quantification of emboli during conventional and endovascular aneurysm repair. *J Endovasc Surg* 1997; **4**: 33–8.

17 Lipsitz EC, Veith FJ, Ohki T, Quintos RT. Should initial clamping for abdominal aortic aneurysm repair be proximal or distal to minimise embolisation? *Eur J Vasc Endovasc Surg* 1999; **17**: 413–18.

18 Parodi JC, La Mura R, Ferreira LM. Initial evaluation of carotid angioplasty and stenting with three different cerebral protection devices. *J Vasc Surg.* 2000; **32**: 1127–36.

Regional Vascular Trauma

33

Vascular Injuries of the Limbs

AIRES AB BARROS D'SA, JOHN M HOOD, PAUL HB BLAIR

INTRODUCTION

Through the millennia and even into the twentieth century the treatment of limb vascular injuries was confined mostly to the staunching of bleeding by cautery, styptics, compression and ligature, in order to save life. The concept of vascular repair aimed at limb preservation was reflected in very few anecdotal reports. In a letter William Hunter records the occasion when Halliwell in 1759 performed the first successful vascular repair on a lacerated brachial artery employing a farrier's stitch. Well over a century later Murphy in Chicago reconstructed a completely transected femoral artery. Encouraging clinical and experimental reports of vein grafting began to emerge from both sides of the Atlantic during the early twentieth century.

In actual practice, however, these vascular repair techniques proved to be largely impracticable when tested during the bitter operational conditions of World War I, in which high explosives and missiles accounted for an amputation rate of 72.5 per cent.[1] During World War II attempts at vascular repair were seen to be demonstrably superior to ligation, lowering the amputation rate to 35.8 per cent.[2] This was at a time when the incidence of popliteal and crural artery injury was estimated to be approximately 20 per cent for each site[2] and when the delay between injury and admission was approximately 10 hours. Despite the average lag time of just over 6 hours between injury and repair in the Korean War, the formal application of well documented methods of vessel reconstruction dramatically reduced lower limb amputation rate to 13 per cent.[3]

During the Vietnam War this striking upturn in limb salvage was maintained at 12.7 per cent.[4–6] The significantly improved long term results of vascular repair in battle casualties in Vietnam, as documented in the Vietnam Vascular Registry, were attributed to evacuation by helicopter within 3 hours of injury, operation by surgeons experienced in vascular repair and the liberal use of autogenous vein grafts. Experimental work on the wounding capacity of missiles has been of immense value to clinicians managing gunshot wounds.[7,8]

> **Wartime rate of amputations**
>
> - World War I – 72.5 per cent
> - World War II – 35.8 per cent
> - Korean War – 13.0 per cent
> - Vietnam War – 12.7 per cent

Lessons from military experience were progressively applied to the rising incidence of limb vascular injuries in urban American civilian practice,[9–15] a quarter of these involving the upper extremity. These injuries inflicted by knives and handguns are increasingly caused by automatic weapons and assault rifles in parallel with the mounting culture of gangsterism and the booming traffic in illicit drugs. Sadly, many of these assailants are juveniles and it could be argued that the portrayal of gratuitous violence or the glamorisation of brutality in the media and films, as if they were a necessary ingredient of human existence, may well play a part in influencing the young mind. Democratic governments and caring societies deservedly place great weight on free expression and libertarian values but they also have a responsibility to ensure that those ideals are tempered by the tenets of a universal sense of morality enshrined in appropriate legislation.

In some parts of the world, such as in Northern Ireland, where terrorists, fuelled by easy access to sophisticated weaponry and poorly detected explosives, and trained in manufacturing massive crude bombs and incendiary devices, have prosecuted a sustained and indiscriminate assault on a civilian population for over a quarter of a century and have accounted for a toll of around 3500 dead and 40 000 maimed. The people of this province have endured physical suffering and grief with resilience and dignity, while the very fabric of their lives was being blighted by the systematic destruction of homes and places of work and leisure. Most of the victims resembled military casualties and were treated predominantly in the main teaching hospital the Royal Victoria Hospital, Belfast, which assumed the responsibilities of a front line evacuation centre.[16–21] Vascular injuries treated in the hospital's regional vascular surgery unit, drew on accumulated global experience and introduced innovative approaches in operative care.

A mounting incidence of iatrogenic limb vascular injuries (see Chapters 38 and 39) complicating arterial cannulation reflects the phenomenal proliferation of diagnostic and therapeutic procedures which are a feature of modern medical practice.[22–26]

THE PROBLEM

Recurring regional conflicts, civil wars, terrorism, violence in large conurbations and the ceaseless toll of accidents on the roads and at work, inevitably, indicate that limb vascular injuries are here to stay. Vascular injuries, caused by a host of mechanisms, will continue to challenge the clinical acumen and operative technique of the vascular surgeon. Injuries limited to vessels alone call for sound technique of vascular repair but those that are complex also demand good judgement.

The defining features of limb vascular injury meriting the term 'complex', regardless of aetiology, include some of the following: high energy wounding agent; severe injury of artery and vein; damage to soft tissues including muscle and collaterals possibly with a haematoma under pressure; fractures, especially those with comminution and periosteal stripping; joint dislocation; nerve injury; varying degrees of contamination.[27–30] The literature shows that vascular injuries are present in 10–48 per cent of cases of complex limb trauma and in this group amputations as high as 85 per cent have been reported.[27]

Some defining features of 'complex' limb vascular injury

- Caused by high energy trauma
- Concomitant artery and vein injured
- Transection, avulsion and damage to long vessel segments
- Atherosclerotic artery
- Fracture(s) with comminution, periosteal stripping
- Joint dislocation, closed or open
- Disruption and loss of soft tissue including collaterals
- Pressure haematoma
- Nerve injury
- Contamination of open wound

Limb vascular trauma is often accompanied by substantial blood loss and hypovolaemic hypotension, compounding the complex pathophysiological events caused by ischaemic arrest of flow. These effects, complicated further by impaired drainage due to concomitant vein injury, raise compartment pressure and may lead to the compartment syndrome, ischaemic contractures and amputation. Risk factors such as smoking, diabetes and peripheral atheroma, especially in the elderly casualty, are likely to contribute to a poor outcome. These potential sequelae can be averted by resuscitative measures and vascular repair, and time is of the essence.

Regardless of the aetiology and environment surrounding limb vessel injury, the essential principles of treatment remain the same: emergency aid at the scene, rapid transport to hospital, vigorous resuscitation, accurate diagnosis and definitive operative repair. In the complex limb vascular injury,[28] especially when injuries to other systems coexist, management often demands the involvement of other disciplines. For optimum results, vascular injuries should be treated by surgeons based in hospitals with the necessary facilities and resources, and with experience in vascular reconstruction and trauma.

MECHANISMS OF INJURY

Penetrating

The circumstances surrounding an incident of penetrating vascular trauma of the limbs, namely, the type of wounding agent, the nature of the injury and the lapse of time before evacuation to hospital, will strongly influence management. Limbs are vulnerable to injury by glass splinters, metal shards, bullets, shrapnel and assorted fragments from explosive devices. These injuries range from simple contusion and puncture to complete transection of a vessel.

The upper extremity is particularly vulnerable to stab wounds in which major vessels, and very frequently elements of the brachial plexus lying in close affinity, may be cleanly divided but with minimal other soft tissue injury. The classical self-inflicted butcher's injury by a boning knife, which may involve the external iliac artery, the common femoral artery or its branches, is accompanied by torrential and even fatal haemorrhage.

The wounding energy of a bullet depends on its mass, its muzzle velocity and the distance it travels before impact.[4,7,8] For example, a low velocity missile (approximately 300 m/s or 1000 ft/s) will ordinarily damage structures including blood vessels lying directly in its path. A missile of high velocity (around 750–900 m/s or 2500–3000 ft/s), dissipating its energy at right angles to its trajectory, creates a temporary cavitational effect of approximately 30–40 times the cross-sectional area of the bullet. The huge forces involved exceed the elastic limits of all tissues, including vessels, which are displaced, torn and obliterated well away from the actual path of the bullet. A humerus or tibia, for example, when struck by a high velocity missile will fragment into pieces which then behave as secondary missiles, causing further soft tissue damage (Fig. 33.1). It should be remembered that even low velocity bullets discharged at close range create a degree of cavitation. The very process of cavitation creates a suction force through the entry wound, which draws in pieces of clothing, dirt and bacteria, immediately contaminating the wound. A relatively benign entry wound conceals the severity of disruption within, but a large exit wound ought to alert the clinician.

A concentrated spread of damage by a shotgun discharged at close range produces massive damage over a wide area of soft tissue, which is often underestimated during inspection of the wounds. Shells, rockets, mortars and mines on the battlefield, and bombs and other explosive devices detonated on a busy street by the terrorist, cause injury both by the blast wave moving faster than the speed of sound, and by metal fragments, secondary missiles and falling masonry. The most common iatrogenic source of penetrating vascular trauma complicate transarterial catheterisation procedures undertaken daily by cardiologists and radiologists in modern hospital practice (see Chapter 38). Limb vascular trauma caused by high velocity missiles, bombs and shells naturally account for much higher amputation rates than those resulting from stabbings and handgun injury.

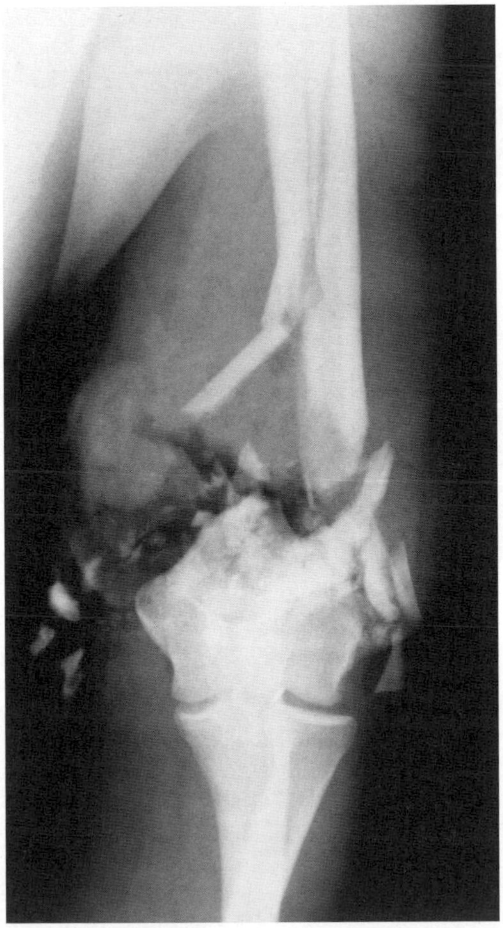

Figure 33.1 *High velocity missile injury: gross comminution of humerus, transection of brachial artery and ulnar nerve (reproduced with permission from Barros D'Sa AAA, in Eastcott HHG (ed).* Arterial Surgery, *3rd edn. Edinburgh: Churchill Livingstone, 1992: 355–411)*

Aetiology of penetrating injury

Sharp object	Assault	Knife
	Accident	Shard of glass, metal
Guns	Handgun	Low velocity bullet
	Rifle	High velocity bullet
	Assault weapon	High velocity bullet
	Machine gun	High velocity bullet
	Shotgun	Shot cluster or spray
Explosive device	Bomb	Shrapnel, secondary missile
	Mine	Shrapnel
	Shell, rocket, mortar	Shrapnel
Iatrogenic	Cannulating instrument	Catheter, stent, milling device
	Sharp instrument	Scalpel, nail, pin, trocar

All penetrating limb wounds in close proximity to main vessels must be viewed with suspicion, whether they occur in civilian practice or as a consequence of terrorism.

Blunt

Blunt vascular trauma of the limbs usually results from sudden deceleration in road traffic accidents and is frequently accompanied by other injuries. Other instances of such injury include falls from heights, lift and scaffolding crashes, as well as air, rail and mining disasters. Such trauma is often of greater severity than that observed on

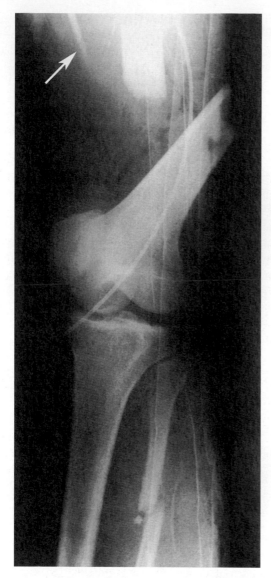

Figure 33.2 *Angiogram shows occluded femoral artery (arrowed) in deceleration injury of the lower limb*

the most severe type IIIc open fractures, extensive damage to bone, soft tissue and long segments of artery, vein and collaterals as well as contamination, combine to bring about the inevitably high amputation rates.[37–39] The severity of the associated bony injury in vascular trauma significantly influences outcome as a result of problems of bony union and of complications such as compartment syndrome and infection, which often lead to amputation.[38]

Amputation rates directly related to multiple crural artery injury are not easily found among available reports,[40–42] which, in most cases, record short term results following arterial ligation rather than repair.[43,44] A low velocity missile such as the plastic bullet has been known to cause non-penetrating lower limb vascular trauma.[45]

The high frequency of associated brachial plexus injury, particularly in blunt avulsive trauma involving the proximal upper limb, may account for a prolonged, and often unsuccessful, functional recovery of the limb.

Aetiology of blunt injury

- Deceleration injury (high velocity)
  - Road traffic accident
  - Rail, air crash
  - Fall
  - Lift, scaffolding collapse
- Torsion, avulsion (low velocity)
  - Sports injury
- Crush injury (falling masonry, etc.)
  - Accident, explosions
  - Mining disaster
  - Natural disaster, earthquake

Crushing

Crush injuries of the limbs caused by falling masonry were sustained, notoriously, during the two world wars, but they have been observed in civilian life following natural disasters such as earthquakes, bombs detonated by terrorists and in road traffic, farm, rail, mining and industrial accidents. The progression of the crush syndrome, significantly causing renal failure, can be accelerated by concomitant injury and thrombosis of the main limb artery, especially if it happens to be atherosclerotic.

Iatrogenic

Iatrogenic injuries in general are dealt with in detail in Chapters 38–40, but the following alludes to those aspects related to limb trauma.

The rising incidence of injuries of the femoral, axillary and brachial arteries, as a consequence of invasive diagnostic and therapeutic procedures, reflects the scale of such

the battlefield and is likely to endanger the limb. Femoral shaft fractures (Fig. 33.2) and fracture dislocations of the knee, for example, carry a 10–40 per cent incidence of vascular injury[31] and the amputation rates are correspondingly of the order of 32–85 per cent.[32,33] The immense shearing forces generated by the sudden violent angulation and fracture of long bones cause disruption of adjacent vessels indirectly at points of relative fixity or directly by sharp bone fragments.[31–35] The avulsive forces in operation, particularly in posterior dislocations of the knee, result in the tearing of all tissues, during which process the layers of the artery, beginning with the intima, disrupt progressively. Notoriously, and not infrequently, such a popliteal injury may not be detected because the examining clinician fails to realise that the dislocated knee tends to reduce spontaneously.

Injuries of the popliteal trifurcation and the crural arteries account for 10 per cent of civilian vascular trauma.[36] In practice in vascular, radiology and cardiology departments over the past two to three decades and accounts for a significant proportion of civilian vascular trauma. Angiography and cardiac catheterisation together are responsible for 60–76 per cent of all iatrogenic vascular injuries,[25,26] which have accelerated in proportion to the steep rise in the number and range of interventional vascular procedures (see Chapters 24, 30–32 and 38–40). Doctors in general, and certainly those undertaking surgical, radiological and other associated disciplines, must be cognisant of the inherent vascular risks and medicolegal implications (see Chapter 10) of those procedures.

These iatrogenic complications may be the result of poor judgement, erroneous or unskilled technique, inaccurate identification of anatomical structures or misinterpretation of X-ray films. In contrast, difficult interventional procedures, such as percutaneous balloon angioplasty, stenting, thrombolysis and atherectomy, represent an increasingly attractive alternative to surgery. The complications include bleeding, thromboembolism, intimal injury and dissection, false aneurysms and arteriovenous fistulae, and catheter retention, all of which are more common in the atherosclerotic femoral artery.

The transaxillary approach, fortunately rarely used, invites the risk of damage to elements of the brachial plexus. The transbrachial approach, still popular in some cardiology units, may cause problems through intimal dissection, thrombosis and later stenosis following repair of an arteriotomy, but an extensive collateral circulation around the elbow protects distal flow. In cases of pre-existing superficial femoral artery occlusive disease, damage to the profunda femoris artery during cannulation, and therefore to the only remaining major source of flow to the lower extremity, may result in amputation. The use of the intra-aortic balloon pump employed in the support of the failing heart, following either acute myocardial infarction or cardiopulmonary bypass, may itself cause iliac and aortic dissection, thromboembolism, perforation and false aneurysm formation.[46]

Damage to the femoral vessels in the groin during surgery for varicose veins occurs recurrently and is attributable either to poor technique or to a lack of awareness of the anatomical anomalies affecting this vasculature. Arterial flow to the legs is also likely to be impaired by iatrogenic injury to the major retroperitoneal vessel trunks during laparoscopic gynaecological interventions, cholecystectomy and herniorrhaphy (see Chapter 40).

A number of orthopaedic procedures, particularly in the elderly and possibly atherosclerotic patient, can cause arterial injury. Chief among these is the ubiquitous total hip replacement, during which the external iliac and common femoral arteries may be injured directly by injudicious retraction of the incised capsule, or indirectly by the exothermic reaction caused by extrusion of the polymer used in preparing the acetabular base. The femoral, and in particular the deep femoral vessels, are also potentially vulnerable to injury during osteotomy for congenital dislocation of the hip, subtrochanteric osteotomy and osteosynthesis of an introchanteric fracture. The popliteal vessels may be damaged during lateral meniscectomy or knee replacement. During lumbar disc surgery lower limb flow may be compromised in the rare event of injury to the aortoiliac and iliocaval systems which may demand immediate intervention.

In all these instances of suspected or evident iatrogenic arterial injury, a vascular surgeon must be sought immediately if serious sequelae are to be averted; these cases are potentially of medicolegal interest and therefore, must be carefully documented.

Irradiation

Arteries within an irradiated field might occasionally undergo dramatic necrosis and potentially fatal rupture of the wall, but this is an unusual complication of excessive dosage and is rarely observed in current practice. More commonly, early injury to the endothelium and internal elastic lamina can be followed over the next few weeks by fibrosis of the media and inflammation of the adventitia.[47] With the passage of time the features of irradiation injury may be indistinguishable from those of atherosclerosis. Irradiation injury to the subclavian–axillary system may complicate treatment of breast cancer, and that of the iliofemoral arterial system during treatment of tumours of the ovary, cervix and testis. Symptoms of impairment of flow and even of critical limb ischaemia may ensue many years later.[48]

MORPHOLOGY OF VESSEL INJURY

It is important to establish precisely the nature of the arterial injury of an extremity for appropriate treatment and repair.[49] Cases of traumatic spasm of an artery are rare, and in most such instances at least some endothelial damage and contusion of the adventitia is present. More importantly, a diagnosis of traumatic arterial spasm engenders inactivity, which can be perilous if a limb-threatening arterial injury exists. Blunt injury of a vessel, or occasionally its proximity to the path of a bullet, may cause thrombosis in continuity. A frequent sequela to injury is intimal fracture, which may progress to an intimal flap developing into a major dissection with intramural bleeding and eventual occlusion, especially if the tear is circumferential.

Bleeding from a laceration, whether clean or ragged, may lead to swift exsanguination because the vessel is unable to contract circumferentially. If bleeding occurs internally, an enlarging haematoma within fascial and bony confines will raise intracompartmental pressure to levels which can occlude the artery. Alternatively, blood may continue to force its way into an organising haematoma to form a false aneurysm lined by endothelium within which thrombus

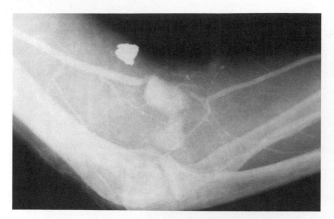

Figure 33.3 *Shrapnel injury to the lower brachial artery resulting in a false aneurysm*

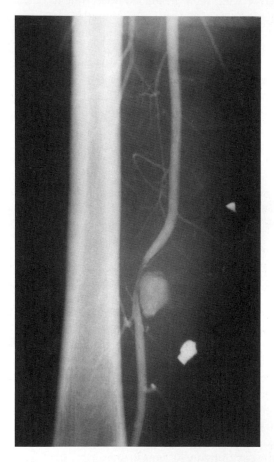

Figure 33.4 *Penetrating injury of the femoral artery with a false aneurysm causing extrinsic pressure on the artery*

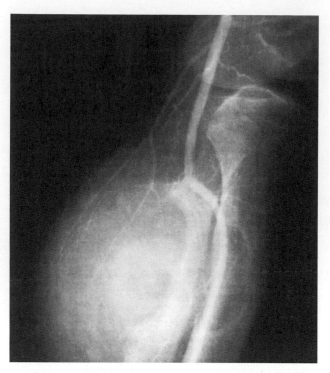

Figure 33.5 *Shell fragment injury of the tibioperoneal trunk with a massive pulsatile false aneurysm in the calf; a healed tibial fracture with a large defect is also seen (reproduced with permission from Borros D'Sa AAB in Eastcott HHG (ed.). Arterial Surgery, 3rd edn. Edinburgh: Churchill Livingstone, 1992: 355–411)*

A false aneurysm may also develop in association with a fistula (Fig. 33.7). If the rate of arteriovenous shunting is marked, a high output cardiac state will manifest itself in due course.

If a vessel is transected, either cleanly by a knife or by a high velocity missile or shrapnel, the free ends constrict, retract and are usually sealed by a plug of thrombus. In a traction injury, classically observed in posterior dislocations of the knee, the avulsive forces involved relentlessly stretch the intima, which then fractures and curls back on itself, to be followed similarly by disruption of the media and adventitia, and as the ends retract, thrombosis ensures occlusion; on clinical examination there may be very little external evidence of the vascular injury.

will form (Figs 33.3–33.5). An expanding false aneurysm may compress surrounding structures, particularly venous channels, and it may eventually rupture. If the penetrating injury involves both artery and adjacent vein, the resulting arteriovenous fistula is often missed on initial clinical examination, although it ought to be recognised by the presence of a continuous thrill and audible bruit[21] (Fig. 33.6). Arterial flow to the limb, and equally drainage from it distal to an arteriovenous fistula tends to be compromised.

Morphology of arterial injury

- Traumatic spasm, contusion
- Intimal fracture, flap
- Dissection, intramural bleeding
- Thrombosis in continuity
- Puncture, laceration
- Occlusion by pressure haematoma
- False aneurysm
- Arteriovenous fistula
- Transection, traction and avulsion

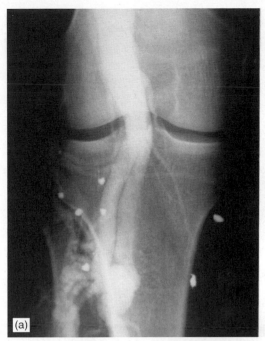 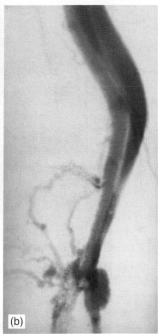

Figure 33.6 *(a) Arteriovenous fistula at the popliteal trifurcation. (b) The digital subtraction film clearly demonstrates the fistulous site*

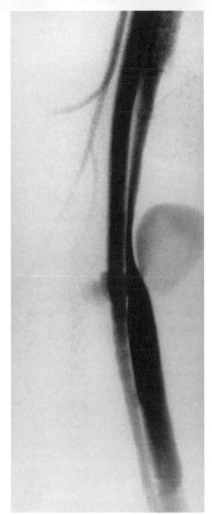

Figure 33.7 *Digital subtraction angiogram showing an arteriovenous fistula of the upper femoral vessels with associated false aneurysms*

PATHOPHYSIOLOGY OF LIMB VASCULAR INJURY

Complex biochemical and cellular pathophysiological mechanisms provoked by limb vascular injury (see Chapter 2) bring about ischaemia-reperfusion injury (IRI) of the muscles.[50–63] Arterial injury arrests distal flow and results in ischaemia, tissue hypoperfusion and hypoxia. Striated muscle is vulnerable to continued warm ischaemia, and after 6–8 hours, depending on level of injury, collateral flow and the degree of hypovolaemic shock leads in most cases to myonecrosis and amputation.[17,56] Adenosine triphosphate (ATP) levels deplete, xanthine dehydrogenase is converted to xanthine oxidase causing a rise in hypoxanthine and xanthine. With reperfusion of ischaemic tissue oxygen free radicals are generated[51–54,57–60] liberating pro-inflammatory mediators which cause neutrophil activation and adhesion, and by lipid peroxidation and directly attacking endothelial cell membranes, the permeability of the microvasculature rises,[58–63] bringing about muscle oedema and the 'no-reflow phenomenon'.[64] Arachidonic acid is metabolised under the action of phospholipase A_2 producing potent vasoactive eicosanoids such as thromboxane A_2, prostaglandins and leucotrienes which strongly mediate in the pathophysiology of IRI.[50] The intensity of this process of IRI is directly proportional to the duration of preceding ischaemia, and will dictate the degree of muscle oedema and consequent necrosis and loss of function.[53,54]

Pathophysiological sequelae of arterial injury

- Ischaemia, hypoperfusion, hypoxia
- Hypovolaemic shock, vasoconstriction
- Ischaemia-reperfusion injury (IRI)
- Systemic inflammatory response syndrome (SIRS)
- Remote injury to gut, lung, heart, kidneys, liver, brain
- Multiple organ dysfunction syndrome (MODS)
- Multiple organ failure (MOF)

The injurious effects of IRI on gut mucosa, where xanthine oxidase is freely available,[53,54,65] produce a general release of cytokines and bacterial translocation.[66] (see Chapters 2 and 3) Portal and systemic endotoxaemia[63,67,68] and the sepsis syndrome[69,70] are not infrequent sequelae. The pulmonary consequences of IRI resemble acute respiratory distress syndrome (ARDS)[71] manifested by raised microvascular permeability and neutrophil sequestration.[58] Cardiac effects include myocardial depression, hyperkalaemic dysrhythmias and even cardiac arrest.[50,72] Oxygen free radicals are also implicated in IRI of cerebral tissue.[57] The remote systemic ramifications of IRI may bring about MODS progressing to MOF and death[73] (see Chapter 4).

Oedema and raised pressures within inelastic fascial compartments rise more steeply in severe bone and soft tissue injury, and may reach levels which obstruct flow through the main arteries. It has been proved clearly at our centre that delay or failure to ensure outflow through an injured vein, either by clamping or ligation, not only exacerbates the effects of IRI in leg muscle, but also causes remote lung injury characterised by non-cardiogenic pulmonary oedema.[74] The sequelae of compartment syndrome, microvascular stasis and thrombosis, aseptic muscle necrosis, ischaemic nerve palsy, Volkmann contracture and amputation inevitably follow[49] unless timely and effective fasciotomy is undertaken.

The adverse effects of IRI can be further aggravated by bacterial contamination, usually by Gram-positive cocci and Gram-negative cocci and bacilli, some of which act synergistically to cause cellulitis or fasciitis, leaving an underlying repair open to breakdown and secondary haemorrhage. The anaerobic environment of ischaemic tissue facilitates the regeneration of clostridial spores (*Clostridium welchii*, *C. novyi* and *C. septicum*) to produce gas gangrene (Fig. 33.8), with its classic features of tense oedema, crepitus, frothy brown watery exudate, brick-red necrotic muscle, toxaemia and cardiovascular collapse. Such an outcome is possible in cases of prolonged ischaemia due to delay in exploration, suboptimal wound care in complex trauma, ligation of vessels and compartmental hypertension.

Superinfection, particularly by *Pseudomonas aeruginosa*, of fasciotomy incisions undertaken to relieve the effects of IRI raises the likelihood of amputation.[11] That is even truer

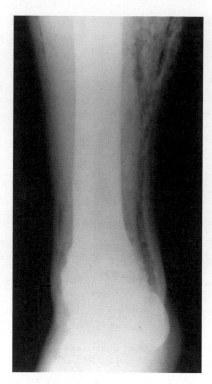

Figure 33.8   *Penetrating trauma causing gas gangrene*

of methicillin-resistant *Staphylococcus aureus* (MRSA) which plagues wound sites in vascular surgical departments around the world.[75]

INITIAL MANAGEMENT

The wounding energy dissipated on impact strongly dictates the nature and extent of injury to blood vessels and other structures and consequently the degree of risk to life, organ and limb. In cases of major injury, survival is determined by speed of resuscitation at the scene, en route to hospital, in the accident and emergency department and in the operating theatre, in concert with definitive surgery.

In the exsanguinating, and especially in the multiply injured patient, standard resuscitative measures are taken to ensure airway, ventilation, and correction of hypovolaemic shock. Control of external bleeding in the upper limb is easy given the superficial anatomical position of the arteries. Digital compression and the use of pad and bandage is the best option in the leg; the blind application of arterial forceps or clamps, particularly by the inexperienced, compounds vessel damage and endangers adjacent nerves. A poorly applied tourniquet will accelerate bleeding and if too tight or not released in time will cause permanent damage to vessel and nerve.

Information should be sought from the patient or associates, for example, about the nature of the wounding agent, the muzzle velocity of a gun and the distance from which it was fired, the amount of blood lost, and the time interval between injury and commencement of treatment. In all penetrating injuries, tetanus toxoid, prophylactic cefuroxime and metronidazole are administered routinely and, if gas gangrene seems likely, specific antitoxin therapy and penicillin may be given. Analgesia is doubly useful: as well as relieving pain, narcotic drugs reduce vasospasm and enhance distal flow to the leg but caution is required in the hypotensive patient.

DIAGNOSIS AND ASSESSMENT

Clinical examination

It is vitally important that clinician should run through a comprehensive mental checklist so as not to miss an arterial injury.

1 If bleeding is continuous, is it mainly arterial or venous?
2 If a haematoma is present, is it expanding or pulsatile?
3 Is there a thrill or an audible bruit indicative of marked stenosis or an arteriovenous fistula?
4 Are the universally recognised 'hard' signs of ischaemia, such as absent distal pulses, pallor, mottling, coolness and numbness, present?
5 If not, are there 'soft' signs, features often overlooked even by the experienced observer, such as transient ischaemia, minimal neurological deficit or a small non-expanding haematoma?[76]

As the lower limb has a poorer collateral network than that in the arm, ankle pulses are less likely to be palpable following vascular injury. Signs of arterial injury may well be obscured in the multiply injured and shocked patient, but it ought to be suspected if, following resuscitation, circulatory recovery in one limb lags behind the other.

In assessing closed fractures caused by blunt injury, the index of suspicion of possible vascular injury tends to be lower than that in penetrating trauma. In most blunt injuries reduction, and therefore correction, of the alignment of long bones, supported by general resuscitation, restores distal flow effectively. If the slightest doubt of arterial injury persists, angiography should be undertaken without delay. The literature is replete with examples of permanent disability or amputation following a presumed diagnosis of spasm which, on subsequent angiographic scrutiny, invariably revealed intimal damage and thrombosis[35] (Fig. 33.9). Notoriously, vascular injury accompanying dislocations of the knee may be missed because of the tendency of the joint to reduce spontaneously, thereby restoring the normal contour of the leg. The absence of signs of bleeding within the tissues owing to constriction of the avulsed ends of the popliteal artery may further induce a false sense of security. This well known pitfall in clinical examination may delay diagnosis, by which time distal thrombosis may have progressed to a point where a distinctly unfavourable outcome is inevitable.

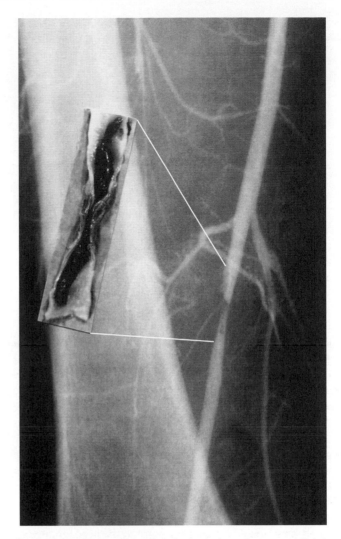

Figure 33.9 *Penetrating injury in proximity to lower superficial femoral artery. Distal pulses were present but were reduced in volume, not by spasm but by mural damage that had progressed to thrombotic occlusion. The thrombus was visible on the angiogram and on the excised segment (inset) (reproduced with permission from Barros D'Sa AAB. A decade of missile-induced vascular trauma.* Ann R Coll Surg Engl *1982; 64: 37–44)*

Ultrasound

Routine Doppler ultrasound examination complements physical examination but calls for an intelligent interpretation of the findings. For example, an audible Doppler signal provides little reassurance that the proximal artery is intact. Much more helpful is the measurement of Doppler pressures and estimation of the ankle:brachial pressure index, which can be compared with that in the contralateral uninjured leg. An ankle:brachial pressure index below 0.90 ought to be viewed with suspicion. Duplex scan imaging can detect and localise injuries of the femoral and popliteal arteries, especially when these vessels lie in proximity to the path of a bullet or knife. Nevertheless, non-invasive investigations take time and are impracticable in the presence of skin loss, fracture deformity and pain. Angiography, however, can demonstrate an arterial injury expeditiously and forms a sound and reliable basis for operative intervention.

Angiography

The competence of preoperative angiography in delineating an arterial injury, or in excluding it, is well established, particularly in penetrating leg injuries[76,77] (see Figs. 33.3–33.7, 33.9). A positive angiogram is almost invariably a mandatory indication for exploration, except for very minor lesions. A non-operative approach in occult injuries requires supervision, possibly further angiography and other studies, and sometimes delayed surgical treatment, all of which can be expensive.[78] A long term study, involving reasonable numbers, appraising the conservative treatment of minor arterial lesions defined by angiography and left unexplored, is awaited. On the other hand, with a few exceptions, a negative angiogram gives the surgeon the necessary confidence not to intervene, thus reducing the incidence of worthless explorations.

In penetrating wounds the yield of arterial injuries detected on angiography located in close proximity to the femoropopliteal system and trifurcation is low,[79,80] and the fact that it is an invasive and expensive procedure becomes an argument for avoiding it.[81] In deciding on the need for angiography, however, the question of the proximity of the wound to the damaged artery is important. For example, in a high velocity missile causing injury well outside its path, the presence of 'soft' signs of arterial injury, and not least the potential medicolegal consequences of limb loss resulting from a missed injury, may point to the need for angiography. Where doubt exists in the stable patient, it might be considered negligent not to obtain an angiogram.

When a surgeon does not have access to angiography and is compelled to rely on clinical acumen, there is no substitute for meticulous and repeated physical examination. Reliance on clinical examination alone to detect arterial injury can be most effective,[82] but if clinical judgement is poor, a vascular injury may well be missed and on occasion operative exploration will be fruitless. Should ischaemia persist after reduction of a femoral fracture, especially in the elderly atherosclerotic patient, timely angiography and the discovery of an injury may help to avert disaster. The high incidence of occult and limb-threatening arterial injury associated with dislocations of the knee, missed at clinical examination, is a compelling argument in favour of mandatory angiography in these cases.

Biplane films defining the site and type of injury assist in planning an operative approach. Fine catheter digital subtraction techniques have largely displaced conventional angiography and permit clear definition of a vascular injury against a background unobscured by bone (see Fig. 33.7). In the absence of such sophisticated equipment, the percutaneous cannulation of the femoral artery for a one-shot, single-plate angiogram similar to the on-table technique is perfectly acceptable.

PREOPERATIVE CONSIDERATIONS

The non–salvageable limb

With the expeditious application of the basic principles of surgery it remains within the skills of the vascular surgeon to salvage some of the critically injured limbs. Successes in such cases may induce a degree of overoptimism in managing the mutilated and irreparable limb. Misdirected zeal may commit both surgeon and patient to a protracted series of injudicious operations on an irretrievably mangled limb, inviting complications such as infection, potentially fatal secondary haemorrhage, poor rehabilitation and eventually amputation of an insensate appendage.

The notion that every limb must be saved at all costs should be questioned: a more objective reappraisal of the condition of a limb on admission is required, and in some cases it may be more prudent to proceed to primary amputation and early rehabilitation with a prosthesis. An equally flawed approach would be to apply rigid guidelines for primary amputation based on the type of wounding agent, the duration of ischaemia, the presence of injuries elsewhere or indeed medicolegal, social or budgetary considerations. The introduction of various scoring systems using clinical criteria aimed at predicting outcome[83,84] have a limited role but may tip the balance when sound clinical judgement is called for in a difficult case. The key reasons for early amputation are irreversible ischaemia, failed vascular repair and sepsis, the latter two of which cannot be reliably predicted, either at admission or intraoperatively.

Dilemmas of this kind do not apply when primary amputation represents no more than the completion of a traumatic amputation or the excision of a severely crushed limb. This scenario is most notoriously illustrated by the injuries resulting from the detonation of antipersonnel mines, which are a feature of so many conflicts and which remain a deadly threat long after the dust of war has settled.[85,86] In these circumstances the surgeon makes every effort to preserve as much viable tissue and skin as possible for delayed closure, at which time a satisfactory stump depends on careful tailoring of the flaps.

The importance of time

An expeditious approach to treating a limb vascular injury is essential as the duration of ischaemia is pivotal to outcome. It may be but one feature of the multiply injured patient and may not deserve priority during resuscitation and definitive surgery for life-threatening injuries of the head, chest and abdomen. Once haemodynamic stability has been restored, attention can be focused on the limb vascular injury. A large survey of severe head injuries in association with concomitant limb bone and vessel trauma[87] has shown that the limb injury may be treated before a head injury except in the case of an extradural haemorrhage which constitutes an absolute emergency.

An assortment of variables has to be taken into consideration, namely the level of arterial injury, the quality of collateral flow, which is much better in the upper limb, the individual patient's tolerance of ischaemia, the degree of hypotension and the extent of associated soft tissue and bone injuries. The relentless progression of warm ischaemia time and its deleterious effect on striated muscle is forewarning of an adverse result, and in some cases limb survival is achieved at the cost of permanent neurological impairment.

In treating limb vascular injuries, and in particular those with severe open wounds, control of bleeding, resuscitation and definitive surgery must be regarded as overlapping rather than sequential stages of management, with the objective of shortening ischaemia time. Nevertheless, a finite period of time is required for the exposure and control of vessels, identification of nerves, debridement and wound care, attention to complex bone injuries and finally the harvesting and preparation of donor vein to be used in arterial and venous repair.

A heightened awareness of the consequences of prolonged ischaemia, and an understandable desire to press on with surgery, may itself cause lapses in surgical principles and in operative technique, with counterproductive results. In this particular climate of urgency, for example, that vascular repair might be performed before a fracture is stabilised, a practice that tends to encourage the use of quick but often flawed repair techniques, including lateral suture and end-to-end anastomosis under tension, both of which may fail. Large venous channels essential to drainage may be ligated simply to save time. There also remains the likelihood that the eventual reduction of a fracture, which often requires the robust manipulation of bone fragments, might disrupt a delicate vascular repair.

Clearly, the merits of reducing a fracture before vascular repair are obvious: damage of soft tissues and vessels by bone fragments is averted, the measurement of vein graft length to restore arterial and venous flow will be optimal, and repair can be undertaken with the confidence that it will not be disturbed. This approach, however, means that stabilisation of one or more fractures will take time. The severity of long bone damage caused by high velocity missiles and bombs demands some form of fixation so that its exact length is established before vascular repair. The consequent prolongation of ischaemia may place the orthopaedic surgeon under some pressure to carry out a hurried, and perhaps technically imperfect, fixation bringing with it the potential immediate risk of compromising a vascular repair and in the longer term raising the possibility of delayed union or non-union.

All these concerns about the order of arterial and bone repair are dispelled if the injured artery and vein are

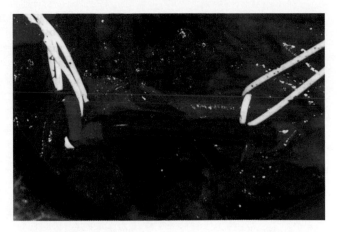

Figure 33.10 *Indwelling shunts: Brener in torn popliteal artery above, and Javid in transected popliteal vein below, preparatory to vein graft replacement of each vessel (reproduced with permission from Barros D'Sa in Greenhalgh RM (ed.).* Limb Salvage and Amputation in Vascular Disease. *London: WB Saunders, 1998: 135–50)*

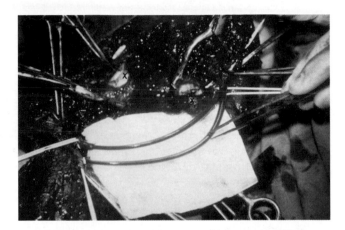

Figure 33.11 *Javid shunt bridging a lengthy gap in the femoral artery and perfusing the distal limb; another such shunt is bridging a similar gap in the adjoining femoral vein and draining the limb. The ends of a fractured femur (XX) are being manipulated prior to fixation (reproduced with permission from Barros D'Sa AAB, Moorehead RJ. Combined arterial and venous intraluminal shunting in major trauma of the lower limb.* Eur J Vasc Surg *1989; 3: 577–81)*

temporarily bridged by the early placement of intraluminal shunts (Fig. 33.10). With shunts in place, vascular and orthopaedic surgeons no longer have to watch the clock anxiously and instead a harmonious multidisciplinary approach is fostered (Fig. 33.11). The presence of shunts allows the implementation of an unhurried logical sequence of manoeuvres, a practice underpinned by over two decades of experience and which has proved helpful in lowering the incidence of compartment syndrome, that of fasciotomy in relieving it, and failing that the incidence of ischaemic nerve palsy, contracture, sepsis, amputation and duration of stay in hospital.[28–30,49,88–93] In the few borderline cases of potential primary amputation, and only when nerve continuity has been confirmed to be macroscopically intact, shunts

Table 33.1 *Comparisons between the pre-shunt (1969–1978) and post-shunt (1979–2000) periods of managing complex limb vascular injuries, penetrating and blunt, in terms of the incidence of fasciotomy, contracture and amputation*

Complex penetrating	Pre-shunt (n = 34)		Post-shunt (n = 57)				
	No.	Per cent	No.	Per cent	P value	OR	95% CI
Fasciotomy	17/30	56.7	13/48	27.1	0.016	3.5	1.3–9.2
Contracture	13/30	43.3	8/47	17.0	0.018	3.7	1.3–10.6
Amputation	11/34	32.4	5/57	8.8	0.009	5.0	1.6–16.0

Complex blunt	Pre-shunt (n = 38)		Post-shunt (n = 49)				
	No.	Per cent	No.	Per cent	P value	OR	95% CI
Fasciotomy	22/35	62.9	16/44	36.4	0.02	3.0	1.2–7.4
Contracture	19/34	55.9	13/45	28.9	0.02	3.1	1.2–7.9
Amputation	15/38	39.5	7/49	14.3	0.012	3.9	1.4–11.0

The incidence of all three parameters was significantly reduced following the introduction of the policy of early intraluminal shunting of artery and vein in 1979 in both the penetrating and blunt injury groups of complex limb vascular injuries. Data were analysed using the statistical package SPSS version 10.0 for windows (SPSS Inc., Chicago, IL, USA). Clinical characteristics of the two study groups were compared and analysed by χ^2 test (Yates' corrected), and Fisher's exact test (when appropriate). Corresponding odds ratio (OR) and 95% confidence interval (95% CI) values were calculated. Variables were considered statistically significant at $P < 0.05$.

may permit more prudent assessment as to whether the limb is salvageable with the prospect of a reasonable functional outcome.

These shunts have made a special contribution to the management of the very challenging subgroup of 'complex' limb vascular injuries, both penetrating and blunt, at our centre. A review of the incidence of fasciotomy procedures undertaken and the outcome in terms of the incidence of contracture and amputation are illustrated in Table 33.1. The incidence of each of these parameters prior to the introduction of shunts (pre-shunt period: 1969–78) was significantly higher than that after the policy of shunting was put into effect (post-shunt period: 1979–2000) in both trauma categories.[28,88]

The problems in treating 'complex' limb vascular injury

- Vessels are injured in 10–48 per cent of limb injuries
- 85 per cent of those limbs are amputated and fatality is not uncommon
- Treatment of damaged artery, vein, bone and soft tissue takes time
- Prolonged ischaemia and impaired venous outflow aggravate IRI
- Intensity of IRI influences outcome
- Compartment syndrome, ischaemic nerve palsy
- Increased need for fasciotomy
- Climate of urgency induces lapses and flaws in operative care
- Greater danger of myonecrosis, contracture, sepsis and amputation

DEFINITIVE SURGICAL TREATMENT

Incisions and exposures

UPPER LIMB

The patient lies supine, the injured upper limb being abducted and extended palm upwards at right angles to the body. Peripheral and central venous lines should not be inserted on this side. The draping should provide an operative field with access to chest, neck and arm, as well as to one lower limb in case donor vein is required.

For stab wounds involving the first part of the axillary artery, it is wise to secure proximal supraclavicular control of the subclavian artery. To approach the axillary artery the incision commences below the clavicle, extending laterally down the deltopectoral groove and continues distally along the course of the brachial artery. Access to the axillary artery is possible either above or below the margins of the pectoralis major, or by separating the fibres of this muscle and dividing the pectoralis minor tendon. The intimate proximity of veins and nerves requires meticulous care during dissection. A standard longitudinal incision will expose an injured brachial artery in the upper arm or at the elbow; the latter is sometimes necessary in dealing with intimal fracture, dissection and thrombosis following diagnostic cannulation. Short longitudinal incisions over the radial and ulnar arteries are quite adequate.

LOWER LIMB

For most lower limb vascular injuries the patient lies supine, both lower limbs being prepared and draped, permitting proximal and distal extension of standard longitudinal incisions in the injured leg, and enabling the procurement of donor vein from the contralateral leg. Vascular injuries of the groin are associated with torrential bleeding, for which control of the external iliac artery has to be established through an oblique muscle-splitting incision for retroperitoneal access above the inguinal ligament. While this is in progress digital pressure is maintained over the bleeding artery and is only released after the external iliac artery has been clamped. A longitudinal groin incision will then enable exposure and control of the common femoral artery, and for injuries at its bifurcation, encirclement and control of the superficial femoral and the profunda femoris artery is essential.

The popliteal artery can be approached medially or posteriorly, the former preserving the adjacent long saphenous vein. External rotation of the thigh supported laterally by a pack of two sterile gowns and some knee flexion provides ideal medial exposure of the popliteal vessels, especially after dividing the medial head of the gastrocnemius. The posterior approach with the patient being prone is rarely used: a gentle S-shaped incision is made in an oblique axis commencing medially above and proceeding laterally downwards to expose the mid-popliteal vessels in the floor of the popliteal fossa, the short saphenous vein and tibial nerve having been identified and preserved. A medial approach is used for access to the popliteal trifurcation, and separate longitudinal incisions are employed in order to expose segments of the crural arteries all the way down to the foot.

In complex injuries requiring orthopaedic intervention the incisional approaches must be such as to facilitate co-operative effort.

Control and preparation of vessels

Exposure of the injured vessels and digital control of bleeding is followed by sharp dissection of the segments of artery and vein above and below the injury before clamping. A sufficient length of artery on either side of the injury is exposed and if necessary trimmed back to a point where the wall is intact.

Release of the upper clamp will usually allow a plug of thrombus to be washed out and occasionally a balloon catheter is required. If ischaemia is prolonged distal balloon exploration will often recover clot, particularly when back bleeding is poor or absent. In the latter circumstance vigorous upward milking of the limb distal to the injury may be helpful in expressing recent propagated clot. The young patient does not possess an adequate collateral circulation and back bleeding is limited; by the same token, arterial repair is imperative if the limb is to be saved. The distal artery is perfused with heparinised saline (20 units/mL); systemic heparinisation is acceptable if there are no other injuries.

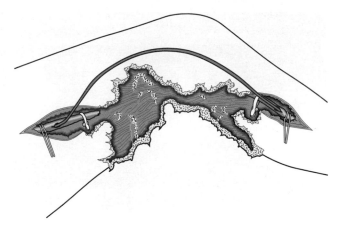

Figure 33.12 *Outlying shunt picking up flow proximal to the injured segment and revitalising the limb distally*

Shunting and operative discipline

The concept of intraluminal shunting has been applied in the past to coronary artery perfusion, is regularly used for carotid endarterectomy, on occasion in replacement of the thoracic aorta, and rarely, in retrohepatic caval trauma. In the proximal upper limb arterial injuries the protective collateral network makes shunts unnecessary. In military trauma of the brachial artery, especially involving the deep brachial artery[6] shunting does have some value.

An indwelling shunt reconnecting the ends of a transected femoral or popliteal artery immediately arrests ischaemia, minimises reperfusion injury, keeps compartment pressure at a level which reduces the need for fasciotomy and consequently buys time for a considered approach to the rest of the operation. In extensive soft tissue injuries with destruction of lengthy segments of vessels long outlying shunts will keep the distal limb alive (Fig. 33.12). If in a multiply injured patient undergoing surgery for life-threatening injuries of the head or torso, space and conditions around the operating table also allow the vascular surgeon to work unobtrusively, injured vessels can be exposed and shunted to keep the limb viable for definitive repair later. In the case of head injuries that timely intervention minimises the local and remote impact of IRI, but if delayed, the sequelae of IRI might represent a formidable further assault on the already traumatised brain.[87]

A severed femoral or popliteal vein cleared of clot is shunted to re-establish drainage, particularly if damage to venous collaterals is extensive (see Figs 33.10 and 33.11). If the main venous channel is clamped rather than shunted, while the distal limb continues to be perfused via an intact or shunted artery, a precarious rise in compartment pressure and remote lung injury will supervene.[74]

One of several commercially available shunts may be employed, but if none is available, silicone elastomer or plastic tubing of suitable consistency, length and calibre is an acceptable alternative provided that the ends are very smoothly trimmed to avoid intimal damage. The ideal design

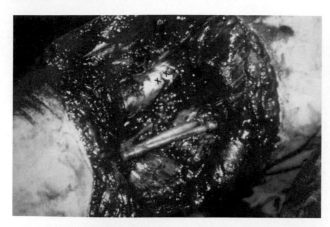

Figure 33.13 *After excision of devitalised muscle, debridement and stabilisation of fracture (XX) interposed vein grafts restore flow through the femoral artery and vein and the deep femoral vein (reproduced with permission from Barros D'Sa AAB, Moorehead, RJ. Combined arterial and venous intraluminal shunting in major trauma of the lower limb. Eur J Vasc Surg 1989; 3: 577–81)*

of a shunt system, purpose-built for vascular trauma,[89] was based on experience in Northern Ireland[27–30,49,74,88–93] and led to useful experimental work on a temporary shunt.[94] The Brener shunt (see Fig. 33.10) in particular has some value in that it has a side arm: placed in an artery, it forms a convenient portal for blood sampling, blood gas estimation and injection of anticoagulants or contrast for on-table angiography; placed in a vein it can act as an outlet for flushing out stagnant blood of low pH, rich in potassium and toxic metabolites, from the distal ischaemic limb and thereby protecting the myocardium in particular.

With both arterial and venous shunts in place, the vascular surgeon has ample time to survey the wound, identify and tag nerves, remove debris and irrigate the tissues. Restoration of flow enables a sharp distinction to be made between viable and dead tissue for more precise excision, and haemostasis is more reliably achieved. Attention can then be focused on the restoration of skeletal integrity using either internal or external fixation: the realigned limb is then ready for definitive vascular repair, which on completion is certain to remain secure and undisturbed (Fig. 33.13). When both the injured artery and vein have been shunted, it is immaterial whether one or other is repaired first, in this way dispelling past debate on priority for repair. Sufficient time is also available to harvest vein graft and, if necessary, compound vein grafts, either of the panel or spiral type, can be fashioned to match the calibre of the host vessel. The shunt offers a further advantage by acting as a stent, which facilitates precise suturing. When an outlying shunt restores distal flow in cases of extensive injury of the limb, time can be taken to construct an extra-anatomic vein bypass through clean, unaffected tissue at some distance from the wound.

Over two decades of experience at our centre has shown that temporary shunting fosters a disciplined and methodical operative routine. The key operative steps are summarised in a simple alliterative *aide mémoire* (Fig. 33.14). The clear

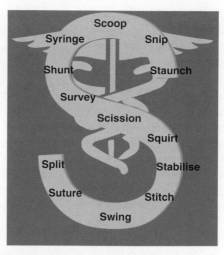

Figure 33.14   Aide mémoire *for the Sequence of Steps in the operative management of complex limb vascular injury:* staunch *the bleeding,* snip *damaged ends of vessels,* scoop *out clot,* syringe *in heparinised saline,* shunt *both artery and vein,* survey *the wound and identify nerve injury,* perform *scission of non-viable soft tissue,* squirt *saline to irrigate wound,* stabilise *fractured bones,* stitch *vessel grafts,* swing *tissue for cover,* suture *the wound (delayed primary if contaminated) and, if necessary,* split *fascia to decompress muscle (redrawn with permission from Barros D'Sa AAB. Complex vascular and orthopaedic limb injuries [editorial]. J Bone Joint Surg (UK) 1992; 74: 176–8)*

dividends accruing from this systematic approach, based on the use of shunts, particularly in the management of complex vascular trauma, are salutary[28] (Table 33.1). They include improved operative technique, lower incidence of complications, better outcome and earlier discharge from hospital.

Benefits of shunting artery and vein
• Immediately restores arterial inflow and venous outflow
• Minimises IRI and its consequences
• Encourages a logical sequence of operative steps
• Buys time for meticulous wound care
• Buys time for ideal method of bone fixation
• Buys time for correct choice of arterial reconstruction
• Vein graft of optimum length harvested for use
• Compound vein graft constructed if required
• Extra-anatomical bypass created if tissue lost/contaminated
• Major vein invariably reconstructed
• Lower incidence of failure of repair/thrombosis
• Reduced need for fasciotomy
• Lowered incidence of sepsis, contracture, amputation
• Fosters harmonious multidisciplinary cooperation

Wound care

A knife wound requires minimal excision of the skin and tissues around its track. The true extent of tissue damage in gunshot wounds, particularly those caused by high velocity bullets, cannot always be reliably gauged from an inspection of the entry and exit wounds. That assessment becomes even more difficult in blunt deceleration injuries, particularly when these are closed injuries. In low velocity wounds, except those caused by guns fired at very close range, only a limited amount of excision is required, whereas in high velocity wounds debridement must be adequate if infection is to be averted. Devitalised muscle, easily recognised by its deep purplish colour and failure to bleed or contract, must be completely excised (see Fig. 33.13). Attached bone fragments, debris, dirt and foreign bodies should be removed meticulously; this should be followed by copious irrigation, preferably pulsatile, to remove remaining contaminants and to lower the concentration of the bacterial inoculum. Cursory care inevitably leads to infection, which remains one of the major causes of amputation.

A contused nerve is simply left alone, but if the transection is clean and the wound is not contaminated, accurate primary repair is advisable. If damage is extensive, the sheath of each nerve end is simply tagged for identification for delayed secondary repair as an elective procedure.

Management of associated fractures

Until the management of combined bone and arterial injuries was streamlined on the basis of shunting, vascular and orthopaedic surgeons at our centre dealt with these complex injuries in random fashion. The policy formulated around the use of intraluminal shunts has established close cooperation between them during the perioperative period and especially in the operating theatre.[27–30] Agreed incisional approaches and adherence to the sequence of steps indicated in Fig. 33.14 has allowed each specialist to work unhindered. Exhortations to repair the artery before bone fixation are attended by the real fears of suture line disruption during the robust manipulations necessary to achieve fracture reduction, and that approach is virtually obsolete at our centre. Those who advocate vascular repair before ensuring skeletal stability cannot reasonably dispute the view that it is sound practice to first stabilise bone, thereby permitting optimum repair of artery and vein, confident in the knowledge that they will not be disrupted (see Fig. 33.13). In turn, particularly in complex limb trauma, the protocol centred on the use of shunts has encouraged harmony between surgeons of different disciplines.

Arterial repair

Damaged minor arteries and veins which do not threaten the viability of the limb may be ligated but in principle all damaged vessels should be repaired. This precept is particularly applicable to the small calibre brachial or femoral artery of a child whose limbs require sufficient blood flow for proper growth and development.

The presumption that axillary or brachial artery ligation will not lead to upper limb amputation due to the protective presence of adequate collateral flow should be dismissed. Brachial artery injuries should not be regarded as innocuous and left to the novice for repair because the opportunities to obtain a good result diminish with each repeated attempt. The Allen test should be used in determining the importance of repairing injured radial and ulnar arteries.

Injury to the tibial or crural arteries is unlikely to result in limb-threatening ischaemia unless more than one artery is involved; in one report limb loss doubled when these arteries were ligated rather than repaired.[36] Neither the literature nor a trawl of vascular surgical opinion offers a standard protocol for the repair of tibial arteries accompanying fractures of the tibia.[95] Although it would be correct in principle to reconstruct injured tibial arteries in order to prevent islands of ischaemia in muscle and bone, in general two are sufficient, if not essential, for limb viability and good function.[95–97] This view is preferable to one which holds that a single Doppler pulse elicited at the ankle is sufficient,[98,99] or to another that either the posterior tibial or anterior tibial should be repaired, but that the peroneal artery may be safely ignored.[100] If any injured tibial artery is exposed, the opportunity should be taken to repair it unless the patient's general condition precludes taking time to do so. This rationale has particular merit in situations of severe damage to soft tissue and collaterals, as for example in type IIIc tibial fractures, when the chances of propagated thrombosis in a partially damaged crural artery may convert an initially viable leg into one that is beyond salvage. The reliance of fractured, and especially denuded bone, on blood supply from adjacent crural arteries cannot be overstated. In recent years an increasing enthusiasm for repair of these vessels has proved rewarding irrespective of the poor circulatory state of the foot.

Various morphological types of vessel injury occur, and in practice different permutations of these may be present in one damaged vessel. The optimal type of repair will depend on the particular circumstances of each case.

LATERAL SUTURE

Closure of small puncture wounds by lateral suture is acceptable, especially if executed transversely using interrupted sutures (Fig. 33.15). Equally, transverse and short oblique lacerations with sharp edges can be repaired in this manner. If, however, the laceration is longitudinal, and particularly if contusion demands excision of the margins, lateral suture simply narrows the lumen (see Fig. 33.15) and encourages thrombosis, notably in critical vessels such as the brachial and popliteal, endangering the extremity.

PATCH ANGIOPLASTY

In order to preserve the calibre of the artery, an angioplasty using a vein patch is usually preferable to a lateral suture (Fig. 33.16). In a closed or uncontaminated injury to a large vessel, such as the iliac or common femoral, it would be quite acceptable to employ a Sauvage filamentous prosthetic patch graft (see Fig. 33.16) in the knowledge that it

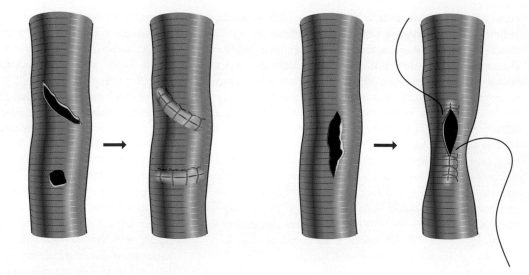

Figure 33.15 *Oblique and transverse suture of small lacerations and puncture wounds. Longitudinal suture may narrow the lumen*

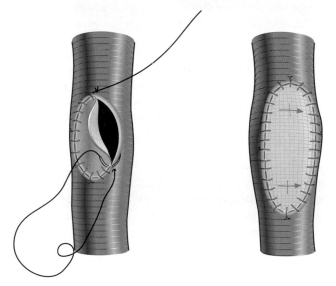

Figure 33.16 *Vein and prosthetic (Sauvage)[101] patch angioplasty*

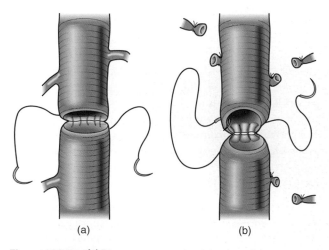

(a)   (b)

Figure 33.17 *(a) Direct anastomosis without tension. (b) Anastomotic tension despite sacrificing branches*

will heal with an endothelialised flow surface within a matter of a few weeks.[101]

DIRECT ANASTOMOSIS

In cases of clean stab wounds of the artery or if there is limited loss of length after excision of the edges, direct end-to-end anastomosis may well be possible (Fig. 33.17). Conversely, if there is any tension at the anastomosis (see Fig. 33.17), thrombotic failure or actual disruption may follow. Of course, a joint should not have to be flexed or major collaterals divided, particularly in an atherosclerotic artery, to enable approximation. These problems are of particular relevance to the axillary and popliteal arteries. In such instances excision and vein grafting is by far the better approach.

VEIN GRAFTS

The attributes of autogenous vein include durability, resistance to infection and an ability to draw nutrient flow from surrounding viable tissue. The long term patency of vein makes it a most desirable graft, a fact which has some resonance with the predominantly younger patient who sustains injury and stands to benefit from it.

The abundant availability of donor vein gives the surgeon the confidence to excise adequate, and sometimes lengthy, segments of damaged vessel in order to leave pristine ends for reconstruction (Fig. 33.18). This is especially relevant to high velocity bullet or traction injuries involving the popliteal vessels in which the outer appearances sometimes belie the true extent of injury to the intima. The long saphenous vein represents the best source for donor vein, the calibre in the upper thigh being ideal for interposition grafting (see Fig. 33.18), while segments further down are better suited to patch angioplasty. In circumstances in which the deep vein of the lower limb is injured, the ipsilateral saphenous vein, which represents a precious drainage channel, ought not to be disturbed; instead, the vein from the opposite leg may be harvested. In the absence of saphenous vein, the cephalic vein may be a reasonable substitute, although its wall is not particularly muscular.

In vessels such as the axillary (Fig. 33.19) and popliteal (Fig. 33.20), the anastomosis is quite simply achieved by using a continuous polypropylene everting suture commenced at diametrically opposite points, which then meet in between, access to each side being attained by rotating the vessel along its axis. An indwelling shunt, with the vein

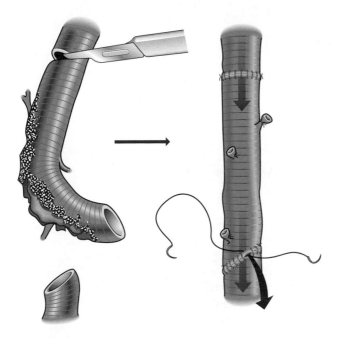

Figure 33.18 *Excision of injured segment back to pristine artery. Reversed interposition vein graft*

graft drawn over it, acts conveniently as a stent and lends itself to disciplined suturing of the anastomoses thus averting 'purse stringing'. When the arterial diameter is less than 3–4 mm, as in the case of radial, ulnar and tibial arteries, and notably the main limb arteries of children, meticulous attention to technique, aided by loupes and fine instruments, is essential to patency. Vasospasm of small arteries is abolished by judicious inflation using a fine, rounded catheter. The ends of the vein graft and host vessel are then cut obliquely and spatulated to prevent stenosis (Fig. 33.21). Good results are obtained by accurate coaptation of intimal surfaces, eversion of the edges to prevent inward protrusion of adventitial strands, and carefully placed tension-free 6-0–8-0 polypropylene sutures, interrupted to accommodate increasing vessel diameter without stenosis as the child grows.

In the older patient damage to a diseased atherosclerotic vessel may necessitate a lengthy vein bypass extending well beyond the injured arterial segment. This is especially important in situations of marked soft tissue loss and especially if severe contamination renders the wound hazardous to vein graft. The trimmed ends of injured artery are ligated back to healthy tissue and an extra-anatomical vein bypass graft, perhaps unreversed but with its valves disrupted, may take the form of a common femoral to anterior tibial bypass tunnelled through clean tissue (Fig. 33.22).

If the calibre of available donor vein is much smaller than that of the host vessel, the discrepancy is likely to lead to graft failure. Such an outcome can be avoided by fashioning a compound vein graft of larger diameter, which will maintain laminar flow. This can be achieved in various ways, and shunts already in place allow ample time for this

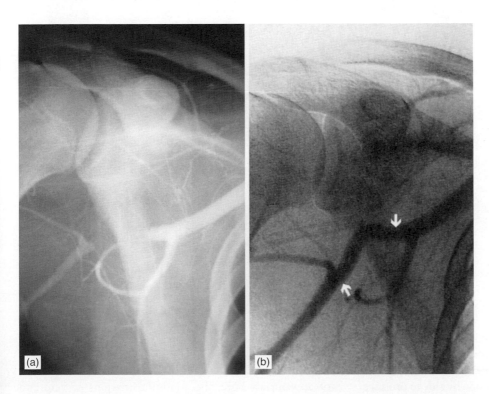

(a)　(b)

Figure 33.19 *Injury to the right shoulder caused by a falling tree, producing a crush injury of the axillary artery and brachial plexus and a humeral fracture. The preoperative angiogram (a) shows a defect in the midaxillary artery. The postoperative angiogram (b) shows interposed vein graft (arrowed) deliberately left lax enough to permit safe adduction (reproduced with permission from Barros D'Sa AAB in Eastcott HHG (ed). Arterial Surgery, 3rd edn, Edinburgh: Churchill Livingstone, 1992: 355–411)*

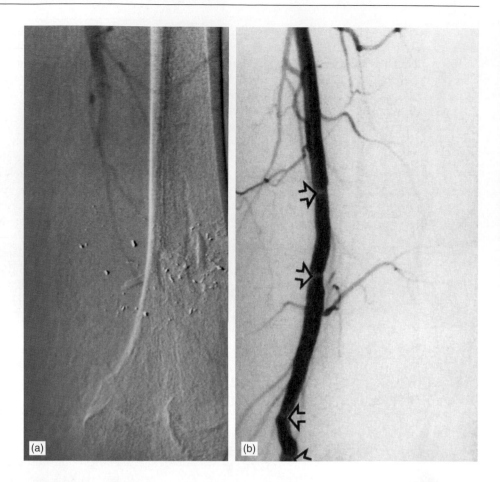

Figure 33.20 *(a) A preoperative angiogram of multiple bullet injuries to the popliteal artery. (b) The postoperative angiogram shows two interposed vein grafts (between arrows)*

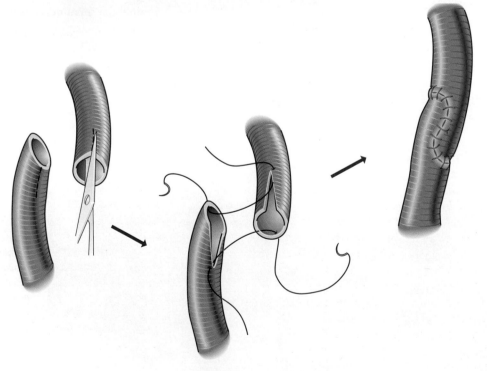

Figure 33.21 *Spatulation of vessel ends to prevent stenosis*

purpose. One technique involves taking two, and if necessary three, equal segments of vein of appropriate length opened longitudinally to form panels; after excising any valves, the panels are sewn together side by side to produce a panelled compound graft (Figs 33.23 and 33.24). Alternatively, a length of vein, slit open longitudinally and bereft of valves, is wrapped spirally over a bridging shunt of appropriate bore; the adjoining margins of vein and

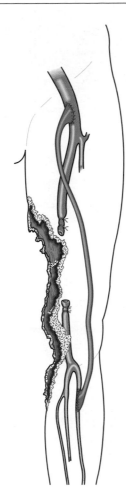

Figure 33.22 *Extra-anatomical vein bypass for extensive contaminated wounds*

host vessel are then approximated by a continuous suture to achieve a spiralled compound graft, a technique suited to larger vessels such as the common femoral artery (Fig. 33.25) and indeed the inferior vena cava.

PROSTHETIC GRAFT

Prosthetic grafts have to be used when saphenous vein is unavailable, either because it has been removed or it is of poor quality. Polytetrafluoroethylene (PTFE) is probably safer and more reliable than Dacron and although the former has been used with some success in closed injuries of the large vessels, its use in highly contaminated wounds should be discouraged. It ought not to be used in preference to vein in the upper limb, in bridging vessels across joints or in replacing damaged vein.

The encouraging reports of the success of prosthetic grafts, and in particular PTFE, in stabbings and low velocity gunshot wounds[21] should not lead to complacency or indeed obscure the inherent risks of infection, secondary haemorrhage and a higher amputation rate when used indiscriminately in dirty wounds. On the occasional instance when substantial loss of tissue leaves a repair inadequately covered or exposed and therefore liable to

necrosis, a prosthetic graft may have some advantage over vein. While sepsis brings about necrosis of the body of a vein graft, such breakdown following the implantation of a prosthetic graft repair tends to affect the anastomoses with the host vessel.[102]

FALSE ANEURYSM

False aneurysm may become apparent soon after diagnostic transfemoral cardiac catheterisation because the common femoral artery lies in a superficial position. In cases of penetrating trauma, however, a false aneurysm of a deeply placed artery may be missed until the aneurysm manifests itself by progressive expansion and pressure effects (see Figs 33.3–33.5, 33.7). For obvious reasons patients in cardiology units undergoing diagnostic cannulation may not be fit for general anaesthesia, and sometimes regional or local anaesthesia may have to be employed. For some years, non-operative, ultrasound guided compression therapy has been successfully used in selected cases.[103]

In those requiring surgical treatment, proximal and distal control is established, the aneurysm opened, thrombus evacuated, the false aneurysm excised and the vessel lumen inspected for intimal damage. Occasionally, proximal control of the external iliac artery is necessary. Back-flow from the profunda femoris may be controlled directly or indirectly by means of a balloon catheter attached to a three-way tap. A loose atheromatous flap in the posterior wall may have to be tacked down with a 5-0 or 6-0 polypropylene suture. The laceration is repaired transversely with interrupted 5-0 double ended sutures, picking upper and lower intimal edges from within outwards. In chronic fusiform aneurysms the opening may be rather large, necessitating patch angioplasty or even segmental excision and graft replacement.

ARTERIOVENOUS FISTULA

Arteriovenous fistulae (see Figs 33.6 and 33.7) are frequently missed on initial examination and even on exploration,[21] most notoriously in shotgun wounds. Consequently, they present much later, usually accompanied by one or two false aneurysms. The use of a sterile stethoscope intraoperatively may be of value in locating fistulae if preoperative angiograms are not available. After control of artery and vein proximally and distally, the fistula is opened and the false aneurysms excised. Reconstruction may take the form of simple lateral suture, vein patch angioplasty and occasionally excision and graft replacement of the arterial segment involved. The vein is easily repaired by lateral suture or by means of a vein patch. In order to discourage recurrence a flap of fascia may be interposed between adjacent suture lines.

On–table assessment of repair

Peroperative evaluation of the quality of repair, in particular of the distal anastomosis, can be achieved simply by assessing the quality of a simulated pulse in the distal artery

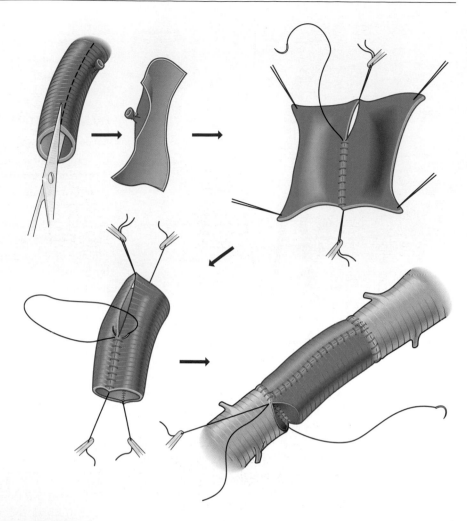

Figure 33.23 *Steps in the construction of a panelled compound vein graft*

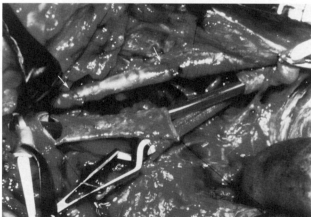

Figure 33.24 *Popliteal artery, above, (previously shunted) repaired using a reversed interposition vein graft (arrowed). Popliteal vein, below, (with shunt in situ) being repaired by a panelled compound vein graft*

produced by forcing heparinised saline from a syringe into it using a cannula. Equally, intraoperative use of a Doppler ultrasound probe placed directly on the vessel wall provides information on functional outcome. Most effectively, an on-table angiogram offers quick visual proof of the technical adequacy of surgery or to identify a defect for immediate correction. This practice provides quality control of repairs of small calibre vessels in the forearm and the lower leg, and is of particular importance in children. In the severely injured hypotensive patient with poor or unrecordable distal pulses and low core body temperature, on-table angiography offers assurance that there is no evidence of distal thrombus. Time consuming angioscopy has been displaced by intraoperative ultrasound in evaluating of the state of the repaired vessel, but our experience so far is limited.

Vein repair

Although a patient may be fortunate not to have a limb compromised by ligation of a major vein, the notion that ligation is not necessarily harmful or that venous repair is of limited importance should be dispelled.[6] Ligation is more than likely to be complicated by deep vein thrombosis, raised compartment pressure and acute oedema as well as by a much higher incidence of fasciotomy than is found following vein repair. Moreover, the likelihood of venous gangrene and amputation in the early stages is increased. In the longer term, post-thrombotic changes may bring about chronic symptoms of obstructive venous insufficiency.

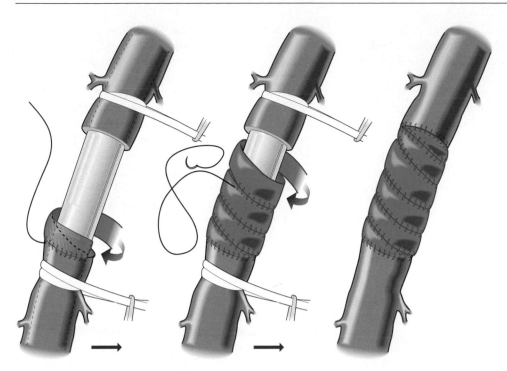

Figure 33.25 *Steps in the construction of a spiralled compound vein graft*

A reconstituted major venous channel will largely prevent these problems and may actually enhance the patency of an adjacent arterial repair.[12] Even if the vein repair fails later, an interim venous collateral network may have developed to the extent that final occlusion of the vein repair may not be associated with chronic oedema.[104] Although grafts fail, there is evidence to show that both the patency of the repair and valve competence within the graft can be maintained in the long term.[105] In the presence of life-threatening injuries elsewhere, vein ligation may be necessary. Lateral suture of a large diameter main venous channel is tolerated very much better than that of the adjacent artery, which has a smaller diameter.[104] Vein graft replacement of a damaged, vein segment is often necessary, but the larger calibre of the host vessel may demand the construction of a compound vein graft of either the panel or spiral variety (see Figs 33.23–33.25). This adds a little time to the operation but with a shunt in place ample time is available for precise work.

In situations in which both vein and artery have been shunted, the order in which each vessel is repaired is immaterial. Alternatively, if neither vessel has been shunted, preliminary vein repair will prevent a serious rise in venous pressure when arterial flow is eventually re-established. Time permitting, an arteriovenous fistula may also be created just distal to the grafted segment to enhance long-term patency.

Fasciotomy

In addition to all the other definitive procedures aimed at restoring flow and drainage in the distal limb, fasciotomy represents an invaluable adjunctive procedure.

Compartmental hypertension resulting from oedema of muscle is largely brought about by reperfusion injury but it is obviously worse in severe trauma or when venous return is impaired due to vein ligation or thrombosis. The temporary insertion of shunts (see Figs 33.10 and 33.11) will abbreviate the period of ischaemia and consequently reduce the severity of reperfusion injury.

Muscle necrosis will inevitably occur unless decompression is timely and adequate. The anterior compartment of the lower leg lies within rigid osseous and fascial boundaries and is therefore the most vulnerable of the four compartments. The muscle compartments of the forearm and palm are also endangered by raised pressure. Palpable distal pulses and reasonable capillary refill are deceptive and may delay fasciotomy beyond the point of irreversible muscle damage. A number of clinical situations call for fasciotomy as a formal procedure: when surgical intervention is delayed beyond a period of 4–6 hours after vessel injury; concomitant injury of main artery and vein; significant injury to distal soft tissues with associated haematoma; obvious oedema and paralysis of muscle with patchy muscle necrosis; plantar flexion of the foot after completion of vascular repair; compartment pressures in excess of 40 mmHg.[17,18,88]

The techniques available for fasciotomy are varied. Percutaneous fasciotomy is generally ineffectual and totally fails to relieve pressure in the deep compartment of the lower leg. If fasciotomy is deemed necessary, the transcutaneous method is most rewarding. The lateral approach, with or without, a mid-third fibulectomy, may enable decompression of the four compartments of the lower leg but this is a rather destructive procedure risking damage to vessels and nerves. The standard two-incision approach, the lateral decompressing the anterior and peroneal compartments and the medial decompressing the superficial and deep posterior compartments, is simple and successful.[106] Severe compression of muscles in the forearm, in both the extensor and flexor compartments, must be relieved, along with that in the thenar eminence of the hand. This is achieved by a longitudinal, centrally placed incision over the extensor compartment and by a further curvilinear incision on the flexor aspect, which commences in the antecubital fossa, identifying and preserving the cutaneous nerves of the forearm, crosses the wrist and extends distally onto the palm along the thenar crease to release the carpal tunnel and thenar muscles, respectively.

Wound closure

The success of any vascular repair is to an extent dependent on the quality of both the vessel and the cover afforded by adjacent soft tissue and muscle, which by inference demands the elimination of any dead space and the prevention of haematoma. The magnitude of soft tissue loss (see Fig. 33.13) may be of a degree which leaves a vein graft exposed and vulnerable to desiccation and degeneration. Prosthetic grafts may be immune to these influences, but if the field is contaminated, suture line dehiscence and catastrophic secondary haemorrhage are very likely to occur.

In instances of soft tissue loss, the superficial muscles of the arm, or the sartorius and gracilis muscles of the leg, can be freed while retaining their blood supply, and swung over in such a way as to ensheath a graft. Various temporary biological dressings, including porcine heterograft and amniotic membrane, have been used in circumstances such as these. Ideally, however, the skills of a plastic surgeon must be brought to the fore in rotating muscle flaps or in the construction of free vascularised musculocutaneous flaps. An alternative approach, of course, is the construction of an extra-anatomical vein bypass (see Fig. 33.22) through clean viable tissue well away from the main wound. The latter then requires debridement followed by split-skin grafting.

Primary suture of the wound is generally successful in closed injuries or in clean stab wounds. In contaminated wounds it is wise to pursue a policy of delayed primary suture 5–7 days later.[17–19] In dirty wounds, and particularly if tissue viability remains questionable, frequent inspections, on a daily basis if necessary, must be undertaken under anaesthesia. Obviously, early attention to wound care and the elimination of devitalised tissue will minimise the morbidity associated with a necrotic and septic focus and expedite closure.

POSTOPERATIVE MANAGEMENT

General measures

In general the injured limb is nursed in the horizontal position, but if it is swollen a little elevation is acceptable. Fluid replacement is essential for good flow through reconstructed vessels and to ensure satisfactory perfusion of the distal bed. In cases of persisting spasm, and only after angiographic confirmation that an arterial injury is not present, selective intra-arterial infusion of tolazoline has been advocated.[107] Low dose heparin is of value in aiding graft patency and also in preventing deep vein thrombosis, although caution is required in the multiply injured patient.

In order to minimise reperfusion injury, a slow mannitol infusion over a 12–24-hour period is helpful in limiting damage. The benefits of mannitol, which were once attributed almost entirely to its osmotic properties, are now increasingly recognised as being achieved largely through the accelerated inactivation of oxygen free radicals, which mediate in reperfusion injury and increased capillary permeability.[58–63] The value of mannitol in combating the effects of reperfusion injury is supported by both experimental[108] and clinical[109] evidence. The timing in instituting such therapy requires considered judgement and care, in particular if the patient is haemodynamically unstable on arrival. Research studies at our centre using ischaemic-preconditioning and the use of recombinant bactericidal/permeability-increasing protein may herald innovative techniques and therapies in attenuating the systemic inflammatory response to IRI and vitiating remote organ injury.[110–113]

Daily dressing of wounds, swab cultures and alertness to early signs of gas gangrene are essential. If gas gangrene is suspected, immediate surgical excision of affected tissue under cover of penicillin and antitoxin therapy may help to counteract its advance; the use of hyperbaric oxygen is controversial but, if available, should be offered in serious cases. In spite of optimal wound care and prophylactic antibiotic therapy, healing may be compromised by impaired tissue perfusion of damaged tissues.

Failure of vascular repair

Continued maintenance of patency of vessels after repair represents a key concern and peripheral flow must therefore be checked by observing pulses, capillary refill time and by using Doppler ultrasound. Close vigilance is necessary and if suspicions of impaired flow and graft failure are aroused urgent angiography is indicated; if the vessel has thrombosed re-exploration and fresh reconstruction are mandatory. Thrombotic occlusion is usually the product of a number of weaknesses of technique, namely, narrowing caused by lateral suture, tension and constriction at the suture line of a direct anastomosis or 'purse stringing' by a continuous tight suture line. Other causes include inadequate excision of a segment with intimal damage, poor coaptation of intima at the suture line or intrusion of the adventitia into the flow surface. When the diameter of the vein graft is small it may fail; when a vein graft is used to restore flow prior to bone fixation, it may well fail if it is either too short, causing anastomotic tension, or too long, resulting in kinking.

In any situation of graft failure, early reoperation will give the limb its best second chance of uncomplicated survival, and when revisiting the wound attention to technique is of crucial importance. Previously sutured ends must be trimmed back, ensuring that there is no residual evidence of the initial injury. Clot is removed both proximally and distally, heparinised saline is infused distally, and a shunt may be inserted at this stage to restore flow. Finally, the new repair must be precise in every respect.

Conclusions

Weapons represent a global health hazard of epidemic proportions, particularly in the hands of irresponsible users and terrorists who target civil populations indiscriminately. As long as such weapons continue to be used surgeons will be confronted by vascular injuries. Limb vascular trauma, particularly when complex, requires some knowledge of the wounding mechanisms and the pathophysiological consequences thereof. The influence of the passage of time on reperfusion injury, compartment hypertension and the potential likelihood of limb loss must be clearly understood. Numerous factors can play a significant role in minimising the complication rate and lowering the incidence of limb loss.

The use of intraluminal shunts in both injured artery and vein, particularly in complex injuries, buys time and introduces a disciplined operative technique which has many advantages. Unhurried and diligent care of the wound, adequate debridement and precise skeletal fixation will create the best conditions for vascular repair of both artery and vein. The avoidance of less desirable techniques of repair in favour of vein grafting and, if necessary, the construction of larger diameter compound vein grafts when the situation demands will promote better results. When necessary, immediate and effective fasciotomy will enhance tissue viability. Postoperatively, alertness to signs of graft failure and, if necessary, re-exploration and fresh reconstruction will improve the chances of limb survival.

Key references

Amato JJ, Billy U, Gruber RP, et al. Vascular Injuries. An experimental study of high and low velocity missile wounds. Arch Surg 1970; **101**: 167–74.

Barros D'Sa AAB, Harkin DW, Blair PHB, et al. The Belfast approach to managing complex lower limb vascular injuries. Eur J Vasc Endovasc Surg (in press).

Menzoian JD, Doyle JE, Cantelmo NL, et al. A comprehensive approach to extremity vascular trauma. Arch Surg 1985; **120**: 801–5.

Mubarak SJ, Owen CA. Double incision fasciotomy of the leg for decompression in compartment syndromes. J Bone Joint Surg (US) 1997; **59A**: 184–7.

Rich NM, Baugh JH, Hughes CW. Acute arterial injuries in Vietnam: 1000 cases. J Trauma 1970; **10**: 359–69.

REFERENCES

1 Ogilvie WH. War surgery in Africa. Br J Surg 1944; **31**: 313.
2 De Bakey ME, Simeone FA. Battle injuries of the arteries in World War II. Ann Surg 1946; **123**: 534–79.
3 Hughes CW. Arterial repair during the Korean War. Ann Surg 1958; **147**: 555–61.
4 Rich NM. Wounding power of various ammunitions. Resident Phys 1968; **14**: 72.
5 Rich NM, Hughes CW. Vietnam vascular registry: preliminary report. Surgery 1969; **65**: 218–26.
6 Rich NM, Baugh JH, Hughes CW. Acute arterial injuries in Vietnam: 1000 cases. J Trauma 1970; **10**: 359–69.
7 De Muth WE. Bullet velocity makes the difference. J Trauma 1969; **9**: 642–3.
8 Amato JJ, Billy U, Gruber RP, et al. Vascular injuries. An experimental study of high and low velocity missile wounds. Arch Surg 1970: **101**: 167–74.
9 Morris GC, Creech O, DeBakey ME. Acute arterial injuries in civilian practice. Am J Surg 1957; **93**: 565–70.
10 Morris GC, Beall AC, Roof WR, et al. Surgical experience with 220 acute vascular injuries in civilian practice. Am J Surg 1960; **99**: 775–81.
11 Drapanas T, Hewitt RL, Weichert RC, et al. Civilian vascular injuries, a critical appraisal of three decades of management. Ann Surg 1970; **172**: 351–60.
12 Perry MO, Thal ER, Shires GT. Management of arterial injuries. Ann Surg 1971; **173**: 403–8.
13 Smith RF, Elliot JP, Hageman JH, et al. Acute penetrating arterial injuries of the neck and limbs. Arch Surg 1974; **109**: 198–205.
14 Lozman H, Beaufils AT, Rossi G, et al. Vascular trauma observed at an urban hospital center. Surg Gynecol Obstet 1978; **146**: 237–40.
15 Feliciano D, Mattox KL, Graham J, Bitondo C. Five year experience with PTFE grafts in vascular wounds. J Trauma 1985; **25**: 71–82.
16 Livingston RH, Wilson RI. Gunshot wounds of the limbs. BMJ 1975; **1**: 667–9.
17 Barros D'Sa AAB, Hassard TH, LivingstonRH, Irwin JWS. Missile-induced vascular trauma. Injury **12**: 13–30.
18 Barros D'Sa AAB. Management of vascular injuries of civil strife. Injury 1982; **14**: 51–7.
19 Johnston GW, Barros D'Sa AAB. Injuries of civil hostilities In: Carter DC, Polk HC (eds). International Medical Reviews Surgery Vol. 1, Trauma. London: Butterworths, 1981.
20 Archbold JAA, Barros D'Sa AAB, Morrison E. Genitourinary tract injuries of civil hostilities. Br J Surg 1981; **68**: 625–31.
21 Graham ANJ, Barros D'Sa AAB. Missed arteriovenous fistulae and false aneurysms in penetrating lower limb trauma: relearning old lessons. Injury 1991; **22**: 179–82.
22 Shaker IJ, White JJ, Signer RD, et al. Special problems of vascular injuries in children. J Trauma 1976; **16**: 863–7.

23 Boontje AH. Iatrogenic arterial injuries *J Cardiovasc Surg* 1978; **19**: 335–40.

24 Natali J, Benhamou AC. Iatrogenic vascular injuries. A review of 125 cases excluding angiographic injuries. *J Cardiovasc Surg* 1979; **20**: 169–76.

25 Mills JL, Wideman IE, Robison JG, *et al*. Minimizing mortality from iatrogenic arterial injuries: the need for early recognition and prompt repair. *J Vasc Surg* 1986; **4**: 22–7.

26 Bergqvist D, Helfer M, Jensen N, *et al*. Trends in civilian vascular trauma during 30 years. *Acta Chir Scand* 1987; **153**: 417–22.

27 Barros D'Sa AAB. The value of shunting in complex vascular trauma of the lower limb In: Earnshaw JJ, Murie JA (eds). *The Evidence for Vascular Surgery*. Shrewsbury: tfm Publishing Ltd, 1999: 189–96.

28 Barros D'Sa AAB, Harkin DW, Blair PHB, *et al*. The Belfast approach to managing complex lower limb vascular injuries. *Eur J Vasc Endovasc Surg* (in press).

29 Barros D'Sa AAB. Shunting in complex lower limb trauma. In: Greenhalgh RM, Hollier L (eds). *Emergency Vascular Surgery*. London: WB Saunders, 1992.

30 Barros D'Sa AAB. Complex vascular and orthopaedic limb injuries [editorial]. *J Bone Joint Surg (UK)* 1992; **74**: 176–8.

31 Connolly J. Management of fractures associated with arterial injuries. *Am J Surg* 1971; **120**: 331–5.

32 Lefrak BA. Knee dislocation. *Arch Surg* 1976; **111**: 1021–4.

33 Alberty RE, Goodfried G, Boyden AM. Popliteal artery injury with fracture dislocation of the knee. *Am J Surg* 1981; **142**: 36–40.

34 Doty DB, Treiman RL, Rothschild PD, *et al*. Prevention of gangrene due to fractures. *Surg Gynecol Obstet* 1967; **125**: 284–5.

35 Smith RF, Szilagyi DE, Elliott JP. Fracture of the long bones with arterial injury due to blunt trauma. *Arch Surg* 1969; **99**: 315–24.

36 Wagner WH, Calkins ER, Weaver FA, *et al*. Blunt popliteal artery trauma: one hundred consecutive injuries. *J Vasc Surg* 1988; **7**: 736–43.

37 Gustilo RB, Mendoza RM, Williams DN. Problems in the management of Type III (severe) open fractures: a new classification of Type III open fractures. *J Trauma* 1984; **24**: 742–6.

38 Lance RH, Bach AW, Hansen ST, *et al*. Open tibial fractures with associated vascular injuries: Prognosis for limb salvage. *J Trauma* 1985; **25**: 203–7.

39 Seiler JG, Richardson JD. Amputation after extremity injury *Am J Surg* 1986; **152**: 260–4.

40 Kelly GL, Eiseman B. Civilian vascular injuries. *J Trauma* 1975; **15**: 507–14.

41 Hartsuck 1M, Moreland HJ, Williams GR. Surgical management of vascular trauma distal to the popliteal artery. *Arch Surg* 1972; **105**: 937–40.

42 Hollemann JH, Killebrew LH. Tibial artery injuries. *Am J Surg* 1982; **144**: 362–4.

43 Menzoian JD, Doyle JE, Cantelmo NL, *et al*. A comprehensive approach to extremity vascular trauma. *Arch Surg* 1985; **120**: 801–5.

44 Pasch AR, Bishara RA, Lim LT, *et al*. Optimal limb salvage in penetrating civilian vascular trauma. *J Vasc Surg* 1986; **3**: 189–95.

45 Best B, Barros D'Sa AAB. Popliteal vessel injury caused by plastic bullets. *Injury* 1987; **18**: 428–9.

46 Pace PD, Tilney NL, Lesch M, *et al*. Peripheral arterial complications of intra-aortic balloon counter-pulsation. *Surgery* 1977; **82**: 685–8.

47 Benson EP. Radiation injury to large arteries. *Radiology* 1973; **106**: 195–7.

48 McCallion W. A, Barros D'Sa AAB. Management of critical upper limb ischaemia long after irradiation injury of the subclavian and axillary arteries. *Br J Surg* 1991; **78**: 1136–8.

49 Barros D'Sa AAB. How do we manage acute limb ischaemia due to trauma? In: Greenhalgh RM, Jamieson CW, Nicolaides AN (eds). *Limb salvage and amputation for vascular disease*. London: WB Saunders, 1988: 135–50.

50 Meerson FZ, Kagan VE, Kozhov YP, *et al*. The role of lipid peroxidation in the pathogenesis of ischaemic damage and the antioxidant protection of the heart. *Basic Res Cardiol* 1982; **77**: 465–85.

51 Halliwell B, Gutteridge SMC. Oxygen toxicity, oxygen radicals, transition metals and disease *Biochem J* 1984; **219**: 1.

52 Korthuis RJ, Granger DN, Townsley MI, Taylor AE. The role of oxygen-derived free radicals in ischaemia-induced increases in canine skeletal muscle vascular permeability *Circ Res* 1985; **57**: 599–609.

53 McCord 1M. Oxygen-derived free radicals in post-ischaemic tissue injury. *N Engl J Med* 1985; **312**: 159–63.

54 Granger DN, Hollwarth ME, Parks DA. Ischaemia-reperfusion injury: role of oxygen derived free radicals. *Acta Physiol Scand* 1986; **548**(suppl): 47–63.

55 Grisham MB, Hernandez LA, Granger DN. Xanthine oxidase and neutrophil infiltration in intestinal ischaemia. *Am J Physiol* 1986; **251**: G567–74.

56 Kuzon WM Jr, Walker PM, Mickle DA, *et al*. An isolated skeletal muscle model suitable for acute ischaemic studies. *J Surg Res* 1986; **41**: 24–32.

57 Armstead WM, Mirro R, Bursija DW, Leffler CW. Post-ischaemic generation of superoxide anion by newborn pig brain. *Am J Physiol* 1988; **255**: H401–3.

58 Anner H, Kaufman RP, Vateri CR, *et al*. Reperfusion of ischaemic lower limbs increases pulmonary microvascular permeability. *J Trauma* 1988; **28**: 607–10.

59 Ernester L. Biochemistry of reoxygenation injury. *Crit Care Med* 1988; **16**: 947–53.

60 Smith JK, Carden DL, Korthuis RJ. Role of xanthine oxidase in post-ischaemic microvascular injury in skeletal muscle. *Am J Physiol* 1989; **257**: H1782–9.

61 Rubin BB, Smith A, Liauw S, *et al*. Complement activation and white cell sequestration in post-ischaemic skeletal muscle. *Am J Physiol* 1990; **259**: H525–31.

62 Beckman JS, Beckman TW, Chen J, *et al*. Apparent hydroxyl radical production by peroxynitrite: implications for endothelial injury from nitric oxide and superoxide. *Proc Nat Acad Sci U S A* 1990; **87**: 1620–4.

63 Kupinski AM, Shah DM, Bell DR. Permeability changes following ischaemia-reperfusion injury in rabbit hind limb. *J Cardiovasc Surg (Torino)* 1992; **33**: 690–4.

64 Allen DM, Chen LE, Seaber AV, Urbaniak JR. Pathophysiology and related studies of the no reflow phenomenon in skeletal muscle. *Clin Orthop* 1995; 122–33.

65 Yassin MM, Barros D'Sa AAB, Parks TG, *et al*. Lower limb ischaemia-reperfusion alters gastrointestinal structure and function. *Br J Surg* 1997; **84**: 1425–9.

66 Yassin MM, Barros D'Sa AAB, Parks TG, *et al*. Lower limb ischaemia-reperfusion injury causes endotoxaemia and endogenous antiendotoxin antibody consumption but not bacterial translocation. *Br J Surg* 1998; **85**: 785–9.

67 Yassin MM, Barros D'Sa AAB, Parks TG, *et al.* Mortality following lower limb ischaemia-reperfusion: a systemic inflammatory response? *World J Surg* 1996; **20**: 961–7.

68 Harkin DW, Barros D'Sa AAB, McCallion K, *et al.* Circulating neutrophil priming and systemic inflammation in limb-reperfusion injury. *Int Angiol* 2001; **20**: 78–9.

69 Glauser MP, Zanetti G, Baumgartner JD, Cohen J. Septic shock: pathogenesis. *Lancet* 1991; **338**: 732–6.

70 Bone RC. The sepsis syndrome: definition and general approach to management. *Clin Chest Med* 1996; **17**: 175–81.

71 Leeman M. Pulmonary hypertension in acute respiratory distress syndrome *Monaldi Arch Chest Dis* 1999; **54**: 146–9.

72 Hoffman MJ, Greenfield LJ, Sugerman HJ, *et al.* Unsuspected right ventricular dysfunction in shock and sepsis. *Ann Surg* 1983; **198**: 307–19.

73 Carrico CJ, Meakins JL, Marshall JC, *et al.* Multiple organ failure syndrome. *Arch Surg* 1986; **121**: 196–208.

74 Harkin DW, Barros D'Sa AAB, Yassin MM, *et al.* Reperfusion injury is greater with delayed restoration of venous outflow in concurrent arterial and venous limb injury. *Br J Surg* 2000; **87**: 734–41.

75 Nassim A, Thompson MM, Naylor AR, *et al.* The impact of MRSA on vascular surgery *Eur J Vasc Endovasc Surg* 2001; **22**: 211–14.

76 Snyder WH, Thal ER, Bridges RA, *et al.* The validity of normal arteriography in penetrating trauma *Arch Surg* 1978; **113**: 424–6.

77 Sirinek KR, Gaskill HV, Dittman WI, *et al.* Exclusion angiography for patients with possible vascular injuries of the extremities – a better use of trauma centre resources. *Surgery* 1983; **94**: 599–603.

78 Frykberg ER, Crump JM, Dennis JW, *et al.* Non-operative observation of clinically occult arterial injuries: a prospective evaluation. *Surgery* 1991; **109**: 85–96.

79 McCormick TM, Burch BH. Routine angiographic evaluation of neck and extremity trauma. *J Trauma* 1979; **19**: 384–7.

80 Reid JDS, Weigelt JA, Thal ER, *et al.* Assessment of proximity of a wound to major vascular structures as an indication for arteriography. *Arch Surg* 1988; **123**: 942–6.

81 Gomes GA, Kreis DJ, Ratner L, *et al.* Suspected vascular trauma of the extremities: the role of arteriography in proximity injuries. *J Trauma* 1986; **26**: 1005–8.

82 Frykberg ER, Dennis JW, Bishop K, *et al.* The reliability of physical examination in the evaluation of penetrating extremity trauma: results at one year. *J Trauma* 1991; **31**: 502–11.

83 Gregory RT, Gould RJ, Peclet M, *et al.* The mangled extremity syndrome (MES): a severity grading system for multisystem injury of the extremity. *J Trauma* 1985; **25**: 1147–50.

84 Johansen K, Daines M, Howey T, *et al.* Objective criteria accurately predict amputation following lower extremity trauma. *J Trauma* 1990; **30**: 568–73.

85 Anderson N, Patha de Sousa C, Paredes S. Social cost of landmines in four countries: Afghanistan, Bosnia, Cambodia and Mozambique. *BMJ* 1995; **311**: 718–21.

86 Coupland RM. The effect of weapons: surgical challenge and medical dilemma. *J R Coll Surg Edinb* 1996; **41**: 65–71.

87 Vara-Thorbeck R, Ruiz-Morales M. Severe head injury combined with orthopaedic and vascular trauma of the limbs. *Langenbecks Arch Surg* 1998; **383**: 252–8.

88 Barros D'Sa AAB. A decade of missile-induced vascular trauma. *Ann R Coll Surg Engl* 1982; **64**: 37–44.

89 Barros D'Sa AAB. Leading article. The rationale for arterial and venous shunting in the management of limb vascular injuries *Eur J Vasc Surg* 1989; **3**: 471–4.

90 Barros D'Sa AAB, Moorehead RJ. Combined arterial and venous intraluminal shunting in major trauma of the lower limb. *Eur J Vasc Surg* 1989; **3**: 577–81.

91 Elliott J, Templeton J, Barros D'Sa AAB. Combined bony and vascular limb trauma: a new approach to treatment. *J Bone Joint Surg* 1984; **66–B**: 281.

92 Barros D'Sa AAB. Upper and lower limb vascular trauma. In: Greenhalgh RM (ed). *Vascular Surgical Techniques.* London: Bailliere Tindall, 1989: 47–65.

93 Barros D'Sa AAB. Leading article. Twenty-five years of vascular trauma in Northern Ireland. *BMJ* 1995; **310**: 1–2.

94 Walker AJ, Mellor SG, Cooper GJ. Experimental experience with a temporary intraluminal heparin-bonded polyurethane arterial shunt *Br J Surg* 1994; **81**: 195–8.

95 Brinker MR, Caines MA, Kerstein MD, Elliott MN. Tibial shaft fractures with an associated infrapopliteal arterial injury: a survey of vascular surgeons' opinions on the need for vascular repair. *J Orthop Trauma* 2000; **14**: 194–8.

96 Keeley S, Snyder WH, Weigelt JA. Arterial injuries below the knee: fifty-one patients with 82 injuries. *J Trauma* 1983; **23**: 285–90.

97 Yeager RA, Hobson RW, Lynch TG, *et al.* Popliteal and infrapopliteal arterial injuries differential management and amputation rates. *Am Surg* 1984; **50**: 155–8.

98 Segal D, Brenner M, Gorczyca J. Tibial fractures with infrapopliteal arterial injuries. *J Orthop Trauma* 1987; **1**: 160–9.

99 Flint LM, Richardson JD. Arterial injuries with lower extremity fracture. *Surgery* 1983; **93**: 5–8.

100 Shah DM, Corson JD, Karmody AM, *et al.* Optimal management of tibial artery trauma. *J Trauma* 1988; **28**: 228–34.

101 Barros D'Sa AAB, Berger K, Di Benedetto G, *et al.* A healable filamentous Dacron surgical fabric. *Ann Surg* 1980; **192**: 645–57.

102 Stone KS, Walshaw R, Sugiyama GT, *et al.* Polytetrafluoroethylene versus autogenous vein grafts for vascular reconstruction in contaminated wounds. *Am J Surg* 1984; **147**: 692–5.

103 Feld R, Patton GM, Carabasi A, *et al.* Treatment of iatrogenic femoral artery injuries with ultrasound-guided compression. *J Vasc Surg* 1992; **16**: 832–40.

104 Meyer J, Walsh J, Schuler J, *et al.* The early fate of venous repair after civilian vascular trauma: a clinical, haemodynamic and venographic assessment. *Ann Surg* 1987; **206**: 458–64.

105 Phifer TJ, Gerlock AJ, Rich NM, McDonald JC. Long term patency of venous repairs demonstrated by venography. *J Trauma* 1985; **25**: 342–6.

106 Mubarak SJ, Owen CA. Double-incision fasciotomy of the leg for decompression in compartment syndromes. *J Bone Joint Surg (US)* 1977; **59**A: 184–7.

107 Dickerman RM, Gewertz BL, Foley DW, Fry J. Selective intra-arterial tolazoline infusion in peripheral arterial trauma. *Surgery* 1977; **81**: 605–9.

108 Buchbinder D, Karmody AM, Leather RP, Shah DM. Hypertonic mannitol. Its use in the prevention of revascularization syndrome after acute arterial ischaemia *Arch Surg* 1981; **116**: 414–21.

109 Shah DM, Naraynsingh Y, Leather RP, *et al.* Advances in the management of acute popliteal vascular blunt injuries *J Trauma* 1985; **25**: 793–7.

110 Harkin DW, Barros D'Sa AAB, McCallion K, *et al.* Ischaemic preconditioning before lower limb ischaemia-reperfusion protects against acute lung injury. *J Vasc Surg* 2002; **35**: 1264–73.

111 Harkin DW, Barros D'Sa AAB, *et al.* Recombinant bactericidal/permeability-increasing protein attenuates the systemic inflammatory response syndrome in lower limb ischaemia-reperfusion injury. *J Vasc Surg* 2001; **33**: 840–6.

112 Harkin DW, Barros D'Sa AAB, Yassin MM, *et al.* Gut mucosal injury is attenuated by recombinant bactericidal/

permeability-increasing protein hind limb ischaemia-reperfusion injury. *Ann Vasc Surg* 2001; **15**: 326–31.

113 Harkin DW, Barros D'Sa AAB, McCallion K, *et al.* Bactericidal/permeability-increasing protein attenuates systemic inflammation and acute lung injury in porcine lower limb ischaemia-reperfusion injury. *Ann Surg* 2001; **234**: 233–44.

34

Vascular Injuries of the Chest

ALASTAIR NJ GRAHAM, KIERAN G MCMANUS, JAMES A MCGUIGAN

THE PROBLEM

The modern city and the highway contribute more major trauma cases daily than do all the declared wars, undeclared wars and terrorist atrocities in the world. The burden of domestic trauma also has enormous implications for healthcare expenditure. In the USA approximately 60 million injuries are recorded annually, 30 million requiring professional care and 3.6 million being admitted to hospital and absorbing much of the health budget. Most importantly, 300 000 permanent disabilities are produced each year and trauma is responsible for more life-years lost than any other cause. Thoracic injuries occur at a rate of 12 per million of the population each day.[1] Major chest trauma is present in 56 per cent of trauma fatalities[2] and is directly responsible for a quarter of all deaths.[3]

Traumatic aortic rupture is an often missed and rapidly fatal condition if not treated judiciously. In examining the full range of thoracic vascular injuries this chapter also addresses cardiac, cervico-mediastinal, pulmonary and chest wall vascular injuries.

Prior to the Vietnam War fewer than 10 cases of injuries to thoracic great vessels had found their way into the world literature[4] whereas in the 1970s they accounted for more than 10 per cent of reported series of vascular injuries.[5] The lessons learned by these military surgeons, used effectively during the recent urban terrorist campaign in Northern Ireland, has been to proceed quickly to surgery without undue attempts at resuscitation. War scenarios produce proportionally fewer thoracic vascular injuries than observed in road traffic accidents, urban violence and terrorist atrocities. The many published series of thoracic trauma experienced in civilian centres have undoubtedly modified treatment on the battlefield. The civilian environment generates large numbers of deceleration injuries as well as calculated close-range handgun attacks.

Management will vary depending on the situation. The patient exsanguinating a mile from a trauma centre may survive if a policy of 'scoop and run', emergency room thoracotomy and 'clamp and sew' repair of the aorta prevails, whereas in the stable, multitrauma patient with contained aortic disruption a more considered approach prior to transfer to a specialist centre would be reasonable.

AETIOLOGY

The traditional division of thoracic injuries into penetrating and blunt is useful in describing aetiology, diagnosis and management as each category displays distinct patterns of progress. The boundaries, however, are frequently blurred as blunt injuries may also have a penetrating component caused by fractured ribs or extraneous objects penetrating the thoracic viscera (Fig. 34.1).

Blunt injuries

In civilian practice most great vessel injuries result from road traffic accidents. For instance, abrupt deceleration from a speed of 48 km/hour (30 mph), unmodified by seatbelt or crumple zone side impact bars, or the anterior chest wall itself, will produce a force of 172 times the force of gravity.[6] The elastic limit of the intima and media of the

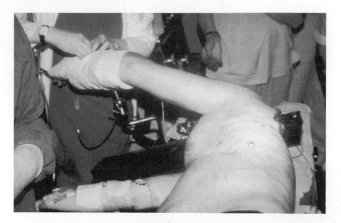

Figure 34.1 *A middle aged man suffered impalement by a wooden fence post after crashing his car. Both penetrating and blunt thoracic injuries were clearly present. A left posterolateral thoracotomy allowed removal of the 'foreign body' followed by thorough debridement and reconstruction of the chest wall. He made a good recovery*

aorta is exceeded by shearing forces as little as 80 G when applied to the mediastinal mass of the heart and adjacent structures. The forces sustained by the occupant of a vehicle involved in a collision, however, are not simple shearing forces but the product of a number of complex forces acting in rapid succession (see box). Similar stresses are placed on the mediastinal vasculature in falls from a great height, in aircraft crashes with the victims sitting in the 'brace' position and in crush injury. The inner layers of the aorta are torn and although the adventitia may contain the rupture for an undefined period of time, rupture will follow in most cases. It is rare for true intimal dissection to occur[7] and the two terms 'rupture' and 'dissection' should not be confused.

Component forces acting on the aorta in severe anterior/posterior deceleration injury

- Horizontal deceleration with 'jerk' deceleration as the chest wall is restrained by a belt or steering wheel leading to a horizontal component of shear stress
- Torsion stress as the heart and its attachments are forced into the left chest and angulation stress as the arch rotates around the isthmus
- Rotational deceleration as the upper torso rotates anteriorly above a belt or steering wheel
- Anteroposterior compression results when the rigid posterior thoracic structures move anteriorly against the already stationary anterior chest wall structures
- Mediastinal structures forcibly displaced superiorly and caudally by abdominal contents compressed by seatbelt or other restraint
- 'Waterhammer' effect on blood within the aorta due to the compression of the heart and abdominal aorta

---

CARDIAC

Blunt trauma to the heart rarely has persistent consequences. The heart is well protected by the sternum, one of the stronger bones in the body. While a sudden praecordial impact can cause dysrhythmias, even ventricular fibrillation, the commonest injury is 'concussion' of the heart. Although the patient may recall a severe crushing central chest pain it is frequently masked by the shock of the situation and associated anterior chest wall pain. Cardiac concussion is most often short lived, underdiagnosed and usually inconsequential. Severe blunt trauma to the heart, however, can result in intimal injury to the anterior descending coronary artery causing infarction and may even lead to the development of a ventricular aneurysm. Coronary artery rupture is rarely seen but when it occurs it is rapidly fatal.[8] Compression of the filled heart against the closed mitral or tricuspid valve has been associated with valvular injury. This may lead to cardiac instability and failure within a few days or may only come to light some months or even years after the event.

AORTIC

The isthmus of the thoracic aorta is immediately distal to the left subclavian artery. It is, as suggested by the nomenclature, the narrowest part of the aorta situated at the junction between the relatively fixed descending aorta and the mobile mediastinal structures attached to the aortic arch and the ligamentum arteriosum. The isthmus, therefore, is the section of the aorta at highest risk of rupture, though it is not the only such site.

CERVICO-MEDIASTINAL

Injuries to the supra-aortic vessels occur in 5 per cent of those investigated after severe blunt thoracic trauma and interestingly, the innominate, left common carotid and left subclavian arteries are equally likely to be affected.[9] These injuries occur most commonly in motor vehicle – car more frequently than motorcycle – collisions and also in crush injuries, falls and similar injuries from a great height.[10] The mechanism of injury is thought to be a combination of traction with violent head and arm movements and scalene muscle compression. Avulsion of the supra-aortic branches can follow the simultaneous anterior impact on the chest driving the arch downwards while accompanying hyperextension of the neck produces long axis traction which can exceed the internal elastic limit of the intima. Injury of the great vessels frequently results in thrombosis and diagnosis is often delayed, but rupture does occur, and most commonly involves the innominate and left subclavian arteries.[11] When these injuries are isolated the patient is usually stable and repair is possible without the use of cardiopulmonary bypass (CPB)[12] (Fig. 34.2).

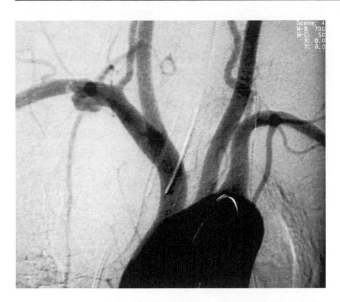

Figure 34.2 *On admission after a crash, a young motorcyclist was found to be haemodynamically unstable. A contrast enhanced computed tomography (CT) scan showed evidence of mediastinal haemorrhage but a discrete vascular lesion could not be seen. Digital subtraction angiography showed that the right internal mammary artery had avulsed from the subclavian artery with acute false aneurysm formation. Surgical repair using an interposition graft gave a good result. If a thoracic vascular injury is suspected because of hypotension, and the CT scan only shows a mediastinal haematoma, angiography becomes mandatory*

PULMONARY VESSELS

Peripheral contusions of the lung involve intrapulmonary tears with alveolar haemorrhage. This low pressure system is easily tamponaded once the lung is reinflated by appropriate chest drain placement. Major central pulmonary vascular injuries tend to be rapidly fatal and are usually only diagnosed at thoracotomy, a procedure generally avoided in blunt trauma.

CHEST WALL VESSELS

Rib fractures caused by blunt trauma will frequently lacerate intercostal vessels. Bleeding from the injured internal mammary artery may be limited initially by vascular spasm but fluid resuscitation may precipitate delayed primary haemorrhage. The likelihood of this outcome may not be apparent from the findings on the initial chest X-ray and emphasises the need for a follow-up study within 6 hours. Appropriate chest drainage will usually expose such bleeding. However, poorly inserted tube thoracostomy may itself result in iatrogenic injury to intercostal vessels.

Penetrating injuries

Unlike the effects of blunt injuries, all great vessels in the chest are vulnerable to penetrating trauma in the form of gunshot wounds or stabbings. While all penetrating missiles, knives and other sharp implements puncture and lacerate vessels and cause blood loss, the degree of damage varies considerably. Ironically, some patients who survive to reach hospital after injuries caused by high velocity bullets, depending on velocity at impact, may have sustained limited vessel injury and not necessarily the classic massive cavitation injury. Nevertheless, even though the patient may be stable, significant arterial wall contusion may have occurred and the risk of subsequent dissection, rupture, false aneurysm formation or thromboembolism is such that any penetrating injury in the vicinity of the great vessels demands arteriography or a similar imaging study.

High velocity injuries to the chest, however, are rarely 'clean through and through' injuries, the rib or other bony structure often being hit, splintering bone and shattering the missile. The resulting injury is more akin to a shotgun blast at close quarters generating multiple secondary missiles. Low velocity missiles have a reputation for dissecting around vessels and major viscera. It may be difficult therefore to predict their track through the tissues. In addition to laceration and bleeding, a special feature of low velocity missiles is their ability to penetrate and embolise within the pulmonary or systemic vasculature.[13] Shotgun injuries vary depending on the distance from which they are fired and the type of shot used. At less than 15 cm the effect is one of a single large, low velocity missile coring a hole in any structure with which it comes into contact. From 15 cm to 3 m, or when clothing or bone has dispersed the shot, the body is peppered with multiple low velocity missiles which cause multiple lacerations. Such injuries to the ascending aorta or pulmonary outflow tract will make surgical repair almost impossible. At distances greater than 3 m shotgun pellets tend to lodge in the subcutaneous tissues with little ill effect.

The effects of stab injuries are usually easier to predict, particularly if the weapon is known. An anterior stab would place the internal mammary arteries at risk causing significant intrapleural blood loss but usually without cardiovascular collapse (see Fig. 34.2). If cardiac injury has occurred and the patient survives to reach hospital the clinical situation is usually one of tamponade rather than exsanguination with the right ventricle or main pulmonary artery usually being the site of injury. The lungs are often injured in wounds to the lateral and posterior aspects of the chest and with posterior wounds the descending aorta is also at risk. Aortic or other vascular injury should always be suspected in stab injuries and a conservative approach is acceptable only if accompanied by repeated clinical reassessment and adequate imaging to exclude vascular injury (Fig. 34.3).

The distribution of major thoracic vascular injuries in one large series from Houston, TX, USA, was as follows: descending thoracic aorta 21 per cent, subclavian artery 21 per cent, pulmonary artery 16 per cent, subclavian vein 13 per cent, intrathoracic vena cava 11 per cent, innominate artery 9 per cent, pulmonary veins 9 per cent.[14] In general, gun shot wounds, secondary blast injuries and stab wounds of the

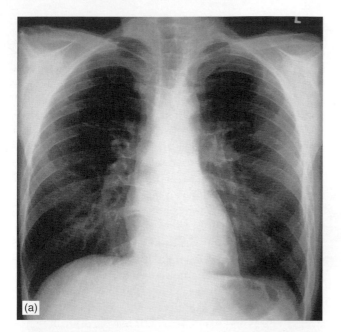

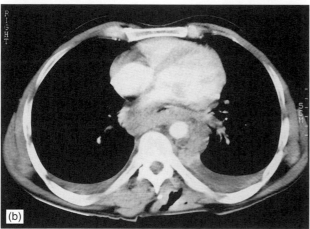

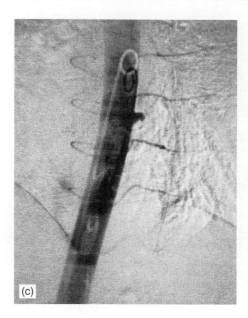

Figure 34.3 *On Christmas Eve a 22-year-old man's wife stabbed him with a kitchen knife. (a) An entry wound was evident 10 cm to the left of the spinous process of the eighth thoracic vertebra. He was haemodynamically stable and the chest X-ray failed to reveal a left pleural effusion. (b) In view of the anatomical site of the entry wound an intravenous contrast enhanced computed tomography scan was performed. The descending thoracic aorta appeared normal but it was surrounded by a large haematoma and small bilateral pleural effusions were also noted. (c) Digital subtraction angiography revealed a false aneurysm of the descending thoracic aorta. It was approached via a left posterolateral thoracotomy and repaired by direct suture*

aorta usually lead to death within 1 hour in 90 per cent of victims. Within the rather limited anatomical space of the thoracic inlet resides a collection of major vessels and any penetrating trauma in this area has a high likelihood of causing vascular injury. While the subclavian artery is most at risk,[15] aortic and innominate artery injuries also occur.[5] The classic sign is an expanding haematoma. It is noteworthy, however, that 8 per cent of patients with great vessel injuries presenting at one centre showed no clinical signs of vascular injury.[16]

Blast injuries

Blast injuries are even more complicated than simple penetrating or blunt trauma, because they are caused by a combination of the blunt effect of the shockwave on the torso, high and low velocity penetrating injuries from secondary shrapnel, deceleration injuries as a result of the body being displaced by the explosion, and finally, the

syndrome known as 'blast lung' which may not be apparent for many hours.

Iatrogenic injuries

One of the commonest mechanisms of iatrogenic vascular trauma is the result of inserting cannulae, either for diagnostic or therapeutic purposes, presenting as a variety of cervico-mediastinal arterial and venous injuries (see Chapters 38 and 40).

PATHOPHYSIOLOGY OF RESUSCITATION

Evidence from laboratory and clinical studies has shown that fluid resuscitation prior to obtaining definitive control of major vessel haemorrhage results in poorer outcomes than those associated with a policy of 'permissive hypotension'.[17–20] Bickell *et al.*,[17] using a swine model in which haemostasis was achieved by the formation of thrombus after aortotomy, compared resuscitation with and without 80 mL/kg of isotonic crystalloid fluid. While all infused animals showed an initial increase in cardiac output and mean arterial pressure, within 30 minutes the levels of these parameters returned to those of untreated animals. Importantly, in the treated animals oxygen delivery was lower and all of them died, whereas the untreated animals survived. A sheep model[19] consisting of a surgically lacerated pulmonary vein with chest drainage, was tested with an infusion of 30 mL/kg of isotonic crystalloid: treated animals were found to have a significantly increased rate, volume and duration of haemorrhage. Similar results were recorded in rat models of uncontrolled haemorrhage.[18]

Clinical studies tend to support inferences from this experimental work. In a retrospective study of 6855 patients from the San Diego County Trauma System, the 56 per cent given a prehospital infusion of crystalloid fluid (620–1554 mL) had a similar mortality rate but a significantly more negative base deficit compared with those not receiving fluid.[21] Other studies have shown that despite fluid resuscitation the oxygen saturation of blood was unchanged and that the lungs were more likely to suffer from fluid overload.[22,23] At the Ben Taub General Hospital, Houston, a prospective randomised trial of resuscitation after penetrating torso trauma was carried out, acknowledging the inherent logistic problems associated with such a study. A group of 289 patients in whom fluid resuscitation was delayed until they arrival in the operating theatre was compared with 309 patients who received immediate fluid resuscitation: the latter had a significantly higher incidence of renal failure, acute respiratory distress syndrome (ARDS) and mortality.[24]

Caution must be employed, however, before replacing old inflexible guidelines with new inflexible guidelines. The results obtained in the above models of major vascular injury may not be applicable to patients with pulmonary parenchymal injury in whom some evidence of benefit from a degree of volume resuscitation with hypertonic solutions is observed.[25] Where surgery is not immediately available[26,27] or indeed appropriate,[28] the withholding of resuscitation when the cardiac index and both oxygen delivery and consumption are low, increases morbidity and mortality.

DIAGNOSIS

While penetrating vascular injuries may be solitary and the diagnosis straightforward, in blunt trauma they rarely occur in isolation. In all multitrauma patients vascular injury must be suspected until proved otherwise, and unless specific vessel injuries are considered in the light of the history, they will not be looked for and therefore will be missed.

A major thoracic arterial injury open to the skin or the pleural cavity usually results in rapid exsanguination. Following a major deceleration injury or gunshot wound to the chest the combination of dullness, reduced air entry and absent or diminished pulses in a patient with severe dorsal thoracic pain strongly suggests major vessel injury with free rupture.

In the conscious patient who has suffered disruption of a major vessel, even of the size of the aorta, hypotension is not a constant finding. Following arterial laceration or dissection, especially when of partial wall thickness, haemorrhage may be protected by spasm or possibly tamponaded by surrounding mediastinal tissues. The clinical picture is one of a contained haematoma as opposed to free rupture so that clinical signs may not be evident. Suspecting and diagnosing such an injury before it progresses to free rupture is the major duty of the trauma surgeon. The clinical triad of a grossly widened mediastinum on chest X-ray, haemothorax and transient haemodynamic instability is highly specific for aortic injury and a marker for impending death from free rupture.[29]

Aortic

Many patients with aortic injury report severe interscapular pain without its significance being appreciated because of the multiplicity of other injuries. Examination of the chest wall is frequently unremarkable and the lung fields may be clear. Systolic bruits are occasionally found in the interscapular area. The left arm pulse and arterial pressure may be less than the right. Lower limb pulses may be difficult to feel despite satisfactory brachial blood pressure and anuria may follow. Paraplegia may result from reduced flow in the anterior spinal artery.

Cervico–mediastinal

Subtle vascular signs may point to a supra-aortic vessel injury. The classic sign is an expanding haematoma which may mask the actual loss of pulses; either in this situation or if a chest X-ray reveals an upper mediastinal haematoma, arch aortography is recommended (see Fig. 34.2).[30]

Pulmonary

Injuries to the venous or pulmonary vessels, which are low pressure systems, can be effectively tamponaded by the lungs, especially if properly positioned chest drains allow them to expand fully. Haemodynamic instability, rather than breathlessness, is a common feature of tension pneumothorax, particularly when accompanied by a significant haemothorax. The 'stony dullness' of a haemothorax only becomes detectable when at least 1 L of blood has been lost.

Cardiac

Cardiac tamponade following ventricular injury represents a special case of containment in which ventricular pressure interferes with venous filling of the low pressure atria, resulting in falling cardiac output and eventual arrest. The patient, if conscious, is extremely anxious, gasping for breath, hypotensive with peripheral shutdown, the upper torso and face are suffused with dilated veins and the neck is oedematous.

Vena caval system

Injuries to the superior vena cava or the innominate veins are manifested either as a tamponaded mediastinal haematoma or as free bleeding into the chest. Injury to the intrapericardial inferior vena cava may result in cardiac tamponade, or alternatively, as in the case of an injured azygous vein, rapid exsanguination into the chest.

INVESTIGATIONS

In the heat of the moment it is important to keep to a routine, checking airway, breathing and circulation, instituting electrocardiographic (ECG) monitoring and reviewing arterial oxygen saturation and central venous pressure.

In the unstable patient, primary survey may indicate the need to perform emergency thoracotomy without further investigation. A single penetrating cardiac injury with tamponade is usually the only major cardiovascular injury which can be salvaged in this situation, and therefore either anterior thoracotomy or median sternotomy would be a suitable approach. Most contained vascular injuries will be detected on secondary survey, which should also include the following investigations: chest and cervical X-rays, arterial blood gases, baseline haematology and biochemistry assessment including electrolytes and glucose, blood alcohol and, if applicable, a pregnancy test.

Evidence of intrathoracic bleeding or pneumothorax may be absent on the initial chest X-ray, which therefore, in the stable patient, should be repeated within 6 hours. While lung contusion or substernal venous bleeding may produce a wide mediastinal shadow, progressive widening of that shadow is strongly suggestive of an aortic rupture (box and Fig. 34.4a).

Radiological signs of traumatic aortic rupture

- Widening mediastinum
- Loss of aortic 'knuckle'
- Apical cap
- Paratracheal stripe
- Depression of the left main bronchus
- Deviation of the trachea/endotracheal tube to right
- Deviation of the oesophagus/nasogastric tube to right

Once a vascular injury is suspected the next decision is whether to employ computed tomography (CT), trans-oesophageal echocardiography (TOE) or angiography and that usually depends on the likely associated injuries. In the multiply injured patient, with potential abdominal or intracranial injuries a CT scan is a useful initial screening investigation. Aortography is more appropriate when cervico-mediastinal injuries are suspected although TOE may be quicker to perform if life-threatening aortic injury is suspected. These imaging techniques should be regarded as being complementary rather than in competition provided that they can be done quickly and effectively. Surgery on unstable patients should not be delayed by unnecessary extra investigations.

Contrast enhanced helical CT scan

The contrast enhanced CT scan, being non-invasive, widely available and vital in excluding intracranial, intra-abdominal and pelvic injuries is an extremely useful initial study. False negative results for thoracic aortic rupture are usually due to the inappropriate interpretation of poor quality scans;[31,32] spiral CT scans with 2 mm slices at the aortic isthmus, with correctly timed injection of contrast, raise sensitivity to 100 per cent.[20,33–35] The improved accuracy and speed of modern CT scanning has led to a trend eliminating the use of other investigations in the haemodynamically unstable patient and in demonstrating signs of aortic injury and periaortic extravasation of contrast[36] (Fig. 34.4b).

Arch aortogram

Aortography may be necessary on some occasions to confirm the nature of the injury before proceeding to surgery, but with the improved quality of spiral CT scans it is required less often. Although aortography may deliver occasional false positives for thoracic aortic rupture, usually due to the presence of atheroma or ductal diverticula, it is usually a reliable indicator of the presence of thoracic aortic rupture (Fig. 34.4c). A recent series comparing aortography and spiral CT showed the incidence of false positive results to be similar at 4 per cent.[36]

Routine angiography has been regarded as mandatory in evaluating all penetrating neck injuries but a predictive value approaching 100 per cent for chest X-ray seen against a negative physical examination of the neck has cast some doubt on this dogma.[30] Nevertheless, angiography remains the investigation of choice when cervico-mediastinal vascular injuries are suspected.

Transoesophageal echocardiography

Interest has recently increased in the use of TOE in assessing the patient at risk of thoracic aortic rupture (Fig. 34.4d).

This quick, portable investigation can be performed simultaneously with other procedures in the emergency room or operating theatre. It detects concomitant valvular disruption, myocardial contusion and pericardial collections accurately and, unlike aortography and contrast enhanced CT scans, does not involve administering potentially nephrotoxic contrast material to patients already volume depleted. Transoesophageal echocardiography, however, is contraindicated in patients with possible cervical spine, oropharyngeal or maxillo-facial injury, oesophageal strictures or diverticula; further, ascending aortic tears may be missed due to the intervening trachea, right main bronchus, and artefactual acoustic shadows from cannulae.[37] It should also be borne in mind that a negative TOE does not always exclude thoracic aortic rupture, even at the isthmus.

Despite the above advantages TOE is very operator dependent[38,39] and should be treated as a screening test in patients whose transfer to the radiology department would be dangerous or present considerable logistical difficulties. The unstable patient with a thoracic aortic rupture diagnosed by TOE should proceed directly to surgical repair but, as false positive diagnoses are made using this test,[40] in the stable patient, confirmatory angiography is advisable prior to surgical exploration (see Fig. 34.4c).[41]

Magnetic resonance angiography

Although magnetic resonance angiography (MRA) has made significant contributions in the investigation of

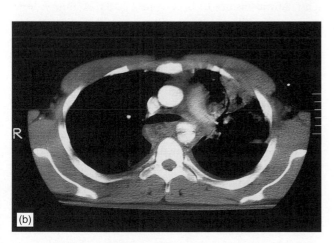

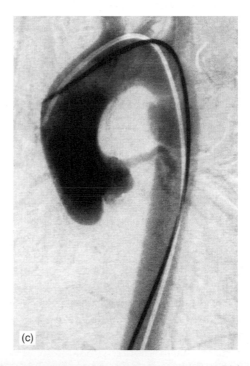

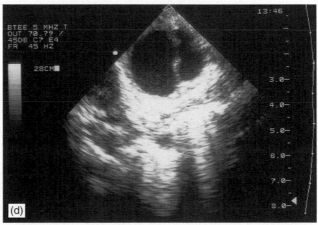

Figure 34.4   *A middle-aged man fell from a roof sustaining multiple injuries. (a) Initial chest X-ray was normal but when repeated it showed widening of the mediastinum. (b) A computed tomography scan showed a haematoma of the mediastinum with an acute false aneurysm at the aortic isthmus. (c) Digital subtraction angiography confirmed the diagnosis. (d) As inotropes were required to maintain adequate blood pressure (in this injury hypertension is the norm), transoesophageal echocardiography was performed and ventricular function was found to be impaired. Good views were obtained of the false aneurysm of the aorta, as shown*

cervical vascular trauma it would not be regarded as a primary study for patients sustaining blunt or penetrating trauma.[42] Magnetic resonance angiography may have a role in excluding diaphragmatic or aortic injury when spiral CT scan or angiography give equivocal results and when differentiating trauma related masses from neoplasia.

GENERAL PRINCIPLES AND PITFALLS IN TREATMENT

The clear aim of the trauma surgeon is to ensure that potentially life-threatening injuries are not missed. A majority of patients with initially stable, but potentially fatal thoracic injuries will have sustained either penetrating cardiac injury or contained rupture of the thoracic aorta. The stable patient with penetrating cardiac trauma is at risk of cardiac tamponade with impaired filling of the right ventricle. Blood loss in these patients is usually of the order of 500 mL, and therefore rapid infusion of several litres of clear fluid will only increase central venous pressure further without a corresponding rise in cardiac output. Stable contained rupture of the thoracic aorta may progress to frank rupture if the blood pressure is suddenly raised by aggressive fluid resuscitation.

PREHOSPITAL MANAGEMENT

In managing patients with thoracic trauma there is no convincing evidence of any benefit from prehospital intervention beyond establishing an airway and relieving tension pneumothorax. Prehospital intervention is contraindicated for haemothorax without respiratory compromise. A modified version of 'scoop and run' with protection of the airway and relief of tension pneumothorax is advisable.

RESUSCITATION

Prehospital care is continued in the accident and emergency department with an assured airway and full oxygenation. Conditions such as tension pneumothorax, cardiac tamponade and bleeding from external wounds are attended to urgently. A systolic blood pressure of 70–80 mmHg, usually sufficient to maintain cerebral perfusion, is acceptable. There is now substantial evidence, laboratory and clinical, that automatic fluid infusion prior to surgery to contend with haemorrhage not only converts a contained haemorrhage into a free rupture but also dilutes coagulation factors and precipitates ARDS, renal failure and fluid overload. Therefore, the emphasis should be on expediting surgical

exploration where deemed appropriate with careful titration of fluid infusion in those whose surgery is delayed or inappropriate.

OPERATIVE MANAGEMENT

The indications for surgical intervention after penetrating thoracic trauma have evolved over some years and remain useful guidelines.

Indications for surgical intervention after penetrating thoracic trauma

- Cardiac arrest
- Significant or sustained haemorrhage (>1 L immediately on drain insertion, >500 mL in first hour or >250 mL/hour thereafter)
- Mediastinal traversing injury
- Major vascular injury
- Sucking chest wound
- Persistent massive air leak
- Diaphragmatic rupture

In unstable patients admitted with gun shot wounds to the chest, thoracotomy is usually undertaken as an emergency in the operating theatre following the steps shown in the algorithm in Fig. 34.5.

Thoracic aortic rupture caused by blunt deceleration trauma is the most common thoracic vascular injury requiring surgery and is associated with an overall mortality of up to 98 per cent.[43] It is traditionally considered to be an extremely unstable injury and its diagnosis and repair have taken precedence over all other injuries.[44] The natural history of blunt thoracic aortic injury, however, is that those patients who actually die due to free rupture tend to do so within 4 hours of injury[45] and deaths beyond this time are principally due to other associated injuries. As the established mode of treatment for nontraumatic acute aortic dissection is pharmacological control of hypertension, principally using β-blockers to suppress myocardial contractility and nitrates to decrease preload and after load, some authorities are now advocating a similar policy in traumatic rupture.[46] If the diagnosis is suspected or confirmed, medical treatment is instituted to control blood pressure and, after other life-threatening injuries have been treated, repair of the aortic injury is carried out on a semi-elective basis.[45] The diminution of the force of ventricular ejection by the use of β-blockers is probably more effective in preventing rupture than the lowering of blood pressure by intravenous nitroprusside.

It was first reported in 1976 that aortic injuries do not all necessarily become more complicated if left surgically uncorrected. Two patients with aortic tears proximal to the

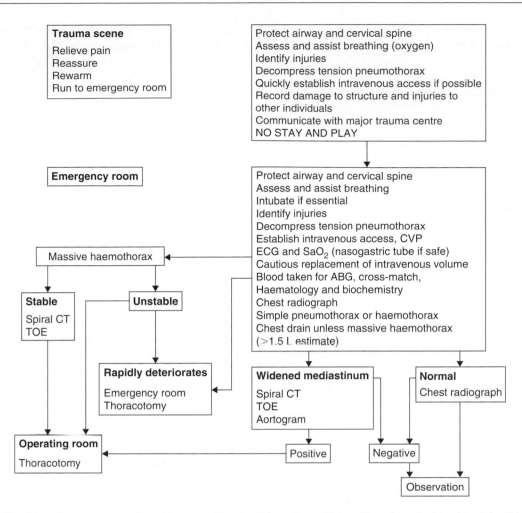

Figure 34.5 *Algorithm of management of chest trauma with potential great vessel injury. **There is no 'golden hour' for this scenario.** ABG, arterial blood gas analysis; CPV, central venous pressure; CT, computed tomography; ECG, electrocardiogram; SaO₂, oxygen saturation; TOE, transoesophageal echocardiography*

isthmus followed-up for up to 2 years showed no evidence of progression of those lesions.[47] Expanding on this experience, Akins *et al.*[48] reported a series of 44 patients with thoracic aortic rupture, 19 of whom received initial pharmacological management without adverse complications. While surgical repair was generally performed within 2–79 days of conservative management, in five cases a long term observational approach was adopted. It is noteworthy that, of the five deaths following immediate surgical repair, two resulting from complications of associated injuries might have been prevented had they been treated definitively before aortic repair. Although this delayed approach in dealing with aortic rupture is now generally accepted as safe,[49,50] prospective randomised trials have yet to be done. In some reports of initial conservative management of these injuries, fatal free rupture occurred within 24–72 hours of injury.[45,51] We feel, therefore, that if a patient presents with a definite diagnosis within 5 days of injury, and even though a 'permissive hypotension' regimen (Table 34.1) might have been

Table 34.1 *'Permissive hypotension' in thoracic vascular trauma*

Patient selection	Diagnosed major vascular injury, or Very high suspicion of major vascular injury
Anaesthesia	Sedated Paralysed Ventilated
Antihypertensive infusion	Esmolol Nipride/labetalol
Monitoring	Urinary catheter Invasive arterial blood pressure Invasive central venous pressure
Arterial blood pressure	Systolic blood pressure <110 mmHg
Urine output	>0.5 mL/kg per minute
'Danger moments'	Induction of anaesthesia Intubation Movement to radiology or operating table

instituted, surgery should not be delayed unless there are specific contraindications to doing so (see below).

Contraindications to immediate aortic repair (after Maggisano *et al.*[51])

- Glasgow Coma Scale less than 6 within 10 days of injury
- Evidence of intracranial haemorrhage on CT scan
- Acute respiratory distress syndrome
- Inability to tolerate one-lung anaesthesia
- Inotropic support required
- Coagulopathy despite adequate treatment
- Sepsis due to other injuries, especially intra-abdominal

Patients diagnosed 5 days or more, but less than 3 months, after injury may be managed with antihypertensives and scheduled for repair within a few days. Patients presenting after 3 months should be considered for elective repair based on the size and expansion rate of the false aneurysm.

Endovascular approaches

There is a growing number of reports of the use of endovascular stents in acute traumatic aortic rupture.[52–58] The left subclavian artery may have to be sacrificed as only a short segment of aorta lies distally within which a stent can be 'landed'. In the young patient surviving such a major injury, collateral perfusion of the arm is usually adequate, but subclavian flow can be augmented either by a bypass in the neck or, via the left cubital fossa, placing a second stent penetrating the main aortic stent.

The procedure is usually performed under general anaesthesia, though these patients are frequently ventilator dependent at the time of induction. Initial imaging is by CT scan with three-dimensional reconstructions which assist in planning a positioning strategy for the stent.[59] Magnetic resonance angiography may provide more accurate and specific images of the anatomy. The femoral artery, usually the left, is cannulated with an 18 or 20 Fr sheath which is passed into the proximal aortic arch where contrast is injected. The stent is passed over a guidewire and positioned using fluroscopy. Endoleak occurs in about 10 per cent of cases[56,57] and can be treated by further stent placement in the majority of cases (see Chapter 30). Long term follow-up is not yet available using this new endovascular technique but it is not free from neurological or other side effects.[60]

Post-traumatic aneurysms have proven to be ideal for endovascular stent placement as they involve a relatively short segment and have a discrete neck. Stenting for supra-aortic injuries has been successful but, until further experience has accrued, should be regarded as experimental.

Surgical approaches

The approach chosen must be based on the principle of securing proximal and distal control of the injured vessel(s). Median sternotomy affords the best access to major cardiac, ascending aortic, cervico-mediastinal and main pulmonary vessel injuries (Fig. 34.6a). For further access to the supra-aortic vessels distally, the median sternotomy can be extended to an oblique cervical or supraclavicular incision, dividing or resecting the clavicle as required, or by adding a third space anterior thoracotomy to create a 'trap-door' incision (see Fig. 34.6a).

In the presence of profound haemodynamic instability, the equipment required for emergency sternotomy may not be available and in these cases an anterolateral thoracotomy sited immediately inferior to the left pectoralis muscle and entering the chest via the fourth intercostal space requires no more advanced equipment than a scalpel (Fig. 34.6b). If further access is required, for example to institute CPB, and if conditions permit, this incision can be easily extended across the sternum into the right chest to create a 'clam-shell' approach (see Fig. 34.6b).

Control and repair techniques

CARDIAC

The pericardium may be opened allowing relief of tamponade and more efficient internal cardiac massage. Emergency control of cardiac injury can be achieved by finger pressure while resuscitation progresses. In some emergency situations the surgeon may just have the time to place the patient on CPB before executing the necessary repairs (Fig. 34.7). Definitive repair usually consists of simple mattress sutures, buttressed by pericardial or prosthetic pledgets. More extensive injuries are often incompatible with survival. Valvular injuries may become evident later and can be dealt with in a semi-urgent manner under CPB.

SUPRA-AORTIC VESSELS

The primary objective is to secure proximal and distal control of a major vessel and the inability to do so swiftly, especially amidst bleeding and a haematoma under pressure, is the most common cause of intraoperative mortality. Immediate compression is essential while adequate exposure is being obtained for clamping. The left innominate vein may be clamped and divided with impunity to gain access to life-threatening arterial bleeding beneath. The occasional anomalous origins of the innominate and the right subclavian must be borne in mind. If the injury

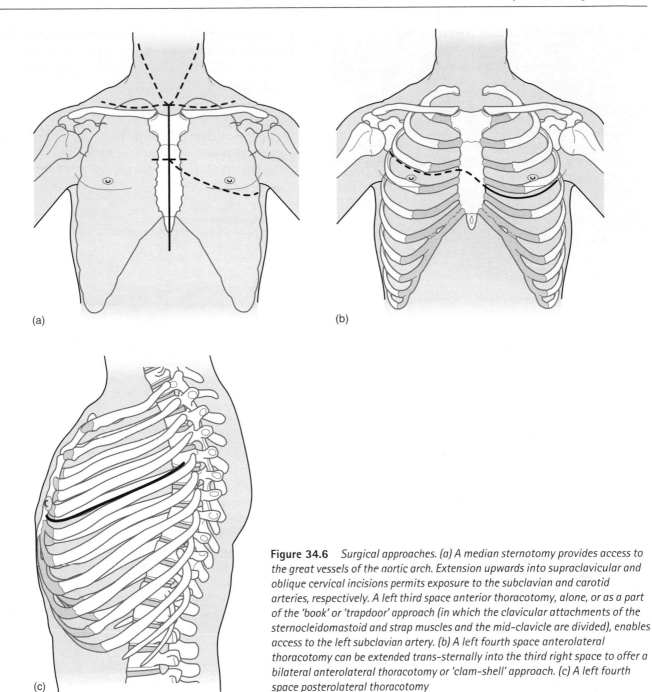

Figure 34.6 *Surgical approaches. (a) A median sternotomy provides access to the great vessels of the aortic arch. Extension upwards into supraclavicular and oblique cervical incisions permits exposure to the subclavian and carotid arteries, respectively. A left third space anterior thoracotomy, alone, or as a part of the 'book' or 'trapdoor' approach (in which the clavicular attachments of the sternocleidomastoid and strap muscles and the mid-clavicle are divided), enables access to the left subclavian artery. (b) A left fourth space anterolateral thoracotomy can be extended trans-sternally into the third right space to offer a bilateral anterolateral thoracotomy or 'clam-shell' approach. (c) A left fourth space posterolateral thoracotomy*

involves the innominate or left common carotid artery at the origin from the aortic arch, an aortic side-biting partially occluding clamp will control bleeding (Fig. 34.8a). Shunting should be instituted where necessary, contributing favourably in ensuring maximal cerebral perfusion in the hypotensive patient. This measure is of particular value in simultaneous injuries to the innominate and left common carotid arteries.

Except for small limited lacerations lateral suture is not easily achieved without tension because the ends retract and patch grafting is preferable. In practice, however, a Dacron softer knitted graft, either bridging the gap or as a

bypass, is required. An injury at the origin of the innominate artery is best dealt with by a 10 mm Dacron aorto-innominate bypass graft taken from a fresh aortotomy on the proximal ascending aorta (Fig. 34.8b); the injury site is closed by lateral suture reinforced with pledgets or by a woven Dacron patch. In order to restore flow to concurrently injured innominate and left common carotid arteries, a bifurcated Dacron graft is ideal (Fig. 34.8c), and from which a 'jump' graft may be taken to a subclavian artery if necessary. Complex tears demand the institution of CPB, induced hypothermic cardiac arrest and graft repair of the aorta.

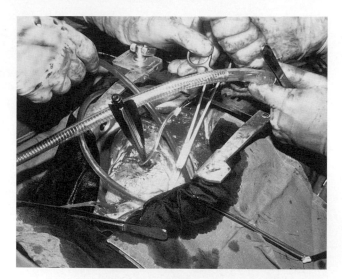

Figure 34.7 *A depressed young man managed to shoot himself in the chest with a crossbow and was admitted with the bolt still lodged in the centre of his sternum. The bolt had transfixed the right and left ventricles, the descending thoracic aorta and the ninth thoracic vertebra. Under full cardiopulmonary bypass, with cardioplegic arrest of the heart, the bolt was removed and the injuries repaired. Cardiac injuries of this nature, requiring cardiopulmonary bypass for repair, are relatively uncommon*

PULMONARY

In the presence of major bleeding from the pulmonary vessels the source of loss may be obscured. Control is achieved either by clamping the pulmonary vessels within the pericardium or by surrounding the hilum, initially manually, until a sloop and 'snugger' can be fashioned. Being a low pressure system the pulmonary vessels can be controlled by oversewing lung tissue. Lobectomy may be necessary to establish control of more centrally placed vascular trauma or of lung tissue obliterated by a shotgun blast or a disintegrated high velocity missile. In these circumstances, pneumonectomy may be the only available course, following which the chances of survival are significantly compromised.

VENA CAVAL SYSTEM

A trans-sternal extension of the anterolateral thoracotomy (see Fig. 34.6b) is necessary to deal with two potentially lethal and rather inaccessible injuries, namely, the posterior aspect of the intrapericardial inferior vena cava and the azygous vein.

CHEST WALL

While chest wall bleeding, particularly from intercostal or internal mammary arteries, may result in dramatic collapse, patients usually respond well to chest drainage and fluid resuscitation. Continued bleeding to a level exceeding 500 mL/hour is an indication for thoracotomy. Repair will usually mean suture ligation, removal of pleural thrombus and drainage. Evacuation of a haemothorax is often possible by minimally invasive thoracoscopy.

AORTIC ISTHMUS

The standard approach is a high left posterolateral thoracotomy, usually at the third or fourth space, and dividing the inferior rhomboids (see Fig. 34.6c). This permits unrestrained access to the aortic arch and subclavian artery for proximal control. It is important, in the heat of the moment, not to make the incision too low as that will limit access.

Findings

A large amount of blood may be lost into the pleural cavity though mostly it tends to form an extrapleural haematoma obscuring the aorta. Opening the pleura may result in free rupture and digital pressure is required until clamps can be applied.

Institution of bypass

Where a form of shunt or bypass is to be used, preparations should be in place before making the skin incision. For partial atriofemoral bypass (Fig. 34.9a), in which the femoral vessels are to be used, the groin should be prepared and the cannulae inserted before turning the patient onto the left lateral position. Access to the left atrium is usually via the atrial appendage or superior pulmonary vein. Alternatively, the inferior pulmonary vein may be cannulated, thereby avoiding opening the pericardium and leaving the cannula outside the operative field. After placement of a purse string, the cannula is inserted and connected to a centrifugal pump ensuring arterial return to the femoral artery. When a shunt, heparinised or heparin bonded, is to be used, purse strings are placed either in the aorta well proximal to the left subclavian or in the apex of the left ventricle (Fig. 34.9b).

Control

Control should precede aortic exploration. As the proximal aorta may be difficult to identify it is worth dissecting the left subclavian artery and following it to the aorta. The proximal clamp is usually placed proximal to and possibly including the subclavian artery. Alternatively, the subclavian can be controlled by clamping or by passing a sloop around it twice. Distal control is usually obtained with ease by clamping relatively normal aorta at the level of the diaphragm. When the level of tear is identified it may be possible to apply the clamp closer to it thereby reducing back-bleeding from intercostal vessels.

Dissection of a haematoma

Once clamps are placed the mediastinal pleura and the aortic adventitia are opened longitudinally and the rupture is exposed. The tear may not be immediately evident if it lies

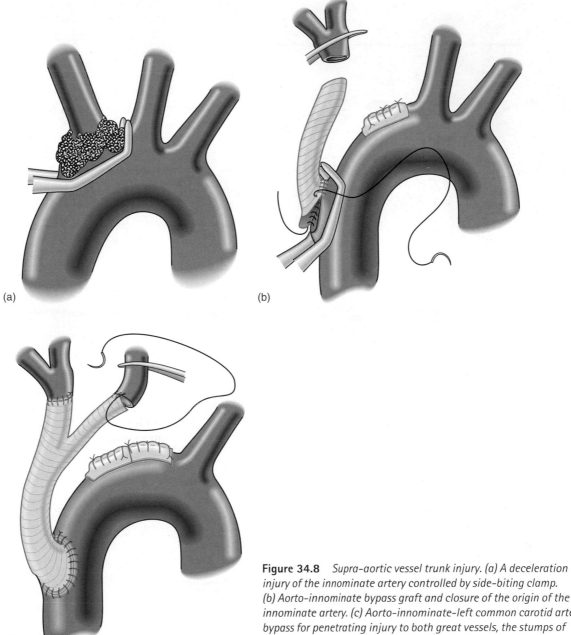

(a)

(b)

(c)

Figure 34.8 *Supra-aortic vessel trunk injury. (a) A deceleration injury of the innominate artery controlled by side-biting clamp. (b) Aorto-innominate bypass graft and closure of the origin of the innominate artery. (c) Aorto-innominate-left common carotid artery bypass for penetrating injury to both great vessels, the stumps of which have been closed*

in the posterior wall. The ends of the aorta will have retracted and apposition to facilitate direct suture may seem possible but it should not be attained at the cost of tension at the point of repair. In most cases an interposition woven Dacron tube graft will be necessary.

Graft and sewing techniques

For minor tears a monofilament non-absorbable suture, knotted on the outside, is commenced from each end of the tear. Before tying, the distal and proximal clamps are released in turn to evacuate air and thrombus. The site is packed while the anaesthetists restore haemodynamic stability and then reinspected for leaks which are oversewn. In

most instances a Dacron graft is necessary (Fig. 34.9c) and should be matched to the size to the aorta prior to crossclamping. A useful tip would be to measure the size of the aorta on the contrast enhanced CT scan and have a suitable graft available in theatre.

Issues of contention in surgery for acute thoracic aortic rupture

Paraplegia after repair of thoracic aortic rupture is a devastating complication and has significant medico-legal consequences. It is present prior to surgery in 2.6 per cent of cases, having been caused by direct spinal cord injury or by injury to the spinal arteries.[61] Although the actual mechanism of

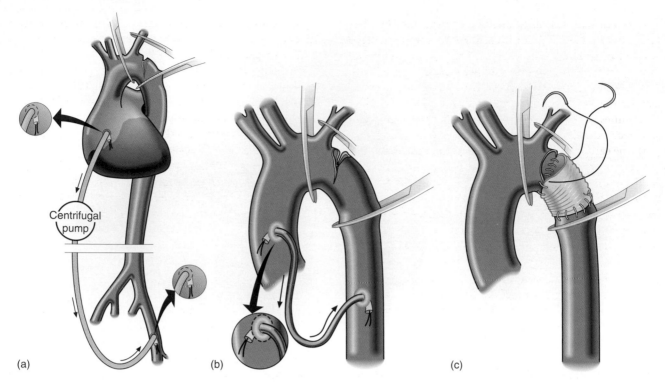

(a) (b) (c)

Figure 34.9 *Deceleration injury of the isthmus of the thoracic aorta. (a) Atriofemoral pump assisted bypass in place prior to aortic repair. (b) Ascending aorta to descending aorta shunt, which may be heparin bonded, preparatory to aortic repair. (c) Aortic 'clamp and repair' using Dacron graft*

postoperative paraplegia is not known it is related to clamp time and duration of ischaemia of the anterior spinal cord. Despite collateral supply, relative hypoperfusion of the distal descending thoracic aorta during the procedure is inevitable. Intercostal artery ligation during mobilisation of the aorta may also be a precipitating factor.

The blood supply to the anterior two-thirds of the spinal cord is from the anterior spinal artery. This vessel is usually well developed in the upper rather than in the lower thorax where it is small, the anterior cord being dependent on variable segmental branches of intercostal arteries. Between T12 and L4 vertebrae the small anterior segmental artery receives flow from the artery of Adamkiewicz, a sub-branch of the intercostals, and, in over 25 per cent of the population, essential to the blood supply of the cord.[62] Therefore, distal thoracic aortic hypotension during aortic cross-clamping may lead to hypoperfusion of the anterior spinal cord.

Amidst conflicting data, there does appear to be evidence, in uncontrolled retrospective studies, of a lower rate of paraplegia when distal circulatory support is available during repair of thoracic aortic rupture. The 'clamp and sew' technique, namely, simple aortic cross-clamping without attempts to perfuse the aorta distally (see Fig. 34.9c), has the advantages of simplicity and the avoidance of systemic heparinisation and its deleterious effects on other injuries. This approach, however, carries a consistent paraplegia rate of 16–20 per cent, compared with 4–6 per cent when some form of distal circulatory support is used,

though mortality rates are almost identical at approximately 15 per cent.[63–65] The risk of paraplegia does rise steeply with the 'clamp and sew' technique once aortic cross-clamp times exceed 30 minutes.[63,65]

Passive shunts, partial or full CPB may be employed to increase perfusion pressure in the descending thoracic aorta and also to prevent left ventricular distension during cross-clamping. Those techniques, however, are associated with several hazards: cardiac tamponade, ventricular fibrillation, atrial fibrillation and phrenic nerve injury,[66] all of which may follow placement of left atrial cannulae. Heparin bonded shunts (see Fig. 34.9c) may not protect against thromboembolism and cerebral infarction.[67] However, the degree of heparinisation required for bypass may exacerbate bleeding from other injuries. Misplacement of the distal end of a shunt with resultant paraplegia has also been reported.[68]

Currently, widespread variation in practice is explained by the lack of prospective randomised studies which are essential in making informed decisions.[69] The experience of major referral centres accepting 'self-selected' stable patients cannot be easily extended to local institutions to which patients may be admitted *in extremis* and where bypass equipment may not be available. In a number of series, including stable and unstable patients and where all techniques were used, the authors concluded that the outcome depended mainly on preoperative clinical status, associated injuries and the timing of surgery.[69,70]

A recent report detailed one case of paraplegia (1.4 per cent) after 71 cases of thoracic aortic rupture were managed without distal circulatory support.[71] In that institution an average of 9.4 cases were treated per year, compared with 2.3 cases in most other large centres, and the mean cross-clamp time was 24 minutes, with only four cases exceeding 30 minutes. It would seem, therefore, that the 'clamp and sew' technique is a safe option in expert hands, and supports the early transfer of stable patients to specialised units. It is the only viable option in those patients who develop frank rupture and are moribund; the likelihood of survival in these cases remains low at 0–6.2 per cent.[63,72] In another large series using the 'clamp and sew' technique no patients developed paraplegia when clamp time was less than 35 minutes; a low but significant paraplegia rate was observed on bypass. The conclusion drawn by the authors probably summarises the current best advice: first, paraplegia can be minimised by 'clamp and sew' where the repair appears straightforward, and second, that bypass should be used when prolonged cross-clamp time is anticipated.[64]

Distal aortic perfusion techniques

Considerable controversy remains regarding the optimal method of distal perfusion were it to be used. The techniques employed have ranged from passive shunts, to partial left heart bypass and to full CPB. The passive shunt most commonly used is the Gott shunt which is a heparin coated purpose designed shunt tapered at either end, although two standard CPB arterial cannulae joined by bypass tubing may be a satisfactory substitute. The shunt is usually inserted connecting the ascending aorta with the distal aorta (see Fig. 34.9b). Access to the former site is readily achieved by a generous posterolateral thoracotomy. Less commonly, the apex of the left ventricle is chosen as the proximal cannulation site. In the meta-analysis by von Oppell,[63] shunting from the ascending aorta was associated with a paraplegia rate of 8.2 per cent, whereas when the left ventricle was used it was 26.1 per cent. The high incidence for the latter technique may reflect the mean cross-clamp time of 40.6 minutes, none being less than 39 minutes. The technique of passive shunting was seldom employed in two recently published large series;[64,72] we feel, however, that it is still a useful technique in situations when systemic heparin has to be avoided in patients undergoing early repair of thoracic aortic rupture in the presence of injuries elsewhere.

Active support of the distal circulation ranges from left heart bypass, i.e. either left atrial to distal aorta or femoral artery using a centrifugal pump (see Fig. 34.9a) or femoral vein to femoral artery bypass without an oxygenator, both of which can be employed without systemic heparinisation, to CPB with full heparinisation. Although the incidence of paraplegia for full CPB is only 2.4–4.5 per cent, the mortality rate of 18.2–22.7 per cent is higher than usually reported[63,72] for all other techniques, and therefore its use in patients with pulmonary or intracranial injuries is unwise.[73] Recent large studies have shown that left heart bypass using a centrifugal pump has the lowest incidence of paraplegia at 0–2.9 per cent and a mortality rate of 11.9–14.5 per cent.[63,72,74]

Although for these reasons left heart bypass using a centrifugal pump is often recommended as the technique of choice,[75] the excellent results of the 'clamp and sew' technique in expert hands[71] and the use of full CPB by others[73] indicates that the best policy has yet to be determined. Nevertheless, the crucial aspects of acute management of thoracic aortic rupture are the institution of 'permissive hypotension' in those in whom the diagnosis is suspected and the transfer of stable patients to the nearest centre wherein appropriate surgical, anaesthetic and intensive care expertise resides.[73]

POSTOPERATIVE CARE

Rapid advances in anaesthesia, monitoring and pain relief have contributed to improved outcomes. In selected patients, i.e. those in whom head injury and intra-abdominal injury have been excluded, the current preferred method for pain control following severe thoracic trauma is epidural analgesia.[76]

The development of regional techniques of analgesia has revolutionised the management of blunt thoracic trauma. It has evolved from a policy of intubation and mechanical ventilation for all patients to one of optimising pain control combined with chest physiotherapy. Although many methods have been used, in carefully selected patients with severe thoracic trauma, epidural analgesia is the preferred technique for pain control.[76] Epidural catheters for continuous narcotic or local anaesthetic administration are both the most reliable and the most effective; once in place they can be easily managed by nurses outside the intensive care setting. Although the benefit in outcome using epidural analgesia has yet to be demonstrated objectively, the parameters of pulmonary function and subjective patient comfort have clearly improved.

RESULTS

The majority of treated thoracic vascular injuries have few long term sequelae but two specific complications of aortic trauma deserve specific mention. Late false aneurysm formation is often the result of untreated rupture caused by apparently trivial trauma, but it may also occur after successful surgical repair. A false aneurysm may come to light when it ruptures but in most cases it is a chance finding on chest X-ray taken for some other purpose. While small asymptomatic false aneurysms can be kept under observation, surgical repair is usually advisable, though endovascular approaches are likely to play an increasing role in management. The importance of follow-up is illustrated by the fact that false aneurysms occasionally develop into aorto-oesophageal or aortobronchial fistulae, the majority of which are fatal. Although definitive surgical repair of major thoracic vascular injuries is often successful, annual lifelong X-ray follow-up is mandatory.

Conclusions

Techniques continue to evolve in the diagnosis and treatment, surgical and endovascular, of major thoracic vascular injuries. Most of the newer modalities are applicable to the stable patient presenting with contained haemorrhage. Injuries presenting with free bleeding call for a 'scoop and run' approach to admission, minimal investigation and resuscitative surgery. Fluid resuscitation prior to surgical control of haemorrhage is counterproductive and increases morbidity in survivors. The stable patient with contained haemorrhage should be managed on a 'permissive hypotension' regimen until essential investigations are undertaken and after attending to other life-threatening injuries.

While CT and three-dimensional reconstruction is replacing aortography as the standard investigation, other modalities such as TOE and MRA are playing an increasingly important role. The aim is to bring a stable patient to surgery in a more controlled manner and to repair or graft the injured vessels, possibly with the aid of appropriate bypass to reduce the incidence of paraplegia, and to prevent renal failure or stroke. The urgency of the situation, however, may still demand a 'clamp and sew' approach.

Surgical repair represents just the commencement of management of patients with thoracic vascular injury. Having suffered major trauma they will generally require prolonged intensive care, months or years of rehabilitation and, given the risk of false aneurysm and fistula formation, follow-up for life.

Key references

Bickell WH, Wall MJ Jr, Pepe PE, *et al*. Immediate versus delayed fluid resuscitation for hypotensive patients with penetrating torso injuries. *N Engl J Med* 1994; **331**: 1105–9.

Fabian TC, Richardson JD, Croce MA. Prospective study of blunt aortic injury: multicenter trial of the American Association for the Surgery of Trauma. *J Trauma* 1997; **42**: 374–83.

Mattox KL. Approaches to trauma involving the major vessels of the thorax. *Surg Clin North Am* 1989; **69**: 77.

Saletta S, Lederman E, Fein S, *et al*. Transesophageal echocardiography for the initial evaluation of the widened mediastinum in trauma patients. *J Trauma* 1995; **39**: 137–41; discussion 141–2.

Symbas PN, Sherman AJ, Silver JM, *et al*. Traumatic rupture of the aorta: immediate or delayed repair? *Ann Surg* 2002; **235**: 796–802.

REFERENCES

1 Besson A, Saegesser F. *Color Atlas of Chest Trauma and Associated Injuries*. Oradell, 1983.
2 Gebhard F, Kelbel MW, Strecker W, *et al*. Chest trauma and its impact on the release of vasoactive mediators. *Shock* 1997; **7**: 313–17.
3 Trunkey DD. Current therapy of trauma. In: Trunkey DD, Lewis FR. (eds.) St Louis, MO: CV Mosby, 1984.
4 Rich NM, Spencer FC. *Vascular Trauma*. Philadelphia, PA: WB Saunders Co, 1978.
5 Reul GJJ, Beall ACJ, Jordan GL, Mattox KL. The early operative management of injuries to the great vessels. *Surgery* 1973; **74**: 862.
6 Marsh CL, Moore RC. Deceleration trauma. *Am J Surg* 1957; **93**: 623.
7 Mimasaka S, Yajima Y, Hashiyada M, *et al*. A case of aortic dissection caused by blunt chest trauma. *Forensic Sci Int* 2003; **132**: 5–8.
8 Straub A, Beierlein W, Kuttner A, *et al*. Isolated coronary artery rupture after blunt chest trauma. *Thorac Cardiovasc Surg* 2003; **51**: 97–8.
9 Chen MY, Regan JD, D'Amore MJ, *et al*. Role of angiography in the detection of aortic branch vessel injury after blunt thoracic trauma. *J Trauma* 2001; **51**: 1166–71; discussion 1172.
10 *Colour Atlas of Chest Trauma*. London: Wolfe Medical Publications, pp. 171–6.
11 Petre R, Chilcott M, Murith N, Panos A. Blunt injury to the supra-aortic arteries. *Br J Surg* 1997; **84**: 606–9.
12 Karmy-Jones R, DuBose R, King S. Traumatic rupture of the innominate artery. *Eur J Cardiothorac Surg* 2003; **23**: 782–7.
13 Khanna A, Drugas GT. Air gun pellet embolization to the right heart: case report and review of the literature. *J Trauma* 2003; **54**: 1239–41.
14 Mattox KL. Approaches to trauma involving the major vessels of the thorax. *Surg Clin North Am* 1989; **69**: 77.
15 Robbs JV, Barker LW. Subclavian and axillary artery injuries. *SA Med J* 1976; **51**: 227.
16 Meredith JW, Trunkey D. *Thoracic Gunshot Wounds in Management of Gunshot Wounds*. New York: Elsevier Science Publishing, 1988.
17 Bickell WH, Bruttig SP, Millnamow GA, *et al*. The detrimental effects of intravenous crystalloid after aortotomy in swine. *Surgery* 1991; **110**: 529–36.
18 Craig RL, Poole GV. Resuscitation in uncontrolled hemorrhage. *Am Surg* 1994; **60**: 59–62.
19 Sakles JC, Sena MJ, Knight DA, Davis JM. Effect of immediate fluid resuscitation on the rate, volume, and duration of pulmonary vascular hemorrhage in a sheep model of penetrating thoracic trauma. *Ann Emerg Med* 1997; **29**: 392–9.
20 Fabian TC, Davis KA, Gavant ML, *et al*. Prospective study of blunt aortic injury: helical CT is diagnostic and antihypertensive therapy reduces rupture. *Ann Surg* 1998; **227**: 666–76.
21 Kaweski SM, Sise MJ, Virgilio RW. The effect of prehospital fluids on survival in trauma patients. *J Trauma* 1990; **30**: 1215–18; discussion 1218–19.
22 Demling RH, Manohar M, Will JA. Response of the pulmonary microcirculation to fluid loading after hemorrhagic shock and resuscitation. *Surgery* 1980; **87**: 552–9.
23 Bickell WH, Barrett SM, Romine-Jenkins M, *et al*. Resuscitation of canine hemorrhagic hypotension with large-volume isotonic

crystalloid: impact on lung water, venous admixture, and systemic arterial oxygen saturation. *Am J Emerg Med* 1994; **12**: 36–42.

24 Bickell WH, Wall MJ Jr, Pepe PE, *et al.* Immediate versus delayed fluid resuscitation for hypotensive patients with penetrating torso injuries. *N Engl J Med* 1994; **331**: 1105–9.

25 Matsuoka T, Hildreth J, Wisner DH. Uncontrolled hemorrhage from parenchymal injury: is resuscitation helpful? *J Trauma* 1996; **40**: 915–21; discussion 921–2.

26 Jacobs LM. Timing of fluid resuscitation in trauma. *N Engl J Med* 1994; **331**: 1153–4.

27 Banerjee A, Jones R. Whither immediate fluid resuscitation? *Lancet* 1994; **344**: 1450–1.

28 Rady MY, Edwards JD, Nightingale P. Early cardiorespiratory findings after severe blunt thoracic trauma and their relation to outcome. *Br J Surg* 1992; **79**: 65–8.

29 Simon BJ, Leslie C. Factors predicting early in-hospital death in blunt thoracic aortic injury. *J Trauma* 2001; **51**: 906–10; discussion 911.

30 Eddy VA. Is routine arteriography mandatory for penetrating injury to zone 1 of the neck? Zone 1 Penetrating Injury Study Group. *J Trauma* 2000; **48**: 208–13.

31 Graham AN, McManus KG, McGuigan JA, McIlrath E. Traumatic rupture of the thoracic aorta. *Ann R Coll Surg Engl* 1995; **77**: 154–5.

32 Durham RM, Zuckerman D, Wolverson M. Computed tomography as a screening examination in patients with suspected blunt aortic injury. *Ann Surg* 1994; **220**: 699–704.

33 Agee CK. Computed tomographic evaluation to exclude traumatic aortic disruption. *J Trauma* 1992; **33**: 876–81.

34 Miller FB, Richardson JD, Thomas H. Role of CT in the diagnosis of major arterial injury after blunt thoracic trauma. *Surgery* 1989; **106**: 596–602.

35 Raptopoulos V, Sheiman RG, Phillips DA, *et al.* Traumatic aortic tear: screening with chest CT. *Radiology* 1992; **182**: 667–73.

36 Downing SW, Sperling JS, Mirvis SE, *et al.* Experience with spiral computed tomography as the sole diagnostic method for traumatic aortic rupture. *Ann Thorac Surg* 2001; **72**: 495–501; discussion 501–2.

37 Lick SD, Zwischenberger JB, Mileski WJ, Ahmad M. Torn ascending aorta missed by transoesophageal echocardiography. *Ann Thorac Surg* 1997; **63**: 1768–70.

38 Saletta S, Lederman E, Fein S, *et al.* Transesophageal echocardiography for the initial evaluation of the widened mediastinum in trauma patients. *J Trauma* 1995; **39**: 137–41; discussion 141–2.

39 Smith DC, Bansal RC. Transesophageal echocardiography in the diagnosis of traumatic rupture of the aorta. *N Engl J Med* 1995; **333**: 457–8.

40 Oxorn D, Towers M. Traumatic aortic disruption: false positive diagnosis in transoesophageal echocardiography. *J Trauma* 1995; **39**: 386–7.

41 Vignon P, Lagrange P, Boncoeur MP, *et al.* Routine transoesophageal echocardiography for the diagnosis of aortic disruption in trauma patients without enlarged mediastinum. *J Trauma* 1996; **40**: 422–7.

42 Mirvis SE, Shanmuganathan K. MR imaging of thoracic trauma. *Magn Reson Imaging Clin North Am* 2000; **8**: 91–104.

43 Richens D, Kotidis K, Neale M, *et al.* Rupture of the aorta following road traffic accidents in the United Kingdom 1992–1999. The results of the co-operative crash injury study. *Eur J Cardiothorac Surg* 2003; **23**: 143–8.

44 Borman KR, Aurbakken CM, Weigelt JA. Treatment priorities in combined blunt abdominal and aortic trauma. *Am J Surg* 1982; **144**: 728–32.

45 Pate JW, Fabian TC, Walker W. Traumatic rupture of the aortic isthmus: an emergency? *World J Surg* 1995; **19**: 119–25; discussion 125–6.

46 Pate JW. Is traumatic rupture of the aorta misunderstood? *Ann Thorac Surg* 1994; **57**: 530–1.

47 Turney SZ, Attar S, Ayella R, *et al.* Traumatic rupture of the aorta. A five-year experience. *J Thorac Cardiovasc Surg* 1976; **72**: 727–34.

48 Akins CW, Buckley MJ, Daggett W, *et al.* Acute traumatic disruption of the thoracic aorta: a ten-year experience. *Ann Thorac Surg* 1981; **31**: 305–9.

49 Symbas PN, Sherman AJ, Silver JM, *et al.* Traumatic rupture of the aorta: immediate or delayed repair? *Ann Surg* 2002; **235**: 796–802.

50 Kwon CC, Gill IS, Fallon WF, *et al.* Delayed operative intervention in the management of traumatic descending thoracic aortic rupture. *Ann Thorac Surg* 2002; **74**: S1892–8.

51 Maggisano R, Nathens A, Alexandrova NA, *et al.* Traumatic rupture of the thoracic aorta: should one always operate immediately? *Ann Vasc Surg* 1995; **9**: 44–52.

52 Ahn SH, Cutry A, Murphy TP, Slaiby JM. Traumatic thoracic aortic rupture: treatment with endovascular graft in the acute setting. *J Trauma* 2001; **50**: 949–51.

53 Lagattolla N, Matson M, Self G, *et al.* Traumatic rupture of the aortic arch treated by stent grafting. *Eur J Vasc Endovasc Surg* 1999; **17**: 84–6.

54 Semba CP, Mitchell RS, Miller DC, *et al.* Thoracic aortic aneurysm repair with endovascular stent-grafts. *Vasc Med* 1997; **2**: 98–103.

55 Orend KH, Kotsis T, Scharrer-Pamler R, *et al.* Endovascular repair of aortic rupture due to trauma and aneurysm. *Eur J Vasc Endovasc Surg.* 2002; **23**: 61–7.

56 Marty-Ane CH, Berthet JP, Branchereau P, *et al.* Endovascular repair for acute traumatic rupture of the thoracic aorta. *Ann Thorac Surg* 2003; **75**: 1803–7.

57 Lamme B, de Jonge IC, Reekers JA, *et al.* Endovascular treatment of thoracic aortic pathology: feasibility and mid-term results. *Eur J Vasc Endovasc Surg* 2003; **25**: 532–9.

58 Bell RE, Taylor PR, Aukett M, *et al.* Results of urgent and emergency thoracic procedures treated by endoluminal repair. *Eur J Vasc Endovasc Surg* 2003; **25**: 527–31.

59 Horike K, Fukata Y, Kanoh M, Kurushima A. Two cases of stent graft repair for thoracic aortic dissection: usefulness of three-dimensional computed tomogram. *Kyobu Geka* 2001; **54**: 573–6.

60 Greenberg R, Resch T, Nyman U, *et al.* Endovascular repair of descending thoracic aortic aneurysms: an early experience with intermediate-term follow-up. *J Vasc Surg* 2000; **31**: 147–56.

61 Sturm JT, Hines JT, Perry JF. Thoracic spinal fractures and aortic rupture: a significant and fatal association. *Ann Thorac Surg* 1990; **50**: 931–3.

62 Adams HD, Von Geertruyden HH. Neurologic complications of aortic surgery. *Ann Surg* 1956; **144**: 574.

63 von Oppell UO, Dunne TT, De Groot MK, Zilla P. Traumatic aortic rupture: twenty-year metaanalysis of mortality and risk of paraplegia. *Ann Thorac Surg* 1994; **58**: 585–93.

64 Hunt JP, Baker CC, Lentz CW, *et al.* Thoracic aorta injuries: management and outcome of 144 patients. *J Trauma* 1996; **40**: 547–55; discussion 555–6.

65 Katz NM, Blackstone EH, Kirklin JW, Karp RB. Incremental risk factors for spinal cord injury following operation for acute traumatic aortic transection. *J Thorac Cardiovasc Surg* 1981; **81**: 669–74.

66 Karmy-Jones R, Carter Y, Meissner M, Mulligan MS. Choice of venous cannulation for bypass during repair of traumatic rupture of the aorta. *Ann Thorac Surg* 2001; **71**: 39–41; discussion 41–2.

67 Duke BJ, Moore EE, Brega KE. Posterior circulation cerebral infarcts associated with repair of thoracic aortic disruption using partial left heart bypass. *J Trauma* 1997; **42**: 1135–9.

68 Verdant A, Mercier C, Page A, *et al.* Major mediastinal vascular injuries. *Can J Surg* 1983; **26**: 38–42.

69 Tatou E, Steinmetz E, Jazayeri S, *et al.* Surgical outcome of traumatic rupture of the thoracic aorta. *Ann Thorac Surg* 2000; **69**: 70–3.

70 DelRossi AJ, Cernaianu AC, Madden LD, *et al.* Traumatic disruptions of the thoracic aorta: treatment and outcome. *Surgery* 1990; **108**: 864–70.

71 Sweeney MS, Young DJ, Frazier OH, *et al.* Traumatic aortic transections: eight-year experience with the 'clamp-sew' technique. *Ann Thorac Surg* 1997; **64**: 384–9.

72 Fabian TC, Richardson JD, Croce MA. Prospective study of blunt aortic injury: multicenter trial of the American Association for the Surgery of Trauma. *J Trauma* 1997; **42**: 374–83.

73 Pate JW. Modern management of traumatic rupture of the aortic isthmus. *Ann Thorac Surg* 1998; **66**: 611–12.

74 Read RA, Moore EE, Moore FA, Haenel RRT. Partial left heart bypass for thoracic aortic repair: survival without paraplegia. *Arch Surg* 1993; **128**: 747–52.

75 Von Oppell UO, Brink J, Hewitson J, *et al.* Acute traumatic rupture of the thoracic aorta. A comparison of techniques. *S Afr J Surg* 1996; **34**: 19–24.

76 Ferguson M, Luchette FA. Management of blunt chest injury. *Respir Care Clin North Am* 1996; **2**: 449–66.

35

Vascular Injuries of the Neck

S RAM KUMAR, FRED A WEAVER

THE PROBLEM

Injury to major vascular structures of the head and neck complicates 25 per cent of cervical injuries. Carotid artery (CA) injuries constitute 5–10 per cent of all arterial injuries, while injuries to the vertebral artery (VA), once thought to be uncommon, account for 30 per cent of all cervical vascular injuries.[1] Penetrating trauma is the leading cause of cervical vascular injury, with less than 10 per cent of injuries following blunt trauma.[2] Despite significant advances in the diagnosis and management of these injuries, mortality remains at 10–30 per cent, and the incidence of permanent neurological deficit approximates 40 per cent.[3–5]

HISTORICAL PERSPECTIVE

Ambroise Paré successfully treated a CA injury by ligation in 1522.[6] Ligation, which resulted in high rates of hemiplegia and death, remained the only mode of management until the twentieth century. The application of techniques of primary arterial repair, first employed during the Korean conflict, to civilian carotid injuries, resulted in significant reductions in neurological injury and mortality. However, following a report by Wylie et al.[7] of intracranial haemorrhage after carotid revascularisation for acute thrombotic stroke, Cohen questioned the wisdom of carotid repair in the neurologically compromised patient.[8] He warned that reconstruction in the presence of a severe neurological deficit could result in a significant incidence of haemorrhagic infarction and death. Bradley's subsequent autopsy report in 1973, detailing haemorrhagic

infarction following CA repair in two neurologically compromised patients supported Cohen's admonition.[9] Ligation was hence considered the procedure of choice in patients who presented with 'significant' neurological deficits. More recent reports, however, of individual and collective experience with CA repairs in the neurologically compromised patient have not demonstrated a significant incidence of intracranial haemorrhage.[3,10] Consequently, contemporary vascular surgical practice dictates repair of CA injuries, regardless of neurological findings.

Until recently, VA injuries were considered uncommon, and usually only recognised at autopsy. This led to the mistaken conclusion by Matas that isolated VA injuries were lethal.[11] Few VA injuries were reported during the world wars or during the Korean and Vietnam conflicts. With the increased use of diagnostic angiography in the management of cervical trauma, however, VA injuries have been increasingly recognised. As with CA injuries, ligation, first reported in 1852 by Maisonneuve,[12] was the only mode of therapy for VA injuries until the second half of the twentieth century. In 1974, Serbinenko reported the use of percutaneous endovascular techniques to manage VA injuries.[13] Endovascular management has now replaced surgical intervention as the treatment of choice for most VA injuries.

MECHANISM OF INJURY

Penetrating cervical vascular injuries result from high velocity projectiles which injure vessels directly in their path (Fig. 35.1), or indirectly, by concussive forces or secondary missiles such as bone fragments. Injuries from low velocity penetrating injuries such as stab wounds are generally confined to the path of penetration.

Mechanisms of injury

- Penetrating
  - Knives
  - Bullets
  - Shrapnel
- Blunt
  - Direct: blow to neck/Skull base fracture – CA
    cervical spine fracture – VA
  - Indirect: hyperextension/rotation of neck – CA
    lateral flexion/rotation of neck – VA

Blunt injuries result from direct blows to the vessel or by bony fragments from basilar or spinal fractures. Biffl *et al.*[14] reported that 39 per cent of blunt VA injuries were associated with a cervical spine fracture the presence of which was an independent clinical predictor of a VA injury. Significant injury may also be caused by seemingly inconsequential cervical hyperextension and rotation. Excessive neck extension or flexion stretches the CA over the transverse process of the second cervical vertebra, which may produce an intimal crack or a mural contusion, typically in the distal internal carotid artery (ICA). The VA is more likely to be injured by bending and axial rotation of the cervical spine than by cervical flexion or extension. The seemingly innocuous activities of chiropractic neck manipulation and roller coaster riding, where axial rotation and lateral bending may be accentuated, have been reported to cause VA injuries.

PENETRATING CAROTID INJURIES

Diagnosis

Carotid artery injuries are classified into one of three anatomical zones (Fig. 35.2):

- I – injuries from the clavicle to the cricoid cartilage
- II – injuries between the cricoid and angle of mandible
- III – injuries above the angle of mandible

A cervical bruit or thrill, a rapidly expanding cervical haematoma and an absent CA pulse are pathognomonic signs of a CA injury (Fig. 35.3). Additional soft signs include a pulse deficit in the superficial temporal artery, signs of air embolism, active bleeding from an oropharyngeal or neck wound, widened mediastinum, ipsilateral Horner's syndrome, or dysfunction of cranial nerves IX–XII. Contralateral neurological deficits may be present, but obscured by associated head injuries, systemic hypotension or the patient's use of psychoactive substances.

The zone or location of the presumed CA injury dictates the diagnostic work-up (Fig. 35.3). For zone II injuries, both primary neck exploration and screening angiography have a low positive yield.[15] Consequently, many surgeons

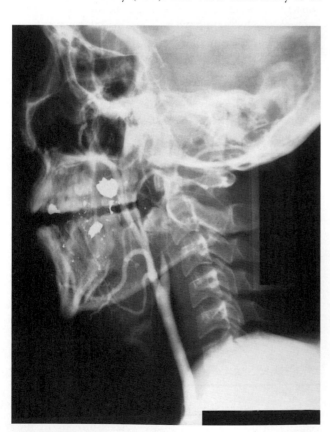

Figure 35.1 *Gunshot wound to the neck causing internal carotid artery occlusion*

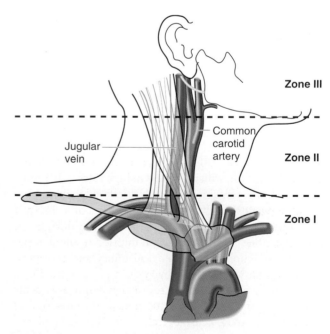

Figure 35.2 *Anatomical landmarks for carotid injuries by zone (redrawn with permission from Donovan A (ed). Trauma Surgery: Techniques in Thoracic, Abdominal and Vascular Surgery. St Louis, MO: Mosby, 1994)*

have increasingly employed duplex scanning as the initial screening assessment. Several studies have documented the accuracy of duplex sonography in the diagnosis and follow-up of cervical vascular injuries when performed by a trained technologist (Table 35.1). Longitudinal and transverse grey scale and colour flow images have been shown to correlate well with angiographic findings in over 90 per cent of injuries. Doppler waveform analysis can reveal turbulent or high resistance flow suggestive of an upstream lesion in the non-visualised distal ICA. It should be emphasised that the accuracy of a duplex evaluation and interpretation relies heavily on a skilled technologist and an experienced reader. If such resources are not available, angiography should be liberally employed despite the small yield.

In contrast to the zone II injury, clinical evaluation and duplex scanning are inadequate for screening zones I

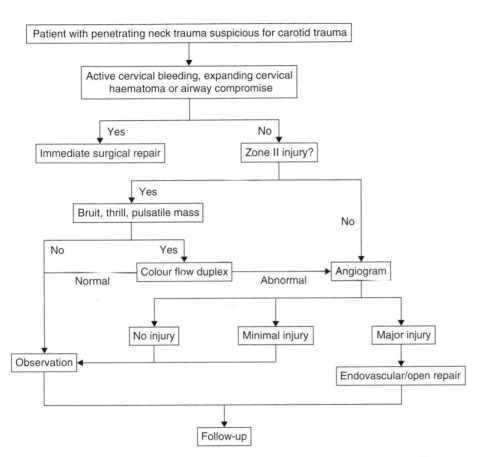

Figure 35.3 *Algorithmic approach to the diagnosis and management of penetrating carotid trauma (redrawn with permission from Kumar SR, Weaver FA, Yellin AE. Cervical vascular injuries – carotid and jugular venous injuries.* Surg Clin North Am *2001; 81: 1331–44, xii–xiii)*

Table 35.1 *Clinical trials evaluating the role of duplex examination in the diagnosis of carotid trauma*

Authors	Year	Findings	Conclusion
Kuzniec et al.[17]	1998	91 per cent sensitive; 100 per cent specific; 96 per cent accurate	Reproduces results of angiography
Ginzburg et al.[18]	1996	100 per cent sensitive; 85 per cent specific	Primary investigation of choice, patient-friendly, cheap
Fry et al.[16]	1994	100 per cent accuracy	As effective as angiography, procedure of choice
Cogbill et al.[19]	1994	86 per cent accuracy	Potential role in diagnosis and follow-up
Bynoe et al.[20]	1991	95 per cent sensitive; 99 per cent specific; 98 per cent accurate	Cost effective, reliable method of diagnosis
Meissner et al.[21]	1991	100 per cent accuracy	Rapid, effective screening tool
Greenwold et al.[22]	1991	94 per cent sensitive; 99 per cent specific; 99 per cent accurate	Accurate screening tool

Reproduced with permission from Kumar SR, Weaver FA, Yellin AE. Cervical vascular injuries – carotid and jugular venous injuries. *Surg Clin North Am* 2001; **81**: 1331–44, xii–xiii.

and III CA injuries. Angiography is mandatory for injuries suspected in these zones (see Fig. 35.3) since bony structures such as the clavicle or mandible obstruct carotid insonation during a duplex evaluation. In addition, knowledge of the anatomy of the vascular tree is essential in planning the surgical approach to these injuries. Angiography also allows for endovascular management of injuries that are not surgically approachable and has the added benefit of detecting unsuspected vertebral, aortic arch, great vessel or contralateral CA injuries.

Brain computed tomography (CT) scans are routinely obtained in patients with high velocity penetrating neck injuries to evaluate associated head trauma, bony injuries and the state of the brain parenchyma. The presence of significant parenchymal ischaemic injury soon after an occlusive CA injury indicates a poor neurological outcome, regardless of therapeutic intervention. The technological advance of helical CT scanning/angiography allows for high resolution information concerning parenchymal injury with the added option of reconstructing an in-continuity image of the cervical vascular tree.[23]

Management

All injuries associated with pulsatile haemorrhage or an expanding cervical haematoma with or without airway compromise mandate immediate surgical attention (see Fig. 35.3). In contrast, low velocity penetrating injuries of the CA may result in angiographically non-occlusive 'minimal injuries', such as small intimal defects, pseudoaneurysms less than 5 mm in size or adherent, or downstream, non-obstructive intimal flaps. A high percentage of these injuries heal without surgical intervention,[24] nevertheless, vessel healing should be documented by follow-up duplex scans or angiography. Patients with a CA occlusion on angiography and a dense neurological deficit due to a large brain infarct on CT scan have a poor outcome regardless of treatment,[4] whereas an occlusive ICA injury in a patient with a normal neurological examination can be managed solely by anticoagulation and avoidance of hypotension. Anticoagulation should be subsequently continued for a minimum of 3 months to prevent thrombus propagation. High zone III injuries, not surgically accessible may best be managed by endovascular means. All other angiographically documented CA injuries require operative repair regardless of neurological status.

SURGICAL THERAPY

Zone II injuries are exposed by a neck incision overlying and parallel to the anterior border of the sternocleidomastoid muscle. Zone I injuries frequently require a median sternotomy for access to the more proximal portions of the common carotid artery (CCA) or to deal with concomitant arch injuries. Zone III injuries may require division of the digastric muscle to provide exposure of the distal ICA. Access to the artery above the digastric may also be facilitated by anterior subluxation of the mandible, which is accomplished by using archbars to fix the mandible in a subluxed position (Fig. 35.4). This converts a narrow triangular space between the skull and the mandibular ramus into a

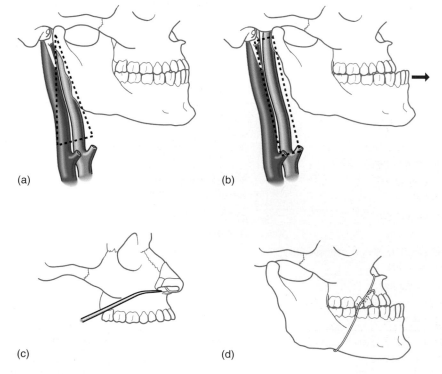

(a)   (b)

(c)   (d)

Figure 35.4   *Technique for gaining access to the distal internal carotid artery (redrawn with permission from Donovan A (ed).* Trauma Surgery: Techniques in Thoracic, Abdominal and Vascular Surgery. *St Louis, MO: Mosby, 1994)*

wider, more rectangular opening, providing exposure to the CA up to the base of the skull. Osteotomy of the angle of mandible, instead of mandibular subluxation, is an alternative method of achieving additional distal exposure.

Vascular control is achieved in the usual fashion before exposing the injury. When encountering a very distal ICA injury, a vascular balloon catheter or a balloon catheter shunt (Inahara–Pruitt) can be used for control by inserting the catheter into the vessel either through the injury itself, or through a proximal arteriotomy. Once control is established, an intraluminal shunt accompanied by anticoagulation is used to maintain antegrade flow for ICA repairs. Routine use of an intravascular shunt instantly improves and maintains ICA cerebral perfusion. If an interposition graft is necessary, the shunt is passed through the lumen of the graft prior to anastomosis to the native artery. The graft is then sewn in place and the shunt removed before placement of the last few sutures. In contrast to injuries of the ICA, and those of the CCA proximal to the bifurcation, a shunt is not mandatory as cross-filling via the external carotid artery (ECA) and circle of Willis is sufficient to maintain cerebral perfusion.

Routine techniques of surgical repair such as lateral arteriorrhaphy, patch graft or excision of the injured area with end-to-end or interposition graft repair are used to manage CA injuries. Autogenous grafts are preferred for zone II and III injuries, while prosthetic grafts are used for zone I CCA injuries. Injuries to the carotid bulb or proximal ICA may be reconstructed with an interposition graft, or alternatively, the distal ICA may be transposed to the proximal stump of the ECA (Fig. 35.5) following distal ECA ligation. Ligation of the ICA is recommended only when the distal vessel has thrombosed and patency cannot be restored or if the injury is so distal and extensive that it is not reconstructible. If ICA ligation is necessary, anticoagulation is continued for at least 3 months to prevent propagation of thrombus. As the ECA is an important collateral for cerebral flow, every effort should be made to repair the isolated simple injury, but ligation is the prudent course when the injury is complex. For all CA repairs, routine completion angiography or duplex examination is mandatory to confirm a technically perfect repair and to assess the distal arterial tree for unsuspected injury or thrombus.

In the presence of associated aerodigestive tract injury or repair, the vascular repair should be protected from saliva and bacterial contamination by the interposition of soft tissue. This can be achieved by rotating the belly of the sternocleidomastoid muscle after having divided it at its mastoid insertion. In the patient with compromised airway, early endotracheal intubation is preferred to tracheostomy, as the latter increases the incidence of contamination of the vascular repair. Aerodigestive tract injury is a relative contraindication to the insertion of prosthetic material. When extensive soft tissue injury hinders cover of an arterial repair, consideration should be given to primary ligation.

ENDOVASCULAR THERAPY

The ability to treat CA injuries at the time of angiography has improved with advances in catheter-based technology. Endovascular delivery of detachable coils, balloons or foam can be used to obliterate a traumatic carotid-cavernous fistula or a false aneurysm in a surgically inaccessible distal ICA segment.[25] If endovascular obliteration is contemplated, the patient's neurological status must be monitored after a temporary test occlusion. If a contralateral deficit develops, a bypass to the middle cerebral artery (CCA-MCA) may be required prior to obliteration. Covered stents have been deployed successfully in treating traumatic false aneurysms of the distal ICA.[26]

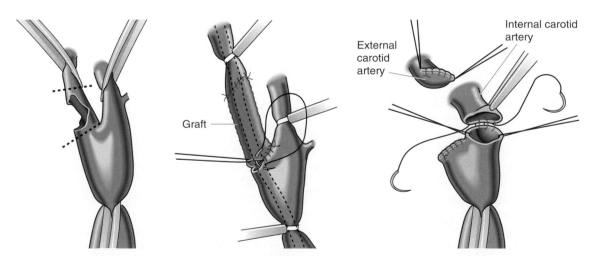

Figure 35.5 *(a) An injury of the proximal internal carotid artery (b) repaired by an interposition graft or (c) external carotid artery transposition (redrawn with permission from Donovan A (ed).* Trauma Surgery: Techniques in Thoracic, Abdominal and Vascular Surgery. *St Louis, MO: Mosby, 1994)*

Table 35.2 *Studies evaluating outcome following surgery for carotid trauma*

Author	Year	Management	Neurological deficit (per cent)		Mortality (per cent)
			At presentation	At discharge	
Mittal et al.[5]	2000	89 per cent repair; 11 per cent ligation	0	0	17
Kuehne et al.[4]	1996	48 per cent repair; 8 per cent ligation; 44 per cent observation	24	12	4
Weaver et al.[3]	1988	68 per cent repair; 11 per cent ligation; 21 per cent observation	34	23	6
Robbs et al.[27]	1983	63 per cent repair; 37 per cent ligation	25	11	7
Brown et al.[10]	1982	80 per cent repair; 17 per cent ligation; 3 per cent observation	27	20	8

Results

Repairs of CA injuries as described result in significant improvement in absolute and relative neurological outcomes.[3] Even in the patient with a neurological deficit, restoration of cerebral perfusion can reverse the electrical failure surrounding the zone of irreversible cerebral injury (see Chapter 5), and result in dramatic neurological improvement. In a retrospective review of 85 CA injuries, we have shown that operative management regardless of initial deficit improves mortality and ultimate neurological status. Several other studies have corroborated these findings (Table 35.2).

BLUNT CAROTID INJURIES

Diagnosis

Blunt CA injuries can pose a significant diagnostic challenge. The severity of trauma causing the carotid artery to fracture may not be evident on physical examination. Furthermore, a specific history or pattern of injury indicative of CA injury cannot be elicited in the majority of injuries. Consequently, a blunt CA injury may be missed in up to two-thirds of patients.

Although a few patients with blunt CA injury may report loss of consciousness or present with abrupt focal neurological deficit at time of injury, in the majority no immediate neurological symptoms are recorded. The classic history of loss of consciousness with a 'lucid interval' of hours to days between the injury and the appearance of lateralising neurological symptoms occurs infrequently. Other less common signs and symptoms include a 'buzzing' sound in the ear, a cervical bruit, Horner's syndrome, neck contusion or haematoma. Mandibular fracture is the most frequently associated injury[28] and occasionally skull fractures are seen.

Although angiography remains the standard diagnostic test, duplex scanning is being used increasingly as a screening tool in patients with blunt neck trauma. Although the accuracy of a duplex scan has not been evaluated prospectively, experience is accruing with its application in this clinical setting. In a multi-institutional study of 60 blunt CA injuries duplex scanning accurately demonstrated 12 out of the 14 injuries studied.[29] Other diagnostic modalities include the use of helical CT scans to define zone III blunt CA injuries and gadolinium enhanced magnetic resonance angiography (MRA) to rapidly image the carotid and vertebral arteries from the aortic arch to the circle of Willis.[30] Until prospective studies evaluating non-invasive methods of diagnosis for blunt CA trauma become available, the demonstrated accuracy and universal availability of angiography make it the primary investigative modality.

Conventional CT scans of the brain parenchyma are helpful in assessing the presence and extent of parenchymal injury, bony spine injury, concomitant intracranial haematomas,[29] cerebral oedema, or cranial vault injuries. A neurological deficit unexplained by CT of the brain raises the suspicion of a CA injury and is an indication for angiography.

Management

Maintenance of haemodynamic stability is critical when a blunt CA injury is suspected. Hypotension promotes thrombus formation and propagation, while hypertension facilitates extension of the intimal dissection when present. The rare, short, symptomatic zone II dissection confined to the cervical CA should be repaired surgically. However, most blunt CA injuries result in intimal disruption with dissection and/or thrombosis involving long segments of the CA (Fig. 35.6). Consequently, systemic anticoagulation, which limits thrombus propagation and distal embolisation, is the preferred treatment for the vast majority of injuries. Heparin therapy is highly efficacious and is associated independently with improved survival and better neurological outcomes.[31] When instituted before the onset of symptoms, heparin therapy can pre-empt

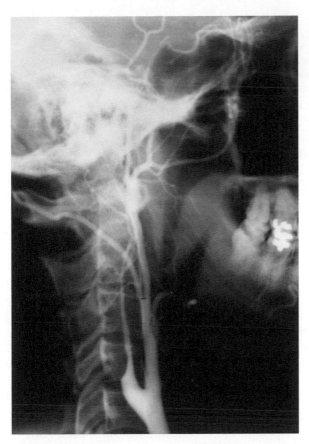

Figure 35.6 *Carotid angiogram demonstrating long segment dissection of the internal carotid artery following blunt trauma*

neurological deterioration.[31] Anticoagulation with warfarin should then be continued for a period of at least 3 months.[32]

Endovascular therapy is being used more frequently for blunt CA injuries, especially in the subgroup of patients with contraindications to anticoagulation. The primary goal of endovascular therapy for CA dissection is restoration of the true lumen and distal blood flow. Stents and stent-grafts have been used successfully to tack down separated layers and obliterate the false lumen in extracranial CA dissections.[25]

Results

The outcome of a blunt CA injury depends primarily on the presence or absence of an initial neurological deficit. A high index of suspicion leading to early diagnosis facilitates early anticoagulation and is associated with improved neurological outcomes.[32] With conservative management, most arteries demonstrate uncomplicated healing in 3 months. Pseudoaneurysms develop in 20–30 per cent of patients treated with anticoagulation, emphasising the need for careful follow-up and sequential imaging studies. When false aneurysms occur, they can often be managed by endovascular means.

VERTEBRAL ARTERY INJURIES

Diagnosis

The majority of VA injuries are clinically silent. Neurological signs following VA trauma are rare because of the collateral flow afforded by the contralateral VA and the circle of Willis. In a series of 25 VA injuries, Blickenstaff *et al.*[33] reported only two (8 per cent) patients with neurological symptoms of vertebrobasilar origin. Other non-neurological findings, such as external haemorrhage, bruits and expanding or stable neck haematomas are found in 10–30 per cent of VA injuries.[1,33] The remaining majority of injuries are an unsuspected additional finding on cerebral angiography performed principally to evaluate the carotid and brachiocephalic vessels.

In the asymptomatic patient, the possibility of a VA injury should be suspected if the trajectory of a penetrating injury crosses the VA or if cervical spine fractures are present (Fig. 35.7).[34] Some authors advocate angiographic evaluation of all patients with blunt cervical spine fractures.[14] Cerebral angiography continues to be the gold standard for the diagnosis, although it may be inaccurate in characterising the true extent of the lesion.[35] Although duplex scanning has been recommended for evaluating the vertebral arterial system, only the first part of the VA is accessible to insonation because the remainder of the artery is encased within the cervical spine and cranium. Computed tomographic scans provide additional information concerning the cervical spine and can be coupled with intravenous contrast enhancement and helical CT technology to detect VA lesions. Gadolinium enhanced MRA permits simultaneous evaluation of the cervical spine and brain parenchyma, but several anatomical factors including inherent arterial asymmetry and flow related venous enhancement limit its accuracy.[36] Furthermore, the use of MR imaging is incompatible with the presence of orthopaedic fixation equipment or residual metallic debris from the offending injury.

Management

The VA contributes less than 10 per cent of total cerebral blood flow and is anatomically unique in that the VAs join to form a single basilar artery. Consequently, a traumatic unilateral VA occlusion is well tolerated except when the contralateral VA is atretic, hypoplastic or absent, which occurs in about 3.1 per cent of left and 1.8 per cent of right VAs (Fig. 35.7). The unique anatomy of the VA permits traumatic occlusion as a situation which, in most cases, does not demand treatment. Non-occlusive 'minimal' injuries such as intimal tears or pseudoaneurysms of less than 5 cm[1,24] can be simply observed.

Intervention is indicated in the following VA injuries: those associated with external haemorrhage and/or an

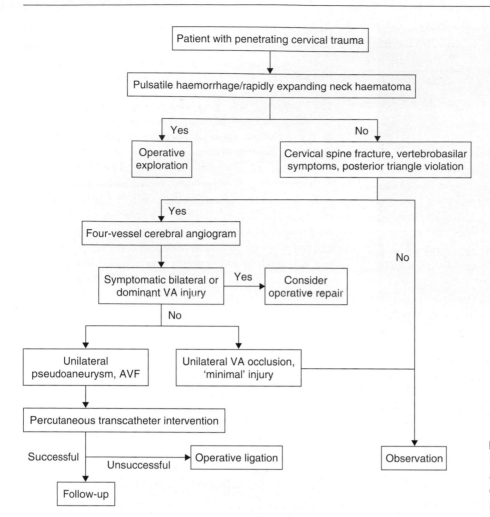

Figure 35.7 *Algorithm outlining the approach to the diagnosis and management of suspected vertebral artery (VA) injury. AVF, arteriovenous fistulae*

expanding haematoma, an angiographically documented high flow arteriovenous fistula or a false aneurysm greater than 5 mm. With the exception of the proximal VA prior to its entrance into the bony cervical canal, exposure of the remainder of the vessel is complicated and potentially hazardous. The technical difficulties associated with operative exploration of the VA and the capability of endovascular methods in managing injuries percutaneously at the time of diagnostic angiography, render catheter-based interventions preferable. The advantages of endovascular interventions are so significant that it is wise, when exploring the neck for other injuries, to leave a stable, known VA injury undisturbed, to be managed by endovascular means in the postoperative period.[33]

Percutaneous transcatheter embolisation with coils or balloons provides adequate proximal and distal control and is sufficient for the treatment of most pseudoaneurysms, arteriovenous fistulae or expanding cervical haematomas. On occasion, occlusion distal to the injury may necessitate a retrograde approach via the contralateral VA. Even when larger pseudoaneurysms or high flow fistulae cannot be completely occluded by embolisation alone, this technique does facilitate subsequent formal VA ligation.[33] Prior to percutaneous embolisation of an injured

VA, it is necessary to demonstrate angiographically that the contralateral VA is of normal calibre and uninjured. Therapeutic anticoagulation following embolisation should be used to limit propagation of distal thrombus.

Although percutaneous endovascular management of VA injuries is possible in most patients, there are limitations. The small calibre of the VA makes the use of stents or covered stents for traumatic pseudoaneurysms difficult.[37] Further, extensive damage to the lumen of the VA following high velocity penetrating injuries can make identification of the true lumen prior to endovascular manipulation challenging.[26] Occasionally, distal VA injuries are situated at branch points making embolisation less attractive. For instance, the need to sacrifice the posterior inferior cerebellar artery in order to control an injury may result in Horner's syndrome.[38]

On rare occasions, patients with acute haemorrhage following VA injury, possibly transection confirmed on angiography, will require emergency surgical exploration (see Fig. 35.7). Simple ligation is the preferred treatment in these instances. In the largest reported series of VA injuries,[35] 41 of 43 arteries were ligated without any neurological sequelae. Both proximal and distal ligation is usually required to arrest haemorrhage effectively.[35] Primary repair of the VA is almost never necessary, and given the technical impediments, could be potentially harmful. Although vertebral revascularisation is sometimes undertaken in patients with non-traumatic vertebrobasilar insufficiency, there are no specific reports of successful surgical repair of a VA injury. Nevertheless, repair may be necessary in the rare patient with posterior circulation neurological deficit and bilateral traumatic VA occlusion or occlusion of a dominant VA. For lesions proximal to the bony canal direct repair may be possible; in most instances however, and particularly in more distal injuries, bypass of the injured segment with interval ligation will be necessary. This requires familiarity with the reconstructive techniques described in respect of the VA.[39,40]

The management of blunt vertebral injuries is less well defined. In a recent, non-randomised study of blunt VA trauma, Biffl et al.[14] found that systemic heparinisation resulted in improved neurological outcomes in 50 per cent of patients in comparison with 20 per cent of the non-treated group. Their results however, did not reach statistical significance. Despite their recommendation for lower target anticoagulation, bleeding in this population continues to be of significant risk, with two haemorrhagic strokes among heparinised patients in their study. Anecdotal reports have also described successful tacking of the dissected layers of VA intima with covered stents.[37]

Results

In a series of 25 penetrating VA injuries, Blickenstaff et al.[33] reported only two (8 per cent) VA associated neurological deficits and no mortality. Demetriades et al.[1] reported a single death due to an isolated VA injury (4.5 per cent), and no neurological sequelae attributable to VA trauma. They also observed angiographic evidence of healing at follow-up 1 month after an intimal VA tear; several other studies have also reported spontaneous healing of most small injuries. In contrast, Biffl et al.[14] reported a death rate of 8 per cent and a 20 per cent incidence of neurological deficit in patients who had sustained a blunt VA injury.

Conclusions

The diagnosis of cervical vascular injuries has evolved considerably over the past two decades. Prompt recognition, timely diagnostic evaluation and a tailoring of surgical and endovascular interventions to the specific vascular injury is the key to minimising adverse events and neurological injury. Further improvement in outcomes will require a concerted multidisciplinary effort by surgeons and interventional radiologists and the appropriate application of evolving endovascular techniques.

Key references

Cogbill TH, Moore EE, Meissner M, et al. The spectrum of blunt injury to the carotid artery: a multicenter perspective. J Trauma 1994; **37**: 473–9.

Fry WR, Dort JA, Smith RS, et al. Duplex scanning replaces arteriography and operative exploration in the diagnosis of potential cervical vascular injury. Am J Surg 1994; **168**: 693–5.

Kuehne JP, Weaver FA, Papanicolaou G, Yellin AE. Penetrating trauma of the internal carotid artery. Arch Surg 1996; **131**: 942–7.

Stain SC, Yellin AE, Weaver FA, Pentecost MJ. Selective management of non-occlusive arterial injuries. Arch Surg 1989; **124**: 1136–40.

Weaver FA, Yellin AE, Wagner WH, et al. The role of arterial reconstruction in penetrating carotid injuries. Arch Surg 1988; **123**: 1106–11.

REFERENCES

1 Demetriades D, Theodorou D, Asensio J, et al. Management options in vertebral artery injuries. Br J Surg 1996; **83**: 83–6.

2 Martin RF, Eldrup-Jorgensen J, Clark DE, Bredenberg CE. Blunt trauma to the carotid arteries. J Vasc Surg 1991; **14**: 789–95.

3 Weaver FA, Yellin AE, Wagner WH, et al. The role of arterial reconstruction in penetrating carotid injuries. Arch Surg 1988; **123**: 1106–11.

4 Kuehne JP, Weaver FA, Papanicolaou G, Yellin AE. Penetrating trauma of the internal carotid artery. Arch Surg 1996; **131**: 942–7.

5 Mittal VK, Paulson TJ, Colaiuta E, et al. Carotid artery injuries and their management. J Cardiovasc Surg (Torino) 2000; **41**: 423–31.

6 Watson WL, Silverstone SM. Ligature of common carotid artery in cancer of the head and neck. Ann Surg 1939; **109**: 1.

7 Wylie EJ, Hein MF, Adams JE. Intracranial hemorrhage following surgical revascularization for treatment of acute strokes. J Neurosurg 1964; **21**: 212–15.

8 Cohen A, Brief D, Mathewson C Jr. Carotid artery injuries. Am J Surg 1970; **120**: 210–14.

9 Bradley EL III. Management of penetrating carotid injuries: an alternative approach. J Trauma 1973; **13**: 248–55.

10 Brown MF, Graham JM, Feliciano DV, et al. Carotid artery injuries. Am J Surg 1982; **144**: 748–53.

11 Matas R. Traumatisms and traumatic aneurysms of the vertebral artery and their surgical treatment, with the report of a cured case. Ann Surg 1893; **18**: 477.

12 Maisonneuve JGF. J Connaissances Med Chir 1852; **2**: 181.

13 Serbinenko FA. Balloon catheterization and occlusion of major cerebral vessels. J Neurosurg 1974; **41**: 125–45.

14 Biffl WL, Moore EE, Elliott JP, et al. The devastating potential of blunt vertebral arterial injuries. Ann Surg 2000; **231**: 672–81.

15 Rivers SP, Patel Y, Delany HM, Veith FJ. Limited role of arteriography in penetrating neck trauma. J Vasc Surg 1988; **8**: 112–16.

16 Fry WR, Dort JA, Smith RS, et al. Duplex scanning replaces arteriography and operative exploration in the diagnosis of potential cervical vascular injury. Am J Surg 1994; **168**: 693–5.

17 Kuzniec S, Kauffman P, Molnar LJ, et al. Diagnosis of limbs and neck arterial trauma using duplex ultrasonography. *Cardiovasc Surg* 1998; **6**: 358–66.

18 Ginzburg E, Montalvo B, LeBlang S, et al. The use of duplex ultrasonography in penetrating neck trauma. *Arch Surg* 1996; **131**: 691–3.

19 Cogbill TH, Moore EE, Meissner M, et al. The spectrum of blunt injury to the carotid artery: a multicenter perspective. *J Trauma* 1994; **37**: 473–9.

20 Bynoe RP, Miles WS, Bell RM, et al. Noninvasive diagnosis of vascular trauma by duplex ultrasonography. *J Vasc Surg* 1991; **14**: 346–52.

21 Meissner M, Paun M, Johansen K. Duplex scanning for arterial trauma. *Am J Surg* 1991; **161**: 552–5.

22 Greenwold D, Sessions EG, Haynes JL, et al. Duplex ultrasonography in vascular trauma. *J Vasc Technol* 1991; **15**: 79–82.

23 LeBlang SD, Nunez DB Jr, Rivas LA, et al. Helical computed tomographic angiography in penetrating neck trauma. *Emerg Radiol* 1997; **4**: 200–6.

24 Stain SC, Yellin AE, Weaver FA, Pentecost MJ. Selective management of non-occlusive arterial injuries. *Arch Surg* 1989; **124**: 1136–40.

25 Hemphill JC, Gress DR, Halbach VV. Endovascular therapy of traumatic injuries of the intracranial cerebral arteries. *Crit Care Clin* 1999; **15**: 811–29.

26 Gomez CR, May AK, Terry JB, Tulyapronchote R. Endovascular therapy of traumatic injuries of the extracranial cerebral arteries. *Crit Care Clin* 1999; **15**: 789–809.

27 Robbs JV, Human RR, Rajaruthnam P, et al. Neurological deficit and injuries involving the neck arteries. *Br J Surg* 1983; **70**: 220–2.

28 Popowich L. Blunt carotid artery trauma associated with maxillofacial injuries: report of three cases. *J Oral Maxillofac Surg* 1984; **42**: 462–5.

29 Cogbill TH, Moore EE, Meissner M, et al. The spectrum of blunt injury to the carotid artery: a multicenter perspective. *J Trauma* 1994; **37**: 473–9.

30 Remonda L, Heid O, Schroth G. Carotid artery stenosis, occlusion, and pseudo-occlusion: first-pass, gadolinium-enhanced, three-dimensional MR angiography – preliminary study. *Radiology* 1998; **209**: 95–102.

31 Fabian TC, Patton JH, Croce MA, et al. Blunt carotid injury. Importance of early diagnosis and anticoagulant therapy. *Ann Surg* 1996; **223**: 513–22.

32 Biffl WL, Moore EE, Ryu RK, et al. The unrecognized epidemic of blunt carotid arterial injuries: early diagnosis improves neurologic outcome. *Ann Surg* 1998; **228**: 462–70.

33 Blickenstaff KL, Weaver FA, Yellin AE, et al. Trends in the management of traumatic vertebral artery injuries. *Am J Surg* 1989; **158**: 101–15; discussion 105–6.

34 Bear HM, Zoarski GH, Rothmann MI. Evaluation of vertebral artery injury from ballistic trauma to the neck. *Emerg Radiol* 1997; **4**: 346–8.

35 Reid JDS, Weigelt JA. Forty-three cases of vertebral artery trauma. *J Trauma* 1988; **28**: 1007–12.

36 Mascalchi M, Bianchi MC, Mangiafico S, et al. MRI and MR angiography of vertebral artery dissection. *Neuroradiology* 1997; **39**: 329–40.

37 Waldman DL, Barquist E, Poynton FG, Numaguchi Y. Stent graft of a traumatic vertebral artery injury: case report. *J Trauma* 1998; **44**: 1094–7.

38 Golueke P, Sclafani S, Phillips T, et al. Vertebral artery injury – diagnosis and management. *J Trauma* 1987; **27**: 856–65.

39 Berguer R, Flynn LM, Kline RA, Caplan L. Surgical reconstruction of the extracranial vertebral artery: management and outcome. *J Vasc Surg* 2000; **31**: 9–18.

40 Edwards WH, Mulherin JL Jr. The surgical management of proximal subclavian-vertebral artery stenosis. *Contemp Surg* 1980; **17**: 11–19.

36

Abdominal Vascular Injuries

JOHN V ROBBS

THE PROBLEM

Discussion on this topic revolves around injuries of the aorta and its major branches namely coeliac, mesenteric, renal and the iliac arteries and their branches. With regard to venous trauma the inferior vena cava (IVC), the iliac veins and the portal system will be discussed. Injuries to the aorta and the IVC and their major branches are relatively uncommon, certainly in the context of those admitted to hospital for surgical management. In our own 15-year database of patients with arterial trauma managed on the vascular service, abdominal vessels were only involved in 5 per cent of the total of 3000 patients. The most frequently involved arteries were the iliac arteries (2.5 per cent).

The mortality for these injuries is high both in the pre-hospital setting as well as following efforts at treatment. The reasons for this are difficulty in controlling haemorrhage prior to admission and the relative inaccessibility of the vessels in the retroperitoneum making rapid access and control difficult. The problem is often compounded by emergency laparotomies being carried out by relatively inexperienced surgeons and under these circumstances the situation can be further aggravated by the release of whatever tamponade exists in attempts to control bleeding with blind clamping, often causing further vascular damage. This is an extremely challenging group of injuries from the technical point of view, often with little reward in terms of patient survival.

AETIOLOGY AND PATHOLOGY

The mechanisms and the pathology of vascular injuries are varied.[1] Penetrating wounds are the most frequently encountered. These may be subdivided into stabs, gunshot, shotgun and iatrogenic injuries. In general, stab wounds cause fairly circumscribed trauma. Low velocity gunshot wounds caused by muzzle velocities of less than 600 m/s, generally show no more damage than that found along the missile track. They also tend to be relatively localised, but the problems lie with tracing the trajectory of the missile. High velocity missile wounds, as encountered in military situations where muzzle velocities exceed 600 m/s, release energy causing extensive damage around the track of the missile; when these wounds traverse the abdomen they are usually incompatible with survival. More detail on the ballistics can be obtained by referring to an appropriate text.[2]

Shotgun wounds at close range caused by multiple pellets deserve special consideration as they usually penetrate the abdominal wall and cause extensive damage. This is almost invariably associated with visceral injury with or without contamination by bowel contents, and the vascular injuries tend to be complex and may even be multiple.[3] It should be borne in mind that as many of these vessels are situated in the retroperitoneum a high incidence of associated hollow visceral injury can be expected.

Iatrogenic injuries may complicate interventional catheter procedures. Operative misadventure is not an infrequent cause of iatrogenic vascular injury. These are beyond the scope of this chapter but are discussed in Chapters 38–40.

The mechanisms encountered in penetrating trauma may involve perforation of the vessel resulting in either free haemorrhage or the formation of a pseudoaneurysm. In this context, a through-and-through perforation, often oblique, can be most challenging, especially when dealing with the IVC or the aorta. Simultaneous perforation of artery and adjacent vein produces an arteriovenous fistula with or without an intervening false aneurysm; the most frequently encountered in our practice have been aortocaval and common iliac fistulae. A false aneurysm may compress adjacent viscera or erode into the bowel or biliary system with resultant gastrointestinal haemorrhage. Penetrating parenchymal injuries involving the liver or the kidney may present with haemobilia or haematuria, respectively.

Blunt trauma involving these vessels is relatively uncommon. One type of injury appears to involve a crushing mechanism such as a pedestrian run over by a vehicle which may result in shearing of the major branches from the aorta. In our experience we have seen distal aortic thrombosis following this type of injury. The fractured pelvis may damage the common iliac vessels when there is disruption of the sacroiliac joint with cephalad displacement of the hemipelvis. Fractures with disruption of the pelvic ring also frequently cause multiple small vessel, predominantly venous, injuries. Acceleration/deceleration trauma frequently involves the renal vessels in which it would appear that the weight of the viscera, with forward momentum, causes marked distraction and applies shearing forces upon the renal pedicle. We have also seen these injuries involving the IVC at the level of the diaphragm, the weight of the liver causing shear stresses where the IVC traverses the diaphragm.

The basic pathology in all blunt trauma is that crushing and distracting forces cause the vessel to tear from its luminal surface outwards. Intima is the least elastic and therefore most vulnerable to tearing. The most elastic and durable element of the vessel wall is the adventitia which may well remain intact although the inner layers are disrupted. Exposure of this extensive thrombogenic surface may bring about thrombosis with occlusion. Partial or total transmural disruption may result in perforation and haemorrhage with false aneurysm formation. In the long term, partial disruption of the vessel wall, with an intact adventitia is likely to lead to a localised aneurysm. These considerable forces cause a high proportion of associated solid and hollow visceral injuries, further compounding the difficulties in diagnosis and management.

CLINICAL PRESENTATION AND DIAGNOSIS

Clinically, patients can broadly be divided into two categories: those in whom the diagnosis is acutely apparent or those in whom the presentation is subtle, manifesting itself days, weeks or even years later.[1]

Acute presentation

HAEMORRHAGE

Patients may present with an obvious major intra-abdominal vascular catastrophe with hypovolaemic shock, poorly responsive to resuscitation and abdominal distension. On occasion patients with major venous injuries respond well initially to volume resuscitation but they may gradually become hypovolaemic once more and require ongoing resuscitation. A more subtle manifestation of vascular injury contained by the retroperitoneum is illustrated by the patient who requires extensive volume resuscitation initially, stabilises, but is then found to have abdominal distension and a low haemoglobin level; this is highly suggestive of a contained major vascular disruption.

LOWER LIMB ISCHAEMIA

Crush injury with iliac or aortic occlusion may present with lower limb ischaemia. It may remain undetected at the time of the primary clinical survey due to hypothermia and shock. This possibility, however, must be considered in any patient with pelvic fracture or significant abdominal crush injury.

It is also likely that when intimal tears occur, thrombosis may follow within hours of the injury, and unless the patient is repeatedly assessed this may be missed, with unfortunate consequences.

ANURIA

Bilateral renal pedicle injuries are relatively uncommon. A patient who fails to pass urine after sustaining acceleration/deceleration trauma, and in whom all other possible lower urinary tract injuries have been excluded, may have developed bilateral renal artery thrombosis. Unilateral renal artery disruption may be extremely difficult to detect and often remains undiagnosed.[1] If some perfusion persists through a partially occluded vessel, the patient may well have microscopic haematuria. The only means of detecting such injuries is to be clinical aware of their possibility and to proceed with basic screening investigations such as an excretory urogram (EUG).

INTRAOPERATIVE DIAGNOSIS

This occurs when laparotomy has been necessary, for example for peritoneal irritation, and a retroperitoneal haematoma is found, which may well mask a significant vascular injury. Under these circumstances it is important to localise the haematoma anatomically, i.e. central, lateral or pelvic, and to assess whether it is stable, expanding or pulsatile.

Acute presentation
• Haemorrhage
• Lower limb ischaemia
• Anuria
• Operative diagnosis

Delayed presentation

PULSATILE MASS

A contained perforation of any of the major arteries often results in pseudoaneurysm formation. This pulsatile mass compresses adjacent viscera and may manifest itself as a duodenal obstruction. These pseudoaneurysms require urgent intervention as their natural history is one of eventual rupture or erosion into adjacent viscera.

GASTROINTESTINAL HAEMORRHAGE

Haemobilia may follow penetrating liver injuries with partial disruption of the hepatic artery branches and the formation of a fistula into the biliary radicles. This may present days to weeks after the injury and is characterised by right upper quadrant pain and episodes of upper gastrointestinal haemorrhage, usually melaena, but less frequently haematemesis.[4] Injury to the peripancreatic vessels may result in erosion into the duodenum of a pseudoaneurysm with intermittent massive gastrointestinal haemorrhage.

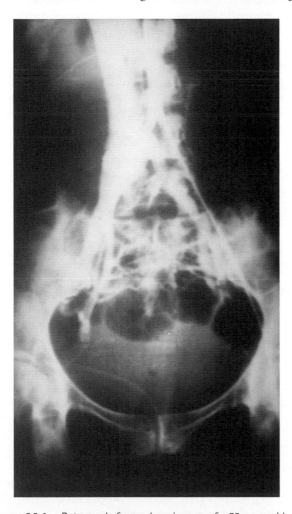

Figure 36.1 *Retrograde femoral angiogram of a 59-year-old man showing an aortocaval fistula following a low velocity gunshot wound to the abdomen*

This outcome is probably associated with an element of traumatic pancreatitis due to activation of proteolytic enzymes. Massive rectal bleeding has also followed the development of false aneurysms involving the internal iliac vessels.[5]

HAEMATURIA

Penetrating renal parenchymal injury with the formation of an intrarenal pseudoaneurysm may result in quite severe intermittent haematuria manifesting itself several days after the original injury.[6]

ARTERIOVENOUS FISTULA

Aortocaval fistula usually presents fairly acutely with the appearance of lower limb oedema and an obvious arteriovenous bruit in the abdomen. Small fistulae may remain undetected until the patient presents months, or even years, later in congestive heart failure caused by a hyperdynamic circulation and marked lower extremity venous hypertension. Iliac fistulae present mainly with signs of lower extremity venous hypertension coupled with an arteriovenous bruit.[3] Figure 36.1 shows the angiogram of a 59-year man who developed an aortocaval fistula following a gunshot injury.

> **Delayed presentation**
>
> - Pulsatile mass
> - Gastrointestinal haemorrhage
> - Haematuria
> - Arteriovenous fistula

INVESTIGATIONS

Angiography

Selective retrograde femoral angiography is the gold standard of investigation. It should be reserved, however, for stable patients in whom vascular injury is strongly suspected on clinical grounds: that group comprises patients with a pulsatile mass, arteriovenous murmur, significant haematuria, gastrointestinal haemorrhage or an ischaemic limb. Angiography should also be performed for patients with stable retroperitoneal haematomas as many of these lesions can be dealt with by interventional techniques. There is no place for angiography in the unstable patient who is actively bleeding.

> **Indications for angiography in a haemodynamically stable patient**
>
> - Ischaemic lower limb(s)
> - Pulsatile mass

- Arteriovenous murmur
- Suspected haemobilia
  - Right upper quadrant pain
  - Jaundice
  - Upper gastrointestinal bleeding
- Suspected renal pedicle injury (acceleration/deceleration)
  - Anuria
  - Delayed/absent function on excretory urography
  - Retroperitoneal haematoma (stable)
  - Lateral (perinephric)
  - Pelvic
- Gastrointestinal bleeding
  - Eroding false aneurysm?

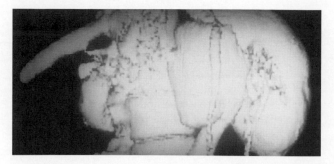

Figure 36.2 *Computed tomography (CT) angiogram showing a pseudoaneurysm arising from the juxtarenal aorta in an 18-year-old man who sustained a gunshot wound to the abdomen. At the time of initial wounding he underwent laparotomy at which several small bowel perforations were repaired. He presented 1 month later with a palpable pseudoaneurysm*

Excretory urography

The EUG is a useful screening test in patients in whom a renal injury is suspected, such as those with haematuria or anuria or those with the appropriate pattern of injury in whom renal injury is likely. Delayed or non-excretion of contrast should provoke selective renal angiography.

Duplex scan

This investigation has limited value in an acute presentation but may be useful in detecting the site of an iliac arteriovenous fistula, or under certain circumstances and in the appropriate patient, in assessing blood flow in the renal artery in someone whose abdomen is not grossly distended or who is relatively thin. Published experience confirms the usefulness of this investigation in the evaluation of neck trauma.[7]

Computed tomography

Computed tomography (CT) and CT angiography are useful in selected situations in which there is localised injury requiring further elucidation.[4] In Fig. 36.2, CT angiography shows a pseudoaneurysm of the juxtarenal aorta following a gunshot injury to the abdomen of an 18-year-old man who presented 3 months after the injury. The aortic injury had not been detected at his initial laparotomy when small bowel perforations had been repaired.

PRINCIPLES OF MANAGEMENT

The text has alluded to the spectrum of clinical presentations. In the unstable shocked patient the standard approach to resuscitation must be followed, namely, maintenance of

airway and insertion of at least two wide bore intravenous cannulae (see Chapter 7B) with monitoring of progress of resuscitation by means of urine output, central venous pressure, systemic blood pressure, core temperature and acid–base status. Those patients with obvious continuing haemorrhage, or in whom there are other indications for urgent exploration such as evisceration or peritonitis, demand urgent operation. In the latter cases occult vascular injury may be present in the form of a contained retroperitoneal haematoma only discovered at operation.

In the second category, that is, those who have been stabilised but in whom a vascular injury is strongly suspected on clinical grounds, further investigations are indicated. The most useful of these is angiography which accurately localises the injury and offers the possibility of some form of endovascular intervention in the appropriate situation. An algorithm of management (Fig. 36.3) can be of assistance.

OPERATIVE MANAGEMENT

Access and control

Once operative management has been decided upon, wide exposure is absolutely of the essence in dealing with these injuries. The patient should be prepared and draped from the nipple line to the knees. This gives access to the chest and to the groin vessels if necessary.

The incision of choice is in the midline extending from the xiphisternum to the pubis (Fig. 36.4) Access may be improved by lateral extension into the loin on either side as required. On occasion a lower sixth or seventh intercostal space thoracotomy or even median sternotomy may be required. The surgeon should not hesitate to extend the incisions to improve access; 'keyhole' surgery invites disaster.

A useful manoeuvre is to obtain control of the aorta at the hiatus. The oesophagus is mobilised and retracted to the patient's left. The liver can then be retracted cephalad

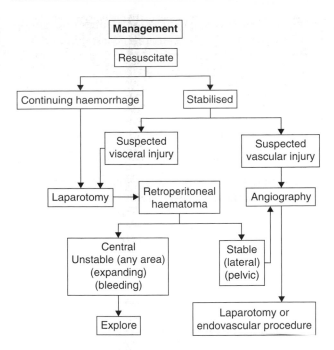

Figure 36.3 *Algorithm of management in patients suspected of having an abdominal vascular injury*

by means of a Deaver retractor, and the aorta can be palpated (Fig. 36.5a). The aorta can be compressed against the spinal column either by manual pressure or with a 'sponge stick', but preferably by clamping, to facilitate which the right crus of the diaphragm overlying the aorta may be divided. The aorta is then straddled using the middle and index finger and a straight aortic clamp can then be applied using the fingers as a guide (Fig. 36.5b). The aorta should not be encircled and snared as that may risk avulsing the lower intercostal vessels.

On opening the lesser sac, access can be obtained to the coeliac and superior mesenteric vessels. If more extensive exposure of the aorta in this region is required a left visceral rotation (Fig. 36.6) can be performed by mobilising the colon, the spleen and the pancreas to the patient's right in a plane anterior to the left kidney. This manoeuvre also provides optimal access to the left renal artery. The infrarenal aorta is readily exposed through the root of the mesentery and the common iliac vessels by opening the peritoneum over the pelvic brim.

The IVC below the liver is best exposed by right visceral rotation in which the ascending colon is mobilised, along

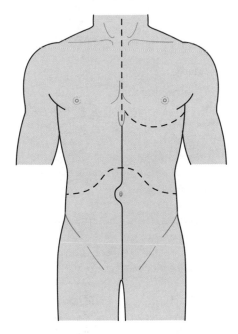

Figure 36.4 *Incisions for access to abdominal vascular injuries*

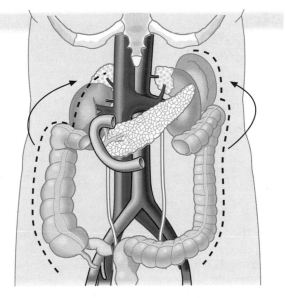

Figure 36.6 *Left and right visceral rotation procedures to gain access to major retroperitoneal vessels*

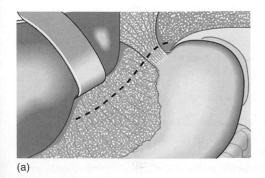

(a)

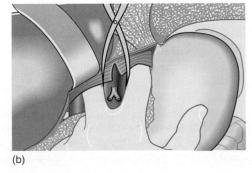

(b)

Figure 36.5 *(a) Exposure for control of the aorta at the diaphragmatic hiatus and (b) control of aorta at the hiatus*

with the duodenum and pancreatic head by the Kocher manoeuvre, and reflected to the patient's left. This exposure also provides optimal access to the right renal vessels.

The visceral rotation procedures are illustrated in Fig. 36.6. Access to the retrohepatic IVC can be gained by dividing the suspensory ligaments of the liver and reflecting the liver to the patient's left. Details are discussed under the appropriate heading below.

Specific vascular scenarios

ACTIVE ONGOING HAEMORRHAGE

The major problem under these circumstances is that the patient is usually extremely unstable, and it is often difficult to localise the source of haemorrhage. The initial step is to 'eviscerate' the abdomen, taking the small bowel out of the abdominal cavity and allowing it to lie on the abdominal wall. It is advisable to use swabs to mop up blood and to restrict use of the sucker; the patient's blood volume may rapidly disappear into the sucker reservoir without the surgeon fully appreciating the extent of the loss, particularly with low pressure venous bleeding.

It is also extremely important to keep pace with volume resuscitation. If possible, tamponade the abdominal cavity and resuscitate before mobilising or exploring haematoma or bleeding sites. If the bleeding is obviously arterial, aortic control at the hiatus is obtained as described. This will usually slow the bleeding down sufficiently to localise its source and appropriate exposure can then be undertaken. Once the injury has been isolated, more localised control is obtained if possible, for example, with side-biting clamps restoring visceral and renal perfusion while resuscitation is completed. Each lesion can then be dealt with on its specific merits. If the bleeding is obviously venous and welling up into the operative field, it may be extremely difficult to identify the source by virtue of its low pressure. The IVC is best exposed by right visceral rotation, or in the case of the retrohepatic IVC by mobilisation of the right lobe of the liver. This will be dealt with more specifically in discussion on IVC injuries.

The major judgement call in this type of patient is whether or not to embark upon a 'damage control' strategy.[8] These patients are more likely to die from 'metabolic failure' than from the actual vascular injury (see Chapter 4). The balance lies between restoring normal anatomy and the fatal triad of hypothermia, acidosis and coagulopathy. The strategy comprises temporising manoeuvres allowing for active resuscitation in an intensive care unit (ICU) setting with subsequent re-exploration for definitive treatment.[9–11] Consideration must be given to adopting this strategy in a patient who has a metabolic acidosis (pH less than 7.25), hypothermia (core temperature less than 34 °C), coagulopathy (non-surgical bleeding) and massive blood transfusion (more than 10 units), and in whom the operation has taken more than one and a half hours.[12]

Principles of damage control involve the arrest of bleeding and limiting contamination. In terms of surgical bleeding non-essential vessels are ligated, and simple suture repair carried out where possible. Consideration can be given to balloon tamponade and the use of temporary shunts for major more essential arteries. For venous or non-surgical bleeding packing should be entertained. All ends may be ligated or stapled and the abdominal wounds closed temporarily. Various strategies have been advocated for this including the use of towel clips to approximate skin edges and meshes or transparent adhesive abdominal drapes to cover exposed bowel.[13]

In the ICU setting active re-warming is commenced using warmed fluids. Coagulopathy is treated, volume restored and acidosis corrected. Bleeding not thought to be due to coagulopathy may necessitate earlier re-exploration but, if planned, it should take place between 24 and 72 hours later. Consideration can be given to the operation once core temperature exceeds 35 °C, serum lactate is less than 2.5 mmol/L and the international normalised ratio (INR) and prothrombin time (PTT) are less than 1.25 times normal.[12,14,15]

The major consideration in the postoperative period, besides the complex metabolic derangements that may continue to occur, is that of the abdominal compartment syndrome.[16–18] This is the situation in which increasing abdominal pressures due to distended bowel, or for whatever reason, results in progressive oliguria, elevated airway pressure, hypoxemia and hypotension due to decreased venous return. It is important to be aware of this problem after all major abdominal injuries. The optimum method of measuring intra-abdominal pressure is by means of an intravesical catheter.[19]

It would appear that a pressure in excess of 22 mmHg necessitates decompression. Abdominal wounds should be reopened and one of the strategies of visceral containment embarked upon.[12] Detailed discussion of this subject is beyond the scope of this chapter except to note that 20 per cent or more patients in this category will develop this complication, which, unless remedied early, will certainly contribute to rapid deterioration.

The damage control strategy is extremely labour intensive and it puts great stress on resource management.[20] The mortality remains in excess of 50 per cent but it is difficult to compare various series due to the heterogeneous nature of the patients and their injuries. The philosophy, in essence, is that some chance is better than no chance.

RETROPERITONEAL HAEMATOMAS

Retroperitoneal haematomas are classified into three zones according to their site (Fig. 36.7), namely central haematomas (zone 1), lateral haematomas (zone 2) and pelvic haematomas (zone 3). Central haematomas may

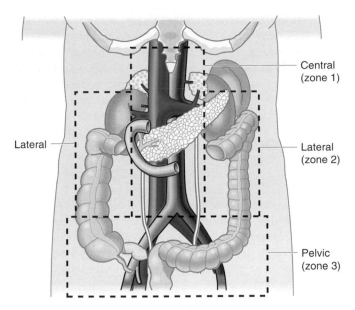

Figure 36.7 *Retroperitoneal haematoma zones*

result from injuries to the great vessels of the abdomen, pancreas and duodenum; lateral haematomas result from injured kidney, renal vessels and ureter, and pelvic haematomas result from damage to the great vessels of the pelvis, bladder, ureters, and the rectum. Combination haematomas are classified as zone 4.[21–23]

All zone 1 haematomas should be explored because of the high incidence of visceral and major vascular injuries.[23–25] The haematoma should not be entered without attempting to resuscitate the patient as far as possible by controlling the bleeding area with pressure packs and volume replacement. This is often easier said than done.

If the haematoma or the bleeding site involves the suprarenal area the aorta should be controlled at the oesophageal hiatus as described. The next step will be to open the lesser sac and to attempt to isolate the injury. If this does not prove possible left lateral visceral rotation should be used. If the haematoma is predominantly infrarenal, or if it is situated at the base of the mesentery, the transverse colon should be retracted superiorly after mobilising the duodenum, so that the aorta can be controlled below the left renal vein before entering the haematoma.[26] An essential principle in managing these injuries is to avoid blind clamping as the IVC, left renal vein and in particular the common iliac veins are fragile and very susceptible to injury. Lacerations of these large vessel trunks can turn a controlled situation into a hopeless blood bath.

If a lateral zone 2 haematoma is expanding or pulsatile, exploration is indicated. The same would apply when there is radiological evidence of major pedicle or parenchymal injury and significant urinary extravasation. The reason for not exploring stable non-pulsatile haematomas is that haemorrhage adequately tamponaded by perinephric fascia may become uncontrollable and result in unnecessary

nephrectomy.[22,26–29] When exploration is indicated, however, the renal pedicle must be controlled before opening the haematoma. Renal artery injuries are repaired on their merits.

Haematomas in the medial portion of zone 2, where the renal pelvis, renal pedicle and lateral duodenum are situated, can be problematic. Much debate has taken place as to whether these should be explored in stable patients by virtue of the morbidity caused by missed injuries, particularly to the duodenum, and a case for routine exploration can certainly be made. These particular haematomas should probably be classified with the central zone 1 group.[30]

With regard to zone 3 pelvic haematomas in general, management depends on whether the injury is actively bleeding or contained. A contained haematoma, if non-expansile and flaccid, should not be opened in the presence of a pelvic fracture, when arterial pulsation in the groin is intact and there is no evidence of urological trauma on urethrography and cystography. Exploration is indicated, however, if a pelvic haematoma has ruptured, if it is rapidly expanding or pulsatile in close proximity to major vessels, if arterial pulsation in the groin is absent or if intraperitoneal rupture of the bladder has occurred.[30–32]

An essential part of controlling haemorrhage in relation to pelvic fracture is urgent fixation and stabilisation of the fracture.[30,31] Deep pelvic haematomas in relation to the internal iliac vessels and their branches even if pulsatile are probably best left undisturbed or treated by tamponade until the precise source of bleeding is elucidated by angiography. Most of these injuries are amenable to endovascular procedures, embolotherapy in particular.[33,34] Details of the management of rectal and urological injuries are beyond the scope of this chapter.

MAJOR ARTERIAL INJURIES

The options available for definitive therapy are lateral suture, patch angioplasty repair, end-to-end anastomosis or interposition grafts. Under certain circumstances ligation may be necessary. Repair follows well established principles[35] such as debridement of the vessel ends to healthy vessel wall, removal of propagated thrombus and flushing of the distal arterial tree with heparinised saline solution. Repairs must be performed with intima to intima apposition without causing luminal narrowing or any tension on the suture line. In general, injuries compatible with survival can usually be repaired by simple techniques. As a general rule, through and through injuries are best managed by transection of the vessel, incorporating both wounds, followed by reanastomosis in an end-to-end fashion.

When an interposition graft or a patch closure is required autogenous material such as the long saphenous vein is probably the best option. This applies particularly when there has been an element of contamination in the operative field. Nevertheless, when there is no contamination, and in the interests of expedience, prosthetic grafts may be required.

Mesenteric injuries

With regard to the superior mesenteric artery, definitive management depends largely upon the anatomical zone involved. Fullen and his colleagues[36] classified these as follows:

- Zone 1 – extending from the aorta to the first major branch, the inferior pancreaticoduodenal artery
- Zone 2 – from the inferior pancreaticoduodenal to the middle colic artery origin
- Zone 3 – the trunk distal to the middle colic
- Zone 4 – segmental branches to the jejunum, ileum or colon.

The chances of bowel ischaemia are maximal for zone 1, minimal for zone 3 and extremely unlikely for zone 4 disruptions. With ligation of the proximal superior mesenteric artery, collaterals may well occur through the coeliac axis and inferior mesenteric artery branches. The patients, however, are invariably shocked and the severe associated vasospasm and hypotension can further perpetuate borderline ischaemia. Ligation of zones 1 and 2 injuries have an extremely high mortality and it is strongly recommended that repair be effected for these. It is probably also advisable to repair zone 3 injuries. For injuries close to the aorta it is probably best to oversew the aortic defect and to restore continuity by means of a graft taken from the side of the infrarenal aorta.[37,38]

Clear guidelines are lacking for the treatment of the associated superior mesenteric venous injury. Such injuries do not seem to influence overall mortality and, in general, a simple injury can be oversewn or reanastomosed, whereas a more complex injury with a wall defect would probably be best treated by ligation.

Coeliac axis injuries

There is little information specifically concerning injuries to this vessel. Our own experience has been to restore continuity of this vessel by simple suture wherever possible, and if not to simply ligate it. It would appear that ligation is well tolerated in the presence of a patent superior mesenteric artery.[38]

Any mesenteric or coeliac artery disruption is potentially likely to result in bowel ischaemia in the postoperative period (see Chapters 3, 4 and 29). There is some debate as to whether a second look laparotomy should be performed as routine in these patients, but no firm guidelines exist.

Renal artery injuries

The basic principles with regard to restoration of arterial continuity apply. In most cases the optimum procedure is to use a saphenous graft which takes its origin from the infrarenal aorta and is anastomosed distally end-to-side or end-to-end to healthy renal artery. Unless there has been partial disruption of the vessel with preservation of some prograde flow the results of renal pedicle avulsion in terms of kidney salvage are extremely poor, mainly due to the delay in making the diagnosis and the poor tolerance of the kidney to prolonged ischaemia.[28,29,39]

MAJOR VENOUS INJURIES

Inferior vena cava injuries

With simple lower IVC injuries avulsion of lumbar veins should be avoided by resisting attempts to encircle and clamp the IVC. It is preferable to obtain control by pressure above and below the laceration using sponge sticks and by digital compression of the lumbar veins against the posterior abdominal wall[26,40] (Fig. 36.8a). For larger injuries indwelling Foley balloon catheters may be used to control bleeding.

For simple anterior puncture wounds a side-biting atraumatic vascular clamp is applied to provide adequate control (Fig. 36.8b). The possibility of an additional posterior puncture wound due to a through and through injury should be excluded. Under these circumstances, the posterior injury is best sutured through an enlarged anterior wound. Attempts to rotate the IVC should be avoided as it invariably results in avulsion of the lumbar veins (Fig. 36.8c).

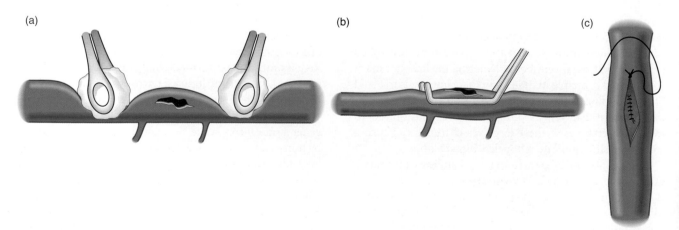

(a) (b) (c)

Figure 36.8 *Infrarenal inferior vena caval injuries: (a) control; (b) side-biting clamp control; (c) transluminal repair of posterior wall laceration*

In the presence of complex injuries which may require interposition grafts, or if there is uncontrollable haemorrhage, ligation is the best option and is extremely well tolerated by most patients. Grafts of the IVC have given uniformly poor results in terms of patency.[40,41]

Juxtahepatic inferior vena cava injuries

This refers to the IVC extending from above the renal veins under the liver to the diaphragm, and by convention, includes injuries to the hepatic veins. The only tributaries entering this segment of the IVC are the hepatic veins, the right adrenal vein and the inferior phrenic veins. Therefore, by clamping the portal vein and the hepatic artery, and controlling the IVC above and below the liver, hepatic flow is effectively arrested and there should be minimal bleeding.

Obviously, occlusion of the IVC at this level seriously compromises venous return to the heart and is doubly challenging in the hypovolaemic patient. This problem led to the development of the concept of the atriocaval shunt, in which an attempt is made to isolate the retrohepatic IVC while allowing venous drainage to continue into the atrium by means of strategically placed apertures within the shunt, once the IVC has been isolated[42] (Fig. 36.9).

The first step entails performing the Pringle manoeuvre, i.e. cross-clamping at the porta hepatis. A total median sternotomy must then be carried out, followed by a pericardiotomy, isolating the intrapericardial IVC. The juxtahepatic IVC is mobilised by right visceral rotation as well as by mobilising the duodenum using the Kocher manoeuvre. The suprarenal IVC is isolated, the auricle of the atrium opened and a 36 Fr chest drain tube is passed into the IVC. Prior to insertion of this tube a side-hole is cut into the proximal end of the tube through which drainage can occur. The position of the tube is confirmed by palpation. The IVC is secured around the tube by means of snares.[42] An alternative that has been described is the use of an endotracheal tube passed from the atrium, inflating its balloon in the infrahepatic segment of the IVC so obviating the need to mobilise it at this level.[43] The technique for insertion of these shunts is difficult and has the potential for further disruption of the injured area by the tip of the tube. Unless the drainage holes are correctly positioned the shunt will have no influence whatever on bleeding. Median sternotomy is also time consuming and there is major potential for initiating further bleeding.[42]

The alternative to using the atriocaval shunt is total occlusion of the IVC and portal system.[40,44,45] As already mentioned this severely reduces venous drainage and can cause marked hypotension. Before attempting it, therefore, the patient must be well resuscitated in terms of volume.

After initiating the Pringle manoeuvre the ligamentum arteriosum and the falciform ligament are divided and the liver is gently pull in a caudad direction. The central tendon of the diaphragm is then divided to gain access to the pericardium, which exposes the intrapericardial IVC (Fig. 36.10a). The infrahepatic IVC is then exposed as described earlier. The liver is then totally mobilised by dividing the right and left triangular ligaments and the anterior and posterior layers of the coronary ligament on the right. The IVC can now be clamped within the pericardium and below the liver. If the blood pressure drops precipitously the aorta can be clamped at the hiatus in order to sequestrate the upper body circulation. The liver can now be rotated to identify the venous injury, which, in most cases can be repaired expeditiously; again most injuries compatible with survival can be dealt with by simple suture (Fig. 36.10b).

The mortality for these injuries is prohibitive and in most reported series exceeds 80 per cent. No patients requiring resuscitative thoracotomy have been reported as survivors.[42] In most experienced hands only about 50 per cent of patients have survived shunt insertion in order to allow repair of the injury. In our own experience, we have attempted atriocaval shunt placement in four patients and have had no survivors; certainly two died due to haemorrhage provoked by attempts to achieve this objective. We have had 10 patients in whom total isolation was performed, of whom seven survived; all these had penetrating trauma with simple lacerations.[40] All patients had some degree of postoperative liver function derangement which resolved within a week or so. The deaths were a direct result of blood loss and the cascade of multiple organ failure[40,44] (see Chapter 4). It is extremely difficult to compare results

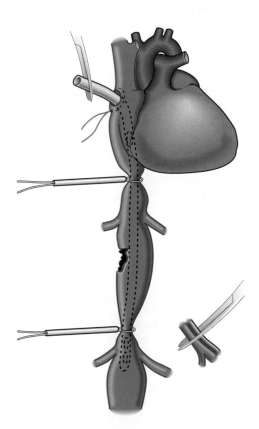

Figure 36.9 *Juxtahepatic inferior vena caval injuries. Use of the atriocaval shunt*

between reported series because they tend to be small and represent an extremely heterogeneous group of patients.

Portal vein injuries

These injuries are seldom if ever isolated and they are surgically inaccessible. A high proportion of patients with these injuries exsanguinate intraoperatively.[45–48]

Access to the portal vein is achieved by means of right visceral rotation with mobilisation of the duodenum and head of pancreas to the right. Occasionally, in order to reach the confluence of the splenic and superior mesenteric vein, it may be necessary to divide the neck of the pancreas.[45] The major problem is to control bleeding while exposure is being established and to this end ingenuity may certainly

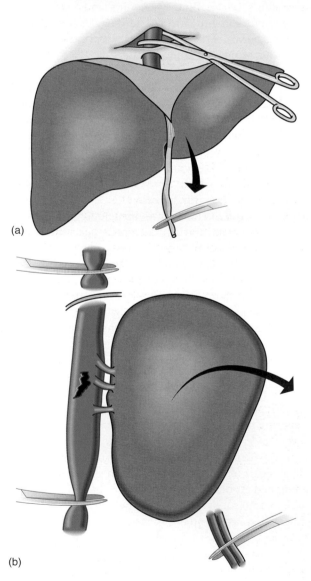

(a)

(b)

Figure 36.10 *Juxtahepatic inferior vena caval injuries – total hepatic isolation. (a) Exposure of intrapericardial inferior vena cava and (b) isolation of retrohepatic inferior vena cava with mobilisation of right lobe of liver*

be tested. As always there is no place for blind application of clamps. Wherever possible one should attempt to control bleeding by compression.

As a general rule in terms of definitive repair, simple lateral suture, or if possible end-to-end anastomosis, is the most feasible. Complex injuries with major vessel wall defects are best treated by ligation.[49–52] Emergency portal–systemic shunt insertion cannot be recommended as it is a complex procedure invariably performed in an unstable patient. In addition, the reported rate of encephalopathy is unacceptably high[53] (see Chapter 46). By the same token various other procedures have been reported, such as the use of interposition grafts using either vein or prosthesis, with the occasional survivor.[9]

Results are uniformly poor in terms of survival and 50–80 per cent mortality is reported.[45–53] The major influences on this outcome are the associated injuries and massive blood loss. In the longer term, there is little information on the patency of attempted repairs. One small study using duplex Doppler showed that long term patency can be achieved following simple venorrhaphy.[48] During the postoperative period there is a relatively small risk of bowel infarction (see Chapters 3 and 29). More frequently reported, however, is the massive sequestration of fluid in the splanchnic bed, particularly after ligation, which calls for significant fluid resuscitation. In the longer term there are no reports related to the incidence of symptomatic portal hypertension. Some authors have advocated a second look procedure within 24 hours to exclude bowel infarction.[45,49,51,52] Our own experience is limited to 15 patients for whom we have records: the mortality was 80 per cent and most of the injured vessels in survivors had been ligated. With regard to superior mesenteric vein injuries no specific reports can be found and the approach advocated is that of simple repair when feasible, and failing that, ligation.

Renal vein injuries

It is well established that the left renal vein can be ligated provided that collaterals through the suprarenal and gonadal vein are preserved. Whenever possible simple repair should be attempted. The right kidney does not tolerate ligation of the right renal vein, as the only collaterals are those via the renal capsule, the gonadal and adrenal veins draining directly into the IVC.

Iliac vein injuries

Diffuse bleeding related to pelvic fractures is probably best treated by packing followed by reoperation for removal of the packs 24 hours later. Common or external iliac vein injuries should be repaired wherever possible but if these are complex, ligation is the best option, and in our experience tolerated well in the short term. Information regarding lower limb venous repairs in the civilian setting indicate a high incidence of occlusion, particularly after complex repairs, but they did not influence limb salvage.[54–57] We have no information of results in the longer term and there are few, if any, studies in the literature.

On occasion, access to a bleeding common iliac vein may be difficult due to the overlying arteries. Under these circumstances the overlying iliac artery may be transected, and once the venous injury has been attended to, reanastomosed. This action is preferable to blind groping with clamps and compounding the situation by further lacerating the fragile iliac venous structures.

Important specific vascular scenarios

- Active continuing haemorrhage
- Retroperitoneal haematomas
- Mesenteric vessel injuries
- Juxtahepatic inferior vena cava injuries
- Portal vein injuries
- Concomitant arterial and colonic injuries

ABDOMINAL ARTERIAL INJURY IN THE PRESENCE OF CONTAMINATION

This scenario is applicable, for example, to the presence of sigmoid colon injury coupled with lower aortic or iliac artery disruption. In the presence of gross faecal contamination it would be unwise to perform arterial repair and in particular interposition grafting (see Chapters 18 and 25). Autogenous tissue tends to disintegrate once infected. Various statements regarding the 'resistance' to infection of certain prosthetic grafts is certainly not borne out by our own experience.[1,58]

In this group of patients it is advisable to ligate the major vessels within the area of contamination and to restore circulation by means of an extra-anatomical bypass. For example, in the presence of a contaminated aortic disruption axillobifemoral bypass may be entertained. Similarly, in the presence of an iliac injury, a femoro-femoral crossover bypass may be used. Once again

ingenuity may be tested in these complex circumstances. Ultimately in-line reconstruction is desirable, especially in young patients, but revision surgery should not be considered before an arbitrary period of about 6 months has elapsed to ensure that all sepsis has resolved.

ENDOVASCULAR TECHNIQUES

Interventional radiological procedures provide an attractive option in the stable patient with trauma involving inaccessible vessels. The value of embolotherapy has been demonstrated in non-essential vessels of the neck, pelvis and the extremities using thrombin pellets and spring coils. No major morbidity has been reported to date, although the literature on this subject is sparse.[34,59–62] Potential hazards with placement of occlusive devices close to the origins of tributaries from major parent vessels must be kept in mind, for instance, migration and distal embolisation of the occluding device.[34] With regard to embolotherapy for arteriovenous fistulae an essential principle is that both the arterial inflow and outflow component must be occluded. Failure to do this almost invariably results in recurrence of the fistula. With larger vessels there is also the danger of migration and embolisation into the venous system through the fistula itself.[34,59]

A specific indication in which embolotherapy has come into its own is in the treatment of traumatic haemobilia.[4,63–67] This usually follows penetrating trauma with the formation of pseudoaneurysms, often quite sizeable, on the branches of the hepatic artery which form fistulae with bile duct radicles.[67,68] In a recent series,[63] 23 patients with traumatic lesions were successfully treated using catheter occlusive techniques. There was one death not specifically related to the embolotherapy and the long term results on these patients have been excellent without recurrence of the problems. Liver function was not compromised.[63] In Fig. 36.11 the results of successful embolisation for traumatic haemobilia are shown. The patient was a

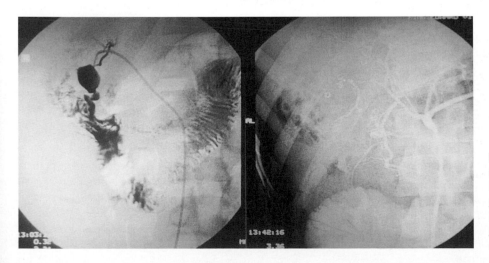

Figure 36.11 *Angiograms before and after embolotherapy to hepatic artery branches in a 29-year-old man presenting with haemobilia in the form of acute episodes of upper gastrointestinal bleeding 1 week after a gunshot wound*

29-year-old man who had sustained gunshot trauma to the liver and presented 2 weeks later with a gastrointestinal bleed. Other peripancreatic pseudoaneurysms with fistulation into the duodenum have been successfully treated by embolic occlusion.[69]

Renal arterial trauma is often associated with intraparenchymal pseudoaneurysms which present with significant haematuria and lend themselves well to selective segmental arterial occlusion. Although segmental infarction of the kidney occurs it does not have long term sequelae in terms of hypertension.[27] Deep-seated pulsatile haematomas associated with pelvic fractures usually arise from the disruption of branches of internal iliac or median sacral vessels and are best dealt with by selective occlusion.[1,59,62]

The role of stent placement in trauma is not well documented and, in general, experience is limited to small series.[70–76] In relation to penetrating trauma, most reports deal with lesions involving the subclavian and carotid vessels for which covered stents were used.[73,76–78] Of particular interest is their successful deployment in cases of arteriovenous fistula.[76]

Few reports exist of blunt trauma of the abdominal vessels. Self-expanding stents have been used successfully in dissections of the abdominal aorta and iliac vessels[70,77–79] (see Chapter 24). This modality of treatment, in selected cases, represents a very attractive alternative to open surgery. Medium term results with stents are good and no major acute complications have been reported. Follow-up ranged from 3 months to 4 years but long term evaluation is essential.

There are very few trauma centres in the world wherefrom meaningful experience with major abdominal vascular injuries can be reported. Much of this information is subjective and relates to experience gained retrospectively or with relatively few patients. Much of what is produced in this chapter is based on personal experience within the vascular service of the University of Natal Hospitals, South Africa. In general, the results remain poor for two main reasons: massive haemorrhage that is difficult to control and the high incidence of associated visceral injuries. Comparative data are difficult to obtain by virtue of the heterogeneous nature of the injuries in these patients, although various trauma scoring systems may assist in producing some evidence-based data.[37,38]

These injuries are probably the most challenging in trauma surgery.

Conclusions

Blunt abdominal vascular injuries are rather uncommon and largely caused by sudden deceleration and the avulsive and shearing forces involved in road traffic and other accidents. Penetrating abdominal vessel injuries inflicted by guns and knives occur much more frequently and early

fatality is attributable to torrential bleeding and delays in securing control due to the relative inaccessibility of some of the main arterial and venous trunks. Continuing haemorrhage and associated organ injury, including contamination from perforated bowel, represent a major challenge which demands timely and experienced intervention.

In the stable patient a CT scan, if necessary complemented by angiography, will assist in planning surgical management and in considering the likely value of endovascular therapies.

Wide exposure is crucial to gaining adequate access both for control and in executing the necessary repairs, a principle of special relevance when a retroperitoneal, possibly pulsatile, haematoma is revealed. In cases of severe trauma requiring prolonged surgery, it may be wiser to aim for 'damage control' as a first step followed by re-exploration and definitive vascular repair when a degree of stability has been achieved in the ICU. Injuries to the juxtahepatic IVC, mesenteric vessels and the portal venous system require specific operative manoeuvres and solutions.

Key references

Burch JM, Oritz V, Richardson RJ, *et al.* Abbreviated laparotomy and planned reoperation for critically ill patients. *Ann Surg* 1992; **215**: 476.

Ghimenton F, Thomson SR, Muckart DJJ, Burrows R. Abdominal content containment: practicalities and outcome. *Br J Surg* 2000; **87**: 106–9.

Hirsberg A, Walden R. Damage control for abdominal trauma. *Surg Clin North Am* 1997; **77**: 813–20.

Parodi JC, Schonolz C, Ferreira LM, Bergan J. Endovascular treatment of traumatic arterial lesions. *Ann Vasc Surg* 1999: **13**: 121–9.

Robbs JV, Costa M. Injuries to the great veins of the abdomen. *S Afr J Surg* 1984; **22**: 223–8.

REFERENCES

1 Robbs JV, Baker LW. *Cardiovascular Trauma. Current Problems in Surgery.* Chicago, IL: Year Book Medical Publishers, Inc, 1984: **XX1**(4).

2 Levien LL. Ballistics of bullet injury. In: Dudley H, Carter D and Russell RCG (eds). *Rob & Smith Operative Surgery. Trauma Surgery Part 1.* 4th edn. London: Butterworths.

3 Robbs JV, Carrim AA, Kadwa AM, Mars M. Traumatic arteriovenous fistula: Experience with 202 patients. *Br J Surg* 1994; **81**: 1296–9.

4 Moodley J, Singh B, Lalloo S, *et al.* Non-operative management of haemobilia. *Br J Surg* 2001; **88**: 1073–6.

5 Mokoena T, Robbs JV. Surgical management of mycotic aneurysms. *S Afr J Surg* 1991; **29**: 103–7.

6 Angorn IB. Segmental dearterialisation in penetrating renal trauma. *Br J Surg* 1977; **64**: 59.

7   Corr P, Abdool Carrim ATO, Robbs JV. Colour flow ultrasound in the detection of penetrating vascular injuries of the neck. *S Afr Med J* 1999; **89**: 644–6.

8   Burch JM, Oritz V, Richardson RJ, *et al.* Abbreviated laparotomy and planned reoperation for critically ill patients. *Ann Surg* 1992; **215**:476.

9   Moore EE. Staged laparotomy for the hypothermia, acidosis, and coagulopathy syndrome. *Am J Surg* 1996; **172**:405.

10 Abramson D, Scalea T, Hitchcock R, *et al.* Lactate clearance and survival following injury. *J Trauma* 1993; **35**: 584.

11 Davis J, Makerise R, Holbrook T, *et al.* Base deficit as an indicator of significant abdominal injury. *Ann Emerg Med* 1991; **20**: 842.

12 Moore E, Burch JM, *et al.* Staged physiological restoration and damage control Surgery. *World J Surg* 1998; **22**: 1184.

13 Ghimenton F, Thomson SR, Muckart DJJ, Burrows R. Abdominal content containment: practicalities and outcome. *Br J Surg* 2000; **87**: 106–9.

14 Martin R, Byrne M. Postoperative care and complications of damage control surgery. *Surg Clin North Am* 1998; **77**: 929.

15 Hirshberg A, Mattox K. Planned reoperation for severe trauma. *Ann Surg* 1995; **222**: 3–8.

16 Burrows R, Edington J, Robbs JV. A wolf in wolf's clothing – the abdominal compartment syndrome. *S Afr Med J* 1995; **85**: 46–8.

17 Meldrum DR, Moore FA, Moore EE. Selective management of the abdominal compartment syndrome: results of a prospective analysis. *Am J Surg* 1997; **174**: 667.

18 Ivatury RR, Diebel L, Porter JM, Simon RJ. Intra abdominal hypertension and the abdominal compartment syndrome. *Surg Clin North Am* 1997; **77**: 783–800.

19 Krohn IL, Harman PK, *et al.* The measurement of intra abdominal pressure as a criterion for abdominal exploration. *Ann Surg* 1984; **199**: 28.

20 Granchi TS, Liscum K. Logistics of damage control. *Surg Clin North Am* 1997; **77**: 921.

21 Madiba TE, Muckart DJJ. Retroperitoneal haematoma and related organ injury – management approach. *S Afr J Surg* 2001; **39**: 41–4.

22 Goins WA, Rodriquez A, Lewis J, *et al.* Retroperitoneal haematoma after blunt trauma. *Surg Gynecol Obstet* 1992; **174**: 281–90.

23 Kudsk KA, Sheldon GF. Retroperitoneal haematoma. In: Blaisdale FW, Trunkey DD (eds). *Abdominal Trauma*. New York: Thieme-Stratton, 1982: 279–93.

24 Streichen FM, Dargan EL, Pearlman DM, Weil PH. The management of retroperitoneal haematoma secondary to penetrating injuries. *Surg Gynecol Obstet* 1966; **123**: 581–91.

25 Costa M, Robbs JV. Management of retroperitoneal haematoma following penetrating trauma. *Br J Surg* 1985; **72**: 662–4.

26 Weil PH. Management of retroperitoneal trauma. *Curr Probl Surg* 1983; **20**: 539–620.

27 Angorn IB. Segmental de-arterialisation in penetrating renal trauma. *Br J Surg* 1977; **64**: 59–65.

28 Corriere JN, McAndrew JD, Bension GS. Intraoperative decision making in renal trauma surgery. *J Trauma* 1991; **31**: 1390–2.

29 Carroll PR, Klosterman PW, McAninch JW. Surgical management of renal trauma: analysis or risk factors, technique and outcome. *J Trauma* 1982; **22**: 285–90.

30 Feliciano DV. Management of traumatic retroperitoneal haematoma. *Ann Surg* 1990; **211**: 108–23.

31 Baumgartner F, White GH, White RA. Controversies in the management of retroperitoneal haemorrhage associated with pelvic fractures. *J Nat Med Assoc* 1995; **87**: 33–8.

32 Brotman S, Soderstorm CA, Oster-Granit M, *et al.* Management of severe bleeding in fractures of the pelvis. *Surg Gynecol Obstet* 1981; **153**: 823–6.

33 Hirsberg A, Walden R. Damage control for abdominal trauma. *Surg Clin North Am* 1997; **77**: 813–20.

34 Naidoo NM, Corr PD, Robbs JV. Angiographic embolisation in arterial trauma. *Eur J Vasc Endovasc Surg* 2000; **19**: 77–81.

35 Robbs JV. Vascular trauma – general principles of surgical management. In: Dudley H, Carter D and Russell RCG (eds). *Rob & Smith Operative Surgery. Trauma Surgery Part II*, 4th edn. London: Butterworths.

36 Fullen WD, Hunt J, Altemeier WA. The clinical spectrum of penetrating injury ton the superior mesenteric arterila circulation. *J Trauma* 1972; **12**: 656–64.

37 Asensio JA, Chahwan S, Hanpeter D, *et al.* Operative management and outcome of 302 abdominal vascular injuries. *Am J Surg* 199; **178**: 235–9.

38 Asensio JA, Britt LD, Borzotta A, *et al.* Multiinstitutinal experience with the management of superior mesenteric artery injuries. *J Am Coll Surg* 2001; **193**: 354–66.

39 McAnnich JW, Caroroll PR. Renal exploration after trauma. Indications and reconstructive techniques. *Urol Clin North Am* 1989; **16**: 203–11.

40 Robbs JV, Costa M. Injuries to the great veins of the abdomen. *S Afr J Surg* 1984; **22**: 223–8.

41 Degiannis E, Velmahos GC, Levy RD, *et al.* Penetrating injuries of the abdominal inferior vena cava. *Ann R Coll Surg Engl* 1996; **78**: 485–9.

42 Schrock T, Blaisdell FW, Mathewson C Jr. Management of blunt trauma to the liver and hepatic veins. *Arch Surg* 1968; **96**: 698–704.

43 Yellin AE, Chaffee CB, Donovan AJ. Vascular isolation in treatment of juxtahepatic venous injuries. *Arch Surg* 1971; **102**: 566–73.

44 Khaneja SC, Pizzi WF, Barie PS, Ahmed N. Management of penetrating juxtahepatic inferior vena cava injuries under total vascular occlusion. *J Am Coll Surg* 1977; **184**: 469–74.

45 Pachter HL, Spencer FC, Hofstetter RS, *et al.* Management of juxtahepatic venous injuries without an atriocaval shunt. *Surgery* 1986; **28**: 1433–8.

46 Sheldon GF, Lim RC, Yee ES, Petersen SR. Management of injuries to the porta hepatis. *Ann Surg* 1985; **202**: 539–45.

47 McFadden D, Lawlor BJ, Ali F. Portal vein injury. *Can J Surg* 1987; **30**: 91–2.

48 Jurkovich GJ, Hoyt DB, Moore FA, *et al.* Portal triad injuries. *J Trauma* 1995; **39**: 426–34.

49 Rao R, Ivatury MD, Manohar N, *et al.* Portal vein injuries-noninvasive follow up of venography

50 Bostwick J, Stone HH. Trauma to the portal venous system. *South Med J* 1976; **68**: 1369–72.

51 Stone HH, Fabian TC, Turkleson ML. Wounds of the portal system. *World J Surg* 1982; **6**: 335–41.

52 Pachter HL, Drager S, Godfrey N, *et al.* Traumatic injuries of the portal vein. The role of acute ligation. *Ann Surg* 1979; **189**: 383–5.

53 Petersen Sr, Sheldon GF, Lim RC Jr. Management of portal vein injuries. *J Trauma* 1979; **19**: 616–20.

54 Fish JC. Reconstruction of the portal vein. Case reports and literature review. *Am Surg* 1966; **32**: 474–8.

55 Nair R, Abdool Carrim ATO and Robbs JV. Gunshot injuries of the popliteal artery. *Br J Surg* 2000; **87**: 602–7.

56 Meyer J, Walsh J, Schuler J, *et al.* The early fate of venous repair after civilian vascular trauma. A clinical haemodynamic, and venographic assessment. *Ann Surg* 1987; **206**: 458–64.

57 Mullins RJ, Lucas CE, Ledgerwood AM. The natural history following venous ligation for civilian injuries. *J Trauma* 1980; **20**: 737–43.

58 Lau JM, Mattox KI, Beall AC, *et al.* Use of substitute conduits in traumatic vascular surgery. *J Trauma* 1977; **17**: 541.

59 Grace DM, Pitt DF, Gold RE. Vascular embolisation and occlusion by angiographic techniques as an aid or alternative to operation. *Surg Gynecol Obstet* 1976; **143**: 469–79.

60 Higashida RT, Halbach VV, Fong YT, *et al.* International neurovascular treatment of traumatic carotid and vertebral artery lesions. *Am J Radiol* 1989; **153**: 577–82.

61 Sclafani AP, Sclafani JA. Angiography and transcatheter embolisation of vascular injuries of the face and neck. *Laryngoscope* 1996; **106**: 168–73.

62 Robbs JV. Basic principles in surgical management of vascular trauma. In: Greenhalgh RM (ed). *Vascular and Endovascular Techniques*. Philadelphia, PA: WB Saunders, 1994.

63 Green MHA, Duell RM, Johnson CD, Jamieson NV. Haemobilia. *Br J Surg* 2001; **88**: 773–86.

64 Fagan EA, Allison DJ, Chadwick VS, Hodgson HJ. Treatment of haemobilia by selective arterial embolisation. *Gut* 1980; **21**: 541–4.

65 Mitchell SE, Schuman LS, Kaufman SL, *et al.* Biliary catheter drainage complicated by haemobilia: treatment by balloon embolotherapy. *Radiology* 1985; **157**: 645–52.

66 Sclafani SJA, Ben-Menachem Y. Embolotherapy in abdominal trauma. In: Neal MP Jr, Tisnado J Cho S-R, (eds). *Emergency Interventional Radiology*. Boston, MA: Little, Brown, 1989: 53–77.

67 Krige JEJ, Bornman PC, Terrblanche J. Liver trauma in 446 patients. *S Afr J Surg* 1997; **35**: 10–15.

68 Olsen WR. Late complications of central liver Injuries. *Surgery* 1982; **92**: 733–43.

69 Baum S, Athanasoulis CA, Waltman AC, Ring EJ. Gastrointestinal haemorrhage – angiographic diagnosis and control. *Adv Surg* 1973; **7**: 149.

70 Brandt MM, Kazanjian S, Wahl WL. The utility of endovascular stents in the treatment of blunt arterial injuries. *J Trauma* 2001; **51**: 901–5.

71 Parodi JC, Schonolz C, Ferreira LM, Bergan J. Endovascular treatment of traumatic arterial lesions. *Ann Vasc Surg* 1999: **13**: 121–9.

72 Ohki T, Veith FJ, Krass K, *et al.* Endovascular therapy for upper extremity injuries. *Semin Vasc Surg* 1998; **11**: 106–15.

73 Marin ML, Veith FJ, Synamon J, *et al.* Transluminal repair of penetrating vascular injury. *J Vasc Intervent Radiol* 1994; **5**: 592–4.

74 Reddy SG, Rothstein CP, Saker MB, *et al.* Placement of a PTFE covered wall stent through a 12Fr sheath for the exclusion of a common iliac artery aneurysm. *Cardiovasc Intervent Radiol* 1999; **22**: 152–4.

75 Strauss DC, Du Toit DF, Warren BL. Endovascular repair of occluded subclavian arteries following penetrating trauma. *J Endovasc Ther* 2001; **8**: 529–33.

76 Du Toit DF, Strauss DC, Blaszczyk M, *et al.* Endovascular treatment of penetrating of thoracic outlet arterial injuries. *Eur J Vasc Endovasc Surg* 2000; **19**: 489–95.

77 Althaus SJ, Keskey TS, Harker CP, Coldwell DM. Percutaneous placement of self-expanding stent for acute traumatic arterial injury. *J Trauma* 1996; **41**: 145–8.

78 Vernhet H, Marty-Ane C, Lesnik A, *et al.* Dissection of the abdominal aorta in blunt trauma; management by percutaneous stent. *Cardiovasc Intervent Radiol* 1997; **20**: 473–6.

79 Sternbergh WK 3rd, Conners MS 3rd, Ojeda MA, Money SR. Acute bilateral iliac artery occlusion secondary to blunt trauma – successful endovascular treatment. *J Vasc Surg* 2003; **38**: 589–92.

37

Limb Replantation

COLIN M MORRISON, MICHAEL D BRENNEN

THE PROBLEM

Replantation represents one of the pinnacles of reconstructive surgery, involving a wide range of tissues and surgical techniques. It has evolved from an experimental procedure in the 1950s and 1960s to a relatively common emergency operation performed throughout the world.[1–5] The first successful replantation of a traumatically severed limb was carried out by Malt at the Massachusetts General Hospital in 1962.[6] Two years later the first microsurgical replantation of a hand was performed by Chen in China.[7] Subsequent improvements in microvascular technique have extended the indications for replantation and now successful thumb, finger, hand, arm and leg replantations are routinely achieved.[2]

Most major amputations occur in the workplace and the causes vary according to local industry. Large machines, chain saws and farming equipment are capable of trapping and amputating an entire limb. In children an alarmingly high percentage of lower limb amputations are caused by lawn mowers. Studies have shown peaks of amputations occurring on a Monday and Thursday at 11 o'clock in the morning, a time at which employees become hungry, irritable and lose concentration.[4] Industrial educational programmes continue to have the greatest impact in reducing the occurrence of this devastating injury.

DEFINITIONS

- **Replantation** is the reattachment of a body part that has been completely amputated.
- **Revascularisation** is the restoration of circulation to a devascularised but not completely amputated part.

The distinction between replantation and revascularisation is important when discussing the methods and results of reattachment of amputated parts. The survival rates following revascularisation are generally better than those of replantation because adequate venous drainage often remains intact in the former.[1]

CLASSIFICATION

The condition of the amputated part and the stump can be classified according to the mechanism of injury, as this influences the management and subsequent outcome. The mechanism of injury determines the zone of tissue damage and remains one of the most critical components in patient evaluation.

Guillotine amputations divide the tissues sharply and create only a localised zone of injury. The outlook is favourable with a good chance of functional return

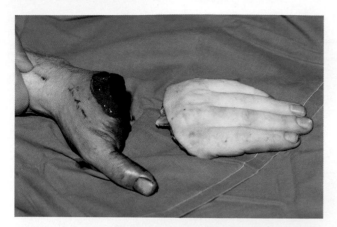

Figure 37.1   *A guillotine amputation at the mid-metacarpal level demonstrating the localised zone of injury*

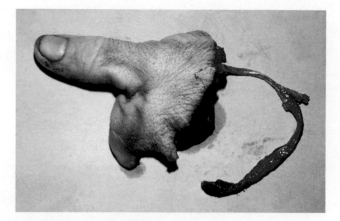

Figure 37.3   *An avulsion injury of the thumb. Note the tendon avulsed from a more proximal level*

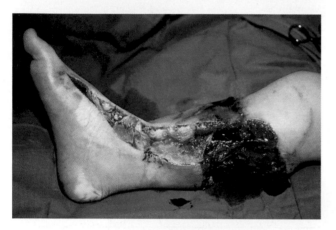

Figure 37.2   *A crush injury with a larger zone of tissue damage*

(Fig. 37.1). **Crushing amputations** result in a larger zone of tissue damage which may not be easily defined (Fig. 37.2). The amount of tissue damage is directly proportional to the size and weight of the object causing the amputation. Crushing amputations often have poor function even if they survive replantation.[1] **Avulsion amputations** are caused by a tearing force and there is usually extensive tissue injury with associated vascular damage extending well beyond the amputation site (Fig. 37.3). A corkscrew appearance of an artery, also known as 'the ribbon sign', suggests that an avulsion force has been applied and this segment of vessel should be excised and replaced by a vein graft.[8,9]

Crushing and avulsion amputations represent relatively poor prospects for successful replantation because extensive tissue resection is required to escape the zone of injury.

EMERGENCY TREATMENT

The patient should receive emergency treatment in accordance with the American College of Surgeons Advanced Trauma Life Support (ATLS) protocol. The immediate priorities are to establish an adequate airway, breathing and circulation. Major life-threatening injuries take precedence over the replantation of an amputated part (Fig. 37.4).[10]

A non-adherent dressing, a firm compression bandage and elevation of the stump are usually sufficient to control bleeding. The use of artery forceps and ligatures should be avoided as these may cause further vessel damage. Tetanus immunisation status should be determined and a booster given if indicated. Broad spectrum antibiotics should be administered if the wound is heavily contaminated or if the patient is diabetic or immunocompromised.

X-rays are taken of the amputated part and the limb suffering the amputation. X-rays of both are important in that they help to determine the best method of bone stabilisation. There may be missing bony fragments and this must be taken into consideration in subsequent management. The amputated part should be wrapped in damp, normal saline gauze and put into a sealed plastic bag. The sealed bag should then be placed in a container containing an ice-saline bath to maintain a temperature of between 4 and 10 °C (Fig. 37.5). *The amputated part should never be directly surrounded by ice or placed into hypotonic or hypertonic solution.*

All accident receiving centres should have telephone access to a replantation centre and should contact the surgeon on call as soon as the patient is admitted. If the patient is a suitable candidate for replantation, then both the patient and the amputated part should be transported to the replantation centre by the most expedient means possible.

Emergency treatment of a patient with a limb amputation

- Establish Airway, Breathing, Circulation
- Rule out other life-threatening injuries
- Control bleeding from the amputation stump

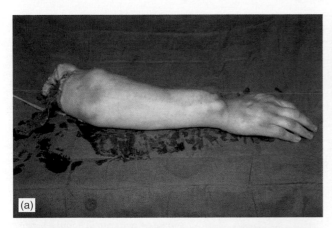

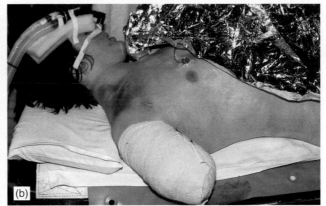

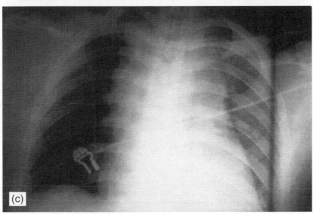

Figure 37.4 *(a) An avulsion amputation of the upper limb in a 22-year-old man caused by a piece of farming equipment. (b) Clinical examination showing marked bruising in the right supraclavicular fossa. (c) A chest X-ray demonstrating widening of the mediastinum. The subclavian artery had been avulsed, requiring operative intervention to control life-threatening haemorrhage*

- Check tetanus immunisation status/administer antibiotics
- X-ray both the amputated part and the limb suffering the amputation
- Cool the amputated part
- Contact the replantation centre

INDICATIONS FOR REPLANTATION

Replantation is not always indicated for patients with limb amputations (Fig. 37.6). In considering a patient for possible replantation the surgeon must weigh the systemic risks against the potential loss of the amputated part.[11] The main factor in patient selection is the potential for the replanted part to become an impediment and success must be measured in terms of the functional outcome rather than limb survival alone. Careful assessment is therefore essential before attempting this difficult and occasionally life-threatening procedure.[12]

All indications for replantation must take into account the status of the amputated part and the patient. Amputated parts that are severely crushed and those with multiple level injuries may have poor function even if they survive

replantation (see Chapter 33). The ischaemic tolerance of an amputated extremity is inversely related to the amount of muscle it contains. A proximal limb amputation can tolerate 4–6 hours of ischaemia before myonecrosis and the release of toxic metabolites results in acidosis, myoglobinuria, cardiogenic shock and renal failure (see Chapters 2 and 4). This is known as the **replantation syndrome**. Replantation of a limb is therefore not recommended if ischaemia time is longer than 6 hours although that period can be prolonged by proper cooling of the amputated part.[13,14]

The smaller vessels of infants make microsurgical repair more difficult but good nerve recovery often leads to excellent return of function. In the elderly, however, nerve recovery cannot be expected with any reliability and any attempt at replantation must be carefully considered. Successful replantation has been reported in an octogenerian, but the functional results were disappointing.[15] In patients with degenerative joint disease, postoperative oedema and splinting can cause stiffness of the whole hand.

Patients who have severe systemic injury or disease may not tolerate the anaesthesia and surgery well. Results with patients who have severe mental disease or suffer from substance abuse (see Chapter 44) may also be poor. Although the technical aspects of replantation in these individuals may

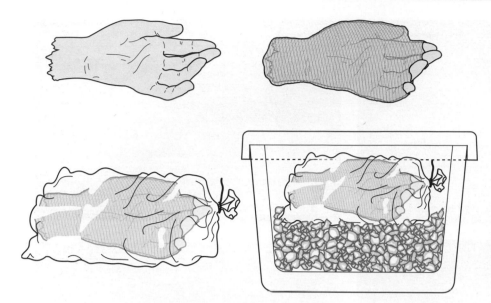

Figure 37.5 *The amputated part should be wrapped in damp gauze and put into a sealed plastic bag. The sealed bag should then be placed in a container containing an ice-saline bath*

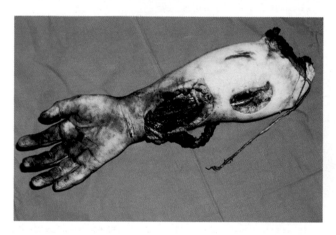

Figure 37.6 *A bomb blast injury of the upper limb. Due to the severe damage and multiple levels of injury replantation was not appropriate*

not present a problem, postoperative compliance is unpredictable and rehabilitation difficult (Fig. 37.7).[3]

The patient's sex, cultural background, occupation and personality may also influence the decision to attempt replantation. The only absolute contraindication to replantation is when the patient's associated injuries or pre-existing medical condition preclude a prolonged surgical procedure.

Replantation strategies

- Indications for limb replantation
  - Amputations at the level of the mid-metacarpal, wrist or distal forearm
  - Amputations at the level of the distal third of the leg
  - Amputations in children
  - Bilateral amputations

- Relative contraindications to limb replantation
  - Severe crush/avulsion injury
  - Multiple levels of injury
  - Prohibitive ischaemia time
  - Significant associated injuries or medical illness
  - Psychiatric instability

MANAGEMENT AT THE REPLANTATION CENTRE

Ideally every replantation centre should have two surgical teams available at all times. One team thoroughly debrides the amputated part under magnification and identifies the various structures while the other team prepares the patient for surgery.

The amputated part

The amputated part is immediately taken to the operating room, where it is cleaned using Hartmann solution. Under loupe magnification the part is carefully debrided and the vessels and nerves identified and labelled with sutures (Fig. 37.8). Labelling of these structures can be very helpful in the later stages of reconstruction when fatigue influences a surgeon's proficiency.[1] The amputated part is then kept cool until required later in the procedure.

The patient

Preparation for surgery should proceed without delay. Repeated preoperative examination of the injured limb

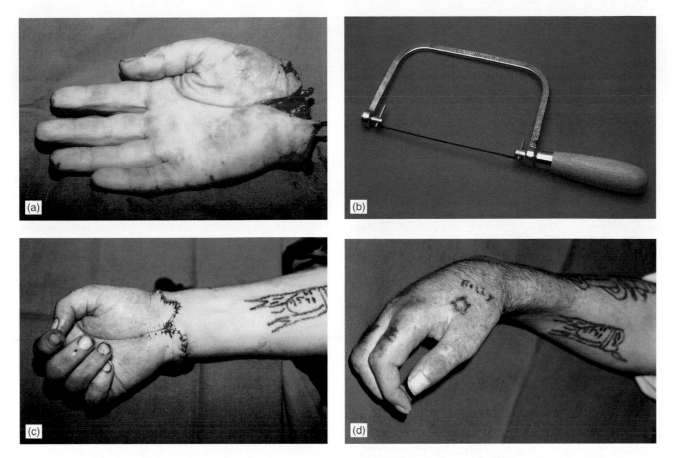

Figure 37.7   *(a, b) A guillotine amputation of the hand caused by a hacksaw. (c) Despite a good immediate postoperative result, the patient failed to comply with rehabilitation. (d) The poor functional result*

should be avoided, as this may increase the risk of vascular spasm. The patient is kept warm and intravenous solutions administered to maintain a hypervolaemic state. A chest X-ray and/or electrocardiogram (ECG) are taken if indicated by the patient's age and associated medical conditions. Blood is taken for a full blood count, blood type and cross-match as the patient may require a blood transfusion.

A thorough history and examination is completed before discussing treatment options and outcomes with the patient and his or her family. Consent should include permission for amputation, vein grafts, nerve grafts, skin grafts, bone grafts and possibly free flaps for soft tissue coverage.

PRINCIPLES OF ANAESTHESIA

Major limb replantation usually lasts many hours and requires general anaesthesia. This can be augmented by regional anaesthesia using indwelling catheters. These provide access for sympathetic nerve blockade aimed at vasodilatation of the limb and for giving continuous analgesia, reducing unnecessary postoperative pain.[16,17]

The patient should be placed on a well padded mattress, for comfort and protection of pressure points and an indwelling urinary catheter inserted. Particular care should be taken when positioning healthy limbs to avoid further injury. The patient should be kept warm and well hydrated. Active warming with a warm air blanket and fluid warmer helps maintain an optimum temperature of 38 °C. Good hydration is essential, allowing for blood loss at the time of injury and during the operative procedure. These measures reduce the incidence of thrombus formation at the vascular anastomosis by avoiding vasoconstriction and hypotension.

Haemoglobin levels should be monitored and maintained at 7–8 g/dL. A low blood viscosity helps promote flow across the site of the anastomosis. Transfusion should be avoided unless the patient becomes symptomatic from anaemia.

RECOMMENDED SURGICAL SEQUENCE FOR REPLANTATION OF AN AMPUTATED LIMB

- Identification of arteries, veins, nerves and tendons
- Wound debridement

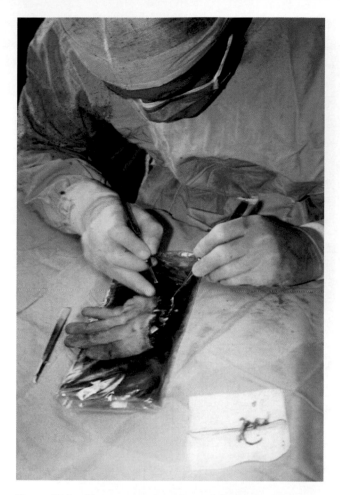

Figure 37.8 *The amputated part is carefully debrided. Vessels and nerves are identified and labelled with sutures*

- Bony stabilisation
- Vascular repair
- Tendon repair
- Nerve repair
- Soft tissue coverage

Identification of arteries, veins, nerves and tendons

Magnifying loupes are worn during the initial dissection and structures to be repaired are identified and marked with sutures. It is extremely important to take great care in isolating vital structures before wound debridement.

Wound debridement

The amputation stump is cleaned and debrided, removing all contaminated, non-viable tissue. Frayed tendon ends and bone fragments are also removed.

Forearm muscles receive most of their blood supply through their proximal half and, therefore, any muscle

present in a distal severed forearm must be carefully evaluated and excised if there is doubt about its future. Similarly, amputations at the metacarpal level require resection of distal avascular intrinsic muscles. The surgeon's haste to re-establish blood flow must not result in neglect of proper wound cleansing and is essential in preventing myonecrosis and subsequent infection.[1,13,14]

Bony stabilisation

Bones may be shortened during replantation to permit better bone contact in comminuted fractures, allow a tension free vascular anastomosis and nerve repair and enable better soft tissue coverage. Rigid fixation also protects the vascular repair and allows early mobilisation of the replanted limb. If possible, the periosteum is repaired to help bone healing and minimise adhesions to flexor and extensor tendons.

Amputations at the forearm level or higher usually result from violent injury in which a large zone of tissue has been affected. Consequently, the amount of bone resected is between 2 and 4 cm. For wrist replantations, however, as little bone as possible is resected in order to preserve mid-carpal or radiocarpal wrist motion. For amputations at the metacarpal level, interosseous wiring through four drill holes at 12, 3, 6 and 9 o'clock in each end of the bone permits two strands of 24 gauge wire to be placed perpendicular to each other. This provides stability, allowing early motion with less chance of angulation and non-union.

For major limb replantation, compression plating is the preferred method of providing bone fixation (Fig. 37.9). However this requires more time and bone exposure, possibly with further damage to soft tissue structures. If contamination is significant, an external fixator may be used to reduce the risk of infection (Fig. 37.10).[18]

Vascular repair

Most amputations of the upper extremity occur at the digit or hand level. Replantation of limbs proximal to the wrist involve greater muscle mass and the duration of avascularity of the detached part is more critical. In replantations proximal to the metacarpal level, arterial inflow must be re-established after initial debridement and rapid bone stabilisation.

If the ischaemia time is prolonged a shunt may be placed between the proximal and distal arteries and veins to perfuse the limb as quickly as possible. The Sundt and Pudenz ventriculoperitoneal shunts are commercially available, but any suitable silastic tubing may be employed as long as great care is exercised during its introduction.[19,20]

Muscles in the hand or forearm inevitably becomes oedematous following reperfusion and therefore prophylactic

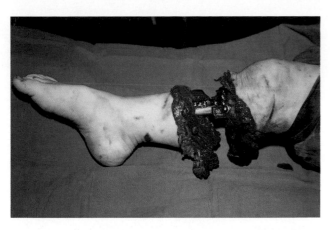

Figure 37.9 *A compression plate used for bony stabilisation*

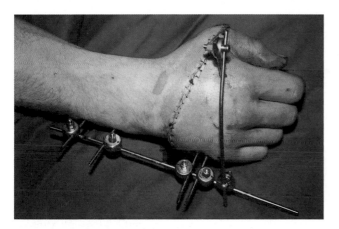

Figure 37.10 *An external fixator applied during replantation*

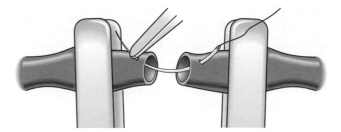

Figure 37.11 *Accurate suture placement is essential when performing the end-to-end anastomosis*

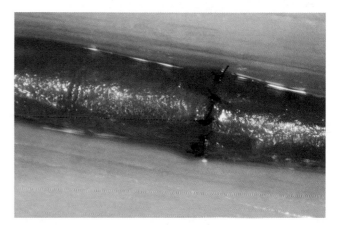

Figure 37.12 *Good arterial flow through the completed anastomosis*

fasciotomy of all muscle compartments in the amputated part should be performed prior to revascularisation. In addition, the carpal tunnel is released if the amputation is proximal to the wrist.

The limb should be re-arterialised before venous repair. Prior to the anastomosis, the tourniquet is released and the vessels debrided back to normal intima, ensuring pulsatile proximal vessel inflow. Small vascular clamps are used to hold both ends of the severed vessels in place and to control bleeding during repair. Loose adventitia is removed and the vessel ends are brought together by sliding the clamps on the holding bar. Heparinised saline solution is flushed into the lumen of the vessels with an irrigating catheter to cleanse and reduce the tendency for platelets to adhere to the intima and anastomotic site. Closed vessel-dilating forceps are inserted into the artery or vein and gently opened, stretching the vessel. This gentle dilatation helps to prevent spasm of the muscle within the vessel wall at the site of vessel repair.

The vascular anastomosis is performed under the operating microscope or loupe magnification. An end-to-end anastomosis is performed enabling accurate opposition of vessels (Fig. 37.11). Fine nylon sutures are used for vessel repair against a yellow polyethylene background to help in localisation of suture placement (Fig. 37.12).[21] *It is imperative to avoid accidentally picking up and suturing together opposite walls.*

The field is kept moist with saline to prevent tissue desiccation. If a tension-free vascular anastomosis cannot be performed an interposition vein graft may be used. Vein grafts are reversed when used for arterial repair so that any valves within the graft do not impede blood flow. The vascular clamps are opened on completion of the anastomosis to allow the release of toxic metabolites into the surgical field and prevent their accumulation in the systemic circulation. Ideally, two superficial veins should be repaired for every arterial anastomosis to maintain a balanced circulation.

Tendon repair

Primary end-to-end repair gives the best opportunity for tendons to regain function. This should be performed without undue tension, after the necrotic or damaged tendon ends have been resected.

Early postoperative mobilisation promotes healing and reduces the tendency of tendons to become adherent to the surrounding tissues. A four strand core suture of 4-0 nylon or braided polyester, together with a 6-0 nylon epitendinous suture provides sufficient strength to allow a flexor tendon to be mobilised, with only a small risk of rupture at the repair site. Extensor tendons only require a core suture but an epitendinous suture may be added to tidy up the tendon ends.

The repaired tendon ends should lie in a healthy soft tissue bed and have good skin and subcutaneous tissue cover. Divided muscle bellies are repaired with 4-0 polyglactin. If tendon damage is too great to allow primary repair a secondary tendon graft or a tendon transfer will be required to restore movement.

Nerve repair

The immediate survival of a replanted part is determined by the success of the vascular anastomosis, but the eventual function of a limb depends on the quality of nerve regeneration. It is vital to identify the extent of nerve damage and to resect the proximal and distal ends back to microscopically normal tissue. In clean cut amputations, primary nerve repair may be possible, especially in cases where bone shortening has been performed. Tension must be avoided and if the nerve cannot be sutured without tension then nerve grafting is required. This can be carried out as a primary procedure in very clean wounds but is normally performed as a secondary operation, when nerve ends are trimmed with a sharp blade and repaired with epineural sutures under magnification.

Nerve regeneration occurs at a rate of 1 mm/day. As a result, there will be no sensory recovery in the fingertips for 9–12 months in amputations at the wrist and for 12–18 months in forearm amputations. Coarse sensation will return but the quality of sensory recovery will be far from normal on formal testing. The results are generally much better in children.

The small muscles of the hand are responsible for fine manipulative movements, positioning and some power but it is rare to get any small muscle recovery following replantation, except in children. Return of forearm function should be expected but secondary surgery, in the form of tendon grafts or tendon transfers, may be required.

Soft tissue coverage

The final and often most important issue in limb replantation is management of the skin and subcutaneous tissue loss. Many surgeons believe that this should be achieved at the time of the first procedure, as exposed bone and neurovascular structures fare poorly if not covered with well vascularised tissue.

If possible, the skin is loosely approximated to prevent vascular constriction when postoperative oedema occurs.

However, local tissue is rarely available for coverage and regional or free flaps may be needed. A split skin graft is usually not appropriate.

Muscle is the best choice for these wounds in terms of vascularity and resistance to infection and adequate tissue should be transferred to fill dead space and afford coverage of deeper structures. The muscle can be raised as a myocutaneous flap or separately and covered with a split skin graft taken from a suitable donor area. The pectoralis major or latissimus dorsi can be very useful as pedicled flaps for coverage of the upper arm but for most forearm injuries a free flap will be required. The surgeon can choose whatever muscle with which he or she is most comfortable.

POSTOPERATIVE MANAGEMENT

Initial dressing

The replanted limb is immobilised to protect the arterial, venous and nerve repairs. A bulky dressing is applied to splint and protect the limb and to maintain it in a position which enhances later mobility. The ideal position of the hand is with the metacarpophalangeal joints in 70 degree flexion, the interphalangeal joints in a neutral position and the thumb in maximum palmar abduction. If this position compromises the vascular repair, an alternative position as close to this ideal as possible should be used. After 48 hours, the thumb and fingers are allowed free to permit early active mobilisation.

Monitoring the circulation

Hypovolaemia and hypotension are prevented by vigorous hydration and the continuous use of adequate analgesia. Vasoconstriction is prevented by keeping the patient warm and by avoiding medication such as caffeine and nicotine. The haemoglobin and electrolyte status are monitored and a blood transfusion administered if required.

Clinical monitoring is the mainstay of postoperative evaluation of a replanted part. The colour, capillary refill, temperature and tissue turgor are carefully and frequently recorded with observations every 30–60 minutes. Arterial insufficiency is manifested by a pale, cool extremity with absent capillary refill and poor tissue turgor. Venous insufficiency is manifested by a congested extremity that has increased tissue turgor and extremely rapid capillary refill.

Needle puncture of the skin is also helpful for assessing circulation. Bright, brisk bleeding is observed if the arterial and venous systems are adequate. If arterial insufficiency is present, the wound will hardly bleed at all. If venous congestion is present, rapid, copious bleeding of dark, deoxygenated blood is seen.

Arterial insufficiency of a limb is treated by lowering it and placing it on a pillow. Venous congestion is treated by elevation, loosening of the dressing and/or removal of sutures to relieve constriction of the vascular repair. *If there is no early response to these measures then re-exploration and revision of the vascular anastomoses should be performed.* Clinical experience has underlined the vital importance of early re-explorations when faced with circulatory complications.

MAINTAINING PASSIVE MOVEMENTS AND ENCOURAGING ACTIVE MOVEMENTS

Once replantation has been successfully accomplished and maintained, the rehabilitation programme can proceed. This begins after 48 hours and the focus is directed towards early control of oedema, passive range of motion and progressive strengthening while avoiding the common problem of joint contracture.

COMPLICATIONS

Early complications include vascular thrombosis leading to circulatory problems, bleeding and infection.[22] Careful postoperative monitoring is necessary to detect early circulatory problems. If initial conservative measures do not restore the circulation rapidly then an early return to theatre is necessary to inspect and re-do the vascular anastomosis. Bleeding may be controlled by elevation but persistent bleeding may also necessitate a return to theatre to find and control the bleeding vessels.

Infection is the main complication of limb replantation. If thorough debridement has not been performed there may be skin necrosis or necrosis of muscle. Antibiotics are not routinely used postoperatively but should be given at the earliest signs of cellulitis and pyrexia. Deeper infection may be due to unrecognised muscle necrosis and further radical debridement may be necessary to eliminate dead tissue and bring infection under control. Such radical debridement may create a situation where flap surgery is needed to maintain soft tissue cover for the anastomosis.

The later complications of limb replantation include those normally expected after trauma to the individual tissues. Fibrosis in the skin and subcutaneous tissues may lead to scar contracture. The tendons may rupture or become adherent. Neuromas in-continuity may develop and cause exquisitely tender spots. Nerve recovery may fail to progress. Non-union and osteomyelitis may require further bone resection and perhaps bone grafting. Painful syndromes may develop and cold intolerance in the replanted part is common.[23]

Complications of limb replantation

- Early
  - Vascular thrombosis
  - Bleeding
  - Infection
  - Loss of the part
- Late
  - Scar contracture
  - Tendon rupture
  - Neuroma
  - Non-union
  - Osteomyelitis
  - Pain
  - Cold intolerance

SECONDARY SURGERY

O'Brien[24] taught that all structures should be repaired primarily to reduce the necessity for secondary surgery. This is usually possible in guillotine or very minimal crush injuries, especially if some bone shortening is performed. Secondary surgery, however, is almost always necessary in major limb replantation.[25] It may not be possible to repair all tendons primarily and secondary tendon repair, grafting or transfer may be needed to restore active movement to a particular joint.

Unless the extent of nerve injury can be accurately assessed it is unwise to perform primary nerve repair. A delayed primary or early secondary repair may be possible if the extent of nerve damage is limited. For larger nerve defects cable grafting, using for example the sural nerve, may be required.

The passive movements of joints adjacent to the site of replantation may be restricted by scar contracture. Release of these will improve the range of movement. Release may require local, distant or free flap coverage to prevent recurrence. Areas of non-union and bone infection are best treated by resection and bone grafting. Arthrodesis may be needed for joints which are severely damaged and/or painful.

REPLANTATION OF THE LOWER LIMB

Amputation of the lower limb is usually secondary to severe trauma and is commonly associated with extensive local tissue destruction and injury to other sites. As a result, there have been few cases of successful outcome following replantation. Magee and Parker are credited with performing the first foot replantation in 1969[26] and sporadic reports have followed.[27–32] Restoration of function remains the primary goal and favourable conditions are a young,

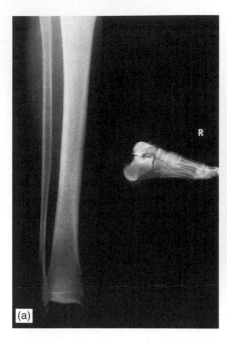
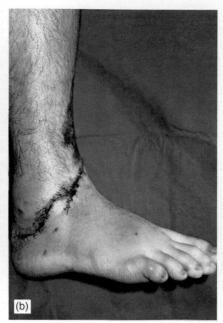
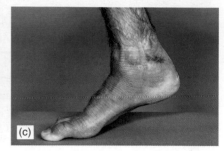

Figure 37.13 *Complete amputation of the foot in a 19-year-old man following a motorcycle accident. (a) X-ray of the limb and the amputated part. (b) Successful replantation. (c) Good return of function*

healthy patient, with a sharp amputation, located in the distal third of the leg (Fig. 37.13).[5]

The contraindications to replantation mirror those of the upper extremity and include life-threatening associated injuries, a crushing or avulsion force and age or illness which precludes a prolonged operation. Due to the larger mass of muscle, myonecrosis and renal failure may follow a significant ischaemic period in this group of patients and particular attention should be paid to this issue.[33] In clinical practice, ideal conditions are rarely encountered and proper patient selection remains the key factor.

CLINICAL RESULTS

Revascularisation of an amputated part should be expected in approximately 80 per cent of patients. Function, however, is the only real measure of success and is usually determined by the quality of sensory recovery. Based on this, success can often be predicted by the level of the amputation (Table 37.1).[3]

A hand replanted from the mid-metacarpal level to the distal wrist offers functional return superior to available prostheses (Fig. 37.14).[12,13,34–36] More proximal amputations need to be considered carefully, as the risk of complications increases while the functional return decreases. At the level of the mid-forearm, reinnervation of the small muscles of the hand is unlikely and this may compromise later performance. At the level of the arm or shoulder, the results are generally poor and the main goal is often the

Table 37.1 *Survival rates following limb replantation*

Authors	Year	Level	Per cent survival
Wang et al.[39]	1981	Upper and lower limb	77
Tamai[4]	1982	Upper limb	94
Wood and Cooney[25]	1986	Above-elbow	71
Daigle and Kleinhert[40]	1991	Upper and lower limb in children	87
Axelrod and Buchler[41]	1991	Upper limb	93

preservation of a functioning elbow for later prosthesis fitting.[37]

Replantation of the lower limb remains controversial. The available lower limb prostheses makes amputation less of a functional problem compared with the upper extremity. The larger mass of leg muscle also tolerates ischaemia poorly, and without adequate sensory recovery, the skin of the foot is at risk of recurrent breakdown.

In children, it is generally believed that replantation should be attempted with almost any part. Viability rates are lower but the functional results are much better than in adults.[36]

THE FUTURE

Composite tissue allotransplantation represents the next frontier in replantation surgery. The recent hand transplants

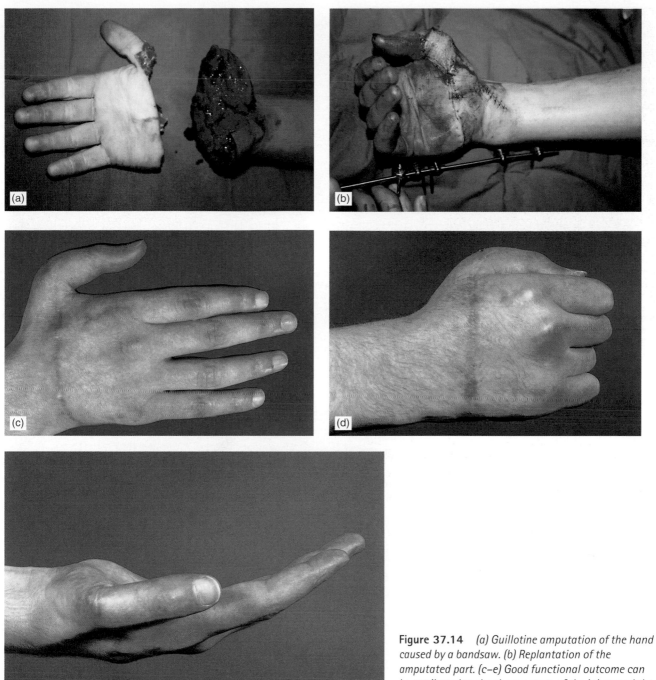

Figure 37.14 *(a) Guillotine amputation of the hand caused by a bandsaw. (b) Replantation of the amputated part. (c–e) Good functional outcome can be attributed to the sharp nature of the injury and the mid-metacarpal level*

performed in Lyon, France and Louisville, KY, USA, have stimulated public interest and heightened the debate about such procedures.

Current replantation literature confirms that significant functional return can be achieved following a hand transplant, provided that the appropriate patient is selected and the procedure and rehabilitation properly implemented. However, composite tissue transplant studies in animal models demonstrate a lack of long term survival data and there is uncertainty about the risk–benefit ratio of lifelong immunosuppression given the potential for organ failure, opportunistic infection and malignancy.

Future successful composite tissue allotransplantation will depend on modalities to induce host tolerance such as major histocompatability complex matching or induction of transplant tolerance by exposing the recipient immune system to donor marrow elements before its maturity.[38]

Conclusions

The primary goal of replantation is to restore function. The surgical team tries to produce a well perfused replanted part which is supple, sensate and capable of active movement. Careful case selection is important. Good results will be achieved with clean amputations relatively distally in the limb in young patients. Crush or avulsion injuries give less favourable results. More proximal amputations usually give poorer functional results. Recovery of sensation in elderly patients is poor and this will compromise the outcome. Replantation in infants is technically difficult but gives excellent results.

As well as the microvascular surgery, skeletal fixation, tendon repair, nerve suture and healthy skin cover must all be given meticulous attention. Postoperative monitoring, dressings and wound care requires specialist nursing and medical care. Physiotherapy and occupational therapy are essential, especially in the upper limb. The patient may also need social and even psychological support.

Good results can be achieved in amputations at or distal to mid-forearm level. The thumb should always be considered for replantation, as should multiple finger amputations. Single finger amputations require special indications for replantation. The aesthetic value of replantation should not be underestimated. Many patients are very pleased to have the part restored even though it is of little functional value.

The indications for replantation in the lower limb, especially with distal amputations is very limited as below-knee prostheses are functionally very good. Replantation should also be considered in scalp avulsions and in amputations of specialised parts such as the ear, nose and penis.

Key references

Goldner RD, Urbaniak JR. Replantation. In Green DP, Hotchkiss RN, Pederson WC (eds). *Green's Operative Hand Surgery*, 4th edn. New York: Churchill Livingstone, 1999: 1139–57.

Kleinert HE, Jablon M, Tsai TM. An overview of replantation and results of 347 replants in 245 patients. *J Trauma* 1980; **20**: 390–8.

Pederson WC. Replantation. *Plast Reconstr Surg* 2001; **107**: 823–41.

Tamai S. Twenty years' experience of limb replantation – review of 293 upper extremity replants. *J Hand Surg* 1982; **7**: 549–56.

Walton RL, Rothkopf DM. Judgment and approach for management of severe lower extremity injuries. *Clin Plast Surg* 1991; **18**: 525–3.

REFERENCES

1 Goldner RD, Urbaniak JR. Replantation. In Green DP, Hotchkiss RN, Pederson WC (eds). *Green's Operative Hand Surgery*, 4th edn. New York: Churchill Livingstone, 1999: 1139–57.

2 Kleinert HE, Jablon M, Tsai TM. An overview of replantation and results of 347 replants in 245 patients. *J Trauma* 1980; **20**: 390–8.

3 Pederson WC. Replantation. *Plast Reconstr Surg* 2001; **107**: 823–41.

4 Tamai S. Twenty years' experience of limb replantation – review of 293 upper extremity replants. *J Hand Surg* 1982; **7**: 549–56.

5 Walton RL, Rothkopf DM. Judgment and approach for management of severe lower extremity injuries. *Clin Plast Surg* 1991; **18**: 525–3.

6 Malt RA, McKhann CF. Replantation of severed arms. *JAMA* 1964; **189**: 716–22.

7 Chen Z-W, Meyer VE, Kleinert HE, Beasley RW. Present indications and contraindications for replantation as reflected by long-term functional results. *Orthop Clin North Am* 1981; **12**: 849–70.

8 van Beek AL, Kutz JE, Zook EG. Importance of the ribbon sign, indicating unsuitability of the vessel, in replanting a finger. *Plast Reconstr Surg* 1978; **61**: 32–5.

9 Cooney WP III. Revascularization and replantation after upper extremity trauma: experience with interposition artery and vein grafts. *Clin Orthop Rel Res* 1978; **137**: 227–34.

10 King C, Kuzon WM. Replantation. In: Jebson PJL, Kasdan ML (eds) *Hand Secrets*. Philadelphia, PA: Hanley & Belfus, 1998: 229–33.

11 Sood R, Bentz ML, Shestak KC, Browne EZ. Jr. Extremity replantation. *Surg Clin North Am* 1991; **71**: 317–29.

12 Hales P, Pullen D. Hypotension and bleeding diatheses following attempted arm replantation. *Anaesth Intensive Care* 1982; **10**: 359–61.

13 Goldner RD, Urbaniak JR. Indications for replantation in the adult upper extremity. *Occup Med* 1989; **4**: 525–538.

14 Goldner RD, Nunley JA. Replantation proximal to the wrist. *Hand Clin* 1992; **8**: 413–25.

15 Leung PC. Hand replantation in an 83-year-old woman – the oldest replantation?. *Plast Reconstr Surg* 1979; **64**: 416–18.

16 Berger A, Tizian C, Zenz M. Continuous plexus blockade for improved circulation in microvascular surgery. *Annals of Plastic Surgery* 1985; **14**: 16–19.

17 Matsuda M, Kato N, Hosoi M. Continuous brachial plexus block for replantation in the upper extremity. *Hand* 1982; **14**: 129–34.

18 Tupper JW. Techniques of bone fixation and clinical experience in replanted extremities. *Clin Orthop Rel Res* 1978; **133**: 165–8.

19 Barros D'Sa AAB. The rationale for arterial and venous shunting in the management of limb vascular injuries. *Eur J Vasc Surg* 1989; **3**: 471–4.

20 Barros D'Sa AAB, Moorehead RJ. Combined arterial and venous intraluminal shunting in major trauma of the lower limb. *Eur J Vasc Surg* 1989; **3**: 577–81.

21 Rasheed T, Gordon D. Plastic innovations: background material for microvascular anastomosis. *Br J Plast Surg* 1999; **52**: 159.

22 Strauch B, Greenstein B, Goldstein R, Liebling RW. Problems and complications encountered in replantation surgery. *Hand Clin* 1986; **2**: 389–99.

23 Russell RC, O'Brien B McCMacLeod AM, *et al.* The late functional results of upper limb revascularization and replantation. *J Hand Surg (Am)* 1984; **9**: 623–33.

24 O'Brien BM. Replantation and reconstructive microvascular surgery. *Ann R Coll Surg Engl* 1976; **58**: 171–82.

25 Wood MB, Cooney WP III. Above elbow limb replantation: Functional results. *J Hand Surg (Am)* 1986; **11**: 682–7.

26 Magee HR, Parker WR. Replantation of the foot: results after two years. *Med J Aust* 1972; **1**: 751–5.

27 Chen ZW, Zeng BF. Replantation of the lower extremity. *Clin Plast Surg* 1983; **10**: 103–13.

28 Fukui A, Inada Y, Sempuku T, Tamai S. Successful replantation of a foot with satisfactory recovery: A case report. *J Reconstr Microsurg* 1988; **4**: 387–90.

29 Lesavoy MA. Successful replantation of lower leg and foot, with good sensibility and function. *Plast Reconstr Surg* 1979; **64**: 760–5.

30 Morrison WA, O'Brien BM, MacLeod AM. Major limb replantation. *Orthop Clin North Am* 1977; **8**: 343–8.

31 Tsai TM. Successful replantation of a forefoot. *Clin Orthop Rel Res* 1979; **139**: 182–4.

32 Usui M, Minami M, Ishii S. Successful replantation of an amputated leg in a child. *Plast Reconstr Surg* 1979; **63**: 613–17.

33 Gayle LB, Lineaweaver WC, Buncke GM, *et al.* Lower extremity replantation. *Clin Plast Surg* 1991; **18**: 437–47.

34 Blomgren I, Blomqvist G, Ejeskar A, *et al.* Hand function after replantation or revascularization of upper extremity injuries: a follow-up study of 21 cases operated on 1979–1985 in Goteborg. *Scand J Plast Reconstr Surg* 1988; **22**: 93–101.

35 Meyer VE. Hand amputations proximal but close to the wrist joint: prime candidates for reattachment (long term functional results). *J Hand Surg (Am)* 1985; **10**: 989–91.

36 Saies AD, Urbaniak JR, Nunley JA, *et al.* Results after replantation and revascularization in the upper extremity in children. *J Bone Joint Surg (Am)* 1994; **76**: 1766–76.

37 Graham B, Adkins P, Tsai TM, *et al.* Major replantation versus revision amputation and prosthetic fitting in the upper extremity: a late functional outcomes study. *J Hand Surg (Am)* 1998; **23**: 783–91.

38 Lee A.WP, Mathes DW. Hand transplantation: pertinent data and future outlook. *J Hand Surg* 1999; **24**: 906–13.

39 Wang SH, Young KF, Wei JN. Replantation of severed limbs – clinical analysis of 91 cases. *J Hand Surg* 1981; **6**: 31–8.

40 Daigle JP, Kleinhert JM. Major limb replantation children. *Microsurgery* 1991; **12**: 221–31.

41 Axelrod TS, Buchler U. Severe complex injuries to the upper extremity: revascularization and replantation. *J Hand Surg* 1991; **16A**: 574–84.

Iatrogenic Injuries

38

Injuries of Arterial Catheterisation

DAVID BERGQVIST, CHRISTER LJUNGMAN

THE PROBLEM

Arterial catheterisation or puncture may cause bleeding, occlusion or stenosis due to thromboembolism or intimal injury, arteriovenous fistula, pseudoaneurysm, arterial wall dissection, and on occasion a foreign body may be left in the arterial system. Toxic injury or allergic reaction caused by contrast media will not be discussed here neither will we review infectious complications.

AETIOLOGY AND TYPES OF INJURY

Haemorrhage

Haemorrhage is common after arterial puncture and is usually localised and of minor degree. Major haemorrhage may be caused by perforation of the back wall of the artery (Fig. 38.1), which is difficult to control with manual pressure, simply because retroperitoneal counterpressure cannot be applied. Such haemorrhage may cause hypovolaemia and shock.

Factors contributing to excessive blood loss are multiple punctures, introducers of large diameter and anticoagulant/antiplatelet therapy. Another factor of importance is puncture through a calcified vessel wall with its lack of contractility. Haemorrhage may also be due to perforation by the tip of the catheter, a risk which is particularly marked in infants whose arteries are fragile.

Thromboembolism

Thromboembolism is the result of two main processes. The first mechanism has to do with the formation of platelet

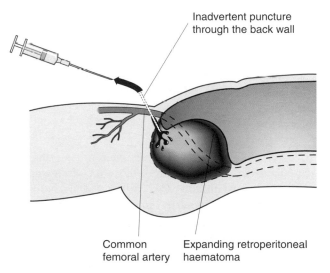

Figure 38.1 *Inadvertent puncture through the back wall of the common femoral artery causing retroperitoneal haemorrhage*

aggregates and fibrin on the surface of the catheter and in the holes on the catheter tip. At catheter pull-out, the fibrin sheath is washed off on the inner side of the vessel, forming a thrombotic plug. This thrombus may occlude the artery, but it usually forms a wall-adherent, non-occlusive thrombus. The thrombus may propagate locally or embolise distally. Heparinisation significantly decreases the amount of thrombotic material on the catheter.[1] The amount of thrombus formed depends on the type of material from which the catheter is made, the length and width of the catheter as well as the duration of catheterisation. Thrombotic material in the holes on the tip of the catheter may embolise if the catheter is flushed leading to occlusion of peripheral arteries and a clinical picture of microembolism.

The second mechanism is intimal rupture and dissection, or dislodgement of thrombotic or atherosclerotic material, either at the place of catheter insertion or caused by the tip of the catheter. Intimal dissection may bring about immediate occlusion or progressive formation of thrombus, resulting in occlusion or embolisation after some time. Fragmentation of the tip of the catheter or guidewire may also occur and in turn these parts of the catheter may embolise.

Arteriovenous fistula

Arteriovenous fistulae are caused by simultaneous perforation of an artery and adjacent vein and these have been well documented.[2–5]

Pseudoaneurysm

Pseudoaneurysms are found around the puncture hole in the artery. They are usually small and are particularly prone to develop if there has been excessive bleeding, and especially when patients are on anticoagulants or antiplatelet drugs.[6,7] The risk increases with the complexity of the procedure.[8] They may occlude spontaneously by progressive development of thrombosis,[9–12] especially those with small flow volumes.[13] The longer the pseudoaneurysm neck the greater the chances that it will close spontaneously.[14] Infected or mycotic aneurysms may occur when the infected tip of a catheter perforates the intima (see Chapters 18 and 44).

Dissection

Dissection of the arterial wall occurs mainly after translumbar puncture or catheterisation of the aorta, when contrast medium is injected intramurally.[15] Intestinal and renal circulation may be compromised by intramural contrast medium.

Types of catheter injury

- Haemorrhage
- Thrombosis – occlusive, non-occlusive, embolic
- Arteriovenous fistula
- Pseudoaneurysm
- Dissection

INCIDENCE

Major complications are usually 'complications threatening life, limb, or the visceral integrity of the patient, or requiring subsequent surgical intervention for diagnosis or treatment, or significantly prolonging the hospital stay of the patient'.[16] Minor complications are 'asymptomatic complication(s) of arteriography detected radiographically or a clinically insignificant transient symptom or sign not endangering the patient or requiring further evaluation'.[16]

A pragmatic way of defining major complications is to include those requiring surgical intervention and those ending in fatality. The registered frequency of these complications obviously depends on the definition and whether the study is prospective or retrospective.

Lang surveyed 11 402 procedures of retrograde percutaneous transfemoral arteriography (Seldinger procedure), collecting data by questionnaires completed by 300 hospital radiologists.[17] There were 81 (0.7 per cent) complications, including thrombosis, requiring surgical intervention, six of which resulted in limb loss. There were five cases of guidewire or catheter breakage and seven cases of major haematoma. Massive retroperitoneal haemorrhage from perforation of a pelvic artery occurred in three cases. These results were compared with those from a survey of 3250 patients undergoing translumbar aortography by Lang,[18] which resulted in only 11 major complications (0.3 per cent). The mortality in the translumbar group, however, was higher (0.28 per cent v 0.06 per cent).

In a survey in 1981, Hessel and co-workers[19] reported on complications arising from 118 591 angiographic examinations from a large number of hospitals, comparing transfemoral, translumbar and transaxillary approaches. The overall complication rates was 1.7 per cent for the transfemoral group, 2.9 per cent for the translumbar group and 3.3 per cent for the transaxillary group. Thirty deaths were reported, with the highest number in the transaxillary group and the lowest in the transfemoral group. In the transaxillary group there were also more neurological complications, including seizures and hemiplegia, but also more cases of haemorrhage, haematoma in the neurovascular sheath, arterial obstruction and pseudoaneurysm. In the translumbar group there were more cases of bleeding and of extraluminal contrast injection. The incidence of puncture-site thrombosis was 0.1 per cent in the transfemoral group, compared with 0.6 per cent in the transaxillary group and 0 per cent in the translumbar group. Emboli occurred in 0.1 per cent of the transfemoral group, 0.1 per cent of the transaxillary group and 0 per cent of the translumbar group. The complication rate was more than four times higher in hospitals doing fewer than 200 angiographies (2.7 per cent) than in those doing more than 800 (0.6 per cent).

There has been an obvious trend during the past 20 years of a decreasing incidence of complications reported after arterial punctures and catheterisations, as suggested by a series of prospective studies.[20] The translumbar technique, although used less frequently today, has also been characterised by a decreased incidence of complications.

The site of catheterisation is of decisive importance in the incidence and type of complication. Several reports have confirmed a high frequency of complications following catheterisation of the axillary artery. Brachial plexus paralysis could be eliminated by meticulous technique and by avoiding delay in surgical exploration once paresis has occurred.

The brachial artery has been used as an alternative to axillary artery catheterisation to avoid the risk of damage

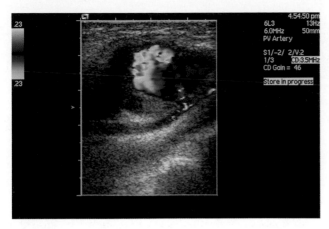

Figure 38.2 *Ultrasound image of pseudoaneurysm of the common femoral artery after percutaneous transluminal coronary angioplasty. The neck of the pseudoaneurysm and the common femoral artery are demonstrated*

to the brachial plexus. These procedures, as with catheterisation of other peripheral arteries, can be done either by the cut-down technique using an open arteriotomy or by a percutaneous technique more commonly used in recent years. The risk of brachial artery occlusion is high, whatever technique is used for brachial artery catheterisation. This is probably due to the fact that the artery is narrow and that the upper limb arteries are more liable to spasm than those of the lower limb. The exact incidence of brachial artery occlusion is unknown, since many patients remain asymptomatic. Gangrene of the fingers is rare, and is probably most often due to peripheral embolic occlusions.

In operating rooms and intensive care units radial artery cannulation is often used to permit repeated arterial blood sampling and pressure recording. The cannulation can be performed either percutaneously or via an open arteriotomy. The catheter is often allowed to remain in place for several days, contrary to most other peripheral artery catheters. Thrombosis in the radial artery, noted as a disappearance of the radial pulse, occurs frequently but clinical symptoms of persisting finger ischaemia are rare. In the majority of patients the thrombosis disappears after removal of the catheter. Nevertheless, persistent finger or hand ischaemia and even gangrene after radial artery cannulation, requiring amputation of the hand or lower forearm has been reported. It is recommended therefore, that the Allen test be carried out before the decision is made to catheterise the radial artery but a negative Allen test does not exclude the possibility of permanent damage.[21] With the introduction of percutaneous transluminal angioplasty (PTA) the frequency of vascular complications seems to have increased, especially after coronary angioplasty when the haemostatic systems are often heavily influenced by pharmacological means.[8,22,23] Pseudoaneurysm formation is the dominating complication of angiography. Messina *et al.*[8] reported a 3.4 per cent incidence of vascular complications after interventional cardiac catheterisation and 0.7 per cent after diagnostic procedures.

In a survey in our institution in 1994, based on the coronary procedure registry, 49 complications occurred in 649 procedures (7.6 per cent), and of these 32 per cent were pseudoaneurysms. Stent usage was associated with 10 per cent of pseudoaneurysms compared with 2.2 per cent associated with percutaneous transluminal coronary angioplasty (PTCA) only (Fig. 38.2). Surgical treatment of haemorrhage was necessary in 10 patients (1.6 per cent). In 34 per cent of haemorrhages a transfusion was necessary. Haemorrhagic complications presented as an obvious expanding haematoma in all except two patients: one with a rectus abdominis sheath haematoma and the other with a retroperitoneal haematoma, respectively. There was no rise in mortality related to complications at the puncture site.

CLINICAL PRESENTATION

Major haemorrhage will cause local or general symptoms. The most common local symptom/sign is at the site of catheter insertion, namely, an expanding painful haematoma. In the axillary artery such a haematoma may cause brachial plexus compression with paraesthesia, paresis, or paralysis of the arm, and in the carotid area, compression of the trachea and oedema of the larynx. Major bleeding may cause general symptoms of hypovolaemic shock. A retroperitoneal haemorrhage is particularly treacherous, because it does not usually reveal itself by local symptoms (see Fig. 38.1). Computed tomography (CT) scanning is essential in diagnosing retroperitoneal haematoma.

Thrombosis at the place of catheterisation may cause peripheral ischaemia. In common femoral artery occlusion there is no pulsation in the groin and peripheral ischaemia is severe. In superficial femoral artery occlusion pulsation is felt in the common femoral artery, but not distally, and ischaemic symptoms are more modest. The thrombus may not always be occlusive. Progression of the thrombotic process will alter clinical symptoms and signs within hours of catheterisation. Repeated investigations are therefore important. Symptoms are basically characterised by the five Ps: pain, paraesthesia, pallor, pulselessness and paralysis.

Emboli to the lower leg from a catheterisation site thrombus may occlude large or medium sized arteries. Showers of microemboli may enter the small peripheral arteries and cause symptoms of an apparent skin rash or the 'blue toe syndrome'.[24] Catheterisation of a severely atherosclerotic aorta may cause massive embolisation or aortic occlusion, a complication which may be fatal.[24]

Arterial occlusion after catheterisation of arteries of the upper extremity usually causes only mild symptoms because of the presence of a rich collateral circulation. Loss or weakening of distal pulses is the most important symptom. Occasionally, pallor and some paraesthesia are evident, but paresis or pain is rare. Some patients do develop symptoms of 'arm claudication' later. Gangrene of fingers or hands is a rare occurrence.

Thromboembolic complications in arteries other than those of the extremity may cause stroke or blindness, myocardial infarction, renal ischaemia with infarction, renovascular hypertension or intestinal infarction. Most of the thromboembolic complications appear while the patient is still being catheterised or soon after catheter withdrawal.

Clinical features suggestive of catheter injury

- Bleeding
- Haematoma
- Ischaemia
- Microembolisation – 'blue toe syndrome', cerebral/ocular symptoms, intestinal/renal ischaemia or infarction
- Pulsatile swelling/thrill/bruit

Arteriovenous fistulae rarely have haemodynamic consequences. They are diagnosed accidentally when a murmur or a thrill is detected. An arteriovenous fistula between the vertebral artery and Batson's vein plexus surrounding the artery manifests itself as a murmur, which is heard by the patient and may be thought to be tinnitus.

A pseudoaneurysm may form at the point of catheterisation and on palpation is felt to be an expanding tumour. It may be difficult to distinguish from a small haematoma. A pseudoaneurysm develops after the haematoma has been established. In contrast to the haematoma, a pseudoaneurysm expands with the pulse wave, can be felt by bimanual palpation and, furthermore, a machinery murmur can be heard. Ultrasound imaging will reveal the extent of the pseudoaneurysm (see Fig. 38.2) and the typical flow profile in its neck (Fig. 38.3). Rupture is rare[25] but the skin circulation may be compromised.[26]

PREVENTION OF CATHETER INJURY

Several measures can be taken to reduce the risk of arterial injury. Angiography should be performed in hospitals with a reasonable workload of such procedures, because the number of complications decreases with increasing experience. Transfemoral catheterisation should be the route of choice. The catheterisation of smaller arteries increases the risk for various types of injury, as does selective catheterisation. The translumbar route is hardly ever indicated. When arterial catheterisation is difficult or expected to be so it is best abandoned or indeed avoided altogether. In these cases other diagnostic methods such as magnetic resonance angiography (MRA) or duplex ultrasonography should be used. The time taken for catheterisation should be short and the catheter used of small calibre. Dextran before and heparin during catheterisation together seem to decrease the risk of thromboembolism.

To diminish the risk of haemorrhage and later of pseudoaneurysm formation many angiographers use some form of compression device such as FemoStop (Radi Medical Systems, Uppsala, Sweden). Another way of decreasing this

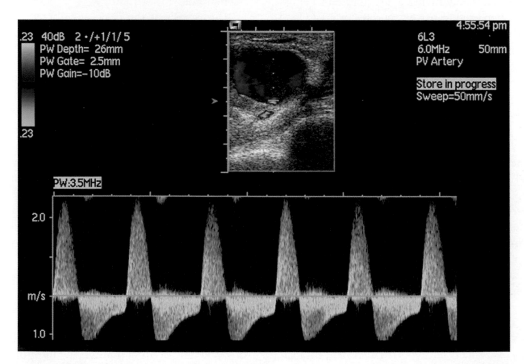

Figure 38.3   *Ultrasound image of pseudoaneurysm of the common femoral artery with spectral Doppler recording. The typical 'to and fro' flow profile in the neck of the pseudoaneurysm is demonstrated*

risk is by the use of a tissue sealant achieved by the deposition of collagen in the extravascular puncture canal,[27–29] although a potential complication is thrombosis when it is accidentally injected into the vessel lumen.

Percutaneous suturing devices to close arterial access puncture sites may prevent bleeding and allow the patient to be mobilised more rapidly.[30–33] The Food and Drug Administration (FDA) has currently approved two suturing devices: Prostar/Techstar and Closer. These devices may be used with a low complication rate but bleeding, thrombosis

and retained devices have been described.[34,35] In a recent report on the use of 3000 percutaneous suturing devices eight complications were recorded (0.03 per cent):[36] thrombosis,[2] haemorrhage (four, with one infection) and retained devices.[2]

Pathways of care are simplified in algorithms for the detection and management of haemorrhage (Fig. 38.4) and of pseudoaneurysms (Fig. 38.5).

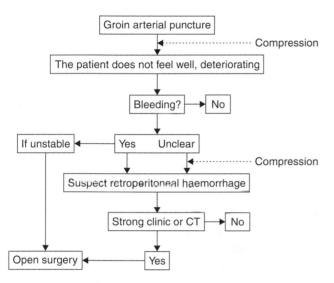

Figure 38.4 *Algorithm of the detection and management of haemorrhage*

> ## Factors which reduce risk of catheter injuries
>
> - Angiographic competence
> - Preferential use of the transfemoral route
> - Use of small calibre catheters
> - Dextran and heparin to reduce thromboembolism
> - Use of FemoStop®, tissue sealant, percutaneous suture

MANAGEMENT OF COMPLICATIONS

Early detection of complications is the key to successful handling. This is particularly important in cases of thromboembolic occlusion. The circulation in the extremities should always be checked before angiography, immediately after removal of the catheter, and before the patient is allowed to leave the hospital. Impaired circulation after catheterisation is often ascribed to 'spasm', but signs of peripheral ischaemia persisting after removal of the catheter should never be ascribed to spasm until arterial

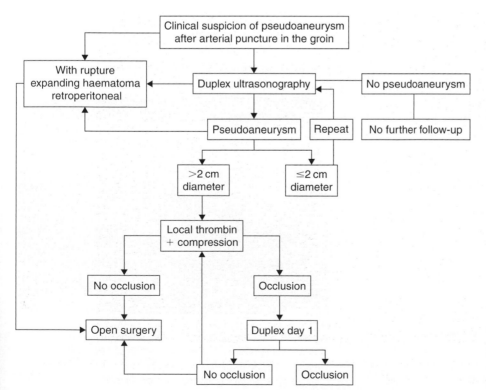

Figure 38.5 *Algorithm of the detection and management of pseudoaneurysm*

thromboembolism has been excluded by clinical means, repeat angiography or preferably duplex scan.

Open surgery

When exploring the femoral artery it is important to make the skin incision proximal enough to allow for control above the hole created by the needle or catheter.[37] The hole is sometimes quite large and lacerated and closure sometimes requires a patch. The use of a Fogarty catheter is essential in **clearing the distal vascular bed**. The peripheral vasculature must be evaluated by angiography or duplex scan while the patient is on the operating table.

The handling of occlusive injuries of the brachial artery after catheterisation (see Chapter 41) is more controversial. Most asymptomatic patients will remain in that state, particularly if they are not active, but as a general rule these injuries should be repaired.

Stroke may be caused by carotid artery occlusion from thrombosis, dissection or embolism. In the former case, immediate exploration and revascularisation may restore cerebral function[6] (see Chapters 5 and 11–14). Haemorrhage should be handled by early diagnosis and early exploration. In cases of carotid artery puncture it is important to observe the patient in order to be aware of the development of laryngeal and tracheal compression by a haematoma. Early exploration and tracheotomy are advisable when there are signs of compression. Early exploration is necessary when bleeding is suspected after axillary artery catheterisation. The patient often experiences some numbness or weakness in the hand after removal of the axillary catheter. Persistence of symptoms or new symptoms such as tingling, pain, decreased sensation, numbness or weakness indicate continued bleeding from the puncture site. Immediate exploration is mandatory. Haemorrhage following arterial puncture is usually easy to treat by simple suture. Occasionally, a patch is necessary.

Most pseudoaneurysms are detected within one to a few weeks after catheterisation when the haematoma has disappeared. A pseudoaneurysm can thrombose and disappear spontaneously, but it may also rupture. It is easy to close the hole with one or two longitudinal stitches. Pseudoaneurysms of the axillary artery may be more difficult to treat surgically but early exploration is also very important. Great care has to be taken to avoid injuring the nerve plexus around the artery, but the neurovascular sheath must be opened to avoid pressure on the nerves.

The use of endografts

Today, catheter or balloon induced lesions such as perforation, dissection, pseudoaneurysm and rupture or arteriovenous fistula may be safely and effectively treated by insertion of a covered endoprosthesis, i.e. a combination of stent and graft, to exclude and seal the entrance of the lesion,[38–41]

thereby also preventing secondary formation of pseudoaneurysms. In case of bleeding preliminary haemostasis can usually be obtained by upstream balloon occlusion.[40]

Non-surgical treatment of pseudoaneurysms

Ultrasound guided compression has been successfully used since the early 1990s.[26,42–46] One drawback is the need for prolonged compression, lasting 30 minutes to more than an hour, which may be painful for the patient and demanding for the clinician.[45,47–49] A modification with the FemoStop compression device to occlude the pseudoaneurysm has been advocated as a substitute for manual compression.[50,51] There is a higher failure rate in patients who are anticoagulated, those with pseudoaneurysms larger than 4 cm[26,44,45] and in pseudoaneurysms associated with an arteriovenous fistula.[52]

Since the report by Cope and Zeit[53] injecting thrombin into the aneurysmal sac, the combination of percutaneous thrombin induced thrombosis and ultrasonographically guided compression has been increasingly used[54–61] (Fig. 38.6). Thrombin is slowly injected into the aneurysmal sac, preferably from the periphery and under ultrasonographic control. The amount of thrombin used is between 100 and 500 units and thrombosis occurs within seconds compared with half an hour or more during compression alone.[62] The rapidity of occlusion has significantly reduced the burden on vascular laboratory resources. Although thrombosis of the native artery has been described,[57,63,64] this complication seems to be extremely rare. To diminish the risk, injection of small amounts of diluted thrombin solutions has been recommended.[62] Another rare complication is allergy and even anaphylaxis after injection of bovine thrombin.[65,66] Also, if topical thrombin has been used previously, i.e. during haemodialysis, IgE mediated anaphylaxis may be induced.[67] The success rate in occluding a

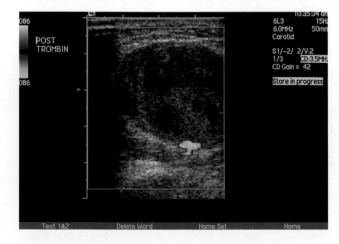

Figure 38.6   *Ultrasound image of pseudoaneurysm of the common femoral artery following injection of 1000 units of thrombin. Visible thrombus formation and the absence of colour confirm there is no flow in the pseudoaneurysm*

pseudoaneurysm by thrombin injection is near 100 per cent. If unsuccessful another percutaneous option is the delivery of coils into the aneurysmal sac.[68] This method is limited by the potential of introducing infection in the process of placing foreign material within a groin haematoma.

A recent approach, which has yet to be evaluated, is the local administration of recombinant activated factor VII.[69]

Conclusions

Arterial catheterisation is an invasive procedure carrying the risk of bleeding, occlusion by various means, thromboembolism, pseudoaneurysm, arteriovenous fistula and the added possibility that a foreign body may be left behind in the vessel. The site chosen for puncture influences the type and the incidence of complications, most of which become apparent during the procedure or soon after catheter withdrawal. The vascular surgeon and the radiologist must be aware of the risks and should be prepared to correct any injury inflicted, while those in other disciplines calling for these interventions should ensure that a vascular team is available on standby.

Key references

Bergentz S-E, Bergqvist D. *Iatrogenic Vascular Injuries*. Berlin: Springer Verlag, 1989. Overview of all types of iatrogenic injuries but not the recent therapeutic options.

Ettles D, Earnshaw J. Complications in interventional radiology and thrombolysis. In: Campbell B (ed). *Complications in Arterial Surgery. A Practical Approach to Management*. London: Butterworth-Heinemann, 1996. Practical guidelines.

Kang S, Labropoulos N. Nonoperative treatment of femoral pseudoaneurysms. In: Yao J, Pearce W (eds). *Practical Vascular Surgery*. New York: Appleton & Lange, 1999. Details on ultrasound-guided treatment.

Messina LM, Brothers TE, Wakefield TW, *et al*. Clinical characteristics and surgical management of vascular complications in patients undergoing cardiac catheterization: interventional versus diagnostic procedures. *J Vasc Surg* 1991; **13**: 593–600.

Takolander R, Bergqvist D, Jonsson K, *et al*. Fatal thrombo-embolic complications at aorto-femoral angiography. *Acta Radiol Diagn (Stockh)* 1985; **26**: 15–19.

REFERENCES

1 Antonovic R, Rosch J, Dotter CT. The value of systemic arterial heparinization in transfemoral angiography: a prospective study. *Am J Roentgenol* 1976; **127**: 223–5.

2 Bergstrom K, Lodin H. Arteriovenous fistula as a complication of cerebral angiography. Report of three cases. *Br J Radiol* 1966; **39**: 263–6.

3 Picus D, Totty WG. Iatrogenic femoral arteriovenous fistulae: evaluation by digital vascular imaging. *AJR Am J Roentgenol* 1984; **142**: 567–70.

4 Heystraten FM, Fast JH. Arteriovenous fistula as a complication of the Seldinger procedure of the femoral artery and vein. Report of 2 cases. *Diagn Imag* 1983; **52**: 197–201.

5 Kron J, Sutherland D, Rosch J, *et al*. Arteriovenous fistula: a rare complication of arterial puncture for cardiac catheterization. *Am J Cardiol* 1985; **55**: 1445–6.

6 Bergentz SE, Hansson LO, Norback B. Surgical management of complications to arterial puncture. *Ann Surg* 1966; **164**: 1021–6.

7 Eriksson I, Jorulf H. Surgical complications associated with arterial catheterization. *Scand J Thorac Cardiovasc Surg* 1970; **4**: 69–75.

8 Messina LM, Brothers TE, Wakefield TW, *et al*. Clinical characteristics and surgical management of vascular complications in patients undergoing cardiac catheterization: interventional versus diagnostic procedures. *J Vasc Surg* 1991; **13**: 593–600.

9 Allen BT, Munn JS, Stevens SL, *et al*. Selective non-operative management of pseudoaneurysms and arteriovenous fistulae complicating femoral artery catheterization. *J Cardiovasc Surg (Torino)* 1992; **33**: 440–7.

10 Rivers SP, Lee ES, Lyon RT, *et al*. Successful conservative management of iatrogenic femoral arterial trauma. *Ann Vasc Surg* 1992; **6**: 45–9.

11 Kotval PS, Khoury A, Shah PM, Babu SC. Doppler sonographic demonstration of the progressive spontaneous thrombosis of pseudoaneurysms. *J Ultrasound Med* 1990; **9**: 185–90.

12 Kent KC, McArdle CR, Kennedy B, *et al*. A prospective study of the clinical outcome of femoral pseudoaneurysms and arteriovenous fistulas induced by arterial puncture. *J Vasc Surg* 1993; **17**: 125–31; discussion 131–3.

13 Paulson EK, Hertzberg BS, Paine SS, Carroll BA. Femoral artery pseudoaneurysms: value of color Doppler sonography in predicting which ones will thrombose without treatment. *AJR Am J Roentgenol* 1992; **159**: 1077–81.

14 Samuels D, Orron DE, Kessler A, *et al*. Femoral artery pseudoaneurysm: Doppler sonographic features predictive for spontaneous thrombosis. *J Clin Ultrasound* 1997; **25**: 497–500.

15 Crawford E, Beall A, Moyer J, DeBakey M. Complications of aortography. *Surg Gynecol Obstet* 1957; **104**: 129–41.

16 Reiss MD, Bookstein JJ, Bleifer KH. Radiologic aspects of renovascular hypertension. 4. Arteriographic complications. *JAMA* 1972; **221**: 375–8.

17 Lang E. Complications of retrograde percutaneous arteriography. *J Urol* 1963; **90**: 604–10.

18 Lang EK. Complications of direct and indirect angiography of the brachiocephalic vessels. *Acta Radiol Diagn* 1966; **5**: 296–307.

19 Hessel SJ, Adams DF, Abrams HL. Complications of angiography. *Radiology* 1981; **138**: 273–81.

20 Babu SC, Piccorelli GO, Shah PM, *et al*. Incidence and results of arterial complications among 16 350 patients undergoing cardiac catheterization. *J Vasc Surg* 1989; **10**: 113–16.

21 Wilkins RG. Radial artery cannulation and ischaemic damage: a review. *Anaesthesia* 1985; **40**: 896–9.

22 Oweida SW, Roubin GS, Smith RB 3rd, Salam AA. Postcatheterization vascular complications associated with percutaneous transluminal coronary angioplasty. *J Vasc Surg* 1990; **12**: 310–15.

23 McCann RL, Schwartz LB, Pieper KS. Vascular complications of cardiac catheterization. *J Vasc Surg* 1991; **14**: 375–81.

24 Takolander R, Bergqvist D, Jonsson K, *et al.* Fatal thrombo-embolic complications at aorto-femoral angiography. *Acta Radiol Diagn (Stockh)* 1985; **26**: 15–19.

25 Graham AN, Wilson CM, Hood JM, Barros D'Sa AA. Risk of rupture of postangiographic femoral false aneurysm. *Br J Surg* 1992; **79**: 1022–5.

26 Feld R, Patton GM, Carabasi RA, *et al.* Treatment of iatrogenic femoral artery injuries with ultrasound-guided compression. *J Vasc Surg* 1992; **16**: 832–40.

27 Camenzind E, Grossholz M, Urban P, *et al.* Collagen application versus manual compression: a prospective randomized trial for arterial puncture site closure after coronary angioplasty. *J Am Coll Cardiol* 1994; **24**: 655–62.

28 Sanborn T, Gibbs H, Brinker J, *et al.* A multicenter randomized trial comparing a percutaneous collagen hemostasis device with conventional manual compression after diagnostic angiography and angioplasty. *J Am Coll Cardiol* 1993; **22**: 1273–9.

29 Henry M, Amor M, Allaoui M, Tricoche O. A new access site management tool: the Angio-Seal hemostatic puncture closure device. *J Endovasc Surg* 1995; **2**: 289–96.

30 Aker UT, Kensey KR, Heuser RR, *et al.* Immediate arterial hemostasis after cardiac catheterization: initial experience with a new puncture closure device. *Cathet Cardiovasc Diagn* 1994; **31**: 228–32.

31 Gerckens U, Cattelaens N, Lampe EG, Grube E. Management of arterial puncture site after catheterization procedures: evaluating a suture-mediated closure device. *Am J Cardiol* 1999; **83**: 1658–63.

32 Baim DS, Knopf WD, Hinohara T, *et al.* Suture-mediated closure of the femoral access site after cardiac catheterization: results of the suture to ambulate and discharge (STAND I and STAND II) trials. *Am J Cardiol* 2000; **85**: 864–9.

33 Carere RG, Webb JG, Ahmed T, Dodek AA. Initial experience using Prostar: a new device for percutaneous suture-mediated closure of arterial puncture sites. *Cathet Cardiovasc Diagn* 1996; **37**: 367–72.

34 Eidt JF, Habibipour S, Saucedo JF, *et al.* Surgical complications from hemostatic puncture closure devices. *Am J Surg* 1999; **178**: 511–16.

35 Gonze MD, Sternbergh WC 3rd, Salartash K, Money SR. Complications associated with percutaneous closure devices. *Am J Surg* 1999; **178**: 209–11.

36 Nehler MR, Lawrence WA, Whitehill TA, *et al.* Iatrogenic vascular injuries from percutaneous vascular suturing devices. *J Vasc Surg* 2001; **33**: 943–7.

37 Rutherford R, Pearce W. Acute problems following diagnostic and interventional radiological procedures. New York: Grune and Stratton, 1987.

38 Nyman U, Uher P, Lindh M, *et al.* Stent-graft treatment of iatrogenic iliac artery perforations: report of three cases. *Eur J Vasc Endovasc Surg* 1999; **17**: 259–63.

39 Formichi M, Raybaud G, Benichou H, Ciosi G. Rupture of the external iliac artery during balloon angioplasty: endovascular treatment using a covered stent. *J Endovasc Surg* 1998; **5**: 37–41.

40 Scheinert D, Ludwig J, Steinkamp HJ, *et al.* Treatment of catheter-induced iliac artery injuries with self-expanding endografts. *J Endovasc Ther* 2000; **7**: 213–20.

41 Thalhammer C, Kirchherr AS, Uhlich F, *et al.* Postcatheterization pseudoaneurysms and arteriovenous fistulas: repair with percutaneous implantation of endovascular covered stents. *Radiology* 2000; **214**: 127–31.

42 Fellmeth BD, Roberts AC, Bookstein JJ, *et al.* Postangiographic femoral artery injuries: nonsurgical repair with US-guided compression. *Radiology* 1991; **178**: 671–5.

43 Cox GS, Young JR, Gray BR, *et al.* Ultrasound-guided compression repair of postcatheterization pseudoaneurysms: results of treatment in one hundred cases. *J Vasc Surg* 1994; **19**: 683–6.

44 Hajarizadeh H, LaRosa CR, Cardullo P, *et al.* Ultra-sound guided compression of iatrogenic femoral pseudoaneurysm failure, recurrence, and long-term results. *J Vasc Surg* 1995; **22**: 425–30; discussion 430–3.

45 Coley BD, Roberts AC, Fellmeth BD, *et al.* Postangiographic femoral artery pseudoaneurysms: further experience with US-guided compression repair. *Radiology* 1995; **194**: 307–11.

46 Schaub F, Theiss W, Heinz M, *et al.* New aspects in ultrasound-guided compression repair of postcatheterization femoral artery injuries. *Circulation* 1994; **90**: 1861–5.

47 Agarwal R, Agrawal SK, Roubin GS, *et al.* Clinically guided closure of femoral arterial pseudoaneurysms complicating cardiac catheterization and coronary angioplasty. *Cathet Cardiovasc Diagn* 1993; **30**: 96–100.

48 Moote DJ, Hilborn MD, Harris KA, *et al.* Postarteriographic femoral pseudoaneurysms: treatment with ultrasound-guided compression. *Ann Vasc Surg* 1994; **8**: 325–31.

49 Khoury M, Batra S, Berg R, Rama K. Duplex-guided compression of iatrogenic femoral artery pseudoaneurysms. *Am Surg* 1994; **60**: 234–6; discussion 236–7.

50 Dangas G, Mehran R, Duvvuri S, *et al.* Use of a pneumatic compression system (FemoStop) as a treatment option for femoral artery pseudoaneurysms after percutaneous cardiac procedures. *Cathet Cardiovasc Diagn* 1996; **39**: 138–42.

51 Trertola SO, Savader SJ, Prescott CA, Osterman FA, Jr. US-guided pseudoaneurysm repair with a compression device. *Radiology* 1993; **189**: 285–6.

52 Kumins NH, Landau DS, Montalvo J, *et al.* Expanded indications for the treatment of postcatheterization femoral pseudoaneurysms with ultrasound-guided compression. *Am J Surg* 1998; **176**: 131–6.

53 Cope C, Zeit R. Coagulation of aneurysms by direct percutaneous thrombin injection. *AJR Am J Roentgenol* 1986; **147**: 383–7.

54 Walker TG, Geller SC, Brewster DC. Transcatheter occlusion of a profunda femoral artery pseudoaneurysm using thrombin. *AJR Am J Roentgenol* 1987; **149**: 185–6.

55 Wixon CL, Philpott JM, Bogey WM Jr, Powell CS. Duplex-directed thrombin injection as a method to treat femoral artery pseudoaneurysms. *J Am Coll Surg* 1998; **187**: 464–6.

56 Liau CS, Ho FM, Chen MF, Lee YT. Treatment of iatrogenic femoral artery pseudoaneurysm with percutaneous thrombin injection. *J Vasc Surg* 1997; **26**: 18–23.

57 Kang SS, Labropoulos N, Mansour MA, Baker WH. Percutaneous ultrasound guided thrombin injection: a new method for treating postcatheterization femoral pseudoaneurysms. *J Vasc Surg* 1998; **27**: 1032–8.

58 Elford J, Burrell C, Roobottom C. Ultrasound guided percutaneous thrombin injection for the treatment of iatrogenic pseudoaneurysms. *Heart* 1999; **82**: 526–7.

59 Brophy DP, Sheiman RG, Amatulle P, Akbari CM. Iatrogenic femoral pseudoaneurysms: thrombin injection after failed US-guided compression. *Radiology* 2000; **214**: 278–82.

60 Vermeulen EG, Umans U, Rijbroek A, Rauwerda JA. Percutaneous duplex-guided thrombin injection for treatment of iatrogenic

femoral artery pseudoaneurysms. *Eur J Vasc Endovasc Surg* 2000; **20**: 302-4.

61 Tamim WZ, Arbid EJ, Andrews LS, Arous EJ. Percutaneous induced thrombosis of iatrogenic femoral pseudoaneurysms following catheterization. *Ann Vasc Surg* 2000; **14**: 254-9.

62 Taylor BS, Rhee RY, Muluk S, *et al*. Thrombin injection versus compression of femoral artery pseudoaneurysms. *J Vasc Surg* 1999; **30**: 1052-9.

63 Lennox A, Griffin M, Nicolaides A, Mansfield A. Regarding 'Percutaneous ultrasound guided thrombin injection: a new method for treating postcatheterization femoral pseudoaneurysms'. *J Vasc Surg* 1998; **28**: 1120-1.

64 Forbes TL, Millward SF. Femoral artery thrombosis after percutaneous thrombin injection of an external iliac artery pseudoaneurysm. *J Vasc Surg* 2001; **33**: 1093-6.

65 Pope M, Johnston KW. Anaphylaxis after thrombin injection of a femoral pseudoaneurysm: recommendations for prevention. *J Vasc Surg* 2000; **32**: 190-1.

66 Sheldon PJ, Oglevie SB, Kaplan LA. Prolonged generalized urticarial reaction after percutaneous thrombin injection for treatment of a femoral artery pseudoaneurysm. *J Vasc Interven Radiol* 2000; **11**: 759-61.

67 Tadokoro K, Ohtoshi T, Takafuji S, *et al*. Topical thrombin-induced IgE-mediated anaphylaxis: RAST analysis and skin test studies. *J Allergy Clin Immunol* 1991; **88**: 620-9.

68 Pan M, Medina A, Suarez de Lezo J, *et al*. Obliteration of femoral pseudoaneurysm complicating coronary intervention by direct puncture and permanent or removable coil insertion. *Am J Cardiol* 1997; **80**: 786-8.

69 Liem AK, Biesma DH, Ernst SM, Schepens AA. Recombinant activated factor VII for false aneurysms in patients with normal haemostatic mechanisms. *Thromb Haemost* 1999; **82**: 150-1.

39

Injuries of Peripheral Endovascular Procedures

AMMAN BOLIA, PETER RF BELL

THE PROBLEM

Since the first description of endoluminal treatment for peripheral vascular disease by Dotter and Judkins in 1964,[1] there has been a substantial increase in the number of patients treated using percutaneous transluminal angioplasty (PTA). Percutaneous transluminal angioplasty in its various forms has been used as an alternative to reconstructive surgery in patients with critical limb ischaemia and, because it is minimally invasive, the threshold for treatment of claudicants has been reduced.

Although the treatment is successful in a large number of patients, it is not without complications and when these occur, many of them require urgent attention by the operator in order to deal with the situation by endovascular or if necessary open techniques. The incidence of complications is dependent on the experience of the operator.[2,3] The majority of these complications can be managed percutaneously at the time of the procedure without the need for major surgery.[4–11] When percutaneous management fails, however, open surgery is required. The incidence of complications requiring surgery ranges between 1 and 4 per cent[2–12] and surgical help should always be available in centres where percutaneous techniques are practised.

The complications of percutaneous endovascular treatments for peripheral vascular disease (PVD) can be categorised as puncture related, perforation, embolic, thrombotic, compromise of important branches at bifurcations, elastic recoil and compromised collaterals as well as accidental dissection. Some of these can lead to severe acute ischaemia and the patient should always be informed about their incidence before consent is obtained.

Complications of percutaneous endovascular treatments for PVD

- Puncture related complications
- Perforation
- Embolic complications
- Thrombotic complications
- Compromise of important branches at bifurcations
- Elastic recoil and compromised collaterals
- Accidental dissection

PUNCTURE RELATED COMPLICATIONS

Main puncture sites

The commonest puncture site for peripheral vascular and other interventions is the common femoral artery. Other sites, for example axillary, high brachial, radial and popliteal arteries may also be used for access in certain situations.

Common femoral artery

The possible complications arising from the common femoral artery (CFA) as a puncture site include groin haematoma, which is usually a self-limiting problem, but it may be progressive and a substantial number may require transfusion or surgical evacuation. Other potential complications are listed below.

Puncture related complications

- Groin haematoma: self-limiting or expanding
- Retroperitoneal haematoma
- Pseudoaneurysm
- Arteriovenous fistula
- Thrombosis
- Femoral nerve damage

Various factors contribute to the development of these puncture related complications, namely, obesity, hypertension, anticoagulant treatment, over-heparinisation, a tendency to bleed, low platelet count, high femoral puncture causing bleeding retroperitoneally, low superficial femoral artery (SFA) puncture leading to pseudoaneurysm formation, the use of large diameter catheters/sheaths and procedure which is prolonged.

Factors contributing to femoral puncture related complications

- Obesity
- Hypertension
- Patient on anticoagulant treatment/over-heparinisation
- Generalised bleeding tendency/low platelet count
- High puncture: retroperitoneal bleeding
- Low puncture: pseudoaneurysm formation
- Large diameter catheters/sheaths

Axillary or high brachial puncture

Access via the axillary or proximal brachial artery is used when a groin approach is difficult due to scarring or infection or when femoral pulses are impalpable and iliac occlusive disease is suspected. The most serious complication from an axillary or high brachial puncture is damage to the brachial plexus, affecting function in the ipsilateral arm and hand. This may lead to permanent damage or to recovery over a period of time. Damage to the nerves can be due to direct injury or a haematoma at the puncture site compressing the brachial plexus. Direct injury usually affects single nerves whereas compression from a haematoma may affect multiple nerves.

MANAGEMENT OF PUNCTURE RELATED COMPLICATIONS

Haematoma

Haematoma at the femoral puncture site is the commonest complication with frequency ranging from 2 to 8 per cent.[3,13–18] Large diameter catheters, hypertension and obesity are likely to increase the chances of haematoma or false aneurysm formation. The majority of haematomas at the common femoral artery puncture site are self-limiting and do not require any specific treatment. Occasionally, however, a large haematoma may require blood transfusion and/or surgical evacuation and repair.[19]

Retroperitoneal haematoma

A high puncture in the common femoral artery may be required to treat either a flush occlusion or disease in the proximal superficial femoral artery. A high puncture increases the risk of a retroperitoneal haematoma. The incidence of this complication is less than 0.1 per cent.[8]

When a high puncture has to be made intentionally, care is required to puncture that part of the common femoral artery which can be compressed against the underlying superior pubic ramus. Bleeding and haematoma formation is likely to occur due to inadequate compression, with pressure in the wrong place, and/or for too short a time. Prolonged and horizontal compression on the puncture site will usually prevent a potentially fatal retroperitoneal haematoma. Patients in whom a high puncture is anticipated should have blood taken for 'group and save' so that, should transfusion be required, blood can be made available quickly. Also, the nursing staff must be informed that a high puncture has been made so that observations are made with care and more frequently, and action taken as soon as there is any evidence of significant blood loss. Should this happen, there will be a rise in pulse rate, a fall in blood pressure and the patient may feel faint and demonstrate features of hypotension. As soon as it is evident that there is blood loss, immediate transfusion has to be started and consideration given to possible surgical repair of the puncture site.

More recently, closure devices of the puncture sites have become available, methods which may be desirable in creating a seal particularly in patients with hypertension or on anticoagulant treatment.

Prevention of retroperitoneal haematoma and its effects

- Blood for 'group and save'
- Choose correct site for puncture, i.e. not too high
- Maintain adequate pressure and for long enough

- Consider using a closure device
- Lower blood pressure if hypertensive
- Inform nursing staff to keep careful observations

Surgical treatment of bleeding or haematoma

Groin haematomas, once false aneurysm has been excluded by duplex, are usually left alone and will settle spontaneously. Patients may benefit from a short course of antibiotics to avoid infection. If, however, the haematoma is large then a small incision under local anaesthesia can be used to evacuate it and avoid risk of infection. Should the patient present with obvious and continuing retroperitoneal bleeding from a high puncture, blood transfusion becomes necessary and surgical intervention should be considered early rather than late. This is a potentially fatal complication. If, in spite of pressure and the replacement of blood, the patient remains haemodynamically unstable then surgical repair is indicated. Using local or general anaesthetic, an incision is made above the inguinal ligament and the iliac artery approached retroperitoneally through the abdominal musculature to expose the puncture site and arrest the haemorrhage with a 5-0 or 6-0 Prolene suture.

False aneurysm (pseudoaneurysm)

The incidence of pseudoaneurysm following common femoral artery puncture ranges from 0.2 to 0.5 per cent for diagnostic procedures and up to 5–8 per cent for coronary stenting procedures.[2,21] This is likely to occur when there has been inadequate compression at the puncture site and particularly when the puncture has been too low, for example in the superficial femoral artery. A puncture in the superficial femoral or profunda femoris artery cannot be adequately compressed as there is no bone immediately behind them at this level.

A false aneurysm presents itself as a pulsatile mass at the puncture site, which may be quite tender. A duplex scan is the easiest way of diagnosing this condition, although computed tomography (CT) and magnetic resonance imaging (MRI) are equally good at establishing the size, shape and extent of the pseudoaneurysm. Ultrasound compression can be effective but it is painful and time consuming, and the operator has to apply prolonged pressure using the ultrasound probe to stop the pseudoaneurysm from filling.[20,22,23] Nowadays, the majority of pseudoaneurysms can be managed by the injection of thrombin, in a 0.5–1 mL of 1 in 500 units/mL concentration, through a 22 gauge needle directly into the pseudoaneurysm.[24] This has the effect of thrombosing blood within the pseudoaneurysm within seconds. The effect of the treatment can be assessed in real time using duplex ultrasound. Some pressure on the probe immediately following the injection of thrombin helps to prevent blood flowing back into the pseudoaneurysm, thus producing more effective obliteration of the aneurysm sac. The use of an inflated balloon catheter across the neck of the pseudoaneurysm, introduced from the contralateral side, has been advocated to isolate the pseudoaneurysm and prevent thrombin overflowing into the systemic circulation. This practice, however, is probably unnecessary.

Surgical treatment of pseudoaneurysms

If pressure or the injection of thrombin fails, surgical treatment is necessary. By the time such an operation takes place the groin is usually fairly indurated with thrombus and the operation can be difficult. It is best to undertake the procedure under general anaesthesia if the patient is fit. The first move should be to gain control of the artery proximal to the aneurysm. This is achieved through a small incision above the inguinal ligament and gaining access to the iliac artery which can then be compressed with the finger or encircled with an appropriate sling for control. An incision is then made directly over the pseudoaneurysm, the sac opened, the clot evacuated if possible and the artery approached. Bleeding can be controlled by compression or clamping of the iliac artery and retrograde bleeding is usually dealt with by suction as dissecting out all the branches of the artery is unnecessary and usually difficult. A single 5-0 suture placed across the needle puncture site in two directions will usually stop the bleeding. It is important to get down to the artery wall and not simply put the suture into superficial layers as this will not usually work. The wound is closed with drainage and a course of antibiotics is given.

Thrombosis at puncture site

Thrombosis may occur at the puncture site particularly when the catheter/sheath has been passed through a stenotic segment and is compromising flow through it. Prolonged procedures in such a situation, despite heparinisation, may result in a thrombotic complication and surgery may be required to treat it.

Possible sequelae of untreated pseudoaneurysm

- Haemorrhage
- Infection
- Rupture
- Peripheral embolisation
- Deep vein thrombosis
- Pressure on adjacent nerves

Surgical treatment of thrombosis

Thrombosis occurs at the site of a puncture or catheter insertion in which the limb becomes acutely ischaemic. The artery should be exposed, using an appropriate incision and the vessel controlled with slings above and below the puncture site. A longitudinal incision into the artery will then allow removal of the thrombus and assessment of the reason for its occurrence. It may be that a plaque has dissected, in which case it needs to be sewn back into place and the arteriotomy closed with a small patch of vein taken from the adjacent area. Alternatively, a small piece of Dacron may be used, under antibiotic cover.

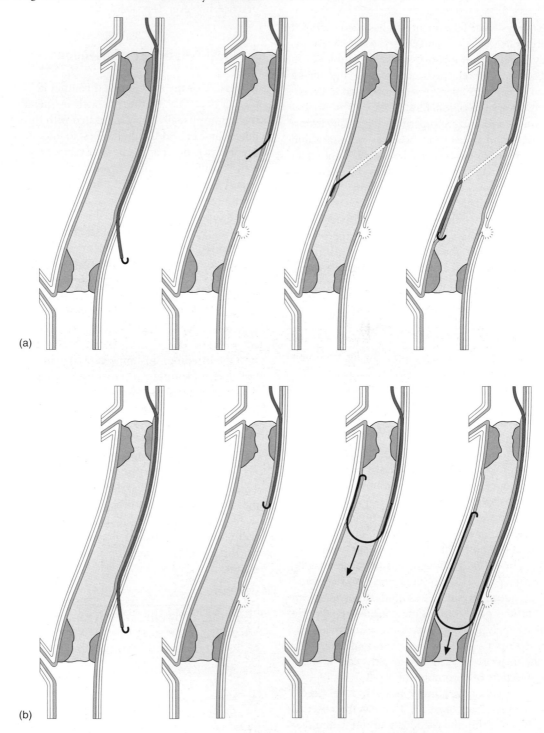

Figure 39.1   *(a) When a perforation occurs with a catheter/guidewire, the combination can be withdrawn out of the perforation site and the wire manipulated to find an alternative dissection. (b) An alternative method of avoiding the perforated site is to manipulate the guidewire into a large loop so that its diameter, being larger than that of the hole at the site of perforation, will not allow it to enter the hole, so preventing dissection along the artery*

It may be better, however, to remember the original problem with which the patient presented and deal with it definitively by an operation using a graft taken from above the area of trauma to the first patent artery distally. If thrombosis occurs during a procedure undertaken for critical limb ischaemia it would be better to resort to a bypass graft rather than try to remove the thrombus. If thrombosis has occurred in a healthy vessel being used for access, then local treatment is usually possible in the way described above. If the limb is not acutely ischaemic, it is often adequate to heparinise the patient and wait and see what happens to the limb under careful observation. In most cases the circulation will be adequate for limb recovery and is dealt with electively rather than as an emergency procedure. Any sign of deterioration, however, should lead to an emergency bypass.

PERFORATION

There are two ways in which a perforation can occur during an endovascular procedure. It may occur as a result of either guidewire/catheter manipulations or inflation of the balloon catheter.

Perforation due to guidewire/catheter manipulations

Perforation is more likely when there is calcification in the artery or when the occlusion is hard and the wire/catheter combination cannot penetrate the occluded segment, instead exiting through the wall of the artery (Fig. 39.1a). Crossing an occlusion with a wire/catheter is usually a painless manoeuvre. Therefore, if the patient experiences sudden pain during advancement of the wire/catheter, perforation is likely to have occurred. Every time the wire enters the perforation, the patient feels pain and this represents useful 'feedback' when managing the perforation. During manipulations to find an alternative path of dissection, this information tells the operator to come out of the perforation and find an alternative route of recanalisation (Figure 39.1b).

When such a perforation occurs in the middle of an occlusion, particularly during subintimal angioplasty, an

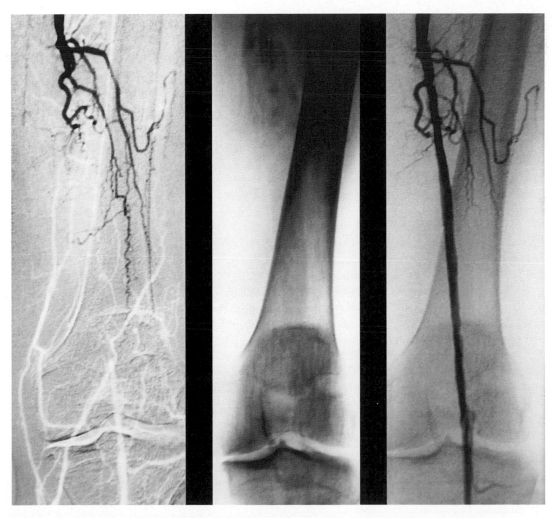

Figure 39.2   *A 10 cm occlusion of the popliteal artery is present. A perforation occurred during attempts at recanalisation and contrast can be seen within the tissues outside the artery. Subsequently, an alternative dissection was found and successful recanalisation achieved*

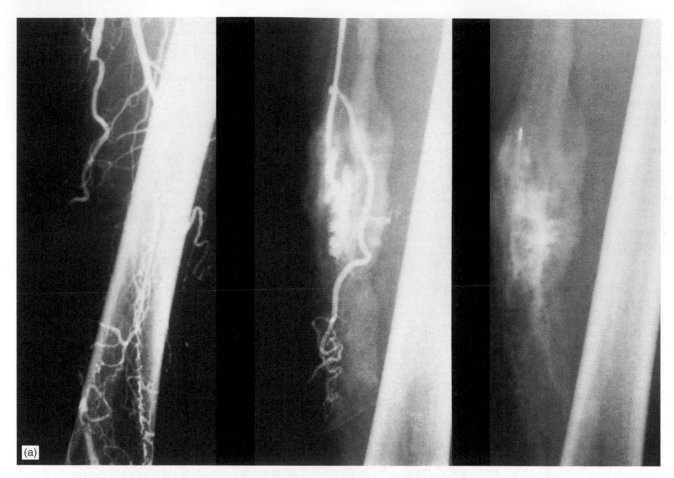

Figure 39.3 *(a) A 10 cm occlusion of the distal superficial femoral artery is present. During attempted recanalisation, a large perforation occurred with substantial extravasation into the tissues. The patient was hypertensive and complained of a significant amount of discomfort. Hence a 3 mm × 1 cm embolisation coil was placed.*

alternative dissection plane can be found in the majority of the cases, and the situation retrieved so that the perforation becomes of no consequence (Figs 39.1b and 39.2). In a small proportion of cases, however, the perforation is so substantial that an alternative dissection plane is difficult to find and the procedure has to be abandoned. If a significant amount of pain is felt due to extravasation of blood, particularly in hypertensive patients, then one may have to consider coil embolisation (Fig. 39.3a). This usually involves placing a 5 mm × 5 cm 0.035 inches coil, at the site of the perforation or just above it. After a few weeks, when the perforation has healed, another attempt can be made to recanalise the occlusion and that usually results in a successful outcome, whether an embolisation coil is present or not (Fig. 39.3b). Perforation in a stenotic segment is extremely unlikely to be due to catheter and wire manipulations but should this occur, then the management would be similar to that when a perforation occurs with balloon dilatation.

Surgical treatment of wire/catheter perforation

This has never been necessary in our practice but is a theoretical possibility. If the use of coils, as described above, or temporary balloon tamponade, fails, the vessel should be exposed and the perforation closed with a single 5-0 Prolene stitch.

Perforation due to balloon dilatation

The incidence of arterial rupture due to balloon dilatation is approximately 0.1 per cent.[25–27] Perforation is diagnosed when, following balloon inflation, the patient feels a sharp and significant amount of pain which does not recede despite balloon deflation. This may be followed by a rise in pulse rate and drop in blood pressure. The patient may look pale, cold and clammy, feel faint and nauseous and yawning is an additional sign of hypotension. A quick injection of contrast will confirm the occurrence of this complication so that treatment can be carried out immediately without any significant blood loss.

This is particularly urgent in situations where the perforation has occurred within a cavity, e.g. the renal or iliac arteries within the abdomen or the subclavian artery within the thorax. In such cases substantial blood loss can occur very quickly and therefore balloon tamponade must be carried out immediately. A drip must be set up and measures taken

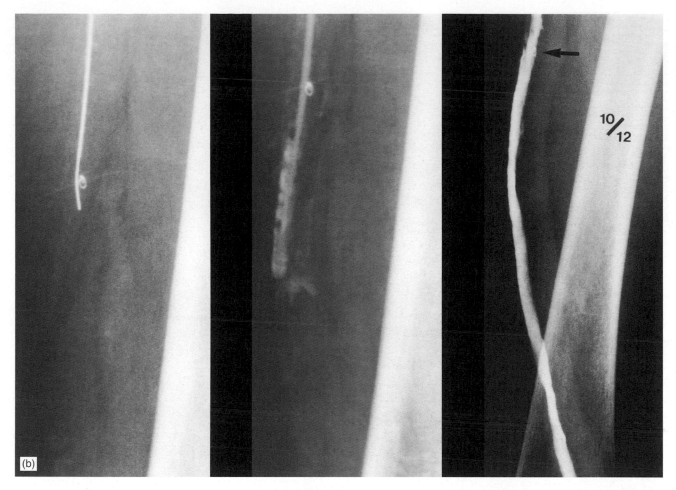

Figure 39.3   *(b) Ten months later an attempt was made at recanalisation. The guidewire found a dissection channel easily and successful recanalisation was achieved, despite the presence of an embolisation coil*

to correct blood pressure mainly with replacement fluids and plasma substitutes while emergency cross-matched blood is awaited. Surgical help must be sought immediately and the patient taken to theatre for emergency repair.

Prevention of perforation due to balloon dilatation

- Do not use balloon of over-sized diameter
- Do not overinflate balloon
- Inflate balloon gradually
- Raise pressure with sequential inflations in tough lesions

When a perforation occurs due to the use of an over-sized balloon, the generation of high pressures rather quickly or balloon rupture, it is usually substantial and may cause a longitudinal split in the artery. Should such a perforation occur within what was previously an occlusion, then the occlusion can be re-created by coil embolisation, ideally placed at both ends of the arterial split so as to isolate the perforated segment. For example, if a perforation in a previously occluded external iliac artery is caused by balloon dilatation, then it may be reasonable to consider re-occluding the artery to stop bleeding. This type of intervention, however, requires experience and speed from the operator to minimise blood loss.

The coils to be used must be opened and ready to be delivered as quickly as possible. This is achieved by locating the tip of the balloon catheter at the intended site of coil placement, the coil being introduced through a partially inflated balloon catheter. When satisfactory placement of this coil has been achieved, the balloon catheter is withdrawn further and the tip positioned at the distal part of the site of the perforation. Once again, another coil is delivered through the same balloon catheter. If the coils are placed satisfactorily, haemostasis will be achieved within minutes of placement and no further blood loss will occur. It must be stressed that only an experienced operator should undertake this manoeuvre because speed is important and any delay in the placement of these coils will result in substantial blood loss, with possible risk of mortality. A less experienced operator would be wise to tamponade the perforation site with a balloon and seek the help of a surgeon immediately.

When a perforation occurs in a previously stenotic segment immediate balloon tamponade is recommended. This

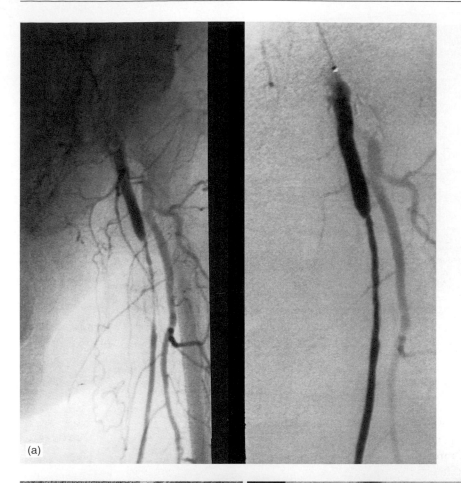

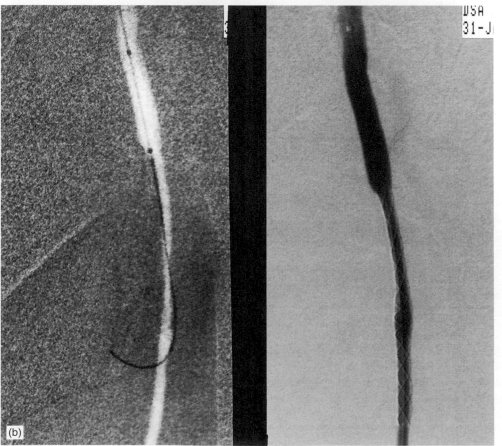

Figure 39.4 *(a) A long tight stenosis is present in the polyfluorotetraethylene (PTFE)/vein composite femoro-popliteal graft. Initial dilatation produced an unsatisfactory result.*
(b) Further balloon inflation with higher pressures ruptured the balloon, causing a perforation in the graft. Note contrast within the tissues and the guidewire tip outside the graft. The perforation was successfully managed with a Wallgraft

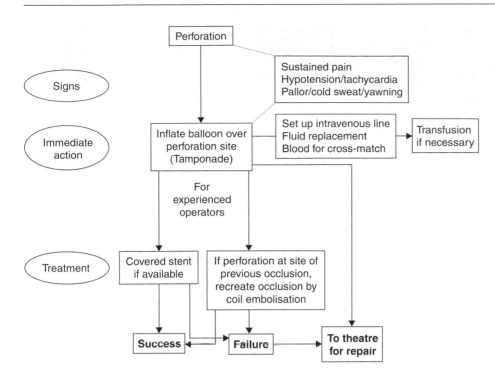

Figure 39.5 *Algorithm of the diagnosis and management of arterial perforation by balloon within a body cavity*

will have the effect of reducing blood loss and allowing the operator some time to think of the best way of managing the situation. With the availability of covered stents, an appropriate sized stent may allow the perforation to be sealed, at the same time establishing flow through the artery without the need for surgery (Fig. 39.4). It should be borne in mind, however, that such a mode of treatment is a temporary measure in the femoral segment where stent-grafts are unlikely to produce long term patency. In the iliac segment, the management of a perforation using a stent-graft is probably the ideal solution to the problem.

Placement of a stent-graft can be a tricky and prolonged procedure putting the patient at risk of substantial blood loss and therefore it should be undertaken with great care. The introduction of a stent-graft will require the use of an appropriately sized large sheath at the ipsilateral puncture site. Introduction of this sheath involves an exchange process during which the tamponade balloon needs to be removed and bleeding continues whilst the exchange is taking place. The stent-graft can then be introduced through the sheath and placed at the site of the perforation. The entire procedure of exchange and placement of the stent-graft can take several minutes during which substantial haemorrhage may occur through the perforation. An alternative and a safer method of management is to introduce another balloon catheter via a contralateral approach to take the place of the tamponade balloon which is then safely removed from the ipsilateral puncture site. The rest of the manoeuvres in introducing the stent-graft from the ipsilateral approach can be carried out safely, but only when the stent-graft is ready for deployment can the contralaterally inserted tamponade balloon be deflated and withdrawn.

It cannot be stressed enough that if the operator has little experience, putting in coils or stent-grafts can be dangerous

and could lead to the death of the patient. Tamponade and surgical intervention is the safest option and the vascular surgeons should be informed as quickly as possible. An algorithm (Fig. 39.5) offers a guide to the diagnosis and management of balloon perforation within a body cavity.

Surgical treatment of perforations

Although balloon tamponade will control the perforation in the short term, immediate surgical treatment is advisable if a solution to the problem is to be found. The approach will depend upon the site of the perforation and whether the artery was patent or occluded at that point. In addition, the reason for the intervention will be important. For example, if a patient complaining of claudication is having an angioplasty, it is probably sensible to simply stop the bleeding and deal with the problem on another day as the leg will be no worse, particularly if the perforation was in an occluded segment. If, however, the leg was acutely ischaemic or becoming worse a bypass graft should be carried out.

Upper limb artery perforations

These are fortunately relatively rare but if they occur it is usually because the arm was being used for the purposes of access (see Chapter 7B). It will be necessary, therefore, to expose the artery and control and repair the perforation with a vein patch taken from an adjacent vein. Subclavian artery perforation is a serious and life-threatening problem as access to the root of the subclavian artery, which is usually where the occlusion lies, is very difficult. Balloon tamponade is an emergency requirement and the lesion has to be repaired surgically. Access can be gained by carrying out either a partial or a complete sternal split and approaching the subclavian artery as it arises from the aortic arch. If the lesion was a stenosis the vessel can be occluded by ligatures and the perforation oversewn without too much detriment to the patient. Any attempt to patch the lesion at this point is dangerous. If the arm becomes ischaemic it can be dealt with by other means, for example a crossover graft in the neck.

Lower limb artery perforations

In the lower limb, the commonest place for perforations is the iliac artery, partly because it is the most frequent site for angioplasty. If the perforation is associated with bleeding and shock, the patient should be taken to the operating theatre rapidly and the situation resolved. In the iliac artery a tamponade balloon will usually be in place and the vessel can be easily exposed retroperitoneally through an iliac muscle-cutting incision leading directly to the perforated artery. The vessels above and below are controlled with clamps and the perforation, if it has occurred in a previously patent artery, repaired, usually with a patch of Dacron or vein taken from the groin. If the artery is perforated in an occluded portion, it can be oversewn. If the vessel is occluded and provided that the patient's condition is satisfactory, it is usually best to place a graft from the normal artery above, such as the common iliac or the aorta, to the groin, in order to obtain symptomatic improvement. If the patient is not well, however, the vessel can simply be ligated. If the procedure is being undertaken for stenosis or occlusion no deterioration will occur and a definitive procedure can be carried out later. If it is impossible to construct an iliofemoral graft then a crossover graft is something which should be considered provided that the inflow is adequate.

For femoral lesions the same rules apply. If the perforated vessel was already occluded and the angioplasty was being done for claudication then simply stopping the bleeding is all that is required, with a view to definitive treatment later. A direct incision down to the bleeding vessel will usually suffice. If, however, the procedure is being performed for rest pain or acute ischaemia then a bypass graft, as will be described later, is necessary (see Chapter 15). For true crural lesions the same rules apply although, generally speaking, the angioplasty would have been undertaken for rest pain or critical ischaemia; under these circumstances some form of bypass will usually be necessary if the leg is to be saved.

EMBOLIC COMPLICATIONS

Cholesterol embolisation (microembolisation)

Excessive catheter manipulation in a diseased aorta is thought to cause this serious complication.[28] When there is

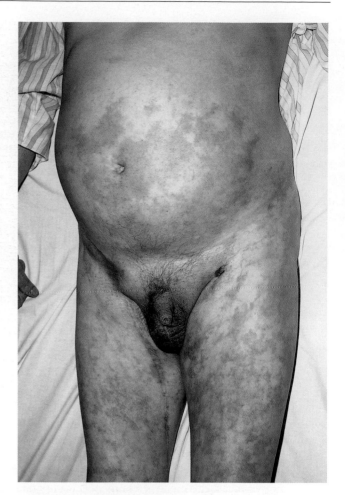

Figure 39.6 *This patient had catheter manipulations within a significantly diseased lower abdominal aorta. It resulted in cholesterol embolisation. An extensive blotchy rash appeared soon after the procedure. The picture shows typical demarcation of the rash at waist level extending downwards*

diffuse and extensive disease within the abdominal aorta, extra care is necessary during catheter manipulation to avoid cholesterol embolisation. Sometimes, and despite all care taken, this complication occurs with relatively minor degrees of manipulation of the catheter in the abdominal aorta. When it does occur, the patient experiences sudden severe back and abdominal pain and some pain in the legs but the most characteristic feature is an extensive blotchy rash which is very well demarcated at waist level and extends all the way down to the feet in a trouser fashion appearing either soon after the procedure or up to a few hours later (Fig. 39.6). Also, characteristically, peripheral pulses are present, despite extensive 'trash' embolisation. 'Trash foot' may eventually be manifested as distal tissue necrosis, frequently requiring amputation.

Treatment is usually conservative. When cholesterol embolisation is higher than waist level, the renal and mesenteric arteries may be involved, in which case there is serious morbidity and possible mortality. Some patients require permanent renal dialysis as cholesterol embolisation

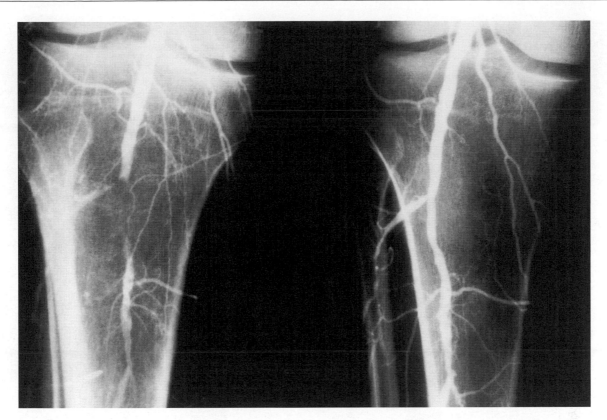

Figure 39.7   *Following recanalisation of the superficial femoral artery, a large embolus from the angioplasty site landed at the trifurcation and it was successfully aspirated*

into the renal circulation causes progressive and often irreversible loss of renal function. Apart from anticoagulation and possibly iloprost infusion there is no treatment for this condition and mortality is high; fortunately, this complication occurs rarely.

Small and large embolisation (macroembolisation)

The commonest sources of such emboli are the iliac arteries, particularly iliac occlusions. When small emboli, up to 3 mm in diameter, are released into the circulation beyond an angioplastied site, they may lodge at the popliteal trifurcation or beyond (Fig. 39.7). When haemodynamically significant, the management of such emboli is, in the first instance, percutaneous aspiration accomplished using a large 50 mL syringe attached to a non-tapered 8 Fr catheter the tip of which is brought into contact with the embolus. When aspirating through this large syringe, a vacuum is created within the catheter, which has the effect of sucking directly on the embolus, which then becomes 'attached' to the catheter tip and is withdrawn along with the catheter through the sheath. Frequently, the embolus becomes detached in the sheath valve and therefore it is important to check that the valve is cleared of any embolic debris before being reattached to the sheath. The majority of emboli of this size can be aspirated percutaneously without difficulty.[29–31]

Some emboli are not haemodynamically significant, affecting one among several run-off vessels supplying the foot. In this situation the embolus may be left alone, particularly if the limb is haemodynamically stable. Other emboli, particularly those larger than 3 mm, may not become 'attached' to the aspiration catheter, despite adequate suction being applied with the large syringe. This may be due to the shape of the embolus which does not allow the rim of the catheter tip to sit uniformly over it and as such, does not allow an adequate vacuum to be created within the catheter. If the embolus is very large, it is difficult to maintain attachment of the embolus to the catheter through suction and in any case, even when the large embolus is attached to the catheter, it may become dislodged at the level of the sheath when attempts are being made to aspirate it. In such a case, if more than one run-off vessel is available, then a compromise situation may be achieved by pushing the embolus into one of them, i.e. 'push and park'[32] (Fig. 39.8). This is achieved by pushing the embolus either with the 8 Fr non-tapered catheter, already there for aspiration attempts, or with an inflated balloon catheter.

Thrombolysis is usually ineffective in embolic complications as, in our experience, the majority of emboli appear to be of hard consistency and therefore unlikely to undergo lysis. Moreover, the length of time it takes to set up thrombolysis and to get it working means that more thrombus is likely to form while flow remains compromised before the treatment takes full effect. It is therefore preferable to

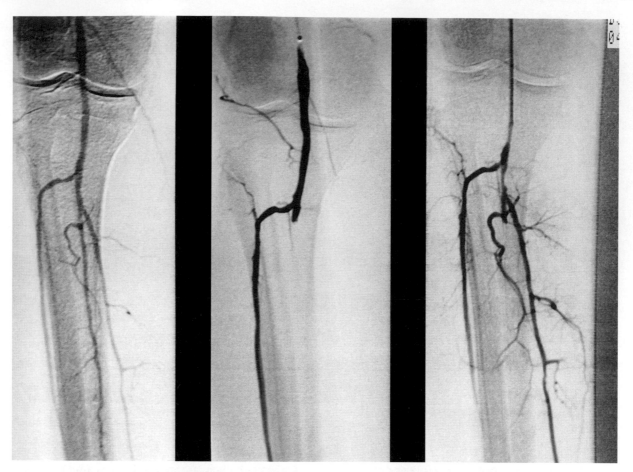

Figure 39.8   *A long femoropopliteal occlusion was undergoing recanalisation but during the procedure, an embolus landed in the tibioperoneal trunk, which could not be aspirated. This embolus was therefore pushed downwards into the peroneal artery. A three-vessel run-off was reduced to two, but this was better than leaving the embolus in the tibioperoneal trunk, which would have meant that only the anterior tibial artery would have been patent*

resolve embolic complication in the way described and establish flow as soon as possible.

Surgery for embolic complications

If the leg becomes ischaemic in spite of attempts to remove the embolus by endovascular means then surgical intervention becomes necessary. As the angiogram is available, the operating surgeon will be aware of the location of the embolus. The embolus is usually in the lower leg in the popliteal artery or trifurcation, and if it is lower than that there is usually one crural vessel still open and the foot is usually not acutely ischaemic. The problem can be approached in one of two ways.

- The femoral artery can be opened in the groin and an embolectomy catheter inserted to remove the thrombus. This is not usually possible if it is done blindly with an ordinary embolectomy catheter. It is best done with an over the wire Fogarty catheter. The wire is inserted first of all under X-ray control using a C-arm and passed beyond the embolus. The catheter can then be passed over the wire and the embolus withdrawn without difficulty. This can be done using local anaesthesia of the groin or under general anaesthesia. A completion angiogram is essential to ensure that the embolus has been retrieved.

- If a groin approach is not possible or fails, then it is necessary to explore the popliteal artery, using a medial below-knee approach, exposing the vessel in the usual way. After the vessel has been controlled proximally and distally it can be opened directly over the area where there is no pulsation and the embolus removed. If this is done the artery should be closed with a vein patch taken from an adjacent vein. If the embolus is in one of the crural arteries then it can be removed with a Fogarty catheter. Completion angiogram is again mandatory.

The algorithm in Fig. 39.9 offers a guide to the management of embolic complications.

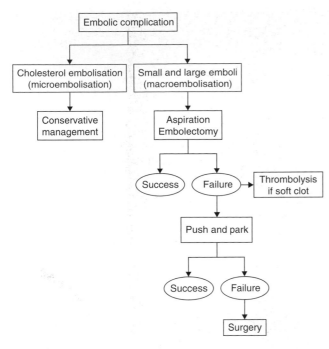

Figure 39.9 *Algorithm of the management of embolic complications*

THROMBOTIC COMPLICATIONS

Thrombotic complications can occur at the site of angioplasty or remote from it, particularly when flow is being obstructed by a catheter or a sheath employed as an access route to some site where angioplasty is being carried out. For example, during renal angioplasty, the catheter/sheath may be obstructing or substantially reducing flow at a diseased external iliac artery site, which is being used as the route for the procedure. Further factors such as inadequate heparinisation, a prolonged procedure and the use of large catheter/sheath sizes may play a part in causing thrombosis. It can also be averted if there is prior knowledge of a lesion on the route to a distant angioplasty site. Further, any significant stenosis along the route can be angioplastied soon after the lesion has been crossed before any further procedures are done at the intended site.

Flow can be compromised at an angioplasty site where there has been a previous stenosis or an occlusion that has been dilated. Such compromise of flow may occur either due to acute thrombosis, elastic recoil or the presence of an intimal flap. In all of these cases, a stent may resolve the situation. In the case of fresh thrombosis, however, thrombolysis may be considered or, alternatively, a stent-graft may resolve the complication.

In some situations, conservative management may be appropriate. For example, when there is adequate collateral circulation around a tightly stenosed segment which then occludes during attempted angioplasty, the collateral flow will allow the lesion to be left alone. One may consider a conservative approach in this situation until such time as the thrombosed segment becomes organised, for example in 3–6 months time, before repeating the angioplasty.

Surgical treatment for thrombosed segments

This would be exactly the same for thrombosis occurring in relation to catheter access as described earlier. If the thrombosis is in a stenosed vessel then a good collateral circulation may be available and an operation is not necessary except for critical ischaemia, in which event a bypass procedure of appropriate type is indicated. This will depend upon the site of the occlusion. It could be iliofemoral, crossover, femoropopliteal or femorodistal.

ELASTIC RECOIL/COMPROMISED COLLATERALS

This complication is specific to subintimal angioplasty where important collaterals become compromised during the dissection and yet adequate flow cannot be achieved due to elastic recoil of the occluding segment (Fig. 39.10). This results in compromised flow to the lower limb. In the past, emergency surgery, which includes balloon embolectomy, thrombolysis and bypass surgery would have been required. More recently long self-expanding stents have been used to resolve the situation. Most cases with compromised flow due to elastic recoil can be resolved with the use of long self-expandable stents, but in a proportion of cases, an emergency bypass operation may still be required. A stent in the infrainguinal arteries is unlikely to have any significant long term patency and therefore bypass surgery may eventually become necessary. The use of a stent in this situation is therefore a temporary measure in order to avoid an emergency operation (see Fig. 39.10c).

Surgery for acutely ischaemic limbs following endovascular intervention

In most circumstances where endovascular techniques are being used for treating claudication, occlusion of the artery or embolisation will not result in acute ischaemia, and watching the limb carefully for an hour or two may allow it to recover sufficiently for a surgical or further endovascular solution to be undertaken later. If the limb is being dealt with for critical ischaemia, however, some form of intervention is necessary as the limb usually becomes worse. This only occurs in a minority, in our experience in less than 1 per cent of cases, and it represents a surgical emergency which needs to be dealt with quickly. In many instances the problem can be dealt with, as described earlier in this chapter, by removal of the thrombus and oversewing the artery with a patch. Occasionally, however, this will not work and further measures are required,

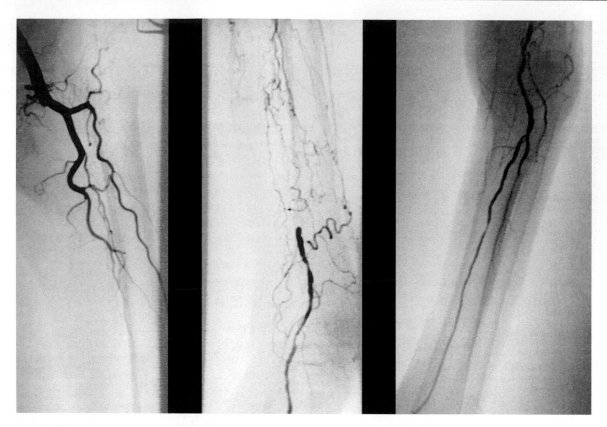

Figure 39.10 *(a) Angiogram showing a full length flush occlusion of the superficial femoral artery*

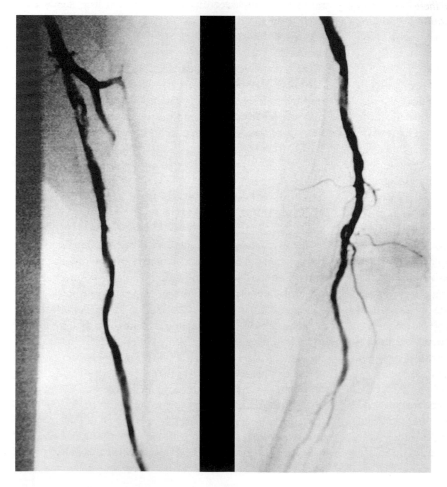

Figure 39.10 *(b) The occlusion was recanalised with subintimal dissection*

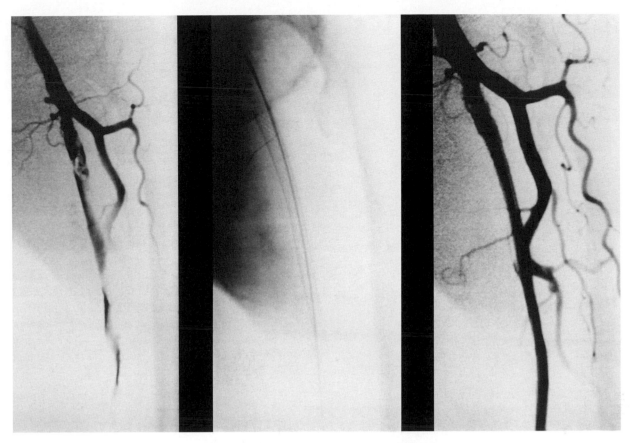

Figure 39.10   *(c) Very soon after recanalisation there was a slowing of flow. Elastic recoil was noted in the upper third of the superficial femoral artery. A long Wallstent was implanted with a successful outcome. Note the 'spiral ribbon' appearance of the dissection channel*

particularly lower down the limb in the crural arteries where subintimal angioplasty is being performed for critical ischaemia. In this situation, as an angiogram will have been done during the procedure, the surgeon will be aware of the condition of the proximal and distal vessels. If the leg becomes painful and pale and if sensation is lost or movement is reduced then urgent treatment is needed.

First of all, the proximal vessel from which the bypass takes off is exposed. This would usually be the femoral artery in the groin or perhaps in the mid-thigh. An on-table angiogram is then carried out to assess the situation and see where a patent distal vessel lies. An appropriate vessel is then exposed for a reversed or *in situ* vein bypass. Before this is done an angiogram of the distal run-off vessels is carried out and if it shows good run-off into the foot then a bypass is created. If however there is a poor run-off into the foot, on-table thrombolysis is necessary. This is achieved using streptokinase, urokinase or tissue plasminogen activator (tPA), made up into a solution of about 100 mL and dripped slowly through a cannula into the distal vessel over a period of 30 minutes or so (see Chapter 16). When that has been done the angiogram should be repeated to ensure that there is now good run-off after which the bypass graft is constructed. This technique will usually take care of most cases of distal embolisation unless it is of the atheromatous variety, in which case nothing more can be done to save the leg.

If no distal vessels can be seen on the first transfemoral angiogram, the popliteal artery should be exposed for on-table angiography to find a vessel which runs into the foot. If no vessel can be found conforming to these requirements then, based on the pre-intervention angiogram, one is chosen and exposed. Again this artery is cleared by on-table thrombolysis and if successful will receive the bypass graft.

This type of acute ischaemia is fortunately rare and its occurrence is a serious situation because only half of the limbs affected by distal embolisation can be salvaged. It is vital, however, to ensure the presence of a vascular surgeon during any intervention as acute deterioration cannot be forecast. The correct approach is to have a vascular team which is multiskilled and able to deal with these situations appropriately. An algorithm offering pathways in the management of compromised collaterals and elastic recoil following attempted subintimal angioplasty is given in Fig. 39.11.

COMPROMISE OF IMPORTANT BRANCHES AT BIFURCATIONS

Any angioplasty at a bifurcation site is at some risk of compromising the adjacent artery. The kissing balloon technique for aortoiliac segment disease has been popular for a long

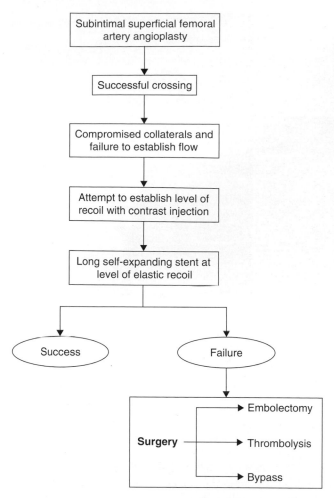

Figure 39.11 *Algorithm of the management of compromised collaterals and elastic recoil following attempted subintimal superficial femoral artery angioplasty*

time and is mainly used for disease extending from the lower abdominal aorta into both common iliac arteries. The same technique, however, applies when there is a solitary stenotic lesion in one of the common iliac arteries, but the lesion is close enough to the origin of the other common iliac artery. Using a single balloon catheter carries a risk of embolisation into the contralateral iliac artery. It is recommended, therefore, that even in a unilateral common iliac origin stenosis, the kissing balloon technique be employed.

At bifurcations of smaller arteries, e.g. the common iliac bifurcation and the common femoral bifurcation, there is some risk of compromise to one of the branches during attempted angioplasty of a lesion in one of these arteries. In such situations too, the kissing balloon technique may be a means of protection.

ACCIDENTAL DISSECTION

Occasionally simple angioplasty of a stenotic lesion may result in an extensive dissection, causing significant dissection flaps. If blood flow is thereby compromised, the management of this complication may include stenting. It has to be stressed, however, that the treatment of atherosclerotic plaques using a balloon catheter does involve creating splits in the intima, which are a form of dissection. In other words, dissection is a part of the process of balloon angioplasty and only when a dissection flap becomes haemodynamically significant, should treatment with a stent be considered. Pressure readings are commonly used to assess any significant gradients and that gradient may be enhanced with the use of adjuvant vasodilators. Such gradients can be reduced to insignificance and indeed eliminated by stent insertion.

An alternative method of improving the haemodynamics in this flow-compromised situation caused by a dissection flap may be to intentionally extend the subintimal dissection until re-entry into the lumen is achieved distally. This is a viable option when the artery distally appears to be disease free, and is a favourable factor in the attempt to achieve re-entry. A standard technique of subintimal angioplasty involves manipulating a hydrophilic guidewire into a loop which can be engaged into the dissection flap, the aim being to extend the dissection, and the same loop can be used to achieve re-entry distally.

OTHER ENDOVASCULAR MANAGEMENT PROCEDURES

There is a chance that materials placed inside a patient may be misplaced, dislodged from the desired position, released or detached prematurely from the delivery device. Utmost care needs to be taken to prevent such an occurrence. In the unlikely event that it does, however, it is important to consider how best to manage this problem and preferably in a minimally invasive fashion.

The ability to retrieve a foreign body can be an important skill for those involved in endovascular procedures. A misplaced stent is not a rare event and when it occurs a rapid solution is required. For example, renal or subclavian artery stenting may result in the stent sliding off from the balloon during the attempted passage of the stent to its precise destination. When a stent has slid off the balloon, an attempt can be made to place it along the route. For example, a renal stent which has come off the balloon catheter may be 'persuaded' to enter the common or external iliac artery where it may be inflated and placed permanently without any significant consequences. Sometimes, however stents embolise distally and need to be removed by open surgery.

One very useful device with which any endovascular operator must become familiar is the Amplatz goose neck snare. It is a clever piece of instrumentation for retrieving foreign bodies in a tubular structure, such as an artery, a vein or even the biliary and urinary tracts (Fig. 39.12). The goose neck snare is designed so that it has a circular loop which is set at 90 degrees to the long axis of the catheter. When the snare is run along a tubular structure, the loop will engage any loose

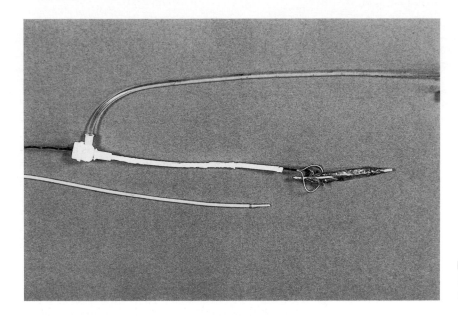

Figure 39.12 *Complete avulsion of the balloon from the catheter successfully retrieved using the goose neck snare*

body present in the tubular structure as long as the size of the snare matches with the diameter of the tubular structure. Small stents which have become dislodged may be engaged into the loop of the snare and pulled out.[33] Embolisation coils are occasionally misplaced or become emboli which can be retrieved with the help of the goose neck snare.

Balloon catheters are designed to burst longitudinally when the designated 'burst pressure' is exceeded. This does not pose any problems during removal. Occasionally, however, a balloon may have a spiral or partial transverse tear. The problem arises when there is a transverse tear, a rare complication due to inflation within a heavily calcified artery. A transversely torn balloon may be difficult to remove because the torn end may fold back when attempts are made to withdraw it. If endovascular removal of that balloon is hard then it is best achieved surgically and the artery repaired with a patch.

Balloon catheters rarely fail but complete avulsion of the balloon from the catheter has occurred in the past and still remains a possibility. It is wise not to inflate the balloon unless there is a wire through it. The presence of the wire helps with any other manoeuvres in dealing with problems that may occur. In the above example of the avulsed balloon, the loop of the goose neck snare can be fed over the wire/catheter in order to engage the avulsed balloon, before pulling it out through the sheath (see Fig. 39.12). A similar manoeuvre can be used with dislodged/ruptured items of catheter, central line or avulsed wire.

Conclusions

Endovascular procedures are carried out in increasing numbers each year in most hospitals and this trend continues year by year. In part, this rise has occurred in tandem with the improved merits of materials and devices, the widening range of indications and the growing experience of radiologists and other operators. The expansion in numbers of PTAs performed correspondingly reflects the incidence of complications that have to be managed by radiologists and vascular surgeons. It is essential therefore that, as part of one's training in endovascular procedures, the trainee is instructed in meticulous technique, is aware of the incidence and types of complications and indeed the care necessary in avoiding them, as well as the best methods available in managing them when they occur. It is equally important that, in the event of failure of endovascular attempts, vascular surgeons are capable of intervening successfully by open surgical means.

Key references

Becker GJ, Katzen BT, Dake MD. Noncoronary angioplasty. *Radiology* 1989; **170**: 921–40.

Belli A, Cumberland D, Knox A, *et al.* The complication rate of percutaneous peripheral balloon angioplasty. *Clin Radiol* 1990; **41**: 380–3.

Matsi PJ, Manninen HJ. Complications of lower limb percutaneous transluminal angioplasty: a prospective analysis of 410 procedures on 295 consecutive patients. *Cardiovasc Int Radiol* 1998; **21**: 361–6.

Morse M, Jeans W, Cole S, *et al.* Complications in percutaneous transluminal angioplasty: relationships with patient age. *Br J Radiology* 1991; **64**: 757–9.

Tegtmeyer C, Hartwell G, Selby B, *et al.* Results and complications of angioplasty in aortoiliac disease. *Circulation* 1991; **83** (suppl I): I-53–60.

REFERENCES

1 Dotter CT, Judkins, MP. Transluminal treatment of arteriosclerotic obstructions: description of a new technic and a preliminary report of its application. *Circulation* 1964; **30**: 654–70.

2 Lewis D, Bullbulia R, Murphy P, *et al*. Vascular surgical intervention for complications of cardiovascular radiology: 13 years experience in a single centre. *Ann R Coll Surg Engl* 1999; **81**: 23–6.

3 Gardiner G, Meyerovitz M, Stokes K, *et al*. Complications of transluminal angioplasty. *Radiology* 1986; **159**: 201–8.

4 Tegtmeyer C, Hartwell G, Selby B, *et al*. Results and complications of angioplasty in aortoiliac disease. *Circulation* 1991; **83**(suppl I): I-53–60.

5 Axisa B, Fishwick G, Bolia A, *et al*. Complications following peripheral angioplasty. *Ann R Coll Surg Engl* 2002; **84**: 39–42.

6 Hayes PD, Chokkalingham A, Jones R, *et al*. Arterial perforation during infrainguinal lower limb angioplasty does not worsen outcome: Results from 1409 patients. *J Endovasc Ther* 2002; **4**: 422–7.

7 Papvavassiliou VG, Walker SR, Bolia A, *et al*. Techniques for the endovascular management of complications following lower limb percutaneous transluminal angioplasty. *Eur J Vasc Endovasc Surg* 2003; **25**: 125–30.

8 Belli A, Cumberland D, Knox A, *et al*. The complication rate of percutaneous peripheral balloon angioplasty. *Clin Radiol* 1990; **41**: 380–3.

9 Morse M, Jeans W, Cole S, *et al*. Complications in percutaneous transluminal angioplasty: relationships with patient age. *Br J Radiol* 1991; **64**: 757–9.

10 Fraedrich G, Beck F, Bonzal T, Schlosser V. Acute surgical intervention for complications of percutaneous transluminal angioplasty. *Eur J Vasc Surg* 1987; **1**: 197–203.

11 Matsi PJ, Manninen HJ. Complications of lower limb percutaneous transluminal angioplasty: a prospective analysis of 410 procedures on 295 consecutive patients. *Cardiovasc Int Radiol* 1998; **21**: 361–6.

12 Becker GJ, Katzen BT, Dake MD. Noncoronary angioplasty. *Radiology* 1989; **170**: 921–40.

13 Starck EE, McDermott J, Crummy AB, Heydwolf AV. Angioplasty of the popliteal and tibial arteries. *Semin Intervent Radiol* 1984; **1**: 296–77.

14 van Andel GJ, van Erp WFM, Krepel VM, Breslau PJ. Percutaneous transluminal dilatation of the iliac artery; long-term results. *Radiology* 1985; **156**: 321–3.

15 Greenfield AJ. Femoral, popliteal, and tibial arteries: percutaneous transluminal angioplasty. *Am J Radiol* 1980; **135**: 927–35.

16 Laerum F, Castaneda-Zuniga WR, Amplatz KA. Complications of transluminal angioplasty. New York: Thieme-Stratton, 1983: 41–4.

17 Zeitler E. Percutaneous dilatation and recanalization of iliac and femoral arteries. *Cardiovasc Intervent Radiol* 1980; **3**: 207–12.

18 Bergquist D, Jonsson K, Weibull H. Complications after percutaneous transluminal angioplasty of peripheral and renal arteries. *Acta Radiol* 1987; **28**: 3–12.

19 Franco C, Goldsmith J, Veith F, *et al*. Management of arterial injuries produced by percutaneous femoral procedures. *Surgery* 1993; **113**: 419–25.

20 Chaterjee T, Do DD, Kaufmann U, *et al*. Ultrasound guided compression repair for treatment of femoral artery pseudoaneurysm: acute and follow-up results. *Catheter Cardiovasc Diagn* 1996; **38**: 335–40.

21 Wixon CL, Philpott JM, Bogey WM, Powell CS. Duplex directed thrombin injection as a method to treat femoral artery pseudoaneurysms. *J Am Coll Surg* 1998; **18**: 464–6.

22 Fellmeth BD, Roberts AC, Bookstein JJ, *et al*. Postangiographic femoral artery injuries: non-surgical repair with US-guided compression. *Radiology* 1991; **178**: 671–7.

23 Kazmers A, Meeker C, Kofz K, *et al*. Nonoperative therapy for postcatheterization femoral artery pseudoaneurysms. *Am Surg* 1997; **63**: 199–204.

24 Owen RJT, Haslam PJ, Elliott ST, *et al*. Percutaneous ablation of peripheral pseudoaneurysms using thrombin: a simple and effective solution. *CardioVasc Intervent Radiol* 2000; **23**: 441–6.

25 O'Keeffe ST, Woods BO, Beckmann CF. Percutaneous transluminal angioplasty of the peripheral arteries. *Cardiol Clin* 1991; **9**: 515.

26 Samson RH, Sprayregen S, Veith FJ, *et al*. Management of angioplasty complications, unsuccessful procedures, and early and late failures. *Ann Surg* 1984; **199**: 234.

27 Weibull H, Bergqist D, Jonsson K, *et al*. Complications after percutaneous transluminal angioplasty in the iliac, femoral, and popliteal arteries. *J Vasc Surg* 1987; **5**: 681.

28 Gaines PA, Cumberland DC, Kennedy A, *et al*. Cholesterol embolisation; a lethal complication of vascular catheterisation. *Lancet* 1988; **i**: 168–70.

29 Murray IG, Brown AL, Wilkins RA. Percutaneous aspiration thromboembolectomy: a preliminary experience. *Clin Radiol* 1994; **49**: 553–8.

30 Cleveland TJ, Cumberland DC, Gaines PA. Percutaneous aspiration thromboembolectomy to manage the embolic complications of angioplasty and as an adjunct to thrombolysis. *Clin Radiol* 1994; **49**: 549–52.

31 Wagner HJ, Starck EE, Reuter P. Long term results of percutaneous aspiration embolectomy. *Cardiovasc Intervent Radiol* 1994; **17**: 241–6.

32 Higginson A, Alaeddin F, Fishwick G, Bolia A. 'Push and park'. An alternative strategy for management of embolic complication during balloon angioplasty. *Eur J Vasc Endovasc Surg* 2001; **21**: 279–82.

33 Gabelmann A, Kramers SC, Tomczak R, Gorich J. Percutaneous techniques for managing maldeployed or migrated stents. *J Endovasc Ther* 2001; **8**: 291–302.

40

Specialty Related Iatrogenic Vascular Injuries

LARS NORGREN

THE PROBLEM

Percutaneous interventions are increasingly used for diagnostic and therapeutic procedures. In vascular surgery, the Swedish Vascular Registry (Swedvasc) between 1987 and 1997 reported an increasing proportion of catheter interventions rising from a third to three-quarters in comparison with open procedures on the aortoiliac segment. In line with this change there seems to be an increasing number of iatrogenic vascular injuries reported. In a Swedish study in 1995 iatrogenic causes accounted for 20 per cent of all vascular injuries reported[1] and an unpublished Swedvasc report valid for the year 2000 found a corresponding figure of 45 per cent. There was also a slightly higher incidence of iatrogenic vascular injuries in larger rather than in smaller hospitals and this is easily explained by the fact that the former treat the more complicated cases.

This chapter gives an overall picture of the kind of damage that can be inflicted on arteries and veins in patients who are not primarily victims of vascular disease. They represent a small proportion of iatrogenic vascular injuries and result from open procedures; these are discussed under the various specialties concerned.

According to Adar et al.[2] iatrogenic complications may be technically classified as the consequences of:

- accident
- faulty technique or routine
- errors in judgement or management
- failure to identify anatomical structures correctly
- failure to interpret X-rays or laboratory findings correctly.

These complications, which are usually treated as emergencies, fall into four groups

- bleeding
- thrombosis
- embolism
- dissection.

A further group of delayed problems includes false aneurysms, arteriovenous fistulae and septic complications but they do not usually need emergency treatment.

Apart from catheterisation procedures there are other specific surgical interventions which give rise to complications. These fall within the three main surgical specialties of orthopaedics, general surgery and gynaecology. Orthopaedic operations on the lumbar disc and on the limbs for various conditions are at risk of producing iatrogenic vascular injuries. Within the broad range of general surgical procedures, certain categories are potentially vulnerable to vascular injury and these include operations in the abdomen, laparoscopic and thoracoscopic interventions, and hernia and varicose vein surgery. Gynaecological operations also place the pelvic vasculature at some risk.

Specialty groups and procedures at risk

- Orthopaedics
  - Lumbar disc surgery
  - Limb surgery
- General surgery
  - Varicose vein surgery
  - Laparoscopic surgery

- Thoracoscopic surgery
- Open abdominal surgery
- Hernia surgery
- Gynaecology

ORTHOPAEDIC VASCULAR COMPLICATIONS

Surgery for lumbar disc herniation, hip arthroplasty and knee operations are all procedures in which vascular problems commonly occur.[3] The overall complication rate for elective orthopaedic surgery varies from country to country. Two Scandinavian studies presented figures showing that only four out of a total of 131[4] and two out of 79[5] vascular injuries were caused by elective orthopaedic surgical procedures. Acute orthopaedic surgery may cause bleeding due to laceration of vessels often associated with the use of nails and pins. Such injuries can also cause delayed complications, mainly bleeding, probably as a result of infection.[6] A German study reported 43 patients with vascular injuries after orthopaedic surgery: 18 were seen after hip surgery, 8 after knee surgery, 2 after lumbar disc surgery and 15 after fracture fixation.[7]

Lumbar disc surgery

The lumbar discs are closely related to the distal aorta, the iliac arteries, the vena cava and the iliac veins. The literature shows that the L4/5 interspace is the most common site for vascular injury. This complication may result in immediate and overt bleeding or the development of a false aneurysm or arteriovenous fistula, the latter commonly presenting much later than the original injury. Such injuries are frequently associated with intraoperative complications. A literature survey of 68 cases with arteriovenous fistulae reported 17 with early signs of bleeding and 16 with a peroperative or postoperative drop in blood pressure.[3] Reoperations are frequently associated with inflammation and a destructive process involving the spinal ligaments contributing to an increased risk of complications.[8]

Treatment of these complications requires a good knowledge of anatomy as well as meticulous technique. Overt bleeding from the operative field is usually a sign of damage to large vessels. If there are signs of severe bleeding, the only effective treatment is to turn the patient and perform an immediate laparotomy. If, with packing, the bleeding ceases, it is imperative to observe the patient extremely carefully during the remaining period of surgery and the immediate postoperative course. Even minimal signs of new bleeding should be considered serious. Ultrasonography, computed tomography (CT) scanning and angiography are occasionally necessary to elicit evidence of a retroperitoneal haematoma.

The surgical procedure is often performed under desperate circumstances with the patient in hypovolaemic shock. On these occasions a gauze pack and manual compression are required while proximal control is being achieved. Even if the bleeding emanates from a large vein, aortic clamping gives much needed respite and a better chance of successful resuscitation. 'Two hands and two eyes' are inadequate in such situations. The management of these injuries depends on the extent of the injury, and, not infrequently, graft replacement is required for distal aortic or iliac artery injury. Venous injuries are certainly not easy to handle and repairs by simple suture, patch, graft replacement or even a ligature may be required. Prompt diagnosis and aggressive treatment of bleeding during lumbar disc surgery may improve the mortality, which currently stands at over 50 per cent.[9]

Anterior approaches to the lumbar spine have become more popular and vascular surgeons are frequently involved in these procedures on an emergency basis. One retrospective study of 102 such lumbar spine procedures reported a 16 per cent incidence of vascular injuries requiring surgical repair.[10]

Arteriovenous fistulae only rarely demand emergency treatment except in instances of heart failure when the indication is obvious and the intervention urgent. This procedure is often difficult technically, necessitating dissection of both proximal and distal artery and vein. If at all possible, a catheter procedure involving embolisation or coiling, the magnitude of which is comparatively limited, should be tried. When adequate resources become available, endovascular treatment of both arteries and veins will probably be the first line of attack. Insertion of a stent-graft at the site of injury is technically demanding but will stop bleeding effectively and relatively atraumatically.

Hip surgery

Case reports on vascular injuries in conjunction with hip replacement indicate an incidence of 0.004–0.25 per cent.[4] The risk of vascular damage is considerably higher during revision than during primary procedures.[11,12] There seems to be a female and left-sided dominance to the problem, which is more often found during hip arthroplasty than hip fracture surgery. The deep femoral artery is more prone to injury during hip fracture surgery and the external iliac artery during arthroplasty. The severity of these iatrogenic accidents is reflected in the incidence of functional sequelae (19 per cent) and mortality (7 per cent).[13]

From a technical point of view the dangerous aspects of hip replacement seem to be twofold: the use of a retractor close to the artery carries a risk of arterial compression or laceration, and manipulation of the femur as the femoral part of the prosthesis is being inserted causes traction of the vessels.[4] The latter may cause thrombosis within vessels already diseased.[12,14] Reoperations are associated with an increased risk of bleeding. The cement used during fixation of the prosthesis may also cause thermal injury to the adjacent vessels. Haemorrhage from the deep femoral artery may sometimes occur at a late stage due to infection at the site of the prosthesis.

Prevention of such complications obviously demands sound surgical technique, and here, as in other instances, a prerequisite is avoiding injury. This is especially relevant in reoperations and in patients with atherosclerotic vascular disease. If bleeding occurs during surgery, the application of clamps and forceps in the wound should be avoided and compression used instead. Control is achieved through a proximal incision over the external iliac artery.

Tachycardia and a drop in blood pressure should be interpreted as signs of retroperitoneal bleeding if the reasons are not otherwise obvious. 'Distal signs', a term coined by hand surgeons, of both ischaemia and neurological deficit should be looked for postoperatively. Bleeding may not be haemodynamically evident, but increasing swelling of the thigh, or on occasions of the gluteal region, along with motor and sensory loss, should be noted; as compartment pressure rises ischaemia may well follow. With more extensive injuries to calcified vessels bypass procedures are usually required, but late bleeding can often be resolved by embolisation of the bleeding source.

Knee surgery

As with other orthopaedic procedures there are no data available establishing the true incidence of vascular injuries during knee surgery. A report from Australia in 1987 described 12 cases after knee arthroplasty during a 10-year period.[15] There were three lacerations of the popliteal artery and seven arterial thromboses. Of these seven cases, five had to undergo major amputation. One false aneurysm and one arteriovenous fistula were also reported. Overall, therefore, the incidence seems to be very low but lesions are found incidentally even after arthroscopy. In an American series of 118 590 arthroscopies, six penetrating injuries of the popliteal artery were registered[3] of which four required amputation. These injuries have also been observed after total knee replacement.[16]

The use of a tourniquet for a bloodless field is controversial in patients with peripheral atherosclerosis as it may well cause arterial thrombosis. Furthermore, traction and manipulation during surgery may cause embolisation of plaque from the popliteal artery.[12]

Fractures and other procedures

It should be emphasised that closed as well as open reduction of fractures, with or without osteosynthesis, may cause compression and injury as well as thrombotic occlusion of arteries, subsequently leading to bleeding or ischaemia. The classic example is the supracondylar fracture of the humerus in children where the brachial artery may be compressed by the fracture and also during closed reduction. Careful observation during and after the procedure is therefore important.

Limb tumour surgery may also involve tackling large vessels and should be performed preferably after preoperative mapping of the main arterial supply and venous drainage.

GENERAL SURGERY

Varicose vein surgery

Injuries in varicose vein surgery are usually caused during dissection of the groin. Two main types of injury are seen: damage to the femoral vein by ligation or resection and damage to arteries by ligation, resection and even stripping of the superficial femoral artery. Even the deep femoral artery has been ligated and resected. Injuries caused by the inadvertent injection of sclerotic agents into arteries, either during surgery or at outpatient varicose vein clinics, have also been reported.[3] During a 20-year period, 15 injuries of groin vessels during varicose vein surgery were reported to the Swedish Board of Health and Welfare; it is impossible to estimate the true incidence of this iatrogenic injury, but it is probably much higher.

In 1986 Cockett described nine cases of iatrogenic arterial lesions, none of which was detected during surgery, and consequently repair was delayed in all cases.[17] A femoral vein injury may be the result of an anatomical mistake during dissection and frequently manifests as bleeding. This type of injury is usually caused by less experienced surgeons. As sclerosing agents are only occasionally injected into the saphenous vein during a 'high tie' the risk of injection into the superficial femoral artery appears minimal. There is, however, a slight risk of percutaneous injection of sclerosant into an artery but this should be small with current techniques of compression sclerotherapy. Even if varicose vein surgery is considered to be rather simple technically, the need for supervised training is as essential as that for more advanced surgical procedures.

As the anatomy of the veins in the groin is variable, careful dissection is mandatory. No attempt to ligate or to introduce a stripper should be made until the anatomy is clear. Even a stripper inserted at ankle level may pass through a perforating vein in the thigh and end up in the femoral vein. Since many of the patients undergoing varicose vein surgery are rather young, dissection of an artery may cause spasm and its pulsation may disappear. Only careful dissection will reveal the true anatomy, a prerequisite to continuing with the operation.

When deep bleeding from the femoral vein occurs unexpectedly, attempts to arrest it using artery forceps is understandable. *This must always be avoided.* The only acceptable measure is to compress the bleeding vein and call for assistance. If the injury has not been worsened by inexpert use of instruments and clumsy clamping, the actual damage is usually found to be quite small, and a simple lateral suture may stop the bleeding. If not, proximal and distal control must be obtained followed by resection and reconstruction.

In the majority of these cases the saphenous vein has already been divided and may well be used for the reconstruction. If the vein has not been divided, it may assist venous return from the leg and should be saved. In such cases the saphenous vein from the other leg should be used. In principle, there are two methods of repairing the femoral vein, which is usually at least twice the diameter of the saphenous vein (see Chapter 33). The first is to take double the length of vein needed and split it longitudinally, divide it into two lengths and suture these side-to-side, thereby doubling the diameter.[18] The second option is to split the vein longitudinally, wrap it spirally over a glass staff and then suture the entire spiral into a tube graft.[19]

The main question, of course, is whether or not this kind of reconstruction stays patent. An arteriovenous fistula can be created as an adjunctive operation. There are no proper studies to prove the results, but even if the reconstruction occludes later, there may be a chance that while it stays open collateral flow will take over. Ligature of the femoral vein is rarely acceptable (see Chapter 33).

Arterial injuries should be repaired immediately but delayed presentation is common. If there is the slightest suspicion of ischaemia, ankle blood pressures are measured and, if damage is still suspected, angiography performed. Reconstructions of these injuries follow general principles of arterial surgery. If possible, a limited resection and end-to-end anastomosis should be carried out or, alternatively, graft replacement, preferably using vein from the contralateral leg.

Intra-arterial injection of sclerosing agents is particularly dangerous and, if the effect is widespread, gangrene and amputation will follow. If the agent has been injected more locally, there is a chance that healing may occur. In either situation it is advisable to give heparin intravenously. If for any reason, pain for example, the complication is suspected and the needle is still in place, heparin-saline and an α-receptor blocker or reserpine should be injected through it. An epidural block might be of value but little scientific proof of its value exists.

Laparoscopic surgery

The tremendous increase in laparoscopic procedures during the past 10 years is reflected in the rise in associated vascular injuries, but the actual number of these cases is small. In a report of 1995 laparoscopies 20 iatrogenic vascular injuries were reported,[20] while in the single-centre experience of 2589 laparoscopic cholecystectomies performed between 1990 and 1996, 0.11 per cent had major vascular injuries.[21] In Sweden, about seven vascular injuries are reported annually to the independent loss adjuster (*PersonSkadeReglering* (PSR)), half of them being injuries

of the large vessels and the other half of the abdominal wall. These figures, however, should not be seen as the true incidence of injuries (PSR, personal communication). The vascular injuries are usually caused by trocar insertion and the most commonly affected are the aorta, iliac arteries and the inferior vena cava. Injuries attributable to the insufflation needle have also been reported.[22] In many countries there are now guidelines on the technique for insufflation and trocar placement.[23]

Taking into consideration the size of the vessels usually damaged during laparoscopic procedures, the mortality risk is high and prompt treatment is required. It is likely that with the current degree of specialisation in surgery, skilled laparoscopic surgeons are not trained to handle vascular problems. Bleeding, revealed at laparotomy, should be immediately controlled by manual compression rather than by a 'trial and error' approach and, in most large centres, experienced vascular surgeons should be available to deal with this catastrophe.

Thoracoscopy

Thoracoscopic sympathectomy has been used increasingly to treat palmar hyperhidrosis. Vascular injuries are not reported frequently and in a study of 940 operations[24] there was only one subclavian artery injury, but there have been occasional reports of mortality.

Open abdominal surgery

Injuries to the portal vein, superior mesenteric vein and concomitant arteries may occur during pancreaticobiliary surgery. For example, vascular injuries have been reported in 3–4 per cent of patients operated for chronic pancreatitis.[25] In pelvic surgery the most commonly injured vessels are the iliac veins.

Cholecystectomy, especially as an acute procedure or after recurrent acute cholecystitis, may be extremely difficult. There are also considerable variations in the anatomy of the arterial supply to the liver and to the gallbladder. When faced with serious bleeding the hepatic artery may be ligated but even if some ischaemia does occur, the risk of liver necrosis is limited. It is not necessary, therefore, to repair the hepatic artery, a quite difficult procedure in any event. If, however, sudden bleeding is experienced during dissection thought to originate from the hepatic artery, the advice, as with all sudden vascular injuries, is to *compress and not to use deep forceps blindly*. The advice 'more hands and more eyes' is usually sufficient to visualise a partially divided artery and to permit lateral repair.

If a pseudoaneurysm results from the injury,[26] a ligature should be applied proximally and distally. Lesions of the superior mesenteric artery and the coeliac axis are rare. The external iliac artery has on occasions been mistaken for the ureter and opened during intended ureterolithotomy operations. Injuries of the inferior vena cava sometimes occur during tumour surgery and also occasionally during aortic surgery.[27] All attempts should be made to repair the vein, but if this proves impossible, a ligature will save the life of the patient.

Hernia repair

Iatrogenic injuries of the femoral artery or femoral vein are not uncommon but are apparently not often reported.[3] The risk attached to an injury is dependent on the type of repair and in principle, the more 'anatomical' the repair the lower the risk. With deep sutures the risk of damage to the common femoral artery increases.[28] The result is either bleeding or, more rarely, thrombosis with embolisation or even the development of a false aneurysm.

Bleeding from an arterial injury is usually best controlled by compression. Compression of the femoral vein and thrombosis seem to occur mainly after hernia repair using the McVay technique.[29] Careful dissection and exact repair of the fascial structures minimises the risks associated with treating these iatrogenic vascular injuries.

GYNAECOLOGICAL SURGERY

Major vascular injuries are reported infrequently. In Sweden the incidence per 10 000 procedures was calculated for the years 1979–83 and found to be 0.93 for laparoscopy, 0.76 for laparotomy and 0.33 for vaginal operations.[30] Laparoscopic complications most frequently involve the aorta and the iliac arteries and should be detected easily by the surgeon. There is, however, at least one report in the literature of carbon dioxide embolism following direct puncture of a major vessel.[31]

During gynaecological laparotomy for pelvic tumour surgery vascular injuries are the most common cause of bleeding,[30] mainly from the iliac vein or iliac artery. Caesarean section has also been reported as the cause of severe vascular problems.[32] Careful handling of instruments inserted during laparoscopy seems to be the most important factor in avoiding injury. If bleeding occurs, an immediate laparotomy has to be performed, if possible with the assistance of a vascular surgeon. The same applies to injuries occurring during laparotomy. It has to be stressed that firm compression and proximal control are the major life-saving measures.

PREVENTION AND TREATMENT

Training and experience are the alpha and omega in preventing injuries. Accidents and misinterpretations of difficult anatomy and pathology, however, cannot be totally avoided. It is important, therefore, to know how to handle complications when they occur. The most devastating complication is abrupt major bleeding occurring during a surgical procedure. This stressful situation may well induce the risk of improper actions, such as the blind use of forceps and clamps. If the source of bleeding is neither absolutely clear nor easily accessible for proper repair, the correct action is to compress the bleeding region firmly with gauze packs. As already emphasised, the assistance of another surgeon would be wise, and in many situations, a necessity. The next step is to achieve proximal and distal control. Established principles of vascular repair are then followed, whether by lateral suture, patching or grafting. Other types of acute vascular injuries resulting in thrombosis, embolism and dissection are treated according to accepted principles. Complications appearing later, such as arteriovenous fistulae and false aneurysms, can usually be treated by endovascular or vascular surgical techniques (see Chapters 33, 38 and 39).

In view of the medicolegal implications (see Chapter 10) detailed note-taking and good communication with patient and family, and, of course, other involved professionals, is particularly important.

Conclusions

Surgeons have to be aware of the potential occurrence of non-catheter induced vascular injuries and be prepared to treat them. Although such injuries are relatively uncommon, bleeding, severe at times, can be a major problem. The possibility of occult bleeding, as for example in lumbar disc surgery, must be considered. The value of simply compressing a bleeding point rather than resorting to hurried and blind clamping cannot be overemphasised. The most worthwhile advice is not to do more harm and to seek assistance whenever possible; an extra pairs of hands may be of crucial importance to outcome. The principles of repairing iatrogenic vessel trauma are the same as those for other vascular injuries. The specialists involved must be willing to improvise as none of these injuries present in a standard manner.

Key references

Adar R, Bass A, Walden R. Iatrogenic complications in surgery. Five years' experience in general and vascular surgery in a university hospital. *Ann Surg* 1982; **196**: 725–9.

Bergentz SE, Bergqvist D. *Iatrogenic vascular injuries*. Berlin: Springer-Verlag, 1989.

Bergqvist D, Källerö S. Reoperation for postoperative hemorrhagic complications. Analysis of a 10-year series. *Acta Chir Scand* 1985; **151**: 17–22.

Jonung T, Pärsson H, Norgren L. Vascular injuries in Sweden 1986–1990; the result of an enquiry. *Vasa* 1995; **24**: 130–4.

Myhre HO, Sahlin Y, Saether OD, *et al.* Vascular complications of elective orthopaedic surgery. In: Greenhalgh RM, Hollier LH (eds). *Emergency Vascular Surgery*. London: WB Saunders, 1992: 353–64.

REFERENCES

1 Jonung T, Pärsson H, Norgren L. Vascular injuries in Sweden 1986–1990; the result of an enquiry. *Vasa* 1995; **24**: 130–4.

2 Adar R, Bass A, Walden R. Iatrogenic complications in surgery. Five years' experience in general and vascular surgery in a university hospital. *Ann Surg* 1982; **196**: 725–9.

3 Bergentz SE, Bergqvist D. *Iatrogenic vascular injuries*. Berlin: Springer-Verlag, 1989.

4 Myhre HO, Sahlin Y, Saether OD, *et al*. Vascular complications of elective orthopaedic surgery. In: Greenhalgh RM, Hollier LH (eds). *Emergency vascular surgery*. London: WB Saunders, 1992: 353–64.

5 Støren G, Holta AL, Myhre HO, *et al*. Arterieskader. *Tidskrift for den Norske Laegeforening* 1976; **23**: 1195–7.

6 Bergqvist D, Källerö S. Reoperation for postoperative hemorrhagic complications. Analysis of a 10-year series. *Acta Chir Scand* 1985; **151**: 17–22.

7 Schlosser V, Kuttler H, Kameda T. Arterial injury during orthopedic and traumatological surgery. *J Cardiovasc Surg* 1987; **28**: 46.

8 Stokes JM. Vascular complications of disc surgery. *J Bone Joint Surg Am* 1968; **50**: 394–9.

9 Sagdic K, Ozer ZG, Senkaya I, Ture M. Vascular injury during lumbar disc surgery. Report of two cases; a review of the literature. *Vasa* 1996; **25**: 378–81.

10 Baker JK, Reardon PR, Reardon MJ, *et al*. Vascular injury in anterior lumbar surgery. *Spine* 1993; **18**: 2227–30.

11 Bergqvist D, Carlsson AS, Ericsson F. Vascular complications of total hip arthroplasty. *Acta Orthop Scand* 1983; **54**: 157–63.

12 Nachbur B, Meyer RP, Verkkala K, Zurcher R. The mechanisms of severe arterial injury in surgery of the hip joint. *Clin Orthop* 1979; **141**: 122–33.

13 Beguin L, Feugier P, Durand JM, *et al*. Vascular risk and total hip arthroplasty: prevention during acetabular revision. *Rev Chir Orthop Reparatrice Appar Mot* 2001; **87**: 489–98.

14 Matos MH, Amstutz HC, Machleder HI. Ischemia of the lower extremity after total hip replacement: report of four cases. *J Bone Joint Surg Am* 1979; **61**: 24–7.

15 Rush JH, Vidovich JD, Johnson MA. Arterial complications of total knee replacement. The Australian experience. *J Bone Joint Surg UK* 1987; **3**: 400–2.

16 McAuley CE, Steed DL, Webster MW. Arterial complications of total knee replacement. *Arch Surg* 1984; **119**: 960–2.

17 Cockett FB. Arterial complications of surgery and sclerosis of varices. *Phlebologie* 1987; **40**: 107–10.

18 Tera H. Emergency repair of femoral vein accidentally divided at operation for varicose veins. *Acta Chir Scand* 1967; **133**: 283–7.

19 Hobson RW, Yeager RA, Lynch TG, *et al*. Femoral venous trauma: techniques for surgical management and early results. *Am J Surg* 1983; **146**: 220–4.

20 Nordestgaard AG, Bodily KC, Osborn RW Jr, Buttorff JD. Major vascular injuries during laparoscopic procedures. *Am J Surg* 1995; **169**: 543–5.

21 Usal H, Sayad P, Hayek N, *et al*. Major vascular injuries during laparoscopic cholecystectomy. An institutional review of experience with 2589 procedures and literature review. *Surg Endosc* 1998; **12**: 960–2.

22 Dixon M, Carrillo EH. Iliac vascular injuries during elective laparoscopic surgery. *Surg Endosc* 1999; **13**: 1230–3.

23 Hanney RM, Alle KM, Cregan PC. Major vascular injury and laparoscopy *Aust N Z J Surg* 1995; **65**: 533–5.

24 Gossot D, Kabiri H, Caliandro R, *et al*. Early complications of thoracic endoscopic sympathectomy: a prospective study of 940 procedures. *Ann Thorac Surg* 2001; **71**: 1116–19.

25 Call FP, Muhe E, Gwohardt C. Results of partial and total pancreaticoduodenectomy in 117 patients with chronic pancreatitis. *World J Surg* 1981; **5**: 269–75.

26 Thomas WEG, May RE. Hepatic artery aneurysm following cholecystectomy. *Postgrad Med J* 1981; **57**: 393–5.

27 Vollmar J. Venous trauma. *Major Prob Clin Surg* 1979; **23**: 191–9.

28 Shamberger RC, Ottinger LW, Malt RA. Arterial injuries during inguinal herniorrhaphy. *Ann Surg* 1984; **200**: 83–5.

29 Klausner JM, Noveck H, Skornick Y, *et al*. Femoral vein occlusion following McVay repair. *Postgrad Med J* 1986; **62**: 301–2.

30 Bergqvist D, Bergqvist A. Vascular injuries during gynecologic surgery. *Acta Obstet Gynecol Scand* 1987; **66**: 9–23.

31 Hanney RM, Alle KM, Cregan PC. Major vascular injury and laparoscopy. *Aust N Z J Surg* 1995; **65**: 533–5.

32 Buri P. Iatrogene Schädigung von Blutgefässen. *Helv Chir Acta* 1971; **38**: 151–5.

Special Acute Vascular Challenges

41

Acute Upper Limb Ischaemic States

KENNETH A MYERS, GREGORY W SELF

THE PROBLEM

Acute ischaemia is less common in the upper than in the lower limbs, but is caused by a wider variety of disease processes and has varied options for treatment. Ischaemia can affect any level from the fingertips to the forearm, and digital ischaemia is a warning that massive occlusion from proximal disease may supervene. Delayed diagnosis and failed salvage leading to amputation is a far greater disaster than loss of the lower limb. This chapter will attempt to provide a plan for diagnostic evaluation and strategies for treatment of acute ischaemia aimed at enhancing successful management of the underlying disease before complications develop.

AETIOLOGY

In contrast to the lower limb, where acute ischaemia virtually always ensues following either embolism from the heart or thrombosis on the basis of underlying atherosclerosis, the causes in the upper limb are much more varied (see Chapter 2).

Less than 5 per cent of peripheral arterial reconstructions are for upper limb arterial disease.[1] The incidence of lower limb arterial reconstruction has progressively risen over the past 20 years,[2] and there are now more operations for thrombosis and fewer for embolism, but whether this is true for the upper limbs is uncertain as the upper limb series are smaller.

Studies of acute upper limb ischaemia have shown that embolism and thrombosis are almost equally responsible, that embolism is commonly due to either cardiac or proximal arterial disease, and that primary occlusive disease is approximately equally due to atherosclerosis or a miscellaneous group of non-atherosclerotic diseases.[3] Other studies suggest that patients with digital ischaemia suffer more often from intrinsic small arterial disease in the hand than proximal major arterial disease.[3] Patients occasionally develop acute thrombosis in essentially normal arteries on the basis of various haematological abnormalities. In the tertiary hospital setting, acute and chronic ischaemia following angiography is increasingly recognised. Accordingly, a long list of possible causes must be kept in mind in any individual patient.

Potential causes of acute upper limb ischaemia

- Embolism
  - Cardiac diseases
  - Proximal arterial diseases
  - Paradoxical embolism
- Intrinsic arterial diseases
  - Occlusive atherosclerosis
  - Atherosclerotic aneurysms
  - Arteritis and autoimmune diseases
  - Fibromuscular hyperplasia
  - Cystic adventitial disease of the brachial artery
- Haematological disorders
  - Hyperhomocysteinaemia
  - Malignant diseases
  - Clotting factor deficiencies
  - Antiphospholipid antibodies
  - Red cell, white cell and globulin disorders
  - Heparin induced thrombosis syndrome
  - Oral contraceptives

- Repetitive external trauma
  - Thoracic outlet syndrome
  - Athletic injuries
  - Axillary crutch injury
- Occupational injuries
  - Trauma to the hands and fingers
- Iatrogenic trauma
  - Arterial catheterisation
  - Anaesthetic arm blocks
  - Intra-arterial injections
  - Thrombosed axillofemoral bypass
  - Irradiation arteritis
  - Ergotism
  - Radial artery fistula steal
  - Harvesting radial artery
- Acute external trauma
  - Blunt injuries
  - Penetrating injuries
  - Intravenous drug abuse
- Non-prescribed drug use
  - Cannabis use

Embolism

Some 10–20 per cent of all emboli are lodged in arteries to the upper extremity, significantly more often on the right side. The most common site is to the brachial artery, less often the subclavian or axillary arteries and uncommonly to arteries below the elbow. The larger proportion come from the heart, particularly in patients with atrial fibrillation or recent myocardial infarction, fewer in rheumatic heart disease and aortic valve prostheses, and rarely from left atrial myxoma. Up to a third originate from disease in the innominate or subclavian arteries owing to atherosclerosis, aortitis and in particular the thoracic outlet syndrome. Paradoxical embolism can also occur.[4]

The clinical features of acute upper limb ischaemia are usually quite evident although delayed in approximately 25 per cent of cases, which is significantly less common than that in the lower limb, so that the proportion treated by embolectomy is higher and the outlook is better. Nevertheless, several studies report amputation rates of 5–10 per cent and mortality rates of 5–15 per cent.[5,6]

Intrinsic arterial diseases

ATHEROSCLEROSIS

Proximal atherosclerosis in the upper limb is more common than is realised, but it may remain relatively asymptomatic because of the abundant collateral circulation around the shoulder. Innominate and proximal subclavian artery disease, which may lead to symptoms of upper limb and cerebrovascular ischaemia, is often revealed by arteriography in the course of assessment of the latter. The Joint Study of Extracranial Arterial Occlusions in more than 6000 patients[7] showed that 17 per cent had aortic arch disease, affecting the left subclavian artery in approximately 15 per cent, the right subclavian artery in 10 per cent and the innominate artery in 5 per cent, and that stenosis was five times more frequent than occlusion. The distribution of upper limb atherosclerotic disease in a more general population has been reviewed, and it appears to affect the subclavian artery in 60 per cent, the innominate in 20 per cent and more distal arteries in 20 per cent.[1] The relative incidence of innominate or subclavian aneurysms compared with thoracic and abdominal aortic aneurysms is not clear.

Occlusions most often cause mild chronic ischaemia, but stenoses can present with multiple microemboli to cause the 'blue finger syndrome', while aneurysms can present with acute ischaemia caused by a major embolus.

ARTERITIS, AUTOIMMUNE AND OTHER DISEASES

A number of uncommon diseases can affect the branches of the aortic arch to cause upper limb ischaemia or cerebrovascular insufficiency, or they may involve the small arteries of the hands to cause digital ischaemia and necrosis.[1,3,8] It is beyond the scope of this chapter to explore each in detail, although they are described more extensively in other reviews.[9,10] They probably have a similar aetiology associated with an immune complex or cell mediated reaction[11] but the precipitating factors are unknown.

Some causes of acute upper limb ischaemia associated with arteritis or autoimmune disorders

- Takayasu's disease
- Buerger's disease
- Giant cell arteritis
- Polyarteritis
- Behçet's syndrome
- Scleroderma
- Hypersensitivity reaction
- Systemic lupus erythematosus

Takayasu's disease affects children and young adults, with a marked female preponderance (see Chapter 43). A panarteritis affects the major aortic branches, leading to weakening of the wall with consequent arterial stenoses, occlusions or aneurysms which are frequently multiple.[12] The condition commences as a non-specific 'rheumatic-like' illness, progressing to become a chronic disease several years later. An elevated erythrocyte sedimentation rate is usual in the acute phase, but the test returns to normal in the 'burned out phase'. The outlook for survival is poor with severe hypertension, cardiac involvement or other risk factors being predictors of death or major complications.[13]

Buerger's disease (thromboangiitis obliterans) usually affects young males who are smokers and is associated with segmental thrombotic occlusions of more distal arteries and veins[14,15] (see Chapter 42). In the acute phase, polymorphonuclear leucocytes infiltrate the vessel wall and thrombus; this is followed by a subacute phase with the appearance of mononuclear and giant cells, and finally a chronic phase of fibrosis and recanalisation. Essentially, this is a clinical diagnosis. Both Japanese and American studies showed that the larger proportion were symptomatic, of whom approximately 60 per cent had only lower limb symptoms, 30 per cent had only upper limb symptoms and 10 per cent had both: this was despite arteriographic findings that showed changes in most lower limb and upper limb arteries, indicating that the disease is much more extensive than can be gauged by symptoms alone.[15,16] The outlook for the limbs is poor, but the prognosis for survival is good in those who stop smoking.[15,16] Regular cannabis smoking can cause changes similar to those of Buerger's disease.[17]

Giant cell arteritis and polymyalgia rheumatica predominantly affect women, occur in most countries and are almost exclusively confined to the white population[18,19] (see Chapter 43). Some 10–15 per cent of patients have clinical involvement of arteries to the extremities[10,20] but a much larger proportion have pathological evidence of disease when studied at postmortem.[20] Major arteries can be affected at any level,[21] but there is usually sufficient time for adequate collaterals to develop. Histological examination reveals lymphocytic infiltration with granulomatous and giant cells, and fragmentation of the internal elastic lamina.

Polyarteritis can be primary or secondary to conditions such as rheumatoid arthritis, Sjögren's disease, cryoglobulinaemia or leukaemia,[22] and the condition predominantly affects the endothelium of small or medium sized arteries so as to cause stenoses, occlusions or small aneurysms.

Behçet's syndrome affects relatively young males from eastern Mediterranean countries or Japan.[23–25] A non-specific vasculitis affects small or large vessels, obliterates vasa vasorum and fragments elastin to cause arterial occlusions or aneurysms which are frequently multiple. The aneurysms are the most frequent cause of death in some 10–25 per cent of patients.[25]

Scleroderma most often affects the small metacarpal and digital arteries in the hands, which can lead to necrosis of the fingertips, but the condition is occasionally also associated with occlusion of the proximal arteries to the upper extremity secondary to severe intimal hyperplasia.[26]

Crohn's disease has been described as causing axillary artery occlusion due to arteritis.[27]

OTHER DISEASES

Fibromuscular hyperplasia has been reported in the brachial artery in a few patients, affecting either sex at various ages.[28] Cystic adventitial necrosis similar to that seen in the popliteal artery has been reported in the brachial artery.[29]

Haematological disorders

A wide variety of conditions can lead to a hypercoagulable state and thrombosis in small or large arteries[30] (see Chapter 2). These include deficiencies of antithrombin III, protein C or protein S, or presence of Leiden factor V, antiphospholipid antibodies, homocysteine or antibodies to heparin causing the heparin induced thrombosis syndrome. Coagulation can be activated by oral contraceptives and in various malignancies. An increase in blood viscosity due to globulin disorders, polycythaemia and various lymphomas or leukaemias predisposes to thrombosis.

Repetitive external trauma

This chapter is not the place to describe acute blunt or penetrating trauma that happens to involve the upper extremity. There are, however, several circumstances which can predispose to specific acute or repetitive arterial trauma with severe consequences to the upper extremity.

THORACIC OUTLET SYNDROME

Neurovascular compression can result from impingement by either soft tissue or bony structures.[31] The clinical picture is mostly one of chronic pain, neurological disturbance or relatively mild vascular symptoms and only a few patients have appreciable arterial insufficiency.[32] Bony abnormalities are a cervical rib or its fibrous extension, congenital abnormalities include the first rib, or a past fractured clavicle.[1]

Cervical ribs are present in less than 1 per cent of healthy individuals, about 50 per cent are bilateral and it would appear that less than 10 per cent of those cause symptoms[33] (see Chapter 22). The cervical rib runs along the anterior border of the scalenus medius muscle immediately under the artery (Fig. 41.1). It can rarely arise at a higher level, i.e. up to the fifth cervical vertebra, and occasionally the rib can pass through the trunks of the brachial plexus. An abnormal first rib is said to be less than one half as common as a cervical rib; the most common severe variant is atresia of the first rib, leaving an exostosis on the second rib at the site where the scalenus anterior muscle is inserted.[34]

Kinking of the artery over a bony prominence or fibrous band can cause turbulent flow, leading to poststenotic dilatation, then intimal disruption and aneurysm formation, finally complicated by thrombosis within the aneurysm or embolism resulting in severe acute ischaemia.

ATHLETIC INJURIES AROUND THE SHOULDER

Athletic activities that require throwing occasionally cause injury leading to thrombosis of the proximal arteries. This

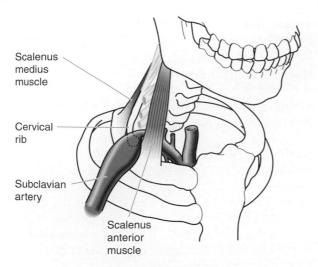

Scalenus
medius
muscle

Cervical
rib

Subclavian
artery

Scalenus
anterior
muscle

Figure 41.1 *A subclavian aneurysm distal to a cervical rib lying on the anterior border of scalenus medius, causing the thoracic outlet syndrome*

has been particularly studied in baseball pitchers and American football quarterbacks;[35,36] other activities include javelin throwing or basketball. Duplex scanning shows that the larger proportion of normal subjects have the potential for this injury, as partial or complete occlusion of the artery does occur in the throwing position.[36] Some are associated with subclavian artery thrombosis due to the thoracic outlet syndrome. Others result in axillary artery thrombosis due to compression by the head of the humerus with the arm abducted and in external rotation, particularly if there is laxity of ligaments around the shoulder joint. It is possible that distal axillary artery thrombosis can result from injury by a hypertrophied pectoralis minor muscle. Once cleared of clot the artery is in most cases found to be essentially normal.

Repeated external **trauma to the axillary artery by the use of a crutch**, though rare, is well recognised and may take the form of acute thrombosis or the gradual development of an axillary aneurysm with secondary thrombosis.[37]

OCCUPATIONAL UPPER LIMB ISCHAEMIA

Occupational activities occasionally lead to acute upper limb vascular ischaemia. These are more often associated with the thoracic outlet syndrome causing neurological or venous syndromes, but arterial complications can occur. Activities include mowing lawns, heavy lifting as a store assistant, installing overhead ducts, or playing sports as described earlier. An occupational history consistent with repetitive external trauma should be sought if the diagnosis is not clear.

TRAUMA TO THE HAND AND FINGERS

Athletic activities that require repetitive catching or striking a ball with the hand can predispose to traumatic

thrombosis of the digital or ulnar arteries.[36] Injuries to the digital arteries particularly involve the index or middle fingers wherein the artery is encircled by ligaments. A condition referred to as the **hypothenar hammer syndrome** occurs particularly in workers who use their hand as a hammer; this includes bricklayers, printers, tilers, mechanics and professional karate experts.[38,39] The ulnar artery is particularly vulnerable to trauma just after it leaves the canal under the hamate bone, where it lies superficial to the tough transverse carpal ligament and is held tight in its course by its deep branch.[38] Trauma can result in either acute thrombosis or aneurysm formation. Ischaemia is particularly likely if the superficial palmar arch is incomplete, but it can also be due to embolism from an aneurysm. Use of vibrating tools can cause distal small artery vasospasm or occlusion. Digital arteries, in particular, become hyperresponsive causing the 'white finger syndrome'.[40]

Iatrogenic trauma

There is a considerable capacity for medical manoeuvres to cause damage to arteries of the upper extremity, often with catastrophic results. Penetrating injuries include **arterial catheterisation** for arteriography or haemodynamic monitoring although the problem is far less common now that most investigations are performed via a transfemoral approach (see Chapter 38). Bleeding from the brachial or axillary puncture site may raise the pressure within the sheath of the neurovascular bundle to such a degree as to cause severe nerve palsies, which are frequently permanent.[41] An **anaesthetic arm block** with accidental intramural injection can cause axillary artery occlusion.[42] A blunt needle technique is recommended, but this does not eliminate the risk. The complication is more likely if the patient is obese or if the artery is already diseased. **Intra-arterial injection** of therapeutic agents such as anaesthetic drugs or of illicit substances by drug abusers may precipitate acute severe extremity ischaemia with permanent damage[43] (see Chapter 44). The difficulties encountered in the treatment of these challenging conditions is frequently compounded by secondary venous thrombosis. **Harvesting the radial artery** for coronary artery bypass surgery fortunately rarely leads to hand ischaemia.[44]

An increasingly common phenomenon is axillary artery thrombosis with or without embolism consequent upon **thrombosis of an axillofemoral prosthetic graft**.[45] Exertion may disrupt the top anastomosis to cause 'the axillary pullout syndrome'.[46] The risk may be increased if the graft is so short that it brings about 'tenting' of the axillary or subclavian artery.[45] Retrograde thrombosis from the upper end of the occluded graft may extend into the subclavian artery, or embolisation down the limb may occur from the cul de sac adjacent to the upper anastomosis.[47] It is possible that the graft may shorten after some years predisposing to thrombosis in the graft and subclavian artery, and it has been suggested that this risk is reduced by making the anastomosis more proximal on the subclavian artery to reduce repetitive movements.[48] The possibility of steal from the arm to a patent graft appears to be unfounded.

Irradiation arteritis of the subclavian, axillary and upper brachial artery, which also compromises collaterals, presents many years after therapy for carcinoma of the breast (see Chapter 33). Vessels occlude due to endothelial damage, disruption of the internal elastic lamina, hyaline thickening of the intima, obliteration of vasa vasorum, and medial and indeed periarterial fibrosis.[49]

Proximal artery vasospasm can result **from treatment with ergot preparations** and leads to severe upper or lower limb ischaemia.[50,51] This complication was responsible for withdrawal of the dihydroergotamine heparin regimen for deep venous thrombosis prophylaxis.

Hand ischaemia can result from **steal induced by an arteriovenous fistula** created for angioaccess in patients requiring dialysis (see Chapter 7B) and the incidence may be as high as 5 per cent.[52] Ischaemic symptoms are not uncommon early on but usually resolve rapidly as collaterals develop. The risk of persisting ischaemia is increased if the ulnar artery supply is inadequate as shown by the Allen test or if, as in diabetic patients, there is pre-existing distal arterial disease. Many access surgeons would now try to avoid the otherwise standard radiocephalic (Cimino) fistula in type 1 diabetic patients in preference to a more proximal fistula which is less likely to steal circulation. Patients undergoing such access must be warned of the symptoms and signs of arterial insufficiency by the surgeon as the problem may not be appreciated or recognised too late by medical and nursing staff in other disciplines.

DIAGNOSIS

Clinical features

It is necessary to discuss all patients presenting with varying grades of ischaemia since many conditions have a potential for sudden complications causing acute ischaemia. Diagnosis must include both the causes and consequences of the diseases. In general, full clinical assessment and various special investigations are appropriate for most patients, considering the wide variety of possible causes, not all of which are immediately obvious. Systemic features associated with the various causes of arteritis and autoimmune disease should be sought in many patients. This requires detailed knowledge of each, which, although beyond the scope of this chapter, is well described in several reviews.[9,10]

Large artery embolism usually presents with acute ischaemia causing pain, pallor, paralysis, paraesthesia, and 'perishing coldness', although in some cases the onset is more insidious (see Chapters 2, 15 and 16). Paralysis is less

frequent than in the lower limb because proximal muscles can perform upper limb movements. The radial pulse is lost and the level of the most proximal pulse usually clearly indicates the site of occlusion. Embolism carries a considerable risk of residual arm claudication, ischaemic neuropathy, ischaemic contracture or even major amputation, usually due to delayed presentation and technical problems at operation.[6] Repeated **microembolism** can cause recurrent episodes of forearm or hand pain with focal areas of discoloration or skin necrosis analogous to the 'blue toe syndrome' of the lower extremity.

The varied presenting clinical features of **chronic large artery disease** may include a palpable aneurysm, forearm claudication, Raynaud's phenomenon, digital necrosis or infarction, or acute ischaemia from the occlusion. Forearm claudication is the least common manifestation because of the rich collateral circulation around the shoulder and because a smaller muscle mass than that in the lower limb has to be supplied. The distal pulse status is far less predictive of chronic proximal disease than is that in the lower limb.[7] A bruit is frequently observed but is not always present. A brachial artery systolic pressure difference between the arms of more than 20 mmHg reliably indicates proximal stenotic or occlusive disease.[53]

A lump representing a **cervical rib** or prominent pulsation of the subclavian artery pushed upwards by the rib is usually diagnostic. The wide variety of physical manoeuvres designed to compromise the pulse in order to establish a diagnosis of thoracic outlet syndrome and the high incidence of false positive results are a testimony to the clinical challenge posed. Harris *et al.*[54] found that 30 per cent of normal subjects showed apparent arterial compression with **thoracic outlet syndrome** provocative manoeuvres, and even this figure may understate the incidence of false positive tests. Nevertheless, a negative test virtually excludes a diagnosis of vascular involvement while a positive test provides confidence to proceed with treatment if a clear history of ischaemia is present. The 'hands-up' manoeuvre is a convenient method of observing whether the pulse disappears, the hand blanches with exercise and a bruit develops as the arm is then lowered (Fig. 41.2).

Small artery disease most commonly presents with Raynaud's phenomenon, digital necrosis or digital gangrene according to the acuteness of onset and extent of disease. The Allen test is very useful for detecting the presence and site of occlusion in small arteries beyond the wrist (Fig. 41.3). It is also used to detect inadequate ulnar artery inflow to the hand prior to radial artery cannulation or the creation of a radial artery fistula (see Chapter 7B).

Haematological investigations

A full blood examination and erythrocyte sedimentation rate would seem to be required in all patients, although the erythrocyte sedimentation rate may not be elevated even

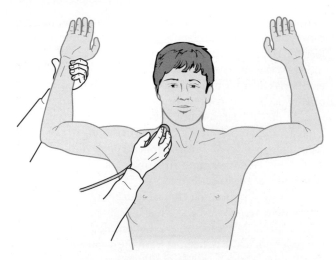

Figure 41.2 *The 'hands-up' manoeuvre to demonstrate arterial obstruction in the thoracic outlet syndrome, observing the hand for pallor after exercising, feeling for loss of the brachial pulse and return with lowering the arm, and listening for a bruit as the arm is lowered*

with florid cases of arteritis.[20] A list of investigations screening for thrombophilia in patients with an uncertain diagnosis[30] is shown below (also see Chapters 2 and 20).

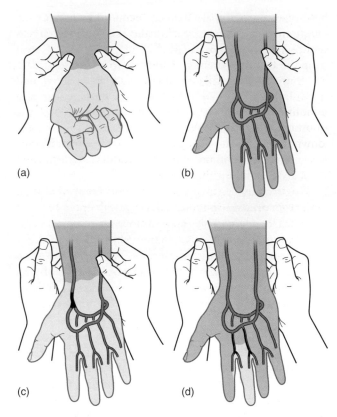

(a)

(b)

(c)

(d)

Figure 41.3 *Allen test: (a) the blanching that occurs after clenching the hand a few times with the radial and ulnar arteries occluded, (b) prompt return of colour after releasing the radial artery, (c) failure of colour to return in the hand if the distal radial artery is occluded or (d) failure of colour to return to a finger if more distal disease affects the metacarpal arteries*

Investigations performed for a thrombophilia screen in a patient with acute upper limb ischaemia with uncertain diagnosis

- Protein C
- Protein S
- Antiphospholipid antibodies
- Antithrombin III
- Factor III
- Factor V Leiden
- Prothrombin mutation
- Homocysteine

Non-invasive investigations

Vascular laboratory techniques can be very useful. Colour Doppler duplex ultrasound scanning has become the preliminary investigation for examining arteries to the upper extremity.[55] The vessels can be visualised from the aortic arch to the palmar arch, but it takes a highly trained ultrasonographer to interpret the results usefully. Duplex scanning has been very well evaluated for the thoracic outlet syndrome.[56] The same cautions over eliciting extrinsic arterial compression by various clinical manoeuvres must be expressed, but at least it can be said that a negative examination by a competent ultrasonographer essentially excludes the diagnosis of vascular compression as a feature of the thoracic outlet syndrome (also see Chapter 22).

Radiology

PLAIN X-RAYS

In patients with suspected thoracic outlet syndrome, a plain X-ray of the neck will detect most cervical ribs and first rib abnormalities. Plain X-rays of the hands and chest may show characteristic features of scleroderma, perhaps leading to a barium swallow.

ARTERIOGRAPHY

Most patients with a clinical diagnosis of disease potentially threatening the upper limb should undergo arteriography. This invasive investigation is frequently required to diagnose the precise site of primary disease and its consequences in the upper extremity. This approach is quite different from that applied to the lower limb where arteriography is usually performed only if intervention is contemplated. Most diseases described in this review have specific arteriographic appearances which will form the basis for appropriate further investigations, even to the point of arterial biopsy to confirm the cause of disease. For example, temporal artery biopsy is required to establish the diagnosis of giant cell arteritis, which in turn may dictate the need for arteriography of the cerebrovascular, visceral or lower limb arteries.

Since the precise site of disease is frequently uncertain, contrast studies usually commence with arch aortography via the groin followed by selective catheterisation of the innominate or left subclavian arteries if required. Digital subtraction arteriography should demonstrate all vessels down to the fingers. This policy is preferable to axillary or brachial artery puncture, the complications of which could further compromise the circulation.

Arteriography may not be warranted and would simply delay treatment in a patient with acute ischaemia due to an embolus which has clearly come from the heart. Arteriography is required, however, if the cause is not clear and if time permits, in order to search for a possible proximal arterial source. There is an increasing role for arteriography in subacute or chronic upper limb ischaemia where time permits the application of various interventional endovascular techniques.

The arteriographic features of atherosclerosis are well known. The absence of atheromatous changes and large plaques in the large arteries, and the demonstration of segments of smooth lesions, should lead to the suspicion of other arterial diseases. Angiography may simply show occlusion and give no indication of the characteristic changes diagnostic of other specific diseases. Takayasu's disease is characterised by a combination of stenotic and occlusive lesions with fusiform or saccular aneurysms which are frequently multiple.[1,57,58] Classic features for Buerger's disease are abrupt occlusion with a 'tree root' configuration of collaterals and 'corkscrew' tortuosity of small distal vessels apparently due to recanalisation[59] (see Chapter 42). Giant cell arteritis shows long, smoothly tapered stenoses or occlusions[1,60] (see Chapter 43). In Crohn's disease, typically a tapering stenosis leads to occlusion.[27] The features of fibromuscular hyperplasia are a characteristic 'string of beads' appearance. In patients with suspected thoracic outlet syndrome, arteriography should include views with the arm abducted and in external rotation, but the cautions expressed as to false positive results hold just as for other diagnostic procedures.

OTHER SPECIAL INVESTIGATIONS

Computed tomography (CT) has been used to evaluate the thoracic outlet syndrome.[61] It was found that if a plain X-ray showed a bony abnormality, a CT scan did not add further information, except in symptomatic patients in whom subtle bony changes were detected. Computed tomography was also found to be accurate in demonstrating non-osseous compression when compared with controls. Nevertheless, the yield from these findings in patients with vascular manifestations is doubtful. The value of magnetic resonance imaging in such cases has yet to be determined.

IMMEDIATE MANAGEMENT

The patient is usually first seen by a general practitioner or at a local district hospital where facilities for diagnosis and vascular surgical treatment may be limited. An arterial ultrasound may have been ordered and its findings might be the reason for a vascular surgical referral. In general, eliciting the cause will require considerable experience, and almost all patients will need urgent intervention to clear the occlusion and to treat the cause. Thus no more than immediate supportive treatment should be instituted before transferring the patient to a vascular service as an emergency. Occasionally, a patient will sustain embolism to both the arm and the brain, and present with simultaneous upper limb ischaemia and a stroke. As the stroke is likely to affect the side contralateral to the ischaemic arm, restoration of flow to this neurologically intact arm becomes even more important.

One important immediate measure is to reduce propagation of distal thrombus by anticoagulation with intravenous heparin. A bolus of 20 000 units or commencement of an intravenous infusion (5000 IU bolus and 1000 IU per hour via a mechanical intravenous pump) should suffice before transferring the patient. Remember to request intravenous cannulation in the contralateral upper limb as use of the veins of the affected limb or of either leg is inappropriate except in critical emergencies. Even in the rare instance where there is concurrent embolism to the brain, anticoagulation is appropriate in most patients to limit intracranial propagation of clot, although this must be discussed with the vascular surgeon prior to transfer.

CONSERVATIVE MEASURES

In general, conservative treatment is considered after the underlying cause of the ischaemia has been corrected, if that were possible. Oral anticoagulation, permanently for thromboembolism due to atrial fibrillation and for a period of a few months in cases of myocardial infarction, will reduce the risk of recurrent embolism.[5] Various vasodilator drugs, prostaglandin or its analogues, antiplatelet agents, and rheological agents such as pentoxifylline have been used in an attempt to improve the distal circulation in patients with large vessel or small vessel disease in the upper extremity. Mills and colleagues[3,62] contend that there is no objective evidence to show that any of these measures improves the outcome, although empirically they do use a calcium blocking agent and pentoxifylline. A randomised study of iloprost, a longer acting prostaglandin analogue given intravenously for 3–4 weeks, showed markedly higher rates of relief of pain and limb salvage in patients with Buerger's disease.[63] Various studies of iloprost for critical ischaemia in the lower limb have shown benefit,[64] and these results may well be extrapolated to the upper extremity. The various causes of arteritis or autoimmune disease generally require treatment with corticosteroids with or without immunosuppressive drugs.[9,19,20,60] Regardless of all these considerations, the patient should stop smoking. Much can be gained from good local care to the hand with minimal debridement, nail excision to drain infection, and skin protection.[3]

A protocol has been described for treatment after intra-arterial injection of drugs by drug abusers,[43] and the measures would seem appropriate for any patient with acute or severe upper limb ischaemia. Treatment includes continuous intravenous heparin and dextran 40 infusion, parenteral dexamethasone, opiates for pain control, elevation of the extremity, and early active and passive movements. Vasodilators such as glyceryl trinitrate (GTN) can be a valuable addition and may be given topically or intravenously as the severity of the situation dictates. Heparin, dextran and GTN have the advantage of easy accessibility in a variety of medical or hospital settings. Iloprost, pentoxifylline, dexamethasone and other vasoactive drugs have a greater role in chronic ischaemic states.

There has been considerable recent interest in the ischaemia-reperfusion syndrome and its management, and this is just as pertinent to the upper extremity as to ischaemia of the lower limbs[65] (see Chapter 2). Mannitol infusion may be required to maintain renal perfusion and limit swelling and raised compartment pressure in the arm, which would further compromise circulation.

RECONSTRUCTIVE SURGERY

Embolectomy

Since most emboli are lodged in the brachial artery, the most favoured approach is to expose this artery at its bifurcation at or just below the elbow in order to allow selective catheterisation of each of the branches through a transverse arteriotomy, with closure by interrupted sutures without a patch.[15,16] If the embolus is arrested more proximally, a higher brachial or even axillary approach may be used, either alone or in combination with the antecubital approach. In some cases the procedure ought to be performed under local anaesthesia in view of the appreciable mortality due to associated heart disease.[6] It is rarely appropriate to manage the problem conservatively (see Chapters 15 and 16).

A personal preference of one author (KAM) is to expose the brachial artery in the mid-portion of the upper arm where its calibre is larger and to perform a longitudinal arteriotomy, which can usually be closed by direct suture without arterial narrowing. The tip of the Fogarty catheter is angled and the balloon is pre-expanded with contrast so that it can easily be seen on fluoroscopy to ensure selective catheterisation of each run-off artery (Fig. 41.4). A study in cadavers showed that a straight catheter passed into the larger of the two outflow arteries in 42 per cent of limbs and into one artery only in 96 per cent of them, whereas positioning an angled tip catheter blindly allowed it to pass down each artery in 87 per cent of limbs.[66] The other author (GWS) prefers a curved incision starting just above the cubital fossa and extending over the bicipital aponeurosis to the tendon of biceps. The brachial artery is well exposed and extension of the incision allows selective catheterisation of the radial and ulnar artery. The affected patient is frequently elderly and often has poorly characterised cardiac disease so the operation is ideally, and easily, performed using local anaesthesia injected by the surgeon with a little supplemental intravenous sedation given by the anaesthetist. Local anaesthesia may be given as 10–20 mL of 1 per cent lidocaine (Xylocaine)

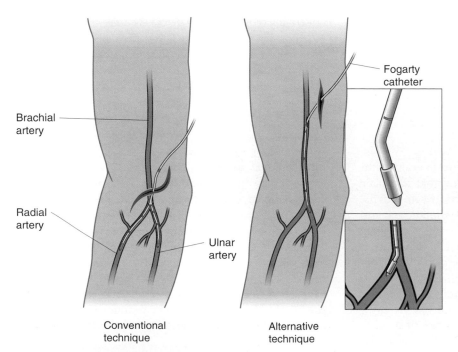

Figure 41.4 *Two techniques for brachial embolectomy to clear the distal arteries (the proximal embolus is removed last): the conventional technique approaches the brachial bifurcation to allow each branch to be dissected out and selectively catheterised; the alternative technique uses a more limited approach to the more proximal brachial artery and uses fluoroscopy to guide the catheter down each branch after angling the tip and filling the balloon with a little contrast*

but a particularly useful solution is 10 mL of 1 per cent lidocaine mixed with 10 mL 0.5 per cent bupivacaine (Marcain) as this provides rapid onset anaesthesia and lasts for a reasonable period of time postoperatively. It is important that the attending surgeon inform the patient's family that the prognosis is grave. The 30-day results of upper limb embolectomy are nearly as bad as those for the lower limb and a reflection of underlying cardiovascular disease.

Fasciotomy of the flexor and extensor compartments should be considered if there is marked residual swelling after reperfusion but is rarely needed due to the usual early recognition of acute limb ischaemia (see Chapter 33).

Occlusive or aneurysmal disease

It is frequently necessary to recommend surgical reconstruction for proximal occlusive or aneurysmal disease because of major or repetitive minor embolism, acute thrombosis causing severe ischaemia, a major risk of such events in the future or associated cerebrovascular symptoms. The older patient with asymptomatic left subclavian artery stenosis, however, is often managed conservatively.

Transthoracic reconstruction is the most direct approach and gives the best long term patency rates of over 90 per cent[67,68] but at the expense of appreciable morbidity and mortality.[1] Endarterectomy (Fig. 41.5) is only suitable for short lesions and is technically more demanding than bypass (Fig. 41.6), which is thus usually preferred. The approach is through a sternal split for the innominate artery or the left third intercostal space for the left subclavian artery (also see Chapter 34). Proximal aneurysms can be resected or an inlay bypass technique can be used.

A range of **extrathoracic reconstructions** is more widely used for occlusive disease. Excellent results have been reported with very low morbidity and mortality rates,

although with slightly lower long term patency rates.[1] Subclavian-carotid transposition (Fig. 41.7) or carotid-subclavian bypass (Fig. 41.8) gives good results for treating subclavian artery occlusions.[69] Axilloaxillary crossover bypass (Fig. 41.9) or femoroaxillary bypass (Fig. 41.10) are reserved for more difficult situations although long term results are satisfactory.[70] It is rarely necessary to use a shunt if the common carotid artery is clamped. A supraclavicular approach, combined with an infraclavicular approach if required, gives excellent exposure and control of the subclavian artery, while appropriate longitudinal incisions are used to expose more distal arteries.

There is preference for synthetic grafts rather than vein grafts for reconstructions involving the subclavian or

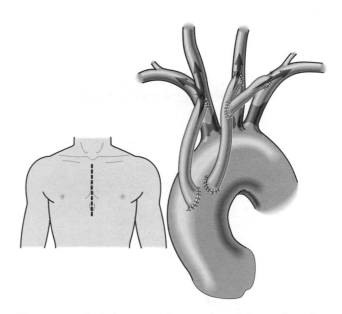

Figure 41.6 *Techniques used for transthoracic bypass from the aorta to the major branches*

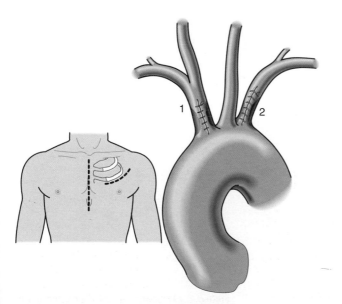

Figure 41.5 *The approaches for transthoracic endarterectomy of the innominate or left subclavian arteries*

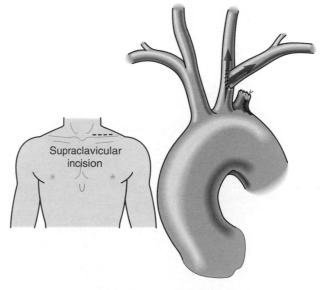

Supraclavicular incision

Figure 41.7 *A technique for extrathoracic subclavian–carotid transposition*

proximal axillary artery[69,71] whereas most prefer autogenous long saphenous vein if the distal anastomosis is to be taken down into the arm (Fig. 41.11).[72–74] A collective review considers that patency rates at 23 years are greater than 80 per cent if the distal anastomosis is proximal to the brachial bifurcation, but closer to 50 per cent if it is distal to that level.[75] Good results can be obtained even with bypass to arteries beyond the wrist.[76]

Takayasu's disease

In patients with Takayasu's disease, bypass is best commenced at the proximal aortic arch to avoid anastomotic stenosis and to achieve quite acceptable late patency

rates.[77,78] Asymptomatic patients in the active phase of arteritis are treated conservatively, tiding them through into the phase of being 'burned out' before contemplating surgical bypass, but the latter option may be appropriate in the acute phase if there are limb-threatening complications.[79]

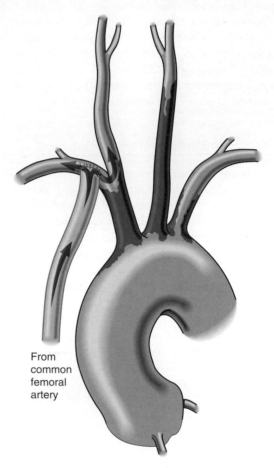

Figure 41.10 *Proximal anastomosis for a femoroaxillary (or femorosubclavian) bypass*

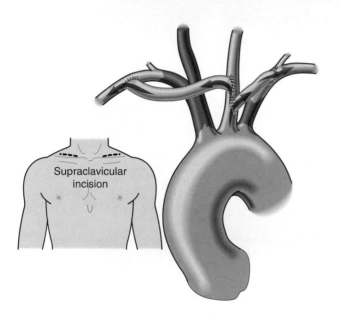

Figure 41.8 *A technique for extrathoracic carotid–subclavian bypass*

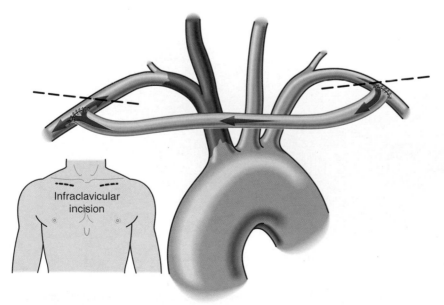

Figure 41.9 *A technique for extrathoracic axilloaxillary (or subclavian-subclavian) bypass*

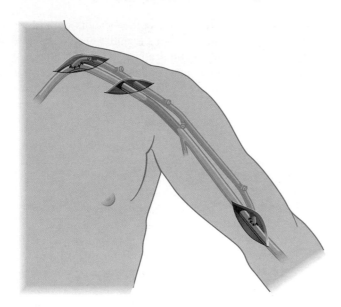

Figure 41.11   *Multiple incisions required for a subclavian–brachial vein bypass graft*

Thoracic outlet syndrome

There is general agreement that constricting structures at the thoracic outlet should be removed if vascular symptoms are present because progressive damage to the subclavian artery and risk of acute thromboembolic complications are probable. There is increasing agreement that, in patients with vascular manifestations, such intervention should routinely involve removing the first rib as well as a cervical rib, dividing all scalene muscle attachments and other fibromuscular bands, in order to avert an appreciable risk of recurrence.[35,80–82] One of several approaches, whether supraclavicular, infraclavicular or transaxillary, will provide the necessary exposure for removal of the first rib. Some favour a combination of the supraclavicular and infraclavicular[80] or the supraclavicular and transaxillary[82] approach to decompressing the outlet, and either combination appears to be essential if arterial reconstruction is required.[80] It should be possible to achieve satisfactory exposure without ever having to divide the clavicle.

Management of arterial complications depends on the findings at operation.[80] The dilated or stenosed segment of artery should be opened and propagated thrombus or embolus removed using a Fogarty catheter. If the intima appears normal, the arteriotomy can be simply closed, taking bites large enough to restore the lumen to a normal diameter. If the intima is ulcerated, limited endarterectomy and closure, primary or using a vein patch, may be sufficient. If damage is too extensive, resection and end-to-end anastomosis will not be feasible without tension, and therefore an interposition graft should be used to replace the damaged segment.

Arterial catheter trauma

This usually affects the brachial artery and almost invariably results from lifting an intimal flap, so that conservative management accepting a diagnosis of arterial spasm is fraught with danger (see Chapter 38). Although the circulation may improve via collaterals, it is usually inadequate, and it is almost invariably better to repair the injury by direct exposure under local anaesthesia. Preoperative arteriography is rarely needed. It may be possible to remove the intimal flap and close the defect with a small vein patch, but sometimes a short interposition saphenous vein graft is needed.

Postmastectomy irradiation arteritis

Critical ischaemia due to occlusion of a long segment of artery years after the injury demands restoration of flow (see Chapter 33). Associated fibrotic damage to the subcutaneous tissues of the anterior chest wall leaves an inelastic, poorly nourished and inhospitable *milieu* for bypass grafting. Instead of forcing a graft through this field, an extra-anatomic carotid-brachial vein bypass graft can be routed well clear of the irradiated area, with excellent long term results.[83]

Radial artery fistula steal

This interesting problem can be resolved by simple ligation of the fistula. Alternatively, ligate the artery immediately distal to the surgical fistula and construct a reversed saphenous vein bypass from the brachial artery proximal to the fistula to the radial artery in the hand (Fig. 41.12).[84]

Hypothenar hammer syndrome

Those with experience of this condition advocate resection of an ulnar artery aneurysm with end-to-end reconstruction by autogenous vein to avoid downstream emboli. Conservative treatment is advocated in most patients if the ulnar artery is thrombosed, reserving bypass for the occasional patient with ischaemia of the ulnar fingers if the palmar arch is inadequate.[39]

ENDOVASCULAR MANAGEMENT

Balloon dilatation or stenting

Several series report results for balloon dilatation of innominate or subclavian stenosis or occlusion, with primary success rates in excess of 90 per cent and acceptable long term results for either atherosclerosis[85–88] or aortoarteritis.[89] Most, however, would now prefer to stent these lesions for better long term outcome, sometimes to resolve problems after balloon dilatation but most often as elective

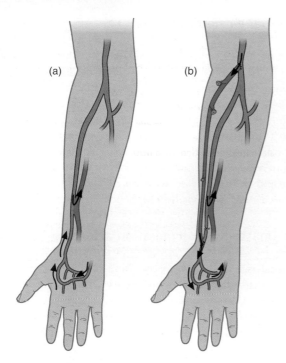

Figure 41.12 *(a) An operation performed for a patient with steal from the hand into a radial artery fistula created for dialysis. (b) The radial artery distal to the fistula is ligated and a vein graft is taken from the brachial to the distal radial artery*

treatment.[90–93] The approach may be from the femoral artery or retrogradely from a cut-down on the brachial artery.[94] There is some early experience with covered stent-grafts for thoracic outlet arterial injuries and aneurysms.[95,96]

Thrombolysis

Thrombolysis, particularly using urokinase, has been extensively used in this context[97] (see Chapter 16). Successful lysis may reveal a stenosis which can then be managed by balloon dilatation, but more extensive disease is frequently present indicating the need for surgical reconstruction. Indeed, some highly respected authorities argue that definitive early embolectomy, thrombectomy or bypass surgery is more effective.[98] Thrombolysis may be effective in clearing emboli lodged distally in the small arteries prior to reconstruction, as for example when such a complication is associated with the thoracic outlet syndrome,[99] and has been successfully used to treat ischaemia from Buerger's disease[100] (see Chapter 42).

Cervical sympathectomy

The literature appears to reveal a growing disenchantment with the idea of adding cervical sympathectomy to a vascular reconstructive procedure in the neck, or of using it for ischaemia caused by small vessel disease in the hands.[3,62]

Surprisingly few authors discuss the benefits of adding cervical sympathectomy to thoracic outlet decompression in patients with vascular complications. Cervical sympathectomy is, however, the mainstay of treatment for Buerger's disease in the upper limbs.[101] As in the lower limb, sympathectomy will be ineffective as the sole treatment of frank tissue necrosis.

Conclusions

For most surgeons, experience with upper limb arterial disease and acute ischaemia in particular, is limited so that the guidelines for successful management are less clear than are those for lower limb ischaemia. The consequences from inappropriate management, however, are likely to be far more serious. Accordingly, it is essential that each patient be carefully assessed even if the presentation appears to be only mildly symptomatic because severe ischaemia can suddenly supervene and an optimal chance for successful treatment will have been lost. Presentation with acute ischaemia almost invariably requires immediate surgical or other effective intervention, as the results of conservative treatment are poor.

Key references

Al-Mubarak N, Liu MW, Dean LS, *et al.* Immediate and late outcomes of subclavian artery stenting. *Catheter Cardiovasc Intervent* 1999; **46**: 169–72. Contemporary experience and techniques for supra-aortic endovascular procedures.

Berguer R, Morasch MD, Kline RA, *et al.* Cervical reconstruction of the supra-aortic trunks: a 16-year experience. *J Vasc Surg* 1999; **29**: 239–46. An experience of a large series of supra-aortic reconstructions.

Nehler MR, Taylor LM, Moneta GL, Porter JM. Upper extremity ischemia from subclavian artery aneurysm caused by bony abnormalities of the thoracic outlet. *Arch Surg* 1997; **132**: 527–32. A comprehensive analysis of arterial lesions in the thoracic outlet syndrome.

Robbs JV, Kadwa AM, AbdoolCarrim ATO. Arterial reconstruction for Takayasu's arteritis: medium to long term results. *Eur J Vasc Surg* 1994; **8**: 401–7. An impressive experience of Takayasu's disease from South Africa.

Roddy SP, Darling RC, Chang BB, *et al.* Brachial artery reconstruction for occlusive disease: a 12-year experience. *J Vasc Surg* 2001; **33**: 802–5. A good overview of results to be expected from bypass grafts in the arm, with some differences from lower limb bypasses being discussed.

Sullivan TM, Gray BH, Bacharach JM, *et al.* Angioplasty and primary stenting of the subclavian, innominate, and common carotid arteries in 83 patients. *J Vasc Surg* 1998; **28**: 1059–65. An excellent review of a large experience of endovascular treatment of upper limb arterial disease from a major American centre.

REFERENCES

1 Fujitani RM, Mills JL. Acute and chronic upper extremity ischemia. I. Large vessel arterial occlusive disease. *Ann Vasc Surg* 1993; **7**: 106–12.

2 Ljungman C, Adami HO, Bergqvist D, *et al.* Time trends in incidence rates of acute, nontraumatic extremity ischaemia; a population based study during a 19 year period. *Br J Surg* 1991; **78**: 857–60.

3 Mills JL, Fujitani RM. Acute and chronic upper extremity ischemia. II. Small vessel arterial occlusive disease. *Ann Vasc Surg* 1993; **7**: 195–9.

4 AbuRahma AF, Downham L. The role of paradoxical arterial emboli of the extremities. *Am J Surg* 1996; **172**: 214–17.

5 Davies MG, O'Malley K, Feeley M, *et al.* Upper limb embolus: a timely diagnosis. *Ann Vasc Surg* 1991; **5**: 857.

6 Vohra R, Lieberman DP. Arterial emboli to the arm. *J R Coll Surg Edinb* 1991; **36**: 835.

7 Fields WS, Lemak NA. Joint study of extracranial arterial occlusion. VII. Subclavian steal: a review of 168 cases. *JAMA* 1972; **222**: 1139–43.

8 Baguneid M, Dodd D, Fulford P, *et al.* Management of acute nontraumatic upper limb ischaemia. *Angiology* 1999; **50**: 715–20.

9 Scott DF, Myers KA, Lord RSA. Nonatherosclerotic diseases causing lower limb ischaemia. In: Myers KA, Nicolaides AN, Summer DS (eds). *Lower Limb Ischaemia.* London: MedOrion 1996.

10 Hunder GG. Vasculitic syndromes. *Curr Opin Rheumatol* 1990; **2**: 479.

11 Lie JT, Buerger's disease and inflammatory aspects of atherosclerosis. *Curr Opin Rheumatol* 1990; **2**: 76–80.

12 Sharma S, Rajani M, Kamalakar T, *et al.* The association between aneurysm formation and systemic hypertension in Takayasu's arteritis. *Clin Radiol* 1990; **42**: 18–27.

13 Sharma S, Rajani M, Shrivastava S, *et al.* Nonspecific aorto-arteritis (Takayasu's disease) in children. *Br J Radiol* 1991; **64**: 690–8.

14 Joyce JW. Buerger's disease (thromboangiitis obliterans). *Rheum Dis Clin North Am* 1990; **16**: 463–7.

15 Shionoya S. Buerger's disease: diagnosis and management. *Cardiovasc Surg* 1993; **1**: 207–14.

16 Olin JW, Young JR, Graor RA, *et al.* The changing clinical spectrum of thromboangiitis obliterans (Buerger's disease). *Circulation* 1990; **82**: 38.

17 Disdier P, Granel B, Serratrice J, *et al.* Cannabis arteritis revisited – ten new case reports. *Angiology* 2001; **52**: 1–5.

18 Brack A, Martinez-Taboada V, Stanson A, *et al.* Disease pattern in cranial and large-vessel giant cell arteritis. *Arthritis Rheum* 1999; **42**: 311–17.

19 Ninet JP, Bachet P, Dumontet CH, *et al.* Subclavian and axillary involvement in temporal arteritis and polymyalgia rheumatica. *Am J Med* 1990; **88**: 13–20.

20 Paice EW. Giant cell arteritis: difficult decisions in diagnosis, investigation and treatment. *Postgrad Med J* 1989; **65**: 743–7.

21 Greene GM, Lain D, Sherwin R, *et al.* Giant cell arteritis of the legs: clinical isolation of severe disease with gangrene and amputations. *Am J Med* 1986; **81**: 727–33.

22 Tsokos M, Lazarou SA, Moutsopoulos M. Vasculitis in primary Sjögren's syndrome: histologic classification and clinical presentation. *Am J Clin Pathol* 1987; **88**: 26–31.

23 O'Duffy JD. Vasculitis in Behçet's syndrome. *Rheum Dis Clin North Am* 1990; **16**: 423–31.

24 Chaillou P, Patra P, Noel S, *et al.* Behçet's disease revealed by double peripheral arterial involvement. *Ann Vasc Surg* 1992; **6**: 160–3.

25 Tuzun H, Sayin A, Karaozbek Y, *et al.* Peripheral aneurysms in Behçet's disease. *Cardiovasc Surg* 1993; **1**: 220–1.

26 Merino J, Casanueva B, Piney E, *et al.* Hemiplegia and peripheral gangrene secondary to large and medium size vessel involvement in CREST syndrome. *Clin Rheumatol* 1982; **1**: 295–9.

27 SheehanDare RA, Goodfield MJD, Wilson PD, Rowell NR. Axillary artery occlusion as a presenting feature of Crohn's disease. *Postgrad Med J* 1989; **65**: 758–60.

28 Reilly JM, McGraw DJ, Sicard GA. Bilateral brachial artery fibromuscular dysplasia. *Ann Vasc Surg* 1993; **7**: 483–7.

29 Wali MA, Dewan M, Renno WM, Ezzeddin M. Mucoid degeneration of the brachial artery: case report and a review of literature. *J R Coll Surg Edinb* 1999; **44**: 126–9.

30 Kottke-Marchant K. Genetic polymorphisms associated with venous and arterial thrombosis: an overview. *Arch Pathol Lab Med* 2002; **126**: 295–304.

31 Nehler MR, Taylor LM, Moneta GL, Porter JM. Upper extremity ischemia from subclavian artery aneurysm caused by bony abnormalities of the thoracic outlet. *Arch Surg* 1997; **132**: 527–32.

32 Gelabert HA, Machleder HI. Diagnosis and management of arterial compression at the thoracic outlet. *Ann Vasc Surg* 1997; **11**: 359–66.

33 Pollak EW. Surgical anatomy of the thoracic outlet syndrome. *Surg Gynecol Obstet* 1980; **150**: 97–103.

34 Baumgartner F, Nelson RJ, Robertson JM. The rudimentary first rib; a cause of thoracic outlet syndrome with arterial compromise. *Arch Surg* 1989; **124**: 109–12.

35 Rohrer MJ, Cardullo PA, Pappas AM, *et al.* Axillary artery compression and thrombosis in throwing athletes. *J Vasc Surg* 1990; **11**: 761–9.

36 McCarthy WJ, Yao JST, Schafer MF, *et al.* Upper extremity arterial injury in athletes. *J Vasc Surg* 1989; **9**: 317–27.

37 Lee AW, Hopkins SF, Griffen WO. Axillary artery aneurysm as an occult source of emboli to the upper extremity. *Am Surgeon* 1987; **53**: 485.

38 Pineda CJ, Weisman WH, Bookstein JJ, *et al.* Hypothenar hammer syndrome. *Am J Med* 1985; **79**: 561–70.

39 Vayssairat M, Debure C, Cormier JM, *et al.* Hypothenar hammer syndrome: seventeen cases with long-term follow-up. *J Vasc Surg* 1987; **5**: 83–8.

40 Bovenzi M. Vibration-induced white finger and cold response of digital arterial vessels in occupational groups with various patterns of exposure to hand-transmitted vibration. *Scand J Worlk Environ Health* 1998; **24**: 138–44.

41 McCready RA. Upper extremity vascular injuries. *Surg Clin North Am* 1988; **68**: 7250.

42 Ott B, Neuberger O, Frey HP. Obliteration of the axillary artery after axillary block. *Anaesthesia* 1989; **44**: 773–4.

43 Treiman GS, Yellin AE, Weaver FA, *et al.* An effective treatment protocol for intraarterial drug injection. *J Vasc Surg* 1990; **12**: 456–66.

44 Royse AG, Royse CF, Shah P, *et al.* Radial artery harvest technique, use and functional outcome. *Eur J Cardiothorac Surg* 1999; **15**: 186–93.

45 Farina C, Schultz RD, Feldhaus RJ. Late upper limb acute ischemia in a patient with an occluded axillofemoral bypass graft. *J Cardiovasc Surg* 1990; **31**: 178–81.

46 White GH, Donayre CE, Williams RA, *et al.* Exertional disruption of axillofemoral graft anastomosis: 'the axillary pullout syndrome'. *Arch Surg* 1990; **125**: 625–7.

47 Cuschieri RJ, Vohra R, Leiberman DP. Acute ischaemia in the donor limb after occlusion of axillofemoral grafts. *Eur J Vasc Surg* 1989; **3**: 267–9.

48 Hartman AR, Fried KS, Khalil I, Riles TS. Late axillary artery thrombosis in patients with occluded axillary femoral bypass grafts. *J Vasc Surg* 1985; **2**: 285–7.

49 Andros G, Schneider PA, Harris RW, *et al.* Management of arterial occlusive disease following radiation therapy. *Cardiovasc Surg* 1996; **4**: 135–42.

50 Glazer G, Myers KA, Davies ER. Ergot poisoning. *Postgrad Med J* 1966; **42**: 562–8.

51 Palombo D, Mirelli M, Peinetti F, *et al.* Spasm of arm arteries due to ergotamine tartrate. *Int Angiology* 1991; **10**: 513.

52 Morsy AH, Kulbaski M, Chen C, *et al.* Incidence and characteristics of patients with hand ischemia after a hemodialysis access procedure. *J Surg Res* 1998; **74**: 8–10.

53 Baxter BT, Blackburn D, Payne K, *et al.* Noninvasive evaluation of the upper extremity. *Surg Clin North Am* 1990; **70**: 87–97.

54 Harris J, Huang W, Tyrer O, *et al.* Clinical and photo-plethysmographic assessment of thoracic outlet arterial compression. *J Vasc Technol* 1989; **13**: 203.

55 Taneja K, Jain R, Sawhney S, Rajani M. Occlusive arterial disease of the upper extremity: colour Doppler as a screening technique and for assessment of distal circulation. *Australasian Radiology* 1996; **40**: 226–9.

56 Longley DG, Yedlicka JW, Molina EJ, *et al.* Thoracic outlet syndrome: evaluation of the subclavian vessels by color duplex sonography. *Am J Radiol* 1992; **158**: 623–30.

57 Matsumura K, Hirano T, Takeda K, *et al.* Incidence of aneurysms in Takayasu's arteritis. *Angiology* 1991; **42**: 308–15.

58 Kumar S, Subramanyan R, Ravi Mandalam K, *et al.* Aneurysmal form of aortoarteritis (Takayasu's disease): analysis of thirty cases. *Clin Radiol* 1990; **42**: 342–7.

59 Mills JL, Taylor LM, Porter JM. Buerger's disease in the modern era. *Am J Surg* 1987; **154**: 123–9.

60 Perruquet JL, David DE, Harrington TM. Aortic arch arteritis in the elderly: an important manifestation of giant cell arteritis. *Arch Int Med* 1986; **146**: 289–91.

61 Bilbey JH, Muller NL, Connell DG, *et al.* Thoracic outlet syndrome: evaluation with CT. *Radiology* 1989; **171**: 381–4.

62 Mills JL, Friedman EL, Taylor LM, Porter JM. Upper extremity ischemia caused by small artery disease. *Ann Surg* 1987; **206**: 521–8.

63 Fiessinger JN, Schafer M. Trial of iloprost versus aspirin treatment for critical limb ischaemia of thromboangiitis obliterans. *Lancet* 1990; **335**: 555–7.

64 Second European Consensus Document on Chronic Critical Leg Ischaemia. *Eur J Vasc Surg* 1992; **6**(suppl A): 18–21.

65 Crinnion JN, Homer-Vanniasinkam S, Gough MJ. Skeletal muscle reperfusion injury: pathophysiology and clinical considerations. *Cardiovasc Surg* 1993; **1**: 317–24.

66 Beckingham IJ, Roberts SNJ, Berridge DC, *et al.* A simple technique for thromboembolectomy of the upper limb. *Eur J Vasc Surg* 1990; **4**: 173–7.

67 Berguer R, Morasch MD, Kline RA, *et al.* Cervical reconstruction of the supra-aortic trunks: a 16-year experience. *J Vasc Surg* 1999; **29**: 239–46.

68 Taha AA, Vahl AC, de Jong SC, *et al.* Reconstruction of the supra-aortic trunks. *Eur J Surg* 1999; **165**: 314–18.

69 AbuRahma AF, Robinson PA, Jennings TG. Carotid-subclavian bypass grafting with polytetrafluoroethylene grafts for symptomatic subclavian artery stenosis or occlusion: a 20-year experience. *J Vasc Surg* 2000; **32**: 411–18.

70 Mingoli A, Sapienza P, Feldhaus RJ, *et al.* Long-term results and outcomes of crossover axilloaxillary bypass grafting: a 24-year experience. *J Vasc Surg* 1999; **29**: 894–901.

71 Ziomek S, QuinonesBaldrick WJ, Busuttil RW, *et al.* The superiority of synthetic arterial grafts over autologous veins in carotidsubclavian bypass. *J Vasc Surg* 1986; **3**: 140–5.

72 Katz SG, Kohl RD. Direct revascularization for the treatment of forearm and hand ischemia. *Am J Surg* 1993; **165**: 312–16.

73 Roddy SP, Darling RC, Chang BB, *et al.* Brachial artery reconstruction for occlusive disease: a 12-year experience. *J Vasc Surg* 2001; **33**: 802–5.

74 Ristow AV, Cury JM, Costa EL, *et al.* Revascularization of the ischaemic hand using *in situ* veins. *Cardiovasc Surg* 1996; **4**: 466–9.

75 McCarthy WJ, Flinn WR, Yao JST, *et al.* Result of bypass grafting for upper limb ischemia. *J Vasc Surg* 1986; **3**: 741–6.

76 Nehler MR, Dalman RI, Harris EJ, *et al.* Upper extremity arterial bypass distal to the wrist. *J Vasc Surg* 1992; **16**: 633–42.

77 Giordano JM, Leavitt RY, Hoffman G, Fauci AS. Experience with surgical treatment of Takayasu's disease. *Surgery* 1991; **109**: 252–8.

78 Weaver FA, Yellin AE, Campen DH, *et al.* Surgical procedures in the management of Takayasu's arteritis. *J Vasc Surg* 1990; **12**: 429–31.

79 Robbs JV, Kadwa AM, AbdoolCarrim ATO. Arterial reconstruction for Takayasu's arteritis: medium to long term results. *Eur J Vasc Surg* 1994; **8**: 401–7.

80 Cormier JM, Amrane M, Ward A, *et al.* Arterial complications of the thoracic outlet syndrome: fifty-five operative cases. *J Vasc Surg* 1989; **9**: 778–87.

81 Colman PD, White GH. Complexities in the management of arterial compromise due to thoracic outlet syndrome. *Aust N Z J Surg* 1990; **60**: 100–2.

82 Thompson JF, Webster JHH. First rib resection for vascular complications of thoracic outlet syndrome. *Br J Surg* 1990; **77**: 555–7.

83 McCallion WA, Barros D'Sa AAB. Management of critical limb ischaemia long after irradiation injury of the subclavian and axillary arteries. *Br J Surg* 78: 136–8.

84 Berman SS, Gentile AT, Glickman MH, *et al.* Distal revascularization-interval ligation for limb salvage and maintenance of dialysis access in ischemic steal syndrome. *J Vasc Surg* 1997; **26**: 393–402.

85 RL, Lambert D, Chamberlain J, *et al.* Percutaneous transluminal angioplasty of the innominate, subclavian, and axillary arteries. *Eur J Vasc Surg* 1990; **4**: 591–5.

86 Hebrang A, Maskovic J, Tomac B. Percutaneous transluminal angioplasty of the subclavian arteries: longterm results in 52 patients. *Am J Radiol* 1991; **156**: 109–14.

87 Millaire A, Trinca M, Marache P, *et al.* Subclavian angioplasty: immediate and late results in 50 patients. *Catheter Cardiovasc Diagn* 1993; **29**: 81–7.

88 Selby JB, Matsumoto AH, Tegtmeyer CJ, *et al.* Balloon angioplasty above the aortic arch: immediate and longterm results. *Am J Radiol* 1993; **160**: 631–5.

89 Tyagi S, Verma PK, Gambhir DS, *et al*. Early and long-term results of subclavian angioplasty in aortoarteritis (Takayasu disease): comparison with atherosclerosis. *Cardiovasc Intervent Radiol* 1998; **21**: 219–24.

90 Harris NJ, Cameron I, Beard JD, Gaines P. Percutaneous stenting of proximal subclavian artery occlusion. *Eur J Vasc Endovasc Surg* 1995; **9**: 479–80.

91 Al-Mubarak N, Liu MW, Dean LS, *et al*. Immediate and late outcomes of subclavian artery stenting. *Catheter Cardiovasc Intervent* 1999; **46**: 169–72.

92 Rodriguez-Lopez JA, Werner A, Martinez R, *et al*. Stenting for atherosclerotic occlusive disease of the subclavian artery. *Ann Vasc Surg* 1999; **13**: 254–60.

93 Sullivan TM, Gray BH, Bacharach JM, *et al*. Angioplasty and primary stenting of the subclavian, innominate, and common carotid arteries in 83 patients. *J Vasc Surg* 1998; **28**: 1059–65.

94 Whitbread T, Cleveland TJ, Beard JD, Gaines PA. A combined approach to the treatment of proximal arterial occlusions of the upper limb with endovascular stents. *Eur J Vasc Endovasc Surg* 1998; **15**: 29–35.

95 du Toit DF, Strauss DC, Blaszczyk M, *et al*. Endovascular treatment of penetrating thoracic outlet arterial injuries. *Eur J Vasc Endovasc Surg* 2000; **19**: 489–95.

96 Park JH, Chung JW, Joh JH, *et al*. Aortic and arterial aneurysms in Behçet disease: management with stent-grafts – initial experience. *Radiology* 2001; **220**: 745–50.

97 Johnson SP, Durham JD, Subber SW, *et al*. Acute arterial occlusions of the small vessels of the hand and forearm: treatment with regional urokinase therapy. *J Vasc Intervent Radiol* 1999; **10**: 869–76.

98 Pemberton M, Varty K, Nydahl S, Bell PR. The surgical management of acute limb ischaemia due to native vessel occlusion. *Eur J Vasc Endovasc Surg* 1999; **17**: 72–6.

99 Widlus DM, Venbrux AC, Benenati JF, *et al*. Fibrinolytic therapy for upper extremity arterial occlusions. *Radiology* 1990; **175**: 393–9.

100 Lang EV, Bookstein JJ. Accelerated thrombolysis and angioplasty for hand ischemia in Buerger's disease. *Cardiovasc Intervent Radiol* 1989; **12**: 957.

101 Sayin A, Bozkurt AK, Tuzun H, *et al*. Surgical treatment of Buerger's disease: experience with 216 patients. *Cardiovasc Surg* 1993; **1**: 377–80.

42

Emergency Aspects of Buerger's Disease

SEKAR NATARAJAN, DHANESH KAMERKAR

THE PROBLEM

Buerger's disease or thromboangiitis obliterans (TAO) is a non-atherosclerotic segmental inflammatory arterial disease which mostly affects small and medium sized arteries. It is most commonly encountered in young adults and is closely identified with tobacco usage. Von Winiwarter, in 1879, was the first to describe Buerger's disease on discovering 'endarteritis' and 'endophlebitis' in an amputated limb. Much later, in 1908, Leo Buerger provided a detailed and accurate description of the disease, differentiating it from atherosclerosis, and called it 'thromboangiitis obliterans'. Even though it has a worldwide distribution the condition is much more common in countries in Asia such as Israel, India and Korea than in the USA or Europe. Cachovan in 1986[1] reported the incidence of Buerger's disease as a proportion of peripheral arterial occlusive disease in different countries (Table 42.1).

Table 42.1 *Geographical incidence of Buerger's disease[1]*

	Country	Incidence (per cent)
Asia	Israel	80.0
	India	45.0–63.0
	Korea	16.0–66.0
Europe	France	1.2–5.6
	Former West Germany	0.5–5.0
	Switzerland	1.0–3.0
	UK	0.25

The incidence of Buerger's disease has been steadily decreasing in the developed nations. At the Mayo Clinic the incidence had regressed from 107 per 10^5 patients registered in 1947 to 12.6 per 10^5 patients registered in 1985.[2] By contrast, the incidence of the disease in women worldwide has been steadily increasing and is a reflection of the rise in numbers of women smokers.[3]

AETIOLOGY

The aetiology of TAO is, in short, still unknown. Although TAO is grouped under the miscellaneous category of vasculitis, it differs from the more commonly encountered variety. Its association with smoking has been well documented but the role of other aetiological factors such as autoimmune mechanisms, genetic factors and hypercoagulability states is not very clear.

There is a very strong association between tobacco usage and TAO. Patients with TAO show a higher incidence of delayed hypersensitivity reaction to tobacco glycoprotein. Papa and colleagues[4] demonstrated a similar response in healthy smokers whereas non-smokers did not respond at all. This effect depends on individual hypersensitivity rather than on the amount of tobacco consumed. Progression of disease and results of treatment are closely linked to the cessation of smoking. Measurement of urinary cotinine and carboxyhaemoglobin in blood can be used to establish whether the patient has really stopped smoking.

In India Buerger's disease is commonly observed in people who are poor and who smoke raw tobacco in the form of 'beedies'[5] but quite unusual in the richer cigarette smokers who seem to develop atherosclerosis. Hence there must be other factors such as nutritional status and infection which may play a role in the pathogenesis of TAO. As only a small number of smokers develop TAO, a lot of work has concentrated on identifying a possible genetic predisposition, but so far no definitive or consistent genetic cause has been detected.

Several studies have confirmed the presence of serum anticollagen, antielastin, antiendothelial cell antibodies and circulating immune complexes[6–9] but a 'cause and effect' relationship remains to be discovered. Chaudhry and colleagues[10] demonstrated that the level of urokinase plasminogen activator was elevated twofold and that free plasminogen activator inhibitor-1 was lower in patients with Buerger's disease – observations indicating some form of endothelial derangement. Makita *et al.*[11] demonstrated impaired endothelium dependent vasorelaxation in the peripheral vasculature of patients with TAO, and it is recognised that vasospasm is a prominent feature of the disease. Attention has now been drawn to the presence of antiphospholipid antibodies and hyperhomocysteinaemia in patients with Buerger's disease but the significance of these findings is still not clear.

PATHOLOGY

Buerger's disease is an inflammatory occlusive disease involving both arteries and veins. It is usually segmental in distribution with characteristic skip lesions. Pathologically, three distinct phases in the course of the disease have been identified.

Acute phase

This is the classic presentation of Buerger's disease and distinguishes it from atherosclerosis. The vessel is swollen with thrombus and the arterial wall and periarterial tissue are oedematous. Characteristically, there is evidence of transmural infiltration by inflammatory cells and of microabscesses with many multinucleated giant cells. Cellular thrombus is unique to Buerger's disease. The adjacent vein may also show similar features with thrombophlebitis. During this stage the patient presents with features of acute ischaemia, tenderness over the artery and inflammatory changes in the skin over the artery.

Intermediate phase

The acute stage is followed by an intermediate phase in which there is progressive organisation of the occlusive thrombus with recanalisation. The microabscesses disappear but giant cell infiltration persists.

Chronic phase

During the chronic stage there is more extensive recanalisation of the thrombus and increased fibrous tissue formation in the media and adventitia. The vessel becomes thin and cord-like. The elastic lamina may show minimal fragmentation but the most important feature is that the general architecture of the arterial wall is well preserved. Calcification never occurs in Buerger's disease (Figs 42.1 and 42.2).

In patients over the age of 40 years, atherosclerosis can coexist with TAO and that has caused some confusion about the exact diagnosis. Progression of the disease can be continuous and creeping or take the form of skip lesions. In the early stages the disease is segmental and starts in the medium and small sized muscular arteries of the extremities. It can also begin in small branches of major proximal arteries such as the iliac gradually extending proximally to

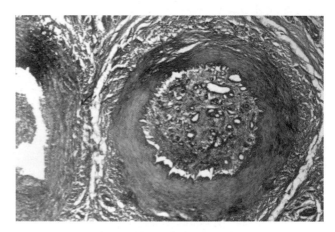

Figure 42.1   *Tibial artery with recanalised thrombus (haematoxylin and eosin × 25). Note vessel architecture is maintained*

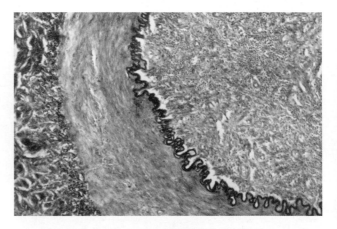

Figure 42.2   *Close-up view of specimen in Fig. 42.1 showing cellular thrombus and exaggerated coiling of internal elastic lamina (haematoxylin and eosin × 160)*

involve major trunks up as far as the aorta. Importantly, therefore, proximal artery involvement should not be viewed as a finding which excludes a diagnosis of Buerger's disease. The involvement of cerebral, coronary and visceral vessels in TAO, a process extending even to vein bypass grafts, has been documented.[12–14]

CLINICAL FEATURES

Buerger's disease predominantly affects young males who are heavy smokers. There is a strong association between smoking and TAO but the disease is also known to occur in non-smokers. The onset of disease is usually before the age of 50 and is now increasingly seen in women who use tobacco.

The disease usually commences in the infrapopliteal vessels and is characterised by acute exacerbations and remissions. As the disease progresses, more proximal arteries become involved, and the symptoms change accordingly. The classic clinical features in the early stages are foot and instep claudication and migratory superficial thrombophlebitis. Rubor and trophic changes are also often observed. Digital ulcers are common but ulceration and gangrene do not always follow the onset of claudication but may actually precede it. Frequently, ulcer or gangrene associated with rest pain is precipitated by trivial trauma or minor surgery such as the removal of a nail.

In an analysis of 112 patients Olin et al.[3] documented the typical pattern and frequency of the clinical features of TAO (Table 42.2), rest pain, ischaemic ulceration and claudication being the most prominent observed.

Very often more than one limb is involved. In Shionoya's report[15] the prevalence of multiple limb involvement was as follows: two limbs in 16 per cent, three limbs in 41 per cent and all four limbs in 43 per cent of patients. Involvement of the upper limb is also quite common but is usually missed because the vessels most frequently involved, namely, the ulnar and palmar arteries, are not always checked. Nonetheless, in most series, the prevalence of upper limb involvement is 45–50 per cent, which is high.

Table 42.2 *Pattern and frequency of clinical features of thromboangiitis obliterans[3]*

Clinical features	Frequency (per cent)
Intermittent claudication	70 (63)
Rest pain	91 (81)
Ischaemic ulcer	85 (76)
Upper extremity involvement	24 (28)
Lower extremity involvement	39 (46)
Both upper and lower extremities	22 (26)
Thrombophlebitis	43 (38)
Raynaud's	49 (44)

In a Cleveland series[3] 63 per cent of patients demonstrated an abnormal Allen's test. Cold sensitivity due to markedly increased sympathetic activity was observed in about 40 per cent of patients but Raynaud's phenomenon has not been noted as often in other series.[16]

ACUTE PRESENTATION

Buerger's disease typically manifests in the form of acute exacerbations triggered by the sudden onset of segmental thrombosis which is usually accompanied by vague systemic symptoms such as low grade fever and malaise. The patient presents with signs of acute ischaemia or a worsening of pre-existing ischaemia. Matsushita et al.[17] found that acute exacerbation is closely associated with high circulating levels of nicotine. It is important to differentiate this picture from embolism, especially as catheter embolectomy for acute thrombosis in Buerger's disease is likely to be unsuccessful and usually followed by a deterioration of the ischaemia. A prior history of claudication and the presence of arterial occlusions in other limbs helps to differentiate it from embolism.

DIAGNOSTIC CRITERIA

The diagnosis of Buerger's disease is primarily based on the clinical picture. Shionoya[15] suggested a set of classic criteria which include:

- onset of disease below the age of 50 years
- a process particularly involving the infrapopliteal vessels but frequently affecting both upper and lower limbs
- migrating thrombophlebitis
- absence of atherogenic risk factors apart from smoking.

Papa et al.[18] suggested a point scoring system and Mills and Porter[19] proposed major and minor criteria for the diagnosis of Buerger's disease. Some confusion has existed in defining these criteria largely because many patients over the age of 50 also display the behaviour and the angiographic findings typical of TAO. Histopathologically, the features of atherosclerosis associated with age have only added to the confusion. Sasaki et al.[20] reported an incidence of associated hypertension in 13.5 per cent, diabetes in 4.4 per cent, and hyperlipidaemia in 7.9 per cent of their TAO patients, and 15 per cent of them were over 50 years of age at the time of diagnosis. In an analysis, Vink[21] identified less than 2 per cent of patients whose symptoms started after the age of 50 years while that was true of 29 per cent of patients in the series reported by Olin et al.[3] Moreover, in addition to infrapopliteal involvement, the disease not uncommonly affects major proximal arteries. In one of our series,[22] 26 per cent of patients presented with aortoiliac disease and 42 per cent with femoropopliteal disease. In India, involvement of the external iliac artery is quite often observed.

LABORATORY TESTS

There are no specific diagnostic laboratory tests for Buerger's disease. Indicators of active inflammation include an elevated erythrocyte sedimentation rate and raised C-reactive protein. Immunological tests such as R factor, anti-nuclear antibody, etc., help to rule out other systematic vasculitic syndromes. Tests for hypercoagulability, including antiphospholipid antibodies and homocysteinaemia, are also of value. Routine electrocardiogram and echocardiogram will help to identify any cardiac illness as well as rule out a possible source of embolism. Angiographic findings are usually pathognomonic of Buerger's disease.

ANGIOGRAPHY

The characteristic findings of TAO on angiography are seen in small and medium sized vessels such as the tibial, pedal, ulnar and palmar arteries, usually with apparently normal large proximal arteries and the absence of atheromatous changes. Key angiographic features are segmental arterial occlusions, interspersed with normal sections; the artery occludes with an abrupt cut-off, from which point leashes of collaterals arise giving a characteristic 'tree root' appearance. The collaterals result in part from the recanalisation of vessels and dilated vasa vasorum which explains their 'corkscrew' shape (Figs 42.3–42.6), sometimes described as 'accordion' or 'corrugated' in appearance. Typically, early venous filling also takes place. In general, the frequency with which abrupt occlusion of arteries of the lower limb is

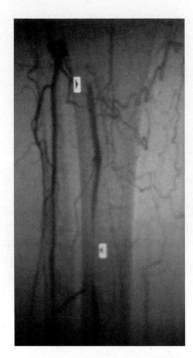

Figure 42.4   *View of distal arterial tree taken from the arteriogram in Fig. 42.3. Note the reformation of tibial vessels with segmental occlusion and 'corkscrew' collaterals*

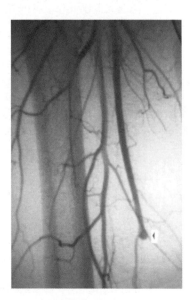

Figure 42.3   *Arteriogram of a 30-year-old man showing abrupt cut-off of superficial femoral artery. Note normal proximal artery*

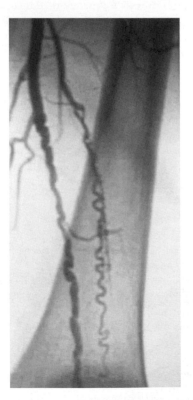

Figure 42.5   *Arteriogram of a 30-year-old man with Buerger's disease. Popliteal and femoral artery showing extensive recanalisation. Note the 'corkscrew' collaterals*

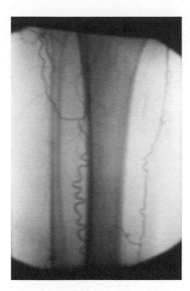

Figure 42.6   *View of arterial tree of mid-lower leg taken from the arteriogram in Fig. 42.5 showing only collaterals*

Table 42.3   *Anatomical prevalence of abrupt arterial occlusion in thromboangiitis obliterans of the lower limbs[15]*

Artery	Incidence (per cent)
Superficial femoral artery	10
Popliteal artery	25
Anterior tibial artery	90
Posterior tibial artery	80
Peroneal artery	50

noted, rises as they ramify distally down the leg. Shionoya[15] reported the prevalence of these angiographic findings in his series (Table 42.3), the aortoiliac segment being involved in 8 per cent, the femoropopliteal segment in 32 per cent, and of the crural vessels the peroneal artery is the least affected (Figs 42.7–42.9).

Classical angiographic findings in TAO

- Small and medium sized vessels diseased (tibial, pedal, ulnar, palmar)
- Segmental occlusion
- Normal proximal arteries
- No atheromatous changes
- Abrupt cut-off with 'tree root' collaterals
- Corkscrew-shaped collaterals
- 'Accordion' or 'corrugated' appearance of vessels affected
- Early venous filling

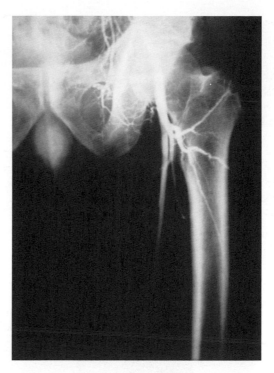

Figure 42.7   *Arteriogram of a 40-year-old man with Buerger's disease. Profunda femoris artery showing early inflammatory changes. Main trunk of profunda occluded*

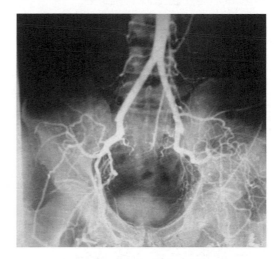

Figure 42.8   *Arteriogram of a 30-year-old man with bilateral external iliac occlusions due to Buerger's disease. Note the extensive collaterals and disease in branches of the internal iliac artery*

NATURAL COURSE

Buerger's disease usually commences in small vessels such as the digital, pedal and palmar arteries and, expectedly, patients present initially with instep claudication and digital ulceration. The disease progresses gradually to involve segments of the crural and popliteal arteries, an advancing process occurring both contiguously as well as by skip lesions. Buerger's disease may also develop in the muscular

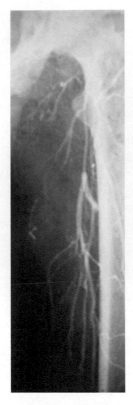

Figure 42.9   *View of segments of a re-formed profunda femoris artery taken from the arteriogram in Fig. 42.8*

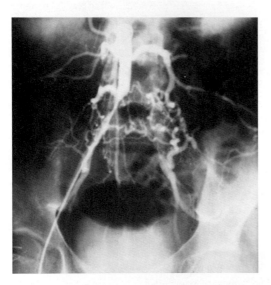

Figure 42.10   *Arteriogram of a 45-year-old man with Buerger's disease showing total occlusion of left common and external iliac arteries with extensive 'corkscrew' collaterals. Note the involvement of a lumbar artery and severe spasm of the right iliac artery*

branches of the proximally situated deep femoral, internal iliac as well as lumbar arteries (Fig. 42.10). Thus, thrombus may form at the ostia of these vessels and progress thence to involve the parent artery. Proximal occlusion may also follow stasis thrombus secondary to more extensive distal disease.

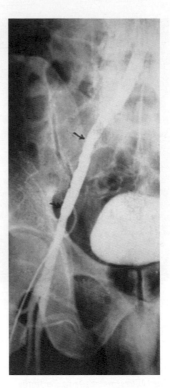

Figure 42.11   *Arteriogram of a 37-year-old smoker presenting with sudden onset of critical ischaemia of both lower limbs showing segmental dilatation of the right external iliac artery with the characteristic 'accordion' appearance (arrow)*

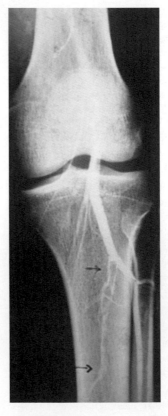

Figure 42.12   *View of popliteal artery and thrombotic occlusion of the left tibioperoneal trunk (arrows) taken from the arteriogram in Fig. 42.11*

Buerger's disease, involving multiple segments with normal skip areas, may manifest as critical ischaemia of sudden onset (Figs 42.11 and 42.12). Progress of disease with typical acute exacerbations is closely associated with heavy smoking. Nevertheless, in spite of stopping smoking, 10 per cent of patients experience recurrence of ischaemic ulceration.[23] As the disease progresses proximally more collaterals occlude, the ischemia worsens and the patient ultimately undergoes major amputation. Long term survival, however, has been shown to be better than that reported for atherosclerosis.

TREATMENT

Modalities of treatment recommended for TAO

- General
  - Abstinence from tobacco
  - Foot care
  - Exercise
- Medical
  - Analgesics
  - Antiplatelet drugs
  - Calcium channel blockers
  - Pentoxifylline
  - Heparin
  - Low molecular weight dextran
  - Prostaglandin
  - Fibrinolytic agents
- Surgical
  - Sympathectomy – chemical; surgical (open, minimal access)
  - Spinal cord stimulation
  - Omentopexy
  - Ilizarov tibial corticotomy
  - Vascular reconstruction
  - Amputation
- Miscellaneous
  - Gene therapy
  - Immunosuppressants

Various treatment modalities have been recommended for Buerger's disease. The mainstay of any advice is the complete abstinence from smoking and patients should be aware that smoking even one or two cigarettes can keep the disease active. In a Cleveland Clinic report,[3] 94 per cent of patients who stopped smoking avoided amputation whereas 43 per cent of those who continued to smoke required it.

Regular walking and exercise helps to improve collateral flow, ensures better distribution and utilisation of circulating blood and assists muscle metabolism. Foot infection should be treated according to its merits with drainage, antibiotics and limited amputation. Antiplatelet drugs and pentoxifylline are used in chronic cases. Vasospasm is prominent feature of Buerger's disease and therefore calcium channel blockers are very useful.

In patients who present with acute symptoms, balloon catheter thromboembolectomy has been tried, but because of the inflammatory nature of the thrombus and the vessel wall, the artery usually re-occludes. Consequently, in these patients, various other treatments such as anticoagulation and lytic therapy have been tried and the former, using heparin, helps in preventing progression of the thrombotic process.

Low molecular weight dextran reduces blood viscosity and enhances the microcirculation. Intra-arterial thrombolytic therapy[24] has been used in patients presenting with gangrenous or pregangrenous lesions with an overall success rate of 58.3 per cent (also refer to Chapter 16). Kubota and coworkers[25] have used superselective infusions of urokinase into the dorsalis pedis artery and demonstrated recanalisation and healing of ischaemic ulcers.

Iloprost, a prostaglandin analogue, has been used successfully by stimulating blood flow through its vasodilatory and platelet inhibitory action. Feissinger and Schafer[26] conducted a prospective randomised double blind study in patients with Buerger's disease presenting with critical ischaemia, comparing a 6-hour daily infusion of iloprost with aspirin. On analysis at the end of the 28-day treatment period 63 per cent of patients given iloprost were entirely relieved of ischaemic rest pain in comparison with 28 per cent treated with aspirin ($P < 0.05$). Also, ischaemic ulcers healed completely in 35 per cent of the study group compared with 13 per cent in the control group. At 6 months the overall response rate in terms of continued pain relief and/or ulcer healing was 88 per cent in the iloprost group and 21 per cent in the aspirin group ($P < 0.05$). The European TAO study group[27] recently completed a double blind randomised trial comparing oral iloprost with placebo in patients with TAO presenting with critical ischemia. Total healing of ulcers was not significantly different between the treatment groups: low dose iloprost was more significantly effective than placebo but in high doses it failed to show any significant beneficial effect. The conclusion was that iloprost was more effective than placebo in the relief of rest pain but not so in ulcer healing. It appears that intravenous iloprost is more effective than the oral form in ulcer healing.

Sympathetic ganglion blockade has been used effectively to relieve rest pain and healing of ulcers. As sympathectomy does not increase muscle blood flow it has no role to play in claudication. Surgical sympathectomy may be reasonable, however, in patients who have severe distal disease where vascular reconstruction is either not possible or has failed. It can also be used adjunctively along with proximal arterial revascularisation in those patients who have extensive distal disease.

Implantable spinal cord stimulators have been used successfully for pain relief and ulcer healing in patients unsuitable for vascular reconstruction.[28] Intramuscular gene transfer of naked plasmid DNA encoding vascular endothelial growth factor has been successfully tried in critically ischaemic patients.[29] It has been beneficial in the relief of rest pain, healing of ulcers and gives a 0.1 improvement in the ankle:brachial index. Angiogenesis has also been confirmed by the appearance of new collateral vessels on magnetic resonance imaging and contrast angiography.

Surgical revascularisation for Buerger's disease is difficult because of multisegmental occlusions, distal location of disease and frequent presence of superficial phlebitis. Sasaki et al.[20] found that only 15.5 per cent of their patients were suitable for vascular reconstruction. Endarterectomy is rarely possible in Buerger's disease because of the inflammatory nature of its pathology, except when the occlusion is caused by stasis thrombus. It follows, therefore, that it can be effective in occlusions of the juxtarenal aorta and the profunda femoris artery. Bypass surgery taking the graft down to patent segments of vessels and even to larger collaterals has been successful and vein is the preferred graft material in these cases (see Chapter 15). Despite the short term patency of these grafts the objectives of ulcer healing, relief of rest pain and limb salvage are served. If the patient can stay away from tobacco the period of remission is likely to last longer. Successful bypasses have been performed to isolated 10–12 cm long segments of tibial arteries even when there was no continuity with the pedal arch (Fig. 42.13).

Sasajima et al.,[30] reviewing their results in 71 bypasses on 61 patients over a period of 18 years, 85 per cent of which were to the crural arteries or to arteries below the ankle, found that primary and secondary patency rates were 48.8 per cent and 62.5 per cent at 5 years, and 43 per cent and 56.3 per cent at 10 years, respectively. The patency rates were 66.8 per cent in non-smokers and 34.5 per cent in those who continued to smoke after surgery; 40 per cent of the secondary failure cases underwent amputation. Shionoya[15] reported cumulative patency rates for femoropopliteal bypass of 70 per cent at 1 year and 60 per cent at 5 years, and for femorocrural bypass 50 per cent at 1 year and 44 per cent at 5 years. In our own large series of 965 patients, 310 (32 per cent) proceeded to vascular bypass procedures: aortoiliac or aortofemoral 11 per cent, iliofemoral 9 per cent, femoropopliteal 34 per cent, femorodistal 36 per cent and upper limb bypass 10 per cent.[22] Lumbar sympathectomy was added as an adjuvant procedure to tibial bypass and when the outflow was poor. Early thrombosis was observed in 28 per cent of patients. The cumulative 2-year and 5-year patency rates for femoropopliteal bypass were 50 per cent and 28 per cent, respectively, and for tibial bypass 30 per cent and 20 per cent, respectively. The overall major amputation rate was 22 per cent. Spasm was a major problem during dissection and anastomosis (Figs 42.14 and 42.15) and therefore gentle tissue handling and the use of vasodilators such as papaverine and dilzem have helped to minimise this problem.

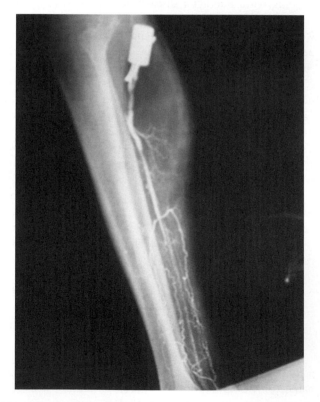

Figure 42.13 *Operative angiogram after popliteo-tibial bypass to a 10 cm long isolated posterior tibial segment and which remained patent for 13 months. Typical 'tree root' and 'corkscrew' appearance of collaterals can be made out. Note the spasm in the posterior tibial artery just distal to the anastomosis*

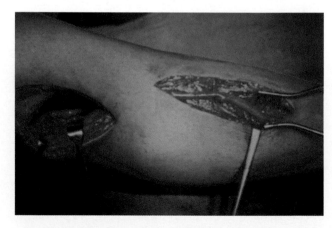

Figure 42.14 *Operative photograph of a 35-year-old man with Buerger's disease presenting with proximal tibial artery occlusion showing a popliteal to posterior tibial reversed saphenous vein graft*

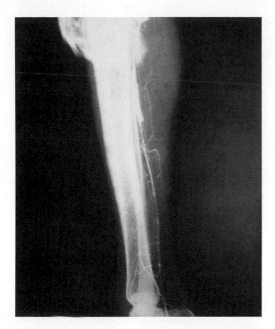

Figure 42.15 *Operative angiogram in Fig. 42.14 showing spasm of the posterior tibial artery. This graft remained patent for 2 years*

There have been reports of indirect revascularisation of ischaemic limbs in Buerger's disease by means of omentopexy, either as free or pedicled grafts, and also of arterialisation of the long saphenous vein with associated claims of ulcer healing and relief from rest pain.[31] Our treatment policy in patients with chronic symptoms is illustrated in Fig. 42.16.

In those patients presenting with acute symptoms, immediate surgery is likely to fail in view of the active inflammatory and immunological response (see Chapter 2). It is better, therefore, to treat these patients medically. The treatment options for acute exacerbation of Buerger's disease are illustrated in Fig. 42.17.

Saha *et al.*[32] recently reported a small non-randomised trial of cyclophosphamide in the treatment of patients with advanced TAO with modest results: improvement in claudication, relief of rest pain and a reduction in the influx of inflammatory cells in thrombus and vessel wall were noted.

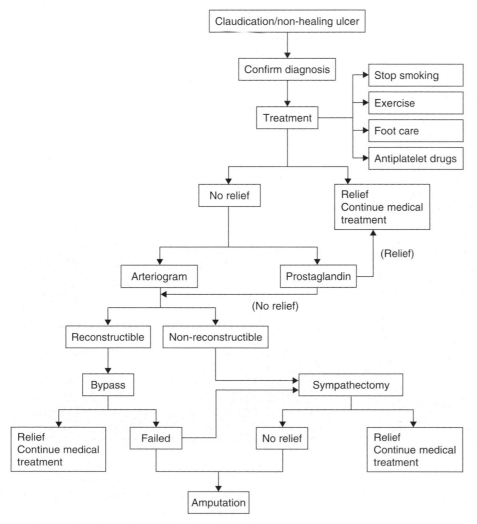

Figure 42.16 *Algorithm of treatment of chronic symptoms of Buerger's disease*

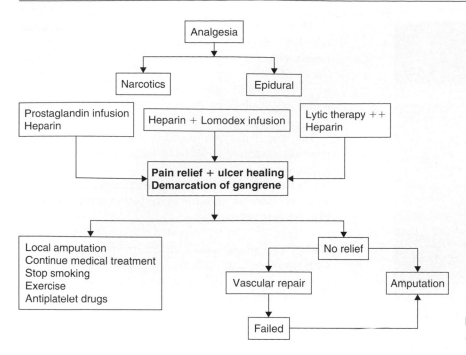

Figure 42.17 *Algorithm of treatment of acute exacerbations of Buerger's disease*

Conclusions

Buerger's disease or TAO is a non-atheromatous, segmental inflammatory arterial disease affecting medium and small muscular arteries of both upper and lower limbs. It is common in young males who are heavy smokers and there is a strong correlation between smoking and progression of disease. Thromboangiitis obliterans usually presents with digital ulcers, gangrene and severe rest pain and this clinical picture is characterised by remissions and relapses. The angiographic findings of segmental occlusion and 'corkscrew' collaterals are pathognomonic of TAO. Complete abstinence from smoking is the mainstay of treatment. In cases of chronic disease exercise and antiplatelet drugs are worth trying. In the acute case anticoagulant and thrombolytic therapy may arrest deterioration. Vascular reconstruction is difficult but can be successfully undertaken with bypasses to patent segments of the artery. Long term patency of these grafts should not be expected but they do relieve rest pain and prevent amputation or minimise the extent of tissue loss, particularly if the patient gives up smoking permanently.

Key references

Olin JW. Name of chapter. In: Rutherford RB (ed).*Thromboangiitis Obliterans (Buerger's Disease) in Vascular Surgery* 5th edn. Philadelphia, PA: WB Saunders 2000: 350–64.

Sasajima T, Kubo Y, Inaba M, *et al.* Role of Infrainguinal bypass in Buerger's disease: an eighteen year experience. *Eur J Vasc Endovasc Surg* 1997; **13**: 186–92.

Shionoya S. Clinical manifestations. In: *Buerger's Disease – Pathology diagnosis and treatment.* Nagoya: The University of Nagoya Press, 1990: 113.

Shionoya S. Thromboangiitis obliterans (Buerger's disease). In: Rutherford RB (ed). *Thromboangiitis Obliterans (Buerger's Disease) in Vascular Surgery* 4th edn. Philadelphia, PA: WB Saunders, 1994: 235–45.

The European Study Group. Oral iloprost in the treatment of thromboangiitis obliterans (Buerger's disease): a double blind, randomized, placebo controlled trial. *Eur J Vasc Endovasc Surg* 1998; **16**: 300–7.

REFERENCES

1 Cachovan M. Epidemiologie und geographisches verteilungsmuster der Thromboangitis Obliterans. In: Heidrich H (ed). *Thromboangiitis Obliterans Morbus Winiwarter – Buerger.* Stuttgart: George Thieme, 1988: 31–6.

2 Lie JT. Thromboangiitis obliterans (Buerger's disease) in women. *Medicine* 1987; **64**: 65–72.

3 Olin JW. Thromboangiitis obliterans (Buerger's disease). In: Rutherford RB (ed). *Thromboangiitis Obliterans (Buerger's Disease) in Vascular Surgery* 5th edn. Philadelphia, PA: WB Saunders 2000: 350–64.

4 Papa M, Bass A, Adar R, *et al.* Autoimmune mechanisms in thromboangiitis obliterans (Buerger's Disease). The role of antigen and the major histocompatibility complex. *Surgery* 1992; **111**: 527–31.

5 Jindal RM, Patel SM. Buerger's disease in cigarette smoking in Bangladesh. *Ann R Coll Surg Engl* 1992; **74**: 436–7.

6 Adar R, Papa M, Halperin Z, *et al.* Cellular sensitivity to collagen in thrombo angitis obliterans. *N Engl J Med* 1983; **308**: 1113–16.

7 Gulati SM, Saha K, Kant L, *et al.* Significance of circulating immune complexes in thromboangiitis obliterans (Buerger's disease). *Angiology* 1984; **35**: 276–81.

8 Roncon A, Delgado L, Correia P, *et al.* Circulating immune complexes in Buerger's disease. *J.Cardiovasc Surg* 1989; **30**: 821–5.

9 Eichhorn J, Sima D, Lindschau C, *et al.* Antiendothelial cell antibodies in thromboangiitis obliterans. *Am J Med Sci* 1998; **315**: 17–23.

10 Chaudhry NA, Pietraszek NH, Hachiya T, *et al.* Plasminogen activators and plasminogen activator inhibitor 1 before and after venous occlusion of the upper limb in thromboangiitis obliterans (Buerger's disease). *Thromb Res* 1992; **66**: 321–9.

11 Makita S, Nakamura M, Murakami H, *et al.* Impaired endothelium dependent vasorelaxation in peripheral vasculature of patients with thromboangiitis obliterans (Buerger's disease). *Circulation* 1996; **94**(suppl II): II-211–15.

12 Donatelli F, Triggiani M, Nascinbene S, *et al.* Thromboangiitis obliterans of coronary and internal thoracic arteries in a young woman. *J.Thorac Cardiovasc Surg* 1997; **113**: 800–2.

13 Hassoun Z, Lacrosse M, De Ronde T. Intestinal involvement in Buerger's disease. *J Clin Gastroenterol* 2001; **32**: 85–9.

14 Lie JT. Thromboangiitis obliterans (Buerger's Disease) in a saphenous vein arterial graft. *Hum Pathol* 1987; **18**: 402–4.

15 Shionoya S. Clinical manifestations. In: *Buerger's Disease – Pathology diagnosis and treatment.* Nagoya: The University of Nagoya Press, 1990: 113.

16 Wysokinski W, Kwiatkowska W, Raczkowska BS, *et al.* Sustained classic clinical spectrum of thromboangiitis obliterans (Buerger's disease). *Angiology* 2000; **51**: 141–50.

17 Matsushita M, Shionoya S, Matsumoto T. Urinary nicotine measurement in patients with Buerger's Disease: effect of active and passive smoking on the disease process. *J Vasc Surg* 1992; **14**: 53–8.

18 Papa MC, Rai I, Adar R. A point scoring system for the clinical diagnosis of Buerger's disease. *Eur J Vasc Endovasc Surg* 1996; **11**: 335–9.

19 Mills JL, Porter JM. Buerger's disease: a review and update. *Semin Vasc Surg* 1993; **6**: 14–23.

20 Sasaki S, Sakumo M, Yasuda K. Current status of thromboangitis obliterans (Buerger's disease) in Japan. *Int J Cardiol* 2000; **75**: 5175–81.

21 Vink M. Symposium on Buerger's disease. *J Cardiovasc Surg* 1973; **14**: 1–51.

22 Hussain SA, Sekar N. Buerger's disease – review article. *Indian J Surg* 2002; **64**: 237–9.

23 Shionoya S. Thromboangiitis obliterans (Buerger's disease). In: Rutherford RB (ed). *Thromboangiitis Obliterans (Buerger's disease) in Vascular Surgery* 4th edn. Philadelphia, PA: WB Saunders, 1994: 235–45.

24 Hussein EA, el Dorri A. Intra-arterial streptokinase as adjuvant therapy for complicated Buerger's Disease early trials. *Int Surg* 1993; **78**: 54–8.

25 Kubota Y, Kichikawa K, Uchida H, *et al.* Superselective urokinase infusion therapy for dorsalis pedis artery occlusion in Buerger's disease. *Cardiovasc Intervent Radiol* 1997; **20**: 380–2.

26 Fiessinger JN, Schafer M. Trial of iloprost versus aspirin treatment for critical ischaemia of thromboangiitis obliterans. The TAO study. *Lancet* 1990; **335**: 555–7.

27 The European Study Group. Oral iloprost in the treatment of thromboangiitis obliterans (Buerger's disease): a double blind, randomized, placebo controlled trial. *Eur J Vasc Endovasc Surg* 1998; **16**: 300–7.

28 Chierichetti F, Mambrini S, Bagliani A, Odero A. Treatment of Buerger's disease with electrical spinal cord stimulation – review of three cases. *Angiology* 2002; **53**: 341–7.

29 Isner JM, Baumbartner I, Rauh G, *et al.* Treatment of thromboangiitis obliterans (Buerger's disease) by intramuscular gene transfer of vascular endothelial growth factor: preliminary clinical results. *J Vasc Surg* 1998; **28**: 964–75.

30 Sasajima T, Kubo Y, Inaba M, *et al.* Role of Infrainguinal bypass in Buerger's disease: an eighteen year experience. *Eur J Vasc Endovasc Surg* 1997; **13**: 186–92.

31 Talwar S, Jain S, Porwal R, *et al.* Free versus pedicled omental grafts for limb salvage in Buerger's Disease. *Aust N Z J Surg* 1998; **68**: 38–40.

32 Saha K, Chabra N, Gulati SM. Treatment of patients with thromboangiitis obliterans with cyclophosphamide. *Angiology* 2001; **52**: 399–407.

43

Acute Limb Vascular Inflammatory Conditions

MATTHEW WALTHAM, KEVIN G BURNAND

ACUTE ARTERIAL INFLAMMATORY CONDITIONS

Vascular inflammatory conditions of the limbs may present in the context of a wide variety of clinical syndromes, including Buerger's disease, scleroderma, systemic lupus erythematosus (SLE), Takayasu's disease and giant cell arteritis. These diseases are characterised by inflammatory cell invasion of arteries causing swelling, luminal obstruction and often thrombosis. Operative and endovascular techniques are rarely indicated in their treatment and should only be used in carefully selected patients. Surgical biopsy of a vessel or muscle may be useful in the diagnosis of vasculitic syndromes.

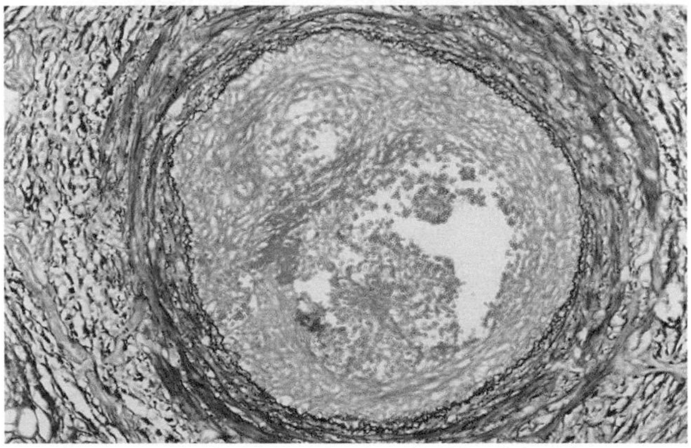

Aetiology and pathology

Thromboangiitis obliterans (Buerger's disease) is characterised by progressive obliteration of distal vessels of the upper and lower limbs (see Chapter 42). The exact pathophysiology is poorly understood, but patients are almost invariably young cigarette-smoking males, although the condition has also been described in cannabis smokers[1] and women. Histological examination of affected vessels shows transmural inflammation with intimal proliferation, surrounded by collagen deposition (Fig. 43.1). Luminal thrombosis occurs within the vessels, and the accompanying veins may also become inflamed leading to superficial and deep vein thrombosis. Progressive ischaemia leads first to digital gangrene and then more major amputation of the limbs becomes necessary if cigarette smoking continues.[2,3]

Systemic autoimmune diseases often cause transmural inflammation of small vessels, affecting individual crural vessels, pedal arch vessels, metatarsal and digital arteries

Figure 43.1 *Cross-section of affected small vessel in Buerger's disease, showing transmural inflammation and luminal thrombosis*

(Fig. 43.2), a process often progressing to arterial occlusion and limb ischaemia. Collateral pathways are less likely to develop with more distal occlusions, which, therefore, are more likely to cause critical ischaemia.

Takayasu's arteritis is an idiopathic systemic inflammatory disease usually involving the aorta and its main branches (see Chapter 41). It is most frequently observed in young women from Far Eastern Asian countries. With early disease there is focal or continuous granulomatous inflammation which leads to fibrosis of the vessel wall. This results in multiple stenoses or occasionally aneurysms.

Giant cell arteritis is the commonest form of systemic arteritis. There is focal inflammation of medium and small arteries, usually affecting the extracranial branches of the external carotid artery. The aetiology of this disease is unknown. Surgery plays no part in treatment but arterial biopsy is often useful in establishing the diagnosis.

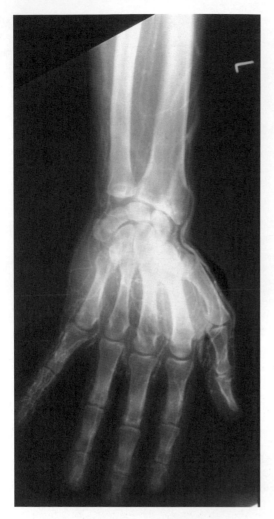

Figure 43.2   *Angiogram showing obliteration of digital vessels in a patient with Raynaud's disease secondary to scleroderma*

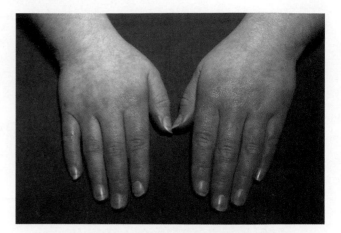

Figure 43.3   *Typical colour changes in the hands of a patient with Raynaud's disease*

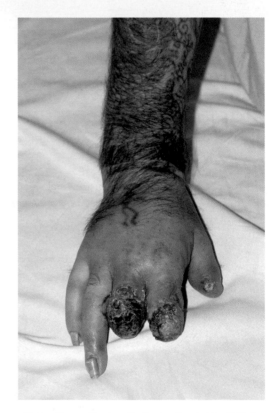

Figure 43.4   *Severe Raynaud's disease has led to digital amputation in this patient*

Diagnosis

CLINICAL

Critical limb ischaemia may present as pain, ulceration or gangrene in the affected limb, which may be preceded by a history of intermittent claudication. Buerger's disease should always be suspected if the patient is a young male smoker. Many of the vasculitides present with severe Raynaud's phenomenon, i.e. digital pallor in response to cold exposure followed by cyanosis and then reactive hyper-aemia (Fig 43.3). This is often intractable and may progress to digital ulceration and even frank gangrene (Fig. 43.4). Affected limbs feel cool, distal pulses are impalpable and ischaemic paronychiae are common around the nails.

Takayasu's disease often begins with non-specific signs and symptoms indicative of a systemic inflammatory response. Specific features of arterial disease may then emerge, either from limb or end organ ischaemia. The clinical features affect the peripheral vascular, neurological, cardiac and pulmonary systems. The course of the disease usually extends over several years and varies in severity and speed of progression.

INVESTIGATIONS

Duplex ultrasound and angiography are indicated to define the anatomical site of disease and to evaluate the possibility of vessel reconstruction. In diseases affecting distal arteries Doppler pressures in pedal vessels are reduced and duplex scanning shows normal blood flow to the popliteal arteries. Duplex scanning is less valuable in

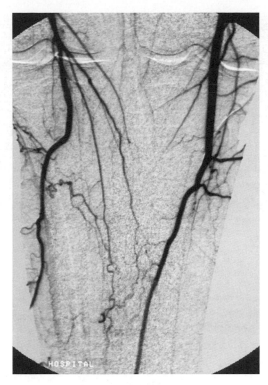

Figure 43.5   *Angiogram showing typical 'corkscrew' collaterals in a patient with Buerger's disease*

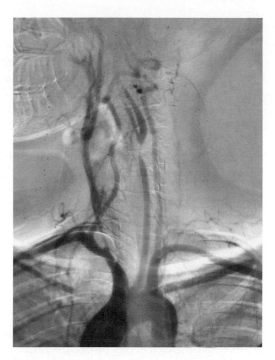

Figure 43.6   *Angiogram showing carotid and subclavian artery disease in a patient with Takayasu's disease*

these cases as it rarely defines disease in the distal vasculature. In Buerger's disease arteriography shows a characteristic pattern of normal proximal vessels and distal occlusions often with many 'corkscrew' collaterals (Fig. 43.5). Occluded vessels may be biopsied to confirm the diagnosis.

In Takayasu's disease the aorta and its main branches are most commonly affected, and these can be easily imaged by intravenous digital subtraction angiography (Fig. 43.6). The diagnosis is based on the clinical features and the presence of typical configurations of affected arteries. The erythrocyte sedimentation rate (ESR) and C-reactive protein (CRP) level may be raised. Disease activity is sometimes difficult to assess as the clinical features or acute phase reactants do not accurately reflect blood vessel inflammation.

Management

GENERAL PRINCIPLES AND PITFALLS

The surgical options for treating occlusive inflammatory arterial disease are sympathectomy, bypass procedures and amputation. Unfortunately, the distal nature of most vasculitides means that surgical options are limited and often have a poor outcome. In most cases surgery is only considered for intractable pain or in cases where there is ulceration or frank gangrene. The majority of cases of arteritis affecting the limbs should be treated with non-surgical methods.

Active Takayasu's disease is treated with high dose corticosteroids alone or together with a cytotoxic agent. Stenoses causing critical limb, or end organ, ischaemia should be treated by interventional radiology or surgical bypass.

MEDICAL OR CONSERVATIVE TREATMENT

In patients with Buerger's disease the long term course of the disease and the frequency and extent of amputations depends almost exclusively on whether the patient continues to smoke. The emphasis of treatment must therefore be to stop the patient smoking.

An attempt should be made to find a cause for Raynaud's phenomenon, such as an underlying connective tissue disorder or a cervical rib. Attacks are often precipitated by a number of triggers, for example cold exposure, and avoidance of these triggers, e.g. the wearing of heated gloves or stopping smoking, can control the symptoms adequately. Vasodilator drugs may also be useful particularly in primary Raynaud's syndrome; nifedipine reduces the frequency and severity of vasospastic attacks. Alternative medication includes naftidrofuryl and inositol nicotinate.

Patients with severe vasospasm may respond to an infusion of prostaglandin, e.g. iloprost. The dose should be titrated to the maximum tolerated without causing significant hypotension, and continued for several days. Vasculitides of large muscular arteries, for example giant cell arteritis and Takayasu's disease, should be treated primarily with corticosteroids. This is almost always successful for giant cell arteritis but 50 per cent of patients with Takayasu's arteritis become refractory to steroids and surgery becomes necessary (see Chapter 41).

SURGICAL TREATMENT

Sympathectomy

The sympathetic nervous system innervates the arterioles and precapillary sphincters in the skin and muscle of the limbs. The cutaneous nerves are mostly vasoconstrictor whereas muscles have both vasoconstrictor and vasodilator fibres. Sympathectomy in a normal limb results in a large increase in blood flow, but its effect in an ischaemic limb is greatly attenuated because maximal vasodilation is already present. Additionally, in diabetic patients peripheral neuropathy has often already effected an 'autosympathectomy'.

Sympathetic vasomotor blockade, however, does result in a redistribution of blood flow with a marked increase in cutaneous flow at the expense of muscular flow. Although this may worsen claudication distance the increased skin blood flow will sometimes allow ischaemic nail folds and ulceration to heal. Blockage of sudomotor activity may also dry up ischaemic and infected ulcers.[4,5] There is also evidence that dividing the sympathetic chain not only affects local neurotransmitter production but also reduces afferent pain fibre transmission in the spinal cord thus reducing or abolishing pain.

Sympathectomy cannot reverse or improve frank gangrene and if present the procedure must be combined with ablation. Although the effects are often short lived, healing of ischaemic areas combined with cessation of smoking may provide long term benefit. Sympathectomy is not indicated in claudication, but may help relieve symptoms in patients with rest pain who are not suitable for reconstructive procedures. Percutaneous sympathetic block may be helpful in identifying patients with residual vasoconstriction. Operative sympathectomy may be beneficial in those whose symptoms are relieved with perhaps some objective increase in skin temperature.

Sympathectomy is achieved either by surgical excision of part of the sympathetic chain or by chemical ablation of the chain. Chemical sympathectomy is performed by injection of phenol around the chain using local anaesthetic and radiographic control. Surgical excision is preferable in patients with vasculitides because recurrence may follow chemical sympathectomy. Salvage surgical sympathectomy following a failed chemical sympathectomy is a very difficult procedure.

The most successful application of sympathectomy is in the treatment of thromboangiitis obliterans or Buerger's disease, perhaps because the condition is characterised by a significant component of vasospasm (see Chapter 42). Sympathectomy often relieves rest pain and may allow small areas of gangrene to heal. Sympathectomy is rarely if ever indicated for Raynaud's phenomenon and most patients can achieve satisfactory symptom control by simply avoiding cold, abstaining from tobacco and wearing warm or heated gloves in the winter. Sympathectomy often produces dramatic early benefit[6] but this is short lived and after a year or two the benefits are marginal.[7,8]

Cervical sympathectomy

The sympathetic fibres to the arm synapse in the second to fifth thoracic ganglia, with the first thoracic ganglion fusing with the inferior cervical ganglion to form the stellate ganglion. Inadvertent injury to this ganglion will result in a permanent Horner's syndrome. Cervical sympathectomy may be performed by anterior cervical,[9] transaxillary[10] or thoracoscopic[11] approaches depending on surgical preference.

Thoracoscopic cervical sympathectomy

The thoracoscopic approach is now well established and has become the standard procedure although complications are not uncommon. Damage to the first cervical ganglion is most easily avoided using this approach as it is not usually possible to get any higher than the second rib from the pleural space.

The procedure is performed under general anaesthesia, preferably using a double lumen tube, with the patient supine and with the arms abducted. The ipsilateral lung is deflated and an artificial pneumothorax established. A 5 mm laparoscope is inserted through the third intercostal space and advanced across the pleural cavity to identify the sympathetic ganglia and chain passing over the necks of the ribs. The appropriate ganglia and interconnecting rami are coagulated using a diathermy probe inserted through a separate incision. This blunderbuss technique fails to remove the sympathetic chain for histological examination and can, if poorly performed, fail to interrupt the chain. For this reason a two port technique with careful excision of the chain is preferable. Care must be taken not to damage the first thoracic ganglion. The lung is reinflated at the end of the procedure, the laparoscope is removed and the wounds closed. A postoperative chest X-ray is taken to identify any residual pneumothorax.

Transaxillary cervical sympathectomy

This operation has largely been replaced by the thoracoscopic procedure. The patient is placed in a lateral position with the operated side uppermost and the axilla widely displayed by abducting the arm and flexing the forearm. An 8 cm oblique incision is made from latissimus dorsi, running forwards and down across the third rib as far as the posterior border of pectoralis major. The periosteum of the rib is exposed, divided with diathermy, and reflected from the superior surface to expose the costal pleura. This is divided along the upper border of the rib and a rib retractor is inserted and opened widely. The apex of the lung is displaced downwards and the ganglia and interconnecting chain identified running beneath the costal pleura over the necks of the ribs. The overlying pleura is opened and the chain and rami lifted and divided above the T2 and below the T5 ganglia. The wound is closed and the lung re-expanded. A postoperative chest X-ray is taken.

Anterior cervical sympathectomy

The traditional access to the sympathetic chain is through a cervical approach. The patient is placed feet down supine with a sandbag under the shoulders and the head turned to the opposite side. A 5 cm incision is placed 1 cm above the clavicle with the medial end just overlying the sternomastoid. The platysma, lateral fibres of sternomastoid and any intervening veins are divided to expose the scalenus anterior. This muscle is divided low down preserving the phrenic nerve on its surface and by reflecting it medially. That exposes the subclavian artery which is retracted upwards or downwards by dividing its branches to expose the costopleural membrane which in turn is incised to expose the apex of the lung. The sympathetic chain is exposed by carefully stripping the lung downwards with a finger. The chain is excised between the stellate and fourth cervical ganglia.

Lumbar sympathectomy

This may be performed either by an open operation or by injecting phenol around the lumbar chain using radiological guidance. The latter has very low morbidity and so has gained popularity, and may be particularly appropriate for treating some elderly patients with ischaemic rest pain. For younger patients surgical sympathectomy should be performed to ensure complete removal of the sympathetic chain. At operation the second and third lumbar ganglia are removed. In males the first lumbar ganglion on at least one side must be retained in order to preserve normal ejaculation.

Patients with distal vessel occlusive disease, and therefore poor candidates for reconstructive procedures, may be suitable for lumbar sympathectomy to relieve rest pain and sometimes rescue critically ischaemic tissue. The major benefit is in the relief of rest pain, but it occurs in only 60 per cent of cases and lasts for up to 3 years. The amputation rate is not affected.[12] Surgical lumbar sympathectomy can be performed either as an open procedure or laparoscopically.

Open lumbar sympathectomy

The lumbar sympathetic chain is approached through a transverse incision lateral to but at the level of the umbilicus on the side to be denervated. The oblique muscles of the abdominal wall are divided to expose the peritoneum. This is freed by blunt dissection from the deep surface of the transversus abdominis muscle and retracted medially to expose the retroperitoneal space. The psoas is found on the posterior wall and the groove between the medial border of this muscle, the lumbar vertebrae and the aorta on the left and the inferior vena cava on the right is defined. The lumbar sympathetic chain can usually be palpated as a firm cord punctuated by a number of swellings lying in this groove on the front of the vertebrae. The chain is picked up with a nerve hook and dissected up to the diaphragmatic crura and down to the pelvic brim. All of the rami that join the ganglia are divided and the first, second and third ganglia are excised. The wound is closed in layers with suction drainage.

Endoscopic lumbar sympathectomy

The technique of laparoscopic lumbar sympathectomy has been described as an alternative to the traditional open approach. This may be performed using either a transperitoneal[13] or a retroperitoneal, balloon-assisted,[14] approach. The benefits of this method have yet to be demonstrated but may combine the advantages of a minimally invasive approach with the certainty of surgical excision of the sympathetic chain.

BYPASS PROCEDURES

Distal revascularisation procedures, either endovascular or by surgical bypass, have a high rate of failure and are rarely indicated. This is largely because the secondary periarteritis is often very severe and makes dissection of the vessels very difficult. Unfortunately, autoimmune vasculitis also tends to affect distal vessels, and distal bypass procedures have a much lower flow rate and patency rate than proximal procedures. Results are therefore poor, and these procedures should only be considered in exceptional cases.

In the presence of ulcers bypass grafting may be useful. Even if the graft only remains patent for a short time, this may allow ulcers to heal. If the graft then fails, the ulcers often do not recur provided that the patient stops smoking.

Bypass procedures in patients with Takayasu's disease

Takayasu's disease and the middle aortic syndrome are diseases that are very amenable to surgical bypass (also see Chapter 41). Takayasu's disease most commonly causes stenosis of the subclavian and innominate arteries and aortic arch followed by the descending aorta and aortoiliac region. The presenting symptoms depend upon the vessels affected but transient ischaemic attacks, visual problems, arm and leg claudication and the subclavian steal syndrome can all occur.[15] The disease may also sometimes cause aneurysms and aortic valve regurgitation.

Surgical intervention should be timed to avoid acute inflammatory episodes, guided by the ESR or CRP. When there is critical ischaemia, and immediate surgical treatment cannot be avoided, it should be accompanied by high dose steroid treatment. Arteriography must be performed to assess the disease in order to plan surgery, and it often demonstrates either a smooth tapering stenosis of the affected vessel or total occlusion. Surgical bypass to normal vessels beyond the limits of the disease is indicated for patients with ischaemic symptoms, aneurysms or significant renal artery disease.[16–18]

Standard operative techniques achieve good results.[19–21] Surgery may take the form of carotid artery reconstruction, carotid–subclavian bypass, thoracoabdominal aortic bypass, renal artery reconstruction or aneurysm repair.[22] If possible the surgery should be performed in one stage to correct all affected vessels, with multiple reconstructions if necessary. Saccular aneurysmal disease has a high rate of rupture and should be treated urgently, whereas fusiform aneurysms can be treated similarly to atheromatous disease. Treatment is by resection and replacement with a synthetic graft.

AMPUTATION

When the above procedures are not indicated or fail then there is often no alternative but to amputate critically ischaemic or gangrenous tissue. Amputation should be as conservative as possible while ensuring that satisfactory healing is achieved. Dead or devitalised tissue or bone must be removed completely.

SURGERY FOR GIANT CELL ARTERITIS

The diagnosis of giant cell arteritis can be confirmed surgically by taking a segment of the superficial temporal artery under local anaesthetic. The incision is placed directly over the vessel. Histological examination shows pronounced intimal thickening, round cell infiltration through all layers of the arterial wall with destruction of the internal elastic lamina and the presence of a few giant cells.

ACUTE VENOUS INFLAMMATORY CONDITIONS

Acute superficial thrombophlebitis is a common problem. It is generally considered to be a benign condition but it is sometimes associated with deep vein thrombosis (DVT) or other underlying pathology.

Aetiology and pathology

Thrombophlebitis usually affects an isolated segment of superficial vein in the leg. The vein becomes acutely inflamed, often to a greater extent than is clinically apparent. The commonest risk factors are the presence of varicose veins, obesity and age. It may be associated with DVT, pulmonary embolism (PE) or autoimmune disease such as SLE or Behçet's disease. Migrating superficial thrombophlebitis or Trousseau's phenomenon is associated with visceral cancer, in particular carcinoma of the pancreas.

Diagnosis

CLINICAL

The diagnosis of superficial thrombophlebitis is primarily clinical. The leg is most commonly affected, presenting with painful inflammation over one or more veins. On examination there may be tender palpable subcutaneous cords along the course of the saphenous veins or their tributaries with associated erythema and oedema.

INVESTIGATIONS

Duplex ultrasound examination of the deep venous system should be performed to identify deep vein thrombosis, particularly if the proximal long saphenous vein is involved. A search for an underlying malignancy or thrombophilia

should be made when Trousseau's phenomenon occurs. The patient should be screened for autoantibodies when there are other features of a connective tissue disease.

Management

In general, thrombophlebitis can be treated successfully with anti-inflammatory drugs.

MEDICAL OR CONSERVATIVE TREATMENT

Superficial thrombophlebitis should be treated with aspirin or non-steroidal anti-inflammatory drugs (NSAIDs). Venous compression stockings may prevent recurrent attacks.

SURGICAL TREATMENT

Surgical stripping of the long saphenous system can be of value in preventing recurrent attacks of above-knee thrombophlebitis.

Conclusions

Surgery has a limited role in treating patients with arterial inflammatory conditions or vasculitides. Sympathectomy is the most commonly performed operation. Bypass procedures are most effective in patients with Takayasu's disease and the mid-aortic syndrome. Amputation may be necessary in patients with gangrene.

Acute superficial thrombophlebitis may complicate varicose veins but deep vein thrombosis or malignancy may have to be excluded before treatment.

Key references

Crawford ES, De Bakey ME, Morris GC, Cooley DA. Thrombo-obliterative disease of the great vessels arising from the aortic arch. *J Thorac Cardiovasc Surg* 1962; **43**: 38–53.

Crawford ES, Snyder DM, Cho GC, Roehm Jr JO. Progress in treatment of thoracoabdominal and abdominal aortic aneurysms involving celiac superior mesenteric and renal arteries. *Ann Surg* 1978; **188**: 404.

Lande A. Abdominal Takayasu's aortitis, the middle aortic syndrome and atherosclerosis: a critical review. *Int Angiol* 1998; **17**: 1–9.

Lupi-Herrera E, Sanchez-Torres G, Marcushamer J, *et al.* Takayasu's arteritis. Clinical study of 107 cases. *Am Heart J* 1977; **93**: 94–103.

Ohta T, Shionoya S. Fate of the ischaemic limb in Buerger's disease. *Br J Surg* 1988; **75**: 259–62.

REFERENCES

1   Schneider HJ, Jha S, Burnand KG. Progressive arteritis associated with cannabis use. *Eur J Vasc Endovasc Surg* 1999; **18**: 366–7.

2 McPherson JR, Juergens JL, Gifford RW. Thromboangiitis obliterans and arteriosclerosis obliterans: clinical and prognostic differences. *Ann Intern Med* 1963; **59**: 288–96.

3 Kinmonth JB. Thromboangiitis obliterans. Results of sympathectomy and prognosis. *Lancet* 1948; **2**: 717.

4 Ohta T, Shionoya S. Fate of the ischaemic limb in Buerger's disease. *Br J Surg* 1988; **75**: 259–62.

5 Kunlin J, Lengua F, Testart J, Pajot A. Thromboangiosis or thromboangeitis treated by adrenalectomy and sympathectomy from 1942 to 1962. A follow-up study of 110 cases. *J Cardiovasc Surg* 1973; **14**: 21–7.

6 Baddeley RM. The place of upper dorsal sympathectomy in the treatment of primary Raynaud's disease. *Br J Surg* 1965; **52**: 426.

7 Gifford RW, Hines, EA, Craig WM. Sympathectomy for Raynaud's phenomenon *Circulation* 1958; **17**: 5.

8 Johnston EN, Summerly R, Birnstingl M. Prognosis in Raynaud's phenomenon after sympathectomy. *BMJ* 1965; **42**: 962–4.

9 Telford ED. The technique of sympathectomy. *Br J Surg* 1935; **23**: 448.

10 Atkins HJB. Peraxillary approach to the stellate and upper thoracic ganglia. *Lancet* 1949; **2**: 1152.

11 Hederman WP. Sympathectomy by thoracoscopy. In: Greenhalgh RM (ed). *Vascular and Endovascular Surgical Techniques*. London: WB Saunders 1994: 281.

12 Cotton LT, Cross FW. Lumbar sympathectomy for arterial disease. *Br J Surg* 1985; **72**: 678–83.

13 Wattanasirichaigoon S, Ngaorungsri U, Wanishayathanakorn A, *et al*. Laparoscopic transperitoneal lumbar sympathectomy: a new approach. *J Med Assoc Thai* 1997; **80**: 275.

14 Elliott TB, Royle JP. Laparoscopic extraperitoneal lumbar sympathectomy: technique and early results. *Aus N Z J Surg* 1996; **66**: 400–2.

15 Lupi-Herrera E, Sanchez-Torres G, Marcushamer J, *et al*. Takayasu's arteritis. Clinical study of 107 cases. *Am Heart J* 1977; **93**: 94–103.

16 Crawford ES, De Bakey ME, Morris GC, Cooley DA. Thrombo-obliterative disease of the great vessels arising from the aortic arch. *J Thorac Cardiovasc Surg* 1962; **43**: 38–53.

17 Crawford ES, Snyder DM, Cho GC, Roehm Jr JO. Progress in treatment of thoracoabdominal and abdominal aortic aneurysms involving celiac superior mesenteric and renal arteries. *Ann Surg* 1978; **188**: 404.

18 Thompson BW, Read RC, Campbell GS. Aortic arch syndrome. *Arch Surg* 1969; **98**: 607–11.

19 Robbs JV, Human RR, Rajaruthnam P. Operative treatment of nonspecific aortoarteritis (Takayasu's arteritis), *J Vasc Surg* 1986; **3**: 605–16.

20 Fraga A, Mintz G, Valle L, *et al*. Takayasu's arteritis: frequency of systemic manifestations (study of 22 patients) and favorable response to maintenance steroid therapy with corticosteroids (12 patients). *Arthritis Rheum* 1972; **15**: 617–24.

21 Weaver FA, Yellin AE, Campen DH, *et al*. Surgical procedures in the management of Takayasu's arteritis. *J Vasc Surg* 1990; **12**: 429–37.

22 Lande A. Abdominal Takayasu's aortitis, the middle aortic syndrome and atherosclerosis: a critical review. *Int Angiol* 1998; **17**: 1–9.

44

Vascular Emergencies Caused by Substance Abuse

RONALD A KLINE, RAMON BERGUER

HISTORY

Recreational drug use has existed for centuries and is present in almost all cultures, be it the opium of ancient China, the coca leaves of the rainforest, or the American Indian use of peyote. Ingestion or inhalation were the usual routes of administration. Although forms of intravenous injection began as early as 1670 it was Charles Gabriel Pravaz and Alexander Wood who are credited with the independent yet simultaneous development in 1853 of a syringe with a hollow needle fine enough to pierce vessels.[1] This revolutionised the administration of narcotics. The application of this new device was in treating pain through the use of opiate injections. Its recreational usage was not intentional.

In the UK, all drugs were legal and reportedly used routinely across society, until 1860.[2] The former Prime Minister William Gladstone and Florence Nightingale used opium, while Queen Victoria used cannabis. Sir Arthur Conan Doyle wrote a graphic description of Sherlock Holmes injecting drugs with a syringe as a normal way of relaxing during the hiatus between cases, much to the chagrin of Dr Watson. The mode of consumption has not changed to date. Illicit substance usage is ingested, inhaled in smoking or snorting or injected.

THE PROBLEM

The adverse effects of substance abuse are dependent upon the agent and the route of administration. Most injected agents are contaminated with diluents. Heroin, naturally a white powder, is rarely obtainable in its street version without being adulterated. This is notwithstanding bacterial or viral contamination of the agent itself or the instruments of delivery. All three vascular systems, lymphatic, venous and arterial can be affected. The resulting injurious effects may be local or systemic.

The spectacular increase in drug consumption over the past 20 years has resulted in a large number of drug related injuries to the vascular system. About half of the acutely injured patients presenting at the level 1 trauma unit of the Detroit Receiving Hospital, MI, USA, test positive for cocaine, heroin or both. In 1998 the National Institute of Drug Abuse estimated that over 21 million Americans have tried cocaine, including three million who had done so within the previous month.[3] Medical examiners in Memphis, TN, USA, noted a 53 per cent increase in drug related homicides with cocaine related deaths being most responsible.[4] This reflects the activities in many large cities. Similar reports come from Salt Lake City, UT, and Tucson, AZ, USA, where cocaine associated violent deaths and poisonings are rising.[5] Substance abuse also extends to the adolescent and childhood trauma scene.[6–9]

The Drug Abuse Warning Network (DAWN) of the US Section of Health and Human Services appears to be underreporting this rising usage to Congress.[10] Whereas DAWN recorded a 5 per cent incidence of cocaine use in patients treated at the Hospital of the University of Pennsylvania in 1992, a prospective internal analysis showed that 20 per cent of blunt trauma and 57 per cent of penetrating trauma victims treated during 1992 tested positive for cocaine.[10] In this study 38 per cent of industrial injury patients had cocaine 'on board'.[10]

Substance abuse agents

- Marijuana
- Cocaine
- Angel dust, PCP
- Amphetamines and such drugs
- Heroin

MARIJUANA

Marijuana is not usually considered a causative agent for problems. Its use in conjunction with other drugs, however, cannot be ignored. While there is debate about the extent of harm caused by marijuana usage, research evidence indicates that more carcinogens are released in marijuana smoke than in cigarette smoke. Baldwin *et al.* at University of California at Los Angeles, USA, examined immune cell response to smoking different drugs[11] and were able to show that alveolar macrophages from marijuana smokers had reduced bactericidal activity against *Staphylococcus aureus*, a common pathogen in drug abusers. The same was not observed in tobacco smokers, cocaine smokers, or non-smokers. Macrophages from non-smokers, cocaine smokers, and tobacco smokers had similar phagocytic activity, whereas those from marijuana smokers demonstrated markedly depressed phagocytic activity. Marijuana smokers have been shown to have depressed cytotoxic and immunoprotective levels of interleukin-6, tumour necrosis factor-α, and granulocyte-macrophage colony-stimulating factor.[12] The combined use of marijuana and other drugs, especially the injected forms, may account for the frequent infections seen in this patient population.

COCAINE

Cocaine is an alkaloid extracted from the *Erythroxylon coca* plant and supplied in powder form. Cocaine is snorted, smoked and injected intravenously. Cocaine may be inhaled in several ways. The cocaine alkaloid can be dissolved in acetone or alcohol, purified to a more potent form, and smoked as the so called 'free base'.[13] This has the danger of causing injury from fire or explosion of the flammable solvent. The alkaloid can be dissolved in hydrochloric acid to form a water soluble salt, available as a crystalline granular powder, which may be inhaled or smoked with a flammable vehicle. 'Crack' cocaine is a neutral form, like 'free base', but is made without solvent extraction. In making crack, an alkali is added to an aqueous solution of cocaine hydrochloride and the resulting alkaloid precipitates from the supernatant.[13] It is from this that the 'rocks' are made and sold as such.

Its usage is the most common cause of myocardial infarction or stroke in young patients in America. It affects arteries of all sizes. This cheap but potent form is smoked in a pipe while the rock is ignited from above with a butane lighter. Crack smokers have found that transpulmonary absorption is increased by the Valsalva manoeuvre, the smoke being blown forcefully into another person's airway as that recipient strongly inhales it. This practice may result in air dissection into the mediastinum, pleural space and pericardium, the sudden mediastinal emphysema causing acute and intense pain in the mid-thorax and shortness of breath.[14] Treatment is supportive until symptoms abate. If the air dissects into the central vessels it can embolise to the carotid or coronary systems.

The physiological effects of cocaine are local anaesthesia and a sympathomimetic action derived from blocking the presynaptic reuptake of noradrenaline and dopamine.[15] Cocaine increases coronary artery reactivity and potentiates the pressor effect of noradrenaline,[16] an effect which is dose dependent. The arterial lesions induced by cocaine derive from two pathological effects. The first is an increase in the product of heart rate and blood pressure ($\Delta p/\Delta t$) which may result in dissection of the thoracic aorta or in rupture of a berry aneurysm and subarachnoid haemorrhage. Figure 44.1 shows the thoracic arteriogram of a 14-year-old boy who, following crack consumption, came to us with an extensive thoracoabdominal dissection starting at the left subclavian artery. The second effect of cocaine is spasm of medium or small sized arteries and intravascular thrombosis, which may be partial or complete.[17]

Unexplained thrombi in arteries of all sizes, including the aorta, have been documented.[15] We have seen patchy thrombosis in the thoracic and abdominal aortas of cocaine

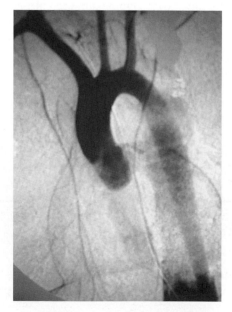

Figure 44.1 *Arteriogram of a 14-year-old boy with cocaine induced thoracoabdominal aortic dissection originating just distal to left subclavian*

users resulting in distal embolisation.[18] Cocaine induced vasospasm is due not only to cocaine but also its metabolites norcocaine and benzoylecgonine.[19] Cocaine may also augment procoagulants by decreasing protein C and antithrombin III levels[20] and by increasing plasminogen activator inhibitor activity, thereby inhibiting thrombolysis.[21] Additionally, cocaine induces platelet activation and aggregation. Long term vascular changes are suggested by the increase in adventitial mast cells and atherosclerosis in chronic abusers.[22] These myriad effects are responsible for the myocardial infarctions,[23] strokes,[24] mesenteric ischaemia,[25] venous thrombosis[26] and acute renal failure[27,28] observed following cocaine intake.

It has been recommended that the treatment of cocaine induced thrombosis be one of heparin anticoagulation unless terminal organ dysfunction requires urgent operative or other intervention.[18] We have seen large intra-aortic thrombi fully resolve with this treatment as long as the patient is cocaine free.

ANGEL DUST, PCP

Cocaine in powder form may be mixed with other agents. Although these diluents are often chemically inert, not infrequently another active agent may be used, one of which is PCP, better known as 'angel dust'.[29] The name PCP is the abbreviation for its chemical name 1-(1-phencyclohexyl) piperidine. On the street, a long list of pseudonyms exists: 'hog', 'squeeze', 'wack' and 'space base' (when mixed with crack cocaine). Although angel dust originally referred to a combination of heroin and cocaine its contemporary nomenclature refers to PCP. The problem of mixing PCP with cocaine is that the two potentiate each other's effects along with decreasing the dose at which toxic and even lethal side effects can occur.

Low doses of PCP (3–8 mg) cause mild intoxication. Users show impaired coordination, slurred speech and erratic eye movement. Larger doses (8–12 mg) increase the low dose effects as well as raising heart rate and blood pressure, and causing fever, sweating, nausea, a blank stare and a shuffling, disjointed gait that some users call 'zombie walking'. Doses above 12 mg can unleash a range of serious effects from profound hypotension to muscular rigidity, convulsions, even coma and death. The titanic muscle activity can result in rhabdomyolysis necessitating fasciotomies. While lower dose effects may only last a few hours, higher dose effects can continue for several days. Treatment is usually supportive until the body has been cleared of the agent.

AMPHETAMINES

Methamphetamine and 'ecstasy' (3,4-methylenedioxymethamphetamine) are two drugs now fashionable among adolescents and young adults. Their presence at 'rave parties' (nocturnal congregations involving dancing, sex, heavy alcohol consumption and drug usage) is almost ubiquitous. Consumption of either of these will result in severe inotropic and chronotropic effects. Like cocaine they result in strokes and aortic dissections.

A general scheme for treating the vascular complications of non-injected substances is presented as an algorithm in Fig. 44.2. Identification of the specific agent is crucial so that substance specific treatment can be instituted. Unfortunately, that is not often forthcoming at the initial presentation of these patients.

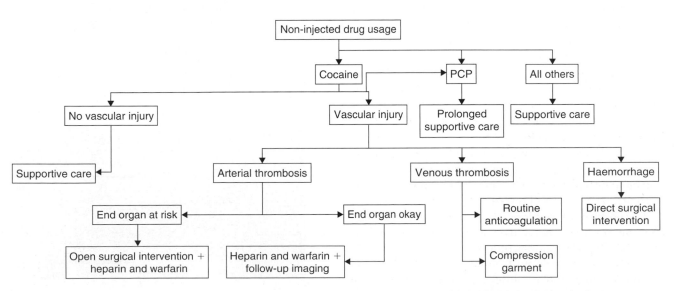

Figure 44.2 *Algorithm for management vascular complications of non-injected substances. PCP, 1-(1-phencyclohexyl) piperidine (angel dust)*

OTHER AGENTS

Anything that can be dissolved or liquefied can and has been injected. Common oral agents that have been used are paracetamol (acetaminophen) with codeine and pentazocine (Talwin). Since these do not fully dissolve a common problem with their usage is particulate embolisation. Even powdered agents such as heroin and cocaine may not fully dissolve or will precipitate in the syringe prior to injection. If an intravenous route is used they are filtered by the pulmonary circulation and are directly responsible for pulmonary complications. If an inadvertent, or even intentional, intra-arterial route is used, terminal vessel occlusion often leads to tissue loss,[30] not uncommonly seen in the hand and frequently leading to digit or forearm amputations. Interdigital injections, used when an intravenous route is no longer possible, will often result in cannulation of the digital arteries. Anticoagulant treatment with heparin, awaiting demarcation to occur, is followed by amputation at the level of viable tissue.[31] If the carotid is used, the particles lodge in the terminal cerebral vessels causing cerebral infarction or seizure and carries the ignoble name of 'huckbucks', referring to the fictional character Huckleberry Finn. This name has arisen from the Kentucky hills where the routine use of pentazocine had been popular.

HEROIN

Heroin derives from the poppy plant *Papaver somniferum*.[32] Morphine is another derivative from it. Heroin use is nearly as old as civilisation itself. The effects of heroin are mediated by the interaction with endogenous opiate receptors which function as neurotransmitters, neurohormones and modulators of neural transmission throughout the central nervous system. Heroin is delivered to the street in powder form where it is generally diluted in water and injected intravenously and almost never in aseptic fashion. If venous access is no longer available then the chronic user often resorts to subcutaneous injections. These frequently lead to dermal ulcerations and scarring referred to as 'skin pop marks' and the practice is referred to as 'skin popping' (Fig. 44.3). The deleterious effects of heroin in the abuser include overdose, vascular aneurysms and myriad infectious complications which impair recovery after injury. These infections may be at the site of injection or anywhere in the body. Endocarditis, both acute and subacute, is frequently observed.

The problem of overdose related death or severe injury after heroin use reflects user ignorance regarding the strength of a particular injection.[33] While heroin is distributed in various levels of purity, pure or almost pure heroin is quite strong and may cause sudden unexpected death when a patient thinks the injectate had been diluted. The dilution or 'cutting' of heroin is done to increase profits during the exchange from one distributor to another. The extent of dilution is unknown unless distributors have developed an excellent reputation for consistency. One locally popular version is called 'mixed jive' and contains the additives of strychnine, talc powder, lidocaine, quinine, sugar, starch and occasionally the 'dust' from the interior of spent fluorescent light tubes. Local purveyors often have custom blends named after celebrities.

The overdosed patient will be somnolent, stuporous or in coma. The breathing pattern is shallow, respiratory rate slowed and minute volume diminished. Cyanosis may occur as heroin reduces the responsiveness of the brain stem to increases in carbon dioxide tension and depresses the pontine and medullary centres involved in regulating respiratory rhythmicity.[32,33] Deaths from opiate overdosage are usually due to respiratory depression. Like morphine, heroin induces peripheral vasodilatation and a decrease in systemic vascular resistance augmented by a concomitant release of histamine. Therefore, opiate intoxicated patients with hypovolaemia exhibit profound hypotension.

Therapy includes establishing an airway and confirming adequate ventilation. During resuscitation, administration of naloxone hydrochloride, a specific opiate receptor antagonist, may be beneficial. Naloxone yields a dramatic reversal of the respiratory depression and peripheral vasodilatation associated with opiate toxicity.[32,33] Intravenous doses of 0.4 mg, repeated every few minutes as necessary, are effective. However, excessive naloxone may precipitate opiate withdrawal, thus complicating therapy. Because the effective half-life of naloxone is shorter than that of most opiates, re-dosing every several hours may be necessary until the circulating opiate is excreted.

In heroin addiction the arterial injury is generally a consequence of failing to cannulate a vein for injection and accidentally injecting the adjacent artery, the slang for this is 'hitting pink'. The arterial damage from heroin is the consequence of the chemical and bacterial contamination of the mixture along with the bacterial contamination

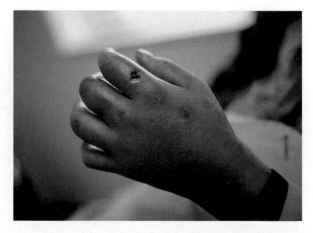

Figure 44.3 *Injection 'pop-marks' on the hand; note the oedema and the resulting flexion of the fingers*

resulting from sharing needles and syringes. An abscess forms in the arterial wall which undergoes necrosis and results in an infected pseudoaneurysm. As crack cocaine usage became popular over the past decade, the incidence of drug induced mycotic pseudoaneurysms at our facility fell precipitously.

Twelve years ago, at the height of the heroin epidemic in the USA, we reviewed our experience with heroin induced arterial injuries. There were 32 upper extremity cases, 136 lower extremity cases and four neck cases. Half of our patients had positive blood cultures on admission and of these, half grew methicillin-resistant *Staphylococcus aureus* (MRSA). It should not come as a surprise that bacterial endocarditis, such as the one shown in Fig. 44.4, was a frequent finding in these patients. Infected false aneurysms of the visceral arteries, such as the coeliac artery aneurysm in Fig. 44.5, are metastatic arising from valvular endocarditis.

In the upper extremity, the most commonly involved arterial sites were the brachial and radial arteries. Patients with upper extremity problems presented with either an infected false aneurysm or with severe hand ischaemia. Those with pseudoaneurysms had severe pain, a palpable mass and cellulitis. Patients with hand ischaemia had mostly hand and forearm pain, neuromuscular deficits in the forearm and gangrenous changes in the fingers. Extensive fasciotomies may be needed, as in the case of massive compartment syndrome following an axillary injection of heroin (Fig. 44.6).

In the neck, the subclavian or common carotid arteries are accidentally hit while the abuser or a friend attempts cannulation of the subclavian or internal jugular veins. The euphemism for this is 'shooting the pocket'. Since this manoeuvre is often difficult to self-perform, a society of fellow addicts known as 'street doctors' has evolved, and for a fee, be it monetary or a portion of the injectate, will administer the injection.

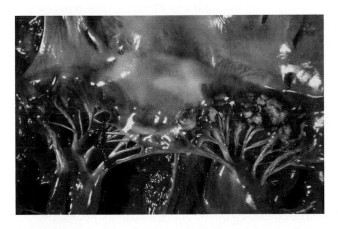

Figure 44.4   *Post-mortem examination of a drug abuse patient showing valvular vegetations from bacterial endocarditis*

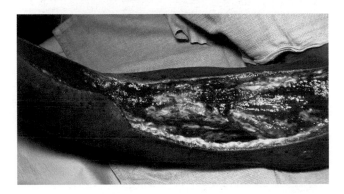

Figure 44.6   *Arm fasciotomy in a drug user who injected into the axillary region*

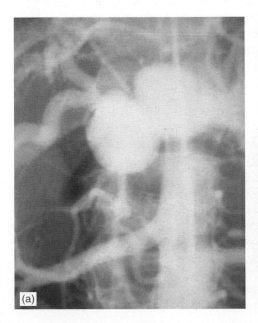

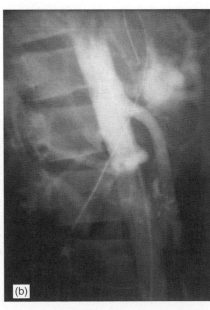

Figure 44.5   *Arteriogram of metastatic mycotic aneurysm of the coeliac artery in an active drug user: (a) anteroposterior view (b) lateral view*

VASCULAR SYSTEM CONSIDERATIONS

Lymphovenous complications

As stated, abscess formation and cellulitis are common soft tissue complications resulting from the use of intravenous drugs obtained on the street. Repeated injections result in fibrosis and destruction of dermal and deep lymphatic tissues.[34] With the destruction of the lymphatics the extremity is prone to additional infections in turn resulting in further lymphatic damage. These repeated injuries coupled with the often associated 'skin popping' results in a chronic woody oedematous limb. The skin develops epidermal hypertrophy termed lichenification (Fig. 44.7), which can harbour fungal infection. These limbs are also prone to necrotising fasciitis (Fig. 44.8) and not infrequently emergency amputation is required for sepsis control.

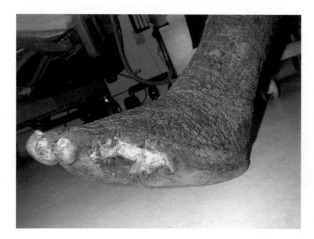

Figure 44.7 *50-year-old man with a 30-year history of intravenous drug abuse required open ray amputation of several toes; note hypertrophy of the skin due to chronic oedema from combined venous and lymphatic obstruction*

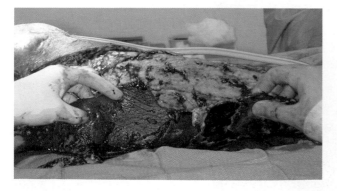

Figure 44.8 *A 42-year-old man, an active intravenous drug addict, with large venous ulcers of the leg, developed necrotising fasciitis; he ultimately required an open knee disarticulation for control of sepsis*

Although the lower extremities and groins are common sites for injection, the upper extremities, the axilla and neck can be involved as well. *Staphylococcus aureus* is again the most common bacterium associated with these injection sites and 40 per cent is MRSA.[34] Abscesses, however, are frequently polymicrobial and include not only oral flora but also *Peptostreptococcus* and *Bacteroides* spp.[31,34]

Although intravenous antibiotic therapy appropriate to the organism identified is required, surgical treatment of any soft tissue abscess is mandatory. This requires incision and drainage and sometimes excision of grossly infected and non-viable tissue. Excision may involve not only the skin and subdermis but also the fascia, muscles and/or major vessels. Such surgery should only be performed in the operating room. Although it is tempting to aspirate infected fluid percutaneously, it is not to be recommended near vascular structures. The risk of rupturing unsuspected pseudoaneurysms and causing torrential bleeding should be borne in mind.[35] If fluid is spontaneously draining from an abscess site, any presence of blood or dark purple staining of the fluid would indicate that a major vessel is involved and the operating surgeon must be prepared to ligate the vessel concerned. It has been our experience that purulent fluid not of this colour is usually not associated with injury to a major vessel. All infected wounds should be left open to heal by secondary intention. If a major vein is thrombosed and infected then the entire length of that vein and its thrombotic material must be removed and excised completely.[34]

Repeated injection into a peripheral or central vein will ultimately result in thrombosis of that vessel. Repeated punctures and the subsequent venous endothelial damage will often cause superficial thrombosis and phlebitis.[36] As injections are usually performed with the dominant hand the contralateral side of the body is most frequently affected. Treatment of superficial venous thrombophlebitis usually involves elevation of the affected extremity in order to reduce oedema, anti-inflammatory medication and warm compresses. Because of the nature of the thrombophlebitis and the infected needles used by the substance abuser, these patients are at high risk of developing either local or systemic sepsis. The choice of antibiotic therapy should be driven by the results of the cultures whenever possible. One must be cognisant of the high incidence of MRSA in this patient population. If a local abscess forms at the site of the superficial thrombophlebitis then the thrombosed vein should be excised in its entirety and the wound left open for secondary healing.

The intravenous user generally selects superficial veins as the early targets of his or her addiction. As these vessels thrombose the individual is forced to use larger and more centrally placed veins, either those in the groin, axilla, subclavian, jugular and then even in the breasts, labia or the dorsal penile vein. It is not uncommon, however, for some drug users to selectively inject into the femoral vein because it is relatively easily accessible as well as because this site lends itself to discretion. The larger veins are no less prone to thrombosis than are the superficial veins and over time these too will thrombose and/or become infected. Since many of these patients develop significant oedema, erythema or pain in the affected extremity physical examination cannot be relied upon to make a diagnosis of deep vein thrombosis (DVT). It is also possible that many of these patients will have chronic DVT with superimposed acute DVT. We have relied for years on duplex imaging of these vessels in making the differential diagnosis. The oedema developing in the extremities from these chronic repeated deep and superficial phlebitic insults will result in massively oedematous legs extending all the way up to the femoral region. These are often lifelong complications. Even those who have not used drugs for decades will be afflicted by chronic leg oedema as well as by very large venous ulcers (Fig. 44.9). These patients are also at high risk of experiencing complications from their DVT which include pulmonary embolism (PE), septic PE and bacterial endocarditis.[34]

Unless there is a specific contraindication, patients diagnosed with acute DVT should be treated with intravenous heparin following standard hospital protocols. Warfarin should be started, usually concurrently, with the heparin in anticipation of outpatient therapy. As in any patient with chronic venous insufficiency and/or acute DVT, oedema control should be one of the goals of treatment. All of these patients should be fitted for good medical grade support hosiery; the degree of compression we most frequently use is between 40 and 50 mmHg, replaced at least every 6 months and worn for life if recurrence of venous ulceration is to be prevented.

We do not recommend the use of thrombolytic therapy for DVT in these patients. They are generally unreliable in giving a history and not infrequently the acute DVT will have occurred superimposed on a chronic DVT, therefore making lytic therapy nearly useless. Thrombolytic therapy also runs the risk of causing bleeding from arteries and/or veins which may have been punctured by the individual

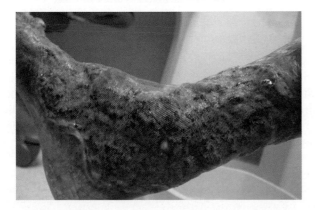

Figure 44.9   *Venous ulcers in a chronic intravenous drug addict are typically quite large*

shortly prior to seeing the physician. Surgical thrombectomy also has a limited role in the care of these patients.

Although mycotic arterial aneurysms are common in patients with repeated intravenous drug use, the entity of mycotic venous aneurysm also exists and usually involves the femoral vein.[34,36] It is usually caused by repeated injections into the femoral vein giving rise to septic phlebitis. The vein may rupture because its wall is weakened by infection or, alternatively, a persistent communication between the skin puncture site and that in the vein leads to adjacent haematoma formation which then becomes infected.[36] The presence of a mycotic venous aneurysm should be suspected in patients who have a non-pulsatile painful groin mass with associated signs of sepsis: pain at the site, fever, leucocytosis. It is reported that half of all these patients have recurrent cellulitis.[31,34] Although the above would be pathognomonic for a mycotic venous aneurysm, many patients are asymptomatic. The diagnosis can be made by venous duplex imaging but in practice it is often made unexpectedly in the operating room during groin exploration for a possible abscess.[36]

Antibiotic treatment should be guided by cultures and sensitivities. Debridement of all infected tissue combined with proximal and distal venous ligation is required. Although the ideal duration of antibiotic therapy is uncertain, a minimum of 2 weeks and up to 6 weeks, blood cultures being positive, is usually recommended. Venous reconstruction is rarely indicated and unlikely to be successful. It is critically important that when ligating the infected vein one resects back to what grossly appears to be normal venous wall. If residual wall infection is left at the site of ligation the ligatures will eventually erode through and massive haemorrhage will ensue.

Intra-arterial injection

Inadvertent intra-arterial injection often results in severe limb ischaemia and tissue loss. The ischaemic changes are thought to be due not only to embolisation of non-solubilised particulate matter but also to arterial spasm, platelet aggregation, thromboxane release, and sympathetic mediated vasospasm.[35] As the particulate matter passes into the capillary system vasospasm occurs in both the arterial and venous side of the tissue bed.[36] This, in addition to the obstruction of the capillary bed by the particles, will result in acute, severe and often unrelenting pain. The extremity will be swollen and quite cool[37] and the digits flexed or claw like (Fig. 44.10). Sensory loss is often observed and occurs despite palpable pulses in the major vessels leading into the limb. Although this clinical picture is usually true of the upper limb it is not at all uncommon to see it in the lower extremities. The ultimate outcome is extensive loss of tissue, and if that does not occur, permanent neurological dysfunction often ensues.[38] We have found arteriography to be of little benefit in the overall care of the patient

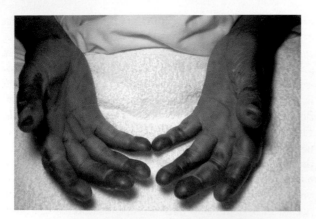

Figure 44.10 *Patient with particle embolisation of hands from intravenous drug use*

because the damage largely affects the digital vessels and the microcirculation.

As one waits for demarcation between the viable and the gangrenous portions of the limb, pain management can be problematic. Although narcotic administration is necessary these patients have a very high tolerance to narcotics and a very low tolerance to pain. Since there is no ceiling on narcotic dosing, medications should be titrated up until adequate analgesia is obtained. In the lower extremity continuous analgesia via epidural catheter can be very beneficial. Intravenous heparin administration in order to achieve a partial thromboplastin time (PTT) of two to three times the control may limit the extent of the thrombotic event. Once a clear line of demarcation occurs then amputation can be planned. Elevation of the affected extremity to minimise oedema with will also aid in reducing the extent of inflammation and thrombosis.[31]

In patients sustaining inadvertent intra-arterial drug injections, Tait *et al.* have reported significant improvement in distal perfusion following an infusion of prostacyclin iloprost.[39] No major complications were associated with the administration of this agent and they believe it helped to control the ischaemic injury; unfortunately they did not report the extent of tissue injury seen at initial presentation.

If a major limb arterial segment occludes and revascularisation is performed, compartment fasciotomy may be required. Since many of these patients have chronic oedema, it is difficult to determine by mere physical inspection whether compartment pressures are abnormal. The measurement of these pressures is advocated, avoiding fasciotomy in those compartments with pressures less than 30 mmHg.[39]

As with any major soft tissue injury involving a muscle compartment, rhabdomyolysis can occur. This may be due to the ischaemic event with subsequent reperfusion (see Chapters 2 and 4) or it may be caused by the dissemination of particulate matter into the capillary bed of the muscle. Renal failure and subsequent haemodialysis is not uncommon.[40] Renal failure may complicate rhabdomyolysis or

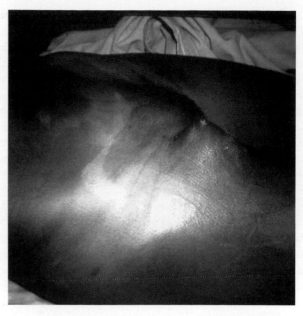

Figure 44.11 *Mycotic femoral aneurysm resulting from intravenous drug use; frequently, purulent eruptions arise from the apex of the infected site*

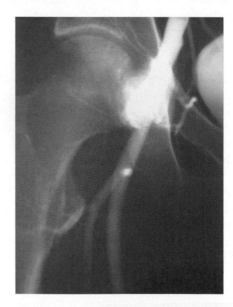

Figure 44.12 *Arteriogram of a drug induced mycotic femoral aneurysm showing extravasation of contrast*

there may be an underlying condition of renal impairment due to the chronic drug abuse itself. Intravenous and intra-arterial injection of illicit drugs will result in chronic endothelial injury and a form of drug induced, possibly systemic, vasculitis.

Arterial mycotic aneurysms

The classic presentation of a mycotic aneurysm is one of a pulsatile mass over a major arterial site associated with a puncture in the area, the presence of a bruit and intact distal pulses.[41] The typical clinical appearance of an infected femoral pseudoaneurysm is seen in Fig. 44.11. The septic patient has a painful pulsatile mass in the groin with some suppuration at the tip where the skin is necrosed. The arteriogram in Fig. 44.12 shows extravasation of contrast through the disrupted wall of the femoral artery. The infection may be induced by inadvertent puncture of the artery and subsequent seeding of the arterial wall or by adjacent spread of bacteria into the arterial wall by a local abscess. In the drug-using population the most common site for a mycotic arterial aneurysm is the femoral artery. Although any artery can be affected, the most common sites in descending order are femoral, brachial and radial.[34,31] Yellin *et al.* report a 5 per cent incidence of unsuspected arteriovenous (AV) fistulae in these patients.[34] A duplex scan will help one determine the degree of tissue involvement as well as identify the artery and/or vein involved and the presence of an AV fistula if one is present. It also will help in documenting thrombosis in the venous system which may be present. Rarely is peripheral arteriography required at this point.

Management of these patients includes intravenous antibiotic therapy, debridement of all infected tissue including the artery and/or vein and removal of the entire infected segment of vessel.[31,34–36,41] Although distal embolisation can occur from these aneurysms, rupture is the most common sequela. If the artery involved is not resected back to healthy tissue delayed rupture will occur. It is often difficult to determine how far one needs to resect until healthy vessel is encountered. A seasoned surgeon will have a sense of what might be termed adequate arterial wall based upon the appearance of the vessel and the sensation of the needle passing through the segment. If the needle punctures very easily it is possible that that segment is abnormal and more distant resection and ligation is recommended.

Revascularisation is not routinely required at the time of ligation of mycotic pseudoaneurysms unless the extremity involved becomes ischaemic. Subsequently, almost all patients experience intermittent claudication, but less than 20 per cent ultimately require revascularisation to prevent major amputation.[31,36,42] In patients with infected mycotic aneurysms, such procedures, when indicated, can be problematic. These patients often have no usable autogenous venous conduit for the repair.

We treated 112 aneurysms and six AV fistulae of the lower extremities secondary to drug injection. The most frequent presentation was a painful, pulsatile mass with extensive cellulitis. Foot ischaemic complications were infrequent. In order to discriminate between a plain groin abscess and an infected pseudoaneurysm we used both ultrasound and angiography. In all cases the aneurysm was dealt with by a direct approach and excision of the infected femoral artery. At the beginning of our experience we used a separate retroperitoneal exposure of the external iliac artery to obtain proximal control. Further into this series,

and for the sake of efficiency, we approached the false aneurysm directly, controlling the bleeding with digital pressure above and below the area of wall destruction. Today, for the occasionally infected pseudoaneurysm we see, and given the very high incidence of HIV and hepatitis in these patients, we have gone back to proximal control to have a tidier and safer field for the surgical team. The femoral artery segment with inflammation or necrosis of the wall is excised. In some cases the excision and simple ligation is limited to the common femoral artery; in others the length of artery excised also demands ligation of the superficial and deep femoral arteries, in other words, triple ligation. When a triple ligation is done severe limb-threatening ischaemia of the leg is much more likely and one cannot predict when it will occur. Our routine is to observe the patient in the recovery room and base our decision upon the appearance of the limb and symptoms at that time.

At the beginning there was debate as to whether one should revascularise these legs following inflow ligation. These patients do not have superficial veins for grafts, these having been ruined by repeated injections and thrombophlebitis. One is therefore limited to the use of a prosthetic bypass which has to be routed away from the contaminated operative field (see Chapter 18). Two atopical or extra-anatomical routes were used for revascularisation of the lower extremity: the lateral femoral route and the obturator route.[35,41,43–45] In the lateral femoral route, after excising the pseudoaneurysm, the patient is prepped clean and using a new set of instruments, the proximal external iliac artery is exposed though a retroperitoneal approach for inflow to the bypass tunnelled lateral to the inguinal ligament into the lateral thigh; from there it is swung medially and anastomosed to a segment of distal superficial femoral artery.

The obturator bypass was introduced in 1963 by Shaw and Baue[46] and later expanded upon by Guida amd Moore in 1969.[47] More contemporary modifications of this technique and their application, not only in drug induced femoral mycotic aneurysms but also for prosthetic graft infections, have been described.[48–53] The common or external iliac arteries are exposed in the pelvis for the proximal anastomosis. The graft is tunnelled through the obturator foramen into the upper or middle thigh where it is joined to the superficial femoral artery. The obturator bypass is not an easy operation in men who have a rather narrow pelvis. More importantly, in most of these patients, the common femoral veins have thrombosed through repeated injections, venous outflow occurring through large collaterals traversing the obturator foramen; serious venous bleeding can arise from these collaterals while tunnelling the graft blindly through the obturator foramen, even if one keeps anteromedial to the obturator vessels as one should. Since these grafts often lie in a subcutaneous location, it is not uncommon for many of these patients, as they remain addicted, to inject the easy-to-locate arterial

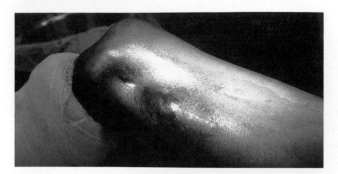

Figure 44.13 *This individual had an obturator bypass to the mid-femoral artery but the graft became infected when it was used as a drug injection site; a perigraft abscess developed requiring explantation of the graft followed by high thigh amputation*

graft. This of course will result in early graft thrombosis and graft infection necessitating another operation for removal of the infected bypass, as seen in Fig. 44.13. A high thigh amputation is required frequently.

Some surgeons in our group performed simultaneous revascularisation if there was evidence of limb-threatening ischaemia or a severe drop in the ankle:brachial index while others did not do so in septic patients. When our collective experience was tabulated, including 118 femoral aneurysms alone,[31] we adopted a general policy of not doing simultaneous reconstructions. Our decision was supported by the following facts. First, few patients need it to preserve their limbs,[31,34,44] and second, among those patients who had undergone revascularisation, a substantial number developed graft infection and ended up with a higher level of amputation than would have been required for the ischaemia subsequent to ligation of the pseudoaneurysm.[31,46] The question of vascular reconstruction is generally raised after a triple ligation. None of the patients undergoing revascularisation suffered immediate amputations. Some patients with triple ligation who did not undergo revascularisation lost their legs. In our series, following excision of an infected pseudoaneurysm, and using either triple or single ligation, 13 patients out of 102 lost their legs. Three months after treatment, however, the percentage of limb loss experienced by patients who underwent simultaneous reconstruction was slightly higher than those who did not, and that was because of infection of the prosthetic graft.

If systemic sepsis is present at the time of initial pseudoaneurysm ligation, we do not advocate routine revascularisation as in these patients limb amputation may be the safest course of treatment. This is in contrast to a report from the New York Medical College where concomitant restoration of blood flow was advocated, but their experience was limited to 15 cases.[54]

In conclusion, for infected femoral pseudoaneurysms secondary to drug injection, we recommend primary

ligation, excision and drainage of the abscess and the use of antibiotics effective against the causative organism, usually MRSA. Once sepsis has cleared and the wound is clean, and if severe ischaemia causing rest pain persists, consideration may be given to carrying out an extra-anatomical bypass (see Chapter 18). This somewhat fatalistic policy has been reaffirmed by other and more recent series.[55]

The presentation of heroin induced arterial injury is different for the upper extremities. In the arm, the common presentation is a compartment syndrome with neuromuscular deficit and hand ischaemia. This almost certainly represents inadvertent intra-arterial injection and has been described above.

Because the practice of 'shooting the pocket' can result in subclavian and/or carotid artery mycotic aneurysms, treatment of these vessels is not too dissimilar from that of the lower extremity. Although duplex imaging can be useful in confirming the diagnosis and in documenting flow into the affected vessel, arteriography may be more accurate in identifying the origin of the aneurysm and in planning the overall operation. Common carotid aneurysms can be ligated and rarely need reconstruction as long as the internal carotid artery is patent and can be perfused by way of reversed flow from the external carotid system.[34] Mycotic aneurysms involving the external carotid system can simply be ligated but those involving the internal carotid artery should undergo, if possible, not only excision but also reconstruction. Again, the use of prosthetic material in this infected site is contraindicated. If an autogenous venous conduit cannot be found, as is usually the case, the superficial femoral artery can be harvested and used as an autogenous arterial conduit followed by replacement of the superficial femoral artery with an appropriate prosthetic graft.[56]

As repeatedly stated, systemic sepsis in these patients is common. Cardiac vegetations from endocarditis can cause septic emboli to disseminate throughout the vascular tree. Pulmonary abscesses and pulmonary mycotic aneurysms do occur. The septic emboli may also affect any peripheral or central artery as well as intracerebral, adrenal, splenic, mesenteric, and renal vessels.[34,35] Ischaemic bowel manifestations may occur due to embolism to the superior mesenteric artery or from resulting mycotic aneurysms which rupture. In these cases treatment involves ligation of the vessel and bowel resection if the segment of bowel perfused by the ligated vessel is non-viable.

Arterial thrombosis secondary to drug use

Intra-arterial injections of drugs can directly result in thrombosis of the vessel with distal embolisation. Self-administration of substances, and as noted above, especially those of cocaine, can, due to their pharmacological

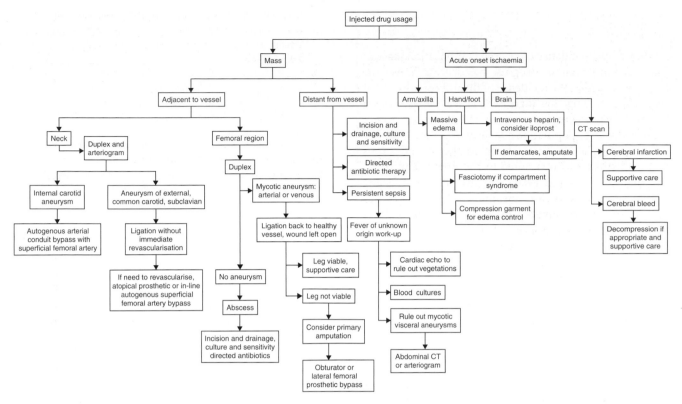

Figure 44.14   *Algorithm for determining the treatment of patients who have injected illicit substances. CT, computed tomography*

properties, cause thrombosis of large central and/or peripheral vessels. This can occur not only in the arterial tree but also in the venous system. Lymphatic obstruction from systemic usage of drugs other than those injected is not well documented. The aetiology of large vessel thrombosis, including that of the thoracic and abdominal aorta, is unclear. It is possible that a prothrombotic state occurs associated with local spasm of the vasa vasorum resulting in a localised thrombotic event. This can occur despite a grossly normal endothelium seen at the time of operation.[18] If the thrombosis occurs in the venous system then routine treatment of either superficial thrombophlebitis or DVT should be instituted. If it involves the arterial tree then treatment is dictated by any complications associated with the thrombosis. If a large thrombus is identified it has been our routine not to operate to remove it unless it has embolised or end organ function is threatened. We have successfully treated large intra-aortic thrombi with intravenous heparin administration keeping the PTT level to 2–2.5 baseline. Heparin should be continued for at least 7–10 days in hospital. Repeat imaging, be it arteriogram, spiral computed tomography or magnetic resonance imaging, has been used to monitor the regression of the thrombosis. These patients, if deemed reliable, will subsequently be started on warfarin, and then discharged for follow-up imaging until the thrombus

fully resolves. It has been our experience that as long as the patient is free of the inciting agent, frequently cocaine in any of its forms, the thrombus will resolve completely and at such a time anticoagulant treatment can be stopped.

If the thrombus or thrombotic event threatens end organ function then standard thrombectomy or lytic therapy can be used depending upon the clinical situation. In those cases where this has been necessary the vessels have appeared grossly normal. We do not recommend long term anticoagulation in these patients, assuming that a work-up for endogenous hypercoagulability is negative. On the other hand, if a demonstrable defect is detected in the coagulation cascade, or if deficiencies of either protein C, S, antithrombin III, lupus anticoagulant, anticardiolipin antibodies, factor V Leiden, PT 20210A, etc., are discovered, then these patients should be kept on lifelong warfarin therapy unless contraindicated by the overall medical condition. Patient counselling is extremely important as is successful antidrug detoxification if complications of anticoagulant therapy are to be avoided.

A decision tree for determining the treatment of patients who have injected illicit substances is presented in Fig. 44.14. This schema can be used as a general guide to therapy but it must be tailored to the individual patient and circumstance.

Conclusions

Although the incidence of arterial complications associated with intravenous drug use has decreased over the past two decades, the incidence of thrombosis associated with cocaine usage has increased. There has also been a recent rise in the recreational use of intravenous heroin in the suburban population as a drug of choice. Whether there will be a concomitant rise in the complications from this usage as was noted in the urban population during the 1970s and 1980s remains to be seen. Many users have access to clean insulin needles, syringes and alcohol swabs obtainable over the counter without prescription; these factors may help to reduce the historical incidence of septic complications. Should that happen, then any complications arising from usage will be dictated by the agent rather than by the route of administration.

Key references

Baldwin GC, Tashkin DP, Buckley DM, *et al.* Marijuana and cocaine impair alveolar macrophage function and cytokine production. *Am J Respir Crit Care Med* 1997; **156**: 1606–13.

Berguer B, Benitz P. Surgical emergencies from intravascular injection of drugs. In: (eds) *Vascular Surgical Emergencies.* New York: Grune & Stratton, 1987: 309–16.

Fuller MG, Diamond DL, Jordan M, Walter MC. The role of a substance abuse consultation team in a trauma center. *J Stud Alcohol* 1997; **56**: 267–71.

Kolodgie FD, Virmani R, Cornhill JE, *et al.* Increase in atherosclerosis and adventitial mast cells in cocaine abusers; an alternative mechanism of cocaine-associated coronary vasospasm and thrombosis. *J Am Coll Cardiol* 1991; **17**: 1553–60.

Webber J, Kline RA, Lucas CE. Aortic thrombosis associated with cocaine use: report of two cases. *Ann Vasc Surg* 1999; **13**: 302–4.

REFERENCES

1 Hypodermic Needle – Syringe Needle. Extract from 'Blood and Blood Transfusions'. Available at http://inventors.about.com/library/inventors/blsyringe.htm (accessed 7 January 2005).

2 Browne A. Drugs in Britain. *The Observer.* 25 March 2001, London.

3 *National Household Survey on Drug Abuse: Population Estimates 1988.* Rockville, MD: National Institute on Drug Abuse, 20857.

4 Harruff RC, Francisco JT, Elkins SK, *et al.* Cocaine and homicide in Memphis and Shelby County: an epidemic of violence. *J Forensic Sci* 1988; **33**: 1231–7.

5 Rogers JN, Henry TE, Jones AM, *et al.* Cocaine related deaths in Pima County, Arizona, 1982–1984. *J Forensic Sci* 1986; **31**: 1404–8.

6 Sloan EP, Zalenski RJ, Smith RF, *et al.* Toxicology screening in urban trauma patients: drug prevalence and its relationship to trauma severity and management. *J Trauma* 1989; **29**: 1647–53.

7 Vogel JM, Vernberg EM. Children's psychological responses to disasters. *J Clin Child Psychol* 1993; **22**: 464–85.

8 Fuller MG, Diamond DL, Jordan M, Walter MC. The role of a substance abuse consultation team in a trauma center. *J Stud Alcohol* 1997; **56**: 267–71.

9 Vogel JM, Vernberg EM. Children's psychological responses to disasters. *J Clin Child Psychol* 1993; **22**: 464–84.

10 Brookoff D, Campbell EA, Shaw LM. The under reporting of cocaine-related trauma: drug abuse warning network reports vs hospital toxicology tests. *Am J Public Health* 1993; **83**: 369.

11 Baldwin GC, Tashkin DP, Buckley DM, *et al.* Marijuana and cocaine impair alveolar macrophage function and cytokine production. *Am J Respir Crit Care Med* 1997; **156**: 1606–13.

12 Tashkin DP, Simmons MS, Sherrill DL, Coulson AH. Heavy habitual marijuana smoking does not cause an accelerated decline in FEV_1 with age. *Am J Respir Crit Care Med* 1997; **155**: 141–8.

13 Pieper B. Physical effects of heroin and cocaine; consideration for a wound care service. *J Wound Ostomy Continence Nurs* 1996; **23**: 248–55.

14 Sands DE, Ledgerwood AM, Lucas CE. Pneumomediastinum on a surgical service. *Am Surg* 1988; **54**: 434–7.

15 Gawin FH, Ellinwood EH. Cocaine and other stimulants. Actions, abuse, and treatment. *N Engl J Med* 1988; **318**: 1173–82.

16 Frishman WH, Karpenos A, Molloy TJ. Cocaine induced coronary artery disease. *Med Clin North Am* 1989; **73**: 475–86.

17 Kolodgie FD, Virmani R, Cornhill JE, *et al.* Increase in atherosclerosis and adventitial mast cells in cocaine abusers; an alternative mechanism of cocaine-associated coronary vasospasm and thrombosis. *J Am Coll Cardiol* 1991; **17**: 1553–60.

18 Webber J, Kline RA, Lucas CE. Aortic thrombosis associated with cocaine use: report of two cases. *Ann Vasc Surg* 1999; **13**: 302–4.

19 Gold MS, Washton AM, Drackis CA. Cocaine abuse; neurochemistry, phenomenology, and treatment. *Natl Inst Drug Abuse Res Monogr Ser* 1985; **61**: 130–50.

20 Chokshi SK, Miller G, Rongione A, Isner JM. Cocaine and cardiovascular diseases: the leading age. *Cardiology* 1989; **III**: 1–6.

21 Moliterno DJ, Lange Ra, Gerard RD, *et al.* Influence of intranasal cocaine on plasma constituents associated with endogenous thrombosis and thrombolysis. *Am J Med* 1994; **96**: 492–6.

22 Kolodgie FD, Virmani R, Cornhill F, *et al.* Increase in atherosclerosis and adventitial mast cells in cocaine abusers: an alternative mechanism of cocaine-associated coronary vasospasm and thrombosis. *J Am Coll Cardiol* 1991; **17**: 1553–60.

23 Fandino J, Sherman JD, Zuccarello M, Rapoport RM. Cocaine-induced endothelin-1-dependent spasm in rabbit basilar artery *in vivo. J Cardiovasc Pharmacol* 2003; **41**: 158–61.

24 Daras M, Tuchman AJ, Koppel BS, *et al.* Neurovascular complications of cocaine. *Acta Neurol Scand* 1994; **90**: 124–9.

25 Boutros HH, Pautler S, Chakrabarti S. Cocaine-induced ischemic colitis with small-vessel thrombosis of colon and gallbladder. *J Clin Gastroenterol* 1997; **24**: 49–53.

26 Lisse JR, Davis CP, Thurmond-Anderle ME. Upper extremity deep venous thrombosis: increased prevalence due to cocaine abuse. *Am J Med* 1989; **87**: 457–8.

27 Sharff JA. Renal infarction associated with intravenous cocaine use. *Ann Emerg Med* 1984; **13**: 1145–7.

28 Wohlman RA. Renal artery thrombosis and embolization associated with intravenous cocaine injection. *South Med J* 1987; **80**: 928–30.

29 Turney L. Angel dust: new facts about PCP. Do It Now Foundation, #123, March 2003.

30 Yeager RA, Hobson RW, Padberg FT, *et al.* Vascular complications related to drug abuse. *Trauma* 1987; **27**: 305–8.

31 Berguer B, Benitz P. Surgical emergencies from intravascular injection of drugs. In: Bergan JJ, Yao ST (eds). *Vascular Surgical Emergencies*. New York: Grune & Stratton, 1987: 309–16.

32 Vilke GM, Sloane C, Smith AM, Chan TC. Assessment for deaths in out-of-hospital heroin overdose patients treated with naloxone who refuse transport. *Acad Emerg Med* 2003; **10**: 893–6.

33 Jaffe JH, Martin WR. Opoid analgesics and antagonists. In: Gilman AG, Goodman LS, Rall TW, *et al.* (eds). *The Pharmacological Basis of Therapeutics*, 7th edn. New York: MacMillan, 1985: 491–531.

34 Yellin AE, Frankhouse JH, Weaver FA. Vascular injury secondary to drug abuse. In: Ernst CB, Stanley JC (eds). *Current Therapy in Vascular Surgery*, 3rd edn, St Louis, MO: Mosby, 1995: 637–44.

35 Yeager RA, Hobson RW, Padberg FT, *et al.* Vascular complications related to drug abuse. *Trauma* 1987; **27**: 305–8.

36 Woodburn KR, Murie JA. Vascular complications of injecting drug misuse. *Br J Surg* 1996; **83**: 1329–34.

37 Silverman SH, Turner WW. Intraarterial drug abuse: new treatment options. *J Vasc Surg* 1991; **14**: 111–16.

38 Treiman GS, Yellin AE, Weaver FA, *et al.* An effective treatment protocol for intraarterial drug injection. *J Vasc Surg* 1990; **12**: 456–66.

39 Tait IS, Holdsworth RJ, Belch JJ, *et al.* Management of intra-arterial injection injury of Iloprost, *Lancet* 1994; **343**: 419.

40 Dodd TJ, Scott RN, Woodburn KR, *et al.* Limb ischemia after intra-arterial injection of temazepam gel: histology of nine cases. *J Clin Pathol* 1994; **47**: 512–14.

41 Feldman AJ, Berguer R. Management of an infected aneurysm of the groin secondary to drug abuse. *Surg Gynecol Obstet* 1983; **157**: 519–22.

42 Cheng SWK, Fok M, Wong J. Infected femoral pseudoaneurysm in intravenous drug abusers. *Br J Surg* 1992; **79**: 510–12.

43 Johnson JR, Ledgerwood AM, Lucas CE. Mycotic aneurysm: new concepts in surgery. *Arch Surg* 1983; **118**: 577–82.

44 Reddy DJ, Smith RF, Elliot JP, *et al.* Infected femoral artery false aneurysms in drug addicts: evolution of selective vascular reconstruction. *J Vasc Surg* 1986; **3**: 718–24.

45 Fromm SH, Lucas CE. Obturator bypass for mycotic aneurysm in the drug addict. *Arch Surg* 1970; **100**: 82–3.

46 Shaw RS, Baue AE. Management of sepsis complicating arterial reconstructive procedures. *Surgery* 1963; **53**: 75–86.

47 Guida PM, Moore WS. Obturator bypass technique. *Surg Gynecol Obstet* 1969; **128**: 1307–16.

48 Tilson MD, Sweeney T, Gusberg RT, *et al.* Obturator canal bypass grafts for sepsis lesions of the femoral artery. *Arch Surg* 1979; **114**: 1031–3.

49 Erath HG Jr, Gale SS, Smith BM, *et al.* Obturator foramen grafts: the preferable alternate route? *Am Surg* 1982; **48**: 65–9.

50 Pearce WH, Ricco J, Yao JST, *et al.* Modified technique of obturator bypass in failed or infected grafts. *Ann Surg* 1983; **197**: 344–7.

51 Nevelsteen A, Mees U, Deleersnijder J, *et al.* Obturator bypass: a sixteen year experience with 55 cases. *Ann Vasc Surg* 1987; **1**: 558–63.

52 Lai DTM, Huber D, Hogg J. Obturator foramen bypass in the management of infected prosthetic vascular grafts. *Aust N Z J Surg* 1993; **63**: 811–14.

53 Sautner T, Niederle B, Herbst F, *et al.* The value of obturator canal bypass: a review. *Arch Surg* 1994; **129**: 718–22.

54 Patel KR, Semel L, Clauss RH. Routine revascularization with resection of infected femoral pseudoaneurysms from substance abuse. *J Vasc Surg* 1988; **8**: 321–8.

55 Welch GH, Reid DB, Pollock JG. Infected false aneurysms in the groin of intravenous drug abusers. *Br J Surg* 1990; **77**: 330–3.

56 Sessa C, Morasch MD, Berguer R, *et al.* Carotid resection and replacement with autogenous arterial graft during operation for neck malignancy. *Ann Vasc Surg* 1998; **12**: 229–35.

45

HIV/AIDS Related Vascular Emergencies

JACOBUS VAN MARLE, LYNNE TUDHOPE

THE PROBLEM

The Joint United Nations Program on HIV/AIDS (UNAIDS) and the World Health Organization estimated that there would be 39.1 million people infected with human immunodeficiency virus (HIV) by the end of 2004. Approximately 96 per cent of people with HIV/acquired immune deficiency syndrome (AIDS) live in the developing world with 64.5 per cent of them in sub-Saharan Africa.[1]

The long latent period of up to 10 years between primary infection and the development of AIDS, an increased awareness of the disease, and advances in earlier diagnosis and treatment with an expectancy of longer survival have together resulted in an ever increasing population who may also require surgery.[2] The reasons for surgical intervention include pathology directly related to HIV/AIDS as well as HIV seropositive patients who present with common surgical conditions unrelated to the underlying HIV infection. The distinction between HIV and AIDS is based on the Centres for Disease Control classification.[3]

AETIOLOGY

The human immune deficiency virus belongs to the family retroviridae, genus lentivirus. There is a huge variation in HIV isolates with two distinct subtypes, namely, HIV-1 and HIV-2, and a high level of genetic diversity in HIV type1 strains.[4] The virus is cytopathic and is found mainly in CD4 T cells because of the affinity of the virus for the cell coat markers.[5] The CD4 T cell has many important immunological functions and destruction of these cells causes a reduction in immune response. The disease runs a chronic course, with approximately 10 per cent of infected subjects progressing to AIDS within 2–3-years, and the remainder developing AIDS within a median of 10 years from the onset of infection. The virus has been isolated from all body fluids and transmission occurs through oral, rectal and vaginal intercourse, blood product transfusion, intravenous needles, occupational acquisition and vertical transmission from mother to child.[6]

VASCULAR PATHOLOGY AND PATHOPHYSIOLOGY

Joshi et al. were the first to report on the association between arterial disease and HIV.[7] They described a fibroproliferative occlusive disease in the coronary arteries. This consisted of inflammation of the endothelium with lymphocytes and mononuclear giant cells which led to fragmentation of elastin fibres and intimal fibrosis resulting in luminal narrowing. Calabrese et al. described a systemic necrotising vasculitis involving the small vessels in patients with HIV infection.[8]

Du Pont was the first to report on aneurysmal disease being associated with HIV, and since then there have been many publications dealing with this issue. A selection of these publications is listed in the references.[9–12] There is also a trend towards multiple aneurysms, atypical location and a predilection for the carotid arteries.[13–15] The histological appearance of HIV related aneurysms has been described by Chetty *et al.*[16] The principal features are involvement of the adventitia by a mixed acute and chronic inflammatory cell infiltrate centred on the vasa vasorum. Occlusion of the vasa vasorum by inflammatory oedema or cellular infiltrate is a prominent feature. The inflammatory process largely spares the media and intima. The presence of HIV protein within lymphocytes in the aneurysm wall has been confirmed through immunohistochemical staining[12] and polymerase chain reaction (PCR) done on aneurysmal tissue confirmed the presence of viral copies in a patient with multiple aneurysms.[14]

Although it is apparent that HIV related aneurysms constitute a distinct clinical and pathological entity with several features distinguishing them from degenerative and infective aneurysms, the precise pathogenesis remains unclear. Failure to demonstrate microorganisms in the majority of aneurysms makes the hypothesis of bacteraemia, as a result of immunosuppression and secondary mycotic aneurysms, less likely.[12] Weakening of the arterial wall resulting in aneurysm formation may be caused by direct action of the HIV itself, an immune complex mechanism or ischaemia of the arterial wall resulting from occlusion of the vasa vasorum.[8,12] Although viral protein has been demonstrated in arterial wall biopsies from aneurysm margins, evidence to support direct viral action leading to destruction of the arterial wall is still lacking.

Nair *et al.* were the first to report on large vessel occlusive disease associated with HIV infection.[17] They found a histological similarity between HIV related occlusive and aneurysmal disease and suggested a leucocytoclastic vasculitis of the vasa vasorum as the common pathogenesis.

There is growing evidence that HIV influences the physiology of vascular endothelium.[18] Certain endothelial cell products which are considered to be markers for endothelial cell dysfunction, are significantly elevated in patients with HIV. These cell products include the von Willebrand factor, tissue plasminogen activator, β_2-microglobulin and soluble thrombomodulin.[19] Markers of thrombin activation (fragment 1 and 2) and D-dimers are used to determine whether HIV infected patients have a prothrombotic state. Plasma concentration of thrombomodulin is assessed to establish whether an endothelial lesion is concurrently present or not. The presence of anticardiolipin antibodies, protein S deficiency and antithrombin deficiency contribute to the hypercoagulable state associated with HIV/AIDS.[20–22]

HIV infection has been associated with hypertriglyceridaemia which may cause endothelial damage and predispose to accelerated atherosclerosis.[23] There are certain class specific metabolic side effects of protease inhibitor therapy which may also contribute to accelerated atherosclerotic disease. These side effects include increased insulin resistance (which is associated with abnormalities in endothelial function, impaired nitric oxide production and diminished vasodilatation) as well as abnormalities in lipid metabolism with elevated levels of total cholesterol and serum triglycerides.[24]

HIV AND SURGERY: PREDICTORS OF OPERATIVE OUTCOME

There are many publications on abdominal surgery in HIV/AIDS patients and mortality and morbidity varies between 0 and 38 per cent and between 7 and 68 per cent, respectively.[25–31] Many factors interact, including the stage of immune deficiency syndrome, preoperative white cell count, serum albumin concentration, nutritional state, the type of operation: clean versus contaminated and emergency versus elective operations, and the presence of opportunistic infections.

Factors influencing outcome

- Stage of immune deficiency syndrome
- Preoperative white cell count
- Nutritional status
- Anaemia
- Type of operation
- Opportunistic infections

Stage of immune deficiency syndrome

Immunodeficiency is a more important cause of perioperative complications than the operation itself.[32] HIV infection leads to reduction in the CD4 T lymphocyte count and patients with a CD4 count of <200 cells/μL are probably at a greater risk of developing a postoperative infection. This includes worsening of preoperative infections as well as newly acquired postoperative opportunistic infections. Yii *et al.*,[29] Savioz *et al.*[30] and Consten *et al.*[33] reported that perioperative CD4 T lymphocyte counts were significantly lower in patients with overall postoperative complications, disturbed wound healing and infections.

Tran *et al.* suggested that a low percentage of lymphocytes and postoperative CD4 lymphocyte counts have a stronger correlation with mortality.[34] As expected, patients with AIDS fare worse than those who are HIV positive, with poorer wound healing, more complications and a higher mortality.[25] It has also been found that there is no significant difference in postoperative morbidity and mortality between symptom-free HIV positive patients and HIV seronegative patients and that if the CD4 T cell count is above 500 cells/μL, the morbidity in clean surgery is comparable to that of HIV negative patients.[30,31,35]

A recent study by Mellors *et al.* demonstrated that plasma viral load was the single best prognostic indicator of clinical outcome and that HIV-1 RNA concentration was highly predictive of the rate of decline of CD4 lymphocyte counts and progression to AIDS and death.[36] Viraemia is indicative of active viral replication with continuous reinfection resulting in the destruction of CD4 lymphocytes and an increase in the total number of virus-producing cells.[36,37]

White cell count

Several studies report significantly improved survival with lower wound complication rates in patients with a higher preoperative total white cell count.[27,34]

Nutritional status

Low serum albumin levels have been associated with poor surgical outcome in HIV patients and are independent prognostic factors in survival studies of AIDS patients.[25,27,38] Whitney *et al.* found a weight loss of >10 per cent to be a significant prognostic indicator. [27]

Anaemia

Binderow *et al.*[38] found a trend in low versus high haematocrit values as a predictor of outcome whereas Yii *et al.*[29] found haemoglobin concentration to be a significant prognostic indicator.

Type of operation

Emergency surgery has a higher mortality than elective procedures in any cohort of patients. Savioz *et al.* found a significant difference between clean and contaminated operations, especially if the CD4 T cell count was ≤200 cells/µL.[31] They recommend that a CD4 cell count <200 cells/µL should be considered a threshold for contaminated surgery and it should only be undertaken when the procedure is considered to be unavoidable. With clean surgery, mainly orthopaedic procedures, the probability of morbidity remains <50 per cent even with a very low CD4 count.

Opportunistic infections

The presence of opportunistic infections implies an immunocompromised state and results in a poorer surgical outcome.[25]

HIV AND VASCULAR SURGERY

Vascular problems in HIV/AIDS patients manifest themselves in three different ways. First, there are those patients who present with the normal spectrum of vascular disease but are incidentally found to be HIV positive, and in whom the vascular condition is *not* related to the underlying HIV infection. Second, there are those who present with vascular disease directly related to HIV/AIDS. Finally, there are some patients who present with complications of hypercoagulability due to HIV/AIDS.

Vascular problems in HIV/AIDS

- Vascular condition unrelated to underlying HIV infection
- Vascular disease directly related to HIV/AIDS
- Complications of hypercoagulability due to HIV/AIDS

Due to the high incidence of HIV/AIDS in South Africa we follow a policy of routine testing for HIV on all admissions to the vascular unit. Patient consent is required for HIV testing and the vast majority of patients comply. The incidence of HIV positivity in our unit is >15 per cent. The majority of patients who present with vascular problems and are found to be HIV positive, present with either occlusive disease, aneurysms or trauma, and are otherwise well, exhibiting no symptoms or signs of immunodeficiency. The spectrum of HIV/AIDS related vascular disease includes fibro-obliterative disease, necrotising vasculitis, aneurysms and the complications of hypercoagulability. Spontaneous arteriovenous (AV) fistula arising from HIV arteritis has recently been described.[39]

There are some clinical characteristics specific to HIV related vascular disease which should alert the treating physician to the possibility of underlying AIDS.

Clinical features suggestive of HIV related vascular disease

- Younger presenting age
- Absence of typical risk factors for atherosclerosis
- Multiple aneurysms
- Atypical location of aneurysms
- Features of immunodeficiency

Five short case descriptions demonstrate the spectrum of disease treated in our unit. All the patients had a positive smoking history but no other risk factors for vascular disease.

Case report 1

A 25-year-old man presented with a large, tender, pulsating mass involving the right axilla and infraclavicular region (Fig. 45.1a). On angiography he was found to have a contained rupture of a right subscapular artery aneurysm (Fig. 45.1b) and multiple aneurysms involving the peripheral arteries and abdominal aorta (Fig. 45.1c and d, respectively). The patient had AIDS with a CD4 count of <200 cells/μL, but due to the fact that the aneurysm was severely symptomatic with pain and restriction of movement and function in the right arm, the decision to operate was made. The aneurysm was evacuated and the subscapular artery tied off. Postoperative recovery was uneventful but the patient died 6 months later due to advanced AIDS.

Case report 2

A 29-year-old man presented with a pulsatile mass on the left side of his neck (Fig. 45.2a). Carotid angiography confirmed an aneurysm of the carotid bifurcation involving both the external and internal carotid arteries (Fig. 45.2b). His CD4 count was <200 cells/μL, but he was otherwise asymptomatic. Due to extensive involvement of the internal carotid artery, arterial reconstruction was not possible. Carotid stump pressure was >50 mmHg and intraoperative electroencephalogram (EEG) as well as transcranial

oximetry remained normal after test clamping of the common carotid artery. The aneurysm was therefore resected and the vessels ligated. Postoperative recovery was uneventful and the patient is being followed-up.

Case report 3

A 60-year-old man presented with a huge pulsatile mass in the left popliteal fossa, venous congestion of the lower limb and limiting claudication (Fig. 45.3a). A computed tomography (CT) scan and angiography confirmed the diagnosis of a huge popliteal artery aneurysm (Fig. 45.3b and c, respectively). The patient's CD4 count was >500 cells/μL. The aneurysm was excised and a femoropopliteal bypass

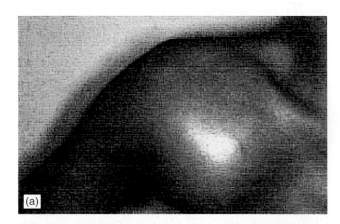

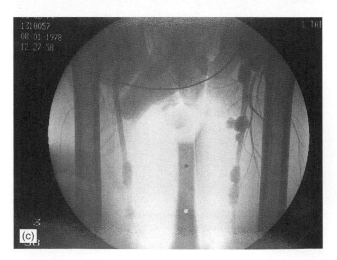

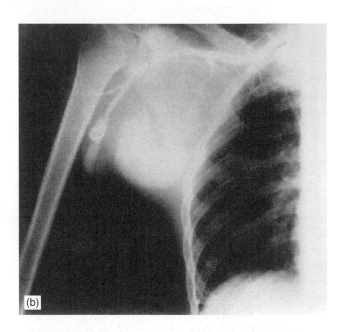

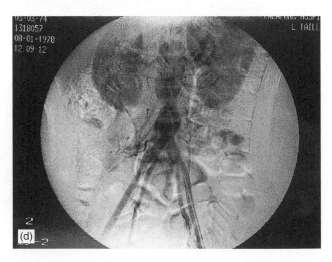

Figure 45.1 *(a) An aneurysm in the right axilla of a 25-year-old man. (b) Angiogram reveals a contained rupture of the subscapular artery. (c) Angiogram also shows multiple aneurysms of the peripheral arteries. (d) Angiogram additionally demonstrates an abdominal aortic aneurysm*

performed using the saphenous vein. The patient had an uneventful recovery and is being followed up.

Case report 4

A 49-year-old man presented with a non-viable left lower limb and a history of having had a right below-knee amputation three years' previously. Angiography confirmed

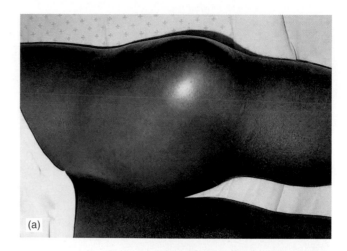

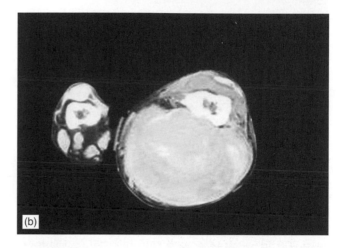

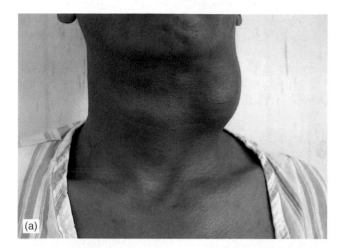

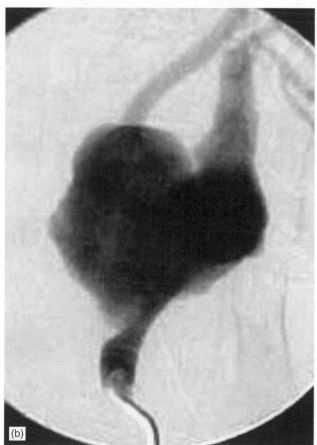

Figure 45.2   *(a) Left carotid artery aneurysm in a 29-year-old man. (b) Angiogram shows the aneurysm of the carotid bifurcation involving both the external and internal carotid arteries*

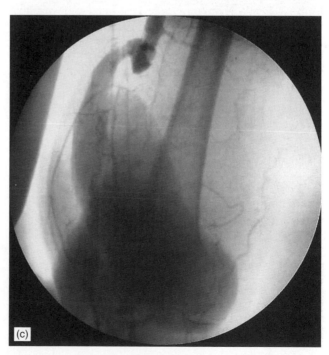

Figure 45.3   *(a) Popliteal artery aneurysm in a 60-year-old man. (b) Computed tomography scan of the popliteal artery aneurysm. (c) Angiogram also shows the popliteal artery aneurysm*

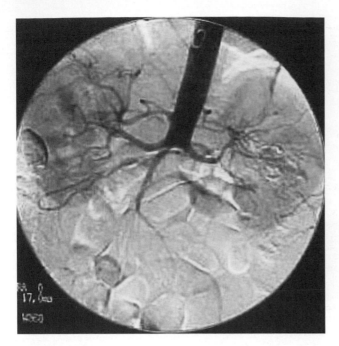

Figure 45.4 *Angiogram showing occlusion of the infrarenal aorta*

complete occlusion of the infrarenal aorta (Fig. 45.4). The CD4 count was 900 cells/μL. A high upper-leg amputation was performed, but due to poor wound healing he required disarticulation of the hip.

Case report 5

A 65-year-old man presented with bilateral critical lower limb ischaemia (Fontaine stage IV), bilateral lower limb swelling and empyema. He had bilateral femoropopliteal occlusive disease on angiography and a venous duplex Doppler study confirmed bilateral deep vein thrombosis. The CD4 count was below 200 cells/μL and anticardiolipin antibodies were positive. He refused amputation and was managed with anticoagulation and general supportive measures. He died within 10 days due to advanced disease.

DIAGNOSIS

In addition to the usual diagnostic work-up required for vascular patients certain **additional** tests are required in the patient with HIV/AIDS. These pertain mostly to predictors of operative outcome and complications.

Additional diagnostic tests in HIV/AIDS patients

- Sexually transmitted diseases
- Tuberculosis
- Hepatitis
- CD4 cell count

- CD4/CD8 ratio
- HIV-1 RNA count
- Hypercoagulability screening

The treating physician must be aware of the systemic effects of HIV/AIDS which may influence anaesthetic technique, operative outcome and postoperative management. These systemic effects include cardiac, pulmonary and central nervous system manifestations as well as hypercoagulability and these conditions should be investigated using appropriate tests. Two excellent review articles discussing these problems in detail are recommended.[40,41] The cardiac and pulmonary manifestations of HIV/AIDS are summarised below.

Cardiac manifestations of HIV/AIDS

- Myocarditis
- Dilated cardiomyopathy
- Pericardial effusion
- Endocarditis
- Coronary artery disease
- Pulmonary hypertension, right ventricular failure
- Drug related cardiotoxicity
- Nutritional cardiomyopathy
- Cardiac involvement in AIDS related tumors

The frequent association between tuberculosis and HIV/AIDS must be kept in mind.[42] Spinal cord involvement, myopathy and peripheral neuropathy may occur with cytomegalovirus (CMV) or HIV infection itself.[43]

Pulmonary manifestations of HIV/AIDS[41]

- *Pneumocystis carinii* pneumonia
  - Respiratory failure
  - Pneumatocoeles
  - Pneumothorax
  - Chronic respiratory insufficiency
- Cavitatory lung disease
  - Pyogenic bacterial lung abcess
  - Pulmonary tuberculosis
  - Fungal infection
  - *Nocardia* infection
- Disseminated tuberculosis
- Respiratory failure due to bacterial pneumonia
  - *Streptococcus pneumoniae, Moraxella catarrhalis, Haemophilus influenzae*
  - *Staphylococcus aureus, Pseudomonas aeruginosa*

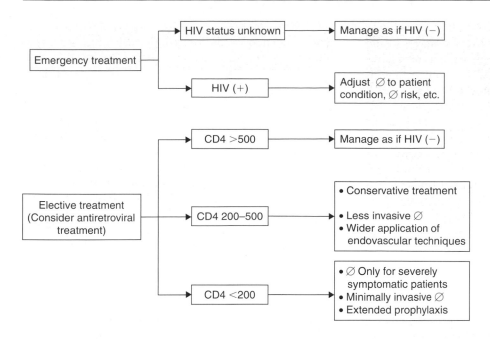

Figure 45.5 *Algorithm for managing vascular problems in HIV/AIDS*

Various factors contribute towards a procoagulant state in HIV/AIDS and deep vein thrombosis has been reported to occur 10 times more frequently in these patients than in the general population.[44] Hypercoagulability may not only cause venous thromboembolism but may contribute to bypass/graft occlusion and therefore the necessary precautions should be taken.

> ### Increased risk for venous thromboembolism in HIV/AIDS
>
> * Hypercoagulability
>   - Anticardiolipin antibodies
>   - Protein S deficiency
>   - Antithrombin deficiency
>   - Procoagulant products of endothelial cell dysfunction
> * Opportunistic infections: cytomegalovirus[45]
> * Intravenous drug abuse
> * Malignancies

MANAGEMENT

Concerns do exist that general anaesthesia and/or surgery may compound immunosuppression in HIV/AIDS patients leading to more rapid progression of the disease. The immune suppression seen postoperatively in HIV seronegative patients is transient and does not affect recovery or prognosis.[46,47] There is no documented evidence that surgery or any related intervention hastens the disease process in HIV/AIDS; these interventions should not be withheld because of HIV status or concern for subsequent complications.[34,41,48]

The algorithm in Fig. 45.5 provides an outline for the management of vascular problems in HIV/AIDS.

Emergency surgery

Surgery for vascular emergencies is performed regardless of HIV status, because seropositivity and degree of immunodeficiency are often only available after completion of surgery. When confirmed HIV positive patients present with life- or limb-threatening vascular conditions, surgery may be adjusted according to the degree of immunodeficiency and the patient's general condition; for example, opting for amputation rather than extensive revascularisation procedures. Our own experience supports that of Carrillo *et al.* that low levels of morbidity and mortality can be achieved with standard surgical care and techniques.[49] Guth *et al.* found that the incidence of complications in trauma patients with HIV was associated with an increase in the injury severity score (ISS) rather than HIV status.[50]

Elective surgery

Asymptomatic HIV seropositive patients as well as those with a CD4 count above 500 cells/μL have no increased surgical morbidity or mortality when compared with HIV seronegative patients and are treated as such.[30,35] For those patients with a CD4 count of <500 cells/μL, a conservative alternative to operation should be strongly considered.[31] This may involve a wider application of endovascular techniques. Patients with AIDS (CD4 $\leqslant$ 200 cells/μL) have a median survival time of 1 year. Surgery, however, should still be offered to severely symptomatic patients with limb- and life-threatening conditions, and in whom symptoms can be alleviated with minimum morbidity. This type of surgery is, essentially, only palliative and should be as minimally invasive as possible. This includes, for example, doing an endarterectomy or a profundoplasty or even a lower limb amputation in preference to an extensive bypass procedure for critical lower limb ischaemia. One may also have to accept, for example, an extra-anatomical bypass which may have lower long term patency than that of a more invasive anatomical procedure. Ligation instead of repair of aneurysms may also be considered in this patient group.

Principles of surgery

The standard principles of vascular surgery apply in HIV positive patients. Diseased arterial segments are excluded or bypassed from the circulation and care is taken to perform anastomoses to macroscopically normal tissue. Autogenous vein is preferred as a bypass conduit wherever possible. Where vein cannot be used, in circumstances where it is either unavailable or when a larger diameter conduit is required, we will resort to polyfluorotetraethylene or polyester grafts.

Where there is a high probability of sepsis, polyester grafts previously soaked in rifampicin or the commercially available silver-coated grafts have been used. Standard antibiotic prophylaxis for vascular surgery consists of a first generation cephalosporin. Savioz et al. found that 35 per cent of infective complications were caused by opportunistic infections outside the range of normal vascular prophylaxis.[31] These complications will require therapeutic antibiotic and antifungal treatment according to culture and sensitivity. Prophylaxis against *P. carinii* pneumonia should be given to all patients with a CD4 T cell count of <200 cells/μL.[3] Similarly, a single dose of fluconazole could probably prevent oral and oesophageal candidiasis.[31]

Endovascular management

There are no published series on endovascular management of vascular problems in HIV/AIDS patients. Our indications for endovascular therapy in asymptomatic HIV seropositive patients (CD4 T-cell count >500 cells/μL) are the same as for HIV seronegative patients. In patients with a CD4 count of <500 cells/μL, more liberal use is made of percutaneous techniques, extending the application of percutaneous transluminal angioplasty (PTA) to SCVIR (Society for Cardio-Vascular and Interventional Radiology) categories III and IV lesions. In AIDS patients, endovascular management should be considered in critical limb ischaemia, aneurysms and trauma in those locations which would require difficult or extensive access, for example, iliac or subclavian arteries. The cost implications of covered stent-grafts and endovascular procedures may limit their use in units or in countries with budgetary constraints.

Antiretroviral therapy

The use of highly active antiretroviral therapy (HAART) has resulted in dramatic declines in morbidity and mortality among HIV infected patients with advanced immune suppression.[51] There is, however, growing concern about patient compliance and the long term adverse effects of therapy. These include impact on quality of life, drug interactions, viral resistance and potential metabolic abnormalities including premature cardiovascular disease. The International AIDS Society has published updated recommendations for antiretroviral therapy.[52] Perioperative use at this stage is limited to patients who require elective surgery that can be postponed for at least 3 months for possible beneficial therapeutic effect. Tran et al., however, found that the presence or absence of antiretroviral therapy and the number of antiretroviral drugs did not affect surgical outcome.[34]

OCCUPATIONAL EXPOSURE AND PROPHYLAXIS

Healthcare workers looking after patients with HIV/AIDS should take the necessary precautions against accidental exposure. This includes double gloving, water resistant surgical gowns, eye protection and careful surgical technique to minimise blood spillage. Guidelines for the management of healthcare worker exposure to HIV and recommendations for post-exposure prophylaxis and therapy have been described in detail.[53,54]

Conclusions

HIV/AIDS is reaching pandemic proportions in the developing world. Therefore, surgeons will encounter an increasing population of HIV seropositive patients presenting with a spectrum of vascular problems. Emergency vascular surgery for trauma is performed regardless of HIV status. Elective surgery is undertaken in patients who are not immunocompromised as it is for HIV seronegative patients. In patients, who are already immunocompromised, a more conservative approach is being adopted, surgery being reserved for patients who are severely symptomatic. Even then, less invasive procedures are preferred. Life expectancy and the condition of the patient should always be weighed against the potential risk of the operation.

There is a need for multidisciplinary care in managing patients with HIV/AIDS and collaboration between different specialists is essential. Management strategies should be developed based on the everchanging understanding of the pathogenesis and treatment of HIV/AIDS and this will ensure optimum treatment of this rapidly expanding patient population.

Key references

Avidan MS, Jones N, Pozniak AL. The implications of HIV for the anaesthetist and the intensivist. *Anaesthesia* 2000; **55**: 344–54.

Barbaro G. Cardiovascular manifestations of HIV infection. *J R Soc Med* 2001; **94**: 384–90.

Nair R, Robbs JV, Naidoo NG, Woolgar J. Clinical profile of HIV-related aneurysms. *Eur J Vasc Endovasc Surg* 2000; **20**: 235–40.

Savioz D, Chilkot M, Ludwig C, *et al.* Preoperative counts of CD4 T-lymphocytes and early postoperative infective complications in HIV-positive patients. *Eur J Surg* 1998; **164**: 483–7.

Trann HS, Moncure M, Tarnoff M, *et al.* Predictors of operative outcome in patients with human immunodeficiency virus infection and acquired immunodeficiency syndrome. *Am J Surg* 2000; **180**: 228–33.

REFERENCES

1 World HIV and AIDS statistics. www.avert.org/wordstats.htm

2 Vipond MN, Ralph DJ, Stotter AT. Surgery in HIV-positive and AIDS patients: indications and outcome. *J R Coll Surg Edinb* 1991; **36**: 254–8.

3 Centers for Disease Control and Prevention. 1993 Revised classification system for HIV infection and expanded surveillance case definition for AIDS among adolescents and adults. *MMWR Morb Mortal Wkly Rep* 1992; **41**: 1–19.

4 Benn S, Rutledge R, Folks TJ, *et al.* Genomic heterogeneity of AIDS retroviral isolates from North America and Zaire. *Science* 1985; **230**: 949–51.

5 McDouglas JS, Kennedy MS, Sligh JM. Binding of HTLV-111/LAV to T4 + T-cells by a complex of 110 K molecule. *Science* 1985; **231**: 382–85.

6 Quinn TC. Global burden of the HIV pandemic. *Lancet* 1996; **348**: 99–106.

7 Joshi VV, Pawel B, Conor E, *et al.* Arteriopathy in children with acquired immune deficiency syndrome. *Pediatr Pathol* 1987; **7**: 261–75.

8 Calabrese LH, Estes M, Yen-Liebermann B, *et al.* Systemic vasculitis in association with human immunodeficiency virus infection. *Arthritis Rheum* 1989; **32**: 569–76.

9 Du Pont JR, Bonavita JA, Di Giovanni RJ, *et al.* Acquired immunodeficiency syndrome and mycotic abdominal aneurysms: a new challenge? Report of a case. *J Vasc Surg* 1989; **10**: 254–7.

10 Sinzobahamvya N, Kalangu K, Hamel-Kalinowski W. Arterial aneurysms associated with human immunodeficiency virus (HIV) infection. *Acta Chir Belg* 1989; **89**: 185–8.

11 Marks C, Kuskov S. Patterns of arterial aneurysms in acquired immunodeficiency disease. *World J Surg* 1995; **19**: 127–32.

12 Nair R, Abdool-Carrim ATO, Chetty R, Robbs JV. Arterial aneurysms in patients infected with human immunodeficiency virus: a distinct clinical pathology entity? *J Vasc Surg* 1999; **29**: 600–7.

13 Nair R, Robbs JV, Naidoo NG, Woolgar J. Clinical profile of HIV-related aneurysms. *Eur J Vasc Endovasc Surg* 2000; **20**: 235–40.

14 Tudhope LE, Van Marle J. Multiple arterial aneurysms in an HIV infected patient: retrovirus positivity established as possible etiology by means of the polymerase chain reaction [abstract]. Vascular Association of SA Conference, Sun City, South Africa, 6–9 August 1999: **2**.

15 Veller M, Pillay J, Abdool-Carrim T, Britz R. Aneurysms in patients with HIV infection: Involvement of the carotid artery bifurcation [abstract]. *Cardiovasc Surg* 2001; **9**(suppl 1): 15.

16 Chetty R, Batitang S, Nair R. Large artery vasculopathy in HIV positive patients: Another vasculitic enigma. *Human Pathol* 2000; **31**: 374–9.

17 Nair R, Robbs RV, Chetty R, Naidoo NG, Woolgar J. Occlusive arterial disease in HIV-infected patients: a preliminary report. *Eur J Vasc Endovasc Surg* 2000; **20**: 353–7.

18 Chi D, Henry J, Kelly J, *et al.* The effects of HIV infection on endothelial function. *Endothelium* 2000; **7**: 233–42.

19 Blann A, Constans J, Dignat-George F, Seigneur M. The platelet and endothelium in HIV infection. *Br J Haematol* 1998; **100**: 613–14.

20 Bloom EJ, Abrams DI, Rogers G. Lupus anticoagulant in the acquired immunodeficiency syndrome. *JAMA* 1988; **256**: 491–3.

21 Lafeuillade A, Alessi MC, Martin-Poizot I, *et al.* Protein S deficiency in HIV infection. *N Engl J Med* 1991; **324**: 1220.

22 Von Kaulla E, Von Kaulla KN. Antithrombin 111 and diseases. *Am J Clin Pathol* 1967; **48**: 69–80.

23 Grunfeld C, Kotler DP, Hamadeh R, *et al.* Hypertriglyceridemia in the acquired immunodeficiency syndrome. *Am J Med* 1989; **86**: 27–31.

24 Behrens G, Dejam A, Schmidt H, *et al.* Impaired glucose tolerance and beta cell function and lipid metabolism in HIV patients under treatment with protease inhibitors. *AIDS* 1999; **13**: F63–70.

25 Diettrich NA, Cacioppo JC, Kaplan G, Cohen SM. A growing spectrum of surgical disease in patients with human immunodeficiency virus/acquired immunodeficiency syndrome: experience with 120 major cases. *Arch Surg* 1991; **126**: 860–6.

26 Binderow SR, Cavallo RJ, Freed J. Laboratory parameters as predictors of operative outcome of major abdominal surgery in AIDS and HIV infected patients. *Am Surg* 1993; **59**: 754–7.

27 Whitney TM, Brunel W, Russel TR, *et al.* Emergent abdominal surgery in AIDS: experience in San Fransico. *Am J Surg* 1994; **168**: 239–43.

28 Bizer LS, Pettorino R, Ashikari A. Emergency abdominal operations in the patient with acquired immunodeficiency syndrome. *J Am Coll Surg* 1995; **180**: 205–9.

29 Yii MK, Saunder A, Scott DF. Abdominal Surgery in HIV/AIDS patients: indications, operative management, pathology and outcome. *Aust N Z J Surg* 1995; **65**: 320–6.

30 Savioz D, Lironi A, Zurbuchen P, *et al.* Acute right iliac fossa pain in acquired immunodeficiency: a comparison between patients with and without acquired immune deficiency syndrome. *Br J Surg* 1996; **83**: 644–6.

31 Savioz D, Chilkot M, Ludwig C, *et al.* Preoperative counts of CD 4 T-lymphocytes and early postoperative infective complications in HIV-positive patients. *Eur J Surg* 1998; **164**: 483–7.

32 La Raja RD, Rothenberg RE, Odom JW, Mueller SC. The incidence of intra-abdominal surgery in acquired immunodeficiency syndrome: a statistical revue of 904 patients. *Surgery* 1989; **105**: 175–9.

33 Consten EC, Slors FJ, Noten HJ, *et al.* Anorectal surgery in human immunodeficiency virus-infected patients. Clinical outcome in relation to immune status. *Dis Colon Rectum* 1995; **38**: 1169–75.

34 Tran HS, Moncure M, Tarnoff M, *et al.* Predictors of operative outcome in patients with human immunodeficiency virus infection and acquired immunodeficiency syndrome. *Am J Surg* 2000; **180**: 228–33.

35 Paiement GD, Hymes RA, LaDouceur MS, *et al.* Postoperative infections in asymptomatic HIV-seropositive orthopedic trauma patients. *J Trauma Inj Inf Crit Care* 1994; **37**: 545–51.

36 Mellors JW, Munoz AM, Giorgi JV. Plasma viral load in CD4+ lymphocytes as prognostic markers of HIV-1 infection. *Ann Intern Med* 1997; **126**: 946–54.

37 Hughes MD, Daniels MJ, Fischl MA, *et al.* CD 4 cell count as a surrogate endpoint in HIV clinical trials: a meta-analyses of studies of AIDS Clinical Trials Group. *AIDS* 1998; **12**: 1823–32.

38 Binderow SR, Cavallo RJ, Freed J. Laboratory parameters as predictors of operative outcome after major abdominal surgery in AIDS- and HIV-infected patients. *Am Surg* 1993; **59**: 754–7.

39 Nair R, Chetty R, Woolgar J, *et al.* Spontaneous arteriovenous fistula resulting from HIV arteritis. *J Vasc Surg* 2001; **33**: 186–7.

40 Barbaro G. Cardiovascular manifestations of HIV infection. *J R Soc Med* 2001; **94**: 384–90.

41 Avidan MS, Jones N, Pozniak AL. The implications of HIV for the anaesthetist and the intensivist. *Anaesthesia* 2000; **55**: 344–54.

42 Drobniewski FA, Pozniak AL, Uttley AHC. Tuberculosis and AIDS. *J Med Microbiol* 1995; **43**: 85–91.

43 Price RW. Neurologic complications of HIV infection. *Lancet* 1996; **348**: 445–52.

44 Saber AA, Aboolian A, La Raja RD, *et al.* HIV/AIDS and the risk of deep vein thrombosis: a study of 45 patients with lower extremity involvement. *Am Surg* 2001; **67**: 645–7.

45 Van Dam-Mieras MC, Bruggemen CA, Muller AD, *et al.* Induction of endothelial cell procoagulant activity by cytomegalovirus infection. *Thromb Res* 1987; **47**: 69–75.

46 Lennard TW, Shenton BK, Borzotta A, *et al.* The influence of surgical operations on components of the human immune system. *Br J Surg* 1985; **72**: 771–6.

47 Tonnensen E, Wahlgreen C. Influence of extradural and general anaesthesia on natural killer cell activity and lymphocyte subpopulations in patients undergoing hysterectomy. *Br J Anaesth* 1988; **60**: 500–7.

48 Ayers J, Howton MJ, Layon AJ. Post-operative complications in patients with human immunodeficiency virus disease. Clinical data and literature review. *Chest* 1993; **103**: 1800–7.

49 Carrillo EH, Carrillo LE, Byers PM, *et al.* Penetrating trauma and emergency surgery in patients with AIDS. *Am J Surg* 1995; **170**: 341–4.

50 Guth AA, Hofstetter SR, Pachter HL. Human immunodeficiency virus and the trauma patient: factors influencing post-operative infectious complications. *J Trauma Inj Infect Crit Care* 1996; **41**: 251–6.

51 Palella FJ, Delaney KM, Moorman AC, *et al.* Declining morbidity and mortality among patients with advanced human immuno deficiency virus infection. *N Engl J Med* 1998; **338**: 853–60.

52 Carpenter CC, Cooper DA, Fischl MA, *et al.* Antiretroviral therapy in adults: updated recommendations of the International AIDS Society – USA panel. *JAMA* 2000; **283**: 381–90.

53 Centres for Disease Control and Prevention. Public Health Service guidelines for the management of health care worker exposure to HIV and recommendations for post exposure prophylaxis. *MMWR Morb and Mort Wkly Rep* 1998; **47**(RR-7): 1–33.

54 Department of Health. *Guidelines on post-exposure prophylaxis for healthcare workers occupationally exposed to HIV.* London: Department of Health, 1997.

46

Portal Hypertension and Variceal Bleeding

ROWAN W PARKS, THOMAS DIAMOND

THE PROBLEM

Although uncomplicated portal hypertension does not require treatment, urgent intervention is obviously indicated once bleeding occurs from oesophageal varices. Several treatment options are available, but the management will ultimately be tailored according to the medical fitness of the patient, and the medical facilities and local clinical expertise.[1] The availability of several non-operative therapies, including pharmacotherapy, balloon tamponade, endoscopic injection sclerotherapy, endoscopic variceal ligation and most recently transjugular intrahepatic portal–systemic **stent** shunt (TIPSS) has relegated emergency surgery to a secondary, yet very important, role in most institutions. Conservative therapy may be unsuccessful, and in this situation surgical intervention may be the only remaining alternative.

Therefore, the challenge is to recognise when non-operative treatments are failing or are unlikely to be successful so that surgery can be performed while the patient still has a chance of survival. Following successful management of an acute variceal bleed, the patient should be considered for definitive long term treatment. This chapter will outline the aetiology and pathophysiology of portal hypertension, the present methods of evaluation and the various therapeutic approaches available.

AETIOLOGY

Causes of portal hypertension can be categorised as pre-hepatic, intrahepatic and posthepatic. The intrahepatic causes can be further subdivided into presinusoidal, sinusoidal and postsinusoidal. Prehepatic portal hypertension is due to portal vein thrombosis, the cause of which is unknown in the majority of cases, but may be secondary to sepsis, trauma or malignant obstruction. By far the most common intrahepatic cause of portal hypertension in the USA and Europe is cirrhosis.[2] The pathogenesis of this sinusoidal obstruction to portal flow is varied and includes alcohol abuse, which is the most common cause, viral hepatitis, primary and secondary biliary cirrhosis and haemochromatosis. In terms of the actual incidence of portal hypertension worldwide, schistosomiasis is probably the most common cause,[3] the parasite producing portal tract fibrosis responsible for the 'pipe-stem' appearance on macroscopic examination. The importance of this presinusoidal block is that liver function is usually normal,[4] accounting for a much improved prognosis.[5] Postsinusoidal or posthepatic causes of portal hypertension result from hepatic vein thrombosis either as a major vein thrombosis (Budd–Chiari syndrome) or small vessel veno-occlusive disease.[6]

PATHOPHYSIOLOGY

Normal portal pressure is 5–10 mmHg with a portal flow in the order of 1–1.5 L/min. Portal hypertension represents a rise in portal pressure exceeding 12 mmHg. Portal hypertension was previously considered to arise solely as a consequence of increased resistance to portal venous blood flow, the 'backward flow' theory. Recent experimental and clinical studies, however, have shown both increased resistance to portal blood flow and increased portal blood flow. The characteristic finding in patients with liver cirrhosis is systemic and splanchnic vasodilatation due to a decrease in vascular tone. Circulating vasodilators, for example nitric oxide, have been implicated in the aetiology of the vasodilatation associated with portal hypertension. The recognition of vasodilatation and hyperdynamic circulation has led to the 'forward flow' theory, which proposes that increased portal venous inflow plays a central role in the pathogenesis of portal hypertension and this is independent of the resistance in the portal venous and collateral circulations.

Patients with portal hypertension characteristically develop portal–systemic collateral channels at sites where the splanchnic and systemic circulations meet, namely the gastro-oesophageal junction, the haemorrhoidal junction, the peri-umbilical veins, the retroperitoneal veins of Retzius and the perihepatic veins of Sappey. The collateral circulation only partially decompresses the portal venous system. In some cases blood may be shunted through the collateral circulation in sufficient quantities to cause a reversal of flow in the portal vein, i.e. hepatofugal or retrograde flow.[7]

Interestingly, it is usually only the lower oesophageal varices that bleed. Although increased portal pressure is essential for the development of varices, the raised hydrostatic pressure alone cannot be the only factor responsible since there is a poor correlation between the height of portal pressure and the risk of bleeding.[8] The two most important risk factors that determine the risk of variceal haemorrhage are the severity of liver disease and the size of the varices.[9] Studies have shown that large varices are more likely to rupture at lower transmural pressures than are small varices.[10] Endoscopic features such as 'red spots' and 'wale' markings have been reported to be important in the prediction of variceal haemorrhage. These features represent changes in variceal wall structure and tension associated with the development of microtelangiectasias.

Varices may also occur in the gastric fundus, but they are a source of bleeding in only 5 per cent of cases. Dilatation of the gastric submucosal veins results in portal hypertensive gastropathy which affects mainly the fundus and body of the stomach and produces an erythematous appearance at endoscopy. An interesting, but rare, form of localised portal hypertension, known as left-sided, segmental, or 'sinistral' portal hypertension, occurs in those with splenic vein thrombosis and should be suspected in patients presenting with bleeding oesophageal or gastric varices and normal liver function.

CLINICAL DIAGNOSIS

Cirrhosis results in two major events, namely hepatocellular failure and portal hypertension. Patients with cirrhosis may have non-specific symptoms such as general malaise,

Table 46.1 *Grading of portal hypertension: Child–Pugh classification*

	Number of points		
	1	2	3
Bilirubin (μmol/L)*	<34	34–51	>51
Albumin (g/L)	>35	28–35	<28
Prothrombin time prolonged by (s)	<3	3–10	>10
Ascites	None	Slight to moderate	Moderate to severe
Encephalopathy	None	Slight to moderate	Moderate to severe

Grade A 5–6 points; grade B 7–9 points; grade C 10–15 points.
* In primary biliary cirrhosis, the point scoring for bilirubin level is adjusted as follows: 1, <68; 2, 68–170; 3, >170.

anorexia or abdominal pain. The clinical signs of chronic liver failure include leuconychia, finger clubbing, palmar erythema, spider naevi, gynaecomastia (or breast atrophy in females), testicular atrophy and loss of secondary sexual hair. The existence of portal hypertension is recognised by splenomegaly and abdominal wall venous collaterals, caput medusa being the classic manifestation.

The main complications of portal hypertension are variceal bleeding, ascites and hepatic failure. Variceal bleeding is the most dramatic of these complications, but hepatic failure is the major determinant of survival.

Disease severity is assessed by a combination of clinical parameters and standard laboratory tests. The Child–Pugh classification is used to standardise the staging of the disease. The combination of ascites and encephalopathy, bilirubin concentration, albumin concentration and prothrombin time are evaluated and scored (Table 46.1).[2] A total score from the five parameters classifies the patient as Child–Pugh grade A (score 5–6), grade B (score 7–9) or grade C (score 10–15).

INVESTIGATIONS

In the acute situation, **blood tests** for the emergency evaluation of haematocrit, haemoglobin, coagulation status and serum electrolytes are essential. Liver function tests and serum albumin concentration give an indication of liver function. Specific serological markers for hepatitis A, B and C may help define the aetiology,[2] while serological assessment of autoimmune disease and primary biliary cirrhosis should be routine.

Although the level of activity of the underlying liver disease may be apparent from standard biochemical tests, **percutaneous needle biopsy** may be used to demonstrate the presence of cirrhosis and to assess its activity.

Upper gastrointestinal **endoscopy** is an essential procedure in the assessment of oesophageal varices. In the patient who is actively bleeding or has just stopped bleeding, it is important to establish the exact diagnosis and source of bleeding by endoscopy but only after adequate resuscitation and restoration of haemodynamic stability. Administration of 10–20 mg metoclopramide intravenously prior to endoscopy may produce a temporary cessation of bleeding permitting blood and clot to be evacuated from the stomach and facilitate the visualisation of all potential bleeding sources. In approximately 10 per cent of all patients presenting with upper gastrointestinal haemorrhage in the Western world, oesophageal varices are the cause of bleeding. In addition, in patients with known portal hypertension and oesophageal varices, or in those in whom the presence of portal hypertension is suspected from the history and examination, non-oesophageal variceal sources will be found in 10–25 per cent.

These sources include gastritis, peptic ulceration, Mallory–Weiss tears, gastric varices or portal hypertensive gastropathy. It is important to recognise these causes of bleeding in determining further therapeutic strategies as some techniques, such as balloon tamponade or sclerotherapy, which would be indicated in patients with oesophageal varices arc inappropriate in those with gastric varices or portal hypertensive gastropathy. When there is difficulty in identifying the exact cause of bleeding, endoscopy should be repeated.[11] In the patient being evaluated in a non-acute situation, the varices should be graded for size, tortuosity, and factors for risk of bleeding. The detailed definition by some groups[12,13] of cherry red spots, varices upon varices, and the size of varices as prognostic risk factors of further bleeding has proved useful.[2]

Radiological studies are an integral part of evaluation. Ultrasound combined with Doppler study of the vessels, computed tomography (CT) and angiography may be indicated.[14,15] The morphology of the liver can be assessed with ultrasound and CT. Ultrasound is also useful in demonstrating the portal and hepatic veins. When ultrasound is combined with Doppler flow measurements, directional flow may be depicted in these vessels. Arteriography and hepatic venography are used to demonstrate anatomy and to measure venous pressures, two mandatory investigations prior to shunt surgery. If the patient's history and laboratory findings suggest cirrhosis secondary to extrahepatic biliary obstruction, cholangiography should be performed.

MANAGEMENT

The management of bleeding oesophageal varices begins with emergency resuscitation and initial control of the bleeding episode and continues with long term treatment to eradicate the varices and reduce the risk of further bleeding. In general, both the emergency and long term

management of these patients is best undertaken in a specialised centre where experienced medical and nursing staff have the necessary facilities.

EMERGENCY RESUSCITATION AND CONTROL OF BLEEDING VARICES

Resuscitation

The initial resuscitation of a patient with bleeding oesophageal varices is similar to that for any patient with upper gastrointestinal haemorrhage. A wide bore (16 gauge) cannula is required for the administration of colloidal fluids, packed red cells and coagulation factors in the form of fresh frozen plasma. Saline infusions should be avoided because of the risk of fluid retention and aggravation of ascites. Central venous and arterial lines are necessary to monitor response and to record the blood pressure. Excessive transfusion or fluid administration should also be avoided as this may increase the risk of further bleeding by overexpansion of the circulating blood volume. Comatose patients and those with massive haematemesis may require endotracheal intubation to prevent aspiration.

Pharmacotherapy

Several pharmacological agents are available for the emergency control of variceal bleeding. Most of these act by lowering portal venous pressure but others are thought to act by constricting the lower oesophageal sphincter, hence strangulating the varices and arresting haemorrhage.

Vasoactive drugs have been widely used for the past four decades in an attempt to control bleeding from oesophageal varices. Vasopressin was the first drug used to induce splanchnic vasoconstriction,[16] but it is effective in only half of the patients treated[17] and its use is associated with the development of major complications in approximately 25 per cent of patients.[17,18] Even the use of an analogue of vasopressin, terlipressin (triglycyl-lysine-vasopressin; Glypressin), or concomitant administration of the hormone with nitrates has failed to produce convincing benefits with respect to both the control of bleeding and reduction of side effects.[19]

The vasoactive peptide hormone somatostatin has a wide spectrum of actions. Although in pharmacological doses somatostatin has only a moderate vasoconstrictive effect on the splanchnic vasculature, it reduces oesophageal variceal pressure and has been shown to be beneficial in the treatment of bleeding varices. The results of several randomised controlled trials suggest that variceal bleeding can be controlled in 65–70 per cent of patients treated, avoiding major complications but without necessarily significantly reducing the mortality.[20,21] Somatostatin has a half-life of less than 3 minutes, necessitating continuous intravenous infusion to achieve a therapeutic response. This short half-life together with its relatively non-specific effects and the rebound hormonal hypersecretion on cessation of infusion, have severely limited its clinical use.

The more recently developed somatostatin analogue octreotide, however, has a much more selective action than somatostatin, is longer acting and is also less expensive. Infusion of octreotide at 25 μg/hour has been shown in one study to be as effective as balloon tamponade of the oesophagus in controlling variceal bleeding in the acute situation and has less associated morbidity and mortality.[22] Five randomised controlled trials have found somatostatin[23,24] or octreotide[25–27] to be equally effective with fewer associated complications than injection sclerotherapy in controlling initial variceal haemorrhage. Furthermore, both somatostatin and octreotide have been shown to be very effective in controlling early postinjection sclerotherapy bleeding, which can occur from the varices themselves, or from oesophageal ulceration or oesophagitis.[28] This observation would suggest that both somatostatin and octreotide are useful as adjuvant treatment to injection sclerotherapy. Vasoactive therapy for control of variceal bleeding remains an attractive proposition since it is the only treatment that can be initiated, without specialist expertise, as soon as the patient enters hospital. Preliminary studies also suggest that octreotide is very effective in controlling severe gastric bleeding in patients with portal hypertensive gastropathy or gastric varices.[29] Octreotide should be administered intravenously as either 500 μg in 500 mL of 5 per cent dextrose over 12 hours, or 500 μg in 60 mL of 5 per cent dextrose over 12 hours via a syringe driver.

Agents that act by a constrictor effect on the lower oesophageal sphincter include pentagastrin and metoclopramide.[30,31]

The risk of encephalopathy is reduced by the administration of neomycin (250 mg–1 g four times daily), to reduce the number of ammonia-producing bacteria in the bowel, and lactulose (10–30 mL three times daily) to increase gut motility and lower faecal pH, hence reducing ammonia absorption. Lactulose may also produce some benefit via an antiendotoxin effect.

Oesophageal tamponade

Balloon tamponade is an effective method of achieving temporary control of variceal bleeding (70–90 per cent) but in view of the high rate of recurrent bleeding (60 per cent) after removal of the tube, it should be reserved for selected situations. These include instances of continued massive bleeding because varices cannot be sclerosed, when surgical intervention is required because acute sclerotherapy has failed, and prior to transfer of a bleeding patient to a specialised centre.

In general it is unwise, and even hazardous, to insert a balloon tube in a patient before a definite diagnosis has been made by endoscopy. If upper gastrointestinal haemorrhage from an oesophageal or gastric neoplasm is mistaken for variceal bleeding, an inexperienced clinician may inflate the gastric balloon within the oesophagus and rupture the latter. With adequate resuscitation and use of pharmacological agents, particularly octreotide, insertion of a balloon tube prior to endoscopy is now rarely necessary. The one exception is possibly the patient with a previous history of varices or a clinical picture strongly suggestive of portal hypertension, presenting with bleeding and haemodynamic instability which does not respond to resuscitation and pharmacotherapy.

The four-lumen (Sengstaken–Blakemore or Minnesota) tube (Fig. 46.1), which is most commonly used, should be stored in a refrigerator to render it less pliable, thus facilitating insertion. Both balloons of a fresh tube are tested for leaks prior to insertion, the nasal route being preferred as it is ultimately more comfortable for the patient. Once in the stomach, the gastric balloon is filled with 200 mL of air and pulled back to impinge on the cardia. The oesophageal balloon is then inflated with air to obtain an intraluminal pressure of approximately 40 mmHg, estimated by using a blood pressure manometer. The tube is strapped to the nares in this position but no traction is necessary. Test aspiration via the gastric lumen of the tube is undertaken approximately every 15 minutes to check for further bleeding, and this lumen may also be used for administration of neomycin and lactulose. A fourth lumen allows aspiration of the upper oesophagus and pharynx in order to reduce the risk of bronchial aspiration. In patients who are stuporous or comatose, the airway should be protected by an endotracheal tube. The use of oesophageal tamponade is a temporary holding measure until definitive therapy is instituted. The oesophageal balloon is generally deflated after 12–24 hours to prevent oesophageal ulceration, but the position

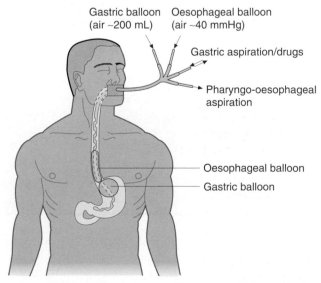

Figure 46.1 *Use of a four-lumen (Sengstaken–Blakemore) tube for oesophageal tamponade*

of the gastric balloon may be maintained. If bleeding recurs the oesophageal balloon may be reinflated but by this stage a more definitive line of therapy should be established. If re-bleeding does not occur within the subsequent 24 hour period, the gastric balloon is deflated and the tube removed, but these patients too will require definitive treatment.

Complications of balloon tamponade occur in about 10–20 per cent of patients[32] and include pressure damage to the surface of the oesophagus causing mucosal ulceration, oesophageal perforation and aspiration pneumonia. Some patients find the tube uncomfortable and often become distressed and agitated.

Injection sclerotherapy

Crafoord and Frenckner first described injection sclerotherapy in 1939 in the management of acute bleeding in a patient with portal vein thrombosis.[33] In 1973 Johnston and Rodgers reported their 15 year experience with 195 administrations of injection sclerotherapy for acute bleeding in 117 patients.[34] Control of bleeding was obtained in 93 per cent of patients, and the hospital mortality was 18 per cent. In the following two decades, endoscopic injection sclerotherapy became the most frequently used form of therapy for both emergency and long term control of variceal haemorrhage.[35]

The technique relies on the obliteration of varices by a process of sclerosis and fibrosis. Several methods are used to achieve this objective, including intravariceal injection of sclerosant, which is the most widely used method,[1,36] and paravariceal or submucosal injection,[37] which aims to produce an area of fibrosis and thickening superficial to the varices. Some sclerotherapists use a combination of the intravariceal and paravariceal methods, in an attempt to combine the advantages of each.[38] Various sclerosing agents are used, including ethanolamine oleate, sodium tetradecyl sulphate, polidocanol, and more recently the tissue adhesive N-butyl-2-cyanoacrylate (Histoacryl).[28,39–41] The fact that several agents are available, and are effective, probably indicates that no one in particular is vastly superior to the others.

Injection sclerotherapy can be performed using either a rigid oesophagoscope or a fibreoptic endoscope. Both have advantages and disadvantages, although the latter is more commonly used nowadays. If one uses the rigid instrument, a general anaesthetic is required, but this gives the reassurance of a protected airway. The technique for the passage of the rigid instrument requires more training and skill. The advantages are that the tip of the rigid instrument can be used to compress any bleeding point and the wide bore channel allows the passage of a large sucker for removal of blood or clot. Rotation of the instrument allows compression of the varix following injection of sclerosant. The flexible instrument is technically easier to pass, carries less risk of

oesophageal damage and general anaesthesia is unnecessary. The main disadvantages are the problem of removing blood efficiently during active haemorrhage and the difficulty in providing adequate compression of the varix after injection to ensure the necessary intimal damage.

Complications of injection sclerotherapy are generally minor and include low grade fever, retrosternal discomfort and oesophageal ulceration or mucosal sloughing. More serious complications, which are generally rare, include oesophageal perforation, oesophageal stricture, pleural effusion and empyema. With repeated injection sclerotherapy sessions, complications become cumulative.[42] If oesophageal ulceration becomes a significant problem either somatostatin[43] or omeprazole[44] or both may be used.

In most centres, the initial sclerotherapy is performed at the time of diagnostic endoscopy, and succeeds in controlling acute variceal bleeding in the majority (over 70 per cent) of patients,[45] while in the remainder, a second sclerotherapy session is necessary. Following either one or two injection sessions, acute bleeding will be controlled in 90–95 per cent of patients.[46,47] Failure of acute sclerotherapy is defined as failure to control acute bleeding after two emergency injection treatments during a single hospital admission.[48,49] Such patients should be controlled with balloon tamponade and should undergo TIPSS or be considered for one of the more major surgical options. These include portal–systemic shunt, oesophageal transection/devascularisation or liver transplantation.

During a 37-year period in Belfast, injection sclerotherapy using the rigid instrument was used for the control of acute variceal bleeding. Between 1958 and 1995, 436 patients had a total of 734 injections during 663 admissions for acute bleeding. Bleeding was controlled in 94 per cent of patients, and only 6 per cent of patients required more than one injection for control. The hospital mortality rate was 15 per cent and, of these, 63 per cent were categorised as Child's grade C.

The results for sclerotherapy in the treatment of acutely bleeding gastric varices have generally been poor, although reports on the use of Histoacryl glue have been very encouraging.[50–52] Injection sclerotherapy is not indicated in patients with bleeding due to portal hypertensive gastropathy. In these cases TIPSS or an emergency surgical procedure is indicated if pharmacotherapy fails.

Variceal ligation

Endoscopic variceal ligation (EVL),[53] introduced in 1988, is based on the same principle as banding of haemorrhoids. The target varix is identified and the scope advanced under direct vision until the banding cylinder is in full contact with the varix. The varix is sucked into a chamber attached to the tip of the endoscope resulting in a complete 'redout' and loss of endoscopic visibility. An elastic 'O' band, mounted on the chamber, is then released over the varix by pulling on a trip wire which runs through the working channel of the endoscope. The engorged varix is strangulated at the mucosal junction. Treatment involves ligation of the most distal variceal columns, commencing with the bleeding varix if present. Subsequent ligations are performed at increasingly higher levels, proceeding in a spiral fashion to avoid circumferential placement of bands at the same level. A mechanism which allows repeated banding and obviates the need to use an overtube for repeated removal of the endoscope has been developed recently. The most impressive advantage of EVL is its simplicity. In contrast to endoscopic sclerotherapy, which requires intensive operator training in order to obtain good results, EVL is relatively easy to learn and perform competently.[54]

The technique has proved successful not only in the treatment of acute variceal bleeding, but also in long term management aimed at eradicating varices, as confirmed in a prospective randomised controlled clinical trial comparing this technique with sclerotherapy.[55] The technique has also been successfully used for patients who failed to respond to injection sclerotherapy.[56] Reports of complications of EVL include bleeding or perforation caused by the overtube,[57,58] bleeding from a band induced ulcer and acute oesophageal obstruction caused by banded oesophageal varices.[59]

Portal–systemic shunt procedures

Until the use of sclerotherapy became widespread in the early 1970s portal–systemic shunts were widely used for the treatment of acute variceal bleeding. Shunt surgery has, however, been associated with high operative mortality of 7–30 per cent and a low 5-year survival, particularly in patients with marked hepatic functional decompensation. For these reasons portal–systemic shunting for acute variceal bleeding is not performed routinely in the vast majority of centres and is reserved for the 5–10 per cent of patients in whom bleeding is not controlled by pharmacotherapy or endoscopic techniques. It also remains a useful treatment in countries with a high incidence of non-cirrhotic portal hypertension that occurs during the second or third decade of life.

Orloff, the main proponent of emergency shunt procedures, reported an operative mortality rate of 20 per cent and a 5-year survival rate of 64 per cent in a series of 94 consecutive unselected patients who underwent surgery within 8 hours of admission to hospital.[60] A controlled trial by Orloff's group comparing routine emergency shunting with conventional medical management followed by elective shunting showed better control of haemorrhage and improved early and late survival in the emergency shunt group.[61] Major criticisms of this trial are, first, that endoscopic sclerotherapy, the gold standard for treatment of acute variceal bleeding in most centres, was not used in the medical treatment arm and, second, crossover to surgical treatment for patients who failed medical therapy was not allowed.

If surgery is required in the acute situation, the quickest and simplest procedure is probably the safest. Many surgeons therefore favour the end-to-side portacaval shunt or the interposition mesocaval shunt.[62] Both these procedures, however, completely divert portal flow away from the liver and thereby tend to cause more frequent episodes of encephalopathy than do those following devascularisation procedures and selective shunts.[63] The high incidence of postoperative encephalopathy, which is often chronic and incapacitating, accounts for the trend away from portal–systemic shunts in recent years despite the fact that they prevent recurrent variceal bleeding in virtually all patients.

Clear indications for emergency surgical intervention in many institutions include persistent variceal bleeding despite non-operative treatment with endoscopic techniques, failure of chronic sclerotherapy or EVL, and bleeding from gastric varices or portal hypertensive gastropathy which is unresponsive to acute pharmacotherapy. In our practice, we virtually never use emergency shunt procedures for acute variceal bleeding.

Transjugular intrahepatic portal–systemic stent shunting

A method for producing an intrahepatic portal–systemic stent shunt via the transjugular route was first described in animals by Rosch et al. in 1969.[64] The first transjugular portal–systemic shunt procedure in a patient was described in 1982 when balloon catheters were inflated to produce a tract between the portal and hepatic vein.[65] The success of metallic expandable stents to improve patency rates since 1989 has resulted in an increasing use of this technique.[66]

The internal jugular vein, usually on the right side, is punctured and a sheath is inserted cannulating the right or middle hepatic vein under radiological screening. Then a transjugular liver biopsy needle or sharp stylet is directed out of the hepatic vein, through the liver parenchyma and into a large branch of the portal vein. After passing a guide wire into the portal vein, an angioplasty balloon catheter is used to expand the tract before inserting a metallic stent (Palmaz or Wallstent) (Fig. 46.2).

At present the main indication for this technique is to control and prevent variceal haemorrhage when endoscopic therapy has failed.[67–69] It has been shown in numerous uncontrolled studies that TIPSS reduces re-bleeding in patients with recurrent variceal haemorrhage.[70,71] A recent meta-analysis[72] evaluated 11 randomised trials comparing TIPSS with endoscopic treatment for prevention of variceal re-bleeding and survival. Transjugular intrahepatic portal– systemic stent shunting was compared with sclerotherapy alone in five studies, with sclerotherapy plus propranolol in three studies and with EVL alone in three studies. Overall, TIPSS significantly reduced the re-bleeding rate but did not improve overall survival rate and was associated with a significantly higher incidence of post-treatment

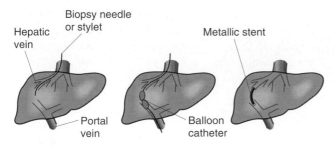

Figure 46.2 *Technique to create an intrahepatic portal–systemic stent shunt*

encephalopathy compared with endoscopic treatment. Although some authors consider TIPSS to be the preferred first line treatment for uncontrolled variceal haemorrhage,[73,74] most support the view that TIPSS should be a rescue procedure for failures of medical/endoscopic treatments.[75,76]

One advantage of TIPSS is that, being an intrahepatic procedure, the extrahepatic venous anatomy is not disturbed and subsequent liver transplantation can, if required, be more easily performed.[74,77] Transjugular intrahepatic portal–systemic stent shunting can also be employed before closure of a surgical portal–systemic shunt which is causing disabling encephalopathy, and it can also be used to relieve intractable ascites.

Transjugular intrahepatic portal–systemic stent shunting is successfully completed in more than 90 per cent of patients, with a procedure related mortality of less than 1 per cent caused mainly by intraperitoneal bleeding.[67] The major side effect of a successfully placed TIPSS is new or worse encephalopathy, which develops in approximately 15–25 per cent of cases.[78] In most cases the symptoms are mild and are readily treated with dietary protein restriction and lactulose therapy.[74] Re-bleeding occurs in 10–20 per cent of patients,[67] and is usually associated with shunt related complications, such as intimal hyperplasia, shunt migration or thrombosis. Therefore, a vigorous surveillance programme is mandatory for the prompt diagnosis and correction of any significant stent dysfunction and to minimise the risk of re-bleeding. Doppler ultrasonography has been used for evaluation of shunt patency, but its sensitivity is inferior to angiography.[79] In cases of shunt occlusion, either a further shunt may be inserted or balloon dilatation of the existing shunt can be carried out.

Oesophageal transection/devascularisation

The alternative to portal–systemic shunting for surgical control of acutely bleeding oesophageal varices is transection of the oesophagus and end-to-end anastomosis using a stapling gun.[49] The aim of this procedure is to remove a segment of the lower 1–3 cm of the oesophagus, which is the most vulnerable in terms of variceal bleeding. Vankemmel

first reported the use of a circular stapling gun to perform oesophageal transection in 1974.[80] It is a relatively simple operation, compared with portal–systemic shunting, but carries a similar mortality. As the portal circulation is not disturbed, postoperative encephalopathy is generally not a problem. The disadvantage of this procedure, however, is that, although acute bleeding may be controlled in over 95 per cent of patients, there is, in contrast to shunt procedures, a significant rate of recurrent variceal bleeding, approximating 30 per cent over the next 5–10 years.

Oesophageal transection (Fig. 46.3) is performed through an upper midline incision. The left gastric venous drainage is ligated in continuity at the upper border of the pancreas in order to interrupt the main connection between the hypertensive portal vein and the varices. The oesophagus is then mobilised, protecting the anterior and posterior vagi. A linen ligature is passed around the oesophagus prior to insertion of the gun. The closed gun is introduced into the lower third of the oesophagus via a small anterior gastrotomy wound, and then slackened off to give a gap of about 3 cm. The linen ligature is then tightened around the oesophagus immediately above the cardia thus invaginating a flange of full thickness wall between the two portions of the head of the gun. The gap in the head of the gun is tightened and the trigger pulled to complete the transection (see Fig. 46.3a). It is necessary to reopen the gap on the head of the gun before withdrawing it through the newly formed anastomosis. The excised portion of oesophageal wall should form a complete 'doughnut', indicating a satisfactory transection.

The incidence of recurrent bleeding may be decreased by a combination of oesophageal transection and devascularisation of the lower oesophagus and upper stomach (see Fig. 46.3b), but this may increase the operative risk. An even more extensive operation involves a thoracoabdominal approach, with oesophageal transection and extensive devascularisation of the oesophagus and upper stomach, including a vagotomy, pyloroplasty and splenectomy (Sugiura operation) (see Fig. 46.3c).[81] This combined procedure, which was used extensively in Japan with excellent reported results in terms of operative complications and re-bleeding,[82] is now less popular there and has never become established in Western practice.

Control of active variceal bleeding

- Resuscitation
  - Insert two 16 gauge peripheral cannulae
  - Correct coagulation abnormalities
  - Central venous access
  - Protect airway by elective intubation if patient has severe uncontrollable variceal bleeding, severe encephalopathy, inability to maintain oxygen saturations above 90 per cent, or aspiration pneumonia

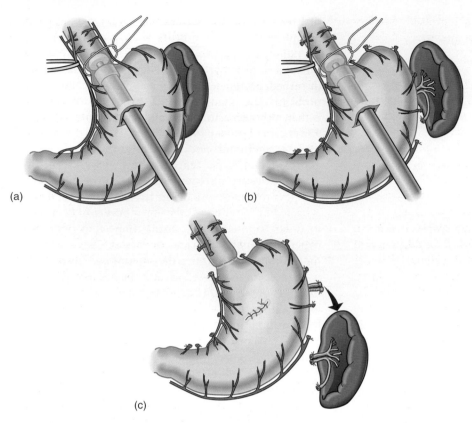

Figure 46.3 *Oesophageal transection/devascularisation procedures: (a) oesophageal transection, (b) oesophageal transection and devascularisation and (c) Sugiura operation*

- Control of bleeding
  - Proceed to upper gastrointestinal endoscopy as soon as patient is haemodynamically stable
  - Variceal band ligation is the method of first choice
  - If banding is difficult because of continuing bleeding, or this technique is not available, endoscopic injection sclerotherapy should be performed
  - If endoscopy is unavailable, vasoconstrictors such as a octreotide or terlispressin should be administered, or a Sengstaken–Blakemore tube should be inserted
- Failure to control active bleeding
  - If bleeding is difficult to control, a Sengstaken–Blakemore tube should be inserted until further endoscopic treatment, TIPSS, or surgical intervention
  - Specialist help should be sought and patient transferred to a specialist centre
  - Choice of TIPSS or other emergency surgical procedure should be decided depending on local expertise

Over a 19-year period, a total of 139 stapled oesophageal transections with devascularisation were performed in Belfast. Twenty-nine procedures were performed as an emergency, with eight deaths, giving a mortality rate of 28 per cent; this compares with a mortality rate of 14 per cent for the 110 patients who underwent elective procedures.

LONG TERM AND DEFINITIVE TREATMENT

During their lifetime some 70 per cent of patients will have a further variceal bleed, the highest incidence and associated mortality rate being during the first few months following the first haemorrhage, and the chance of survival returning to baseline thereafter.[83] There is general agreement that some form of specific long term treatment is usually indicated.

The only form of treatment that cures both the underlying liver disease and the portal hypertension is liver transplantation. Patients presenting with bleeding oesophageal varices nowadays should all be considered for liver transplantation.[84] Only a small percentage will ultimately receive a transplant, but management in possible transplant candidates should subsequently be directed to forms of therapy that will not interfere with any subsequent transplant procedure.

The alternatives to liver transplantation are long term pharmacological management, repeated injection sclerotherapy, repeated variceal ligation, a devascularisation and transection operation, or a portal–systemic shunt procedure.

Long term pharmacotherapy

Although drugs have been used in the treatment of acute variceal bleeding for many years, pharmacotherapy has only recently been investigated and used for the long term prevention of recurrent variceal haemorrhage. The mechanism of action of long term pharmacotherapy is probably a reduction in portal pressure brought about by splanchnic arteriolar vasoconstriction.

Nine published randomised controlled trials have compared β-blockers (propranolol or nadolol) to a placebo for the prevention of recurrent variceal haemorrhage. A meta-analysis of these trials shows a significant reduction in re-bleeding but not in mortality.[85] A number of recent studies have combined administration of isosorbide-5-mononitrate (ISMN) with non-selective β-blockade in preventing variceal rebleeding. Patch *et al.* randomised 102 patients surviving a variceal bleed to EVL or drug therapy using propranolol with the addition of ISMN if target reductions in portal pressure evaluated by the hepatic venous pressure gradient (HVPG), were not achieved at 3 months.[86] Overall, results of drug therapy were similar to those of EVL with no differences in survival or non-bleeding complications. Recent data suggest that reducing HVPG by 20 per cent or more, or reducing portal pressure to 12 mmHg is associated with a marked reduction in the long term risk of developing complications of portal hypertension and is associated with improved survival.[87] 'A la carte' treatment of portal hypertension is being proposed by several authors, suggesting that adaption of medical therapy to the haemodynamic response is important in the management strategy of patients with portal hypertension. Burroughs and McCormick treated 34 patients suffering from cirrhosis and portal hypertension with propranolol and measured HVPG after a median of 4 days.[88] Target HVPG reductions were achieved in 13 'responders'. Isosorbide-5-mononitrate was added in the 21 'non-responders' and HVPG measured again. Seven further patients achieved target HVPG reduction. Bleeding rates were lower in responders than in non-responders. The authors concluded that the haemodynamic response to drug therapy identified patients who were efficiently protected from variceal re-bleeding and suggested that alternative treatment should be considered for non-responders.

Other agents currently being investigated for use in long term pharmacotherapy include calcium channel blockers such as verapamil, serotonin antagonists and octreotide. Drug therapy, however, has disadvantages, such as the cost of lifelong medication, problems with compliance in alcoholic patients and potential side effects.

Repeated injection sclerotherapy

Repeated injection sclerotherapy is currently the most widely used technique for the treatment of recurrent oesophageal variceal bleeding. If a programme of repeated sclerotherapy is thought to be the most appropriate long term therapeutic option, repeat injection sessions usually begin 1–2 weeks after the initial emergency session and are continued every 1–2 weeks until the varices have been completely eradicated. The interval between injection sessions varies in different centres; injections at weekly intervals produce earlier obliteration of varices but may be associated with a higher incidence of oesophageal mucosal sloughing and ulceration than injections at 2- or 3-weekly intervals. Once the varices have been eradicated, follow-up endoscopy is advised every 3–6 months.

The efficacy of long term sclerotherapy in eradicating varices, to prevent recurrent bleeding and ultimately improve survival, has been the subject of several trials. Meta-analysis of eight randomised controlled trials comparing sclerotherapy with a medically treated control group for the prevention of recurrent variceal bleeding has shown that the rebleeding rate is lower in patients who underwent injection sclerotherapy.[85] However, 45–60 per cent of patients treated by injection sclerotherapy will re-bleed some time later.[89] Many of these patients are successfully managed with subsequent sclerotherapy sessions, but the eventual failure rate of injection sclerotherapy is as high as 35 per cent.[90,91]

Failure of long term sclerotherapy is defined as massive bleeding requiring resuscitation and blood transfusion, or two or more bleeding episodes during the injection programme. In this situation a shunt procedure or possibly a devascularisation and transection operation should be considered.[47,92,93] In terms of improvement of overall survival it is generally perceived that sclerotherapy, while effective in treating acute variceal bleeding and reducing the risk of recurrent bleeding, does not improve long term survival. This is thought to be related to the fact that it is only a palliative procedure and does not alter the progression of the underlying disease process. However, a meta-analysis of the controlled trails comparing chronic sclerotherapy with conventional medical therapy shows a statistically significant survival advantage with the former technique.[94]

Repeated variceal ligation

Repeated EVL is an effective procedure for the eradication of oesophageal varices. Seven published trials comparing EVL with endoscopic injection sclerotherapy have been combined in a meta-analysis which included 547 patients.[95] This concluded that EVL carried a significantly lower rate of recurrent variceal bleeding, a decreased mortality rate and reduced complications such as oesophageal stricture, while fewer sessions were required to achieve variceal obliteration. Endoscopic variceal ligation is now considered in many centres to be the endoscopic treatment of choice for patients with bleeding oesophageal varices.[95,96]

It has been the experience of some, that the frequency of recurrence of oesophageal varices is higher following EVL and therefore a combination of EVL and injection sclerotherapy may prove to be a useful option – using EVL to treat large varices followed by a course of injection sclerotherapy for small varices and to achieve fibrosis of the inner wall of the oesophagus.[97] The additive effect of sclerotherapy to patients receiving repeated EVL has been shown in a prospective randomised trial to be safe and results

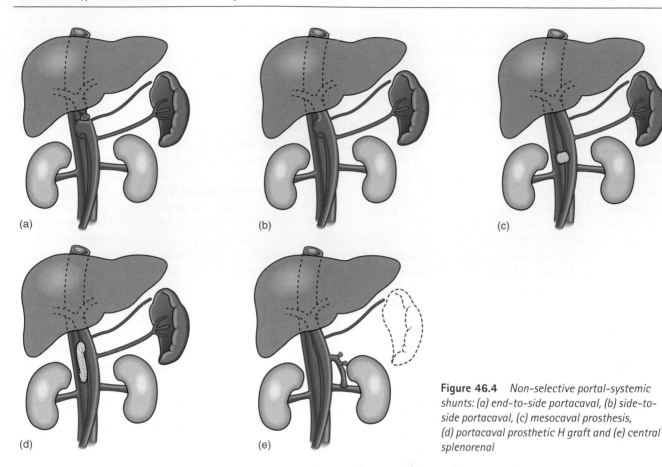

Figure 46.4 *Non-selective portal-systemic shunts: (a) end-to-side portacaval, (b) side-to-side portacaval, (c) mesocaval prosthesis, (d) portacaval prosthetic H graft and (e) central splenorenal*

in a significant reduction in the re-bleeding rate.[98] Other authors, however, have not shown any significant benefit of combination therapy and have reported that it is associated with a greater morbidity.[99–101]

Elective oesophageal transection/devascularisation

Transection/devascularisation procedures are being used less frequently for the elective or long term management of patients with variceal bleeding. This is probably related to the fact that, although they have the advantages of being relatively simple to perform and not associated with encephalopathy, they are associated with a high incidence of recurrent variceal bleeding (approximately 30 per cent). They may continue to have a limited role in some countries, where access to liver transplantation is not available and where the patient is unsuitable for a shunt procedure, namely, elderly patients, patients with advanced liver disease, diabetic patients, patients with schistosomiasis and those with previous encephalopathy.

Of the 139 stapled oesophageal transections with devascularisation in Belfast carried out between 1976 and 1995, 110 were elective operations, often performed during the same hospital admission but usually within a few weeks of the onset of bleeding. There were 23 operative deaths in the total series, 10 of these occurring in patients with Child's

grade C disease. Fifteen patients in the series required oesophageal dilatation because of stricture formation. Of the 117 patients who survived to leave hospital, 46 developed recurrent haemorrhage during a follow-up period ranging from 3 months to 19 years. In 30 patients recurrent varices were identified and treated with post-transection injection sclerotherapy. Often recurrent haemorrhage was of a minor nature, and only seven of those 46 patients died as a result of the bleeding. The overall 5-, 10- and 15-year cumulative survival rates for the whole series were 49 per cent, 32 per cent and 28 per cent, respectively.

Elective portal–systemic shunts

Although many types of portal–systemic shunt have been developed, they fall into two main groups, namely non-selective and selective. Non-selective shunts decompress the entire portal system and as a result the incidence of retrograde portal blood flow and the risk of postoperative encephalopathy are high. The diversion of portal flow away from the liver and the consequent loss of hepatotrophic factors, is thought to cause a deterioration of hepatocellular metabolism and function. Examples of these non-selective shunts include the standard end-to-side portacaval shunt, the side-to-side portacaval shunt, the mesocaval shunt using a prosthetic graft, the portacaval prosthetic H graft and the central splenorenal shunt (Fig. 46.4).

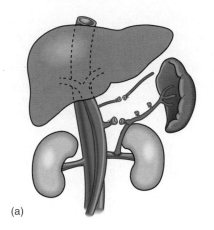 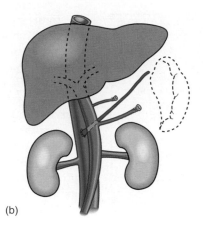

(a)   (b)

Figure 46.5 *Selective portal-systemic shunts: (a) Warren distal splenorenal and (b) Inokuchi left gastric–inferior venacaval*

One of the non-selective shunts, the portacaval prosthetic H graft, is worth further consideration. It has been suggested that by using a small diameter prosthesis, approximately 10 mm in diameter, the resistance of the shunt could be increased, thus decreasing the flux across the shunt and maintaining prograde or hepatopedal portal flow. The effect of the 'partial' shunt is not only to decompresses the portal system sufficiently to prevent recurrent variceal bleeding, but also to maintain prograde portal flow and prevent encephalopathy and deterioration in hepatocellular function;[102] the results have been encouraging in a few centres.[103–105] Other advantages are that it is a relatively easy shunt to construct and, as dissection in the area of the hepatic pedicle is minimal, subsequent orthoptic liver transplantation is not compromised.[104]

Selective shunts aim to decompress only a part of the portal system, namely the oesophago-gastric venous network, to prevent variceal bleeding while still maintaining portal venous pressure and prograde portal flow to avert encephalopathy.[106] Examples include the Warren distal splenorenal shunt and the Inokuchi left gastric–inferior vena caval shunt (Fig. 46.5). The Warren shunt is the most widely used and is reported to be associated with a much lower incidence of encephalopathy than that following non-selective shunts.[107] Nevertheless, not all patients maintain prograde portal perfusion after construction of the shunt, and this is particularly true of alcoholic patients with cirrhosis. In addition, it is thought that, in a significant number of patients with this shunt, prograde portal perfusion may not be maintained in the long term.[108] Shunting continues to have a small but definite role in the management of young patients with minimal hepatic impairment and who do not have a history of diabetes, encephalopathy, active hepatitis or acute bleeding.[109] It may also have a place in the treatment of patients with portal hypertensive gastropathy, in whom reduction of portal pressure may be the only successful form of treatment.

Liver transplantation

As the results of liver transplantation have improved, the operation has become more widely available and represents another treatment option for some patients with recurrent variceal bleeding.[84] In practice, economic factors and a restricted supply of donor organs limit its availability, and in any case a significant percentage of patients are not candidates for this procedure because of advanced age, active alcohol or drug abuse, or advanced disease in other organ systems. Similarly, patients with extrahepatic portal vein thrombosis and schistosomiasis are not transplant candidates because hepatic functional reserve is maintained indefinitely in these conditions. Transplantation, however, is the treatment of choice in patients who have endstage liver disease. Bismuth *et al.* have reported a 4-year survival rate of 73 per cent in Child's grade C patients undergoing liver transplantation,[110] while survival rates among patients with comparable hepatic risk managed by primary shunt or sclerotherapy were 31 per cent and 59 per cent, respectively. This evidence, confirmed by other investigators,[84,111] suggests that, in the absence of any contraindications, patients with end-stage liver disease should undergo liver transplantation. It may also be required as the treatment of choice in patients with a poor quality of life and suffering from encephalopathy, asthenia and fatigue but whose disease is not end stage. Those patients with good hepatic function and static or slowly progressing disease are best treated in the interim by methods other than transplantation. If future transplantation is anticipated, the technique of surgical treatment should be considered carefully: non-shunt operations do not adversely affect subsequent transplantation and, if a shunt is required, the distal splenorenal, mesocaval or portacaval prosthetic H shunts, with which dissection in the area of the hepatic pedicle is minimal, are most suitable. End-to-side and side-to-side portacaval shunts should be avoided, but these techniques have been largely superseded by TIPSS.

Secondary prophylaxis of variceal bleeding in patients with cirrhosis

- Endoscopic variceal band ligation
  - Following control of active variceal bleeding, the varices should be eradicated using endoscopic methods. The method of first choice is band ligation
  - It is recommended that each varix is banded with a single band at weekly intervals until completely eradicated
  - The use of an over-tube should be avoided as it is associated with increased complications
  - Following successful eradication of varices, patients should undergo endoscopy at 3- to 6-monthly intervals
  - Recurrent varices should be treated with further variceal eradication
- Endoscopic injection sclerotherapy
  - If banding is not available, injection sclerotherapy should be used
  - The sclerotherapy agent used may vary between institutions
- Non-selective β-blocker with or without endoscopic therapy
  - Non-selective β-blockade may be used alone or in combination with endoscopic techniques
- TIPSS
  - TIPSS is more effective than endoscopic treatment in reducing variceal re-bleeding but does not improve survival and is associated with more encephalopathy
- Portal–systemic shunt formation
  - Continues to have a small but definite role in the management of young patients with minimal hepatic impairment who do not have a history of diabetes, encephalopathy, active hepatitis or acute bleeding

PROPHYLACTIC THERAPY

The aim of prophylactic therapy is to prevent a first episode of variceal bleeding and thereby reduce subsequent complications and mortality. As bleeding from documented oesophageal varices will occur in only 30 per cent of patients with cirrhosis,[112,113] many authors recommend observation until the first variceal bleed occurs. Nevertheless, the high mortality of over 50 per cent in poor-risk Child's C patients associated with the first bleed is reflected in controlled trials of prophylactic treatments including pharmacotherapy, injection sclerotherapy, portal–systemic shunt procedures and extensive devascularisation and transection operations.

Initial studies of prophylactic shunt procedures during the 1960s showed increased morbidity and mortality in the shunt groups[114–116] and they were therefore abandoned. A more recent multicentre study from Japan, comparing prophylactic portal non-decompressive surgery with conventional management, has shown significantly improved survival and reduced re-bleed rates in the shunt group at 5 years.[117] This study remains to be repeated in Western countries, where the aetiology of portal hypertension largely differs from that in Japan, and where major prophylactic shunt surgery of this nature is currently unjustified outside controlled trials.

Although initial controlled trials[118,119] reported that prophylactic sclerotherapy reduced the risk of first variceal haemorrhage and improved survival, these results were not borne out by a meta-analysis of 19 randomised trials assessing the effect of prophylactic sclerotherapy for oesophageal variceal haemorrhage.[120] This meta-analysis showed a significant benefit for sclerotherapy in the prevention of the initial variceal haemorrhage, but as there was significant heterogeneity in the results, the authors concluded that the overall results were equivocal. The authors of another meta-analysis of randomised controlled trials concluded that prophylactic sclerotherapy should not be widely applied at present owing to insufficient documentation of benefit.[121] There is even a danger that injection treatment might precipitate the first variceal bleed, which may prove fatal.[122]

Endoscopic variceal ligation, which has an inherently low complication rate and brings about rapid obliteration of varices, may be a better option for primary prophylaxis of variceal haemorrhage. At least two groups have reported a significantly reduced initial variceal bleeding rate and mortality after prophylactic EVL compared with no treatment.[123,124] The results of these two trials which have demonstrated efficacy of EVL for primary prophylaxis do not yet justify a conclusion that this treatment should be recommended for patients with varices that have not bled and further study is needed.

The most widely used form of prophylaxis is pharmacotherapy, particularly β-blockade with propranolol. There have been nine controlled studies on the prevention of initial variceal haemorrhage in patients with cirrhosis and oesophageal varices. Propranolol was the active agent used in seven studies and nadolol in two. Three meta-analyses,[120,125,126] one based on individual data from four randomised controlled trials,[126] have been published. All three concluded that the risk of initial haemorrhage was significantly reduced and there was a trend towards improved survival in cirrhotic patients with oesophageal varices. A recent cost-effectiveness analysis of variceal bleeding prophylaxis with propranolol, sclerotherapy, and shunt surgery in cirrhotic patients concluded that, at present, propranolol is the only cost-effective modality for prophylaxis of initial variceal bleeding.[127] Most workers in the field agree that patients with large varices who have not bled and presumably carry a high risk of haemorrhage should be offered prophylactic β-blocker therapy. There are as yet insufficient data to make recommendations for small varices.

Isosorbide mononitrate has been shown to be as effective as propranolol in the prevention of first variceal bleeding with no difference in survival.[128] Merkel *et al.* have also reported that a combination of ISMN with nadolol was of greater benefit than nadolol alone;[129] however, Garcia-Pagan *et al.* reported that the addition of ISMN did not further lower the risk of bleeding in patients already receiving propranolol.[130] Long acting nitrates may be a reasonable alternative for patients who have contraindications to, or are unable to tolerate β-blockers, or they could be prescribed as an additional therapy for primary prophylaxis in high risk patients.

Primary prophylaxis

- Methods
  - Pharmacological therapy with propranolol is the best available modality
  - If propranolol is contraindicated or there is intolerance, variceal band ligation is the treatment of choice
  - If neither propranolol nor variceal band ligation can be used, ISMN is the treatment of first choice
- Diagnosis
  - All patients with cirrhosis should undergo endoscopy at the time of diagnosis
  - If at the time of first endoscopy no varices are observed, the patient with cirrhosis should undergo endoscopy at 3-yearly intervals
  - If small varices are diagnosed, the patient should undergo endoscopy at yearly intervals
  - If patients have grade 2 varices and Child's B or C disease, they should have primary prophylaxis
  - If grade 3 varices are diagnosed, patients should have primary prophylaxis irrespective of severity of liver disease

---

It is evident that further studies are required and only time will tell whether pharmacotherapy, variceal ligation, or perhaps a combination of these therapies, may be the most appropriate approach for prophylaxis of oesophageal variceal haemorrhage.

RESULTS AND PROGNOSIS

The prognosis in an individual patient depends on the severity of the bleeding episode and underlying liver function.[122] Patients with non-cirrhotic portal hypertension or cirrhosis with good liver function have good short and long term prognosis. In patients with established cirrhosis, the presence of alcoholic hepatitis, hepatocellular carcinoma and/or portal venous thrombosis may adversely affect prognosis. Operative mortality rates are also more dependent on the status of the liver disease at the time of surgery, rather than the procedure performed.

Conclusions

The initial management of a patient with bleeding oesophageal varices is similar to that for any patient with upper gastrointestinal haemorrhage, and subsequent treatment follows a protocol with generally agreed indications for each therapeutic option (Fig. 46.6). Immediate resuscitation involves administration of fluids and blood, preferably guided by measurement of central venous pressure, and correction of coagulation deficits. Emergency endoscopy is necessary to confirm that the patient is bleeding from oesophageal varices. Pharmacotherapy, either with somatostatin or octreotide, may be used if necessary. Oesophageal tamponade may be necessary on rare occasions: in a patient who has massive variceal bleeding which disallows acute sclerotherapy, when sclerotherapy fails in a patient waiting for surgery and in transporting an acutely bleeding patient to a specialised centre.

Once variceal bleeding has been confirmed, immediate injection sclerotherapy or band ligation should be performed. Using one or sometimes two endoscopy sessions, acute variceal bleeding will be controlled in 90–95 per cent of patients. Acute endoscopy techniques are deemed to have failed when two sessions have been unable to control the acute bleeding episode.

In the 5–10 per cent of patients in whom emergency endoscopic techniques fail, an emergency surgical or radiological procedure is indicated. The available options are a portal–systemic shunt (including TIPSS) and oesophageal transection, with or without devascularisation. The indications for each of these options and their relative merits remain controversial. In general, emergency portal–systemic shunting produces a definite arrest of haemorrhage and prevents recurrence but is associated with a high incidence of encephalopathy and a high operative mortality. If an emergency portal–systemic shunt is contemplated, TIPSS is now the procedure of choice. Alternatively, an oesophageal transection can be performed. This is associated with a lower incidence of encephalopathy but a higher incidence of recurrent bleeding.

In general, therapeutic options for long term control of variceal bleeding are palliative procedures designed to prevent recurrent bleeding and do not improve overall

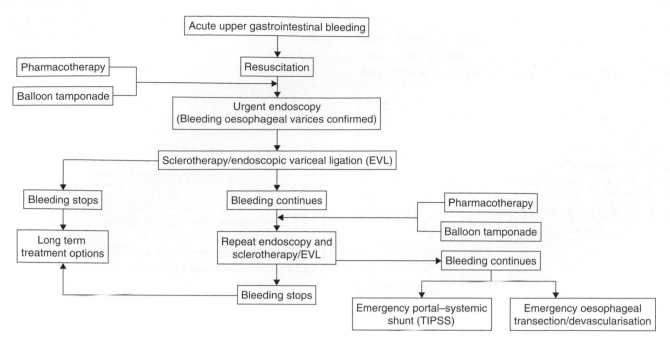

Figure 46.6   *Algorithm for acute management of a patient with bleeding oesophageal varices. TIPSS, transjugular intrahepatic portal-systemic stent shunting*

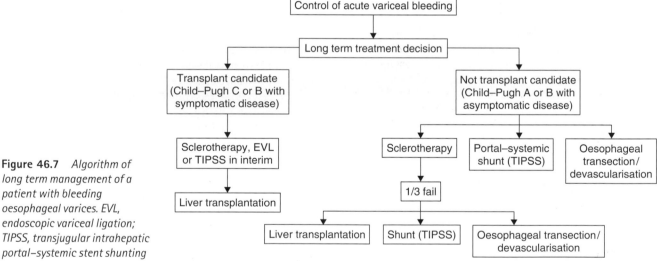

Figure 46.7   *Algorithm of long term management of a patient with bleeding oesophageal varices. EVL, endoscopic variceal ligation; TIPSS, transjugular intrahepatic portal–systemic stent shunting*

survival. The only treatment which addresses the underlying pathology and improves survival is liver transplantation. When considering the appropriate therapeutic option for each patient, it is useful to first consider whether the patient is a candidate for transplantation (Fig. 46.7). Patients with advanced liver disease are best treated by transplantation. Patients with moderate liver dysfunction but who are symptomatic, for example those with encephalopathy, asthenia, fatigue or a poor quality of life, are also probably best treated by transplantation. Those awaiting a suitable liver graft should undergo sclerotherapy, EVL or TIPSS in the interim period.

Only β-blockers have been clearly shown to be of benefit in the prevention of initial variceal bleeding. All patients with established cirrhosis should undergo screening endoscopy to assess the presence of varices. Although data concerning the best time intervals for repeat screening sessions are lacking, several established liver centres have adopted a policy of screening patients every 2–3 years. Patients with large varices and/or endoscopic signs for risk of bleeding should be placed on treatment. Whether treating patients with small oesophageal varices is cost-effective or clearly influences survival is unknown.

Key references

D'Amico G, Pagliaro L, Bosch J. The treatment of portal hypertension: a meta-analytic review. *Hepatology* 1995; **22**: 332–54.

Jalan R, Hayes PC. UK guidelines on the management of variceal haemorrhage in cirrhotic patients. *Gut* 2000; **46**(suppl III): iii1–15.

Rosch J, Keller FS. Transjugular intrahepatic portosystemic shunt: Present status, comparison with endoscopic therapy and shunt surgery, and future prospectives. *World J Surg* 2001; **25**: 337–46.

Tait IS, Krige JEJ, Terblanche J. Endoscopic band ligation of oesophageal varices. *Br J Surg* 1999; **86**: 437–46.

Teran JC, Imperiale TF, Mullen KD, *et al.* Primary prophylaxis of variceal bleeding in cirrhosis: a cost-effectiveness analysis. *Gastroenterology* 1997; **112**: 473–82.

REFERENCES

1 Johnston GW. Bleeding from oesophageal varices. In: Imrie CW, Moosa AR (eds). *Gastrointestinal Emergencies.* Edinburgh: Churchill Livingstone, 1987: 24–45.

2 Henderson JM. Portal hypertension and shunt surgery. *Adv Surg* 1993; **26**: 233–57.

3 Ryley NG, McGee JO'D. Cirrhosis and portal hypertension: pathological aspects. In: Blumgart LH (ed). *Surgery of the Liver and Biliary Tract.* 2nd edn. New York: Churchill Livingstone, 1994: 1589–602.

4 Warren KS, Reboucas G. Blood ammonia during bleeding from esophageal varices in patients with hepatosplenic schistosomiasis. *N Engl J Med* 1964; **271**: 921–6.

5 Mohamed AE, al Karawi MA, al Otaibi R, Hanid MA. Results of sclerotherapy in 100 patients comparison of the outcome between schistosomiasis and hepatitis B. *Hepatogastroenterology* 1989; **36**: 333–6.

6 Tilanus HW. Budd-Chiari syndrome. *Br J Surg* 1995; **82**: 1023–30.

7 Rector WG, Hoefs JC, Hossack KF, Everson GT. Hepatofugal portal flow in cirrhosis; observations on hepatic hemodynamics and the nature of the arterioportal communications. *Hepatology* 1988; **8**: 16–20.

8 Lebrec D, De Fleury P, Rueff B, *et al.* Portal hypertension, size of esophageal varices and risk of gastrointestinal bleeding in alcoholic cirrhosis. *Gastroenterology* 1980; **79**: 1139–44.

9 Jalan R, Hayes PC. UK guidelines on the management of variceal haemorrhage in cirrhotic patients. *Gut* 2000; **46**(suppl III): iii1–15.

10 Mahl TC, Groszmann RJ. Pathophysiology of portal hypertension and variceal bleeding. *Surg Clin North Am* 1990; **70**: 251–66.

11 Bornman PC, Krige JEJ, Terblanche J. Management of oesophageal varices. *Lancet* 1994; **343**: 1079–84.

12 Beppu K, Inokuchi K, Koyanagi N, *et al.* Prediction of variceal hemorrhage by esophageal endoscopy. *Gastrointest Endosc* 1981; **27**: 213–18.

13 The Italian Liver Cirrhosis Project. Reliability of endoscopy in the assessment of variceal features. *J Hepatol* 1987; **4**: 93–8.

14 Burns P, Taylor K, Blei AT. Doppler flowmetery and portal hypertension. *Gastroenterology* 1987; **92**: 824–6.

15 Oliver TW, Sones PJ. Hepatic angiography: Portal hypertension. In: Bernardino ME, Sones PJ (eds). *Hepatic Radiology.* New York: Macmillan Publishing Co., 1984: 243–75.

16 Kehne JH, Hughes FA, Gompertz LA. The use of surgical pituitrin in the control of varix bleeding. *Surgery* 1956; **39**: 917–25.

17 Westaby D. The management of active variceal bleeding. *Intensive Care Med* 1988; **14**: 100–5.

18 Rector WG. Drug therapy for portal hypertension. *Ann Intern Med* 1986; **105**: 96–107.

19 Walker S. Vasoconstrictor therapy and bleeding oesophageal varices. *Hepatogastroenterology* 1990; **37**: 538–43.

20 Burroughs AK, McCormick PA, Hughes MD, *et al.* Randomised, double-blind, placebo-controlled trial of somatostatin for variceal bleeding. *Gastroenterology* 1990; **99**: 1388–95.

21 Jenkins SA, Shields R. Variceal haemorrhage after failed injection sclerotherapy: the role of emergency oesophageal transection. *Br J Surg* 1988; **76**: 49–51.

22 McKee R. A study of octreotide in oesophageal varices. *Digestion* 1990; **45**(suppl): 60–5.

23 Shields R, Jenkins SA, Baxter JN, *et al.* A prospective randomised control trial comparing the efficacy of somatostatin with injection sclerotherpay in the control of bleeding oesophageal varices. *J Hepatol* 1992; **16**: 128–37.

24 Planus R, Quer JC, Boix J, *et al.* A prospective randomized trial comparing somatostatin and sclerotherapy in the treatment of acute variceal bleeding. *Hepatology* 1994; **20**: 370–5.

25 Sung JJ, Chung SC, Lai CW, *et al.* Octreotide infusion or emergency sclerotherapy for variceal haemorrhage. *Lancet* 1993; **342**: 637–41.

26 Freitas DS, Sofia C, Pontes JM, *et al.* Octreotide in acute bleeding oesophageal varices: a prospective randomized sudy. *Hepatogastroenterology* 2000; **47**: 1310–14.

27 Sivri B, Oksuzoglu G, Bayraktar Y, Kayhan B. A prospective randomized trial from Turkey comparing octreotide versus injection sclerotherapy in acute variceal bleeding. *Hepatogastroenterology* 2000; **47**: 168–73.

28 Jenkins SA, Shields R, Jaser N, *et al.* The management of gastrointestinal haemorrhage by somatostatin after apparently successful endoscopic injection sclerotherapy for bleeding oesophageal ulcers. *J Hepatol* 1991; **12**: 296–301.

29 Jenkins SA, Baxter JN, Rennie MJ. Acute and long-term treatment of oesophageal varices. *Br J Intensive Care* 1993; **3**: 65–72.

30 Kleber G, Sauerbruch T, Fischer G, *et al.* Reduction of transmural oesophageal variceal pressure by metoclopramide. *J Hepatol* 1991; **12**: 362–6.

31 Taranto D, Suozzo R, de Sio I, *et al.* Effect of metoclopramide on transmural oesophageal variceal pressure and portal blood flow in cirrhotic patients. *Digestion* 1990; **47**: 56–60.

32 Vlavianos P, Gimson AES, Westaby D, Williams R. Balloon tamponade in variceal bleeding: use and misuse. *BMJ* 1989; **298**: 1158.

33 Crafoord C, Frenckner P. New surgical treatment of varicose veins of the oesophagus. *Acta Otolaryngol* 1939; **27**: 422–9.

34 Johnston GW, Rodgers HW. A review of 15 years' experience in the use of sclerotherapy in the control of acute haemorrhage from oesophageal varices. *Br J Surg* 1973; **60**: 797–800.

35 Terblanche J. Portal hypertension management. *Surg Endosc* 1993; **7**: 472–8.

36 Rose JDR, Crane MD, Smith PM. Factors affecting successful endoscopic sclerotherapy for oesophageal varices. *Gut* 1983; **24**: 946–9.

37 Paquet KJ, Oberhammer E. Sclerotherapy of bleeding oesophageal varices by means of endoscopy. *Endoscopy* 1978; **10**: 7–12.

38 Terblanche J. Has sclerotherapy altered the management of patients with variceal bleeding? *Am J Surg* 1990; **160**: 37–42.

39 Gottlib JP. Endoscopic obturation of oesophageal and gastric varices with a cyanoacrylic tissue adhesive. *Can J Gastroenterol* 1990; **4**: 637–8.

40 Feretis C, Tabakopoulos D, Benakis P, Xenofontos M, Golematis B. Endoscopic hemostasis of esophageal and gastric variceal bleeding with Histoacryl. *Endoscopy* 1990; **22**: 282–4.

41 Kahn D, Jones B, Bornman PC, Terblanche J. Incidence and management of complications after injection sclerotherapy: a 10 year prospective evaluation. *Surgery* 1989; **105**: 160–5.

42 Dhiman RK, Chawla Y, Taneja S, *et al.* Endoscopic sclerotherapy of gastric variceal bleeding with N-butyl-2-cyanoacrylate. *J Clin Gastroenterol* 2002; **35**: 222–7.

43 Kind R, Guglielmi A, Rodella L, *et al.* Bucrylate treatment of bleeding gastric varices: 12 years' experience. *Endoscopy* 2000; **32**: 512–19.

44 Gimson A, Polson R, Westaby D, Williams R. Omeprazole in the management of intractable esophageal ulceration following injection sclerotherapy. *Gastroenterology* 1990; **99**: 1829–31.

45 Terblanche J, Krige JEJ, Bornman PC. The treatment of esophageal varices. *Annu Rev Med* 1992; **43**: 69–82.

46 Terblanche J, Bornman PC, Kahn D, *et al.* Failure of repeated injection sclerotherapy to improve long-term survival after oesophageal variceal bleeding. *Lancet* 1983; **ii**: 1328.

47 Terblanche J, Burroughs AK, Hobbs KEF. Controversies in the management of bleeding oesophageal varices. *N Engl J Med* 1989; **320**: 1398–8.

48 Bornman PC, Terblanche J, Kahn D, *et al.* Limitations of multiple injection sclerotherapy sessions for acute variceal bleeding. *S Afr Med J* 1986; **70**: 34–6.

49 Burroughs AK, Hamilton G, Phillips A, *et al.* A comparison of sclerotherapy with staple transection of the esophagus for the emergency control of bleeding from esophageal varices. *N Engl J Med* 1989; **321**: 857–62.

50 Mostafa I, Omar MM, Nouh A. Endoscopic control of gastric variceal bleeding with butyl cyanoacrylate. *Endoscopy* 1993; **25**: A11.

51 Pretis G, de Comberlato M, Guelmi A, *et al.* N-butyl-cyanoacrylate in bleeding oesophageal (EBV) and gastric (GBV) varices: experience in 135 cirrhotic patients. *Endoscopy* 1993; **25**: A14.

52 Thakeb F, Abdel Kader S, Salama Z, *et al.* The value of combined use of N-butyl cyanoacrylate and ethanolamine oleate in the management of bleeding esophagogastric varices. *Endoscopy* 1993; **25**: A16.

53 Stiegmann G, Sun JH, Hammond WS. Results of experimental endoscopic esophageal varix ligation. *Am Surg* 1988; **54**: 104–8.

54 Binmoeller KF, Vadeyar HJ, Soehendra N. Treatment of esophageal varices. *Endoscopy* 1994; **26**: 42–7.

55 Stiegmann GV, Goff JS, Michaletz-Onody PA, *et al.* Endoscopic sclerotherapy as compared with endoscopic ligation for bleeding esophageal varices. *N Engl J Med* 1992; **326**: 1527–32.

56 Saeed ZA, Michaletz PZ, Wincester CB, *et al.* Endoscopic variceal ligation in patients who have failed endoscopic sclerotherapy. *Gastrointest Endosc* 1990; **36**: 572–4.

57 Johnson PA, Campbell DR, Antonson CW, *et al.* Complications associated with endoscopic band ligation of esophageal varices. *Gastrointest Endosc* 1993; **39**: 119–22.

58 Goldschmiedt M, Haber G, Kandel G, *et al.* A safety maneuver for placing overtubes during esophageal variceal ligation. *Gastrointest Endosc* 1992; **38**: 399–400.

59 Saltzman JR, Arora S. Complications of esophageal variceal band ligation. *Gastrointest Endosc* 1993; **39**: 185–6.

60 Orloff MJ, Orloff MS, Rambolt M, Girard B. Is portosystemic shunt worthwhile in Child's class C cirrhosis? *Ann Surg* 1993; **216**: 256–66.

61 Orloff MJ, Bell RH, Greenberg AG. A prospective randomized trial of emergency portacaval shunt and medical therapy in unselected cirrhotic patients with bleeding varices. *Gastroenterology* 1986; **90**: 1754.

62 Rikkers LF, Jin G. Surgical management of acute variceal hemorrhage. *World J Surg* 1994; **18**: 193–9.

63 Rikkers LF, Jin G. Variceal hemorrhage: surgical therapy. *Gastroenterol Clin North Am* 1993; **22**: 821–42.

64 Rosch J, Hanafee W, Snow H. Transjugular portal venography and radiologic portacaval shunt. An experimental study. *Radiology* 1969; **92**: 1112–14.

65 Colapinto RF, Stronell RD, Birch SJ. Creation of an intrahepatic portosystemic shunt with a Gruntzig balloon catheter. *CMAJ* 1982; **126**: 267–8.

66 Richter GM, Palmaz JC, Noeldge G, Rossle M. The transjugular intrahepatic portosystemic stent-shunt. A new nonsurgical percutaneous method. *Radiology* 1989; **29**: 406–11.

67 Jalan R, Redhead DN, Hayes PC. Transjugular intrahepatic portosystemic stent shunt in the treatment of variceal haemorrhage. *Br J Surg* 1995; **82**: 1158–64.

68 Rosch J, Keller FS. Transjugular intrahepatic portosystemic shunt: Present status, comparison with endoscopic therapy and shunt surgery, and future prospectives. *World J Surg* 2001; **25**: 337–46.

69 Ring EJ, Lake JR, Roberts JP, *et al.* Using transjugular intrahepatic portosystemic shunts to control variceal bleeding before liver transplantation. *Ann Intern Med* 1992; **116**: 304–9.

70 Helton WS, Belshaw A, Althaus S, *et al.* Critical appraisal of the angiographic portacaval shunt (TIPS). *Am J Surg* 1993; **165**: 566–71.

71 Rossle M, Haag K, Ochs A, *et al.* The transjugular intrahepatic portosystemic stent-shunt procedure for variceal bleeding. *N Engl J Med* 1994; **330**: 165–7.

72 Papatheodoridis GV, Goulis J, Leandro G, *et al.* Transjugular intrahepatic portosystemic shunt compared with endoscopic treatment for prevention of variceal rebleeding: a meta-analysis. *Hepatology* 1999; **30**: 612–22.

73 McCormick PA, Dick R, Panagou EB, *et al.* Emergency transjugular intrahepatic portasystemic stent shunting as salvage treatment for controlled variceal bleeding. *Br J Surg* 1994; **81**: 1324–7.

74 Jalan R, John TG, Redhead DN, *et al.* A comparative study of the transjugular intrahepatic portosystemic stent-shunt (TIPSS) and oesophageal transection in uncontrolled variceal haemorrhage. *Am J Gastroenterol* 1995; **11**: 1932–6.

75 Merli M, Salerno F, Riggio O, *et al.* Transjugular intrahepatic portosystemic shunt versus endoscopic sclerotherapy for the prevention of variceal bleeding in cirrhosis: a randomized multicenter trial. Gruppo Italiano Studio TIPS (GIST). *Hepatology* 1998; **27**: 48–53.

76 Escorsell A, Banares R, Garcia-Pagan JC, *et al.* TIPS versus drug therapy in preventing variceal rebleeding in advanced cirrhosis: a randomized controlled trial. *Hepatology* 2002; **35**: 385–92.

77 Sternbeck M, Ring E, Gordon R, *et al.* Intrahepatic portocaval shunt: a bridge to liver transplantation in patients with refractory variceal bleeding. *Gastroenterology* 1991; **100**: 801.

78 Stanley AJ, Jalan R, Forrest EH, *et al.* Long-term follow-up of transjugular intrahepatic portosystemic stent shunt (TIPSS) for the treatment of portal hypertension: results in 130 patients. *Gut* 1996; **39**: 479–85.

79 Ferguson J, Jalan R, Redhead DN, *et al.* The role of duplex Doppler in monitoring shunt function following transjugular intrahepatic stent shunt. *Br J Radiol* 1995; **68**: 587–9.

80 Vankemmel M. Resection-anastomose de l'oesophage sus-cardial pour rupture de varices oesophagiennies. *Nouv Presse Med* 1974; **5**: 1123–4.

81 Sugiura M, Futagawa S. A new technique for treating oesophageal varices. *J Thorac Cardiovasc Surg* 1973; **66**: 677–85.

82 Sugiura M, Futagawa S. Esophageal transection with para-esophagogastric devascularization (the Sugiura procedure) in the treatment of esophageal varices. *World J Surg* 1984; **8**: 673–9.

83 Burroughs AK, Mezzanotte G, Phillips A, *et al.* Cirrhotics with variceal hemorrhage: the importance of the time interval between admisssion and the start of analysis for survival and rebleeding rates. *Hepatology* 1989; **9**: 801–7.

84 Iwatsuki S, Starzl TE, Todo S, *et al.* Liver transplantation in the treatment of bleeding esophageal varices. *Surgery* 1988; **104**: 697–705.

85 D'Amico G, Pagliaro L, Bosch J. The treatment of portal hypertension: a meta-analytic review. *Hepatology* 1995; **22**: 332–54.

86 Patch D, Sabin CA, Goulis J, *et al.* A randomized, controlled trial of medical therapy versus sendoscopic ligation for the prevention of variceal rebleeding in patients with cirrhosis. *Gastroenterology* 2002; **123**: 1013–19.

87 Abraldes JG, Tarantino I, Turnes J, *et al.* Hemodynamic response to pharmacological treatment of portal hypertension and long-term prognosis of cirrhosis. *Hepatology* 2003; **37**: 902–8.

88 Burroughs AK, McCormick PA. Prevention of variceal rebleeding. *Gastroenterol Clin North Am* 1992; **21**: 119–47.

89 Rikkers LF, Jin G, Burnett DA, *et al.* Shunt surgery versus endoscopic sclerotherapy for variceal hemorrhage: late results of a randomized trial. *Am J Surg* 1993; **165**: 27–33.

90 Henderson JM, Kutner MH, Millikan WJ Jr, *et al.* Endoscopic variceal sclerosis compared with distal splenorenal shunt to prevent variceal hemorrhage in cirrhosis. A prospective, randomized trial. *Ann Intern Med* 1990; **112**: 262–9.

91 Terblanche J. The surgeon's role in the management of portal hypertension. *Ann Surg* 1989; **209**: 381–95.

92 Terblanche J, Kahn D, Borman PC. Long-term injection sclerotherapy treatment for esophageal varices: a 10-year prospective evaluation. *Ann Surg* 1989; **210**: 725–31.

93 Infante-Rivard C, Esnaola S, Villeneuve JP. Role of endoscopic variceal sclerotherapy in the long-term management of variceal bleeding: a meta-analysis. *Gastroenterology* 1989; **96**: 1087–92.

94 Laine L. Ligation: endoscopic treatment of choice for patients with bleeding oesophageal varices. *Hepatology* 1995; **22**: 661–5.

95 Bureau C, Peron JM, Alric L, *et al.* 'A La Carte' treatment of portal hypertension: adapting medical therapy to hemodynamic response for the prevention of bleeding. *Hepatology* 2002; **36**: 1361–6.

96 Tait IS, Krige JEJ, Terblanche J. Endoscopic band ligation of oesophageal varices. *Br J Surg* 1999; **86**: 437–46.

97 Hashizume M, Ohta M, Ueno K, *et al.* Endoscopic ligation of esophageal varices compared with injection sclerotherapy: a prospective randomized trial. *Gastrointest Endosc* 1993; **39**: 123–6.

98 Lo GH, Lai KH, Cheng JS, *et al.* The additive effect of sclerotherapy to patients receiving repeated endoscopic variceal ligation: a prospective, randomized trial. *Hepatology* 1998; **28**: 391–5.

99 Saeed ZA, Stiegmann GV, Ramirez FC, *et al.* Endoscopic variceal ligation is superior to combined ligation and sclerotherapy for oesophageal varices: a multicentre prospective randomised trial. *Hepatology* 1997; **25**: 71–4.

100 Iso Y, Kawanaka H, Tomikawa M, *et al.* Repeated sclerotherapy is preferable to combined therapy with variceal ligation to avoid recurrence of oesophageal varices: a prospective randomised trial. *Hepatogastroenterology* 1997; **44**: 467–71.

101 Al Traif I, Fachartz FS, Al Jumah A, *et al.* Randomized trial of ligation versus combined ligation and sclerotherapy for bleeding esophageal varices. *Gastrointest Endosc* 1999; **50**: 1–6.

102 Rypins EB, Mason RG, Conroy RM, Sarfeh IJ. Predictability and maintenance of portal flow patterns after small-diameter portacaval H-grafts in man. *Ann Surg* 1984; **200**: 706–10.

103 Sarfeh IJ, Rypins EB, Moussa R, *et al.* Serial measurement of portal haemodynamics after partial portal decompression. *Surgery* 1986; **100**: 52–8.

104 Adam R, Diamond T, Bismuth H. Partial portacaval shunt – renaissance of an old concept. *Surgery* 1992; **111**: 610–16.

105 Rosemurgy AS, Serafini FM, Zweibel BR. Transjugular intrahepatic portosystemic shunt vs. small-diameter prosthetic H-graft portacaval shunt: extended follow-up of an expanded randomized prospective trial. *J Gastrointest Surg* 2000; **4**: 589–97.

106 Rikkers LF. Definitive therapy for variceal bleeding: a personal view. *Am J Surg* 1990; **160**: 80–5.

107 Warren WD, Millikan WJ, Henderson JM, *et al.* Ten years' portal hypertensive surgery at Emory. Results and new perspectives. *Ann Surg* 1982; **195**: 530–42.

108 Maillard J, Flamant YM, Hay JM, Chandler JG. Selectivity of the distal splenorenal shunt. *Surgery* 1979; **86**: 663–71.

109 Helton WS, Maves R, Wicks K, Johansen K. Transjugular intrahepatic portasystemic shunt vs surgical shunt in good-risk cirrhotic patients: a case-control comparison. *Arch Surg* 2001; **136**: 17–20.

110 Bismuth H, Adam R, Mathur S, Sherlock D. Options for elective treatment of portal hypertension in cirrhotic patients in the transplantation era. *Am J Surg* 1990; **160**: 105–10.

111 Millikan WJ, Henderson JM, Stewart MT, *et al.* Change in hepatic function, hemodynamics and morphology after liver transplantation. Physiological effect of therapy. *Ann Surg* 1989; **209**: 513–25.

112 Grace ND. Prevention of initial variceal hemorrhage. *Gastroenterol Clin North Am* 1992; **21**: 149–61.

113 Kleber G, Sauerbruch T, Ansari H, Paumgartner G. Prediction of variceal hemorrhage in cirrhosis: a prospective follow-up study. *Gastroenterology* 1991; **100**: 1332–7.

114 Conn HO, Lindenmuth WW, May CJ, Ramsby GR. Prophylactic portacaval anastomosis. A tale of two studies. *Medicine* 1972; **51**: 27–40.

115 Jackson FC, Perrin EB, Smith AG, *et al.* A clinical investigation of the portacaval shunt. ii Survival analysis of the prophylactic operation. *Am J Surg* 1968; **115**: 22–42.

116 Resnick RH, Chalmers TC, Ishihara AM, *et al.* A controlled study of the prophylactic portacaval shunt. A final report. *Ann Intern Med* 1969; **70**: 675–88.

117 Inokuchi K, Cooperative Study Group of Portal Hypertension in Japan. Improved survival after prophylactic portal nondecompressive surgery for esophageal varices: a randomized controlled trial. *Hepatology* 1990; **2**: 1–6.

118 Paquet KJ. Prophylactic endoscopic sclerosing treatment of the oesophageal wall in varices: a prospective controlled randomized trial. *Endoscopy* 1982; **14**: 4–5.

119 Witzel L, Wolbergs E, Merki H. Prophylactic endoscopic sclerotherapy of oesophageal varices: a prospective controlled trial. *Lancet* 1985; **i**: 773–5.

120 Pagliaro L, D'Amico G, Sorensen TIA, *et al.* Prevention of first bleeding in cirrhosis. A meta-analysis of randomised trials of nonsurgical treatment. *Ann Intern Med* 1992; **117**: 59–70.

121 Van Ruiswyk J, Byrd JC. Efficacy of prophylactic sclerotherapy for prevention of a first variceal hemorrhage. *Gastroenterology* 1992; **102**: 587–97.

122 Santangelo WC, Dueno MI, Estes BL, Krejs GJ. Prophylactic sclerotherapy of large esophageal varices. *N Engl J Med* 1988; **318**: 814–18.

123 Sarin SK, Guptan RK, Jain AK, *et al.* A randomised controlled trial of endoscopic variceal band ligation for primary prophylaxis of variceal bleeding. *Eur J Gastroenterol Hepatology* 1996; **8**: 337–42.

124 Lay CS, Tsai YT, Teg CY, *et al.* Endoscopic variceal ligation in prophylaxis of first variceal bleeding in cirrhotic patients with high-risk esophageal varices. *Hepatology* 1997; **25**: 1346–50.

125 Hayes PC, Davis JM, Lewis JA, *et al.* Meta-analysis of value of propanolol in prevention of variceal haemorrhage. *Lancet* 1990; **336**: 153–6.

126 Poyard T, Cales P, Pasta L, *et al.* and the Franco-Italian Multicentre Study Group. Beta-adrenergic antagonist drugs in the prevention of gastrointestinal bleeding in patients with cirrhosis and esophageal varices: an analysis of data and prognostic factors in 589 patients from four randomised clinical trials. *N Engl J Med* 1991; **324**: 1532–8.

127 Teran JC, Imperiale TF, Mullen KD, *et al.* Primary prophylaxis of variceal bleeding in cirrhosis: a cost-effectiveness analysis. *Gastroenterology* 1997; **112**: 473–82.

128 Angelico M, Carli L, Piat C, *et al.* Isosorbide-5 mononitrate versus propanolol in the prevention of first bleeding in cirrhosis. *Gastroenterology* 1993; **104**: 1460–5.

129 Merkel C, Martin R, Enzo E, *et al.* Randomised controlled trial of nadolol alone or with isosbide mononitrate for primary prophylaxis of variceal bleeding in cirrhosis. *Lancet* 1996; **348**: 1677–81.

130 Garcia-Pagan JC, Morillas R, Banares R, *et al.* Propranolol plus placebo versus propranolol plus isosorbide-5-mononitrate in the prevention of a first variceal bleed: a double-blind RCT. *Hepatology* 2003; **37**: 1260–6.

Cold Injury

PER-OLA GRANBERG

THE PROBLEM

Humans are tropical beings but, unlike most other mammals, we lack an effective hairy covering. Our adaptation to a cold environment was primarily an intellectual event. Thus, cold induced injuries are almost exclusively a result of our inability to protect ourselves adequately against our environment.

Serious injuries caused by cold are in most cases preventable, occurring only sporadically in civilian life. Despite populations of about 100 million at risk in areas where subzero temperatures are commonplace, injuries caused by cold are surprisingly unusual or rare.[1] On the other hand such injuries are of major significance to military personnel operating in the cold and to populations involved in cataclysms. For example, during World War I, 115 000 British soldiers suffered cold injuries, with morbidity rates ranging from 27 to 33 per cent for the years 1914 and 1915.[2] The corresponding figures for the French and Italian armies were 80 000 and 38 000, respectively. During World War II, 10 per cent of American soldiers, i.e. more than 90 000, suffered cold injuries.[3] The great losers in this respect, however, were the Germans; in their case figures exceeding 600 000 victims have been presented. The numbers could be much higher if one included the common combination of war wounds and hypothermia. Often the cold is an enemy worse than the opposition themselves. During the Fenno–Russian War of 1940, 9000 Swedish volunteers enlisted in the Finnish army, and of these 130 had to be sent back to Sweden as a result of cold injuries; this contrasts with 33 who were killed and 50 who were wounded.

THERMOREGULATION

The human body tries to maintain thermal equilibrium between heat production and heat loss with a core temperature of 37 ± 2 °C. Basal heat production under conditions of thermal comfort is around 70–100 W. Body temperature is regulated in the hypothalamus. Thermosensitive endorgans in the skin, and possibly elsewhere, transmit cold perception via the lateral hypothalamic tracts.[4]

Various mechanisms regulate heat loss. *Depending on both temperature and humidity*, radiation accounts for 60 per cent of total heat loss, convection for about 18 per cent, conduction for 3 per cent and evaporation for 20–30 per cent. When thermoregulation is impaired and core temperature starts to decline, the affected individual suffers cold stress, which can deteriorate into hypothermia.

Mechanisms of regulating heat loss

- Radiation: heat loss – 60 per cent
- Convection: heat loss – 18 per cent
- Conduction: heat loss – 3 per cent
- Evaporation: heat loss – 20–30 per cent

In a cold environment one is obliged to prevent heat loss by wearing clothing which produces a subtropical microclimate. If, however, such protection is inadequate, physiological adjustment to cold is accomplished by two main mechanisms. Heat loss by conductance is limited by increased cutaneous vasoconstriction mediated by unmyelinated sympathetic constrictor fibres with noradrenaline as the transmitter.[5] Furthermore, heat production can be augmented by voluntary muscular activity, also by involuntary muscular tensing, but most of all by muscular shivering. Heat production is also influenced by the secretion of thyroxine and catecholamines, the so-called thermogenic hormones.[6,7]

Cold injuries may be either systemic or localised. The latter injuries most often precede systemic hypothermia. The local injuries described in the next two sections constitute two clinically different entities: freezing cold injuries (FCIs) and non-freezing cold injuries (NFCIs). The final section of this chapter deals with systemic hypothermia *per se*.

Broad types of cold injury

* Localised
  - Freezing cold injuries
  - Non-freezing cold injuries
* Systemic
  - Hypothermia

FREEZING COLD INJURIES

Freezing cold injuries occur when the temperature drops below freezing point and there is *true freezing of the tissue*. Normally, human flesh freezes at $-2\,°C$, but supercooling is common if the skin is dry. Skin wetness is conducive to frostbite, as it allows crystallisation to terminate supercooling.[8] Pathogenic mechanisms thought to contribute to tissue heat loss due to FCIs include a direct cryogenic insult to the cells and vascular damage with decreased perfusion and tissue hypoxia.

Pathophysiology

The adrenergic vasoconstriction of cutaneous vessels is of great importance in the origin of frostbite. The skin's normal blood flow far exceeds its nutritional requirements. In peripheral structures such as hands, feet, nose and ears, the flow can vary considerably owing to wide arteriovenous shunts. In a warm environment the hands, for example, are superperfused and the tips of the fingers are even warmer than the lips. Only about *10 per cent of the flow to the hands, however, is needed for tissue oxygenation; the rest creates warmth, thereby facilitating dexterity*. Local cooling of the skin occludes these shunts even in the absence of any decrease in core temperature. When skin is exposed to an extreme cold environment for a longer period of time, even the nutrition begins to suffer. Fingernails grow more slowly in arctic climates than in temperate zones.

In order to protect the viability of the peripheral parts of the extremities early *during cold exposure, an intermittent cold induced vasodilatation (CIVD) takes place*. Cold induced vasodilatation is a result of the opening of arteriovenous anastomoses, occurring every 5–10 minutes. This alternating constriction and dilatation, known as the 'hunting response', was described by Sir Thomas Lewis as long ago as 1930.[9] Cold induced vasodilatation is a compromise in the human physiological plan to conserve heat and yet intermittently preserve the function of hands and feet. It is perceived by the patient as periods of prickling heat, and it becomes less pronounced as body temperature decreases. Great individual variations in the degree of CIVD might explain differing susceptibility to local cold injury. Importantly, people indigenous to a cold climate present a more pronounced CIVD.

In contrast to cryopreservation of living tissue when *crystallisation* occurs intracellularly and extracellularly, the clinical congelation with a slow rate of freezing produces only extracellular ice crystals. The process is an exothermic one, liberating heat, for which reason the temperature of the limb remains at freezing point until freezing is complete. Not until then does the limb temperature start to decline to the ambient level.[10]

When water in the extracellular spaces is transformed into ice, the osmolality of this space will increase and lead to a passive diffusion of water from the intracellular compartment.[11] Cell hydration alters protein structures, membrane lipids and cellular pH, leading to destruction incompatible with cell survival.[12] Resistance to freezing injury varies in different tissues. Skin is more resistant than are muscle and nerves, possibly owing to a lower water content, both intracellularly and intercellularly, in the epidermis.

Indirect haemorheological factors also influence the pathophysiology, but their role is debatable. These factors start to influence matters during the prefreeze phase, with sympathetic vasoconstriction, which causes transendothelial plasma leakage. The increased intravascular viscosity retards flow and causes sludging. This indirect vascular effect was earlier interpreted as similar to that found in NFCIs. Recent studies on rabbit ears[13–15] however, have shown that freezing causes intimal lesions in the microvasculature prior to any evidence of damage to other skin parenchymal elements. The earliest and most severe lesions were found in the intima of the arterioles, but venules and capillaries subsequently demonstrated the same changes. The endothelial cells shrank and separated from the elastic internal lamina, and this event was present in samples removed immediately after freezing, which proves that blood reflow could not be responsible for the changes. These findings provide evidence that the rheological part of the pathogenesis of FCI is also dependent on a cryobiological effect. Other studies confirm these results.[16]

When frostbitten tissue is rewarmed, ice crystals melt as an endothermic reaction, absorbing the previously lost heat of crystallisation.[10] This means that the temperature of the frozen area levels out at around $-2\,°C$ until all the ice crystals have melted. Rediffusion of water to the dehydrated cells then starts, leading to intracellular swelling. The thawing further induces a maximal vascular dilatation, causing hyperaemia. The endothelial cell injury increases fluid extravasation, leading to oedema and blister formation. The mechanical stability of red corpuscle aggregates increases, and showers of emboli pass along the microvessels. The disruption of the endothelial cells exposes the basement membrane and provides an opportunity to initiate platelet adhesion, which in turn starts the coagulation cascade.[17] Blood flow then stagnates, and progressive thrombosis culminates in anoxia.

Cells that are damaged by direct freezing injury with dehydration, and those that succumb due to microcirculatory congestion and anoxia, cannot be saved. However, in an intermediate, pivotal zone of injury located between the distal frostbitten tissue and the unaffected limb, various forms of therapy might affect the survival of tissue. Progressive dermal ischaemia due to the increased enzyme activity of vasoconstricting metabolites of arachidonic acid possibly plays a role in the pathogenesis in this zone.[18,19] Free radicals may also act in this context. Manson et al.[15] succeeded in improving viability in frozen rat ears by administering superoxide dismutase (SOD) at the time of thawing, pointing to a reperfusion injury in both FCIs and NFCIs[20] (see Chapter 2).

Environmental factors

The development of an FCI *depends upon ambient temperature and duration of exposure*. However, many other factors influence the course of events. Experiences from polar expeditions have taught that when the ambient temperature falls below −60 °C, human flesh may freeze within a minute. It is the heat loss to which the exposed tissue is subjected which determines the damage, and in this respect *windchill is an important factor*. In calm weather a normothermic person is surrounded by a thin layer of warm air next to the skin. As wind velocity increases, more heat is lost and the danger of possible cold injury increases. Thus the temperature feels 'much colder' when the wind is blowing as is obvious from the windchill chart.[21] Any movement of air past the body has the same effect. Thus, running, skiing, skijoring and riding in open vehicles must be considered in addition to direct wind. During World War II the US army suffered more than 90 000 injuries due to cold, and heavy bomber crews suffered more FCIs than all other injuries combined.[3] However, exposed flesh will not freeze as long as the ambient temperature is above the freezing point, even at high wind velocities.

Clothing, wet with perspiration, rain or melted snow *increases conductive loss* because of reduced insulation. Moreover, water as a thermal conductor is superior to air by a factor of about 25.[21] Use of alcohol and tobacco products, as well as poor nutrition and fatigue, are also factors predisposing to frostbite. Previous cold injury increases the risk of subsequent frostbite owing to an abnormal sympathetic response.

Cold metal, when grasped with the bare hand, can rapidly cause an FCI owing to high conductive heat loss. Most people are aware of this but often do not realise the risk of handling *supercooled liquids*. Petrol cooled down to −30 °C will freeze exposed flesh almost instantly as evaporative heat loss combines with conductive loss. Such rapid freezing causes both extracellular and intracellular freezing, with destruction of cell membranes, primarily on a mechanical basis.[22] Similar FCIs have been reported following spilling of liquid propane directly on to the skin.[23,24] This gas is usually transported as a liquid under pressure at −64 °C and has been shown in experimental animals to cause dermal necrosis after spraying for as little as 12 seconds.[25]

Clinical picture

As with a thermal injury, FCI has been classified into first, second, third and fourth degree injuries. However, in the initial stages it is certainly difficult to predict the extent of a frostbite according to such a scheme. *Freezing cold injuries are therefore better subdivided into superficial and deep frostbites*.[26] The superficial injury is limited to the skin and the immediately subcutaneous tissues. A stinging, pricking pain is often the first symptom. In a snowstorm, however, this sensation of pain is often absent. The affected skin turns pale or waxy-white, becomes numb and will indent when pressure is applied to it, as the underlying and surrounding tissues are still viable and pliable (Fig. 47.1). If, however, the frostbite extends into a deep injury, the skin turns white and marble-like, feels hard and adheres to the adjacent tissues. One must bear in mind, however, that even a superficial FCI on the extremities may appear to be frozen solid due to the freezing alone.[26]

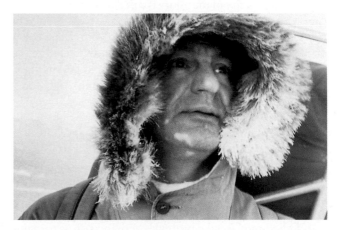

Figure 47.1 *A superficial local cold injury is limited to the skin, which turns pale or waxy-white. The injury should be treated as early as possible in order to avoid deep frostbite. (Photo courtesy of Anders Holmström)*

Treatment

FIRST AID TREATMENT

The golden rule of treatment is to *take care of the local cold injury at once*. This prevents a superficial frostbite from turning into a deep one. If the victim cannot be taken indoors, they must be protected from the wind by the shelter of companions, wind sac or similar makeshift refuge. The frostbitten area should be thawed by passive transmission of heat from a warmer part of the body, for example by placing the warm hand against the face or the cold hand into the axilla or groin. The victim is often under cold stress, with peripheral vasoconstriction, and therefore a warm comrade can provide excellent therapy. *Massage and rubbing the frostbitten part with snow or a woollen muffler is contraindicated.* The tissue is filled with ice crystals and such mechanical treatment aggravates the injury. Similarly, *rewarming with dry heat in front of a camp fire or a camp stove should never be considered in any circumstances* as the heat does not penetrate to any depth, the area is partly anaesthetised and treatment may even end up in a burn injury.

Frostbitten feet give warning signals of pain when the local temperature falls to around +15 °C. This sensation of pain disappears before the actual freezing takes place, as nerve conductivity is abolished at +8 to +7 °C.[27] The paradox is that the last sensation one feels is that one does not feel anything at all. In the field frostbitten feet are best treated by rewarming them in a comrade's armpit in the lee of natural shelter. Under extreme conditions, when evacuation from cold requires travel on foot, one should avoid thawing. Walking on frostbitten feet does not appear to increase the risk of tissue loss, whereas refreezing of a local cold injury certainly does.

If conditions allow, *the most effective treatment for a frostbite is thawing in warm water at +40 °C to +42 °C*, a temperature just tolerable on the back of the hand. One should not, however, postpone thawing by time-consuming transportation, as the severity of the injury is a product of low temperature and time. The temperature of the bath should be checked frequently to prevent the water from falling below 40 °C. The thawing procedure should continue until sensation, colour and tissue softness return. Rapid rewarming in warm water often ends up in not so much a pink, but more a burgundy, hue due to venous stasis (Fig. 47.2).

Out in the field it is important to be aware of the fact that treatment requires more than local thawing. *The correct treatment includes the whole individual*, as frostbite is often the first sign of creeping hypothermia. More clothes should be put on and a warm, nourishing beverage given. The victim is often apathetic and unwilling to do anything. Should victims be forced to stay in the open, they should be urged to take muscular activity such as trudging through the snow and buffeting their arms against their sides. Such manoeuvres open the peripheral arteriovenous shunts in the extremities.

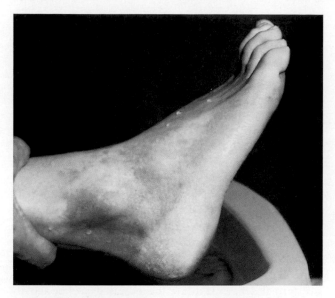

Figure 47.2 *If available, rapid re-warming in warm water at +40 °C to +42 °C has been found to give the best results. Thawing is continued until the flush has extended to the tips of the toes. The thawed area develops a burgundy hue and the patient needs analgesics as this rapid thawing is painful*

FCIs: first aid treatment

- Protection from the wind or trudge through snow buffeting arms against sides
- Warm clothes, warm nourishing beverage
- Thawing of area by passive transmission of body heat of victim or comrade
- Thawing in warm water maintained at +40 °C to +42 °C

HOSPITAL TREATMENT

If thawing with passive warmth transfer proves unsuccessful after 20–30 minutes, a deep frostbite is present and the patient should be sent, properly protected, to the nearest hospital. If delay is likely because of transportation problems, it is better to get the patient into the nearest housing and thaw the injury in warm water. After complete thawing the patient should be put to bed with the injured area elevated (Fig. 47.3). Prompt transportation should then be arranged to the nearest hospital, where warm water thawing is recommended, provided that the injury is still in the frozen state. The best clinical results are obtained, paradoxically, by rapid rewarming, raising the tissue temperature without a simultaneous rise of blood flow and oxygen access. This emphasises the cryobiological aetiology of frostbite as the most important one, at least in the early stages. Frozen tissue appears to withstand hypoxia better than intracellular dehydration. There is evidence to suggest that if the whole individual is immersed in a warm water bath, the thawing process can be accelerated.[28]

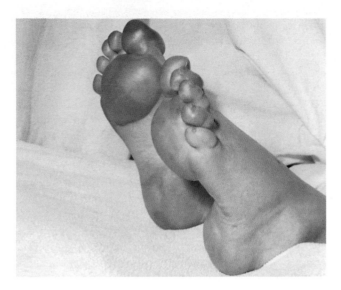

Figure 47.3 *The thawed extremity is placed in an elevated position. Interdigital specimens are taken for bacterial growth. Tetanus toxoid is given, and the extremities are kept on sterile sheets under cradles. (Photo courtesy of Ejnar Eriksson)*

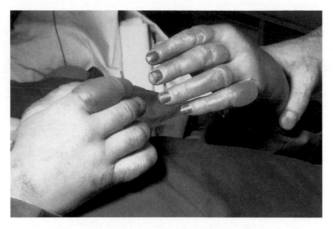

Figure 47.4 *Six to 12 hours after thawing, blisters appear. Every precaution should be taken to avoid their rupture. (Photo courtesy of Ejnar Eriksson)*

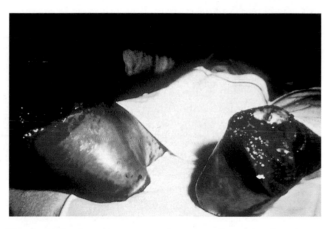

Figure 47.5 *Premature surgery is malpractice and ends up in infection, delay in healing and unnecessary tissue loss*

Rapid rewarming gives moderate to severe pain of a burning quality, and the patient will often require an analgesic. If ibuprofen is at hand 600 mg should be given as soon as possible and the medication repeated every 6 hours if transportation is prolonged. The capillary damage causes leakage of serum, with local swelling and blister formation during the first few days. Blistering is more common on the back of the fingers, hands and feet, where the tissues are more lax than on the palms or the soles (Fig. 47.4). Clear blisters are most common. Haemorrhagic blister fluid reflects structural damage to the subdermal plexus. In order to prevent infection *the blister should be kept intact and debrided only if infected.* Tetanus prophylaxis is indicated. Antibiotics should be given only if there is clinical evidence of infection (Fig. 47.4).

Further hospital *treatment should be open and non-occlusive* (Fig. 47.3). Placement of sterile cotton pledgets between the toes and fingers is helpful. Daily treatment in a whirlpool bath at normal skin temperature cleanses the wounds gently, removes bacteria, aids circulation and provides physiological debridement. Patients are encouraged to exercise the affected digits in the whirlpool.[26] Such treatment frightens many surgeons, who imagine that this may well transform a dry gangrene into a wet one. However, unlike that in atherosclerosis, gangrene due to frostbite is essentially superficial and the necrotic tissue may extend to a depth of no more than a few millimetres. Escharotomy on the dorsum or the dorsolateral part of the fingers should be performed if joint motion is limited.[26]

Being a thermogenic injury, frostbite is often compared with burn injuries. The inappropriateness of classifying cold injuries as burn injuries was mentioned earlier. It is even more inappropriate, however, to compare these two entities when dealing with surgical therapy. In a burn injury the border between living and dead tissue is established within a few days, whereas this takes months in frostbite, in which *it is difficult to predict the amount of non-viable tissue at an early stage.*

A conservative approach is to be recommended. 'Frostbite in January, amputate in July' and 'Hurry up and wait before you ablate' are dictums to be remembered by the over-zealous surgeon (Fig. 47.5). The only indication for early amputation is septicaemia; this is a rarity. Efforts to establish the borderline between living and dead tissue in order to decrease the duration of inpatient hospitalisation have through the past decades been numerous. The multiplicity of procedures recommended, e.g. plain X-rays, venous radioisotopic scanning, angiography, digital plethysmography, laser Doppler, thermography, technetium scintigraphy, triple-phase bone scanning, magnetic resonance imaging and angiography speak for themselves and show that, so far, there is no accurate method for early detection of viability. The appropriate level of amputation

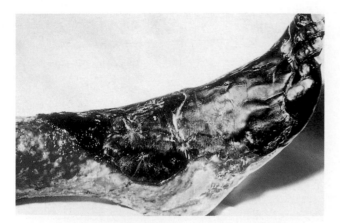

Figure 47.6   *The blackened carapace acts as a protective covering for tissue regeneration (photo courtesy of Ejnar Eriksson)*

is not clear until the tissue declares itself. *Local frostbite is still a 'wait and see injury'.* Even if early recognition should prove possible, thereby sparing days of hospitalisation, clinical experience has shown that surgical intervention should be minimal. The blackened carapace acts as a protective covering for tissue regeneration and will separate by itself without intervention (Fig. 47.6). Premature surgery most often ends up in infection, unnecessary tissue loss and delay in healing, rather than the reverse.[1,29] If amputation must be performed, a modified guillotine procedure is recommended at the lowest level, with later secondary closure.[26]

FCIs: hospital treatment

- Prompt transportation
- Rapid warm water thawing if area affected is still frozen
- Analgesia: ibuprofen 600 mg, repeated every 6 hours
- Tetanus prophylaxis
- Antibiotics only if infection present
- Blisters kept intact and debrided only if infected
- Cotton pledgets placed between toes and fingers
- Daily whirlpool baths at normal skin temperature
- Dorsal or dorsolateral escharotomy if finger joint movement limited
- Avoid premature debridement/amputation

ADJUVANT THERAPY

Considerable interest has been focused on treatment with various anticoagulants believed to prevent progressive microvascular thrombosis and tissue loss. Treatment with heparin was used in Korea but proved ineffective. In order to be of value the therapy should be given early, as intravascular cellular aggregation, stasis and thrombosis occur soon

after thawing. Conversely, it has been shown in experimental studies on frostbite in rabbits that there was very little deposition of fibrin after thawing.[13] Marzella *et al.* have confirmed these findings and conclude that this observation was consistent with the lack of efficacy of heparin administration in experimental frostbite.[14]

Low molecular weight dextran has often been used in the treatment of local frostbite in order to reduce sludging and thrombosis in the small blood vessels. Clinical results are far from encouraging, and in animal experiments, dextran, like heparin, has to be administered in the early postoperative period.[30] Some investigators find that infusion of the rheological substance may actually increase the oedema.[31]

Early sympathectomy is of doubtful value. Experimental evidence has shown that sympathectomy performed within the first few hours of injury exacerbates oedema, blister formation and tissue destruction.[17,32] 'Medical sympathectomy' with intra-arterial reserpine has frequently been used as the first choice of treatment. The drug causes significant depletion of arterial wall noradrenaline content for up to 4 weeks.[33] However, in a multiarmed experimental study comparing slow re-warming combined with intravenous low molecular weight dextran, intra-arterial reserpine or tolazoline, all the drug treatments were superior to slow thawing. Rapid re-warming, however, was as effective as any of the drug treatments.[34] Randomised multicentre studies are indicated to evaluate these adjuncts in the treatment of deep FCIs.

More recently, a combination of systemic antiprostaglandin therapy in the form of ibuprofen and the topical agent aloe vera has been used to inhibit localised thromboxane production, which has been implicated as a cause of progressive dermal ischaemia.[19] Such antiprostaglandin treatment was reported to reduce both hospital stay and morbidity in patients with frostbite. The study, however, was not randomised and it lacked patients with severe injuries. The breakdown products of arachidonic acid were first implicated in burn injuries,[35] but treatment with antiprostaglandin agents has now been abandoned at most burns centres. One must remember, however, that a burn injury and frostbite differ in many respects, which is why antiprostaglandin therapy may yet have a place in the treatment of frostbite. Contrary to recommended protocols[19] we prefer to administer systemic antiprostaglandin whenever possible, even before thawing the local injury.

FCIs: adjuvant therapy

- Anticoagulant therapy – heparin if given early
- Low molecular weight dextran
- Early sympathectomy, 'medical sympathectomy' using intra-arterial reserpine/tolazoline
- Systemic antiprostaglandin therapy as ibuprofen plus topical aloe vera

NON-FREEZING COLD INJURIES

This form of local cold injury almost exclusively affects legs and/or feet. The aetiology of NFCIs is multifactorial. *Prolonged exposure to cold and wet conditions is a pre-requisite*, combined with immobilisation causing venous stagnation due to unnatural posture or constricting foot-wear. Dehydration, inadequate food and stress, intercurrent illness or injury, and fatigue are also important contributory factors. The recognition of this type of cold injury has remained rather unusual because it seldom occurs in civilian life. In the military context, however, NFCI has been and seems to be a serious problem, most often due to being unaware of the condition and the slow and indistinct first appearance of symptoms.

Non-freezing cold injury was not distinguished from frostbite until World War I. The injury was then called 'trench foot' as it occurred in soldiers on trench duty. During World War II the syndrome was seen in the survivors of ships sunk in arctic waters who had spent time in water-logged boats or rafts, and this injury was therefore called 'immersion foot'. Other names for the disorder include swamp foot, tropical jungle foot, paddy-field foot and foxhole foot. Non-freezing cold injuries can occur in any condition where the environmental temperature is lower than body temperature. The exposure time necessary to produce NFCIs lengthens with increasing temperature of the wet medium. Wrenn has suggested that the single term 'immersion foot' should be applied to this syndrome.[36] In connection with the more severe effects of immersion at temperatures below 15 °C, the subcategory 'cold water immersion foot' should be used. The more benign variant occurring at temperatures above 15 °C should be called 'warm water immersion foot'.

Pathophysiology

While experimental studies on FCIs have been numerous over the years, there are scarcely any such studies on NFCIs in the literature, and the true genesis of this type of cold injury is still far from resolved. As in FCIs, sympathetic constrictor fibres, together with the cold itself, induce prolonged vasoconstriction. The contributory effect of cold reduces the rate of reuptake and metabolism of noradrenaline at the nerve endings.[37]

Endrich et al. presented interesting findings concerning the microvascular ultrastructure in the NFCI.[38] In an animal model, using a transparent chamber implanted into a dorsal skin fold in Syrian hamsters, they studied the integrity of the subcutaneous microcirculation during repeated non-freezing local cold exposures. Endothelial damage was prominent in the true capillaries and venous vessels, while arterioles remained unaffected. Smaller vessels were often completely clogged with blood cells and with leucocytes integrated into

the endothelial wall. In contrast, fibrin was never observed within the occluded vessels. Later, increased permeability leading to tissue oedema was demonstrated by extravasation of FITC-dextran. In the light of this Endrich et al. considered that the initial event in NFCI is rheological in nature and resembles that observed during ischaemia-reperfusion injury (see Chapter 2). Iyengar et al.[39] drew the same conclusion from experiments in rabbits, where they found that free radicals (OH⁻) generated after cooling increased significantly upon re-warming.

Wrenn adds other interesting observations to our understanding of the pathophysiology of NFCI.[36] Thus, in addition to the duration of temperature of the medium, the susceptibility of the victim is important. The pathological hallmark of immersion foot is waterlogging of the thick stratum corneum on the soles of the feet. Absorption of 1–2 g of water per hour by the foot has been reported.[40,41] The amount of absorption depends on the salinity of the medium: fresh water causes much greater absorption. The absorbed liquid passes into the circulation but some is always retained in the stratum corneum. The thicker sole is more prone to injury than the thinner skin on the dorsum of the foot.

The pathological changes thus induced affect many tissues. Fat degenerates early on and is replaced by fibrous tissue. Muscles undergo degeneration, necrosis and fibrosis and ultimately atrophy, similar in appearance to that seen in chronic denervation.[42] Osteoporosis is an early event, probably caused by vascular disturbances.

Of special interest is the pathophysiology of the nerves, as *it is nerve damage which accounts for the pain, prolonged dysaesthesia and hyperhidrosis.* Denny-Brown et al.[43] reported from experiments on cats that, in NFCI, large myelinated fibres suffered injury most likely mediated by ischaemia. On exposing the tibial nerve in rabbit, Kennet and Gilliat[44] found local failure of conduction at the site of cooling (1–5 °C for 2–4 hours), which persisted after re-warming. This was followed by distal degeneration of the affected fibres. The fastest conducting motor and afferent axons were particularly affected. Histology revealed primary axonal damage, particularly in large-diameter fibres. The changes are similar to those described after ischaemic injury.[45] The hypoxic theory, however, seems less probable in cooling nerve tissue, as the duration of cooling was too short for ischaemic injury to occur. By immersing the hind limb of the rabbit in a water bath at +1 °C for 10–14 hours, Kennet and Gilliat[46] reported subsequent persistent nerve damage to the tibial nerve, with distal degeneration of the affected fibres. Evidence of persistent conduction block, however, was not seen. The study also showed that pure cold neuropathy occurred in the absence of histological abnormalities in blood vessels or muscles. This is an interesting observation as, in milder cases of NFCI, neurological symptoms appear to predominate, with minor involvement of other tissues. The involvement of autonomic fibres in NFCI is of particular importance. The post-traumatic hyperhidrosis and cold sensitivity are similar to the effects of postganglionic sympathetic denervation.[47]

Clinical picture

Compared with an FCIS, NFCIS have an insidious onset. As the symptoms are vague victims realise the imminent danger only when it is too late. The feet become cold and swollen and feel heavy, woody and numb. Clinically, the condition reveals a cool, painful, tender, white foot with wrinkled soles and most often pulseless pedal arteries on palpation. Brawny oedema, scaling, maceration, erythema and abrasions over pressure points from shoes or socks may also be seen. This first, ischaemic phase can last for hours up to a few days and is followed by a hyperaemic phase of 2–6 weeks, during which time the feet are warm, with bounding pulses and increased swelling. Anaesthesia is replaced by tingling and aching pain, now and then intensified by intermittent throbbing. There may be blistering and ulceration, which in severe cases may culminate in gangrene.

Treatment

The treatment of NFCIs is basically supportive. *Out in the field the feet should be dried carefully but, in contrast to freezing injuries, kept cool.* The whole body, however, should be warmed. Plenty of warm beverages should be given. In hospital the patient is put to bed with the feet elevated. The local injuries should not be actively warmed. Treatment with 40–42 °C warm water as used for FCIs is contraindicated. Warm water is only allowed when ice crystals are present in the tissue.

The feet should be carefully washed, dried and cooled with a fan.[48] Tetanus toxoid should be given. Non-steroid anti-inflammatory agents (NSAIDs) may be beneficial, but most often analgesics are required to mitigate the pain. Heparinisation and the use of low molecular weight dextran may be of value, but convincing reports are still awaited. Early surgical sympathectomy should be avoided, and the value of chemical sympathectomy is controversial.

As a rule treatment should be conservative. Nevertheless, fever, an elevated creatinine phosphokinase level, signs of disseminated intravascular coagulation, and liquefaction of affected tissues indicate early surgical intervention. In most reported cases antibiotics have played a minor role in recovery, even in the presence of fever and lymphadenopathy.[49] In severe cases, however, coverage for both streptococcal and staphylococcal species should be given until the results of cultures become available.[37] Patients suffering from NFCI injuries later complain of cold sensitivity, hyperhidrosis, swollen tender feet and sometimes contractures of their toes.[50]

> **NFCIs: treatment**
>
> - Generally conservative
> - Wash and dry the feet and keep them cool (no active warming)
> - Bed rest in warm clothes with feet elevated
> - Warm beverages
> - Tetanus toxoid
> - Analgesic and/or NSAIDs
> - Heparin/low molecular weight dextran
> - Antibiotics if indicated
> - Amputation when injury irreversible

Prevention

As the treatment of NFCI is often passive and relatively ineffective, prophylaxis is extremely important. Adequate foot care with time to dry the feet is crucial, as also are dry socks, rest with the feet elevated and hot beverages if at all possible. NFCI is almost exclusively a war phenomenon. The British Army learned the lesson from World War I and showed that this form of injury was preventable. For example, the 10th British Corps, which formed an integral part of the 5th US Army, had, during their Italian campaign, a ratio of 1:45 between cold injuries and battle casualties; the corresponding ratio for the US corps was 1:4.[51]

Ahle *et al.*[51] reinvestigated Argentinian soldiers with trench foot injuries in the Falklands war. Passive re-warming of the cold-water stressed foot was evaluated in 33 trench foot patients who had recovered and in 15 uninjured subjects. Poor re-warming was noted in all injured subjects, compared with five uninjured patients but 14 normal subjects failed to re-warm normally following the cold stress, and this group was statistically indistinguishable from the injured group. This could mean that a large proportion of a normal population are at great risk of suffering NFCI under appropriate conditions.

HYPOTHERMIA

The human body strives to maintain thermal equilibrium between heat production and heat loss, with a core temperature of 37 ± 2 °C. When thermoregulation is impaired and core temperature starts to decline, the individual suffers cold stress, but not until the central temperature reaches 35 °C is the victim considered to be in a hypothermic state.

Physiological reactions to decreased core temperature

During cold stress an intense adrenergic vasoconstriction redirects blood from skin to deeper areas, i.e. from the shell to the core, thereby preventing heat conduction from the core to the skin. This physiological reaction increases the insulating capacity sixfold.[52] The vasoconstriction is most pronounced in the extremities.[27] The arms and legs constitute around 30 per cent of body weight and half of the body surface. Such a 'physiological amputation' of the extremities means a tremendous reduction in heat loss. *Adrenergic vasoconstriction does not occur in the head and neck region.* A bare headed person loses around half of their resting heat production at −4 °C and this loss increases to 75 per cent at −15 °C.[53]

Good health, good physical fitness and adaptation to cold improve the tolerance to the lowered temperature; cold stress raises the respiratory rate. Immersion in cold water can increase ventilation fourfold and induce hypocapnia. Further, cold induces shivering, which is preceded by increased muscular tone. Shivering is believed to result from feedback oscillations of the stretch reflex mechanism and can increase the metabolic rate four- to sixfold. Of importance also is good nutrition and last but not least adequate fluid balance. Dehydration is often neglected in this connection.

A hypothermic victim has almost always been fighting with the cold, the snow and the wind. Cold stress elevates the catecholamines released from the sympathetic nerve terminals, which induces peripheral vasoconstriction, centralises blood volume and increases blood pressure and cardiac output.[54] These events lead to diuresis. This cold induced increase of urine flow is an osmolal diuresis with sodium and chloride as the main constituents independent of the antidiuretic hormone. Cold diuresis decreases the blood volume leading to a reduced physical working capacity.[55] The kidney is only a magnifying mirror in this context. Increased filtration is general and fluid also moves into the extracellular and intracellular spaces. Working in the cold furthermore induces increased water loss via respiration due to the low water vapour pressure of cold air which also disguises loss via perspiration. Most insidious, however, is the victim's peculiar lack of thirst despite dehydration[56] and the difficulties of getting hold of enough water in a wintry environment. A decreased capacity for work, increased peripheral vasoconstriction and raised blood viscosity are all factors which multiply the risk for local cold injuries as well as general hypothermia!

Under such circumstances leaders of groups should be aware of the problem and see to it that members stay well hydrated. The order should be: 'Drink your fill and double that volume'. In forced situations it is wise to use every member's own 'autoanalyser': let them pee into the snow! Clear, pale, yellow urine indicates adequate hydration while dark, orange and reddish-brown marks in the snow tells you that somebody is in trouble.

When core temperature is lower than 35 °C the human body begins to lose its ability to generate enough heat to maintain bodily functions. Between 35 and 32 °C, the hypothermia is classified as mild, between 32 and 28 °C it is moderate and below 28 °C, severe. As temperature decreases cardiac output and blood pressure may be markedly depressed by the negative inotropic and chronotropic effects of hypothermia and further depressed by the concomitant hypovolaemia.

At 33–32 °C systole is prolonged more than diastole. Atrial irritability in early hypothermia often induces atrial fibrillation. J waves or Osborne waves are observed at temperatures lower than 32 °C.[57] This electrocardiographic abnormality is a secondary wave following the S wave. At lower temperatures ventricular extrasystoles are common. Death supervenes at temperatures from 28 °C and lower, most often resulting from ventricular fibrillation, but asystole may also occur.[58] The lowest known adult accidental hypothermia was a 13.7 °C core temperature,[59] and the lowest infant hypothermia was 15.2 °C.[60]

Hypothermia depresses the central nervous system. Cerebral metabolism decreases 6–7 per cent per degree Celsius.[61] Lassitude and apathy are early signs of decreasing temperature. Sluggish cerebration impairs judgement, causes bizarre behaviour and ataxia and often ends in lethargy and coma between 30 and 28 °C. At 28–27 °C there are no muscle reflexes, no response to pain and no pupillary light reflex. The corneal reflex disappears below 25 °C.[62] The electroencephalogram flattens out at 20–19 °C.

Exposure to an environmental temperature colder than one's body temperature is the basic prerequisite for the occurrence of hypothermia. Extremes of age are risk factors. Neonates with an increased surface area to body mass ratio, as well as elderly persons with impaired thermoregulatory function and reduced muscle mass and insulating fat layer, run a greater risk of suffering hypothermia.

Victims dying of hypothermia are often found in a total or partial undressed state. This phenomenon has been named 'paradoxical undressing'. This peculiar behaviour had already been observed in 1719. When the Swedish King Charles XII was killed during his war against Norway, General Armfeldt, who had tried to capture Trondhjelm, decided to beat a retreat. With 6000 men he went over the border mountains but his army was caught in a horrible snowstorm. More than 3000 soldiers froze to death. In an effort to find out whether any equipment was salvageable the surviving soldiers discovered to their surprise that many of the dead were more or less naked. Historians have later claimed that those who survived were such cruel bastards that they robbed their comrades of their clothing. Those who made such a statement had never experienced a snowstorm.

The reasons why a person starts to undress in the cold have been difficult to establish. Hallucinations and neurochemical changes in the brain have been suggested.[63] A cold induced paralysis of the arterial nerves with 'warm' core blood perfusing the skin seems possible. Some of the reported victims, however, had been walking quite a distance while undressing, and as these individuals were hypovolaemic, vasodilation would promptly lead to syncope.

Recent studies have thrown a new light on this phenomenon. It is well known that when a patient gets an infection their central temperature set-point is raised and shivering begins until body temperature has reached the new set-point. In analogy the set-point is lowered in deep hypothermia and the victim experiences warmth and starts to undress. The phenomenon has been named 'anapyrexia' or 'reversed fever'.[64] In this context it is worth mentioning that in animal experiments alcohol has been shown to induce anapyrexia,[65] a finding which might explain why drunken hypothermic victims are often lucid at temperatures where sober individuals are unconscious.

It is of utmost important to recognise this phenomenon to avoid misinterpretation of the cause. If a person in a cold environment is found partly undressed or with severe disordered clothing, especially a woman or child, the police will often interpret the situation as the result of a sexual attack. The police officer is not competent to diagnose death and most often cordons the area in order to collect evidence. Not even for a medical practitioner is it always possible to determine whether such a victim is dead or not. The patient should, however, be brought to a hospital as soon as possible.

Different forms of hypothermia

There are many classifications of hypothermia, but from a practical point of view the three subdivisions given in the box below are useful.

> ### Forms of hypothermia
>
> - Accidental hypothermia
>   - Acute immersion hypothermia
>   - Subacute exhaustion hypothermia
> - Subclinical chronic hypothermia
> - Hypothermia of major surgery and trauma

Accidental hypothermia is a major cause of death in people engaged in outdoor recreational activities. Acute immersion hypothermia occurs when a person falls into cold water. This medium has a specific heat 4000 times that of air and a thermal conductivity approximately 25 times greater.[66] The core temperature, therefore, decreases rapidly even if heat production is maximal. Hypothermia sets in before the victim becomes exhausted.

Accidental subacute exhaustion hypothermia happens to skiers, climbers and walkers in the mountains. Muscular activity maintains the body temperature as long as energy sources are available, but when hypoglycaemia ensues, the victim is in a hazardous situation. Furthermore, prolonged exposure to cold induces increased loss of body fluids due to cold diuresis, augmented insensible loss of water from skin and airways and sequestration of water in the intercellular and intracellular compartments, all events leading to hypovolaemia and decreased capacity for physical work. The haematocrit rises by around 2 per cent per degree Celsius decline in temperature.

Subclinical chronic hypothermia is most often found in elderly persons, often in association with malnutrition, inadequate clothing and restricted mobility. Acute or chronic alcoholism, acute intoxication and chronic metabolic diseases, as well as psychiatric disorders, are contributory causes in this form of hypothermia.

Hypothermia is a common complication in patients undergoing major surgery. The anaesthetic agents interfere with thermoregulation by reducing the metabolic rate[67,68] and depressing the thermostatic reflexes. Muscle paralysis abolishes muscle tone and eliminates shivering,[69] and furthermore anaesthesia nullifies the sympathetic vasoconstrictory response to cold. A fall in central core temperature is common during surgery. All patients undergoing major abdominal surgery and no less than two-thirds of patients undergoing minor abdominal surgery are found to become hypothermic.[70]

Hypothermia is an ominous complication in patients who have sustained major trauma. The critically injured patient is unable to maintain body temperature in the immediate postinjury period. Heat loss may be exacerbated by infusion of unwarmed fluids and by removal of clothing. Patients in shock who become hypothermic have a higher mortality than do normothermic victims.[71,72] The critical temperature seems to lie around 32–33 °C. Severely traumatised patients whose core temperature falls below 32 °C have even been considered non-salvageable.[73] The duration of environmental exposure is a primary factor in accidental hypothermia. A heated rescue vehicle, heated intravenous fluids and warm blankets can reduce the amount of initial heat loss. A heated trauma room at the accident and emergency department, where the victim is promptly undressed for multiple examination, is of importance in this context. Evaporative heat losses can be restricted by avoiding volatile solutions for skin cleansing. Warming and humidification of inspired gases is also important.

Treatment

IN THE FIELD

The main principle of primary care of a patient suffering from hypothermia is to prevent further heat loss. If the patient is conscious, they should be moved indoors or at least into shelter. They should be kept in a lying position and wet clothing should be removed. Now and then there may be difficulties in undressing a wet, stiff victim and if that is the case, it would be appropriate to put that individual into a plastic bag, ensuring as much insulation as possible and remembering to cover their head. A fire may be built or a stove lit, but the patient should not be exposed close to its radiant heat which may cause a burn injury. A conscious patient who has been well cared for can be given a warm, nourishing beverage. Transportation to the nearest hospital should then be arranged.

If the victim is comatose from hypothermia then this is a 'true medical emergency, but an emergency in slow motion'.[74] People die slowly in the cold. Mills has likened the hypothermic victim to a 'metabolic icebox' where the low temperature to a large degree protects certain core organs.[26] It is mandatory to handle patients gently to minimise the risk of possible ventricular fibrillation (VF). Mouth-to-mouth respiratory support should be tried in apnoeic patients. The positive pressure often produces gasping respiration, which indicates the presence of some cardiac function.[48]

If available, the unconscious victim should be given warm, moist oxygen and an intravenous infusion of glucose at 37–40 °C. Electrocardiographic (ECG) monitoring is an advantage in the prehospital setting. One must be aware, however, that adhesive pads for monitor leads will not stick to the skin and needle electrodes may have to be inserted. Shivering often obscures the interpretation of the ECG.

The scenario out in the field generally lacks all these facilities. The primary treatment on these occasions is to insulate the victim and attempt to re-warm them; this often comes down to minimising further decreases in temperature. *Do not try to prewarm a patient in chronic hypothermia out in the field without physiological control.* Transportation of a hypothermic person is far less risky than enthusiastic attempts to re-warm in the field where it is difficult to treat complications.

In contrast, when hypothermia is due to cold water immersion, the cooling occurs rapidly and the extreme metabolic derangements seen in exhaustion hypothermia are absent. This set of circumstances provides the only situation in which the victim may be treated with rapid immersion re-warming, even out in the open, if that is feasible.

It is often difficult, even for trained medical personnel, to determine whether or not a hypothermic person is alive. Apparent cardiovascular collapse may actually be represented only by depressed cardiac output. Palpation or auscultation for at least a minute to detect spontaneous pulses may be necessary. Pressure on the neck, which may trigger the vagus nerve, should be avoided. The femoral arteries in the groin should be checked instead.

In the field, the decision as to whether administer cardiopulmonary resuscitation (CPR) should be administered, is difficult. The problem is more often governed by the situation rather than medical circumstances. If there is any sign of life at all, CPR is contraindicated, as prematurely performed chest compressions may induce VF. Cardiopulmonary resuscitation is not indicated when there is a major threat to the rescuers, but it should be initiated immediately after a cardiac arrest is witnessed, when the patient is in a stable environment and the procedure can be performed reasonably and continuously. In normothermia, CPR induces blood flow from phasic alterations[75] in the intrathoracic pressure rather than from cardiac compression. Althaus et al.[76] reported three cases of prolonged hypothermic cardiac arrest without neurological sequelae after prolonged closed chest compression. In one patient at 22 °C they found the heart to be hard as stone and impossible to compress. The role of a 'thoracic pump' with the heart as a passive conduit seems to be a plausible hypothesis in hypothermia as well.[77]

The maxim 'No one is dead until warm and dead', when dealing with a hypothermic victim, should be completed with 'unless serum potassium is greater than 10 mmol/L' because severe hyperkalaemia carries an adverse outcome. Furthermore a core temperature of less than 12 °C must also be considered low enough to declare a person dead. Thermometers for measuring tympanic temperature are now available for use in the field.[78,79] Resuscitation under such circumstances has proved to be a waste of resources.

Hypothermia: treatment in the field

- Move patient into sheltered area and place in supine position
- Handle gently to avert VF
- Avoid neck pressure to detect pulse as it may trigger vagus nerve
- Mouth-to-mouth support if apnoeic
- CPR for cardiac arrest but avoided if situation threatens lives of rescuers
- CPR contraindicated if signs of life present as chest compression may induce VF
- Remove wet clothing, if impossible use plastic bag and ensure good insulation
- If conscious give warm nourishing beverage
- Light fire or stove but do not expose to its radiant heat
- If available warm moist oxygen, intravenous glucose at 37–40 °C, ECG monitoring (needle electrodes)
- Rapid immersion re-warming only if cold water immersion is the cause
- Arrange transportation to hospital

HOSPITAL MANAGEMENT

If not previously instituted, warm, humidified oxygen should be administered by face mask and, after preoxygenation, by endotracheal tube. Continuous core temperature (T°) and ECG monitoring should be instituted. An intravenous infusion of isotonic dextrose in saline at 35–45 °C should be given. Solutions containing lactate are unsuitable as the liver cannot metabolise lactate at lower temperatures. Colloids should only be administered to patients not responding to crystalloids. A central venous pressure (CVP) catheter is often useful for registering fluid overload and imminent pulmonary oedema. Laboratory evaluations should include arterial blood gases (ABGs) uncorrected for body temperature, full blood and platelet counts (FBP), blood sugar, electrolyte (Es), creatinine (Cr), serum calcium, serum magnesium and serum amylase levels, prothrombin (PT) and partial thromboplastin times (PTT) and fibrinogen (F) levels. A toxicology (Tox) screen, thyroid function tests (TFTs) and cardiac isoenzymes (CIs) should be considered if the level of unconsciousness does not correlate with the actual core temperature. Remember also that a warm skin on a cold patient is possibly due to a vasodilatatory drug or sepsis.[80]

Re-warming can be performed with different techniques, passive and active, depending on whether heat is or is not added. Active re-warming may be delivered by external means or by core re-warming. Each has its advantages and disadvantages. The method used will often depend on local factors. The accessibility of resources can differ widely, between, for example, a hypothermic skier found in the mountains who may be many miles from a well-equipped hospital, and in contrast, an urban, homeless alcoholic found in the street.

Hypothermia: hospital management

- Warm humidified oxygen by face mask/endotracheal intubation
- Monitoring of core temperature (T°), ECG, CVP
- Intravenous isotonic dextrose in saline at 35–45 °C
- Blood for ABGs, FBP, sugar, Es, Cr, calcium, magnesium, amylase, PT, PTT, F
- If level of unconsciousness does not correlate with core T°, Tox screen, TFTs and CIs
- Re-warming – passive, active (external or internal)

PASSIVE RE-WARMING

Re-warming without adding heat takes place as a result of metabolic heat created by shivering. Measures such as removing wet clothes and covering the patient in layers of warm blankets are less effective at lower temperatures, as shivering ceases at around 30 °C. Passive rewarming is the method of choice in haemodynamically stable and otherwise healthy patients with a core temperature above 30–32 °C.[81] The rate of rewarming varies greatly with most series, reporting increases of around 0.5 °C per hour; the lower the body temperature, the slower the rate. If the rise in body temperature is much slower, a complicating disease such as hypothyroidism should be suspected. Generation of heat requires energy and will quickly deplete muscle glycogen stores, and this loss must be

compensated. Passive re-warming is physiologically sound. It avoids the rapid cardiovascular derangements often encountered in patients in chronic hypotension when treated with active methods. Passive re-warming is often recommended for elderly patients with intravascular volume contraction.[82]

ACTIVE EXTERNAL RE-WARMING

Patients with temperatures below 32 °C require *more active re-warming* by direct transfer from an exogenous source to the surface of the body.

Examples of achieving this objective include electric re-warming blankets, heating pads, radiant heat sources and trunk immersion. It has been stressed that the re-warming should be confined to truncal areas and too rapid a re-warming of the extremities with its consequent 'afterdrop' should be avoided. This afterdrop is a paradoxical decrease in core temperature of 2–3 °C occurring soon after the start of shell re-warming.[82] This complication is believed to be initiated by peripheral vasodilatation and shunting of stagnant, cold, acidotic blood to the core, thus further chilling the heart and possibly inducing potentially fatal ventricular fibrillation. The significance of this statement has been disputed. Studies on humans have shown afterdrop, affecting both oesophagus and rectum, without any increased blood flow in the extremities.[83] The **afterdrop phenomenon** may therefore merely be due to the slow conductive heat transfer from the shell to the core during aggressive re-warming.[84]

In active surface re-warming, however, the problem of plasma volume depletion may be exacerbated by peripheral vasodilatation, resulting in hypotension. Furthermore, CPR is difficult to perform when the victim is immersed. The hot bath is not recommended for the elderly.[85,86] The method has been advocated when hypothermia is combined with local frostbite.[26]

The Royal Danish Navy has adopted a field model of re-warming in mild to moderate hypothermia proposed by Vanggard and Gjerlof.[87] It is a simple technique supplying exogenous heat by immersing hands, forearms, feet and lower legs in water at 44–45 °C. When the distal extremities are warmed, the arteriovenous anastomoses in the fingers and toes are opened which greatly increases the venous return to the heart via the superficial venous route in the forearms and lower legs. This raised perfusion of the skin surface enhances the delivery of heat to the core with minimal countercurrent heat exchange as the superficial veins are not in close proximity to the arteries. The hypothesis has recently been tested on volunteers cooled in water to around 35 °C. The postcooling afterdrop in oesophageal temperature after such a treatment was decreased compared with the shivering alone procedure.[88] The extremity immersion rewarming method does not require any specialised equipment or expertise and can be performed in the field and on board smaller ships without sophisticated means of heat donation.

This model of extremity re-warming has been refined and tested on hypothermic subjects during recovery from general anaesthesia.[89] The re-warming was performed by a water-perfused blanket (45–46°C). In a test group the blood vessels in the hand were distended by exposing the distal part of the arm to subatmospheric pressure (−30 to −40 mmHg). Compared with controls this procedure, with maximum vasodilatation, resulted in a 10-fold increase in re-warming rates. This promising method has been confirmed on cold-stressed (<36°C) healthy volunteers.[90] The combined application of heat and subatmospheric pressure increases local subcutaneous blood flow thereby allowing heat to be transferred subcutaneously directly from the skin of the extremity to the critical body core despite the central drive for vasoconstriction.[87–89]

Hypothermia: active external re-warming

- Re-warm trunk only (to avoid afterdrop) – electric blankets, heating pads, radiant heat sources
- Hot bath immersion – contraindicated in the elderly and if CPR required
- Extremity re-warming (can be effected with water-perfused blanket 45–46°C)

ACTIVE INTERNAL RE-WARMING

In comatose victims active internal re-warming should take precedence over external methods. A variety of techniques are available for this, the most invasive type of treatment of hypothermia. These options include irrigation of body cavities, gastric and/or colonic lavage, airway re-warming, diathermy and extracorporeal blood rewarming or cardiopulmonary bypass (CPB).

Peritoneal lavage is most widely used because it is practical, inexpensive and easy to administer at any medical facility.[90,91] The method involves lavage using a dialysate of warmed standard fluids (40–42.5°C) which is best performed via two catheters and allows fluid values up to 10–12 L/hour. This method also facilitates the management of drug intoxication and renal failure, and improves liver function and drug detoxification by directly re-warming the liver. Contraindications to peritoneal irrigation include abdominal trauma and recent abdominal surgery.

Pleural lavage has the advantage of re-warming the heart directly. Two thoracotomy tubes are inserted, one in the fifth intercostal space in the posterior axillary line and the other in the second or third intercostal space in the midclavicular line.[90,91] A flow rate up to 0.5 L/min can be achieved. An adequate outlet for the fluid, however, is mandatory in avoiding increasing intrathoracic pressure, with the consequent risk of depressed pulmonary and cardiac function. Pleural lavage may also be used in combination with a thoracotomy for open cardiac massage in a haemodynamically unstable, severely hypothermic patient.[76]

Gastric and/or colonic re-warming is used less often nowadays. Anatomical proximity to the heart and to the liver is an advantage in gastric lavage but the actual surface area for heat exchange is small.[90] Tube insertion may cause ventricular fibrillation and prolonged lavage causes severe electrolyte imbalance. In order to prevent the latter disadvantage, a modified Sengstaken tube has been used.[92]

Diathermy is a technique in which core temperature is increased by using ultrasonic, short wave or microwave irradiation. The great advantage is that the re-warming takes place below the skin and subcutaneous tissues without requiring any invasive procedure. Even though studies in dogs have revealed a re-warming speed comparable to that of peritoneal lavage,[93] reports on its clinical use are anecdotal.[94] There are numerous contraindications to this form of re-warming, for example haemorrhage, malignancies, pregnancy, tuberculosis and implanted devices such as arthroplasty and pacemakers, most of which are difficult to identify in a comatose patient.[90]

Extracorporeal re-warming by means of CPB and/or haemodialysis is the most reliable way to maintain cardiovascular function in severely hypothermic patients, especially when cardiac activity is absent. The bypass is performed by cannulation of one or both femoral veins. The blood is oxygenated, warmed and returned by a mechanical pump to the femoral artery.[95,96] Cardiopulmonary bypass re-warms at four times the rate of conventional core re-warming.[97] It is superior to other re-warming techniques because it possesses the ability to oxygenate the blood and provides haemodynamic support even in total circulatory failure. The method rapidly increases myocardial temperature and improves microcirculatory flow.[98]

The drawbacks of CPB are the risk of heparinisation, haemolysis, arterial injury and air embolism. Significant trauma constitutes the main contradiction to CPB, owing to anticoagulation. A heparin-coated bypass is now available and seems to be preferable even in non-traumatised patients as systemic anticoagulation will exacerbate the coagulopathy induced by hypothermia.[99] Furthermore, this technique is available only in larger hospitals. Endothelial leakage during reperfusion needs massive volume supplementation during bypass. Patients with simultaneous deep frostbite may develop compartmental syndromes requiring fasciotomy.[100] In smaller units, an interesting option for extracorporeal re-warming has been reported by Gregory et al., using a venovenous rewarmer.[98] The blood is removed through a central venous catheter, warmed to 40°C through a warming column and returned to a second central or peripheral venous catheter at a flow rate of 150–400 mL per minute. The device can be set up in about 10 minutes and without the subsequent use of heparin.

Hypothermia: active internal re-warming

- Irrigation of body cavities
  - Peritoneal lavage – best in non-arrests, detoxifies, improves renal and liver function
  - Pleural lavage – also re-warms heart directly
  - Gastric/colonic lavage – dangers are tube induced VF and electrolyte imbalance
- Airway re-warming – using hot, moist gas
  - Diathermy – ultrasonic, short wave or microwave; these have numerous contraindications
- Extracorporeal re-warming
  - Cardiopulmonary bypass – femoral vein(s) to femoral artery. Fast and reliable if hypothermia severe and no cardiac activity, oxygenates blood, gives haemodynamic support; but it has drawbacks
  - Veno-venous – from CVP line via warming column and back into a peripheral vein
- Amino acid infusions

The use of amino acids is a new, interesting contribution to the re-warming of hypothermic patients. A balanced mixture of amino acids has been proven to prevent anaesthesia induced hypothermia and shivering. Three-quarters of the heat production occurred in extrasplanchnic tissue, possibly partly in the muscles. These findings are of importance when dealing with accidental hypothermia. Amino acid infusions ought to be included in the therapeutic arsenal.[101]

Of course, many of the techniques described can be used synchronously. Air re-warming with inhalation of hot, moist gas and administration of warmed intravenous fluids should be a matter of course in every hypothermia case. For patients with a non-arrest rhythm, peritoneal irrigation is often preferable. It usually takes around 1 hour at best to start up CPB, and during that time the abovementioned options should be instigated and combined with CPR if the patient shows haemodynamic instability.

Patients suffering from hypothermia, especially of the chronic exhaustion type, are dehydrated. The combination of cold diuresis, peripheral vascular leakage and increased losses from skin and airways while fighting the cold in the cold dry air makes these losses greater than would be expected. Intravenous infusions of warm solutions are more than necessary, but one must pay attention to CVP. Pulmonary oedema is a frequent complication in elderly patients at temperatures lower than 27 °C. This hazardous event is usually encountered during re-warming. The aetiology of this non-cardiac oedema is debatable: decreased ciliar activity,[102] destruction of surfactant from anoxic pulmonary damage[103] and circulatory elements have all been incriminated as possible agents. Pulmonary oedema in connection with decreased cardiac output is also found in hypertensive crises in patients suffering from phaeochromocytomas and in connection with severe head trauma.[104,105] Pulmonary oedema is mediated via a massive sympathetic discharge, producing an intense but transient vasoconstriction with a resultant shift of blood from the high resistant systemic circulation to the low resistant pulmonary circulation. Catecholamine levels in the unconscious victim are low during re-warming, but noradrenaline and adrenaline levels rise rapidly, indicating some kind of depot effect.[106,107] This kind of oedema is well controlled by positive end-expiratory pressure.

Conclusions

When dealing with cold injury it is important to distinguish between the different aetiologies. In the early stages of cold injury physical signs are unreliable and the relevant history from the patient or witnesses is therefore the key to treatment. It is only when the likely the aetiology has been established that specific treatment can begin.

Key references

Althaus V, Aeberhard P, Scheupback P, *et al.* Management of prolonged accidental hypothermia with cardiorespiratory arrest. *Ann Surg* 1982; **195**: 492–5.

Francis TJR, Golden FStC. Non-freezing cold injury: the pathogenesis. *J R Nav Med Serv* 1985; **71**: 3–8.

Hamlet MP. Human cold injuries In: Pandolf KB, Sawka MN, Gonzales RR (eds). *Human Performance Physiology and Environmental Medicine at Terrestrial Extremes.* Indianapolis: Buchmark, 1988: 435–66.

Jolly BT, Ghezzi KT. Accidental hypothermia. *Emerg Med Clin North Am* 1992; **10**: 311–27.

Mills WJ Jr. Out in the cold. Frostbite. A discussion of the problem and a review of an Alaskan experience. *Alaska Med* 1993; **35**: 29–66.

REFERENCES

1 Ward M. Frostbite. *BMJ* 1974; **1**: 67–70.

2 Grattan HW. *General History of Medical Services Hyiene of War.* Vol II. London: HMSO 1931.

3 Whayne T, DeBakey M. *Cold injury ground type.* Washington, DC: US Government Printing Office, 1958.

4 Spray DC. Cutaneous temperature receptors. *Annu Rev Physiol* 1986; **48**: 625–9.

5 Francis TJR. Non-freezing cold injury: a historical review. *J R Nav Med Serv* 1984; **70**: 134–9.

6 Le Blanc J. Effect of reserpine on increased sensitivity to noradrenaline of cold adapted rats. *Am J Physiol* 1966; **204**: 520–2.

7   Jansky L. Non-shivering thermogenesis and its thermoregulatory significance. *Biol Rev* 1973; **48**: 85–132.

8   Smith DJ Jr, Robson MC, Heggers JP. Frostbite and other cold-induced injuries. In: Auerbach PS, Geehr EC (eds). *Management of Wilderness and Environmental Emergencies*. St Louis, MO: CV Mosby, 1988: 101–18.

9   Lewis T. Observation upon the reaction of vessels of the human skin to cold. *Heart* 1930; **15**: 177–208.

10 Vogel JE, Dellon AL. Frostbite injuries of the hand. *Clin Plastic Surg* 1989; **16**: 265–76.

11 Merryman HT. Tissue freezing and local cold injury. *Physiol Rev* 1957; **37**: 233–51.

12 Mazur P. Causes of injury in the frozen and thawed cells. *Federation Proc* 1965; **24**(suppl 14–15): 3.

13 Bourne MH, Piepkorn MW, Claryton F, Leonard LG. Analysis of microvascular change in frostbite injury. *J Surg Res* 1985; **40**: 26–35.

14 Marzella L, Jesudas RR, Manson PN, *et al*. Morphological characterization of acute injury to vascular endothelium of skin after frostbite. *Plastic Reconstr Surg* 1989; **83**: 67–75.

15 Manson PL, Jesudass R, Marzella L, *et al*. Evidence for an early free radical mediated reperfusion injury in frostbite. *Free Radic Biol Med* 1991; **10**: 7–11.

16 Daum PS, Bowers WD Jr, Tejada J, *et al*. Cooling of heat of fusion (HOF), followed by rapid rewarming, does not reduce the integrity of microvascular corrosion casts. *Cryobiology* 1991; **28**: 294–301.

17 Wheatherly-White RCA, Sjöström B, Paton BC. Experimental studies in cold injury: The pathogenesis of frostbite. *J Surg Res* 1964; **4**: 17–22.

18 Robson MC, Heggers JP. Evaluation of hand frostbite blister fluid as a clue to pathogenesis. *J Hand Surg* 1981; **6**: 43–7.

19 McCauley RL, Hing DN, Robson MC, Heggers JP. Frostbite injury: a rational approach based on the pathophysiology. *J Trauma* 1983; **23**: 143–7.

20 Knize DM. *Cold Injury in Reconstructive Plastic Surgery, General Principles*, Vol. 1, 2nd edn. Philadelphia, PA: WB Saunders, 1977.

21 Dinep M. Cold injury: a review of current theories and their application to treatment. *Medicine* 1975; **39**: 8–10.

22 Artursson G. The tragedy of San Juaurico – the most severe LPG disaster in history. *Burns* 1987; **13**: 87–102.

23 James NK, Moss ALH. Cold injury from liquid propane. *BMJ* 1989; **299**: 950–1.

24 Wegener EE, Barraza KR, Das SK. Severe frostbite caused by freon gas. *South Med J* 1991; **84**: 1143–6.

25 Hicks LM, Hunt JL, Baxter CL. Liquid propane cold injury: a clinicopathologic and experimental study. *J Trauma* 1979; **19**: 701–3.

26 Mills WJ Jr. Out in the cold. Frostbite. A discussion of the problem and a review of an Alaskan experience. *Alaska Med* 1993; **35**: 29–66.

27 Vanggard L. Physiological reactions to wet cold. *Aviat Space Environ Med* 1975; **10**: 235–41.

28 Renström B. Brrr ... klarar kroppen kampen mot kylan. *Quantum Satis* 1991; **4**: 24–7.

29 Edlic RF, Chang DE, Birk KA, *et al*. Cold injuries. *Compr Ther* 1989; **15**: 13–21.

30 Webster DR, Bourn G. Low molecular weight dextran in the treatment of experimental frostbite. *Can J Surg* 1965; **8**: 423–7.

31 Welch GS. Frostbite. *Practitioner* 1974; **213**: 801–4.

32 Golding MR, De Jong P, Sawyer PN, *et al*. Protection from early and late sequelae of frostbite by regional sympathectomy: mechanism of 'cold sensitivity' following frostbite. *Surgery* 1963; **53**: 303–8.

33 Porter J, Lindell T, Leung B, *et al*. Effect of intra-arterial injection of reserpine on vascular wall catecholamine content. *Surg Forum* 1972; **23**: 183–5.

34 Snider RL, Porter JM. Treatment of experimental frostbite with arterial sympathetic blocking drugs. *Surgery* 1975; **77**: 557–61.

35 Artursson G, Hamberg M, Johnsson CE. Prostaglandin in human burn blister fluid. *Acta Physiol Scand* 1973; **87**: 270–6.

36 Wrenn K. Immersion foot. A problem of the homeless in the 1990s. *Arch Intern Med* 1991; **151**: 785–8.

37 Francis TJR, Golden FStC. Non-freezing cold injury: the pathogenesis. *J R Nav Med Serv* 1985; **71**: 3–8.

38 Endrich B, Hammersen F, Messmer K. Microvascular ultrastructure in non-freezing cold injuries. *Res Exp Med* 1990; **190**: 365–79.

39 Iyengar J, George A, Russel JC, Das K. Generation of free radicals during cold injury and rewarming. *Vasc Surg* 1990; **24**: 467–74.

40 Beuttner KJK. Diffusion of liquid water through human skin. *J Appl Physiol* 1959; **14**: 261–8.

41 Schenplein RJ, Blank IH. Permeability of the skin. *Physiol Rev* 1971; **51**: 702–47.

42 Blackwood W. Injury from exposure to low temperature: pathology. *Br Med Bull* 1944; **4**: 138–41.

43 Denny-Brown D, Adams RD, Brenner C, Doherty MM. The pathology of injury to nerve induced by cold. *J Neuropathol Exp Neurol* 1945; **4**: 305–23.

44 Kennet RB, Gilliat DM. Nerve conduction studies in experimental non-freezing cold injury. I. Local nerve cooling. *Muscle Nerve* 1991; **14**: 553–62.

45 Nukada H, Dych PJ. Acute ischemia causes axonal stasis, swelling, alteration and secondary demyelination. *Ann Neurol* 1987; **22**: 311–18.

46 Kennet RB, Gilliat DM. Nerve conduction studies in experimental non-freezing cold injury. II Generalized nerve cooling by limb immersion. *Muscle Nerve* 1991; **14**: 960–7.

47 Emmelin N, Trendelenburg V. Degeneration activity after parasympathetic and sympathetic denervation. In: *Reviews of Physiology*. Berlin: Springer Verlag, 1972.

48 Hamlet MP. Human cold injuries In: Pandolf KB, Sawka MN, Gonzales RR (eds). *Human Performance Physiology and Environmental Medicine at Terrestrial Extremes*. Indianapolis: Buchmark, 1988: 435–66.

49 Akers WA. Paddy foot: a warm water immersion foot syndrome variant. I. The natural disease, epidemiology. *Military Med* 1974; **139**: 605–12.

50 White JC, Warren C. Causes of pain in foot after prolonged immersion. *War Med* 1944; **5**: 6–13.

51 Ahle NW, Buroni JR, Mark W, *et al*. Infrared thermographic measurement of circulatory compromise in trench foot – injured Argentine soldiers. *Aviat Space Environ Med* 1990; **61**: 247–50.

52 Burton AC. The pattern of response to cold in animals and the evolution of homeothermy. In: Hardy JD (ed). *Temperature: its Measurement and Control in Science and Industry*, vol. 3. New York: Book Corporation, 1963: 363–7.

53 Froese G, Burton AC. Heat loss from the human head. *J Appl Physiol* 1957; **10**: 235–41.

54   Hayward JS, Eckerson JD, Kemna D. Thermal and cardiovascular changes during three different methods of resucitation from mild hypothermia. *Resucitation* 1984; **11**: 21–33.

55   Lennqvist S, Granberg PO, Wedin B. Fluid balance and physical working capacity in humans exposed to cold. *Arch Environ Health* 1974; **20**: 241–9.

56   Hamlet MP. Fluid shifts in hypothermia. In: Pozoz RS, Wittmers LE (eds). *The Nature and Treatment of Hypothermia.* London/Minneapolis, MN: Croom Helm/University of Minnesota Press, 1983: 94–9.

57   Treviko A, Razi B, Beller BM. The characteristic electrocardiogram of accidental hypothermia. *Arch Intern Med* 1971; **127**: 470–3.

58   Fergusson NV. Urban hypothermia. *Anaesthesia* 1985; **40**: 651–54.

59   Gilbert M, Busund R, Skagseth A, et al. Resuscitation from accidental hypothermia of 13.7°C with circulatory arrest. *Lancet* 2000; **355**: 375–6.

60   Nozaki R, Ishibaski K, Adaski N, et al. Accidental proformed hypothermia. *N Engl J Med* 1986; **315**: 1680.

61   Ehrmanntrant WR, Ticklin HE, Faxerkras JF. Cerebral haemodynamics and metabolism in accidental hypothermia. *Arch Intern Med* 1957; **99**: 57–61.

62   Enander A. Performance and sensory aspects of work in cold environment – a review. *Ergonomics* 1984; **27**: 365–78.

63   Lloyd EL. *Hypothermia and Cold Stress.* London: Croom Helm, 1986.

64   Cabanac M, Brinnel H. The pathology of human temperature regulation: thermiatrics. *Experimentia* 1987; **43**: 19–27.

65   Granberg PO. Alcohol and cold. *Arct Med Res* 1991; **50**(suppl 6): 43–7.

66   Nadel ER. Energy exchanges in water. *Undersea Biomed Res* 1984; **11**: 149–52.

67   Burton AC, Edholm OE. *Man in a Cold Environment.* London: Edward Arnold, 1955.

68   Mackenzie A. Hazards in the operating theatre; environmental control. *Ann R Coll Surg* 1973; **52**: 361–5.

69   Holdcroft A. *Body Temperature Control in Anaesthesia, Surgery and Intensive Care.* London: Baillière Tindall, 1981.

70   Joackimsson PO. *Prevention and Treatment of Intraoperative Hypothermia. Acta University Uppsalianis,* no. 109. Uppsala: Faculty of Medicine, 1987.

71   Steineman S, Shackford SR, Davies JW. Implications of admission hypothermia in trauma patients. *J Trauma* 1990; **30**: 200–2.

72   Luna GK, Maier RV, Paolin EG, et al. Incidence and effect of hypothermia in seriously injured patients. *J Trauma* 1987; **27**: 1014–18.

73   Jurkovich GJ, Greisen WB, Luterman A, Curreri PW. Hypothermia in trauma victims: an ominous predictor of survival. *J Trauma* 1987; **27**: 1019–24.

74   Fritz RL, Perrin DH. Cold exposure injuries: prevention and treatment. *Clin Sports Med* 1989; **8**: 111–29.

75   Neimann JT. Blood flow without cardiac compression during closed chest CPR. *Crit Care Med* 1981; **9**: 380–3.

76   Althaus V, Aeberhard P, Scheupback P, et al. Management of prolonged accidental hypothermia with cardiorespiratory arrest. *Ann Surg* 1982; **195**: 492–5.

77   Danzl DF, Pozos RS. Multicenter hypothermia survey. *Ann Emerg Med* 1987; **178**: 1042–55.

78   Walpoth BH, Galdiskas J, Leupi F, et al. Assessment of hypothermia with a new 'tympanic' thermometer. *J Clin Monit* 1995; **10**: 91–6.

79   Helm M, Lampl L, Hauke J, Bock KH. Akzidentelle Hypothermie bei Traumapatient. *Anaesthesist* 1995; **44**: 101–7.

80   Fitzgerald FT, Jessop C. Accidental hypothermia: a report of 22 cases and review of the literature. *Adv Med* 1982; **27**: 150–3.

81   Ledingham IMcA, Mone JG. Treatment of accidental hypothermia. A prospective study. *BMJ* 1980; **280**: 1102–5.

82   Miller JW, Danzl DS, Thomas DM. Urban accidental hypothermia: 135 cases. *Ann Emerg Med* 1980; **9**: 456–61.

83   Savard GK, Cooper KE, Veale WL, et al. Peripheral blood flow during rewarming from mild hypothermia in man. *J Appl Physiol* 1958; **58**: 4–13.

84   Webb P. Afterdrop of body temperature during rewarming: an alternative explanation. *J Appl Physiol* 1986; **60**: 385–90.

85   Lloyd EL. *Hypothermia and Cold Stress.* London: Croom Helm, 1986.

86   Moss J. Accidental severe hypothermia. *Surg Gynecol Obstet* 1986; **162**: 501–13.

87   Vangaard L, Gjerloff CC. A new simple method of rewarming in hypothermia. *Int Rev Navy Air Force Med Serv.* 1979; **52**: 427–30.

88   Vanggard DE, Eyolfson D, Xiaojiang X, Weseen G, Giesbrecht CG, Immersion of distal arms and legs in warm water (AVA Rewarming) effectively rewarms mildly hypothermic humans. *Aviat Space Environ Med* 1999; **70**: 1081–8.

89   Grahn D, Brock-Utne J, Watenpaugh DE, Heller HC. Recovery from mild hypothermia can be accelerated by mechanically distending blood vessels in the hand. *J Appl Physiol* 1998; **85**: 1643–8.

90   Jolly BT, Ghezzi KT. Accidental hypothermia. *Emerg Med Clin North Am* 1992; **10**: 311–27.

91   Paton JF. Accidental hypothermia: a matter of turning the scoreboard around. *Med Post* (*Canada*), 1983; **23**: 4–5.

92   Kristensen G, Gravesen H, Benveniste D, Jordening H. An oesophageal thermal tube for rewarming in hypothermia. *Acta Anaesthesiol Scand* 1985; **29**: 846–8.

93   White JD, Butterfield AB, Greer KA, et al. Controlled comparison of radiowave regional hyperthermia and peritoneal lavage after immersion hypothermia. *J Trauma* 1985; **25**: 989–93.

94   Huang Z, Sun QY, Shen MJ. Rewarming with microwave irradiation in severe cold injury syndrome. *Chinese Med J* 1980; **93**: 119–20.

95   Philips SJ, Zeft RH, Kungathorn C, et al. Percutaneous cardiopulmonary bypass: applications and indication for use. *Ann Thorac Surg* 1989; **47**: 121–3.

96   Kugelberg J, Schuller H, Bey B, Kallum B. Treatment of accidental hypothermia. *Scand J Thorac Cardiovasc Surg* 1967; **1**: 142–6.

97   Splittgerber FH, Talbert JG, Sweezer WP, et al. Partial cardiopulmonary bypass for core rewarming in profound accidental hypothermia. *Am Surgeon* 1986; **52**: 407–12.

98   Gregory JS, Bergsten JM, Aprehamiam C, et al. Comparison of three methods of rewarming from hypothermia: advantage of extracorporeal blood warming. *J Trauma* 1991; **31**: 1247–51.

99   von Segessen LK, Garcia E, Turina M. Perfusion without systemic heparinisation for rewarming in accidental hypothermia. *Ann Thorac Surg* 1991; **52**: 560–1.

100 Hauty MG, Essig BC, Hill JG. Prognostic factors in severe accidental hypothermia: experience from the Art. Hood tragedy. *J Trauma* 1987; **27**: 1107–12.

101 Selldén E, Bränström R, Brundin T. Augmented thermic effect of amino acids under general anaesthesia occurs predominantly in extra-splanchnic tissues. *Clin Sci* 1996; **91**: 431–9.

102 Håkansson CH, Toremalm NG. Studies on the physiology of the trachea. I. Ciliar activity indirectly recorded by a new 'light beam reflex' method. *Ann Otol Rhinol Laryngol* 1965; **74**: 954–69.

103 Dubas F. Mountain rescue and treatment of deep accidental hypothermia. In: Cooper KE, Lomax P, Schönbaume, Veale WL (eds). *Homeostasis and Thermal Stress*. Basel: Karger, 1986: 49–54.

104 Baigelman W, O'Brian JC. Pulmonary effect of head trauma. *Neurosurgery* 1991; **9**: 729–40. Predominantly in extra-splanchic tissues. *Clin Sci* 1996; **91**: 431–9.

105 Popp AJ, Shak DM, Berman RA, *et al.* Delayed pulmonary dysfunction in head-injured patients. *J Neurosurg* 1981; **57**: 784–90.

106 Wayne D. Medical afteraction conference Mount Hood. *Bypass rewarming report T 10–88. US Army Research Institute*. Natick: US Army Research Institute, 1986.

107 Wilkersson JE, Reven PB, Boldman NW, Horwath SM. Adaptations in men's adrenal function in response to acute cold stress. *J Appl Physiol* 1974; **36**: 183–99.

Index

WG 170 OSA

This book is due for return on or before the last date shown below.